Nursing Care of the Critically Ill Child

Nursing Care of the Critically Ill Child

Mary Fran Hazinski, R.N., M.S.N.

Clinical Specialist,
Cardiovascular Surgery,
Children's Memorial Hospital,
Chicago, Illinois

Original artwork by
MARILOU KUNDMUELLER

with 268 illustrations

AMERICAN ASSOCIATION OF CRITICAL-CARE NURSES

The C. V. Mosby Company

ST. LOUIS • TORONTO • PRINCETON   1984

Editor: Michael R. Riley
Assistant editors: Sally Gaines, Terry Young
Manuscript editors: Sylvia B. Kluth, Gayle May, Jennifer Collins
Design: Kay M. Kramer
Production: Carol O'Leary, Patricia A. Carlock, Judith Bamert, Ginny Douglas

Printed in the United States of America

The C. V. Mosby Company
11830 Westline Industrial Drive, St. Louis, Missouri 63146

Library of Congress Cataloging in Publication Data
Main entry under title:

Nursing care of the critically ill child.

   Bibliography: p.
   1.   Pediatric intensive care.   2.   Pediatric nursing.
3.   Intensive care nursing.   I.   Hazinski, Mary Fran.
II.   American Association of Critical-Care Nurses.   [DNLM:
1.   Critical care—In infancy and childhood—Nursing texts.
2.   Pediatric nursing.   WY 159 N9739]
RJ370.N87   1984   610.73′62   83-21956
ISBN 0-8016-2125-9

A/VH/VH 9 8 7 6 5 4 3 2   03/C/331

Contributors

JUDY HARR, R.N.

Nurse Educator, Critical Care,
University of California at San Francisco,
San Francisco, California

MARY FRAN HAZINSKI, R.N., M.S.N.

Clinical Specialist,
Cardiovascular Surgery,
Children's Memorial Hospital,
Chicago, Illinois

JEANETTE KENNEDY

Dialysis Nurse,
Good Samaritan Hospital,
Portland, Oregon

LINDA A. LEWANDOWSKI, R.N., M.S.

Pediatric Clinical Nurse Specialist,
Yale–New Haven Hospital,
Assistant Professor of Yale University School of Nursing,
New Haven, Connecticut

DEBORAH RIFFEE MILLER, R.N., M.S.N.

Formerly Clinical Nurse Specialist in Gastroenterology,
Children's Hospital of Philadelphia;
Pediatric Clinical Nurse Specialist,
South Mountain Family Practice Center,
Bethlehem, Pennsylvania

JANET SNOW, R.N., M.N.

Doctoral Candidate,
Rush University College of Nursing,
Vice President, Minor Emergency Centers, Inc.,
Chicago, Illinois

HOLLY WEEKS WEBSTER, R.N., M.S.

Cardiovascular Clinical Specialist,
Primary Children's Hospital,
Salt Lake City, Utah

Dedication

FOR TOM AND MICHAEL

NOTE: The indications for and dosages of medications recommended conform to practices at the present time. References to specific products are incorporated to serve only as guidelines; they are not meant to exclude a practitioner's choice of other, comparable drugs. Many oral medications may be given with more scheduling flexibility than implied by the specific time intervals noted. Individual drug sensitivity and allergies must be considered in drug selection.

The authors and the publisher of this book have made every effort to ensure accuracy and appropriateness of drug selection and drug dosages. New investigations and broader experience may alter present dosage schedules, and it is recommended that the package insert for each drug be consulted before administration. Often there is limited experience with established drugs for neonates and young children. Furthermore, new drugs may be introduced, and indications for usage may change. The clinician is encouraged to maintain expertise concerning appropriate medications for specific conditions.

Foreword

The most important problem facing pediatric intensive care units in 1984 is not a lack of sophistication in either medical therapeutics or applicable technology for management of small infant children. These aspects of critical care have advanced rapidly during the past decade and have caught up with therapeutics and technology in the world of adult intensive care. The most important problem in having truly functional and effective pediatric intensive care units is the number and quality of pediatric intensive care nurses. In addition to educating nurses about the specific disease entities seen in the pediatric intensive care unit setting, certain aspects of technology and care that are concerned with the differences between children and adults must be given proper attention. The administrators and supervisors of such units assume that these two factors will be taught to and understood by pediatric intensive care nurses. What has been most elusive is the ability to provide nurses with confidence in a strong background of physiology, anatomy, pharmacology, and technology in order that, on the basis of this knowledge, they perform independent nursing care. A unit without a cadre of nurses whose independence is based on con-

fidence in their knowledge and skills will never provide first-class care. This text by Mary Fran Hazinski and her co-workers will go a long way in providing that background. Most importantly the text is by nurses for nurses. The relatively brief listing in the table of contents does an injustice to the almost encyclopedic coverage of material. The text presents a thorough review of physiology, anatomy, pharmacology, psychodynamics, technology, and management plans. The language is specific and instructional, and the coverage of each area is thorough. In addition to being well written and well organized the text is readable and available for easy reference as well as thorough review. Pediatric intensive care unit nurses should know the material presented here by Mary Fran Hazinski and her co-workers. If they do, I believe that we cannot help but see a significant development in the quality of pediatric intensive care nursing and level of care in our units.

DANIEL L. LEVIN, M.D.
Medical Director, Pediatric Intensive Care Unit,
Children's Medical Center of Dallas,
Dallas, Texas

Preface

Today's critical-care nurse must be both a generalist and a specialist. The nurse must possess proficiency in clinical assessment, hemodynamic monitoring, physiology, pathophysiology, pharmacology, and mechanical support of cardiopulmonary function. However, in many of these areas, infants and children are unique and cannot be considered "little adults." Thus the nurse caring for the critically ill child and family must also be a pediatric specialist, possessing a thorough knowledge of pediatric nutrition, fluid therapy, and normal growth and development. The pediatric critical-care nurse must also be instinctively attracted to the care of children and must be able to support the child and family through the physically and emotionally stressful critical-care period.

Pediatric critical-care nurses often have the primary responsibility for recognizing and interpreting changes in the child's condition and for instituting appropriate changes in drug therapy or mechanical support. Since the child's normal circulating blood volume, cardiac output, urine production, and ventilatory volumes are much smaller than those of the adult, quantitatively smaller variations in the child's vital signs or urine or cardiac output may indicate qualitatively more significant changes in the child's condition. Such changes must be immediately recognized by the nurse.

Until recently, pediatric critical-care nurses often learned necessary skills piecemeal at the bedside and from a variety of medical and nursing journals and texts. This book attempts to collect information about physiology, pathophysiology, pharmacology, and nursing care needed to care for the seriously ill child. The contributors have been selected because of their experience and expertise as well as for their skills in teaching pediatric critical-care nurses. Most chapters include extensive, current reference lists so that the nurse can obtain more detailed information from original sources. Many tables and charts have been included for bedside use. Whenever possible, information provided in each chapter is complete; thus the bedside nurse will not be forced to spend valuable time flipping through the book for cross-references. In addition, essential tables, such as calculation of maintenance fluid requirements in children, are included in several chapters of the book.

The first chapter, "Children are Different," provides an introduction and summary of the major ways that children differ from adults. Even though psychosocial aspects of particular diseases are discussed in each chapter, the entire second chapter is devoted to consideration of normal pediatric cognitive and emotional development, the effects of life-threatening illness on the pediatric patient and family, and the staff stresses in the critical-care unit.

The book is organized with a systems approach, so that the nurse can select a particular body system for review. One chapter each is devoted to the cardiovascular, pulmonary, neurologic, renal, and gastrointestinal systems. These chapters are divided into the following five sections:

1. Essential anatomy and physiology
2. Common clinical conditions
3. Postoperative/postprocedure care
4. Specific diseases
5. Diagnostic tests

Each chapter begins with a review of relevant anatomy and physiology. Clinical conditions common to most diseases of each system are then presented. This section includes potential *problems* the nurse should anticipate when caring for a child with a disorder of that body system, regardless of the child's specific diagnosis. For example, if the child develops low cardiac output secondary to a cardiomyopathy or myocarditis, the nurse can readily identify the important information about assessment and treatment even before the child's diagnosis is confirmed.

The chapters dealing with body systems include postoperative or postprocedure care of the child. In addition, nursing care plans are presented in table form for quick reference; they contain complete information about the nursing process.

Specific diseases are discussed in the fourth section of each chapter, including information about etiology, pathophysiology, clinical signs and symptoms, treatment, and nursing care. The final section of each body system chapter includes information about specific diagnostic procedures or tests such as cardiac catheterization, the sampling of arterial blood, transcutaneous blood gas measurements, and urinary electrolyte measurements. For each test, the indications, complications, and nursing responsibilities are discussed.

A separate chapter has been devoted to a discussion of instrumentation used in the pediatric critical-care unit. As recently as 5 years ago, pediatric critical-care equipment was largely borrowed from adult units. Now, however, pulmonary, hemodynamic, and neurologic monitoring and support equipment have been designed to provide for the specific needs of children. Since the child's cardiovascular, pulmonary, or neurologic function often depends on the proper performance of each piece of equipment used in his care, it is imperative that each nurse be familiar with the use of such equipment and with the interpretation of equipment data. This final chapter reviews principles of monitoring devices and then presents the purpose, function, and potential problems of these devices.

The Appendix provides information about transport and stabilization of the injured child. In addition, many useful reference tables, such as dosages and effects of frequently used pediatric drugs, and continuous infusion "drip" charts have been included.

This text specifically addresses care of the critically ill *child*. Since neonatal intensive care is usually regarded as an entirely different specialty, this text does *not* include problems or diseases *unique* to the neonatal period. Some disorders, such as congenital heart disease or chronic lung disease, may be common to the neonate as well as the child; thus such disorders are included. Some neonatal disorders cause chronic disease, requiring frequent hospitalizations as the child grows older. In these cases a brief description of the underlying neonatal disorder has been provided.

Although nurses and patients obviously may be male or female, we have used the female pronoun when necessary to refer to nurses and the male pronoun when referring to patients. This usage does not intend to disregard male nurses or female patients but is employed for simplicity and consistency.

With the use of sophisticated monitoring devices and computerized data collection and analysis, it is becoming easier for physicians and nurses to spend less and less time at the patient's bedside. Although these devices are important and may improve the efficiency of care, they cannot take the place of accurate measurements, astute observations, and personal warmth provided by a competent, compassionate pediatric critical-care nurse. We have tried to emphasize the importance of such observations and of direct nursing care throughout the text.

MARY FRAN HAZINSKI

Contents

CHAPTER ONE

Children are Different

MARY FRAN HAZINSKI

The purpose of this chapter is to review the similarities and differences between critically ill children and adults. Many of the clinical signs and symptoms of diseases or organ system failure are the same in all patients. Normal values of serum electrolytes and normal arterial blood gases (beyond the neonatal period) are identical for children and adults. However, because the child is growing and developing emotionally and physically, the nurse must be prepared to modify assessment skills and intervention techniques so that they are suitable for the care of children. Children have a higher metabolic rate per unit of body weight than adults; this requires a greater gas exchange, fluid and caloric intake, and urine volume per kilogram body weight than that required by adults.[18,22] However, since children are smaller than adults, the absolute quantity of their fluid requirements, urine volume, cardiac output, or minute ventilation will be less. Because of the child's small size and immaturity, some diseases or complications are more likely to occur in children. Since this chapter highlights the similarities and differences between children and adults, the reader will be referred to other chapters in the text for further details.

■ PSYCHOSOCIAL DEVELOPMENT

Because children are usually emotionally and intellectually immature, their comprehension of and response to critical illness will be different than that of adults. The child's communication skills are less refined than the adult's, so the nurse must be able to anticipate the child's needs and concerns, and to understand the child's nonverbal communication. Since the family constitutes such an important part of the child's support system, the nurse must be able to establish rapport with the family as well as with the child. The nurse must be able to provide emo-

tional support for all members of the family, since the family's anxiety can quickly be communicated to the child. Specific information about the child's emotional and intellectual development and the response of the child and family to the child's illness is included in Chapter 2.

■ GENERAL ASSESSMENT

Every critical-care nurse must develop a systematic method of determining the severity of the patient's condition, making both *qualitative* and *quantitative* evaluations. Often the nurse's impression of how the patient looks is more important than the numbers recorded on the patient's vital sign sheet. This systematic approach to nursing assessment is necessary whether the critically ill patient is a child or an adult.

When attempting to determine the severity of the child's condition, the nurse should observe the level of the child's activity. The critically ill child is usually very irritable or very lethargic, either sleeps a lot or is too irritable to sleep, and is often not interested in eating. In addition the child is usually not playful and thus not easily distracted by toys. The parents or primary caretaker should be asked to describe the child's normal activity level and activity during illness, so the nurse can better evaluate the child's behavior and response to the environment.

The nurse should form an opinion about the degree of distress the child is demonstrating whenever she approaches the patient's bed. This opinion will be based on color, facial expression, position of comfort, and apparent respiratory effort. The child who is pale with mottled skin and retractions and who is lying still with fists clenched and eyes closed certainly would seem to be in more distress than the child with pink mucous membranes who is sitting up and giggling at a story the nurse is reading. Before disturbing the child, the nurse should obtain whatever "resting" information or measurements are needed, including respiratory rate and effort, heart rate and rhythm (obtained from the cardiac monitor), arterial and venous pressures, and environmental and rectal or skin temperature, if these are displayed on a monitor. It is important to make these assessments before the child is disturbed, and then to compare this information to that obtained when the patient is awake and more active. The child with upper airway obstruction may breathe comfortably when asleep, yet demonstrate increased respiratory effort while awake and active. If, on the other hand, the child has tachypnea and severe retractions even during sleep, these signs of more significant respiratory distress should be reported to a physician immediately. If the child requires mechanical ventilatory assistance, increased inspired oxygen concentration, cardiac pacing, or other mechanical support, the nurse should be able to assess the function of the equipment and the child's dependence on it at a glance.

The child normally has a faster heart rate and respiratory rate and a lower arterial blood pressure than the adult's. As a result, smaller *quantitative* changes in the vital signs may be *qualitatively* more significant in the child than the adult. For example, if the adult's systolic blood pressure falls 15 mm Hg from 140/80 mm Hg to 125/80 mm Hg, the mean arterial blood pressure falls from approximately 100 to 95 mm Hg. This change represents an insignificant fall of 5% in the mean arterial blood pressure. If, on the other hand, the infant's systolic blood pressure falls 15 mm Hg, from 72/42 mm Hg to 57/42 mm Hg, this produces a fall in mean arterial blood pressure from 52 to 47 mm Hg. This change represents a significant fall of approximately 10% in the child's mean arterial blood pressure and may be associated with decreased systemic perfusion. The nurse must be familiar with the normal vital sign ranges for each major pediatric age-group, as well as that particular patient's usual vital sign ranges.

It is important to remember that *normal* vital signs are not always *appropriate* vital signs for the patient. The child with severe congestive heart failure is expected to be tachypneic; if the child's respiratory rate is normal, the child may be tiring and may require some ventilatory assistance. Normal vital sign ranges for children of different ages are provided in Tables 1-1 to 1-3; the nurse must be able to use these ranges and her knowledge of the child's condition to determine the appropriate vital signs for the patient.

Table 1-1 Normal heart rates in children*

Age	Beats per minute
Infants	120-160
Toddlers	90-140
Preschoolers	80-110
School-aged children	75-100
Adolescents	60-90

*Your patient's normal range should always be considered. Also, the heart rate will normally increase in the presence of fever or stress, and will decrease during sleep or vagal stimulation.

Table 1-2 Normal respiratory rates in children*

Age	Rate (breaths per minute)
Infants	30-60
Toddlers	24-40
Preschoolers	22-34
School-aged children	18-30
Adolescents	12-16

*Your patient's normal range should always be considered. Also, the child's respiratory rate is expected to increase in the presence of fever or stress.

Since fear can increase the child's heart rate, respiratory rate, and distress, the nurse must be able to differentiate between anxiety caused by emotional stress and that produced by hypoxia or poor systemic perfusion. If the nurse has developed a rapport with the child, she may be able to calm the frightened child with soothing words and gestures.

Table 1-3 Normal pediatric blood pressure ranges*

Age	Systolic (mm Hg)	Diastolic (mm Hg)
Newborns-12 hr (less than 1000 gm)	39-59	16-36
Newborns-12 hr (3 kg)	50-70	25-45
Newborns-96 hr	60-90	20-60
Infants	74-100	50-70
Toddlers	80-112	50-80
Preschoolers	82-110	50-78
School-age children	84-120	54-80
Adolescents	94-140	62-88

*The above ranges are taken from the tenth to ninetieth percentile ranges determined by the following studies: de Swiet, M., Fayers, P., and Shinebourne, E.A.: Systolic blood pressure in a population of infants in the first year of life: the Brompton study, Pediatrics **65:**1028, 1980; National Heart, Lung, and Blood Institute's Task Force on Blood Pressure Control in Children, 1978; and Versmold, H., and others: Aortic blood pressure during the first 12 hours of life in infants with birth weight 610-4220 gms, Pediatrics **67:**107, 1981.

■ **GENERAL CHARACTERISTICS**
■ **Thermoregulation**

Because infants and young children have a large surface area–to–volume ratio, they lose more heat to the environment through convection and evaporation than do adults. Cold-stressed neonates and infants (less than 6 months of age) cannot shiver to generate heat; as a result, they must break down brown fat in a process called "nonshivering thermogenesis." This process requires energy, increasing the infant's oxygen consumption. Therefore when an infant is subjected to cold stress, the infant will attempt to maintain a rectal temperature of 37° C through the breakdown of brown fat[35]; this will increase the infant's

oxygen consumption. Regeneration of the brown fat requires good nutrition; if the infant's caloric intake is inadequate, brown fat will not be made to replace that used and the infant will be less able to maintain body temperature when subjected to a cool environment.

Although the normal infant may be able to tolerate the increase in oxygen consumption that occurs during nonshivering thermogenesis, the critically ill infant may not be able to effectively increase oxygen consumption. As a result, cold stress can produce hypoxemia, lactic acidosis, and hypoglycemia. Cooling of the neonate can also produce pulmonary vasoconstriction and increased right ventricular afterload. Therefore if the infant already has a cardiovascular problem, cold stress can produce signs of increased heart failure or right-to-left intracardiac shunting.[19]

The "neutral thermal environment" is that environmental temperature at which the infant maintains a rectal temperature of 37° C with the lowest oxygen consumption. The neutral thermal environment temperature ranges for babies of different ages and weights have been determined and should be readily available in the critical-care unit (see Appendix G). The nurse is responsible for providing a neutral thermal environment throughout the infant's care, especially during transport and diagnostic tests.

Children with low cardiac output may demonstrate changes in skin or rectal temperature. Most patients with low cardiac output have cool skin as the result of adrenergic secretion and peripheral vasoconstriction. The very young infant may also demonstrate a fall in core body (rectal) temperature when systemic perfusion is poor. The older infant or child with low cardiac output typically demonstrates a low skin temperature with an increased core body temperature, since heat generated by metabolism cannot be lost through the skin.[17] As a result, both the skin and rectal temperature of the critically ill infant or child should be closely monitored.

■ **Fluid and caloric requirements**

The daily fluid requirement of the child is larger per kilogram body weight than that of the adult because the child has greater insensible water losses per unit of body weight. Children have a larger surface area–to–volume ratio than adults, so children lose relatively greater amounts of fluid to the environment through evaporation. Since the child also has a higher metabolic rate than the adult, the child requires proportionately more water per unit of body weight. As in the adult, the child's insensible water losses are increased with fever (by approximately 50 to 75 ml per degree centigrade elevation in temperature),[25,36] diaphoresis, and congestive heart failure.[20,30] Because use of radiant warmers and phototherapy will also increase the infant's insensible water losses,[6] these factors must be considered when the child's maintenance fluid requirements are calculated (Table 1-4).

Although the child's fluid requirements are higher than those of an adult per unit of body weight, the absolute amount of fluid required by the child is small. As a result the nurse must carefully total the volume of all fluids given to the child to avoid excessive fluid administration. Fluids used to flush monitoring lines or to dilute medications, including continuous infusions of vasoactive drugs, may be sources of inadvertent fluid overload. Comparison of the child's total fluid intake and total fluid output should be made several times daily to aid in evaluation of the child's fluid balance.

If the child's fluid intake is adequate, his urine volume should average 0.5 to 1.0 ml/kg/hour. Since the absolute volume of normal urine output is small in children, a small reduction in urine volume can indicate a significant change in renal perfusion or function.

All sources of fluid loss should be totaled carefully when the child is critically ill. Blood drawn for laboratory analysis, blood lost in pleural drainage, or fluid lost through vomiting, diarrhea, or gastric suctioning can produce net fluid loss in the critically ill patient. If fluid output exceeds fluid intake, the physician should be notified so that fluid administration can be increased if needed.

Daily measurement of the child's weight will aid evaluation of the fluid balance. Since the child's weight may be low, even small errors in measurement must be avoided. To ensure accuracy, the child should be weighed on the same scale at the same time of day (preferably by the same nurse). If any intravenous (IV) lines are inserted or any dressings changed, the dressings and armboard should be weighed before they are placed on the child. If this is impossible, similar materials can be weighed to provide an approximate idea of their contribution to the child's weight. Even small daily weight changes may be significant. A weight gain or loss of 50 gm/day in an infant, 200 gm/day in a child, or 500 gm/day in an adolescent should be discussed with a physician.

The child has relatively more total body water than the adult. In addition a larger proportion of the infant's free water is extracellular; approximately one half of this extracellular fluid is exchanged daily.[24] Because the infant and young child have a high daily fluid requirement and because a large proportion of the child's fluid is extracellular, decreased fluid intake or increased fluid losses can quickly produce dehydration. During the first 1 to 2 years of life, the kidneys are less able to concentrate urine; as a result, dehydration can develop and progress rapidly at this age.[24,29]

Signs of dehydration are approximately the same in all patients, regardless of age. All patients will demonstrate dry mucous membranes, decreased urine volume, and increased urine concentration. With moderate dehydration, children and adults will demonstrate weight loss; with severe dehydration, all patients will demonstrate signs of circulatory compromise. The dehydrated infant will also have a sunken fontanelle and poor skin turgor (the skin will remain "tented" after it is pinched).[7]

IV fluids are often the sole source of fluid intake for the critically ill patient. Since children have small vessels, small catheters are used for venous cannulation. Because these catheters can kink and clot easily, they require careful handling and uninterrupted flush infusion to maintain patency. In addition the catheter and tubing should be sutured or taped securely so that they will not be dislodged or disconnected if the child moves vigorously. Since the insertion of any vascular

Table 1-4 Calculation of maintenance fluids in children

Child's weight	Kilogram body weight formula
Newborns (0-72 hr old)	60-100 ml/kg
0-10 kg	100 ml/kg (may increase up to 150 ml if renal and cardiac function adequate)
11-20 kg	1000 ml for the first 10 kg + 50 ml/kg for each kg over 10 kg
21-30 kg	1500 ml for the first 20 kg + 25 ml/kg for each kg over 20 kg

line in a critically ill child may be difficult, is usually painful, and may be associated with blood loss, the lines should be carefully maintained to avoid the need for frequent reinsertion.

The child requires more calories per kilogram body weight than the adult because the child's metabolic rate is higher than that of the adult (Table 1-5). Since a larger portion of the child's maintenance calories are required for basal metabolism and growth, the critically ill child may still require most of the normal maintenance calories, even if he is immobile.[21] If a child has a fever, his caloric requirements are increased by approximately 12% per degree centigrade elevation in temperature.[37] The child usually cannot obtain sufficient calories from 5% or 10% glucose parenteral solutions, so parenteral alimentation or gavage feedings should be planned if the child will not receive oral feedings for several days.

■ **Electrolyte balance**

Normal serum electrolyte concentrations are the same for both adults and children, and renal and cellular mechanisms for maintaining serum electrolyte balance are relatively the same. However, some forms of electrolyte imbalance are more likely to occur in children than in adults or are more likely to

cause complications during childhood. Serum glucose, calcium, and potassium are three electrolytes that should be monitored very closely in the critically ill child, because imbalances of these electrolytes may be observed frequently.

Adults under stress often become *hyperglycemic,* because epinephrine and glucagon secretion stimulate glycogen breakdown and result in increased blood glucose levels.[10] Since infants have a high metabolic rate, they have high glucose needs. However, because the infant also has low glycogen stores, he can rapidly become *hypoglycemic* during periods of stress. Hypoglycemia can, in turn, depress the infant's cardiovascular function. Hypoglycemia or hyperglycemia may be an early sign of sepsis in the infant, and glycosuria may be an early sign of infection in the child. Therefore the critically ill infant's serum glucose concentration should be monitored closely, and hypoglycemia should be treated promptly. The diagnosis of sepsis or localized infection should be considered if unexplained hypoglycemia or hyperglycemia develops in an infant or if glucosuria develops in a child. In many critical-care units, a 10% glucose solution is administered as IV maintenance fluid for any infant less than 6 months of age. Since 5% or 10% glucose solutions do not provide maintenance calories, parenteral alimentation should be considered for any child who is not able to receive oral feedings for several days (see Chapter 8).

Regulation of serum ionized calcium concentration is influenced by parathyroid hormone, calcitonin secretion, glucocorticoids, thyroid function, sex hormones, and growth hormone[34]; this regulation process is less precise in the infant than in the older child or adult. Since stress stimulates the secretion of growth hormone during infancy, and growth hormone, in turn, increases calcium deposition in bone, hypocalcemia can develop in the critically ill infant.[3] The administration of citrate-phosphate-dextran (CPD) blood will produce precipitation of serum ionized calcium.[2] Therefore the critically ill infant who requires frequent transfusions is especially at risk for the development of hypocalcemia. Since hypocalcemia can depress cardiovascular function, the infant's serum calcium concentration should be monitored closely, and calcium supplements should be administered as needed to maintain a normal serum ionized calcium concentration.

Changes in the serum potassium concentration are known to occur with changes in acid-base status, use of cardiopulmonary bypass, and administration of diuretics. Since hypokalemia can cause cardiac arrhythmias and perpetuate signs of digitalis toxicity, it should be avoided in the critically ill patient. The

Table 1-5 Calculation of caloric requirements in children*

Age	Daily requirements
High-risk neonate	120-150 calories/kg
Normal neonate	100-120 calories/kg
1-2 yr	90-100 calories/kg
2-6 yr	80-90 calories/kg
7-9 yr	70-80 calories/kg
10-12 yr	50-60 calories/kg

*Ill children (with disease, surgery, fever, or pain) may require additional calories above the maintenance value, and comatose children may require fewer calories (because of lack of movement).

critically ill child does not seem to be as sensitive to hypokalemia as the adult, so cardiac arrhythmias related to hypokalemia are often not seen in children until the serum potassium is less than 3 mEq/L.[12] Ventricular fibrillation does not occur in pediatric patients frequently, but it may result from severe hypokalemia or hyperkalemia.

■ CARDIOVASCULAR FUNCTION

Normal cardiac output varies with the patient's age and weight and is higher per unit body weight in the child than in the adult. The cardiac output at birth is initially 400 ml/kg/minute; it falls to approximately 200 ml/kg/minute within the first weeks of life, and to 100 ml/kg/minute by adolescence.[31,32] Since it can be confusing to calculate the normal cardiac output for patients of different ages and sizes, the "cardiac index" is usually used. The cardiac index is equal to the cardiac output per square meter of body surface area and is usually 3.5 to 4.5 L/minutes/m² for children and adults. A cardiac index of less than 2.1 to 2.5 L/minute/m² is considered low cardiac output in a patient of any size.[23,28]

In patients of all ages, the cardiac output is the product of heart rate and ventricular stroke volume. In the child the heart rate is usually higher and the stroke volume smaller than in the adult. Tachycardia is usually the most efficient method of increasing cardiac output during childhood. As a result the child with cardiorespiratory distress or fever is expected to be tachycardic. If the heart rate exceeds 180 to 200 beats per minute, however, diastolic filling time can be compromised and stroke volume and cardiac output can fall.

Transient bradycardia may be normal in the infant or child, particularly during periods of sleep or times of vagal stimulation (such as that produced by suctioning, defecation, or feeding). Persistent bradycardia is very poorly tolerated in the infant, because cardiac output is influenced more by heart rate than stroke volume.[9,23] Profound bradycardia in the critically ill child most commonly results from hypoxemia, severe hypotension, or acidosis.

Cardiac output can be affected by changes in the ventricular stroke volume. The stroke volume increases with age; the newborn's stroke volume is less than 10 ml, and the adolescent's stroke volume is greater than 80 ml.[31] The stroke volume is affected by cardiac *preload, contractility,* and *afterload*; in any patient, cardiac output rises when preload or contractility are increased, and cardiac output can fall when afterload is increased. Volume administration is usually the most effective method of increasing cardiac

preload, yet there is evidence to suggest that the neonate with low cardiac output is less responsive to volume administration than the adult. This poor response to volume therapy is thought to result from the fact that the neonate's myocardium is less compliant and contains proportionately less contractile mass than adult myocardium.[8,15] In addition the neonate seems particularly sensitive to increases in ventricular afterload, so cardiac output can fall significantly if systemic or pulmonary vascular resistance increase.[8] As a result use of inotropic agents and afterload reduction are probably the most effective ways to increase cardiac output in critically ill neonates.

Signs of low cardiac output or poor systemic perfusion are generally the same in any patient, regardless of age. Most patients develop tachycardia, cool skin, pallor, and decreased urine output. Peripheral pulses are difficult to palpate, and metabolic acidosis develops. Hypotension is a late sign of low cardiac output. The child may also develop a high rectal temperature, because profound peripheral vasoconstriction results in reduced skin blood flow (so the heat generated by metabolism cannot be released through the skin).

Signs of congestive heart failure are also similar in the adult and the child. Most patients with congestive heart failure develop tachycardia, decreased urine output, peripheral vasoconstriction, and hepatomegaly. The infant or child with congestive heart failure may demonstrate periorbital edema, and the infant may have a full fontanelle. The jugular venous distention observed in the adult with congestive heart failure is usually not noted in the younger child, because the child's neck is shorter and fatter. Children with congestive heart failure do not often develop ascites or dependent edema, unless congestive heart failure is severe or chronic.

Tachypnea is another sign of congestive heart failure noted in both children and adults. The child also usually develops signs of increased respiratory effort, including retractions, nasal flaring, and grunting. The adult may demonstrate use of accessory muscles of respiration. Although rales are frequently noted when the adult has congestive heart failure, they may not be noted in the young child, and although the adult may demonstrate signs of either right or left ventricular failure (systemic or pulmonary venous engorgement respectively), the child usually demonstrates signs of biventricular failure. As a result signs of systemic and pulmonary venous engorgement are present.[11] (See Chapter 3 for more information.)

The child's circulating blood volume is larger

Table 1-6 Calculation of circulating blood volume in children

Age of the child	Ml/kg body weight
Neonates	85-90
Infants	75-80
Children	70-75
Adults	65-70

per unit of body weight than the adult (Table 1-6); however, the absolute blood volume of the child is still relatively small. As a result, hypovolemia can develop with even small quantities of blood loss in the child. For example, if 25 ml of blood is drawn for laboratory analysis in the 70 kg adult patient, this represents less than 0.6% of that adult's total circulating blood volume. That same 25 ml blood loss in a 7 kg infant would represent nearly 5% of that child's circulating blood volume. For this reason, the child's total circulating blood volume should be calculated on admission to the critical-care unit, and all blood lost or drawn for laboratory analysis should be totaled and considered as a portion of the child's total circulating volume. Blood replacement should be considered when the blood loss totals 5% to 7% of the child's total blood volume. Whenever blood is drawn for laboratory analysis the nurse should consult with the laboratory technicians to determine the smallest volume required for the studies; often, several studies can be performed from the same blood sample.

■ **RESPIRATORY FUNCTION**

During childhood, the airways and alveoli are growing, and the size and configuration of the chest wall is changing; as a result, many causes and symptoms of respiratory distress and respiratory failure are unique to children. Since the incidence of respiratory failure during childhood is highest during infancy,[27] information in this section of the chapter emphasizes aspects of the infant's respiratory anatomy, physiology, and symptomatology that are different than the adult's.

Because the sternum and ribs are cartilagenous,

the infant's chest wall is soft. The infant's ribs are horizontally oriented and the intercostal muscles are poorly developed, so the infant's rib cage moves easily inward or outward. When the infant's lung compliance is decreased and when greater intrathoracic pressure is generated during inspiration, the infant's chest wall may move *in* instead of out during inspiration; this causes *retractions.* When retractions are severe, it is more difficult for the infant to produce an increase in intrathoracic volume during inspiration. Retractions are, therefore, an early sign of increased respiratory effort in the infant,[4] and they may compromise the infant's ability to generate an adequate tidal volume.[26,27] By comparison, the adult's thoracic cage is fairly rigid, so retractions are noted infrequently.

Since the accessory muscles of respiration are poorly developed during early childhood, they do not contribute to the movement of the chest wall during inspiration. For this reason, the infant and young child are much more dependent on effective diaphragmatic function, and anything that compromises diaphragmatic function (such as major abdominal surgery, abdominal masses, body casts, or diaphragmatic paralysis) can dispose these patients to the development of respiratory failure. During spontaneous inspiration in the supine position, the infant's diaphragm tends to draw the lower ribs inward, because the diaphragm inserts horizontally in infants. When the infant is in the supine position, the abdominal contents tend to press against the diaphragm, limiting diaphragmatic excursion. As a result, small children with respiratory distress who are breathing spontaneously should be nursed in the upright position whenever possible.[26] Since the accessory muscles of respiration are well developed in the adult, they will be able to contribute to movement of the chest wall when more negative intrathoracic pressure must be generated. The nurse may observe contraction of the adult's sternocleidomastoid or intercostal muscles during inspiration. Because these muscles are more effective, the adult is less sensitive to compromise of diaphragmatic function. The adult's lung volume is also increased in the upright position and decreased in the supine position. However, the insertion of the adult's diaphragm is more oblique, so there is less tendency for the diaphragm to draw the lower ribs inward.[26]

The infant's larynx is structurally different than the larynx of the adult. The cartilage of the infant's larynx is soft; as a result, the infant's airway can be compressed if his neck is flexed *or* hyperextended. Whenever the critically ill infant is breathing spontaneously, a linen role should be placed under the shoulders, so the infant's neck is extended; this maximizes airway size and minimizes resistance to airflow. The cricoid cartilage is the narrowest portion of the infant's larynx, providing a natural seal around an endotracheal tube. The small size of the cricoid cartilage makes the use of cuffed endotracheal tubes in critically ill children unnecessary and often harmful. Subglottic edema or stenosis can result from prolonged or traumatic endotracheal intubation during childhood, particularly if frequent tube movement is allowed because the tube is inappropriately anchored.

Because they are easily transmitted through the thin chest wall of the young child, breath sounds may be heard over an area of atelectasis or pneumothorax as they are referred from other areas of the lung. Therefore the nurse must note changes in the *quality* of breath sounds as well as in the *quantity* of breath sounds. Often the breath sounds heard over an area of atelectasis or pneumothorax will be different in pitch if not in intensity.

When evaluating effectiveness of the child's ventilation, the nurse must also note the movement of the child's chest wall. Since the chest wall of the infant and small child is so soft, the chest wall should expand during inspiration, especially with positive pressure ventilation. If the child's chest wall is not expanding with hand or mechanical ventilation, the ventilation is ineffective, and the cause should be remedied immediately. The child's endotracheal tube may be malpositioned or occluded or the child may have developed significant atelectasis or a pneumothorax. Often the nurse can quickly assess chest wall movement by standing at the foot of the child's bed and comparing the expansion of the child's right and left chest during inspiration; if one side of the chest wall is not moving, it may be apparent immediately.

The infant is an obligatory nose-breather for approximately the first 4 weeks of life. Therefore anything causing nasal obstruction (such as choanal atresia) can produce respiratory distress.

The airways of the infant and child are smaller than the airways of the adult. Since resistance to airflow is inversely proportional to the fourth power of the airway radius, a small reduction in the child's airway radius (produced by edema or mucous) can tremendously increase resistance to airflow. For example, 1 mm of circumferential muccosal swelling in the 4 mm subglottic airway of the infant will halve the radius of the airway and increase the resistance to airflow by a factor of 16. That same 1 mm circumferential subglottic mucosal swelling in the 10 mm airway of the adult will reduce the radius of the trachea by only 20% and increase the resistance to airflow by a factor of 2.4.

Peripheral airway resistance constitutes a greater portion of total airway resistance in the infant than in the adult.[4] For this reason, diseases that also produce upper airway obstruction (such as croup or epiglottitis) produce greater respiratory embarrassment in the infant than in the adult. Since the smaller bronchioles provide relatively more resistance to airflow, the alveolar units served by the bronchioles require a longer time to fill and to empty. As a result, the duration of expiratory time during mechanical ventilation becomes extremely important; if inadequate expiratory time is provided, the alveoli may become overdistended and emphysema, alveolar rupture, and pneumothorax may occur.

Elastic tissue in the septae of the alveoli that surround the smaller airways helps support the airways so they remain open. Since the child has less alveoli than the adult, there is a greater tendency for the child's small airways to collapse,. The collateral pathways of ventilation (such as the intraalveolar Kohn's pores and the bronchoalveolar canals of Lambert) are incompletely developed during infancy. As a result, airway obstruction is more likely to produce significant compromise of gas exchange in the young child than in the adult. By later childhood and adolescence, the terminal airways are larger and have greater support from surrounding alveoli, so there is less tendency for airway collapse. Airway obstruction can cause less respiratory distress in the adolescent or adult because collateral ventilation may allow ventilation of alveoli distal to the obstruction.[27]

There is some clinical evidence that neonates may be more susceptible to the development of pulmonary edema than older infants or adults. Because increases in the neonate's pulmonary artery pressure and left atrial pressure seem to be easily transmitted to the pulmonary capillary bed, pulmonary edema may develop rapidly with pulmonary arterial or venous hypertension. For this reason, fluid restriction and possible diuresis are often necessary during the care of the critically ill neonate. Most neonates require only 50 to 60 ml/kg/day maintenance fluids if they are nursed in a well-humidified environment (so that evaporative water losses are minimized). For further information about clinical assessment of respiratory function and respiratory failure during childhood see Chapter 4.

■ **NEUROLOGIC FUNCTION**

At birth the infant's neurologic system functions largely at a subcortical level,[16] so brainstem functions (including cardiorespiratory function) and spinal cord reflexes (such as the sucking reflex) are normally present, but cortical functions (such as memory and fine motor coordination) are incompletely developed. The autonomic nervous system is intact but immature; the infant has a limited ability to control body temperature with changes in environmental temperature, and sympathetic nervous system innervation of the heart is incomplete (so the infant's heart rate is particularly sensitive to the effects of parasympathetic stimulation).[9]

At birth the brain is 25% of its mature adult weight. By 2½ years of age, the brain has achieved 75% of its adult size, and by 6 years of age, the brain is 90% of the adult weight.[33] The growth in brain size is largely the result of an increase in nerve fibers and of development of nerve tracts (between areas of the brain), rather than the result of the growth of additional neurons. Because of the tremendous growth that does occur during the first years of life, it is difficult to predict the long-term consequences of neurologic insults (such as intraventricular hemorrhage) that occur during infancy. The child may recover with less sequelae than anticipated because other areas of the brain begin to compensate for the injured areas. Subtle late signs of neurologic sequelae may manifest themselves as learning disabilities when the child enters school.

The infant's skull is not the rigid structure present in the adult. The bones of the cranium are normally not fused until approximately 16 to 18 months of age. As a result, a gradual increase in intracranial volume during infancy will usually produce an increase in the head circumference. While enlargement of the head occurs most readily before the cranial bones have fused, the sutures may separate up to 12 years of age if a significant and gradual increase in intracranial volume occurs. Cranial enlargement may allow accommodation of an increase in intracranial volume (e.g., hydrocephalus) without an increase in intracranial pressure. For this reason, the nurse should measure the infant's head circumference daily (or more frequently) if neurologic disease or injury has been noted.

Since the fontanelles are not covered by skull, palpation of the fontanelles may provide information about intracranial pressure or volume. The fontanelles should feel flat and firm; if they are bulging and tense, the infant's intracranial pressure or volume is probably increased. The fontanelle will typically bulge with any condition that causes an increase in superior vena caval pressure (including vigorous cry, congestive heart failure, and the supine position). If the fontanelle is sunken, significant dehydration may be present.[33]

Since the infant demonstrates primarily reflexive behavior, a large part of the neurologic examination will be evaluation of normal reflexes. It is important to note that a positive Babinski's reflex (fanning of the toes and dorsiflexion of the great toe when the sole of the foot is stroked) is normally observed in the infant, but it is abnormal after the infant has begun to walk. An abnormally positive Babinski's reflex is usually indicative of pyramidal tract disease.[1,5,14] Because all the cranial nerves are intact from birth, examination of cranial nerve function is possible throughout infancy and childhood. Since peripheral neurons are not myelinated until later in infancy, evaluation of fine motor skills is not possible during the first months of life.

Since the infant is unable to understand and respond to questions, evaluation of the level of consciousness is based largely on the infant's alertness, response to the environment, level of activity, and cry. Extreme sensitivity to stimuli usually indicates irritability, and extreme irritability or lethargy is abnormal during infancy. Infants with neurologic disease or injury often develop a high-pitched abnormal cry. The normal infant will usually look at bright objects or faces; the critically ill infant will often not focus visually on any object.

Once the child is old enough to comprehend and answer questions, it will be possible to determine his level of consciousness and orientation to time and place. It is helpful if the nurse records on the nursing care plan names of the child's family members and favorite pets or friends, so any nurse caring for the child can question the child about familiar people and will be able to determine the accuracy of the child's responses. The child's arousability will also be important to determine, although it may be difficult to differentiate between drowsiness caused by fatigue and that caused by neurologic insult. For example, if a 5-year-old child is brought to the emergency room in the middle of the night because he fell out of bed and struck his head, he may normally be very drowsy because his sleep has been interrupted. If, on the other hand, the same child is unresponsive when a venipuncture is performed, he has an inappropriate level of consciousness, which should be reported to a physician immediately.

Evaluation of the child's muscle tone is also an important part of a neurologic examination. The infant usually demonstrates significant dominance of flexor muscles, so extremities are flexed even when the infant is sleeping. The child also demonstrates dominance of flexor muscles (as does the adult), although the child may sleep with extremities extended or flexed. As in the adult, hypotonia or paralysis is nearly always abnormal. Small tremors may be noted during the first months of life in the normal infant, but clonic or tonic-clonic jerks (seizures) are abnormal.

Signs of increased intracranial pressure are basically the same in infants, children, and adults. They include[13]:

1. Deterioration in the level of consciousness
2. Pupillary changes (increase in size and decreased constrictive response to light)
3. Alterations in blood pressure (initially an increase in systolic blood pressure with a widened pulse pressure is noted, then a fall in blood pressure occurs—this is a *late* clinical sign)
4. Alterations in the heart rate (tachycardia may occur initially in infants and children, but bradycardia ultimately develops as a *late* sign)
5. Alterations in respirations (the respiratory rate and rhythm becomes irregular; apnea or respiratory arrest is a *late* sign)
6. Alterations in temperature (either hypothermia or hyperthermia may be noted in infants, and hyperthermia is usually noted in older children or adults)
7. Loss of motor or sensory function
8. Papilledema (this usually does not develop before 48 hours, so is not helpful as an acute sign)
9. Headache (this may be difficult to assess in infants or young children)
10. Vomiting (this may be an early sign of increased intracranial pressure in infants, but is rarely seen in adults)

For further information regarding neurologic assessment and neurologic disease during childhood, see Chapter 6.

■ **CONCLUSION**

Care of the critically ill child is generally very similar to care of the critically ill adult. However, some modifications of nursing assessment techniques and interventions are necessary as a result of the child's physical and emotional immaturity. This chapter has highlighted the ways that a critically ill child is similar to and differs from the critically ill adult. For further information about specific pediatric problems and diseases, symptomatology, treatment, and nursing interventions, the reader is referred to subsequent chapters.

REFERENCES

1. Alexander, M.M., and Brown, M.S.: The neurologic examination. In Pediatric history taking and physical diagnosis for nurses, ed. 2, New York, 1979, McGraw-Hill Book Co.
2. Behrendt, D.M., and Austen, W.G.: Management of infants undergoing cardiac surgery. In Patient care in cardiac surgery, ed. 3, Boston, 1982, Little, Brown & Co.
3. Benawra, R.S., and Mangurten, H.: Neonatal hypocalcemia, Q. Pediatr. Bull. Lutheran General Hosp. **5**:97, 1979.
4. Bryan, A.C., Mansell, A.L., and Levison, H.: Development of the mechanical properties of the respiratory system. In Hodson, W.A., editor: Development of the lung, New York, 1977, Marcel Dekker, Inc.
5. Conway, B.L.: Techniques in assessment. In Pediatric neurologic nursing, St. Louis, 1977, The C.V. Mosby Co.
6. Dreszer, M.: Fluid and electrolyte requirements in the newborn infant, Pediatr. Clin. North Am. **24**:537, 1977.
7. Finberg, L.: Diarrheal dehydration. In Winters, R.W.: The body fluids in pediatrics, Boston, 1973, Little, Brown, & Co.
8. Friedman, W.F.: The intrinsic physiologic properties of the developing heart. In Friedman, W.F., Lesch, M., and Sonnenblick, E.H., editors: Neonatal heart disease, New York, 1973, Grune & Stratton, Inc.
9. Friedman, W.F., and others: Sympathetic innervation of the developing rabbit heart, Circ. Res. **23**:25, 1968.
10. Guyton, A.C.: Metabolism of carbohydrates and formation of adenosine triphosphate. In Textbook of medical physiology, ed. 6, Philadelphia, 1981, W.B. Saunders Co.
11. Hazinski, M.F.: Critical care of the pediatric cardiovascular patient, Nurs. Clin. North Am. **16**:671, 1981.
12. Hazinski, M.F., and Weinberg, M., Jr.: Care of the surgical pediatric cardiac patient. In Neville, W.E., editor: Intensive care of the surgical cardiopulmonary patient, ed. 2, Chicago, 1983, Year Book Medical Publishers, Inc.
13. Hickey, J.V.: Increased intracranial pressure. In The clinical practice of neurological and neurosurgical nursing, Philadelphia, 1981, J.B. Lippincott Co.
14. Hickey, J.V.: The neurological physical exam. In The clinical practice of neurological and neurosurgical nursing, Philadelphia, 1981, J.B. Lippincott Co.
15. Hoffman, J.I.E.: Factors affecting shunting and the development of heart failure. In Heymann, M.A., and Rudolph, A.M., editors: The ductus arteriosus, Columbus, 1978, Ross Laboratories, Inc.
16. Huttenlocher, P.R.: Evaluation of the child with neurologic disease. In Behrman, R.E., Vaughan, V.C., and Nelson, W.E., editors: Nelson textbook of pediatrics, ed. 12, Philadelphia, 1983, W.B. Saunders Co.
17. Idriss, F.S., and others: Postoperative management of the pediatric cardiac surgical patient. In Beal, J.M., editor: Critical care for surgical patients, New York, 1982, Macmillan Publishing Co., Inc.

18. Johnson, T.R., Moore, W.M., and Jeffries, J.E.: Children are different: developmental physiology, ed. 2, Columbus, Ohio, 1978, Ross Laboratories, Inc.

19. Klaus, M., Fanaroff, A.A., and Martin, R.J.: The physical environment. In Klaus, M.H., and Fanaroff, A.A., editors: Care of the high-risk neonate, ed. 2, 1979, Philadelphia, W.B. Saunders Co.

20. Kraus, A.N., and Auld, P.A.M.: Metabolic rate of neonates with congenital heart disease, Arch. Dis. Child. **50:**539, 1975.

21. Laupus, W.E.: Nutritional requirements. In Behrman, R.E., Vaughan, V.C., and Nelson, W.E., editors: Nelson textbook of pediatrics, ed. 12, Philadelphia, 1983, W.B. Saunders Co.

22. Leifer, G.: Some unique aspects of pediatrics. In Principles and techniques in pediatric nursing, ed. 4, Philadelphia, 1982, W.B. Saunders Co.

23. Loomis, J.C.: Care of the pediatric patient following cardiovascular surgery. In Ream, A.K., and Fogdall, R.P., editors: Acute cardiovascular management, anesthesia, and intensive care, Philadelphia, 1982, J.B. Lippincott Co.

24. Metheny, N.M., and Snively, W.D.: Fluid disturbances in infants and children. In Nurses' handbook of fluid balance, ed. 3, Philadelphia, 1979, J.B. Lippincott Co.

25. Metheny, N.M., and Snively, W.D.: The role of nursing observations in the diagnosis of body fluid disturbances. In Nurses' handbook of fluid balance, ed. 3, Philadelphia, 1979, J.B. Lippincott Co.

26. Muller, N.L., and Bryan, A.C.: Chest wall mechanics and respiratory muscles in infants, Pediatr. Clin. North Am. **26:**503, 1979.

27. Newth, C.J.L.: Recognition and management of respiratory failure, Pediatr. Clin. North Am. **26:**617, 1979.

28. Pan, G.V.S., Blackstone, E.H., and Kirklin, J.W.: Cardiac performance and mortality early after intracardiac surgery in infants and young children, Circulation **51:**867, 1975.

29. Rahill, W.J.: Renal physiology-clinical variations. In Rubin, M.P., and Barratt, T.M., editors: Pediatric nephrology, Baltimore, 1975, The Williams & Wilkins Co.

30. Rickard, K., Brady, M.S., and Gresham, E.L.: Nutritional management of the chronically ill child: congenital heart disease and myelomeningocele, Pediatr. Clin. North Am. **24:**157, 1977.

31. Rudolph, A.M.: Changes in the circulation after birth. In Congenital diseases of the heart, Chicago, 1974, Year Book Medical Publishers, Inc.

32. Rudolph, A.M.: General discussion. In Heymann, M.A., and Rudolph, A.M., editors: The ductus arteriosus, Columbus, 1978, Ross Laboratories, Inc.

33. Whaley, L.F., and Wong, D.L.: The normal neonate. In Nursing care of infants and children, ed. 2, St. Louis, 1983, The C.V. Mosby Co.

34. Widdowson, E.M., and McCauce, R.A.: The metabolism of calcium, phosphorus, magnesium, and strontium, Pediatr. Clin. North Am. **12:**595, 1965.

35. Williams, J.K., and Lancaster, J.: Thermoregulation of the newborn, MCN: Am. J. Mat. Child Nurs. **1:**355, 1976.

36. Winters, R.W.: Maintenance fluid therapy. In The body fluids in pediatrics, Boston, 1973, Little, Brown, & Co.

37. Winters, R.W.: Maintenance requirements. In Principles of pediatric fluid therapy, ed. 2, Boston, 1982, Little, Brown & Co.

ADDITIONAL READING

Godfrey, S., and Baum, J.D., editors: Clinical paediatric physiology, Oxford, 1979, Blackwell Scientific Publications.

Psychosocial Aspects of Pediatric Critical Care

LINDA A. LEWANDOWSKI

The hospitalization of a child for even a minor illness is a stressful experience for both child and family. When the child is critically ill, however, the strain is magnified. With sensitive, caring staff, some of the most stressful aspects can be mitigated and the experience made more positive and perhaps even growth-promoting for patient and relatives.

Especially important is the role played by the pediatric critical-care nurse. Nurses spend the most time with the child and family and thus have greatest opportunities for assessment and intervention. Nurses can also influence the approaches of other members of the health-care team to the child and family. A nurse who focuses only on the physiologic and technologic aspects of critical care will be meeting only part of her responsibility. Lack of attention to each child's and family's special abilities, needs, and fears will result in a negative experience for the child and family and may actually contribute to deleterious psychologic effects. Children and their families are in need of understanding and support since the hospitalization experience often represents a crisis period in their lives.

It is impractical to discuss a child and his reactions without also discussing the child's parents. Parental support is an extremely important part of the child's coping skills. Robertson states that, during hospitalization, a child's relationship with his mother governs the patient's level of emotional tension. This is also true of the child's relationship with the father. Robertson further states that this relationship is a prime factor in determining whether changes in the child's emotions and behavior during hospitalization will be detrimental or beneficial to treatment and recovery.[115]

Sullivan[140] describes an emotional linkage or empathy between the child and significant adults. There is evidence of this emotional contagion long before the child shows signs of any comprehension of emotional expression. Thus high anxiety in the parents will lead to high anxiety in the child; a calm, nurturing, and supportive attitude on the part of the parents, on the other hand, will help the child to cope effectively with the situation. Therefore the child's parents and other significant people in the child's life (e.g., siblings) must also be a focus of nursing care and concern. Nursing support is important not only for the sake of the family members but also because of their effect on the child's stress level and recovery.[24,79,134,151,159]

In addition to the physical trauma the child may be experiencing, psychologic stress itself may lead to physiologic complications.[131] The release of catecholamines (i.e., epinephrine and norepinephrine) and their metabolites is one of the most reliable indicators of stress. Increases in blood pressure and pulse rate are early responses of the cardiovascular system to stress. Cardiac glycogen tends to be depleted during periods of stress, and release of vasopressin may result in a decrease in urine output. Stress can accelerate blood coagulation and increase fibrinolysis.[131] Since the basal metabolic rate may increase, body temperature regulation may be made more difficult by the increase in heat production and concomitant increase in heat loss. Adrenocorticotropic hormone (ACTH) is released, causing increased secretion of glucocorticoids, which in turn may lead to hyperglycemia, suppressed immune and inflammatory reactions, thymus shrinkage, and atrophy of lymph nodes. Stress ulcers, increased catabolism, and loss of body weight can occur.[131] Critical illness itself would seem to pose more than enough physiologic problems for the child, without the added physiological effects that accompany acute stress—effects that could be decreased by reducing the child's stress and increasing his ability to cope with the stressful experience.

This chapter explores the psychosocial, emotional, and developmental aspects to be considered when caring for critically ill children in each major age-group. It reviews children's ability to understand and cope with what is happening to them, their major fears, reactions to pain, requirement for play, concept of death, and need for their parents' support, as well as attendant implications for the pediatric critical-care nurse. The chapter also summarizes some reactions of family members to the critical-care unit and some of their special needs during the time the child is critically ill or dying. Finally, both stressful and rewarding aspects of the role of the nurse in a pediatric critical-care unit are reviewed.

■ THE CRITICALLY ILL INFANT

In recent years, much has been discovered regarding the amazing and exciting capabilities of the neonate. At one time infants were regarded as passive recipients of care, unable to see, hear, or interact. We now know that the normal infant comes into the world fully able to establish eye contact, to respond to and discriminate among various sounds, and to initiate social interactions with his parents.[40,50,117,147] A wide range of individual differences in infants with respect to neurobehavioral maturity and control, temperature, and styles of behavior and communication is now recognized by investigators.[*]

■ Developmental tasks

To provide optimal care for the critically ill infant, the nurse must understand some of the special characterisics, needs, and behavioral cues exhibited during this stage of development. Erikson[38] has identified eight crises that must be resolved at major stages of human development. The developmental crisis of infancy is to acquire a sense of basic trust while overcoming a sense of mistrust. To acquire a sense of trust, the infant must develop confidence that his physical needs will be met. The infant also must develop a sense of physical safety. Once this sense of trust is achieved, unfamiliar or unknown situations can be tolerated with a minimum of fear.[157] The quality of the parent-infant interaction and the parents' ability to interpret the infant's cues are highly important to the development of trust.

*References 18, 19, 20, 39, 50, 65, 144.

When an infant is repeatedly frustrated in attempts to make his needs known and have them met, distrust and pessimism about the world may develop.

Both Erikson and Freud have identified infancy as the oral phase of development. Sucking is of primary importance to the infant; it is the infant's major source of gratification and of tension release.

When an infant is hospitalized, particularly in a critical-care unit, the potential for frustration is extremely high. Illness disrupts many of the child's physiologic processes. In addition normal routines and rhythms—eating, sleeping, and exercise—are disrupted. The infant is placed in an unfamiliar environment with unfamiliar caretakers who are not as sensitive as the parents to the infant's cues. The presence of an endotracheal tube or restraints may prevent the infant from sucking, eliminating one of the major sources of gratification and comfort.

The parents are usually best able to teach the nurse about their infant's individual cues, needs, and responses. As a result, their presence during the hospitalization can be extremely helpful in ensuring that the baby's needs are met.

Although infants are unable to verbally express their feelings and needs, they do give indications of their need for more attention or stimulation. And, perhaps more important, they communicate when they are becoming overstimulated and need a rest.

Infants do in fact give signals at a behavioral level often before an irreversible catastrophe to their physiologic stability. Depending on the relative fragility or stability of their physical condition and neurologic maturity, infants use skin color changes, fluctuation and disintegration of movement controls, respiratory irregularities, changes in activity levels, postural shifts (e.g., turning away from the source of stimulation), gaze aversion, facial muscle tone and expression, hiccoughs, yawns, and disturbances in sleep/wake cycle to warn caregivers of impending overload to their nervous system. Tuning of caregiving procedures relative to infant state behavior seems to predict positive or negative sequelae.[50]

It is crucial that the nurse who is planning and providing care constantly assesses the infant's tolerance of these care measures. Many nurses attempt to perform a great number of procedures all at once so that the patient has longer periods of uninterrupted rest. This may work very well for older children but may not be optimal for an infant. Too much stimulation at one time can tax the sick infant's already diminished coping resources, resulting in adverse physiologic reactions such as vomiting, respiratory distress, apnea, or bradycardia.[50]

Gaze aversion is a behavioral cue nurses and parents sometimes miss.

Three-month-old Jamie underwent surgery for ligation of a patent ductus arteriosus. On the second postoperative day, Jamie was being held by his nurse after feeding. She repeatedly tried to establish eye contact with him, but he continued to look away from her. Each time Jamie looked away the nurse spoke encouragingly to him and turned his body or bent her head so that they were again in a position to have eye contact. After several gaze aversion attempts on Jamie's part, he finally vomited his feeding.

Since the nurse had not understood the first cue that Jamie was becoming overstimulated and could not tolerate eye contact at that point in time, the stimulation continued and led to a more extreme response.

■ States of consciousness

The infant's state of consciousness exerts a powerful influence on the way he will respond at any given time.[13] Two sleep states and four awake states have been identified in full-term infants: deep sleep, light sleep; drowsy, quiet alert, active alert, and crying.[13,103,111,160]

During *deep sleep* the infant is still except for occasional startles or twitches. There are no eye or facial movements except for occasional sucking movements at regular intervals. The infant's threshold to stimuli is very high. Only very intense and disturbing stimuli will arouse infants in this state. Although shaking the infant or flicking the bottom of his foot may arouse him briefly, usually he will then return to sleep. The nurse will generally be frustrated in attempts to feed an infant in this state or to arouse him to an alert state. It is generally more effective to wait until the baby moves to a more responsive state. It is important for the nurse to be aware that this deep sleep state exists normally and that the inability to arouse an infant may result from this state rather than from neurologic abnormalities such as increased intracranial pressure.

Light sleep accounts for the highest proportion of an infant's sleep. During this state, some body activity, rapid eye movements (fluttering of eyes beneath closed eyelids), and irregular breathing are observed. Infants are more responsive to stimuli and more easily arousable during this period.

During the *drowsy* state, a variable activity level, irregular breathing, and delayed response to sensory stimuli are present. The infant's eyes appear heavy lidded and have a dull, glazed appearance. Infants in this state can often be aroused to the more interactive quiet alert state by providing them with something to see, hear, and suck. Such intervention may be helpful in facilitating parent-infant interaction in the critical-care unit.

It is during the *quiet-alert* state that the infant can be the most fun and provide the most positive feedback to parents or other caretakers. Infants in this state have wide, very bright eyes, regular breathing, and minimal body activity. They are interested in their environment and focus attention on their caretakers, moving objects, or other stimuli. It can be gratifying and comforting for parents to see their very ill infant in this state since the parents are able to smile at and talk to the baby.

Infants in a critical-care unit may spend a large portion of their awake time in an *active-alert* state. This is characterized by much body activity with periods of fussiness. Breathing is irregular. The infant's eyes are open but are not as bright as in the quiet alert state, and there is much facial movement. The infant becomes increasingly sensitive to and upset by disturbing stimuli such as hunger, noise (prevalent in most critical-care units), and excessive handling. As the infant gets more and more active and upset, intervention is often necessary to bring the infant to a lower state and avoid escalation into a crying state.

Crying is one of infant's major methods of communication: a way the infant communicates that his limits have been reached.[13] The infant shows increased body activity, grimaces, eyes that are open or tightly closed, and more irregular breathing. Although the infant's color may change to bright red, very sick patients or those with cyanotic heart disease may demonstrate circumoral or more generalized cyanosis. Sometimes the infant can bring himself to a quieter state by instituting self-consoling behaviors such as sucking on fingers, fist, tongue, or endotracheal tube or by paying attention to voices or faces nearby or changing position.[13] However, self-consoling maneuvers often are not effective in stressed, ill infants, who often need assistance from their caretakers. Some soothing maneuvers the caretaker can try include changing the infant's diaper or feeding him when necessary; bringing her face close to the infant; talking to the infant in a calm, soft voice; holding both infant's arms close to his body; swaddling, picking up, and rocking the infant; and giving the baby a pacifier. It is important to realize that infants frequently are highly upset when uncovered or wrapped loosely but become calm and drowsy when they are swaddled.[13,101,107,157] Swaddling a critically ill infant snugly is often very difficult or

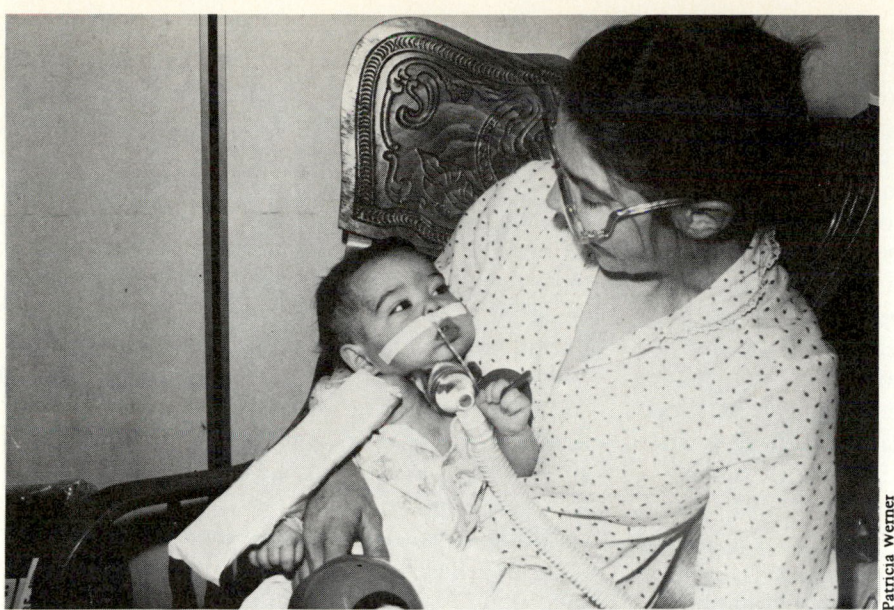

Fig. 2-1 Rocking in mother's lap is very comforting for the sick infant and for his mother.

impossible. However, wrapping or covering the baby as tightly as possible or placing rolled towels[120] or blankets on each side of the torso may be calming. A combination of verbal and tactile (such as patting, stroking, holding, rocking) stimuli is generally more effective in alleviating distress in hospitalized infants than verbal stimuli alone.[146] Rocking seems to bring comfort and build trust between the infant and caretaker.[89] Use of a rocking chair can also relax the parent or nurse as well as the patient (Fig. 2-1).

Touch is extremely important to infants, who need to be caressed, stroked, cuddled, held, hugged, and loved in order to feel secure and develop normally. Many studies have shown the detrimental long-term effects of lack of tactile stimulation during infancy.[112,138]

■ **Cognitive development in infancy**

Cognitive or intellectual development in normal children has been observed and described in detail by the Swiss psychologist, Jean Piaget. Piaget has identified five major phases in a child's development of logical thought.[42,107] The pediatric critical-care nurse must have an understanding of these phases to communicate effectively with children and to understand the basis of their perceptions, fears, and misunderstandings.

Piaget calls the period of infancy and early toddlerhood (from birth to approximately 2 years) the *sensorimotor* phase. There are six stages in this phase of intellectual development. From birth to 1 month, the infant generally uses reflexes like sucking, grasping, and crying. The infant is completely self-centered and cannot differentiate self from others. Infants in this stage show little or no tolerance for frustration or delayed gratification.

In the second stage (approximately 1 to 4 months), the use of reflexes is gradually replaced by voluntary activity. Infants begin to recognize familiar faces and objects such as a bottle, and they show awareness of strange surroundings. They begin to differentiate self from other people and to discover parts of their own body. Young infants delight in playing with their fingers, hands, and feet. These infants seem to believe that an object or person exists only while within their range of vision. If an object falls to the floor or is hidden, the infant immediately loses interest and will not search for it. If a person leaves the room, or even moves out of sight, the infant acts as though that individual no longer exists.[43] Infants in this stage show no anxiety around strangers, and they seem to become bored when left alone for more than a few minutes.

In sensorimotor stage three (approximately 4 to 8 months), causality, time, deliberate intention, and appreciation of separateness from the environment are beginning to develop.[157] During this stage the infant begins to develop the concept of *object permanence*[3]; that is, objects and people exist even when they cannot be seen. The infant will search for partially hidden objects and will look for objects that have disappeared from view,[43] realizing that his parents are present even when they are not in his visual field.[157] Once the infant develops object permanence, attachment to parents or primary caretakers is obvious and strong. The baby demonstrates stranger anxiety and can be expected to protest when his parents depart. He is beginning to be able to postpone gratification and awaits anticipated routines with happy expectation.[153] He is developing an association between objects and events. For example, the infant may begin to cry when a nurse comes forward with a syringe and prepares to administer an injection. Not yet able to take constructive action (such as withdrawal) to try to prevent the painful event, the baby "simply cries to let you know he doesn't like being the victim of your aggressive act."[17]

During the fourth sensorimotor stage (approximately 9 to 12 months), the infant's concept of object permanence develops further. The baby learns that hidden objects still exist, and he can take action (such as retrieving an object from under a blanket) to make the object reappear.[43] This is the beginning of intellectual reasoning. The infant begins to understand the meaning of some words and simple commands and begins to associate gestures with events. For example, waving means someone is going "bye-bye." The presence of the infant's mother is extremely important to the infant's sense of security, and the threat of her departure is met with protests. A sense of independence in feeding and locomotion is developing, and the infant begins to venture away from his mother for short periods to explore the surroundings. The infant now responds to his name and inhibits behavior when told "no, no." By the end of this stage the infant is jabbering expressively, verbalizing words that mean his parents, and saying a few other simple words.

It is during this period that the infant may adopt a favorite blanket, pillow, or stuffed animal as a *transitional object*,[158] which provides comfort and a sense of security during the parent's absence. The "Peanuts" comic strip character, Linus, is known by his transitional object, his blanket.[75] Absence of the transitional object, particularly during times of stress, will cause the child more anxiety. Thumb sucking, genital play, and need for a transitional object are all means by which the child attempts self-consolation in the absence of the parent.[73] Nine-month old Maria calmed herself after a stressful experience by covering her head with her special blanket. Under the security of this tattered friend, she was able to escape from the threatening world outside.

The last two stages in the sensorimotor phase are discussed in the toddler section.

■ The infant in the critical-care environment

The young infant admitted to a critical-care unit may be most affected by the strange environment and disruption of normal routines. The infant's usual sleep/wake cycles are interrupted or interfered with by procedures, lights, alarms, or other noxious stimulation. Often there are attempts to arouse the infant regardless of the sleep state. Sensory deprivation because of a lack of meaningful stimulation is also a hazard of the critical-care unit for children of all ages. Constant, rhythmic sounds such as the "whooshing" of a ventilator and the "beeping" of a cardiac monitor need to be broken by more meaningful, varying sounds such as talking, humming, or singing to the infant or by playing records, tapes, or radio with soft, soothing music. Some hospitals have music therapists on their staff who can help break the sound monotony. It must be kept in mind, however, that too much noise (such as loud laughing or talking at the nurses' desk or very loud, fast music) may be highly disturbing to a critically ill child. Infants or older children who receive paralytic agents such as pancuronium (Pavulon) are hypersensitive to bright lights, loud music, and voices.[99] Since they are not able to move, they may become extremely anxious. The nurse must maintain a soothing and reassuring environment for these children.

The often stark, sterile environment of the critical-care unit can be made more comforting by the use of natural lighting, color on the walls and curtains, and bright mobiles.[58] Colorful blankets, toys, or stuffed animals from home can help make the environment more attractive. The infant's parents can tape pictures of themselves or other family members on the infant's crib in his line of vision to give their child something to look at (infants particularly enjoy looking at faces) and to give the parents the opportunity to personalize the environment.

■ Major fears of infancy

From approximately 6 months of age through the preschool period, separation anxiety is by far the infant's major source of fear. Separation from the mother (or father if he has been a primary caretaker) is extremely stressful. Since separation is so traumatic and painful, it is helpful for a parent to stay with the hospitalized infant as much as possible. Most hospitals now have facilities for parents to room-in with young children. Though it may be impossible to provide space or facilities for parents to remain with their children throughout their critical-care stay, it is extremely beneficial to maintain flexible visiting opportunities around the clock for parents.

Robertson[115] has identified three distinct phases in the crisis of separation: protest, despair, and denial. During the *protest* phase the child cries loudly and screams for his parents while visually searching for them. The infant will tightly cling to the parent if the adult shows signs of leaving. Attention from others is rejected and may even intensify the protest of a child who is experiencing stranger anxiety. Such a patient may seem inconsolable, sometimes quieting only when exhausted. This anxiety, which may last from several hours to several days depending on the child's energy and level of illness,[115] can only add to the child's stress in the critical-care unit. The baby who is demonstrating protest behavior may be frustrating to care for but still needs closeness and acceptance from the nursing staff. By providing consoling gestures, conversation, and objects (such as a pacifier or transitional object) the nurse may succeed in comforting the child. If the nurse takes the time to get acquainted with the patient while the parent is present, that nurse may seem "safe" to the infant, who may, as a result, be more receptive to that nurse's attempts at consolation. It may also be helpful to attempt to distract the infant with a colorful toy or musical mobile.

The second phase of the separation crisis is the phase of *despair.* In this phase the child continues the mourning process but becomes more passive and withdrawn. He seems disinterested in play, food, or the environment and looks sad, lonely, isolated, apathetic, and depressed.[157] Some of the child's activities during this phase may be thumb sucking, masturbation, head banging, rocking, fingering locks of hair, sitting quietly, or clutching a toy.[120] The child continues to watch for the parents' return. When they do come, he may ignore them or act angry but will usually cling ferociously to them if they show signs of leaving again. The child's depression is thought to be a result of increasing hopelessness, grief, and mourning; the child is losing hope that the parents will return for him.[157]

The last phase of the separation crisis is *denial* or *detachment.* The child seems to have adjusted at last, appearing friendly and interested in the environment and other people. He is more receptive to strangers and accepts caretaking from many people. This phase may be interpreted by inexperienced staff as a positive sign that the child is "settling in," getting over his anxiety,[157] and now becoming a "good patient." This behavior is not a sign of contentment, however, but of resignation. The child detaches from the parent to escape the pain of separation.[115] He denies longing for the parent's presence. The child who has advanced to this stage of denial may react with indifference when the parent returns or may

seem to prefer the nurse or another staff member.

Since the parent's presence occasionally seems to upset the hospitalized child, uninformed staff may feel justified in restricting parental visiting privileges.[157] If the parents do not understand the basis of the child's distress, they may be extremely upset. They may restrict their time with the child in an attempt to minimize his distress; this, however, will only reinforce the child's fears. It is important for the nurse to explain the child's behavior to parents and to encourage parents to spend as much time as they can with their child. The nurse needs to assure the parents that they are welcome in the unit and that they are helping their child to cope effectively with the frightening critical-care unit environment. By minimizing the parent's distress, the nurse will be helping to maintain the child's best support system.

■ The infant and pain

The infant's response to pain varies with his stage of development. Although the degree of pain an infant perceives is still not known, it is now widely accepted that infants do feel pain.[4,110] The neonate's physical response to pain is generalized total body movement with a brief period of crying that ceases with distraction (holding, cuddling, or being given a pacifier).[110] Because the young infant cannot verbalize discomfort and because distraction effectively comforts the infant when the painful procedure is completed, some health-care personnel perform painful procedures on infants without the administration of pain medication or local anesthetics. The long term physiologic effects of such exposure to pain in the young infant are not known. In general, painful procedures such as chest tube or central line insertion should not be performed until the infant receives an analgesic. Many times nurses do not medicate infants postoperatively because they do not believe infants perceive pain in the same way older children do; but infants do, in fact, perceive pain. The nurse must be alert to behavioral cues of the infant's discomfort, such as irritability, restlessness, lethargy, poor feeding, disturbed sleep patterns, tachycardia, or increased respiratory distress.

Between 3 and 10 months of age the infant can localize existing pain (e.g., he will attempt to withdraw a leg following an injection). Before 6 months of age, infants do not seem to remember previous painful experiences.[70] After 6 months of age, however, the child's response to pain is influenced by memory of past painful experiences and the anxiety of the parents during the procedure (via the emotional contagion that occurs). Therefore preparation of the infant and parent before any procedure should also be aimed at decreasing the parent's anxiety to improve the infant's response to the procedure.[155]

■ Preparation of the infant for procedures and surgery

See the box on pp. 43-45.

Older infants react intensely to potentially painful situations. They are uncooperative and may refuse to lie still, attempting to push the threatening person away or to escape. Distraction is not as effective as it is with younger infants. The best technique to decrease the fear and resistance of the older infant is to familiarize him with some of the equipment beforehand (e.g., letting the older infant play with a stethoscope), to perform the procedure as quickly as possible, and to maintain parent-child contact.[157] Advance warning of a painful procedure is essential. Painful procedures should *never* be performed on a sleeping child. Belmont[10] describes a situation in which a nurse removed the blanket from a sleeping infant and plunged an intramuscular injection into his buttock without awakening him. The child awoke screaming whenever anyone approached his crib for many weeks thereafter.

■ Play in infancy

Play is critical for development, providing an important way for infants to learn about the world.[28] The first of the three types of play during infancy is *social-affective* play, where the infant interacts with people.[157] The baby learns to imitate adult actions, such as coughing or sticking out his tongue, at a very young age.[23] The second type is *sense-pleasure* play, where the infant derives pleasure from objects in the environment such as lights and colors, tastes and odors, textures and consistencies. Body motion—such as rocking, swinging, or bouncing—and pleasant sounds also provide pleasurable experiences.[157] *Sensorimotor* activity is the third category of play during infancy. Infants first begin to play with their bodies, bringing hands and feet into their mouths; oral testing is one of the most important means of exploration at this time. Motor activity is highly enjoyable for infants, and they take great pleasure in kicking their feet and waving their arms.[153] Between 7 and 10 months of age, the infant is able to enjoy throwing things out of the crib onto the floor.[56] This game seems to be an endless source of fun for the infant; parents and nurses tire of it long before the infant does.

It is very frustrating for the infant to have his feet and arms restrained, particularly when he is accustomed to being very active. Therefore restraints should be used in the critical-care unit only when absolutely necessary.[30] When restraints are necessary, they should still allow the infant as much movement as safety permits.

Pediatric critical-care nurses sometimes need to use a great deal of creativity in facilitating the play of these very ill little patients. Toys that are appropriate for the baby's age should be available, and the nurse should encourage the parents to bring toys from home. The older infant may benefit from watching the nurse play with puppets or dolls or draw pictures at the bedside. This form of passive play may provide the infant with a pleasant distraction from discomfort and fear.

■ The infant and death

Death, *per se*, has no meaning for the infant. The infant's reactions to fatal illness will be based on the degree of discomfort involved and on the parents' reactions. Emotional empathy exists between parents and children,[11,140] which allows for a special kind of communication that makes the feelings of each transparent to the other. Parents serve as the frame of reference for the child, and parental attitudes and feelings are clearly transmitted, even when words may not be fully understood by the child. Therefore if the parents are helped to deal with their strong feelings of anxiety, they will be able to be more calm and supportive with their child; this will decrease the infant's anxiety. Since separation from parents is the most stressful event that can happen to an infant, even highly anxious parents should not be kept away from their child.

■ THE CRITICALLY ILL TODDLER

Ideally, hospitalization of older infants and toddlers (ages 1 to 3) should be avoided since this is the age-group at greatest risk for permanent emotional problems related to the experience of hospitalization.[115] Admission to a critical-care unit can be an even more terrifying experience for a toddler than hospitalization on a pediatric floor. The pediatric critical-care nurse can be instrumental in making this experience less traumatic and more productive for the toddler and his parents.

■ Emotional and psychosocial development of toddlers

The major developmental task for toddlers is beginning the development of autonomy or self-control.

Toddlers are increasingly independent and able to do things for themselves as much as possible. They can be a bountiful source of enjoyment and satisfaction for any caretaker as they take delight in exploring and discovering new things, and they are often liberal with expressions of affection such as engaging smiles, hugs, and kisses. However, their reputation as the "terrible twos" is also well-deserved, and a great deal of patience and understanding is necessary when caring for them. This is the "no" stage, and this newly learned word is often adamantly stated even when the toddler may want to say "yes" (a word and concept that is not learned until later). Resistive behavior results as the toddler struggles to assert independence and gain control of the environment. Frequent temper tantrums can result from the toddler's low frustration tolerance and need to test the limits of acceptable behavior. Dawdling behavior is common during this period, particularly at mealtime.

The toddler is very attached to and dependent on his parents. Parents represent safety and security. As the toddler grows more aware of separateness from the mother, he seeks more attention from her and greater closeness to her. The child is now able to form relationships with his parents, rather than simply requiring their presence.[75]

Although the toddler is now able to tolerate some physical distance from a parent and will venture away to explore and play, he will need to run back to find the parent or call to the parent at short intervals. Separation from the parents for prolonged or unexpected periods is very difficult, particularly when the toddler is also faced with other stresses. Older toddlers are more able to accept symbols, such as mommy's purse or daddy's keys, as an indication that the parent will return. The toddler may also be more able to accept caretaking and consolation from another person if given an opportunity to become familiar with that individual over a period of time and if that person is observed by the toddler to have the parent's approval.

Freud refers to the toddler years as the "anal stage," since elimination and retention are areas of concern. Toilet training begins during this period. Since this is a newly acquired skill for the toddler, it may easily be lost when the toddler is stressed, for example, by admission to the critical-care unit.

■ Cognitive development of the toddler

The toddler makes massive strides in intellectual development, beginning to "think" and "reason," although in a way that is different from adult cognition. During Piaget's fifth sensorimotor stage of intel-

lectual development (approximately 13 to 18 months) the toddler further differentiates himself from other objects and will search for an object where it was last seen to disappear. Early traces of memory also begin to develop during this period. The child in this stage is beginning to be aware of causal relationships and can understand that flipping a switch will cause a machine to make noise. However, the child is not able to transfer that knowledge to new situations and will not be aware that turning a switch of another machine may have the same outcome. The toddler must continuously examine the same object every time it appears in a new place or under changed conditions. Thus a stethoscope is something new to be investigated each time it is brought to the bedside by a new person.

During the final stage of the sensorimotor period (approximately 19 to 24 months), egocentric and magical thinking begin. Toddlers view themselves as the center of the universe and can appreciate no point of view but their own. As toddlers become aware of their thoughts, they believe that others must also be aware of them and believe that events happen because of their activity, thoughts, and wishes.[153] Thus the toddler will believe that his anger made mommy or daddy go away or that his being bad made him get sick.

The toddler is extremely ritualistic and takes comfort from consistency of environment and daily activities. The global organization of thought that is characteristic of this period causes the child to recognize experiences or events as parts of a whole. As a result, if even small changes in the environment or schedule are made, the child usually requires time for readjustment.[153]

The toddler is beginning to develop a sense of time. The child understands some temporal relationships, such as "in a minute" or "after lunch," although specific time intervals, such as "3 hours" or "2 weeks" are meaningless. The toddler's attention span, which is very limited, is characterized by a sense of immediacy and concern for the present.[157] Language abilities increase, and the toddler can now understand simple directions or requests.

From approximately 2 to 4 years of age, the child demonstrates the preoperational or preconceptual phase of cognitive development. Vocabulary and language development markedly increase during this period. Magical thinking and egocentricity are still prevalent during this phase, giving the child feelings of omnipotence and supreme authority. This also places the child in the position of feeling guilty and responsible for events he believes his bad thoughts have caused. The child's inability to reason the cause and effect of illness or accidents makes these events especially stressful.[157]

The toddler will begin to demonstrate *animism,* a process in which life-like qualities are attributed to inanimate objects. For example, the child may blame a glass of milk for falling or believe that an x-ray machine or elevator is a monster.

Instead of using deductive reasoning (from the general to the particular) or inductive reasoning (from the particular to the general), the toddler reasons *transductively* (from the particular to the particular). The child will frequently believe that there is a causal relationship between any two events that occur at the same time or are contiguous to each other in time and space. The color of an object may explain its floating; the need for sleep makes it dark outside, or kicking a pillow off the bed on to the floor made his chest start hurting again.

■ The toddler in the critical-care environment

Toddlers can become terrified in a critical-care unit. They are in a new place where they see, hear, smell, and feel frightening things. There are lots of strangers around who sometimes do scary and painful things to them. Often, toddlers are restrained and unable to move about as they would like. Gone is the security of their familiar surroundings and routines. They are often separated from their parents, and they may be uncomfortable or in pain. As a result of egocentric thinking, toddlers may think that their bad behavior caused their hospitalization.

Parental presence and support are more crucial than ever to the toddler during this period of high stress. When a parent is not present, the toddler may believe that he is being punished through abandonment. The toddler fears that the parent is angry, and he is terrified of complete desertion. Thus cries of "I want my mommy; I be good!" may be heard from the toddler. The toddler may exhibit the same three stages of protest, despair, and denial that the infant does[115] but is now able to be more verbal and assertive in his protest. The toddler may call for the parent and may verbally reject consolation and care from others. Physical aggression, hostility, fighting, kicking, hitting, pinching, and biting may all be displayed by the toddler during this period. If nurses are not familiar with a child's particular rituals for comfort, nursing care or attempted comfort measures may add to the child's confusion and distress.

The best way to minimize the toddler's anxiety is to minimize the toddler's separation from his parents during the hospitalization. For this child, perhaps more than any other, every effort should be made to make arrangements for one parent (or even another familiar adult) to stay with the child as much as possible. It is important for the nurse to convey to the parents that they are welcome in the unit as much as possible and that they are seen as very important and necessary supports for their child. The pediatric critical-care unit is no place for restrictive visiting hours that may benefit the staff but add to the anxiety of the child or the parents.

Rooming-in or frequent regular visiting by the parent decreases the possibility that the child will enter the despair phase of separation anxiety. The child who moves into the despair state may become listless, anorexic, uncommunicative, and withdrawn. Regression to an earlier stage of development usually is demonstrated as loss of sphincter control, reduced verbal communication, or passivity.[153] When the parent returns, the toddler often cries or expresses anger, distrust, or rejection. If the parent attempts to depart again, however, the child may cling very tightly, crying and begging the parent to remain. If the toddler progresses to the denial stage, his behavior is similar to the infant's. The toddler appears to be happier and more interactive but may be more disturbed.

It is important that only a small number of nurses consistently care for the hospitalized toddler in order to minimize the variety of schedules and personalities to which the child must adapt. In addition, the child who has the opportunity to build trust in a few nurses may be able to take comfort from them when a parent is not present. If primary nursing is practiced in the hospital, the consistency of care provided by the primary and associate nurses can increase the toddler's sense of trust.

Physical restraint or restriction, altered routines and rituals, and enforced dependency represent a loss of bodily control to the toddler who is striving for more autonomy. The toddler who is restrained or is forced to lie supine will probably become frightened and resistant.[157] By allowing toddlers as much movement and independence as possible the nurse can increase their cooperation and decrease their fears and frustrations. Children often can be allowed to sit up or remain on their parent's lap during frightening procedures. Physical restraints may not be required if the child is given the opportunity to handle the equipment being used. For example, the toddler often enjoys listening to his chest (or to that of a doll, teddy bear, or another person) with the stethoscope. If the nurse is at the bedside within an arm's reach of any vital tubes, the child may be left unrestrained, with cautions not to touch the tubes. When physical restraints *are* necessary, lost activity should be replaced with another form of activity whenever possible.[87]

Often the child's hands may need only to be mittened so the youngster is unable to grasp vital tubes.

Loss of the toddler's familiar rituals and routines decrease his sense of control, predictability, and security.

Terry's mother always put him to bed at night at home by laying him on the bed, stroking him while she quietly sang a lullaby, then kissing him on both cheeks, pulling his favorite blanket up against his cheek and then turning out the light *in that order.* To 2-year-old Terry, this whole routine was part of "going to sleep."

Encouraging his mother or nurse to carry out this same routine in the hospital will help give Terry a sense of familiarity and security. Routines and rituals that are most important to the toddler must be recorded as part of the nursing history and incorporated into the child's care plan.

All children need limits to feel secure, and they will be frightened without them.[153] This is particularly true of toddlers who have not yet mastered a great deal of control over their own impulses. They need to feel that there is someone close who will protect them from injuring themselves, others, or the environment. Setting limits can help children channel strong feelings into safe, socially acceptable, pleasurable activities. To prevent children from hurting themselves, others, or property, they should be temporarily restrained or removed from the situation with an explanation of why they cannot be allowed to continue their behavior. They then need to be redirected into an activity that will help them learn what behavior *is* acceptable to discharge the strong emotions they are feeling.

Carrie, age 2½, began angrily thrashing about and kicking after her nurse took her blood pressure. Her actions threatened the safety of the IV cutdown in her left foot and several other tubes. Carrie's nurse gently but firmly restrained Carrie's legs and told her: "No, Carrie, I know that you are very angry, but I can't let you kick and move all over like this. You'll hurt yourself. I know what you can do though. I have something fun for you to play with. Stop kicking and I'll show you." After about a minute of this, Carrie settled down and looked expectantly at the nurse. The nurse then produced a hammering board and showed Carrie how she could pound on it—a much more constructive way for Carrie to discharge her anger and one that she seemed to enjoy.

Adults need to acknowledge the child's feelings and then direct the youngster into an acceptable way of dealing with these emotions.

The immature thought processes of toddlers may contribute to their anxiety. Egocentricity, magical thinking, transductive logic, and animism can magnify fears of known events and make unknown or unfamiliar situations terrifying. Sinister characteristics may be attributed to machines and hospital personnel. Toddlers, thinking their misbehavior caused their illness, may not understand their parents' inability or unwillingness to rescue them. Toddlers need very frequent reassurance that they are not bad, that they are not being punished, that they are loved, and that they will get better (if this is true) and be able to walk and talk and go home again. The toddler may not understand the concept of returning home but will be comforted by the concern and reassurance demonstrated by the nurse. Calkin[22] has developed a tool that may be useful in assessing the toddler's response to hospitalization (Table 2-1).

■ **The toddler and pain**

Any real or perceived painful experience will be met by the toddler with extreme emotional distress and physical resistance. Since the toddler has a poorly defined concept of body integrity, any intrusive procedures—even painless ones such as measurement of temperature or examination of the ears—may provoke an intense reaction. Memory of past experiences, physical restraint, separation from parents, emotional reactions of others, and lack of preparation are all factors that influence the child's reaction to a painful procedure. Toddlers can understand only very simple explanations. Prolonged or detailed explanations or explanations given too far in advance may only cause the toddler more anxiety (see the box on pp. 43-45). When it is necessary to perform painful procedures on a toddler, lengthy discussions or provisions of choices are best avoided. It is best to provide a brief explanation, assure the child that you will be with him, perform the procedure as quickly as possible,[157] and then comfort the child.

While the presence of parents is very important to a toddler's sense of security, parents who are extremely anxious may reinforce or accelerate the toddler's anxiety. This does not mean that anxious parents should be asked to leave but that the nurse must try to decrease their anxiety by preparing them for the procedure and by suggesting ways to comfort the child during the procedure. If the child must be held immobile during the procedure, the parents must not be asked to help restrain him, since this may make the child confused, hurt, and angry. The parent would also probably find this role a difficult one. Therefore, during painful procedures, the parent should support, encourage, and reassure the child by speaking in soothing tones or stroking the child and hugging and cuddling the child following the pro-

Table 2-1 Scales for assessing a toddler's behavior

Behavior	Demonstration of lack of autonomy and decreased or absent trust	Demonstration of autonomy with trust	Demonstration of psuedo-independence; hyper-activity; marked aggression; decreased or absent trust
Toileting	• No bowel or bladder control. Is not bothered by wet diapers and is unsuccessful in using potty. • Bowel training is started. May be successful in using the potty when a familiar person encourages it. Does not signal his need to use potty. Wets diapers night and day and has occasional bowel movements in them.	• Urinates in potty when placed on it at intervals. Uses the potty for bowel movements. Wets some diapers daily and is wet at night. Does not ask to go to the potty with any consistency and needs help with clothing. • Dry during the day with occasional accidents when involved in play. Wets at night occasionally but may awaken to void. May need help with clothing and accepts it. May need to be reminded to use the potty. • May tell a familiar person that he is going to the toilet and does so by himself unless he needs help with his clothing. Retains bowel and bladder control almost all the time.	• Does not tell anyone when he needs to go to the toilet. Shows annoyance when helped with his clothing by wiggling and perhaps reaching for an object nearby. Sits on the potty when placed before it, but immediately gets off it to keep moving. Hence he wets the floor or his clothing. • Never tells anyone he has to go to the toilet. Resists physically and/or has a temper tantrum when he is placed on the potty even when he has been dry during the preceding two hours. Struggles to prevent help in being redressed. Wets or soils immediately or soon after being redressed.
Eating	• Does not appear hungry and eats poorly. Shows little interest in feeding himself meals or snacks. May prefer bottle-feeding to cup-feeding and to feed self to a very limited degree.	• Eats well. Drinks from a cup at meals. Feeds self with fingers and sometimes uses utensils. Accepts help with preparation of foods for eating, but doesn't ask for it.	• Tends to be greedy and aggressive during snacks and meals. Actively resists limits being set on his behavior or help offered in preparing his food. May be finicky and actively resist new foods in his diet as well as refuse things in his daily diet (e.g., milk, meat, bread).

Modified with permission from Calkin, J.D.: Are hospitalized toddler's adapting to the experience as well as we think? MCN: Am. J. Matern.-Child Nurs. 4:18-23, 1979.

Table 2-1 Scales for assessing a toddler's behavior—cont'd

Behavior	Demonstration of lack of autonomy and decreased or absent trust	Demonstration of autonomy with trust	Demonstration of psuedo-independence; hyper-activity; marked aggression; decreased or absent trust
Eating—cont'd	• Eats small amounts of meals and snacks and does not ask for second helpings. Does not ask for food between meals except for pop or sweets. Needs some help with feeding (e.g., drinking fluids from a cup) as well as with preparation of food for eating.	• Accepts meals and snacks readily. May have some food dislikes, but they do not affect his daily diet. Shows independence and delight in eating and readily accepts help in preparation of his food. • Eats a great deal and appears very hungry as shown by requests for second helpings and snacks. May initially resist eating at meals or snacks, but follows this by an active interest in eating. Will accept help with the preparation of food from familiar person; may reject assistance from unfamiliar persons.	• Appears unable to sit still for meals or snacks without messing in food, getting up to play or wander, or interfering with others who are eating. May respond to attempts to place reasonable limits on his activities with hyperactivity, temper tantrums or similar behavior.
Resting and sleeping	• Passively accepts being placed in bed. Uses self-comforting devices such as rocking, sucking, or rubbing when placed in bed for rest or sleep. Does not seek people for comfort but may use a familiar object, such as a blanket or shoe, for comfort. May assume a watchful vigil and sleep only when very tired. • Dawdles when rest or sleep is mentioned and does not participate in getting ready for bed. Uses self-comforting devices or familiar objects when placed in bed. Turns away from adults who attempt to comfort him.	• May need comforting when placed in bed for rest or sleep but settles easily and sleeps well. May awaken and call for attention but settles readily if soothed. • Goes to bed willingly and settles easily for sleep. May awaken for attention or toileting but returns to sleep readily. • Protests going to bed by crying and/or calling to get up, but usually settles in 15-20 minutes. Sleeps well although he may awaken for toileting or attention. May protest briefly at this time, but does go to sleep again.	• Shows a great deal of resistance to going to bed for rest or sleep by crying, screaming, and/or trying to get out of bed. May awaken during the night and, when he does, has difficulty returning to sleep. • Resists going to bed even when tired and protests loudly by trying to get out of bed and/or tantrums. External controls (e.g., gentle but firm holding of body or limbs) may be needed to help him rest or he may sleep when exhausted without this help.

Continued.

Table 2-1 Scales for assessing a toddler's behavior—cont'd

Behavior	Demonstration of lack of autonomy and decreased or absent trust	Demonstration of autonomy with trust	Demonstration of psuedo-independence; hyper-activity; marked aggression; decreased or absent trust
Separation from and return of a familiar person	• May cry mournfully and assume a mute and watchful vigil when familiar person leaves. Seeks familiar objects for comfort and/or uses self-comforting behaviors in preference to people. Exploratory activity is minimal. Passively accepts changes in environment without seeking support. When a familiar person returns, does not reach out for comfort but accepts comforting passively or turns away. • Becomes more tense when separated from a familiar person and then turns to objects or self-comforting behaviors for a while in preference to people. Does not make eye contact with adults in his environment. May also attach himself to any person in the environment without showing overt distress when separated from the familiar person. Unable to play without the support of a familiar person. Responds to return of familiar person by ignoring her advances briefly and then actively seeking comfort.	• Protests separation from a familiar person but returns in time to playing with toys. May involve self in separation play (e.g., hiding and finding objects) when familiar person is prepared to leave or does so. Will gradually accept the support of other persons following separation. May reject familiar person on her return (especially mother) if she has been absent for more than a day. • Able to protest separation from a familiar person and to grieve. Initially rejects all unfamiliar persons who attempt to comfort him. May attempt to master separation in play. Able to greet and accept the return of familiar person following absence and protests any subsequent separation, however brief. • Protests loudly any separation from familiar person and tries to prevent person from leaving. Can let person go after some explanation and will return to play or activity. May attempt to master separation through play. Shows delight at the return of the familiar person.	• Protests separation from familiar person or becomes tense and hyperactive. Spends much time exploring the environment during separation and is very active. Often rejects support offered by unfamiliar adults and acts as if he is self-sufficient even when he is in need of care and comfort; may continue this briefly on the return of familiar person. • Protests separation from familiar person and becomes hyperactive and may be aggressive. Acts as if he wants to do everything by himself and protests any interference by unfamiliar adults even when energy is markedly decreased and he needs comfort. Usually continues hyperactivity and pseudoindependence for some time after the return of the familiar person.

Table 2-1   Scales for assessing a toddler's behavior—cont'd

Behavior	Demonstration of lack of autonomy and decreased or absent trust	Demonstration of autonomy with trust	Demonstration of psuedo-independence; hyper-activity; marked aggression; decreased or absent trust
Indications of independence or emotional dependence on adults	• Quiet and withdrawn. Unable to use help or physical comfort from unfamiliar people in order to play or relax. Instead he uses familiar inanimate objects or self-comforting behavior. When with a familiar person, clings constantly and wants help in activities that he can do himself. • Quiet and tense; shows little interest in play and may use self-comforting behavior or inanimate objects rather than unfamiliar persons for support. Follows a familiar person around much of the time, seeking attention when person is not obviously busy.	• Avoids eye contact and interaction with un-familiar persons. Will seek comfort from familiar person. Accepts help with problems (such as dressing) but may not actively seek it. Able to play and will explore his environment when familiar person is close by. • Overtly expresses anger, fear, or discomfort to familiar person. Seeks familiar person for comfort when unhappy or tired. Plays for long periods near other children or with adults. Attempts to please familiar adults. Able to wait for short periods for pleasure or satisfaction. • Overtly expresses anger, fear, or discomfort to any nearby person. Relatively self-sufficient but seeks help when he needs it. Plays for long periods by self or near other children. Will confidently explore environment with a familiar person, accepting or asking for help when needed.	• Shows marked provocative behavior toward familiar and unfamiliar persons. Better able to play and carry on daily activities when clearly stated limits are set for him. Rejects support of adults (at least initially) with an air of bravado even when he needs it. Hyperactive and his attention span is not long. • Shows almost constant activity until ex-hausted and resists support offered by adults. Plays aggressively and may strike out at other children or adults. Unable to use adult support to reduce his need for activity or to help himself relax. Does not tolerate setting of limits. Reacts to reasonable limits with increased activity or temper tantrums.

cedure. In the rare situations in which the parents are too anxious to be supportive or feel they are unable to stay, they should not be made to feel guilty and should be reassured that the nurse will remain with the child to provide support.

Toward the end of the toddler period, children are usually able to communicate the fact that they are in pain; they can usually localize it but not qualify or quantify it. Spontaneous complaints of pain by toddlers should always be taken seriously because they rarely imagine or fake discomfort.[157] Caution must be exercised when trying to elicit information about pain from toddlers, since they may not understand the questions or may respond with "yes" or "no" inconsistently. Behavioral signs of pain in a toddler (such as pulling at his ear or crying when you touch his stomach) are generally more reliable than verbal responses.

■ **Preparation of the toddler for procedures and surgery**

See the box on pp. 43-45.

■ **Play and the toddler**

Most of the toddler's time is normally spent in some type of play activity. Play is a major way toddlers learn about the world, communicate their feelings, overcome boredom, and develop motor skills and independence. The toddler's need for play continues during periods of illness. Through play the toddler can find a constructive, acceptable outlet for fears, frustrations, anxieties, and anger. Familiar toys can be comforting and usually provide a sense of security (Fig. 2-2). Play can serve as a diversion from pain and fear, and it can become a replacement for mobility. It can also provide some feeling of autonomy and independence by giving the toddler control over something.[87]

For the very ill child, play may have to be quite passive. This requires creativity in finding activities that are meaningful for the toddler and that provide positive sensory stimulation to break the monotony of the intensive care unit (ICU) sights and sounds. Bright, colorful mobiles, posters, stuffed animals, and toys can provide visual stimulation. Musical mobiles,

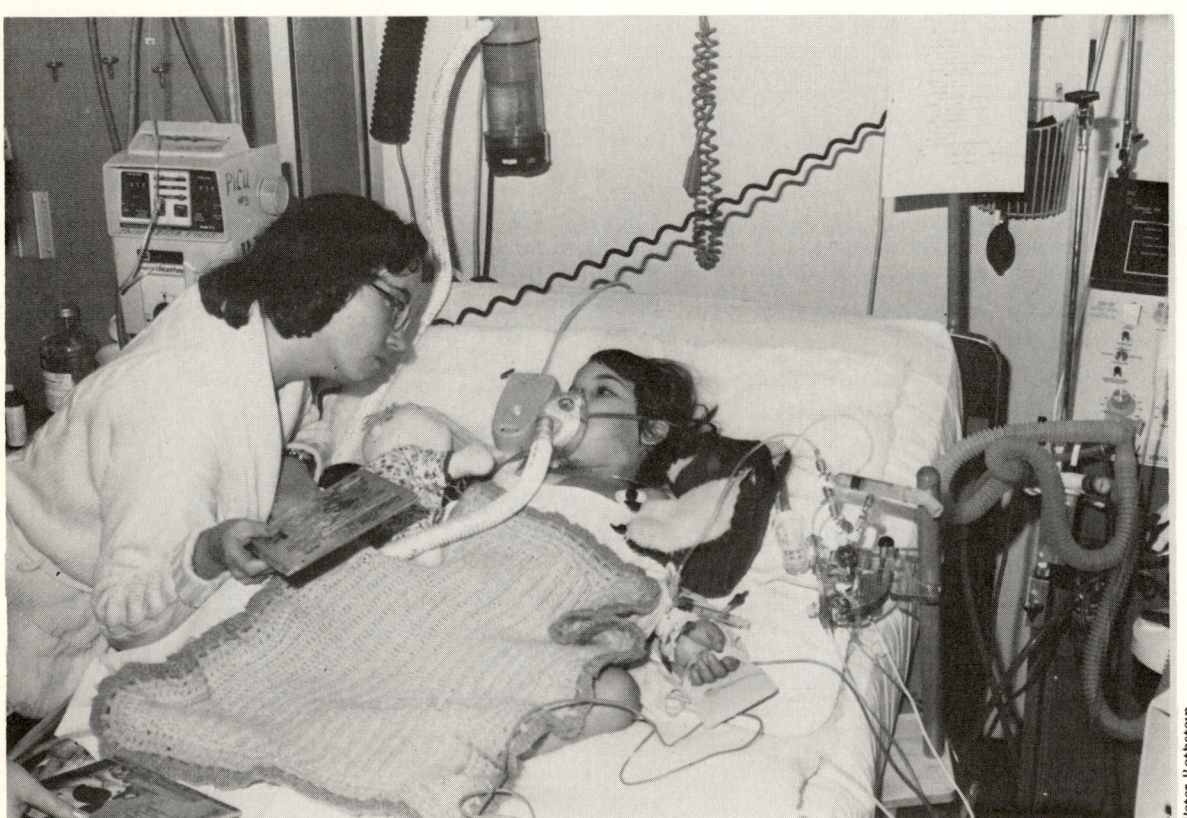

Fig. 2-2 Transitional objects, such as a special blanket and a doll, the familiarity of a favorite storybook, and the presence of a parent, can provide security and decrease fear for a critically ill toddler.

CHAPTER 2 *Psychosocial Aspects of Pediatric Critical Care* ■ 27

records, talking story books, transistor radios, tape recordings made by the child's parents or other family members, and visits from the music therapist can all help substitute pleasant and meaningful sounds for hospital noises. Favorite cartoons or television shows can help bring a sense of familiarity into the critical-care unit. A book of fabrics and other materials with various textures can be stimulating for the child. Any of these activities will be especially comforting if shared with the child's parents.[58]

When the toddler is less ill, more active play can be introduced. Hammering or pounding boards, punching balloons, water play, and active toys such as a "busy box" are all meaningful outlets for the toddler who is immobilized or confined to bed rest. "Peek-a-boo" is still a game that is enjoyed at this age and reinforces the toddler's learning that things (and people) go away but they come back. The child may also enjoy "talking" puppets or dolls. Several books are available with other suggestions for the hospitalized toddler.[51,56,87,105]

■ **The toddler and death**

The toddler's egocentrism, lack of a concept of infinite time, and inability to distinguish between fact and fantasy make it impossible for him to understand absence of life and the permanence of death. Although the toddler may repeat what sounds like a definition of death (e.g., "People who die go to heaven"), he is unable to comprehend what this means.[157] Death may mean separation from the love objects the toddler needs and depends on.[59,124,135,156] The most frightening aspects of hospitalization for the toddler usually include pain, anxiety, and separation from parents, but they do not include anxiety about death. The dying toddler will respond with fear or sadness to the anxiety, sadness, depression, or anger expressed by his parents[157] rather than to the fear of death.

■ **THE CRITICALLY ILL PRESCHOOL CHILD**
■ **Emotional and psychosocial development of the preschooler**

The preschooler (ages 3 through 5) has come a long way in development of motor, verbal, and social skills. This is a time of enthusiastic and energetic learning and exploration. The chief developmental task of the preschooler is creating a sense of initiative.[38] The child's tolerance of frustration is still limited but is better developed. Guilt feelings result when the child is not able to live up to his own or other's expectations of appropriate behavior. The pre-

schooler's conscience is fairly primitive, likely to be overzealous and uncompromising, and may be unnecessarily cruel.[38,44,136] Thoughts about "being bad" or wishing for "bad things" to happen to other people can also lead to feelings of guilt and anxiety. Painful treatments, isolation, separation from parents, loss of autonomy, and immobilization are likely to be interpreted as deserved punishments for real or imagined wrongdoing.

During the preschool years, the child begins the process of sex-role identification. Freud has termed this period the "phallic" stage. Initially, in the oedipal phase of this stage, the child turns toward the parent of the opposite sex and away from the parent of the same sex. Late in the preschool period the child begins to strongly identify with and seeks to imitate the parent of the same sex. It is during this time that children discover that boys and men have penises and girls and women do not. For some children, seeing another child naked in the critical-care unit may be their first experience with this discovery. During this period boys have a fear of castration as punishment for real or imagined misdeeds, and urinary catheterization or other procedures near the genital area may cause them a great deal of anxiety, provoking frantic resistance. Careful explanation of exactly what will and will *not* happen during such procedures is important to decrease the child's fear and increase his cooperation.

The development of the superego or conscience is also a major task for the preschooler. The child begins to learn right from wrong and good from bad. While preschoolers cannot comprehend the reasons why something is acceptable or not acceptable, they learn appropriate behavior through reward and punishment and from the examples set by their parents or other adults. Preschoolers are more aware of danger and can usually be relied on to obey simple limits or rules that have been explained to them.[157]

The preschooler is generally able to tolerate brief separations from his parents with little or no protest if given explanations of where the parents will be and when they will return. He is also less frightened and more trusting of strangers and thus able to relate well to unfamiliar people.[157] Serious illness is likely to cause regression in the preschooler, however, and the need for parents may once again become very strong (Fig. 2-3). Thus the preschooler may manifest some or all of the stages of separation anxiety experienced by the infant and toddler, but the older child's protest behaviors are usually more passive and subtle than those of the infant or toddler. The preschool child may ask his parents over and over when they will return, cry quietly for them, refuse to eat,

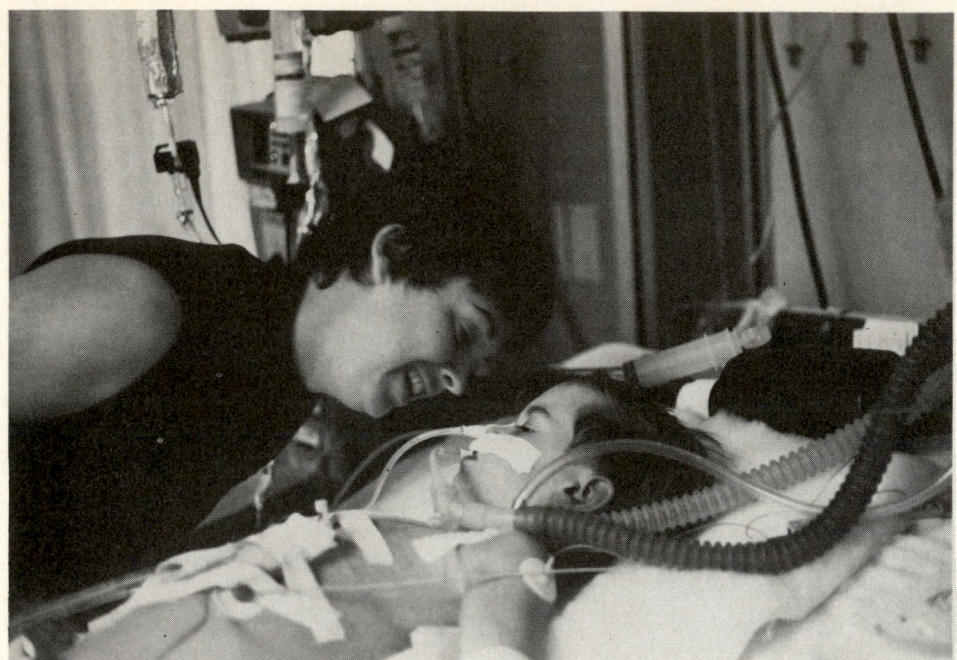

Fig. 2-3 Although the preschooler has gained a lot of independence since the toddler years, he still needs his parents nearby during hospitalization.

be unable to fall asleep, throw things, break a toy, or refuse to cooperate in activities he had performed in the past.[157] The critical-care staff must be alert to these signs and provide the child with reassurance regarding the parents' return and other comforts and interventions as necessary.

■ **Cognitive development of the preschooler**

The preschool child continues in the preoperational phase of intellectual development until approximately age 4. An egocentric view of the world continues, and magical thinking remains. As the imagination develops during this period, the preschool child has a difficult time differentiating reality from fantasy, thus increasing the potential for misunderstanding. Transductive reasoning—association of two events that occur at the same time—remains.[42,106]

The preschooler's magical, egocentric, and transductive thinking, combined with a developing conscience, strengthens the child's view that illness and hospitalization are punishment for misbehavior. This view presents a special problem if the child received an injury while engaged in some forbidden activity such as playing with matches or crossing the street alone. If the child was involved in an accident in which others were injured, particularly if family members were more seriously injured or were killed, the patient may feel inordinate guilt regarding the accident and anxiety concerning his survival. This is particularly true if the child had preaccident fantasies or wishes for injury to or death of his parents or siblings. The child may be terrified when it appears that his fantasies have come true. If these fears are extreme, the child may require psychiatric intervention.

Global organization of thought still ties the early preschooler to rigid routines and the familiar patterns of the rituals of daily activities, which provide the child with a sense of security.

Preschoolers want to know both the cause and the purpose of everything; to them, nothing happens by chance. Questions like, "Why am I here?"; "Why are you doing that?"; "Why is she crying?" may be incessant. Because preschoolers believe that there must be a reason for everything that happens, they are troubled by the purpose of many events.[153] The child is now beginning to generalize his thinking. For example, after getting stuck with a needle by a person in a white coat, the child may believe that everyone approaching him in a white coat is going to stick him with a needle. Although the preschool child may *perceive* an event correctly, the *interpretation* of the event may be faulty.[153]

From ages 4 through 6 years, the child is in the

stage of intellectual development called the *intuitive* phase. "Why" questions persist. The child has a larger vocabulary but tends to define objects in terms of their functions. For example, "A bed is to sleep in." When the preschooler asks "why?" simple answers beginning with "to" and followed by the function may be best understood. The child's attention span and concept of time increase. Toward the end of this period the preschooler's rigidity and ritualism begin to decrease, allowing him more flexibility and fewer negative reactions to changes in environment and routines.[153]

While complex preparation for an event is likely to cause more anxiety in toddlers, explanations in advance are vital to decrease the preschooler's anxiety about a procedure and increase his cooperation (see box on pp. 43-45). It is important, however, that explanations be simple and concrete. Purely verbal explanations may not be enough for preschoolers who cannot abstract or synthesize beyond what their senses tell them.[106,157] Explanations should include mention of what the child will see, hear, feel, smell, and taste.[63] The use of drawings, pictures, slides, videotapes, actual or miniature equipment, and rehearsal of procedures on dolls, teddy bears, or puppets help to prevent serious misinterpretations. Misunderstandings and faulty interpretations may still occur, however, even with careful preparation, since children do not readily admit that they do not understand. Preschool children are extremely literal. They interpret words according to their very narrow range of experience. For example, "IV" may be interpreted as the ivy that grows on the chimney, and the "dye" of x-ray studies may be interpreted as "die."[58] The nurse must be careful to avoid using homonyms (words with several meanings) and must be alert to any cues the child may provide about his interpretation of the explanation. Following any explanation, the child should be asked to reexplain the purpose and technique of the procedure. Anxiety may interfere with a child's ability to understand and remember explanations. It should never be assumed that since a procedure has been explained once that the child will remember the explanation for the next time. The patient should be prepared for each procedure each time it is performed.

It is extremely important to be honest when explaining procedures to children. It is unfair to tell the child a painful treatment will not hurt because this approach deprives the child of an opportunity to prepare himself in advance. Dishonest explanations, changes in plans, unfulfilled promises, and deviations from the procedure as explained may also threaten the child's trust in the staff. When changes are unavoidable, these must be acknowledged and explained to the child. Explanations should also emphasize that staff members care about the child and do not have hostile intent and that the purpose of the procedure is not to punish but to help the child get well.[153]

■ **The preschooler in the critical-care environment**

Five-year-old Timmy had been in the ICU for 3 days; he was intubated, in renal failure, and in need of peritoneal dialysis. Timmy was literally surrounded by equipment and intravenous lines. There were no toys, stuffed animals, or anything nonmedical near him. All of Timmy's extremities were restrained. Although he was receiving morphine, he was fairly alert. Two nurses talked over Timmy's bed about the equipment needed to start his dialysis. Timmy moved about restlessly on the bed and occasionally set off his ventilator alarm. Although Timmy's mother spent much time with him, she was not present at this time. His nurse, appearing harried after what had apparently been a busy morning, put a blood pressure cuff on Timmy's arm and started to pump it up. This increased the child's activity, and the nurse told him, "It's okay, Timmy, settle down now." This "reassurance" did not calm Timmy. The nurse tried to hold Timmy's arm still and after attempting three times to obtain a blood pressure, she stood up, sighed, and began adjusting the IV line. The resident and a medical student entered. The resident took hold of Timmy's other arm and began locating a vein from which to draw blood while explaining Timmy's case to the medical student. The doctor asked the student to hold Timmy's arm; the child's protest activity had markedly increased as the resident placed the tourniquet and "slapped" up a vein. Before the doctor inserted the needle, he said in Timmy's direction, "There's going to be a stick now." Those were the only words spoken to Timmy during the whole procedure. The procedure completed, the resident and medical student left the room. While Timmy continued fighting the ventilator, his restraints, and his situation, the two nurses conferred about the dialysis procedure. A few minutes later the resident returned, watched Timmy for a short time, and told the nurse, "His last gas wasn't terrific and he's really agitated. Let's give him some pancuronium." The nurse agreed that would be a good idea and administered the drug. Timmy was not told that he would soon be unable to move. Very shortly, Timmy lay quietly in his bed with only his increased heart rate to indicate his anxiety.

Although this is an extreme situation, it is a true one. None of the staff members showed empathy for Timmy or tried to decrease his anxiety before deciding to paralyze him—a solution that makes care easier for the staff but that may be terrifying to an awake child. It is sometimes too easy for busy professionals to forget that the struggling patient in the bed in front of them is a frightened child.

To the preschool child who has difficulty separating fantasy from reality, the critical-care unit can provide plenty of material for the child's very active imagination. The environment and personnel in the critical-care unit can appear threatening or hostile to a child who is already frightened, in pain, sleep deprived, and uncomfortable. The preschooler believes in supernatural beings such as ghosts, monsters, and cartoon characters and may develop an explanation for a strange sight or noise involving one of these characters. For example, the child may ascribe sinister explanations to the gurgling of a suction machine behind the curtain next to him, to the clapping sounds of a postural drainage treatment on the other side of the unit, or to strange smells.[94] Overheard snatches of conversation can also be frightening or misleading.

The preschool child also has fears of the unknown, of the dark, and of being left alone. The nurse who reminds the child that she will always be close by and that a light will be left on while the child is sleeping may be able to eliminate some of the child's fears. Much creativity and understanding are necessary on the part of staff and parents if the preschooler is to feel safe and secure in the critical-care unit.

Since preschoolers have primitive ideas about their bodies,[47] major fears of bodily injury and mutilation can cause many misconceptions and a great deal of anxiety about hospitalization. Any intrusive procedure, whether painful or not, is highly threatening to the preschool child. The child not only fears the pain of an injection but may also worry that the puncture or wound site will not close and that all of his "insides" or all of his blood will leak out.[47,157] Band-Aids are a great source of comfort because many preschoolers feel that a Band-Aid will "hold everything in." The nurse should anticipate the child's concern if Band-Aids, dressing, or stitches are removed. This is particularly true for the youngster who believes that a large dressing or many stitches are holding a large part of him together. Assuring the child that the dressing will be replaced or that the skin has healed (if this is true) may decrease his fear and resistance. When it is time for a bandage to be removed, it may be helpful to explain that the "hurt" is better and to show the child that nothing is leaking and that his skin is holding him together now. Bandaging and unbandaging a doll or stuffed animal may help the child work through such fears.

When explaining surgical procedures to preschoolers, it may be best to tell them that something will be "fixed" rather than "removed" or "taken out,"[101] since the threat of losing a part of their body may be very frightening. If anesthesia is described as "being put to sleep," it may invoke images of the way the neighbor's dog died. This can be frightening, and the child should be assured repeatedly that he will wake up after the operation is over.[101] The nurse should avoid promising the child that he will feel better after surgery, since he will undoubtedly feel worse in the immediate postoperative period.

It is very stressful for the critically ill preschooler to lose control of his body or his emotions. While the critically ill child cannot control most aspects of his care, realistic choices should be offered whenever possible. The nurse might allow the child to select which Band-Aid he would like or to decide if he would prefer chest physical therapy or a bath first in the morning; these small choices will help give the child some feeling of control.[29]

Since the preschooler has a great need for movement and large muscle exercise, immobility at this age presents a special problem. Waechter and Blake[152] observed that prolonged use of restraints and immobilization may cause concerns about death in preschoolers, since they equate movement with life.

The preschooler may employ various coping strategies to deal with the stress of critical illness. Regression is most commonly seen because young children usually abandon their most recently acquired skills first.[150] A reappearance of such self-comforting behaviors as thumb sucking, a loss of previously acquired body control, or increased need for physical comfort may disturb the child's family.[153] Parents will require reassurance that such behavior is the child's temporary way of dealing with a stressful situation and that the child will regain lost skills once he has recovered. Since the child needs these behaviors, it is important to accept the regressed behavior and support the child rather than press the child to "act his age" or admonish the child for "bad" behavior such as thumb sucking.

Other coping strategies preschool children may display include projection (they attribute their own feelings, wishes, or behavior to other people or objects), repression, denial, withdrawal, aggression, fantasy, and motor activity.[150] Children may also identify with the aggressor during their play and assume the role of the nurse or physician or other perceived aggressor. In this way they attempt to reduce their fear and anxiety by assuming some of the characteristics of these all-powerful adults and thus, vicariously, feel more control over their situation. McBride and Sack[82] present an excellent case study that provides the nurse with helpful examples of methods allowing the child to maintain some control over his critical care.

■ The preschool child and pain

After age 4, children seem to be able to gain more self-control during painful procedures.[155] However, it is still essential to explain procedures in advance to decrease the child's fears and misconceptions. The idea that a painful procedure is to "help you get better" is difficult for preschoolers to understand. They have a hard time differentiating a "good hurt" (caused by the therapy) from a "bad hurt" (caused by the illness or injury).

Even when a child wants to cooperate, holding still during a painful or frightening procedure may be an extremely difficult task. Thus it is almost always a good idea to have assistance from another staff member. However, while some children may benefit from assistance in holding still, other children react negatively to being held down and are better able to maintain self-control when left on their own with only verbal support. The nurse should be careful to avoid linking evaluation of the child with any specific behavior patterns (e.g., that good boys hold still and bad boys cry), since this will create feelings of guilt for the child who is unable to cooperate. To help the child realize it is not wrong to express pain the nurse should explain that it is acceptable to cry or yell loudly during the procedure. It is also important to keep the child appraised of the progress of the procedure; it can be very comforting to know that a painful process is almost finished. Occasionally, the child may be so caught up in the event itself that he does not realize it is actually over.[81]

Assessment of pain in the preschool child is often very difficult, and some researchers believe children are often undermedicated for pain.[83] The frightened child is often not able to communicate pain clearly. If the nurses repeatedly equate goodness with cooperation or bravery, the child may be intimidated into denying pain or controlling behavioral expressions of it, which can be exhausting and stressful. Verbal expressions of pain by the young child are not always reliable, since they depend on the sophistication of the child's language development. The nurse should be alert for behavioral and physical cues of pain such as flushing of the skin, diaphoresis, increased pulse and respiration, pallor, restlessness, movement or rigidity of extremities, dilation of the pupils, and vomiting.[84,136] Since many of these behaviors and responses may also indicate fear or anger, it is important to differentiate the cause of the behavior before intervening.[157] Other indications of pain in a preschooler are irritability, lowered frustration tolerance, aggressive behavior, dependent behavior, withdrawal, and refusal to eat, drink, or take medi-

cine. Smith[136] has developed an inventory of pain indicators that provides a systematic method for assessing a preschooler's pain.

The nurse should avoid offering an injection at the same time she asks the child about pain since the child may deny pain because of fear of the injection. Intravenous and oral analgesics are usually much less stressful methods of pain control.

■ Preparation of the preschooler for procedures and surgery

See the box on pp. 43-45.

■ The preschooler and play

During therapeutic play, stressful situations, fears, and disturbing facts of life can be repeatedly dramatized until the experience is assimilated and the fear or strong feeling is mastered. This type of play is a way for children to communicate what they cannot yet express verbally, and it is an acceptable outlet for negative feelings.[153] The preschool child may assume the roles of others and may involve other people, often adults, to whom he may assign roles.[29]

The preschooler's play reflects finer motor coordination, increased verbalization, and a longer attention span.[29] The preschooler has a need for large muscle movement during play.

Robby was a 4½-year-old who was admitted to the ICU after a motor vehicle accident. He was immobilized on a Stryker frame and could not move his legs or head. He was free to move only his arms. Robby's nurse recognized his anger and need for activity. She attached a beach ball suspended from a string to the curtain bar above Robby's bed. She told Robby that he could punch the ball if he wanted to whenever he felt like it. While the nurse stood at his bedside, he hesitantly touched the ball, then withdrew and looked away from the nurse. While the nurse was occupied across the room, Robby began to slowly hit the ball. After a few minutes he was punching the ball with more vigorous strokes. Thereafter, Robby spent a great deal of time punching his ball, and its location was occasionally switched so that he could punch it with his other hand and arm.

Therapeutic play periods are a very important part of any critically ill child's plan of care. Petrillo and Sanger[105] have identified eight general rules to guide the staff member in initiating effective play.

1. *Reflect only what the child expresses.* The play should for the most part be nondirective. The staff member should try not to reflect the child's nonverbal expressions or try to explain the child's behavior to him.[51]

2. *Supply materials that stimulate play.* Play

materials must be appropriate to the child's age. Although hospital equipment is valuable play material, in some cases it should be supplemented with materials such as toys, books, and games, so the child can have a choice of play type and content. The child may wish to escape from the realities of the hospital, may not yet be able to deal with potentially threatening equipment or fears, or may just prefer another toy. Art materials are particularly suitable for the hospitalized child, since they allow the patient to express internal emotions and thoughts (Fig. 2-4).

3. *Allow enough time for the child to play without interruption.* The child must feel safe to play freely. Often there is too much activity at or near the child's bed for him to relax enough to play without reservation. It is important for the nurse to allot a specific time for undisturbed play and to ensure that this period is respected—barring life-threatening emergencies—by all members of the health-care team.

4. *Permit the child to proceed at his own pace.* The child should not be pushed to approach frightening ideas before he is ready to deal with such topics. Many times this does not happen until after the child has left the hospital.

5. *Determine when it is appropriate to go beyond the child's expression.* Occasionally, it is appropriate to say things to the child in play beyond what the child is expressing superficially. Such discussion may give an anxious or fearful child the opportunity to see that it is possible to talk about a frightening topic. The nurse or play therapist may give the child a sense of security by remaining friendly and letting him know that it is okay to share fears. The third-person technique (i.e., attributing feelings to a puppet or to other children) may be used as a less direct way of expressing feelings the child is afraid to discuss. The third-person technique also lets the child know he is not alone in his feelings.[105]

6. *Play for the child who cannot play by himself.* Many times children in critical-care units are physically unable to play. In these cases staff members must initiate play for the child and take cues from the child's expressions or verbalizations regarding the issues the child needs to resolve.

7. *Allow direct play for the emotionally strong child.* Some children are able to tolerate thematic expressions that are very close to an emotionally charged reality. These children should be allowed to express themselves, and discussion of subjects such as death should be allowed.

8. *Use knowledge of child growth and development as a guide to professional clinical judgment.* The nurse must ensure that the materials and equipment are appropriate for the child's cognitive development and motor skills. Many hospitals have child-life specialists or play therapists who can assist the child with therapeutic play activities.

■ The preschool child and death

The preschool child views death as a temporary, reversible condition.[124] Nagy[93] states that children under the age of 5 "variously view death as reversible, a departure, a state of sleep, separation, a change of environment, or as a form of limited life." Magical thinking and egocentrism lead the preschooler to believe that his naughtiness, anger, or bad thoughts caused this bad thing that is happening to him now[59]; he feels guilty and believes that he is being punished.

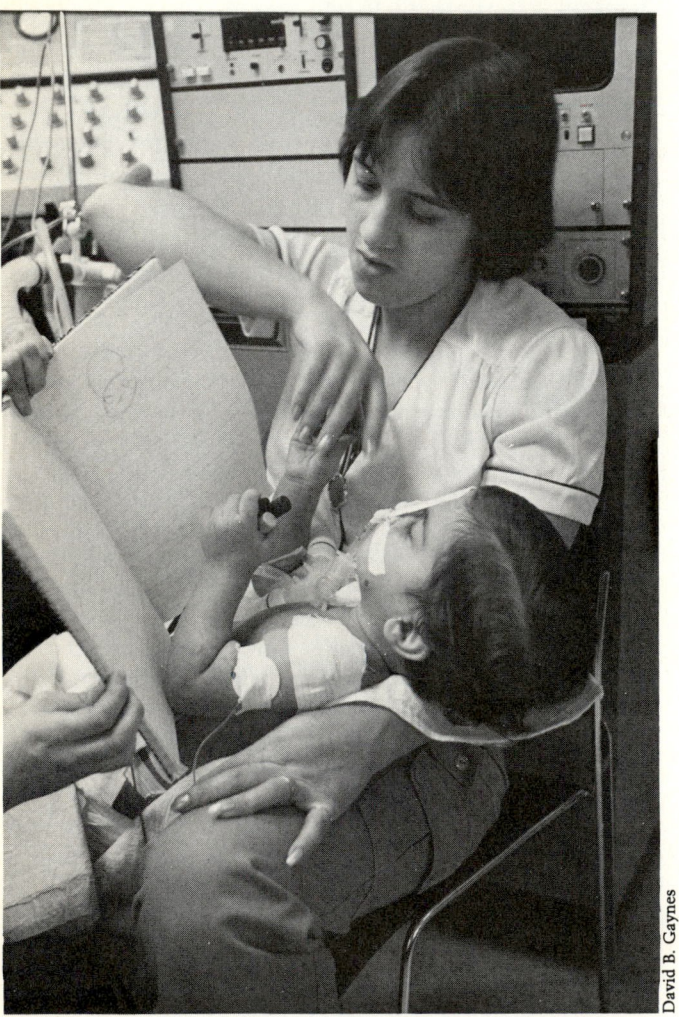

Fig. 2-4 The critically ill child may be able to express fears, frustration, or anger when supplied with simple art materials in a secure environment.

David B. Gaynes

The child needs a great deal of reassurance that he is not being punished and that he is not responsible for his plight.

Much of a preschool child's experience with death consists of the sight of dead birds, dogs, cats or other animals that are often mutilated in death. In addition, the child has fears regarding bodily injury during this period. As a result the preschooler may view death as mutilation or prolonged torture.[31] Pain, restraints, and intrusive procedures that the critically ill child experiences may lend credence to the child's fantasies. It is important to explore the child's view of death, to dispel misconceptions, and to decrease the patient's anxiety. Simple reassurances are often not helpful.

The child's view of death is also affected by past experiences, such as the death of a family member. A 5-year-old child who has been told that her aunt died because she was tired and went to sleep may then fear becoming tired and going to sleep.[157] The child may identify with the illness or death of characters portrayed on television programs or the evening news and may come to view death as "being killed."

Preschool children think of death more often than most adults are aware; the fear of death may begin as early as 3 years of age.[14] Death should be discussed with the preschooler in a simple, honest way, with consideration given to the child's cognitive development and previous experiences.[157] Children often understand *how* things are said better than *what* is said; therefore, the mood and amount of anxiety conveyed may be more important than the actual words used.[98] When children ask if they are going to die, it is important to discover the meaning of the term "die" to the child and the child's perception of his prognosis. The nurse might ask, "What does it mean 'to die' "? or "What do you think is going to happen?" Lengthy explanations are rarely necessary or helpful at this age. If the child does ask a direct question, an appropriate response might be, "Yes, we are all going to die someday, death makes us sad, but we will be with you so it won't hurt".[52] Later, the child can be reassured that if he has pain, he will be helped to feel better.

■ **THE CRITICALLY ILL SCHOOL-AGE CHILD**
■ **Emotional and psychosocial development**

During the school-age period (ages 6 to 12), the child develops a sense of industry.[38] This is the age of accomplishment,[157] increasing competence and mastery of new skills. The child takes pride in the ability

to assume new responsibilities; as he becomes more independent, he begins to develop self-esteem. If the child experiences repeated failures or frustrations in attempts at achievement during this period, however, he may instead develop a sense of inadequacy or inferiority.

As peer relationships and peer-group approval become important, the child becomes less dependent on the family. In the course of the school year the child often becomes a member of a clique, club, or gang and frequently has a best friend. Most peer-group interactions take place with members of the same sex, and children of the opposite sex often are viewed with distaste. This attitude begins to change as the child enters preadolescence at approximately 11 to 13 years of age.

Rejection by a peer group can be devastating to the child during this stage of development. Chronic illness, or illness that causes a visible disability, can set the child apart as different from his peers and may make the child the object of ridicule. Separation from the peer group is often a significant and difficult consequence of illness and hospitalization during school years. The child should be allowed to receive visits, letters, telephone calls, or recorded messages from peers whenever possible. Such messages will help the child to maintain contact with friends. Since school is a very big part of the child's life, the parents might request the child's teacher to have the class send cards and letters to the hospital.[150] Often children may be able to read or do some uncomplicated schoolwork while in the critical-care unit (Fig. 2-5). Some children will be comforted by the fact that they can still do their homework, while other children will prefer the freedom from schoolwork.

The school-age child is also an integral part of a family. Since separation from siblings may be particularly difficult at this time, every attempt should be made to continue contact with the child's siblings through visits, phone calls, letters, or exchange of photographs.

School-age children are able to tolerate separation from their parents and usually do not react to such separations with the intensity of the younger child. Older school-age children may even enjoy periods away from their parents. During periods of critical illness and hospitalization, however, the child's need for parental support and involvement may be increased.

The school-age period marks the beginning of a major change in the parent-child relationship. Children begin to realize that the parent is not the omnipotent, omniscient being they thought during earlier childhood. They discover that the parent is some-

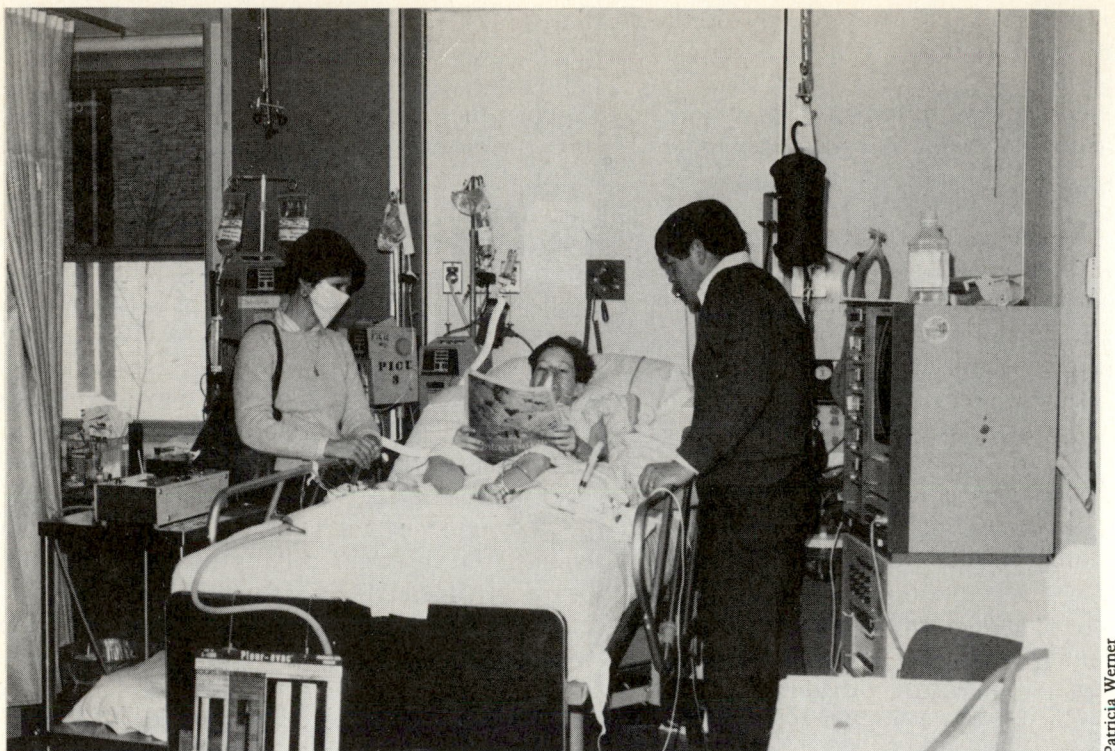

Fig. 2-5 It is important for the hospitalized school-age child to continue participation in favorite activities, such as reading the sport's section of the paper with Dad.

times wrong and will not always be able to protect them from injury or pain, and they begin to question their parent's judgment. Relationships with other authority figures during this period may influence how the child will perceive and relate to authority figures throughout his lifetime.[153] The child is trying to find a balance between increased need for independence and control and continued desire for parental support and guidance. This conflict will intensify as the child approches adolescence.

The parents may already be having some difficulty relinquishing some of their control of the child during this period. The parents need to be particularly patient and sensitive in order to support the child appropriately during illness and hospitalization, yet avoid forcing the child into a dependent role. The parents' response may be complicated by inconsistencies in the child's behavior as he alternates between dependent and independent behavior. The parents may need assistance in understanding their child's behavior in order to decrease potential feelings of hurt, anger, or frustration. The older school-age child will often criticize his parents in an attempt to declare his independence from them.[153]

■ **Cognitive development in the school-age child**

At approximately 7 years of age, the child enters the period of concrete operations. This marks the beginning of logical thought.[43,106] Although the child still functions very much in the present, he is able to use deductive reasoning and to see the relationship of parts of the whole. As a result the child becomes more flexible and may no longer require absolute consistency in daily routine. The school-age period is a time, however, of magical rituals that help children cope with stressful situations and give them security.[153] Rituals such as "crossing my fingers and toes" and incantations like "step on a crack and break your mother's back" help school-age children feel some sense of control over the world and their situations. The child's concepts of time, space, and causality are more sophisticated and realistic. True cooperation becomes possible because children are now able to differentiate their viewpoint from that of others, and they are able to value and respect both their personal autonomy and the viewpoints and opinions of other people.[153]

As school-age children learn to tell time, read, write, and do arithmetic, a whole new world opens to them. They are able to understand events happening in the past, present, and future. They are generally very receptive to the acquisition of knowledge and eager to learn new things.

Moral judgment becomes further developed during this period. Preschool and early school-age children follow rules set down by others because they believe rules are unalterable and imposed from above.[108] They learn to judge the rightness or wrongness of an act by its consequences, rewards, or punishment rather than by its motives.[21] Although young school-age children know the rules and what they may or may not do, they do not understand the reasons behind them. They see behavior as either totally right or totally wrong and believe everyone else sees it that way too. Children of 6 or 7 years of age are still likely to interpret accidents, illness, or other misfortunes as punishments for misdeeds.[157]

Older school-age children no longer view rules as rigid and unchangeable but recognize that rules are established and maintained through social agreement.[108] They also realize that rules are sometimes flexible or changeable based on specific circumstances. They no longer judge an act solely on its consequences but on the motivation and intentions behind the act and the context in which it appears. Although older school-age children can view rule violation in relation to the total situation and the perceived morality of the rule itself, it is not until adolescence or later that they will be able to view morality on an abstract basis with sound reasoning and principled thinking.[157]

The school-age period has been described by Freud[45] as the period of latency. During this period little awareness or concern over bodily matters is normally seen.[48] The child who is hospitalized for a serious illness or injury, however, centers his attention on his body and its functions. The child generally takes a very active interest in his condition but may be very self-conscious when the attention of the health-care team is focused on his body.

It has been shown that children's ideas about illness and body construction and functioning are often nonexistent, very vague, or false.[16,47,104] The nurse cannot assume that the child truly understands the location or function of even commonly discussed organs such as the heart, lungs, or stomach. Older school-age children and adolescents will often nod and seem to understand explanations or words when in reality they have either no idea or a distorted idea of what is being explained to them. They are often reluctant to ask questions or admit they do not know something they believe they are expected to know. To verify the child's comprehension, the nurse should ask the child to explain his illness to another person or to draw a picture of his body and what is wrong with it.

Children may be able to repeat information about their condition just from listening attentively to all that is said around them; however, their interpretations of what they overhear may not always be accurate. They are quick to pick up contradictions and will often request factual information. Cognitive mastery provides one way they are able to maintain a sense of control over what is happening to them.[157] With their newly acquired ability for logical thought and deductive reasoning, they are better able to understand the relationships among their illness or injury, its symptoms, and the treatments that are or will be instituted. School-age children also are more aware of the significance or prognosis of various illnesses, the indispensibility of certain body parts, the potential hazards of treatments, the life-long consequences of permanent injury, and the meaning of death.[157]

Advance preparation for all procedures as well as explanations during the procedure are very important to the school-age child's ability to cope effectively with the situation, to cooperate during the procedure, and to comply with the prescribed treatment regime (see box on pp. 43-45). Such explanations increase the chances that the situation will be a growth-producing rather than a detrimental experience for the child.[149] The nurse may use a doll or human figure outlines to discuss the function of the body and explain procedures and operations. Some older children object to being seen looking at a doll (even if it is described as a teaching doll or dummy), and in those cases, body outlines can be used. School-age children enjoy learning scientific terminology and handling equipment that will be used in their treatment. These methods of preparing children for procedures have been more extensively described in the literature.[33,151,159]

■ The school-age child in the critical-care environment

Most school-age children respond to their experiences in the critical-care unit with negative impressions. Barnes[6,7] has explored the school-age child's perceptions and recall of the ICU using observations, drawings, and interviews. She discovered the children demonstrated a high degree of sensitivity to their surroundings and a detailed recall of events that happened not only to them but to other children as well. Frequently, the child's recollections represented distortion of reality. Most children reported that they could not sleep at night because of the noise or because they were disturbed for procedures. The children also experienced fatigue, sadness, pain, anger, boredom, time disorientation, confusion, and an awareness and fear of death. Barnes concludes that the health-care team must attempt to reduce stimuli whenever possible, must be more sensitive to the awareness levels of children, and must provide periods of undisturbed rest. She emphasizes the importance of repeated clarification and explanation of procedures to eliminate subjective reactions.[7]

Fears during the school-age period are more realistic, although some degree of anxiety based on magic and fantasy is maintained throughout life. Loss of control is a major concern of school-age children who are struggling to become independent. They are in a strange place, subjected to many procedures and examinations by large numbers of unfamiliar people. Physical examinations in open areas without privacy can lead to feelings of resentment and anxiety because the child has acquired feelings of modesty and shame concerning nakedness.[92] The hospitalized child is forced to depend on others (usually strangers) for assistance with basic personal needs such as taking a bath, voiding, and having a bowel movement. It is important to respect the child's privacy and modesty and to give the child choices in scheduling care activities whenever possible.

Fears regarding possible mutilation and bodily injury or harm are prevalent during this period. School-age children begin to show concern about the benefits, hazards, and techniques of procedures.[157] School-age children often fear anesthesia and surgery. They may fear that the physician will start the operation before they are asleep or that they will awaken during the surgery. In addition, they usually fear the helplessness of anesthetized sleep, afraid that they may not wake up again and that they may die.[101] Older school-age children are usually concerned about the consequences of the procedure or operation, including the postoperative appearance of the wound.

The school-age child may not always wish his parents to be present during procedures, and individual preference for parental support or privacy should be respected. When their presence is not desired by the child, the parents may need help understanding this as an assertion of their child's growing independence. The child's preference and needs may change, however, and will have to be ascertained on an ongoing basis.

The school-age child may fear disgracing himself or disappointing parents or other significant adults by losing control. School-age children, especially boys, are often given the message that they are expected to be brave and not act like a baby. It is important to realize that school-age children frequently exhibit the greatest amount of bravado when they are feeling the most helpless and are most in need of support and reassurance.[153] Parents and staff should let the child know that it is all right to be frightened, angry, or upset and that crying may help decrease some anxiety.[74]

David was a 10-year-old who found himself suddenly hospitalized in a critical-care unit with the possible diagnosis of meningitis. It was obvious to the nurse how frightened he was during a lumbar puncture procedure and how much difficulty he was having maintaining control of his emotions. The nurse told him that she realized how frightening this all was for him, that he hurt and was uncomfortable, and that it was okay for him to cry if he felt like it. David loudly responded, "No, I can't; my dad told me not to!" David's father had deprived his son (most likely unwittingly and unintentionally) of a constructive outlet for his pain, fear, and anger. Instead he had given David another major stress to cope with, that is, his father's expectation that he "take it like a man." Parents sometimes need help understanding that crying and protest behavior are healthy and often very helpful outlets for the child facing extremely stressful situations and are not indications of weakness or failure on the part of the child or parents.

One method of helping the child anticipate and communicate his feelings is a "feelings wheel" (Fig. 2-6).[2] This is a particularly useful tool to use with children who are intubated or otherwise unable to communicate verbally, since it provides an alternative means of conveying what they want and how they feel by turning the wheel or pointing to their message. Such a wheel is easy to use and can be designed by the parent with the child's assistance. For younger (prereading) children, pictures such as faces with different expressions (such as happy, sad and crying) or common conversational objects can be cut out and pasted on a larger wheel. As the child's condition or treatments change, a new wheel can be made or new phrases added.

■ Pain and the school-age child

Because of their increased cognitive and verbal skills, school-age children are better able to describe their pain in terms of its onset, location, quality, and intensity.[84] It is important to remember, however, that fears of pain and bodily injury are heightened during the school-age period, so that even slight injuries or pain may be exaggerated.[129]

School-age children are better able to under-

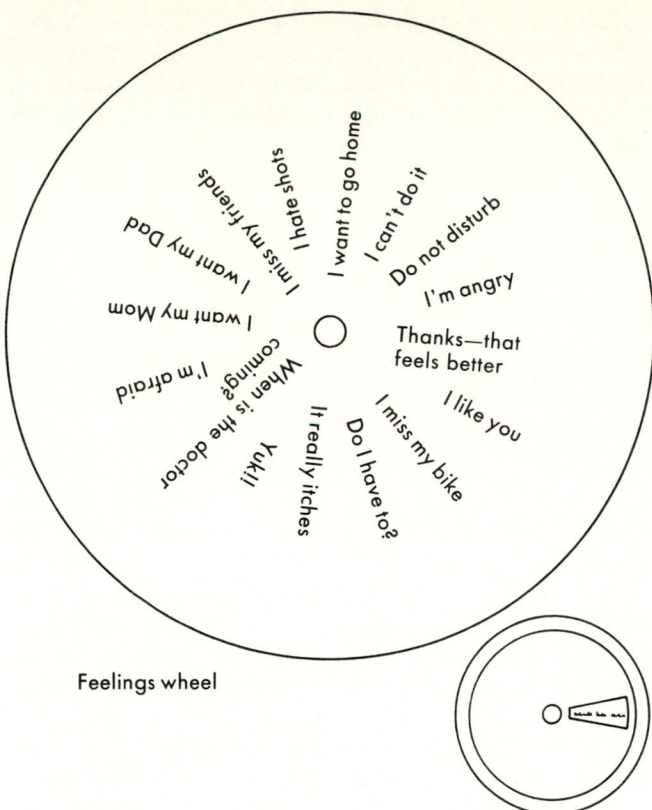

Feelings wheel

Fig. 2-6 The "feelings wheel" may provide a useful tool to aid in communication with older hospitalized children who cannot (or will not) speak. The child can point to the word or phrase that best describes the way he feels. A windowed cover can be made and attached to the center of the wheel (as shown in the lower right corner), so the child can turn the cover of the wheel to make his "feelings" visible.

From Association for the Care of Children's Health: A child goes to the hospital (pamphlet). Reproduced with permission from the Association for the Care of Children's Health, 3615 Wisconsin Avenue, N.W., Washington, D.C. 20016.

or teeth, and trying to act bravely. Overt resistance such as biting, kicking, pulling away, trying to escape, crying, screaming, or plea-bargaining are often denied later for fear of losing status with their peer group or parents.[157]

Savedra[122] describes various strategies that were used by severely burned children for coping with pain. Some of these same strategies may be employed by children experiencing other types of pain. *Reduction of threat* is used when pain is anticipated and the child makes attempts to lessen the expected pain. Such comments as "Don't pull too hard," "Be real careful," and "I want the other nurse to do it 'cuz she knows how to do it so it doesn't hurt so much" are all examples of this strategy. Attempts to *postpone the event* are also frequently employed with pleas of "Wait a minute," "Do it after I'm through with this game," or "I have to go to the bathroom first!" Some postponement may give the child time to gather together his coping resources and to gain a sense of control, but prolonged postponing only increases the child's anxiety. Some children may try to *bypass* the event by telling the nurse, "Just tell them you did my dressing, but don't really do it, okay?" or by assuring the nurse that "The nurse before you did it so you don't have to." More mobile children may try to *create distance between self and threat* by attempts at physical resistance and withdrawal. Emotional withdrawal and detachment from the situation may also be a way for children to distance themselves from what is happening.

Some children, however, *do* need to remain very close to what is happening to them. Many children have a strong need to watch everything that is happening as a means of maintaining their autonomy and control; the child should be given a choice. Well-meaning staff members who tell the child "don't watch" or who literally turn the child's head away may be doing a disservice to the child who desperately needs to watch.[74]

The child may also be helped to cope by *dividing attention or distraction*. The child should be given the option of having a support person whose sole function is to support the child during the procedure. This person can be the patient's eyes if he chooses not to watch (or cannot because of position). The adult can also answer questions and provide distraction, tell the child how much longer, or just give the patient a hand to hold and squeeze.[74] *Sleep* may also be used as a method of avoiding a painful situation.

One other method of coping with stressful, painful events employed by the older school-age child is *intellectualization*. The child may avoid focusing on

stand that painful procedures may be necessary to help them get better, but, again, they need to be well-prepared before the procedure begins. Fear of the unknown is sometimes the worst part of a procedure for children. If the child must be awakened for procedures, it is imperative that he become fully oriented and prepared so that the painful procedure is not remembered as something frightening or painful begun during sleep.

Generally, by the age of 9 or 10 years, most children are fairly cooperative and show little fright or overt resistance to pain or procedures. They generally use more passive methods of coping with the discomfort such as holding rigidly still, clenching their fists painful, threatening aspects of a situation by asking questions about the mechanics of the equipment to be used, the scientific principles involved, or the results of laboratory or diagnostic tests.

Occasionally, children will respond to pain and anxiety with complete submission, compliance, and apparent apathy.[10] These children are often completely focused on frightening fantasies about their illness or treatment and thus require much support, understanding, and reassurance. Younger school-age children may regress to earlier patterns of behavior.

Pain relief may be achieved through administration of analgesics or through supportive measures, which include the following: (1) establishment of a supportive, caring relationship with the child and parents, (2) teaching about pain and various pain-relief measures the child and/or parents might try (3) distraction techniques that involve the senses, rhythm, and imagery such as coached breathing techniques, (4) cutaneous stimulation such as massage or rhythmic rubbing of the painful area or the contralateral extremity (if appropriate), (5) relaxation techniques such as deep breathing and conscious relaxation, or (6) desensitization and "fading in" behavior therapy techniques.[83] The latter approaches may be used with children in chronic or severe pain, although they require a great deal of practice and effort on the part of the nurse and patient.

■ **Preparation of the school-age child for procedures and surgery**

See the box on pp. 43-45.

■ **The school-age child and play**

Once a school-age child begins to recover from a critical illness, boredom may result. Play can serve not only as a means of entertainment and distraction but also as temporary escape from the stresses of serious illness and as a vehicle for resolving emotions. These children have a longer attention span and increased cognitive abilities. They particularly enjoy playing with hospital equipment, and their own accurate use of this equipment reflects their keen observations of protocol, procedure, and technique. They often combine very dramatic reenactments of procedures and situations with active exploration of the equipment.[29] Role reversal with members of the health-care team not only provides the child with the opportunity to exert some control but gives the hospital staff valuable insight into the child's interpretations of and feelings about his illness and care.

It is often difficult or impossible to arrange peer interaction in a critical-care unit, but it might be possible for a visiting sibling or young friend to play with the patient. Competitive games are particularly enjoyable during the school-age years, and it is very important to the child that the rules (often made up by the child) be obeyed. School-age children also enjoy ordering and collecting things. Older school-age children begin to engage in daydreaming.

■ **The school-age child and death**

The child from 5 to 7 years utilizes a superstitious and investigational approach to understanding death.[135] During these years death is often personified as a ghost, skeleton, boogeyman, or devil, and the child may believe that death will come to take him away from his parents and friends. Nightmares and fear of the dark are common at this time, and it is often helpful for the nurse to leave a dim light burning near the child's bed at night. If convinced that there will be nurses nearby throughout the night, the child will often be able to relax and fall asleep, confident that the nurses will protect him.

The finality of death is not yet fully appreciated, since the school-age child has not yet fully grasped the quality of time.[14] Epstein[37] believes that by the time a child is 7 years old, he probably suspects that he himself will die one day. Nagy,[93] however, describes the child's belief that "the only people who die are those who get caught and do not get away."

After the age of 8 or 9 years, the child begins to develop a more permanent view of death, since, at this time, he has a more complete concept of time. The child realizes that his parents are not omnipotent, that they are powerless to avert death, and that ultimately everyone will die.[14] The child of this age often uses symbolic language such as drawings or stories to express his needs and fears.[66]

In the next few years, the child's concept of death is elaborated by cultural and religious experiences. The adult concept of death as final, irreversible, and inevitable is reached between the ages of 11 and 13 years.[14]

Terminally ill school-age children are often aware of their fatal prognosis without being told.[153] They are acutely aware of nonverbal cues and often understand much more of what they overhear than the staff and their parents realize. Attempts to shield the child from knowing he is fatally ill may be done with good intention; however, such an approach is rarely beneficial for the child.

Children can see through false cheerfulness, through the smile that is not reflected in the eyes. When their questions are met with silence, tears, or changes of subject, children recognize adults' evasiveness, and a child may conclude that discussing his illness is wrong, or that what he is experiencing is even more terrible than he had supposed. He learns to believe that discussion is taboo and may even result in separation from his loved ones. His concerns become distorted, he faces even greater fears, and he faces them all alone.[98]

The death of another child in the unit may also be a source of stress for the child. School-age children are often able to describe in detail the events surrounding the death of other children in the ICU.[6] Older children may identify with the deceased child, particularly if their diagnoses or problems are similar.[78] Children need honest explanations to their questions about what happened to the other child, since nervous or evasive answers will only heighten their anxiety. If possible, other children should be reassured that the deceased child did not have the same problem or prognosis. They often have many questions that should be answered as simply and honestly as possible. If staff members (or parents) feel uncomfortable answering the child's questions, a clinical nurse specialist, social worker, chaplain, or physician with particular skill in discussing death with children should be asked to see the child and help the youngster to work through some of the anxiety this event has engendered. Parents often experience a good deal of frustration and helplessness when faced with their child's questions about death and may need assistance in dealing with their anxiety.[64,78]

■ **THE CRITICALLY ILL ADOLESCENT**

Adolescence is a time of profound physiologic, physical, and psychologic change. Because of the turmoil of the adolescent years, critically ill adolescents are often the most challenging patients. Supporting them and meeting their needs require patience, creativity, and understanding on the part of the critical-care unit staff.

■ **Emotional and psychosocial development**

The major tasks of the adolescent period include separation from parents, adaptation to a rapidly changing body, the development of a sexual identity, and acquisition of a sense of identity and autonomous function.

The behavior of the adolescent is frequently inconsistent and unpredictable. It is often bewildering to others and even to the adolescent himself. Many of the behaviors such as mood swings, depression, periodic regression to childhood, and mild antisocial behavior that are normal during adolescence would be potentially pathologic if they were exhibited by a child or an adult.[157]

Adolescence can be divided into three stages— early, middle, and late adolescence—although the boundaries of these stages are quite indistinct.[60] During early adolescence, body image issues are of primary concern. This period extends from approximately 12 to 14 or 15 years in girls and from approximately 13 to 15 or 16 years in boys. The younger teenager is extremely preoccupied with the changes and sensations within his body. He is acutely aware of every possible flaw or imperfection and believes that others are also aware.[35] The peer group continues to grow in importance and becomes the standard against which the adolescent measures his acceptability. During this time the most intense relationships outside the home are with best friends of the same sex. Separation from parents normally increases during this time; the teenager spends more time away from home but is still quite willing to adhere to parental wishes, to communicate with parents, and to be accountable to them. The parent-child relationship still remains relatively intact. Young adolescents who become ill are primarily concerned with how the illness or injury will affect their appearance, function, and mobility.[60]

Midadolescence is generally the most difficult and trying time.[60] Conflicts over issues of autonomy, accountability, and self-determination raise considerable tension between the teenager and his parents. The teenager often rejects and rebels against parental support and control while continuing to depend on them. Midadolescents are still highly egocentric and narcissistic and are very preoccupied with their appearance, attraction to the opposite sex, and ability to meet gender role expectations. Peer reactions and relationships determine the teenager's body image and behavior. With the peer group the teenager tries out and experiments with new roles and behaviors.[60] Since illness or injury would result in enforced dependency and perceived loss of control over everything in his life, hospitalization may be almost intolerable to a child during midadolescence. The hospitalized midadolescent will be extremely anxious about changes in physical appearance that could make him different from or unacceptable to his peer group.

The late adolescent, approximately ages 17 to 22, is normally fairly secure in self-esteem, inner controls, independence, and heterosexual relationships. The adolescent now functions at a very independent level. He listens to parental advice but then makes his own decisions. During this period his primary concern is defining and achieving role definition in terms of education, career, marriage, or life-style. Serious illness or injury during this period is most threatening in its potential for affecting the realization of career and life-style goals or forcing changes in vocational plans.[60]

■ Cognitive development in the adolescent

During adolescence Piaget's fourth and last stage of cognitive development, that of formal operations, is attained. The adolescent develops the ability to think abstractly and is now able to project to the future and see the potential, long-term consequences of actions and illnesses.[42] Although the adolescent is now able to understand other's opinions, feelings, and points of view, there is much self-preoccupation during this period. The adolescent discovers the ability to interpret observations, to develop broad concepts, and to find truths that are uniquely his own.[60] These increased cognitive abilities allow the adolescent to have a greater understanding of his condition, treatment, and prognosis. This means that the teenager is quite capable of being a participant in planning and initiating his treatment.[60]

It is important to realize that the adolescent perception of illness and its significance may be distorted. Illness or injury are often viewed in terms of how it will alter appearance or level of activity.[60] Therefore an adolescent may react more negatively to an insignificant but visible or restrictive illness or injury than to an invisible but potentially life-threatening one.[157]

Magical thinking still exists to some degree during the adolescent years. Teenagers often believe that they are to blame for their illness or injury and sometimes believe that they are being punished for rebellion against parents, forbidden fantasies, or for homosexual or heterosexual activities.[35,157] Thus, while coping with the physical aspects of their illness, they may also be dealing with feelings of guilt and shame. Frequently, adolescents *are* responsible for injuries they receive, since they often take enormous risks and engage in foolhardy feats to convince themselves and others of their bravery and invincibility. When such behavior results in serious injury to themselves or others, the guilt, grief, and mourning may lead to extreme depression or other serious reactions.[60]

■ The adolescent in the critical-care environment

When the adolescent is first admitted to a critical-care unit after a serious injury or sudden illness, he may be in a state of emotional and physical shock, concerned about the terrible insult to his body and the associated pain. At first the teenager may feel protected while in the critical-care unit and thus may have little or no anxiety about being there.[60] However, as this initial shock phase subsides, the period of critical illness may become terrifying or humiliating.

The major threats to seriously ill adolescents are loss of control and of identity, altered body image, and separation from their peer group. Illness and hospitalization constitute a major situational crisis for the adolescent.[157]

Helplessness is much more threatening to adolescents than it is to younger children, even though adolescents have more sophisticated coping mechanisms. They are extremely concerned that others will discover their inadequacy, dependency, and confusion; therefore, they hide it from everyone including themselves.[157]

Adolescents do not wish to be passive recipients of care but rather active participants in planning and implementing their care. Preparation for procedures reduces fear of the unknown and helps the teenager maintain some feelings of control (see box on pp. 43-45). Adolescents react not only to what they are told but also to the manner in which the information is given.[157] They are often very reticent to admit that they do not understand explanations, and their fears may be manifested as an overconfident, conceited, or pretentous attitude.[157] Many adolescents have little understanding of the structure and workings of their body. Thus the nurse must carefully (and tactfully) evaluate the teenager's knowledge of his disorder and individualize each teaching program, since the adolescent will resent any hint of condescension.

Even minor injuries and illnesses are often magnified and can affect a teenager's body image; consequently, a critical illness may be terrifying. Adolescents need much assistance and reassurance in trying to gain a more realistic, nondistorted view of their illness. Since they are facing many unique problems during their hospitalization, they need help identifying their strengths and effective coping mechanisms.

Because of their heightened body awareness and developing sexuality, privacy is of paramount importance to teenagers. Every attempt should be made to keep the critically ill adolescent's body, particularly the genital areas, covered during examinations and treatments. If the critical-care unit does not contain private rooms, many adolescents will prefer to have the curtains drawn around their bed to maintain privacy. It is extremely embarrassing and traumatic for an adolescent to lie exposed while several members of the health-care team examine and discuss his body. Lack of respect for and inattention to these needs may cause the adolescent even greater stress than any existing physical pain.[157]

Although separation from parents may be welcomed and appreciated during this time, separation from peer-group support may be extremely disturbing. Peer-group contact should be maintained and facilitated as much as possible. While some adolescents benefit greatly from visits from their peers, others may not wish to be seen by friends if they believe they look disfigured or will be seen as being different. Such determinations need to be made on an individual basis.

While the adolescent may initially use denial to cope with stress, he may also feel a need to regress. He may become demanding of staff and parents and may be afraid to be alone. Such regression enables the adolescent to return to the more dependent state of early childhood, allowing him to set aside the burden of dealing with tasks he is physically and emotionally unable to handle at that time.[123]

The teenager may also use other coping strategies, for example, varying degrees of withdrawal. In addition, intellectualization may be useful to adolescents who wish to deal with the objective facts about their condition rather than the emotional aspects. High scholastic achievers in particular may utilize this strategy, requesting information and reading material to supplement their knowledge. Intellectualization may be a helpful coping strategy unless the information provided is distorted by the adolescent's fears and fantasies. The staff should support the patient's attempts at cognitive mastery, while frequently verifying the accuracy of his perceptions.[60] Other strategies include reaction formation, projection, and displacement. For example, Schowalter and Lord[128] found that much adolescent anxiety was displaced into complaints about food.

Some of the adolescent behaviors that are most distressing to staff members include manipulative strategies, verbal abuse, physical attacks, sexual suggestiveness, and refusal to cooperate with the plan of care.[123] Schowalter and Anyan[126] found that ill adolescents behave in a way characteristic of the latency period and that sexually aggressive behavior is rarely seen. The adolescent who views staff members as parental authority figures may also be sullen and uncooperative.[153]

■ The adolescent and pain

Because of increased cognitive and verbal skills, adolescents are able to describe verbally and more completely the pain they are experiencing. They are usually hyperresponsive to pain and other abnormal sensations, however, and their reactions may seem quite out of proportion to their actual physical condition. It is unrealistic to expect that the adolescent will react to pain in ways that would be appropriate for children and adults.[60,123]

Unless they are totally unprepared, adolescents generally try to accept pain and painful procedures with a high degree of self-control.[157] When adolescents are unable to react to pain with stoicism, they often are ashamed of their behavior and may need reassurance that their feelings and behavior were appropriate.[17] It is important to show acceptance and understanding because an adolescent's self-image is not only based on how he perceives his actions but also on how *others* react to his body and behavior.[53]

Psychosomatic complaints such as fatigue, abdominal pain, headache, or backache occur frequently during adolescence, and they may be difficult to differentiate from genuine symptoms caused by illness. The adolescent may perceive secondary gains from the sick role, which may prolong or intensify adverse reactions to illness or injury.[157]

The potential for drug abuse during the adolescent period is a real one in today's society. Narcotics received in the critical-care unit may provide the teenager's first experience with euphoric drugs. The nursing staff or even the patient may fear development of patient addiction to these drugs. Yet even the potential for later abuse does not justify withholding analgesics from an adolescent who is in pain. It does mean, however, that such drugs should be used judiciously and their medicinal purposes emphasized to the teenager.[157] In addition, the patient should be reassured that addiction will not develop with short-term narcotics use during critical illness. The staff can also teach the adolescent nonpharmacologic methods of pain relief and request his participation in these strategies. Use of such methods as cutaneous stimulation or relaxation techniques may help the adolescent realize some degree of control over his body and decrease feelings of helplessness.

■ Preparation of the adolescent for procedures and surgery

See the box on pp. 43-45.

■ The adolescent and play

Although the idea of play may seem more appropriately applied to the care of younger children, adolescents also need the opportunity for a temporary escape from their situation, an outlet for strong feelings, and meaningful stimulation that will decrease the possibility of sensory deprivation or overload. Familiar activities, such as watching television or listening to favorite tapes through an earpiece on a tape recorder, may be appropriate and meaningful activities even for a critically ill adolescent. As the adolescent recovers, reading (particularly sports or beauty magazines), schoolwork, puzzles, or even a punching bag setup may be pleasurable (Fig. 2-7). Some adolescents may enjoy writing a diary as a way of venting thoughts and feelings in a private way. Others may benefit from the opportunity to share these thoughts and feelings with an adult they trust and admire.

Daydreaming is a useful occupation for adolescents. It helps them decrease feelings of loneliness, master fears, establish a new identity, solve current problems, test themselves imaginatively in situations they have never experienced, and focus on the future. It also provides a safety valve for the expression of strong feelings.[153] Common roles assumed by the adolescent in daydreams are the martyr who is misunderstood and mistreated by everyone and the hero who is admired by all.[157]

■ **The adolescent and death**

Adolescents have a great deal of difficulty coping with the idea of their own death. The time in their life when they are striving to establish their own identity and make plans for their future is the most difficult period to face the fact they have no future.

Such a realization of death-before-fulfillment adds further turmoil to the troublesome adolescent stage.

Although adolescents have the intellectual capability to understand death on the adult level, they most often do not view death in the same way that adults do. Since remnants of magical thinking still persist during adolescence, the teenager may view fatal illness as punishment and may feel guilty. The adolescent may be unable to totally accept the finality of death because of a belief in his own invincibility. This belief (or denial) may be responsible for some self-destructive or daring behavior, which may result in accidents, drug abuse, and suicide.[85]

Adolescents need to be highly involved in decisions about their own care and treatment. They also need to take part in plans for their own death. Kübler-Ross states that patients should not be told that they are dying but that they should be told that they are seriously ill. She states that:

> When they are ready to bring up the issue of death and dying, we should answer them, we should listen to them, and we should hear the questions, but do not go around telling patients they are dying and depriving them of a glimpse of hope that they may need in order to live until they die.[67]

The critical-care nurse must be alert to non-verbal cues and unasked questions when caring for critically ill adolescents unable to speak because of

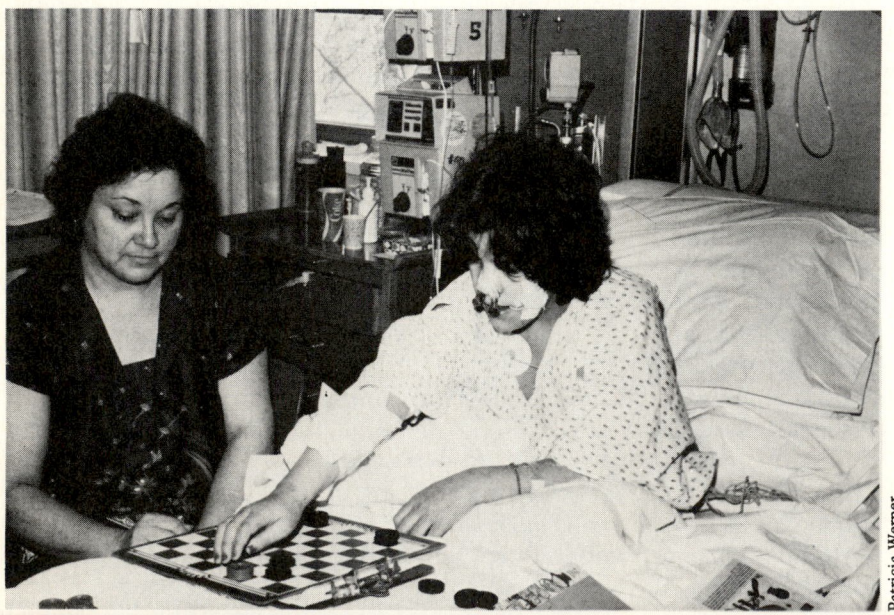

Fig. 2-7 Engaging in games helps alleviate the boredom of the adolescent in a critical-care unit.

PREPARATION OF CHILDREN AND ADOLESCENTS FOR PROCEDURES AND SURGERY

Infants
Major fears

1. Separation
2. Strangers

Preparation

1. *Provide consistent caretakers.*
2. Decrease parents' anxiety, since it is transmitted to infant.
3. Minimize separation from parents.

Toddlers
Major fears

1. Separation
2. Loss of control

Characteristics of toddlers' thinking

1. Egocentric, primitive, magical (inability to recognize views of others)
2. Little concept of body integrity

Preparation

1. Prepare child a few hours or even minutes before some procedures, since preparation too far in advance produces even more intense anxiety.
2. Keep explanation *very* simple, and choose wording carefully, avoiding words with double meanings and other connotations.
3. Let the toddler play with equipment, put mask on teddy bear, and so on.
4. Minimize separation from parents; keep security objects close by.
5. Recognize that *any* intrusive procedure (e.g., rectal temperature or ear examination) is likely to provoke an intense reaction (the problem is not pain but fear of injury).
6. Use restraints judiciously, since being held down may provoke more fear or protest than the actual procedure.

Preschoolers
Major fears

1. Bodily injury and mutilation
2. Loss of control
3. Unknown, dark, being left alone

Characteristics of preschoolers' thinking

1. Preoperational: egocentric, magical, animistic, transductive
2. Tendency to repeat and use words they do not really understand, providing their own explanations and definitions
3. Highly literal interpretation of words
4. Inability to abstract
5. Primitive ideas about their bodies (e.g., fearing that all their blood will leak out if a bandage is removed)
6. Difficulty in differentiating a "good" hurt (beneficial treatment) from a "bad" hurt (illness or injury)

It is important to remember that the child's psychosocial developmental stage may not always match his chronologic age. Particularly in chronically ill children, development may be delayed. For example, an adolescent who is delayed in development may need to be approached more like a school-aged child. When preparing children and their parents, it should be remembered that siblings also need preparation and reassurance. They may have fantasies about what is happening to their sibling, and they may fear that they caused what happened (the illness or injury) or that the same thing will happen to them. It is vital to discuss these issues with parents who may not realize what the siblings are experiencing; they may not know how to approach the preparation.

Continued.

PREPARATION OF CHILDREN AND ADOLESCENTS FOR PROCEDURES AND SURGERY—cont'd

Preschoolers—cont'd
Preparation

1. Prepare the preschooler days in advance for major events (hours for minor ones), since advance preparation is important.
2. Keep explanations simple and concrete, and choose wording carefully; do not use words like "cut," "take out," and "dye."
3. Emphasize that the child will wake up after surgery, since anesthesia described as "being put to sleep" may be frightening.
4. Use pictures, models, actual equipment, or hospital play, since verbal explanations are not enough.
5. Emphasize that the procedure or surgery is to help the child be healthier.
6. Repeat many times that the child has not done anything wrong and is not being punished.
7. Use explanations that include what the child will see, hear, feel, smell, and taste.
8. To check understanding, ask the child to reexplain the information to another person or doll.
9. Reexplain things every time they happen; do not assume the child remembers.
10. Listen to what the child says when playing; look at what the child draws.
11. Be honest! Explain deviations from routines, unfulfilled promises, changes in plans.
12. Do not tell the child he will feel better after surgery, since he will undoubtedly feel worse in the immediate postoperative period.
13. Since the child has a very limited concept of time, tie explanations to known events (e.g., "after your nap" or "after lunch")
14. Give child choices whenever possible.
15. Reassure the child that the room will not be dark and that there will always be someone close by.
16. Do not tie evaluations of the child to behavior during the procedures (e.g., he is not "a good boy" for holding still but rather "That was good holding still")

School-age children
Major fears

1. Loss of control
2. Bodily injury and mutilation
3. Not being able to live up to expectations of important others
4. Death

Characteristics of thinking of school-age children

1. Concrete operational period
2. Beginning of logical thought but continuing tendency to be literal
3. Vague, false, or nonexistent ideas about illness and body construction and functioning
4. A tendency, particularly in older children, to nod with understanding when in reality they do not understand
5. Ability to listen attentively to all that is said without always comprehending
6. Reluctance to ask questions or admit not knowing something the child thinks he is expected to know
7. Better ability to understand relationship between illness and treatment
8. Increased awareness of the significance of various illnesses, potential hazards of treatments, life-long consequences of injury, and the meaning of death

PREPARATION OF CHILDREN AND ADOLESCENTS FOR PROCEDURES AND SURGERY—cont'd

Preparation

1. Prepare days to week in advance for major events because it is extremely important to the child's ability to cope effectively, to cooperate, and to comply with treatment; in addition preparation gives the child a greater sense of control.
2. Have the child explain what he understands.
3. Use body diagrams, pictures, and models, since these children enjoy learning scientific terminology and handling actual equipment because their thinking is concrete (although some older school-age children object to being seen looking at a doll).
4. Since these children are beginning to assert more independence, give them a choice of whether they want their parents present during the procedure.
5. Since the peer group is now important, stress that this contact can be maintained.
6. Since the child does not want to be seen as different, emphasize the "normal" things the child will be able to do.
7. Give as many choices as possible to increase the child's sense of control.
8. Reassure the child that he has done nothing wrong and that necessary procedures and surgery are not punishments.

Adolescents

Major fears

1. Loss of control
2. Altered body image
3. Separation from peer group

Characteristics of adolescent thinking

1. Beginning of formal operational thought and ability to think abstractly
2. Existence of some magic thinking (e.g., feeling guilty for illness) and egocentrism
3. Tendency toward hyperresponsiveness to pain; thus reactions are not always in proportion to the event, and even minor injuries and illnesses are usually magnified
4. Little understanding of the structure and workings of their body

Preparation

1. Allow adolescents to be an integral part of decision-making about their care, since they can project to the future, see long-term consequences, and thus are able to understand much more.
2. Since advance preparation is *vital* to adolescents' ability to cope, cooperate, and comply, prepare them in advance—preferably weeks before major events.
3. Give information sensitively, since adolescents react not only to what they are told but to the manner in which they are told.
4. Explore *tactfully* what adolescents know and what they do not understand, since they are extremely concerned that others will think they are "dumb" or will discover their feelings of inadequacy, dependency, and confusion.
5. Stress how much adolescents can do for themselves and how important their compliance and cooperation are to their treatment and recovery; be honest about the consequences.
6. Allow the adolescent as many choices and as much control as possible.
7. Respect the adolescent's need to exert independence from parents, and remember that he may alternate between dependency and a wish to be independent.
8. For the importance of the peer group, see *steps no. 5* and *6* in the section on school-age children.

intubation or other impedances. These patients may need to write or draw to express their feelings and questions.

Some adolescents may request that their treatment be discontinued and that they be allowed to die. Each situation must be handled individually. Schowalter and associates point out that adolescents can have the cognitive understanding of death without the emotional maturity that is necessary to make final decisions regarding their own life. They add that, on the other hand, older adolescents really can appreciate their own suffering and fatigue and can understand that all life holds for them is continued disability, doubt, and suffering.[127] Certainly, all adolescents should be involved in decisions about continuation or discontinuation of therapy.

■ FAMILY MEMBERS AND THE CRITICAL-CARE UNIT

A child is a member of a family and has roles to play as a son, daughter, brother, sister, grandson, niece, cousin, or friend; these roles continue despite the child's hospitalization. A child's critical illness may cause massive disruption and disharmony in the established roles, rules, and functions of the family system. The way the family responds to this disruption and potential crisis may drastically affect the outcome for the sick member.[100]

Parents and children need each other, and children belong to their families, not to the critical-care unit staff. No matter how caring and attentive the nursing staff, it cannot replace the love and support of the child's own family (Fig. 2-8). It is absurd to talk about *allowing* parents the *privilege* of visiting their child; parents have the right to be involved in their child's care. Other family members may also be very important to the child. A grandparent, favorite aunt or uncle, a sibling, or the child's usual baby-sitter may provide a special form of comfort and security for the child. Family members often feel frustrated because they are not able to contribute to the child's treatment; it is extremely important that they be allowed to remain with the child because they are providing vital emotional support.[46] This knowledge may ease their frustration. Family members may need to actually see the ill child to be reassured or to realize that the child's prognosis is grave. Relatives of critically ill patients have cited the need to be near the patient and the need to feel that there is hope.[88,148] Visits by family members often help the child to feel that he is still a part of the family.[46]

Visiting policies should be liberal and geared to the requirements of the child. The ICU should be open 24 hours a day to those individuals significant to the child. Certainly, space limitations may affect the number of people who visit at one time, but any restrictions should be flexible.

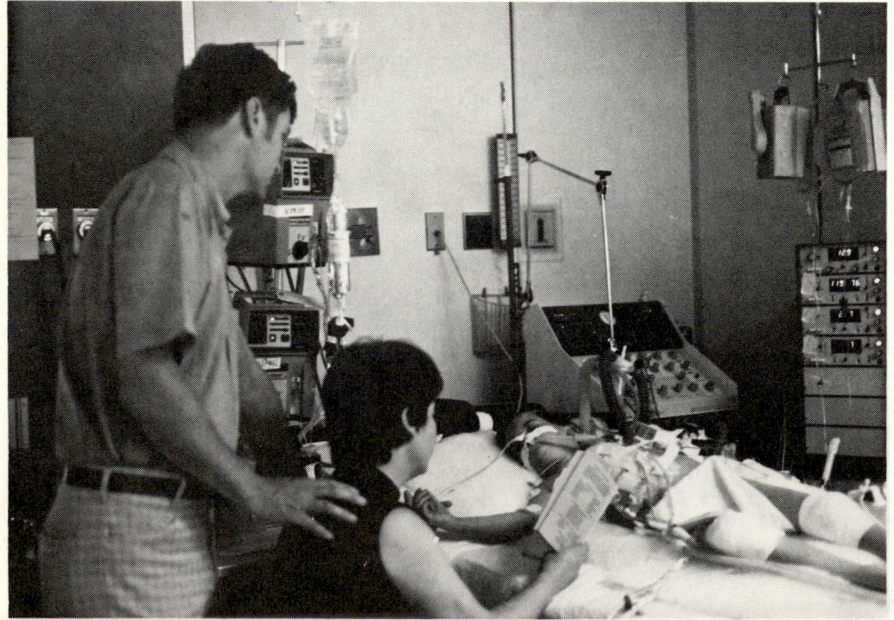

Lani Guzman

Fig. 2-8 Parents make special contributions to their child's care that cannot be duplicated by the staff.

Frequently, nurses have ambivalent feelings about the families of their critically ill patients. Although intellectually they recognize that families are an important source of support to the child, nurses often feel that family members should be kept out of the ICU because visits increase family anxiety.[86] It is possible that nurses find care of the critically ill child so emotionally taxing that they have no energy left to support family members and, therefore, prefer not to have them present. Newer staff nurses may feel uncomfortable performing procedures while family members watch. Often, however, parents who are allowed to remain at the bedside are reassured by the competence of the nurse. Parents who are asked to leave may feel the nurse lacks confidence in her skills or in the validity of the procedure being performed. In most instances parents should be given the option of remaining at the bedside during procedures, since their presence is often comforting to the child and their participation will help them feel more involved in their child's care. Older children may be given the option of asking their parents to remain. Some procedures such as endotracheal suctioning are very difficult for family members to tolerate; the nurse needs to be sensitive to their cues and help them make the best decision for them *and* their child.

Sometimes nurses develop attitudes about family members before they have gathered adequate information about the family relationships. Factors such as the family member's age, sex, demeanor, or appearance may trigger a range of feelings in the nurse—from suspicion, dislike, antagonism, and fear to affection and admiration. Often this process may be only partially conscious.[133] Judgmental feelings about family members serve no useful purpose and may be detrimental to the nurse-family relationship. Although the nurse often cannot prevent such feelings from forming, she can be aware of their presence and try to keep them from interfering in the child's care. However, strong negative feelings are almost impossible to hide from the family members, since so much of what we communicate is nonverbal. In these cases it is better that another nurse care for the child—one who is more able to establish a therapeutic relationship with the family.

■ **The parents**

Parents of children at different ages. Some of the concerns and reactions of parents of critically ill children will vary, depending on the child's age. Parents of the critically ill neonate have a myriad of feelings related to their new status as parents. Often they have awaited the arrival of their child with such high hopes that feelings of inadequacy, failure, and guilt may accompany the parents' discovery that they have failed to keep their child healthy. They may need assistance in developing their parenting roles and in recognizing their importance to their child's care. Parents should be encouraged to participate in their infant's care as much as possible. Activities in which the family can participate, such as stroking, holding, calming, singing, diapering, and feeding, are all very important aspects of the infant's care.

Parents of toddlers need to be encouraged to continue their central role in their child's life. Their presence is very important, as it can help alleviate much of their child's distress. If the toddler has been hospitalized because of accidental injury or ingestion, parents may have to deal with extreme guilt. Parents sometimes blame one another for an accident and require support and assistance in resolving some of their angry feelings. They will often benefit from performing purposeful activities that will help their child. Parents of toddlers are also valuable interpreters of the child's beginning verbal and nonverbal communication, routines, and rituals.

During the preschool period attitudes about discipline, masturbation, and beginning sexual curiosity may influence parental concerns in the hospital. The parents may also be anxious about their child's regression during hospitalization. In addition, the child's relationship with his parents may be affected by the oedipal complex during these years. In general, parents of preschool children can be very helpful in explaining procedures and treatments in language the child can understand, and parental participation in comforting and caretaking activities such as reading and playing games remains important to the child.[137]

During the school-age period, the parent-child relationship changes as the child develops independence and relationships outside of the home. Parents may feel guilt at having allowed independent activity that led to an accident. The child's regression may be difficult for the parents to accept, particularly for fathers who want their sons to be brave. Parents may need assistance in interpreting their child's alternating demanding and rejecting behavior. Family members can dispel some of the child's loneliness and boredom by engaging him in activities within the limits placed by the illness. It is important to help the patient keep abreast of news from home, school, and friends during this period. Parents can also assist in providing comfort and explanations for the child. However, older school-age children may prefer that caretaking activities be performed by the nurse.

Adolescence is often a trying time for the parent-child relationship. Any disagreements or arguments that preceded the adolescent's hospitalization may cause the parents guilt and remorse once the adolescent becomes critically ill. If the adolescent was injured in an accident, the parents may feel guilty or frustrated because they could not prevent the accident. The adolescent often demonstrates both dependent and independent behavior, which can be very confusing to parents. Parents often do not expect regression from their teenagers and need to be prepared for this behavior and reassured that it is normal and temporary. Parents should be encouraged to include the adolescent in decisions about his care. Visits from other family members and friends are particularly important to encourage so that the adolescent will maintain contact with his peer group.

Stresses facing parents of critically ill children. Stress is a condition or situation that imposes on a person demands for adjustment.[49] Parents of critically ill children are faced with a great number of such conditions or situations. The stress associated with their child's critical illness or injury may be monumental, particularly if it was sudden or unexpected. The hospital environment may cause other sources of stress that require adjustment, for example, lack of privacy in the hospital waiting room, a strange environment with unfamiliar people who might be crying or talking loudly, and disrupted sleeping and eating patterns.[69]

Sources of stress from outside the hospital may also exist. Parents may be worried about the care or problems of other children at home or the cost of transportation, babysitters, lodging, food, hospitalization, and time lost from work. Other family members may be ill at the same time the child is hospitalized; this will further increase the parents' stress.[69] If the child is hospitalized at a great distance from family and friends, the parents will be forced to stay in a strange city, away from support systems. At such times, relatively small associated stresses, such as trying to find a parking place, may become intolerable.[72] Family problems that may have existed before the child's illness may become accentuated during this time, particularly if one member is held responsible for the child's illness or injury.

Of all the stresses the parents may face, the critical-care environment itself may cause the most stress. If the child requires "intensive care," most people will assume that this means the child is seriously ill and close to death. Most nonmedical family members, however, cannot imagine how complex or busy the unit is. Just entering a critical-care unit may be overwhelming for lay people, who may initially feel like they have entered forbidden territory.[114,154] Hay and Oken graphically describe the atmosphere a parent encounters:

> A stranger entering an ICU is at once bombarded with a massive array of sensory stimuli, some emotionally neutral, but many highly charged. Initially, the greatest impact comes from the intricate machinery with its flashing lights, buzzing and beeping monitors, gurgling suction pumps, and whooshing respirators. Simultaneously, one sees many people rushing around busily performing life-saving tasks. The atmosphere is not unlike that of a tension-charged strategic war bunker.[57]

Parents often are shocked at the first sight of their child in the ICU (Fig. 2-9). Despite tours and preoperative teaching, parents of pediatric open-heart surgery patients have reported being overwhelmed at the sight of the tubes and equipment surrounding their child. Most of them expressed feelings of helplessness and powerlessness at the loss of their accustomed caretaker and protector roles.[72]

Working with individuals under stress. People under stress are often unable to function at their usual levels. Sedgwick[130] identified seven responses of individuals under stress that are important to understand when working with families of critically ill children. Behavior that would otherwise be inappropriate may be a normal response to stress.

1. *Reduced ability to utilize incoming information.* There is a constant need for repetition. The parent may ask the same question over and over of different staff members, searching for good news. It is essential the *content* and the *wording* of any information given to parents always be consistent, since parents often think they are being given different or inconsistent information when staff members use different words to describe the same condition.[119] If parents are given short written summaries of important information (composed by the primary nurse and physician and documented in the child's care plan), the parents can refer to this information later when they are able to digest it. This documentation will also ensure that consistent terms are used in explanations. People under stress can only absorb a small amount of threatening information at any one time.[9] When explaining treatments and equipment, the nurse should give brief explanations about their *normal* use for particular types of patients and problems. Although the family may hear only fragments of the explanations, they will hear the word "normal."[11] Family members sometimes act surprised at new developments and state that the doctor or nurse did not inform them. Before reacting to such a statement, it is

important to investigate the possibility that the family member *was* in fact told the information but was unable to assimilate it or even hear it at the time. A parent may unconsciously cause or aggravate nursing-staff discord by comparing information or nursing care provided by nurses of different shifts. If inconsistencies in the quality of care are present, these should be investigated and corrected. However, nurses should avoid discussion of minor variations in nurses' personalities or styles with parents.

2. *Decreased ability to think clearly and to problem solve.* Individuals under stress often describe confusion. Their ability to organize their thoughts or questions and to draw conclusions from obvious evidence is limited. The parent may be unable to sort out information and may respond identically to small or large stresses. The mother may appear to be as distressed about the fact that the infant's head was shaved (for insertion of a peripheral intravenous line) as the infant's sudden need for intubation and emergency medical treatment. This inability to prioritize concerns reflects extreme stress.

3. *Reduced ability to master tasks.* This response is related to an altered perception of the environment, a narrowed perceptual field, and an inability to mobilize one's own resources. Even simple tasks such as completing the admission process may be beyond the parent's ability at that time. The nurse should assess the parent's ability to function and provide assistance as needed.

4. *Decreased sense of personal effectiveness.* This may be reflected by feelings of loss, bewilderment, incompetence, failure, worthlessness, helplessness, or humiliation. Relationships with others may suffer. A sense of personal ineffectiveness is perhaps the most frustrating response to stress. All parents feel a sense of helplessness when their child is critically ill. They need to be told what they can do to help. They need to be able to start with small tasks, such as rubbing the child's back, and to progress to more difficult ones as they are able.

5. *Reduced ability to make effective, constructive decisions.* Often parents are asked to give consent for emergency procedures or surgery before they see their child or even understand what has happened.[62] Events are often distorted and exaggerated in their minds, with gaps in memory filled with semifactual information. It is important to help the parent sort out and understand the significant facts that they need to make an informed decision and, if possible, to allow the parents adequate time to assimilate this information.

6. *Heightened or decreased sensitivity to self.* Often body functions become a preoccupation, and

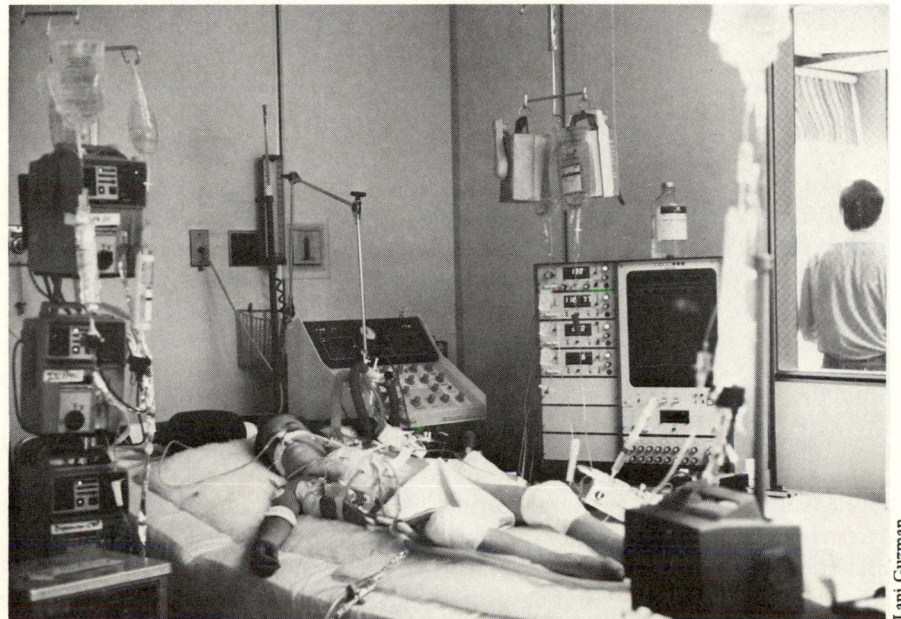

Fig. 2-9 The sight that confronts parents on their first visit to their critically ill child can be overwhelming.

somatic symptoms such as constipation, headache, or backache occur. People under a large amount of stress are easily distracted and annoyed and may be generally irritable. Benign events such as the sound of a tapping pencil in the waiting room may become disproportionately annoying. On the other hand, some parents seem to become totally wrapped up in their child and completely oblivious to themselves. They may need to be reminded and encouraged to eat, to take a break, or to get some rest.

7. *Decreased sensitivity to the environment.* Stressed individuals may be somewhat oblivious to things happening around them. Because of this, they may miss cues from their child, spouse, or the staff. Since subtleties often are not picked up, straightforward communication is best.

Entering a crisis state. An individual who is highly stressed is in danger of entering a crisis state, which is characterized by an inability to use coping mechanisms to deal effectively with an actual or an emerging problem.[15,25] What may constitute a crisis for one person will not necessarily be a crisis for another or, for that matter, may not be a crisis for the same person at another time.[8] Aguilera and Messick[1] have identified three balancing factors that influence an individual's vulnerability to crisis: a realistic perception of the events, adequate situational support, and adequate coping mechanisms.

It is important to determine the individual's *perception of the stressful event.* Often families do not have a realistic perception of the situation; this must be achieved if they are to deal adequately with it. Problem solving will probably not be successful until the real issue is identified. It is important to correct the family's misconception as tactfully as possible.

The presence of *adequate situational supports* is also very important. A person experiencing a crisis is more dependent than usual. It is important that the nurse obtain information about the family structure and relationships, religious affiliations and beliefs, and other possible support systems. If family members are too stressed to support the patient or one another, the assistance of the health-care team will be vital to the family's constructive resolution of the crisis.

Coping can be described as any attempt to master a problem or a new situation.[90] *Coping strategies* are behaviors an individual usually demonstrates when stressed. They are highly individualistic, and the individual may not even be aware of them. Difficulty arises when previously used strategies are not sufficient to solve the current problem. It is important to remember that the behavior displayed repre-

sents the individual's method of coping with that particular situation at that particular time.[90] Coping strategies may include behavior appropriate during periods of stress but inappropriate under normal circumstances. Family members or staff may be concerned about such behavior and may require assurances that the behavior is appropriate during stress.

Coping with the child's critical illness. Parents usually go through various stages in their reactions to their child's admission to a critical-care unit. These stages are similar to the stages of the grieving process.[36] Initially, most parents experience a period of shock, disbelief, and denial. These reactions are characterized by comments such as, "This can't be happening to us; it only happens to other people," "He *can't* be dying!" or "It's not that serious, he'll be OK." For most parents this initial stage passes during the first day, but it may last several days if the child remains unstable or unresponsive.[119] Denial is often necessary to the parent's ability to function. While unrealistic expectations should not be supported, the staff should not attempt to remove all hope. Parents often understand the seriousness of the situation but are not yet able to admit it to themselves or others. As this stage progresses, the parents usually experience feelings of helplessness and guilt as they blame themselves for the child's illness or injury.

Anger is another frequent reaction. Although the anger may be directed at the child for getting sick or injuring himself, or at God for allowing this to happen, neither of these are acceptable targets. Family members are usually not safe targets for anger either, since the parent feels a need for support from these individuals. Anger is often displaced onto the staff with complaints about the child's care. Some parents, however, are afraid to criticize staff members for fear of reprisals against the child. Parents sometimes need help in recognizing the true source of their anger and in finding constructive outlets for their strong feelings.

Depression is common and may indicate that the parent is attempting to deal with the strong feelings the situation has triggered. A supportive listener is usually helpful to the parent during this stage. Eventually, the parents may be able to reach a stage of resolution and acceptance in which they are able to make plans and decisions and can discuss the situation realistically.

Parents may experience all of these reactions and more. Rarely do both parents react in the same way at the same time; these differing reactions may also cause more stress for each of them.

Preparation for the critical-care unit. Various methods can be utilized for preparing parents for their child's critical-care experience. If the admission to the critical-care unit is planned, for example, following major elective surgery, advance preparation is useful. Verbal explanation is probably the most common method of preparation. The extent and accuracy of the information given, however, often varies a great deal, and some information may inadvertently be left out. Some parents who had been prepared by this method emphasized that no matter how much they were *told* about the ICU, they still did not feel prepared for actually *seeing* all of the equipment surrounding their child.[71] Demonstrations using miniature or even full-sized equipment on a doll or teddy bear are useful for preparing children but still do not serve the purpose of giving the parents a realistic view of what to expect.

Tours of the ICU are helpful in familiarizing the parents with the physical characteristics of the unit and in giving them a more accurate idea of what their child will look like. It is usually impractical to depend on tours as the sole method of preparation, however, since there may not always be a stable child in the ICU with the kind of equipment to provide a demonstration that will be adequate, yet not anxiety provoking. In addition, parents often are reluctant to look at other patients, thereby invading the privacy of other children and families.

Books with color pictures of equipment and children with various types of equipment in place may be a useful supplement to the tour. The nurse can use these illustrations to explain the purpose of the various pieces of equipment. Another supplement to the tour might be a standardized film, videotape, or slide-tape program that shows pictures of the hospital staff and the ICU. This information should coincide with the information included in a standardized preoperative teaching plan. With the use of a standardized medium, the parents have an opportunity to see and hear actual sights and sounds from the critical-care unit, information is not inadvertently left out, and the staff is aware of the exact information given the parents. It is important that a staff member view the program with the parents, since some of the sights and information may be upsetting when seen and heard for the first time and may generate many questions. The nurse should then document the specific information presented and the parents' questions and concerns in the preoperative nursing care plan so that the information can be consistantly reinforced.

Coping with the environment. It is extremely important for the parents to visit their child as soon as possible after the admission to the ICU, since they need to see for themselves that their child is in fact still alive. If at all possible, the child and area around the bed should be neat and cleaned of any blood before the parents enter. When time is short, a clean sheet can be placed over the child or the bed. The most important function of the first visit for the family is to reaffirm that the form on the bed is still a living, warm human being who greatly needs their love and support.[69]

The first visit to the child is extremely important and may determine how the parents will cope with the situation. The thought of seeing the child may be very frightening. *No one should ever be brought into a critical-care unit without some preparation for what he or she is about to see.* Even in emergency situations, some on-the-spot preparation at the door can provide information about the most striking aspects of the ICU. These explanations will necessarily be brief, and all of the information given may not be heard at that time. Family members *should always be accompanied by a staff member* on their first visit. The staff member can answer questions, explain events that are happening, and correct major misconceptions about the child's care or equipment. A professional must, of course, be present to react quickly to correct the problem if a monitor or other alarm should sound and to reassure the parents that everything is all right. Parents can be saved some unnecessary anxiety if they realize that alarms often sound when there is no problem. When the child is unconscious or unresponsive, this first visit is even more difficult for the parents.

The nurse may be most helpful to the parents if she simply provides silent support at the child's bedside to allow the parents time to digest the sights and sounds of the ICU. Supportive gestures (such as patting the mother's arm) may be far more needed at that moment than information about the child's ventilator or intravenous lines. The nurse should allow time after the parents' initial visit to assess their response to the environment and to answer additional questions.

During their visits in the critical-care unit, parents may use a variety of coping strategies.[72,90] Immobilization may be the first reaction. The parents may stop a few feet from the child's bed and just stare at the child and equipment. This may be a way of reducing through delay the initial impact of a situation.[90] Parents sometimes just need time to pull their thoughts together before they can move in and support their child. The conscientious nurse who, with all good intentions, takes parents by the arm and brings them closer, saying, "It's OK for you to move up closer to the bed; here, you can hold his hand," may actually be doing the parents a disservice. That approach may not be best for the parents. Seeing the child in this situation may be very frightening, and the parents may not be ready to move closer yet. Since it takes some parents time to be able to accept the situation, restricting visiting privileges to 5 or 10 minutes per hour may not allow some parents time to relax enough to approach their child and interact with him.

Visual survey is another way of becoming familiar with new situations. Some parents seem to pay attention to everything but their child. Their child is the most threatening aspect of the ICU, and the parents may need to become familiar with the environment before they are able to focus on their child. The nurse must wait before giving explanations until the parent is able to focus on what the nurse is saying.

The parents may also use withdrawal as a coping strategy. Some parents withdraw emotionally and seem to be unresponsive or detached; others may leave the ICU after a very brief 1- or 2-minute visit. These parents may need some immediate intervention and explanation. Parents' needs for periods of withdrawal should be respected and sometimes encouraged throughout the child's ICU stay, and nurses should be judicious in timing and methods of intervention.

The parents may restrict the complex situation and focus in on only small details, such as a piece of tape that seems too tight or a small area of blood on the sheet. Such concerns may seem to be inappropriate in light of the child's critical condition, but they may be the only things the parents feel they can change. Such interventions can help parents cope with their feelings of powerlessness by giving them some feeling of control over their child's care.[102]

Another strategy parents use is intellectualization. The workings of machinery or numbers are factors that are often more familiar than other aspects of the situation. Even though parents may not really understand what an arterial oxygen tension of 82 torr means, they may realize that it is higher or lower than before, and such information may be easier to deal with than the possibility of their child's death. The nurse may help the parents to master some of their anxiety by attempting to answer the parents' questions on an intellectual level. This method of coping is sometimes carried to extreme, however. One father used a stopwatch to time his child's ventilator and hurriedly informed the nurse when it delivered 59 rather than the desired 60 breaths per minute. Intervention was necessary to assist this father in identifying and discussing his real fears and concerns.

It is hard to imagine how terrifying it can be to have a child in a critical-care unit. Sympathetic expressions of "I know how you feel" are untrue and inappropriate unless, in fact, the staff member has had a critically ill child. What nurses say to parents is usually not as important to them as the attitude conveyed. The nurse should not feel inadequate or uncomfortable if she cannot think of something profoundly supportive to say during each parental visit. As one pediatrician stated, "Sometimes parents just need to hear from us that we care and that we're sorry that whatever has happened to their child has happened." Parents do not expect staff members to have all of the answers all of the time, but they do expect them to be honest and to care.

■ Siblings

The effect of a child's illness on other siblings in the family has been gaining more attention in recent years.[27,54,142,143] When a critical illness or injury strikes one child, often the other, healthy children in the family feel left out or forgotten because of the large amount of time parents spend at the hospital. Young siblings may fear that their wishes made the ill child get sick. Attempts to shelter siblings from unpleasant information only increases their fears and fantasies. They know something is wrong with their brother or sister but have only their own imagination to draw on for explanations. It may be helpful for siblings to visit their critically ill brother or sister, since it may decrease such fears and fantasies.

Often the parents are extremely concerned about the effect of this situation on their other children but are not sure what to do about it or what to tell the children. Nurses should inquire about other siblings and attempt to help the parents discuss ways of reducing sibling anxiety. Parents may also need to be encouraged to remain at home for several hours or a day to spend time with other family members.

■ When the child is dying

The death of one's child is tragic. Major psychologic adjustment is usually required, since the parents must relinquish their dreams and hopes for the child.[161] When a child's death has been expected, the parents often have had an opportunity for some anticipatory mourning; this allows them to progress through some of the stages of grief in preparation for the child's death.[36,66,68,76] In cases where open communication with the parents has been established and maintained, the nurse may wish to broach the topic of funeral arrangements or the child's burial. Parents often report that such advance planning minimizes confusion and allows them to be spared these decisions following the child's death.[80]

Occasionally, fatally ill children make dramatic recoveries. If the family has gone through the grieving process and has begun to adjust to a life that will not include the child, the Lazarus syndrome[32] may result when the child recovers. The family may feel that they cannot completely readjust to the child's recovery and may have difficulty accepting the child's return to the family. They may be angry at the medical staff or feel guilty that they began to emotionally draw away from the child. The Lazarus syndrome is more likely to occur if the parents' hope has been prematurely destroyed. If the child does recover unexpectedly, the family may require professional assistance in renegotiating their family relationships.

Very often, death in the critical-care unit is a sudden, unexpected occurrence. If the child was previously healthy, death after even several days in the ICU may be regarded as sudden and unexpected. If the child has been injured or has become ill suddenly without the parent's knowledge, the parents are usually notified by emergency room personnel; occasionally, however, it is necessary for the call to be made from the pediatric critical-care unit. This phone call is crucial to the parents' perception of and response to the child's death. Usually, the parents should not be told over the phone that their child has died. This information is best conveyed in a controlled, supportive environment after the parents have arrived at the hospital. Rinear[113] suggests one method of handling such phone calls. After identifying herself and the name of the hospital, the staff member should verify the person's relationship to the child. The family member can then be told generally what has happened, given a general statement about the injuries, and informed that everything possible is being done to help the child. If the relative seems extremely upset, the staff member can suggest that another family member or friend might bring the relative to the hospital or that a taxi be used. A similar approach might be used in calling a family if a child who has been a patient in the ICU suddenly deteriorates. The family members should be urged to drive carefully to the hospital. Family members may be involved in serious automobile accidents because they were speeding to the hospital to see a child who has already died.

Parents of children who have died suddenly report a surge of intense, disruptive, and almost intolerable feelings. Having had little or no time to prepare for the loss, the parents experience the child's death as a major insult, which results in extraordinarily strong feelings of shock and disbelief that may persist for weeks or months.[161] After arriving at the hospital,

the parents need time to begin to assimilate what has happened. It is very important that someone such as a nurse, social worker, or member of the clergy be available to stay with the parents during this time. If a clergy member is not present, the parents may wish to have one called.

If the parents are present at the hospital when their child has a fatal cardiopulmonary arrest, it may be helpful to prolong the code or attempted resuscitation of the child to allow the parents time to be prepared in stages for their child's death. During the unsuccessful resuscitation efforts, the parents should be given periodic reports of what is happening; each report should contain progressively more pessimistic information. The parents may initially be told that the child's heart stopped but that artificial massage and breathing are being performed and drugs are being given to help the heart recover. As the resuscitation continues, the parents should be told that the heart is not responding and that the longer resuscitation efforts are unsuccessful, the more pessimistic the child's outlook. A short time later, the parents may be told that nearly every medication has been given and the heart still has not recovered. Parents often raise the question of brain death or damage to other organs during prolonged resuscitation; if they do not, this may be appropriate for the nurse or physician to mention. When the parents seem ready, they should be told that the resuscitation will not be continued for much longer. Then the primary nurse and physician should inform the parents of the child's death. If this information is provided in careful sequence and is reinforced by a consistent physician and nurse, the parents will be better prepared for news of the child's death. They may even be able to discuss favorite memories of the child or begin planning for funeral arrangements while awaiting the final news of the child's death.

Whenever possible, the news of the child's death should not be given to a lone parent. If the spouse cannot be present, the parent may be told that the situation is very serious and the chances for the survival are extremely slim; a supportive friend or family member can then be summoned.[52] If a support person is unavailable, this role may fall to a staff nurse, clinical specialist, social worker, or chaplain.

Parents ultimately should hear from a physician that the child died, since the physician is the person that the public traditionally associates with diagnosis and treatment. The family needs to know that a physician was present when their child died and that everything possible was done to try to save the child. If a physician does not speak to the parents, they may have lingering doubts about the care their child received.[113] The parents and support person(s) should then be taken to a quiet, private place where the family can grieve alone.

The staff should be prepared for a variety of family reactions when a child dies. It is imperative that the staff recognize that most of this behavior represents a desperate attempt to cope with an unbelievable reality.[145] Comforting measures such as touching, holding a hand, putting an arm around the stricken individual, or hugging may be helpful and appreciated. After being told of the child's death, the parents need time to regroup and assimilate what has happened. Often the parents will want to see the child. This last good-bye is extremely important to their later ability to resolve their feelings about the child's death. The child should be bathed and equipment removed (if hospital policy permits, tubes should be removed). Often the parents will want to hold the child, and they should be given the privacy and time to do so. Sometimes parents may need several hours before they are ready and able to give their child up. Sometimes the parents will wish a staff member to be present while they see their child for the last time in the hospital.[52]

The parents may request that other support persons be called. A parent should not leave the hospital alone after the death of his or her child[113]; if possible, someone else should drive the family members home. They should be given the phone number of someone they can call at the hospital if they have more questions or are in need of further support.

Perhaps one of the most difficult types of death for parents to cope with occurs when the decision is made to withdraw life support from a child. It is difficult for the parents to understand that their child who is warm and pink and has a heartbeat is really dead. He may look no different than he did yesterday when they were told he was still alive; yet now he is dead. They may need repeated statements about the reality of the child's death and may require time to assimilate the fact before life support is withdrawn from the child. Although the parents' opinions, beliefs, and readiness should be taken into account, family members should never feel that they are being asked to make the decision to withdraw support,[119] since they may later translate this into feeling responsible for the child's death. The decision should always be seen as one made by the health-care team. Although such decisions are ultimately the responsibility of the attending physician, they should be made with input from those members of the critical-care team (nurses, house staff, social worker) who are most closely involved in the child's care.

Parents should be allowed to choose whether or not to be present when support is withdrawn. Some parents will wish to hold the child while the heart stops, or they may ask the nurse or other staff member to do so. They may wish to have specific support people present. Whenever possible, their wishes should be honored. It is often helpful for the parents to make funeral arrangments before support is withdrawn, so that they will not have to deal with this after the child dies. Once the child's heart has stopped, parents may need more time to say good-bye.

A follow-up conference with parents is often beneficial approximately 6 to 8 weeks after the child's death. Such conferences may involve the primary physician, primary nurse, the social worker, the parents, and any other family members the parents may wish present. These conferences give parents the opportunity to come back to the hospital and ask questions or clear up any concerns they may still have regarding their child's death. At this time the physician may explain the autopsy results. The staff has the opportunity to assess the family's adjustment and make referrals to appropriate resources if indicated. Both the family and the staff have an opportunity to say their good-byes to individuals who shared a very special and often intimate experience.

■ PSYCHOSOCIAL ASPECTS OF PEDIATRIC CRITICAL-CARE NURSING

A critical-care unit is not only an intense and stressful experience for patients and families but also for the staff who work there. If the demands, tensions, and stresses of pediatric critical-care nursing are not dealt with in a constructive manner, they can escalate and lead to "burn-out" and increased nursing staff turnover. The nurse can control this situation, however, by understanding the sources of stress and by using stress reduction techniques. Many aspects of pediatric critical-care nursing are extremely positive and rewarding; it is these challenges that often keep the staff going.

■ Stresses of pediatric critical-care nursing

Much has been published in recent years regarding the stress involved in critical-care nursing.[61,139] Most of these stresses can be divided into four main categories: interpersonal relationships, coping with the system, patient care, and miscellaneous stressors.

Interpersonal relationships. In a nation-wide study of 1800 critical-care nurses,[139] interpersonal conflict was identified as the greatest source of stress in critical-care units. The most frequently cited and intense stressors were nurse-physician problems. Other areas of interpersonal conflicts identified in this study were nurse-supervisor and nurse-nurse problems. Another type of interpersonal conflict, nurse-family problems, has already been discussed.

Nurse-physician relations. The complex and often life-threatening situations found in the pediatric critical-care unit require good communication, respect, support, cooperation, and teamwork among all members of the health-care team. However, this high level of functioning may not always be achieved. Lack of communication or cooperation and disrespect for the expertise and contributions of others can only lead to conflict and disharmony. This ultimately reduces the quality of care delivered to the children and their families. Many nurses do not believe that a collegial relationship exists between nurses and physicians; they feel physicians neither respect nor listen to their suggestions or opinions.[139] This source of stress can be intensified when the nurse believes that the physician is ineffectively or incorrectly managing the patient's condition.

Critical-care nurses are expanding their level of knowledge and practice and are beginning more and more to function in areas that have traditionally been within the realm of the physician. With experience, the critical-care nurse's knowledge and skills sometimes exceeds that of the beginning resident.[118,132,139] However, traditional lines of authority remain unchanged.[132] In our health-care system, the physician retains ultimate authority and ultimate accountability in patient-care matters. The nurse, however, is held accountable for providing a quality of care consistent with her level of expertise. She is responsible for questioning physicians' orders that appear to be incorrect. In fact the nurse is now legally classified as a "competent observer," capable of assessing medical procedures and making judgments about their propriety.[132] This paradox of the nurse's great responsibility but limited authority, status, and power highlights one of the major sources of role conflict and impedance to communication between nurses and physicians.

The approach the effective nurse must take in dealing with physicians has been described as "suggesting, reminding, urging, and then [if needed] bypassing."[132] This type of informal communication system requires delicacy and tact, since it may be necessary to give the physician a clear message that his or her performance is inadequate in a way that will not be threatening or damaging to professional identity and ego. Obviously, this is not always easy and can require time and patience from already busy and harried nurses. Once a good working relationship has been established, the residents often rotate, and new relationships must be formed and role delineations reestablished.

Frustration with the nurse-physician relationship is not unique to the nurse. Residents often believe that the nurses in critical-care units are highly critical of new physicians and intolerant of change. An intimidating nurse can make a highly competent resident feel insecure and appear hesitant and indecisive. Nurses sometimes bypass house-staff members and seek the advice of senior physicians, thus preventing the residents from keeping appraised of the status of their patients. At times nurses act as though the critical-care unit is their territory, which they are reluctant to share with house-staff physicians. Since several consulting services are often involved in the care of the critically ill child, communication problems are often multiplied. The many consulting services may provide conflicting orders, leaving the nurse caught in the middle and forced to choose which orders to follow. Mutual respect and cooperation must be present among all members of the health-care team if quality care is to be provided. It is imperative that open communication channels be established and maintained between nurses and physicians in critical-care units. The hospital administration may provide guidelines for physician's orders (e.g., who is allowed to write orders for which patients). Head nurses, medical directors, and nurse educators need to consistently model appropriate professional behavior.[132] Both nursing and medical directors must be strong and supportive leaders who are able to solve actual and potential conflicts.[12,26,57]

Staff meetings attended by nursing and medical staff and other professionals should be scheduled regularly and as needed to facilitate communication and mutual support. Differing ideas about treatment plans can be discussed so that all members of the staff feel they are able to contribute to decisions.

Nurse-supervisor relations. A leadership role in a critical-care unit can be difficult. Although it is exciting to work with a staff of predominantly young, intelligent, independent, assertive nurses, it also can be very stressful. Critical-care nurses are expected to take a lot of responsibility for the quality of patient care, so they wish to participate in the decisions being made about that care. Since critical-care units are usually organized with internal standards and controls, high degrees of autonomy and independence, and specialized skills,[73] a participative management approach[96] seems to work best. If a supervisor seeks to impose a more hierarchial, bureaucratic structure, staff stress and resentment usually result.

Some of the anger and criticism directed at nursing supervisors by staff nurses is scapegoating.[26,57] The intense feelings of anger and frustration the critical-care nurse experiences may sometimes be more safely directed toward nursing leadership than at patients, families, co-workers, or physicians. Staff-development instructors and orientation nurses seem to be particularly subject to such scapegoating. Since they usually do not have line authority, control over assignments, or responsibility for performance evaluations, they are even safer targets than the head nurse or charge nurse.

A head nurse may find it difficult to meet staff-nurse expectations. If she provides more direct patient care in response to staff complaints, other nurses may feel she is interfering. If the head nurse utilizes her administrative role to win better working conditions for staff nurses, she may be criticized for being absent from the unit too often for meetings.[26] In addition, the head nurse often is forced to defend unpopular administrative decisions to the nursing staff. Close communication with the staff and sharing of ideas, feelings, difficulties, and solutions are important in reducing or preventing such conflicts. It is vital to discover the real problems causing dissatisfaction. Often, apparently minor complaints provide clues to more serious problems. For example, staff complaints about the unit orientation may actually represent staff frustration with high staff turnover and nursing shortages.

Lack of positive feedback is also very stressful for nurses, particularly when they are working under stressful conditions. Too often, mistakes are widely discussed, while positive behaviors go unnoted. Feedback from supervisors is necessary and important, but supervisors are not the only source of feedback. Both positive and negative feedback can be shared directly among other health professionals. A good way to begin to receive feedback is to start giving positive strokes to others when their performance warrants it. Rewards are important to everyone but are essential to new staff members who are insecure in their new roles and want to be accepted and respected by their co-workers and supervisors.

The types of behaviors for which a nurse is rewarded indicate the value system of the person giving the feedback. It is important to identify the kinds of things for which nurses are rewarded, since behavior that is reinforced will be repeated. Often nurses are rewarded for attention to and knowledge of part-tasks, for example, knowing a particular laboratory result when a physician asks, observing an arrhythmia, or functioning appropriately in an emergency situation. Rarely are nurses rewarded for practicing total patient care, for developing a comprehensive care plan, and for paying attention to the child's special needs and to the needs of the family.[73] It is important that nurses are aware of what type of behaviors are being rewarded in their particular units and make sure that those are the behaviors they *want* repeated.

Nurse-nurse relations. Peer conflicts frequently are not recognized as sources of stress for nurses. Even though staff nurses do not exercise much power or restraint over one another,[61] competitive feelings and envy are often present. Nurses may compete for mastery of technical skills or the most challenging patient assignments. Sometimes the nurse who asks too many questions or admits her fears may be viewed as less than competent by her peers.[12] Offers of help may be viewed as threats to one's competence. A critical-care unit, however, is a place where mutual assistance, support, and interdependence are crucial to the delivery of high-quality care. Staff and leadership nurses in critical-care units need to be sensitive to occasions when competition is winning out over cooperation, and they should take steps to discuss and remedy such situations.

Types of patients and patient care. The pediatric critical-care nurse is faced with many special challenges and stressful situations with which she must cope. Some of these stresses involve working with parents and children in special and often unpleasant circumstances. It may be emotionally exhausting to care for a comatose child. Caring for any unresponsive child for several days can lead to feelings of vulnerability, frustration, anger, sorrow, and anxiety. It is also difficult to support the family during this period.[91,141] It can be particularly stressful to care for children who have been abused or are victims of violent crimes, since the nurse may have strong feelings of revulsion or anger that anyone could so seriously harm a child. Nurses must try to avoid the temptation of assigning guilt, taking sides, and acting out anger they feel toward abusive parents.[95]

Caring for neurologically damaged children may raise questions about the quality of patient life that is being salvaged. It is always extremely stressful for the health-care team to decide to withdraw life support. The nurse may feel frustrated and powerless when her views are not considered, or she may feel a share in the heavy responsibility if she participates in the decision. Enormous amounts of emotional energy may be required to support family members through this experience.

The pediatric critical-care nurse has frequent encounters with death. The nurse not only has to deal with her feelings about the child's death but may receive the brunt of parental anger and anxiety because she is the most available and most involved individual during the child's critical illness.[125] Each patient the nurse cares for represents an investment of her time, energy, and technical skills. The nurse often becomes attached to and involved with her patients, and this emotional bond makes it more difficult for the nurse when the child dies. It is this same emotional bond that allows the nurse to provide the most sensitive support to the family. It is also important that the nurse be able to maintain her therapeutic relationship with the family. If the nurse becomes overwhelmed by her grief, she will be unable to support the family.[67]

Coping with the system. Although the nursing shortage has eased, some critical-care units remain understaffed. The critical-care nurse must bear the increased work load, double shifting, and the stress of working with "floats" and registry nurses who may not be familiar with the skills and activities required in critical-care nursing. Staffing shortages may necessitate frequent schedule changes and postponement of vacations; these only further increase stress.

The lack of well-developed educational programs in the critical-care unit may be particularly stressful during busy times. It is difficult for experienced staff, already feeling taxed and overburdened, to orient many new nurses. If a specific preceptor is identified for each new orientee, the entire nursing staff does not have to feel responsible for the orientation process. In addition, the preceptor can become familiar with the specific qualifications and experiences the orientee still requires; this provides the new nurse with a more consistent, goal-directed orientation and an advocate among the experienced staff.

Nurses have also expressed insecurity about their own knowledge and dissatisfaction with the lack of opportunity for continuing education.[139] Clinical specialists, physicians, nursing instructors, nursing administrators, and staff nurses should all take part in clinical teaching. If physicians are asked to present brief conferences, this not only provides the physician with the opportunity to explain his or her philosophy and preferences for patient care, but it gives the physician an appreciation of the nurses' knowledge of and interest in specific patient-care problems. The nurses may also take such an opportunity to raise questions or suggest alternative care techniques in an environment conducive to exchange of ideas. When patient census is low, the staff nurse may be relieved of patient-care responsibilities to research a clinical problem and deliver a brief summary of her findings to other staff. This allows each staff member to develop specific areas of expertise and

helps staff nurses to gain respect for (and respect from) colleagues.

Equipment malfunctions, cramped facilities, noisy environment, and lack of supplies may add to stressful working conditions. Nursing salaries and benefits often are not commensurate with the responsibility nurses must accept.[139]

Other sources of stress. Other sources of stress for the nurse may arise from events in her personal life. Such concerns outside of the unit cannot be allowed to compromise the nurse's ability to function effectively.

Coping with staff stress. By far the most significant factor in reducing stress in the critical-care unit is supportive relationships with other members of the staff. A hospital unit with a nursing staff that has a close, positive relationship usually has very high morale. Shared, intense, emotional, and stressful experiences can breed a camaraderie, closeness, and an understanding for the feelings of other members of the health-care team. All members of the health-care team need to support one another. This may mean recognizing that a co-worker is reaching a low tolerance level and relieving her so that she can get away for a few minutes. Emotional empathy and reassurance from those with whom one works closely is highly meaningful. Sometimes we need to hear that someone realizes how we feel and recognizes the intensity of our efforts. Physical contact is important, too. As one nurse stated, "Sometimes you just need a hug, and it's nice to work with people who realize that and feel comfortable giving you one!" The benefits of supportive physical contact in the professional setting are now being recognized.[121] Praise from co-workers can be especially satisfying. It is important to take a moment to tell a co-worker that he or she did something especially well.

When the nurse supports a grieving family while the child dies, she needs time to grieve and regroup; she is not ready to pick up another assignment the moment the family leaves the ICU. If the nurse has empathized with the family's sorrow, it will be difficult for her to abandon or suppress those feelings and immediately form a new relationship with another child and family. Nurses need to be sensitive to the feelings and needs of those with whom they work and be sure that they are giving their colleagues time, understanding, and support.[77]

The use of humor is an effective technique to reduce stress. Through the use of humor, the staff can gain a sense of relief and a feeling that the situation is not overwhelming. Tears of laughter are much less threatening than tears of loss and frustration.[34,57] Obviously, the use of humor may be perceived by families as a sign of flippancy and lack of concern for the patients; thus its use is usually best reserved for times when family members are not present.

Group meetings can provide a constructive outlet for feelings and can be a means of sharing and discovering mutual concerns. A staff psychologist may be invited to coordinate the meetings. Such meetings can foster open communication and can be used for problem solving and conflict resolution.[34,118] Such meetings may also facilitate the use of humor in an appropriate setting.

Regular physical activity has been found to be helpful in reducing stress on a long-term basis.[55,162] Relaxation techniques are also helpful stress reducers. An easy five-step technique may be used when things have been particularly hectic and stressful.[55]

1. Find a comfortable place to sit.
2. Place feet flat on the floor.
3. Close your eyes.
4. Breathe steadily and with purpose for about 5 minutes.
5. Take particular notice of the parts of the body that feel tense and will them to relax.

This technique is beneficial in relaxing the body and leaving the mind free to identify what is really needed or wanted from the present situation. After utilizing this technique, the nurse may then have the energy to obtain it.[55]

■ Rewards of critical-care nursing

So often we focus on the stresses and the negative aspects of critical-care nursing, ignoring the reasons that nurses want to be involved in this type of nursing. The major rewards in critical-care nursing are often the same as the major stressors: the nature of direct patient care, interpersonal relationships, and the acquisition of knowledge.[139] It is very exciting to watch a critically ill child progress and recover, especially when the nurse knows that she is partially responsible for that recovery. It is gratifying to visit children after they have been transferred from the ICU—to see the child who was close to death now resuming normal activities.

It can be highly rewarding to assist children and their families through an extremely difficult and sometimes devastating experience and to be allowed to share very personal, intense feelings. Supporting a family through a child's death should also be considered a major, significant, positive activity. It should be seen as an opportunity to help someone through what must be one of the worst tragedies a human can face.[5] The nurse may end up with more

prolonged, intense, positive relationships with these families than with any other. Such opportunities are very special.

The critical-care nurse is able to deliver total patient care and to have close involvement with one or two patients and families. This is not always possible with large numbers of patients in less acute nursing-care units. The nurse is often able to take more initiative and to make more independent decisions in the critical-care unit.

The close working relationships that develop among nurses, physicians, and other co-workers in the critical-care unit can also be rewarding. Teamwork is often evident in these units. Critical-care nurses are usually recognized for their specialized knowledge and competence. The challenge, fast pace, excitement, stimulation, and opportunities for learning are all seen as other positive aspects of the critical-care setting.

■ CONCLUSION

This chapter has discussed some of the psychosocial and emotional considerations for the child, family, and staff in the pediatric critical-care unit. Such considerations are an integral and extremely important aspect of pediatric critical care. They present special challenges for the nurse who cares for critically ill children and their families.

The environment and dynamics of a pediatric critical-care unit may create a great deal of stress for the child, family, and staff. This chapter has discussed some of the psychosocial and emotional considerations that are an extremely important aspect of pediatric critical care. Particular skill and attention are required to prevent these considerations from getting lost in the requirements of technology, physical care, and repetitive routines. A knowledgeable, sensitive, and caring nurse can help to prevent the critical-care experience from becoming a terrifying time for the child and family.

ACKNOWLEDGMENTS

The author wishes to thank Dr. Roberta Ballard, Chief of Pediatrics, Mount Zion Hospital and Medical Center, San Francisco, California, and Patricia Werner, Pediatric Instructor, Yale-New Haven Hospital, for their helpful comments and suggestions regarding this chapter.

REFERENCES

1. Aguilera, D.C., and Messick, J.M.: Crisis intervention: the theory and methodology, St. Louis, 1974, The C.V. Mosby Co., p. 66.
2. Association for the Care of Children's Health: A child

goes to the hospital, Washington, D.C., 1981, The Association.

3. Ault, R.: Children's cognitive development, New York, 1977, Oxford University Press, Inc.

4. Ausubel, D.P., and Sullivan, E.V.: Neonatal and early infant behavior and capacities. In Theory and problems of child development, ed. 2, New York, 1970, Grune & Stratton, Inc.

5. Ballard, R.: Personal communication, March 1980.

6. Barnes, C.M.: School-age children's recall of the intensive care unit. In ANA Clinical Sessions, American Nurses Association, New York, 1974, Appleton-Century-Crofts, p. 73.

7. Barnes, C.M.: Levels of consciousness indicated by responses of children to phenomenon in the intensive care unit, Matern. Child Nurs. J. 4(4):215, 1975.

8. Barrell, L.M.: Crisis intervention: partnership in problem-solving, Nurs. Clin. North Am. 9:6, March 1974.

9. Baudry, F., and Wiener, A.: The family of the surgical patient, Surgery 63:421, 1968.

10. Belmont, H.S.: Hospitalization and its effects upon the total child, Clin. Pediatr. 9:472, 1970.

11. Benedek, T.: The family as a psychologic field. In Anthony, J.B., and Benedek, T.: Parenthood: its psychology and psychopathology, Boston, 1970, Little, Brown & Co., p. 109.

12. Bilodeau, D.C.: The nurse and her reactions to critical care nursing nursing, Heart 2:358, 1973.

13. Blackburn, S.: Sleep and awake states of the newborn. In Barnard, K.E., and others, editors: Early parent-infant relationships, White Plains, N.Y., 1978, The National Foundation for March of Dimes, p. 17.

14. Blake, F., Wright, F.H., and Waechter, E.H.: Nursing care of children, ed. 8, Philadelphia, 1970, J.B. Lippincott Co., p. 41.

15. Bloom, B.L.: Definitional aspects of the crisis concept. In Parad, W.J., editor: Crisis intervention: selected readings, New York, 1965, Family Service Association of America, p. 304.

16. Blos, P.: Children think about illness: their concepts and beliefs. In Gellert, E., editor: Psychosocial aspects of pediatric care, New York, 1978, Grune & Stratton, Inc.

17. Brandt, P.A., and others: IM injections in children, Am. J. Nurs. 72:1402, 1972.

18. Brazelton, T.B.: Infants and mothers: differences in development, New York, 1969, Dell Publishing Co., Inc.

19. Brazelton, T.B.: Neonatal behavior assessment scale, Philadelphia, 1973, J.B. Lippincott Co.

20. Brazelton, T.B.: Behavioral competence of the newborn infant, Semin. Perinatol. 3:35, 1979.

21. Brazelton, T.B., Holder, R., and Talbot, B.: Emotional aspects of rheumatic fever in children, J. Pediatr. 63:339, 1953.

22. Calkin, J.: Are hospitalized toddlers adapting to the experience as well as we think? MCN: Am. J. Matern. Child. Nurs. 4:18, 1979.

23. Call, J.: Games babies play, Psychol. Today 3:34, 1970.

24. Callahan, S.C.: Parenting: principles and politics of parenthood, Baltimore, 1973, Penguin Books, p. 109.

25. Caplan, G., Mason, E.A., and Kaplan, D.M.: Four studies of crisis in parents of prematures, Community Ment. Health J. 1:149, 1965.

26. Cassem, N.H., and Hackett, T.P.: Stress on the nurse and therapist in the intensive care unit and the coronary care unit, Heart Lung 4:252, 1975.

27. Craft, M.J.: Help for the family's neglected "other" child, MCN: Am. J. Matern. Child. Nurs. 4:297, 1979.

28. Crocker, E.: Play progress on pediatric settings. In Gellert, E., editor: Psychosocial aspects of pediatric care, New York, 1978, Grune & Stratton, Inc., p. 97.

29. Doak, S., and Wallace, N.: The doctors wear pajamas. Assoc. Care of Child. Health J. 20:8, 1975.

30. Dowd, E.L., Novak, J.C., and Ray, E.J.: Releasing the hospitalized child from restraints, MCN: Am. J. Matern. Child. Nurs. 2:370, 1977.

31. Duton, H.D.: The child's concept of death. In Schoenberg, B., and others, editors: Loss and grief, New York, 1970, Columbia University Press.

32. Easson, W.M.: The Lazarus syndrome in childhood, Med. Insight 4:44, 1972.

33. Eckhardt, L.O., and Prugh, D.G.: Preparing children psychologically for painful medical and surgical procedures. In Gellert, E., editor: Psychosocial aspects of pediatric care, New York, 1978, Grune & Stratton, Inc., p. 75.

34. Eisendrath, S.J., and Dunkel, J.: Psychological issues in intensive care unit staff, Heart Lung 8:756, 1979.

35. Elkind, D.: Children and adolescents: interpretive essays on Jean Piaget, New York, 1970, Oxford University Press, Inc.

36. Engel, G.L.: Grief and grieving, Am. J. Nurs. 64:93, Sept. 1964.

37. Epstein, C.: Nursing the dying patient, Reston, Va, 1975, Reston Publishing Co., Inc., p. 102.

38. Erikson, E.H.: Childhood and society, ed. 2, New York, 1963, W.W. Norton & Co., Inc.

39. Escalona, S.: The roots of individuality, Chicago, 1968, Alseine Publishing Co.

40. Field, T.M.: Interaction patterns of pre-term and term infants. In Field, T.M., editor: Infants born at risk, New York, 1979, Spectrum Publications.

41. Fitkin Globe, Pediatric Division Newsletter, Yale-New Haven Hospital, New Haven, Conn.

42. Flavell, J.H.: The developmental psychology of Jean Piaget, New York, 1963, Van Nostrand Reinhold Co., Inc.

43. Flavell, J.H.: Cognitive development, Englewood Cliffs, N.J., 1977, Prentice-Hall, Inc.

44. Fraiberg, S.H.: The magic years, New York, 1968, The Scribner Book Companies, Inc.

45. Freud, A.: The role of bodily illness in the mental life of children. In Psychoanalytic study of the child, vol. 7, New York, 1952, International Universities Press, Inc., p. 69.

46. Geary, M.C.: Supporting family coping, Supervisor Nurse 10:59, March 1979.

47. Gellert, E.: What do I have inside of me? How children view their bodies. In Gellert, E., editor: Psychosocial aspects of pediatric care, New York, 1978, Grune & Stratton, Inc., p. 19.

48. Gellert, E., Gircus, J.S., and Cohen, J.: Children's awareness of their bodily appearance: a developmental study of factors associated with the body percept, Genet. Psychol. Monogr. **84:**109, 1971.

49. Goldenson, M.: The encyclopedia of human behavior: psychology, psychiatry and mental health, Garden City, New York, 1970, Doubleday & Co., Inc., p. 1263.

50. Gorski, P.A.: Interaction influences on development—identifying and supporting infants born at risk. Presented at the annual meeting of the American Academy of Child Psychiatry, Chicago, Oct. 19, 1980.

51. Green, C.S.: Understanding children's needs through therapeutic play, Nursing '74, **4:**31, Oct. 1974.

52. Gyulay, J.E.: The dying child, New York, 1978, McGraw-Hill Book Co.

53. Hammar, S.L., and Eddy, J.: Nursing care of the adolescent, New York, 1966, Springer Publishing Co., Inc., p. 33.

54. Hardgrove, C., and Warrick, L.H.: How shall we tell the children? Am. J. Nurs. **74:**448, 1974.

55. Hartl, D.E.: Stress management and the nurse, Adv. Nurs. Sci. **1:**91, 1979.

56. Hartley, R.E., and Goldenson, R.M.: The complete book of children's play, New York, 1963, Thomas Y. Crowell Co.

57. Hay, D., and Oken, D.: The psychological stresses of intensive care unit nursing, Psychosom. Med. **34:**110, 1972.

58. Hedenkamp, E.A.: Humanizing the intensive care unit for children, Crit. Care Q. **3:**63, 1974.

59. Held, M.D.: The dying child: the importance of understanding, Med. Insight **6:**13, 1974.

60. Hofmann, A.D., Becker, R.D., and Gabriel, H.P.: The hospitalized adolescent, a guide to managing the ill and injured youth, New York, 1976, The Free Press.

61. Huckabay, L.M.D., and Jagla, B.: Nurses' stress factors in the intensive care unit, J. Nurs. Adm. **9:**21, 1979.

62. Jay, S.: Pediatric intensive care: involving parents in the care of their child, Matern. Child Nurs. J. **6:**195, 1977.

63. Johnson, J.E., Kirchhoff, K.T., and Endress, M.P.: Altering children's distress behavior during orthopedic cast removal, Nurs. Res. **24:**404, 1975.

64. Karon, M., and Vernick, J.: An approach to the emotional support of fatally ill children, Clin. Pediatr. **7:**274, 1968.

65. Korner, A.F.: Individual differences at birth: implications for early experience and later development. In Westman, J., editor: Individual differences in children, New York, 1973, John Wiley & Sons, Inc.

66. Kübler-Ross, E.: On death and dying, New York, 1969, The MacMillan Co.

67. Kübler-Ross, E.: Questions and answers on death and dying, New York, 1974, Collier Books.

68. Kübler-Ross, E.: Living with death and dying, New York, 1981, MacMillan Publishing Co., Inc.

69. Kuenzi, S.H., and Fenton, M.V.: Crisis intervention in acute care areas. Am. J. Nurs. **75:**832, 1975.

70. Levy, D.N.: The infant's earliest memory of inoculations, J. Genet. Psychol. **96:**3, 1960.

71. Lewandowski, L.A.: Effects of realistic expectations of an event on the anxiety levels and supportive behavior of parents of children undergoing open-heart surgery, master's thesis, San Francisco, 1977, University of California.

72. Lewandowski, L.A.: Stresses and coping styles of parents of children undergoing open-heart surgery, Crit. Care Q. **3:**77, 1980.

73. Lewandowski, L.A., and Kramer, M.: Role transformation of special care unit nurses: a comparative study, Nurs. Res. **29:**172, 1980.

74. Lewis, N.: The needle is like an animal: how children view injections, Child. Today **7:**18, 1978.

75. Lidz, T.: The person—his and her development through the life cycle, New York, 1968, Basic Books, Inc., Publishers, p. 149.

76. Lindemann, E.: Symptomatology and management of acute grief, Am. J. Psychiatry, **101:**141, 1944.

77. Lobsenz, N.M.: How to give and get more emotional support, Women's Day, p. 73, Sept. 1977.

78. Lonetto, R.: Children's conception of death, New York, 1980, Springer Publishing Co., Inc.

79. Mahaffy, P.R.: The effects of hospitalization on children admitted for tonsillectomy and adenoidectomy, Nurs. Res. **14:**13, 1965.

80. Martinson, I.: Caring for the dying child, Nurs. Clin. North Am. **14:**467, 1979.

81. McBride, M.: Can you tell me where it hurts? Assessing children with pain, Pediatr. Nurs. **3:**8, 1977.

82. McBride, M.M., and Sack, W.H.: Emotional management of children with acute respiratory failure in the intensive care unit: a case study, Heart Lung **9:**98, 1980.

83. McCaffrey, M.: Pain relief for the child: problem areas and selected nonpharmacological methods, Pediatr. Nurs. **3:**11, 1977.

84. McGuire, L.: A short, simple tool for assessing your patient's pain, Nursing '81, **11:**48, 1981.

85. McIntire, M.S., Angle, C.R., and Struempler, L.J.: The concept of death in midwestern children and youth, Am. J. Dis. Child. **123:**527, 1972.

86. Michaels, D.R.: Too much in need of support to give any, Am. J. Nurs. **7:**1932, 1971.

87. Miles, M.S., and Olsen, S.: Effects of illness on the toddler. In Scipien, G.M., and others, editors: Comprehensive pediatric nursing, ed. 2, New York, 1979, McGraw-Hill Book Co., p. 270.

88. Molter, N.C.: Needs of relatives of critically ill patients: a descriptive study, Heart Lung **8:**332, 1979.

89. Montagu, A.: Touching, New York, 1971, Harper & Row, Publishers, Inc.

90. Murphy, L.B., and others: The widening world of childhood: paths toward mastery, New York, 1962, Basic Books, Inc., Publishers.

91. Myco, F., and McGilloway, F.A.: Care of the unconscious patient: a complementary perspective, J. Adv. Nurs. **5:**273, 1980.

92. Nagera, H.: Children's reactions to hospitalization and illness, Child Psychiatry Hum. Dev. **9:**3, 1978.

93. Nagy, M.: The child's view of death. In Feifel, M., editor: The meaning of death, New York, 1969, McGraw-Hill Book Co.

94. Nahigian, E.G.: Effects of illness in the preschooler. In Scipien, G.M., and others, editors: Comprehensive pediatric nursing, ed. 2, New York, 1979, McGraw-Hill Book Co., p. 379.

95. Neill, K., and Kauffman, C.: Care of the hospitalized, abused child and his family: nursing implications, MCN: Am. J. Matern. Child Nurs. **1:**117, 1976.

96. Neissner, P.: Participative management in the ICU, Supervisor Nurse, **9:**41, 1978.

97. Noble, M.A.: Communication in the ICU: therapeutic or disturbing? Nurs. Outlook **27:**195, 1979.

98. Northrup, F.C.: The dying child, Am. J. Nurs. **74:**1066, 1974.

99. O'Connor, C.T.: Curare in patient care, Am. J. Nurs. **72:**913, 1972.

100. Olsen, E.H.: The impact of serious illness on the family system, Postgrad. Med. **47:**169, 1970.

101. Oremland, E.K., and Oremland, J.D.: The effects of hospitalization on children, Springfield, Ill., 1973, Charles C Thomas, Publisher.

102. Parfit, J.: Parents and relatives, Nurs. Times **71:**1512, 1975.

103. Parmelee, A.H., and Stern, E: Development of states in infants. In Clemente, C., Purpura, D., and May, F., editors: Sleep and the maturing nervous system, New York, 1972, Academic Press, Inc.

104. Peters, B.M.: School-aged children's beliefs about causality of illness: a view of the literature, Matern. Child Nurs. J. **7:**143, 1978.

105. Petrillo, M., and Sanger, S.: Emotional care of hospitalized children: an environmental approach, ed. 2, Philadelphia, 1980, J.B. Lippincott Co.

106. Phillips, J.L.: The origins of intellect: Piaget's theory, San Francisco, 1975, W.H. Freeman & Co. Publishers.

107. Piaget, J.: The origins of intelligence in children, New York, 1952, International Universities Press, Inc.

108. Piaget, J.: The moral judgement of the child, New York, 1965, The Free Press.

109. Piaget, J.: The language and thought of the child, ed. 3, New York, 1967, Humanities Press, Inc.

110. Poznanski, E.O.: Children's reactions to pain: a psychiatrist's perspective, Clin. Pediatr. **15:**1114, 1976.

111. Prechtl, H.F.R.: The behavioral states of newborn, Brain Res. **76:**185, 1974.

112. Provence, S., and Lipton, R.C.: Infants in institutions, New York, 1967, International Universities Press, Inc.

113. Rinear, E.E.: The nurses challenge when death is unexpected, RN, **38:**52, 1975.

114. Roberts, S.L.: Behavioral concepts and the critically ill patient, Englewood Cliffs, N.J., 1976, Prentice-Hall, Inc., p. 367.

115. Robertson, J.: Young children in hospitals, New York, 1969, Basic Books, Inc., Publishers.

116. Robinson, M.E.: The emotional impact of hospitalization. Paper presented at the Children's Hospital National Medical Center, Washington, D.C., Nov., 1975.

117. Robson, K.S., and Moss, H.A.: Patterns and determinants of maternal attachment, J. Pediatr. **77:**976, 1970.

118. Rosini, L.A., and others: Group meetings in pediatric intensive care unit, Pediatrics **53:**371, 1974.

119. Rothstein, P.: Psychological stress in families of children in a pediatric intensive care unit, Pediatr. Clin. North Am. **27:**613, 1980.

120. Salamaha, C., and others: Growth and development. In Oakes, A.R., editor: Critical care nursing of children and adolescents, Philadelphia, 1981, W.B. Saunders Co.

121. Saltzman, J.: Hug therapy, Scene section, San Francisco Examiner, p. 1, April 20, 1980.

122. Savedra, M.: Coping with pain: strategies of severely burned children, Can. Nurs. **73:**28, Aug. 1977.

123. Savedra, M.: The adolescent in the hospital. In Mercer, R.T., editor: Perspectives on adolescent health care, Philadelphia, 1979, J.B. Lippincott Co., p. 177.

124. Schowalter, J.E.: When a child must die . . ., Med. Insight **6:**37, 1974.

125. Schowalter, J.E.: The reactions of caregivers dealing with fatally ill children and their families. In Sahler, O.J.Z.: The child and death, St. Louis, 1978, The C.V. Mosby Co.

126. Schowalter, J.E., and Anyan, W.R.: Experience on an adolescent in-patient division, Am. J. Dis. Child. **125:**212, 1973.

127. Schowalter, J.E., Ferholt, J.B., and Mann, N.M.: The adolescent patient's decision to die, Pediatrics **5:**97, 1973.

128. Schowalter, J.E., and Lord, R.D.: On the writings of adolescents in a general hospital ward, Psychoanal. Study Child **27:**181, 1973.

129. Schultz, N.V.: How children perceive pain, Nurs. Outlook **19:**670, 1971.

130. Sedgwick, R.: Psychological responses to stress, J. Psychiatr. Nurs. **13:**20, 1975.

131. Selye, H.: Stress in health and disease, Boston, 1976, Butterworth Publishers.

132. Sexton, M.J., Kahn, M.: Communication patterns in the neonatal intensive care unit: an analysis of the effect of role and organizational structure on communication in the neonatal intensive care unit. In Simon, N.M., editor: The psychological aspects of intensive care nursing, Bowie, Md., 1980, Robert J. Brady Co.

133. Simon, N.M., and Poelker, G.: A family affair: dealing with families of ICU patients. In Simon, N.M., editor: The psychological aspects of intensive care nursing, Bowie, Md., 1980, Robert S. Brady Co.

134. Skipper, J.K., Leonard, R.C., and Rhymes, J.: Child hospitalization and social interaction: an experimental study of mother's feelings of stress, adaptation, and satisfaction, Med. Care **6:**496, 1968.

135. Smith, A.G., and Schneider, L.T.: The dying child— helping the family cope with impending death, Clin. Pediatr. **8**:3, 1969.

136. Smith, M.E.: The preschooler and pain. In Brandt, P.A., Chinn, P.L., and Smith, M.E., editors: Current practice in pediatric nursing, vol. 1, St. Louis, 1976, The C.V. Mosby Co.

137. Soupios, M., Gallagher, J., and Orlowski, J.P.: Nursing aspects of pediatric intensive care in a general hospital, Pediatr. Clin. North Am. **27**:628, 1980.

138. Spitz, R.A.: Hospitalism: an inquiry into the genesis of psychiatric conditioning in early childhood. In Fenechel, D., and others, editors: Psychoanalytic studies of the child, vol. 1, New York, 1945, International Universities Press, Inc., p. 113.

139. Steffan, S.M.: Perceptions of stress: 1800 nurses tell their stories. In Claus, K.E., and Bailey, J.T.: Living with stress and promoting well-being, St. Louis, 1980, The C.V. Mosby Co.

140. Sullivan, H.S.: Conceptions of modern psychiatry, New York, 1953, W.W. Norton & Co., Inc.

141. Surveyor, J.A.: The emotional toll on nurses who care for comatose children, MCN: Am. J. Matern. Child Nurs. **1**:243, 1976.

142. Taylor, S.C.: The effect of chronic childhood illness upon well siblings, Matern. Child Nurs. J. **9**:109, 1980.

143. Taylor, S.C.: Siblings need a plan of care, too, Pediatr. Nurs. **6**:9, 1980.

144. Thomas, A., and Chess, S.: Temperment and development, New York, 1977, Bruner/Mazel, Inc.

145. Thornton, D.S.: Grief: a pediatrician's concerns, feelings and their medical significance, Ross Lab. **21**:17, 1979.

146. Triplett, J.L., and Arneson, S.W.: The use of verbal and tactile comfort to alleviate distress in young hospitalized children, Res. Nurs. Health **2**:17, 1979.

147. Tronick, E.D., Als, H., and Brazelton, T.B.: Mutuality in mother-infant interaction, J. Commun. Spring 1977.

148. Vaillot, N.C.: Hope: the restoration of being, Am. J. Nurs. **70**:268, 1970.

149. Vernon, D.T.A., and Schulman, J.L.: Hospitalization as a source of psychological benefit to children, Pediatrics **34**:694, 1964.

150. Vipperman, J.F., and Rager, P.M.: Childhood coping: how nurses can help, Pediatr. Nurs. **6**:18, 1980.

151. Visintainer, M.A., and Wolfer, J.A.: Psychological preparation for surgical pediatric patients: the effect on children's and parents stress responses and adjustment, Pediatric **56**:187, 1975.

152. Waechter, E.H.: Children's awareness of fatal illness, Am. J. Nurs. **71**:1168, 1971.

153. Waechter, E.H., and Blake, F.G.: Nursing care of children, ed. 9, Philadelphia, 1976, J.B. Lippincott Co.

154. Wallace P.: Relatives should be told about intensive care—but how much and by whom? Can. Nurse **67**: 33, 1971.

155. Watson, J.: Research and literature on children's responses to injections: some general nursing implications, Pediatr. Nurs. **2**:7, 1976.

156. Wessel, M.A.: Death of an adult and its impact upon the child, Clin. Pediatr. **12**:29, 1973.

157. Whaley, L.F., and Wong, D.L.: Nursing care of infants and children, ed. 2, St. Louis, 1983, The C.V. Mosby Co., p. 430.

158. Winnicott, D.W.: Transitional objects and transitional phenomena: a study of the first "not me" possession, Int. J. Psychoanal. **34**:89, 1953.

159. Wolfer, J.A., and Visintainer, M.A.: Pediatric surgical patients' and parents' stress response and adjustment, Nurs. Res. **24**:244, 1975.

160. Woolsey, S.F., Thornton, D.S. and Friedman, S.B.: Sudden death. In Sahler, O.J.Z., editor: The child and death, St. Louis, 1978, The C.V. Mosby Co., p. 100.

161. Zindler-Wernet, P.: Regulating stress through physical activity. In Claus, K.E. and Bailey, J.T.: Living with stress and promoting well-being, St. Louis, 1980, The C.V. Mosby Co., p. 101.

ADDITIONAL READINGS

The following books may be extremely helpful for nursing staff and parents coping with the death of a child.

Donnelly, K.F.: Recovering from the loss of a child, New York, 1982, Macmillan, Inc.

Grollman, E.A.: Talking about death: a dialogue between parents and child, Boston, 1976, Beacon Press.

Miles, M.S.: The grief of parents when a child dies, Oakbrook, Ill., 1978, The Compassionate Friends, Inc.

Sahler, O.J.Z.: The child and death, St. Louis, 1978, The C.V. Mosby Co.

Schiff, H.S.: The bereaved parent, New York, 1977, Penguin Books.

CHAPTER THREE

Cardiovascular Disorders

MARY FRAN HAZINSKI

All children admitted to a critical-care unit require thorough assessment of cardiovascular function. Congestive heart failure, low cardiac output, arrhythmias, and hypoxemia are among the most common cardiovascular problems seen in critically ill children. Congestive heart failure is most frequently the result of congenital heart defects. Low cardiac output can result from cardiac dysfunction, arrhythmias, fluid, electrolyte, or acid-base imbalances, hemorrhage, infection, drug toxicity, or pulmonary or neurologic dysfunction. Arrhythmias may result from congenital conduction tissue anomalies, surgical injury to conductive tissue, hypoxia, or electrolyte or acid-base imbalance. Hypoxemia can be caused by respiratory insufficiency (see Chapter 4), cyanotic congenital heart defects, or pulmonary hypertension.

This chapter begins with a brief review of cardiac embryologic development, physiology, and hemodynamic principles. Care of the child with congestive heart failure, low cardiac output, arrhythmias, and cardiac hypoxemia is also discussed. The third section of the chapter highlights common postoperative complications and nursing care responsibilities. The etiology, pathophysiology, clinical signs and symptoms, and medical, surgical, and nursing treatment of specific congenital heart defects and inflammatory diseases of the heart are then discussed. The chapter concludes with a discussion of diagnostic tests frequently required by the pediatric cardiovascular patient.

■ Essential Anatomy and Physiology

The cardiovascular system delivers oxygenated blood and other nutrients to the body. The blood is pumped by the heart, carried by the pulmonary arteries to the lungs for oxygenation, carried by the sys-temic arteries to the tissues, and returned to the heart by the veins. Adequate systemic perfusion requires an adequate cardiac structure, effective cardiac function, adequate circulating blood volume, appropriate arterial and venous tone, adequate oxygen and nutrient supply, appropriate cellular function, and adequate feedback mechanisms.

■ CIRCULATORY DEVELOPMENT
■ Embryology

Epidemiology of congenital heart defects. The majority of fetal cardiac development occurs between the fourth and seventh weeks of fetal life; errors occurring during this time are responsible for the majority of congenital heart defects. It is during this time that the heart is most susceptible to teratogenic agents—any agent or factor that causes fetal malformation. Although we know several factors *associated* with an increased incidence of congenital heart defects, there are very few agents known to *cause* congenital heart defects. Although the link between maternal drug ingestion and fetal malformations has been given a great deal of media attention, very few drugs have been consistently linked in large epidemiologic studies with the development of congenital heart defects.[212] The only well-documented pharmacologic teratogens are maternal thalidomide, trimethadione, and hydantoin ingestion.[219,244,309,310]

Despite frequent attempts to link maternal illness during pregnancy with increased incidence of congenital malformations in offspring, few maternal health factors are associated with an increased risk of congenital heart disease. If the pregnant woman contracts rubella during the first 8 weeks of pregnancy, there is a 50% risk that her baby will have congenital rubella syndrome.[5] This syndrome can include patent ductus arteriosus and/or pulmonary artery branch stenosis.[346] Approximately 10% or more of infants of

Table 3-1 Cardiac anomalies commonly associated with congenital diseases or syndromes[309,310]

Disease or syndrome	Associated cardiac anomaly
Trisomy 13 (Patau's syndrome)	Patent ductus arteriosus and/or ventricular septal defect with pulmonary hypertension
Trisomy 18 (Edward's syndrome)	Ventricular septal defect; patent ductus arteriosus
Trisomy 21 (Down's syndrome)	Endocardial cushion defect; ventricular septal defect; patent ductus arteriosus
Turner's syndrome	Coarctation of the aorta
Mosaic Turner's syndrome (XO/XY)	Pulmonary valvular stenosis
Marfan's syndrome	Aortic or mitral valve abnormalities; dissecting aortic aneurysms; myocardial disease
Holt-Oram syndrome	Atrial septal defect or single atrium; severe pulmonary vascular disease; total anomalous pulmonary venous return; arrhythmias
Ellis-van Creveld syndrome	Single atrium or large atrial septal defect
Williams elfin facies syndrome	Supravalvular aortic stenosis; peripheral pulmonary stenosis
Laurence-Moon-Bardet-Biedl syndrome	Aortic or pulmonary valvular stenosis; tetralogy of Fallot; ventricular septal defect
Hunter's syndrome	Abnormalities of the mitral or tricuspid valves or coronary artery obstruction
Hurler's syndrome	Abnormalities of the mitral or tricuspid valves or coronary artery obstruction
Friedreich's ataxia	Cardiomyopathy
Neurofibromatosis	Pulmonary valvular stenosis
DiGeorge syndrome	Interrupted aortic arch
Rubella syndrome	Patent ductus arteriosus; peripheral pulmonary stenosis
Fetal alcohol syndrome	Ventricular septal defect; atrial septal defect; tetralogy of Fallot
Maternal thalidomide ingestion	Tetralogy of Fallot; truncus arteriosus
Fetal trimethadione syndrome	Ventricular septal defect; tetralogy of Fallot
Maternal diabetes (insulin-dependent)	Transposition of the great vessels; ventricular septal defect

insulin-dependent diabetic mothers have congenital heart disease, appearing most commonly as transposition of the great vessels, ventricular septal defect, or hypertrophic cardiomyopathy.[170,450] Nearly 50% of infants with fetal alcohol syndrome have congenital heart disease (Table 3-1).[310]

Teratogens account for only a tiny proportion of congenital anomalies. Most congenital heart defects are thought to result from a complex interaction of genetic and environmental or intrauterine factors; this is referred to as *multifactorial inheritance.* This theory seems to be confirmed by the observation that concordance for congenital heart disease is not complete in monozygotic twins. Since monozygotic twins have the same genetic and intrauterine influences during fetal development, there must be some additional, unknown factor(s) contributing to the development of the cardiac malformation in only one twin.

Because most congenital heart defects are transmitted through multifactorial inheritance, there is a slightly higher risk (2.5% to 16%) of congenital heart disease among children with one parent or one previous sibling who have congenital heart disease than among children of noninvolved families (0.8% to 1.0%).[219,288,311,443] Some congenital heart defects have shown an unusual familial distribution. Until recently, children with complex congenital heart disease did not survive to reproductive age; therefore recurrence risks of congenital heart disease in their offspring has only recently been available. These recurrence risks may be higher than those of simple congenital heart defects.[61,443] Mothers with left ventricular outflow tract obstruction (such as coarctation of the aorta or aortic stenosis) seem to have the highest incidence of congenital heart disease in offspring.[443]

Some congenital heart defects are associated with chromosomal anomalies or syndromes. Approximately 30% to 50% of infants with Down's syndrome (trisomy 21) have congenital heart disease, and there is an increased incidence of congenital heart disease among infants with trisomy 13 or trisomy 18; pulmonary hypertension may also be present in infants with trisomy 13. The relationship of congenital heart disease with other common chromosomal anomalies is included in Table 3-1.

Congenital heart disease is associated with extracardiac anomalies in 20% to 45% of involved infants.[159,435] The incidence of extracardiac anomalies is highest among low-birthweight infants and infants with combined cardiac septal defects and lowest among infants with transposition of the great vessels.[435]

Approximately 16% of children with congenital heart defects have anomalies of the skeleton, skin, and muscles. Gastrointestinal anomalies occur in approximately 15% of infants with congenital heart disease[435]; conversely, approximately 15% of infants with tracheoesophageal fistula and 25% of infants with congenital diaphragmatic hernia have congenital heart disease.[156,157] Renal and urogenital anomalies occur in approximately 15% of children with congenital heart disease, and heart disease is frequently present when the child has malformation or agenesis of one or both kidneys.[158]

There is a well-documented association between congenital heart disease and asplenia or polysplenia. These infants have a wide variety of visceral and cardiac malformations and malpositions. The infant with asplenia commonly becomes cyanotic in the first days of life as a result of complex cyanotic heart disease. These infants may also demonstrate cardiac malpositions such as dextrocardia and abnormalities of systemic venous return. Anomalous pulmonary venous drainage or transposition of the great vessels may also be present. These children often demonstrate bilateral symmetry of organs (including lung lobes and abdominal organs) with a normal, left, or transverse location of the liver and gallbladder; the stomach is most frequently located on the right side of the abdomen, and total situs inversus may be present.[363]

Infants with polysplenia often have less severe cardiac anomalies; atrial and ventricular septal defects and anomalous pulmonary venous drainage are often noted. Cardiac malpositions may also be present, and anomalous systemic veins, such as bilateral superior vena cavae and absent inferior vena cavae, may be present.[281]

Development of the heart and great vessels. The heart begins development as a tube inside the pericardial cavity. As the tube elongates it begins to coil to the right (this is referred to as dextral or D-looping). This looping occurs by approximately the twenty-eighth day of gestation and once accomplished, the ebb and flow of blood through the heart occur (Fig. 3-1). Malrotation during this period of cardiac development may cause various cardiac malpositions (including dextrocardia) and malformations (including L-transposition).

Cardiac septation occurs during the sixth and seventh weeks of gestation. In the atria, two septa develop and are modified so they will ultimately form a flapped orifice, the foramen ovale. Two mesenchymal cushions, the *endocardial cushions,* fuse together in the middle of the heart and influence this septation process. At the end of the fourth week of fetal life the *septum primum* begins to grow from the

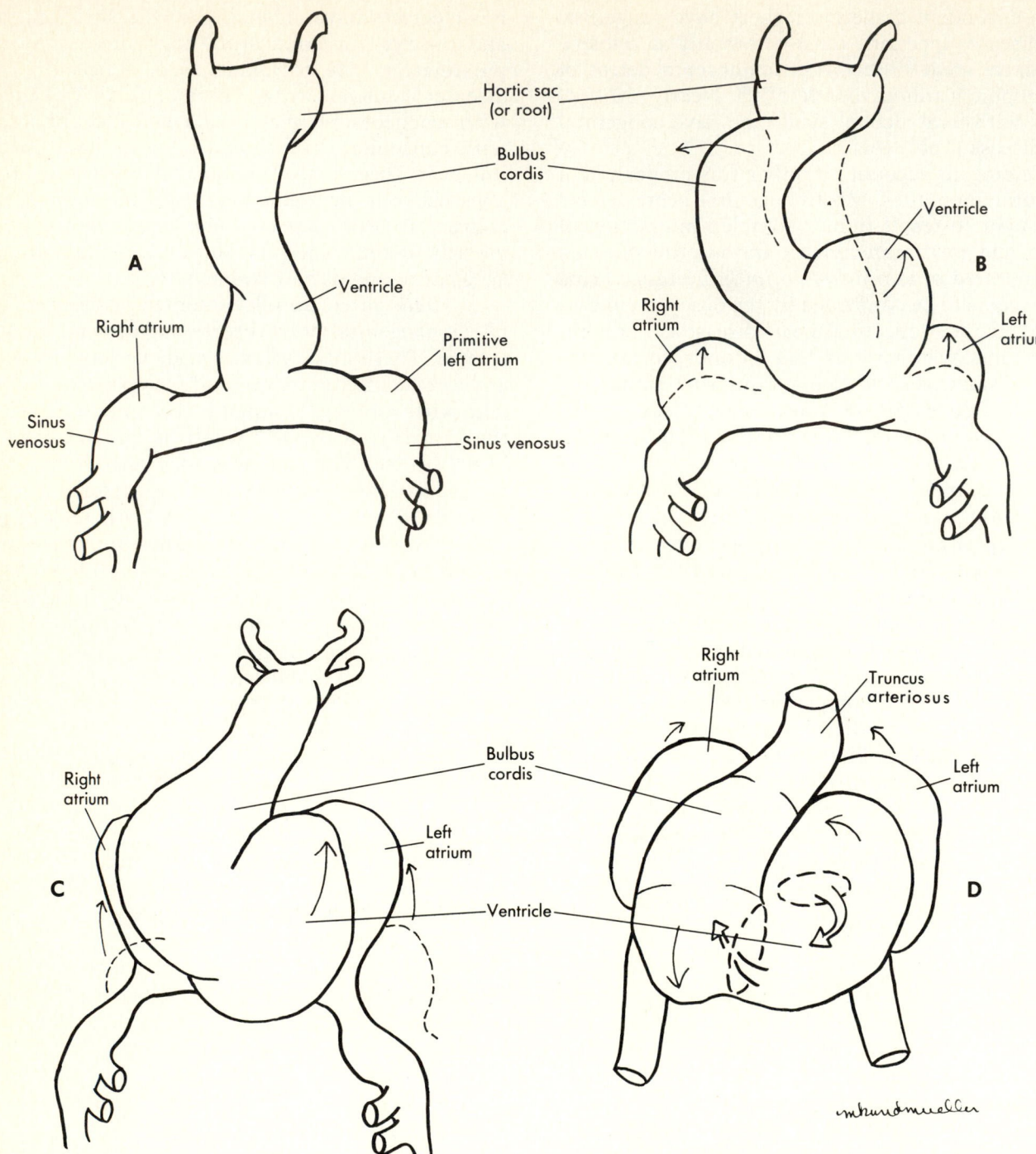

Fig. 3-1 Cardiac embryologic development—coiling of the cardiac tube. At approximately the twenty-first to twenty-second day of life, the two lateral endothelial heart tubes fuse to form a single endocardial cardiac tube, **A.** Between the twenty-second and twenty-eighth days of life, the heart tube thickens and coils to the right, **B** and **C.** By approximately the twenty-eighth day of life, the tube is completely coiled, and major chambers can be distinguished, **D.** At this time, blood is flowing through the heart, and septation of the heart and great vessels can occur.

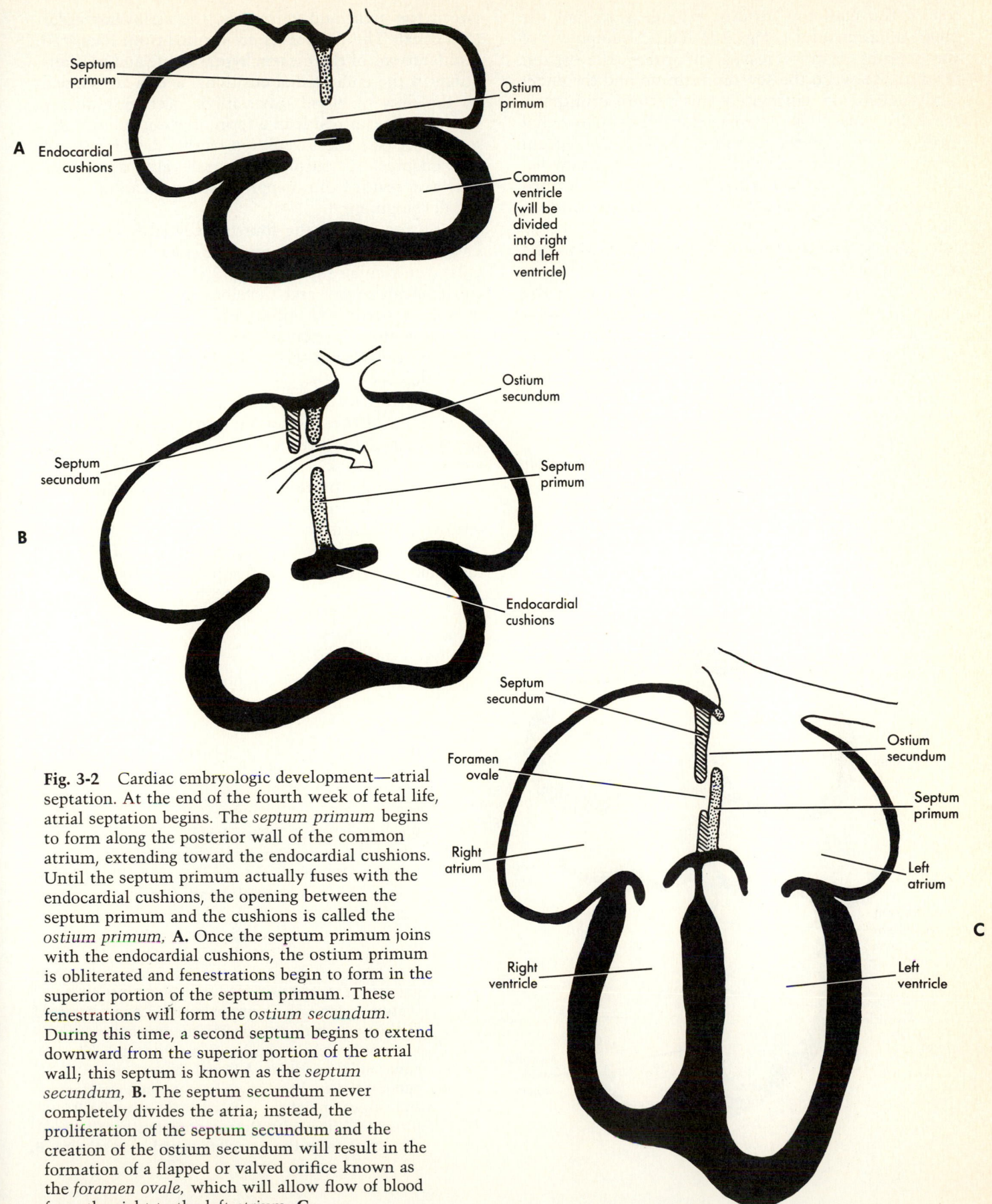

Fig. 3-2 Cardiac embryologic development—atrial septation. At the end of the fourth week of fetal life, atrial septation begins. The *septum primum* begins to form along the posterior wall of the common atrium, extending toward the endocardial cushions. Until the septum primum actually fuses with the endocardial cushions, the opening between the septum primum and the cushions is called the *ostium primum,* **A.** Once the septum primum joins with the endocardial cushions, the ostium primum is obliterated and fenestrations begin to form in the superior portion of the septum primum. These fenestrations will form the *ostium secundum.* During this time, a second septum begins to extend downward from the superior portion of the atrial wall; this septum is known as the *septum secundum,* **B.** The septum secundum never completely divides the atria; instead, the proliferation of the septum secundum and the creation of the ostium secundum will result in the formation of a flapped or valved orifice known as the *foramen ovale,* which will allow flow of blood from the right to the left atrium, **C.**

top of the common atrium, extending toward the endocardial cushions (Fig. 3-2). The development of the septum primum leaves an orifice, the *ostium primum*, between the septum primum and the endocardial cushions. Ultimately this ostium primum is normally closed by extensions of the endocardial cushions, and a perforation forms high in the septum primum so there will still be communication between the right and left atria. The perforation formed in the septum primum is called the *ostium secundum* (see Fig. 3-2).

The second septum that develops within the atria is called the *septum secundum*. This septum also forms with a perforation[242]; the positions of the foramen ovale and the ostium secundum form a valved orifice between the atria. When pressure is higher in the right atrium, this valved orifice allows flow of blood from the right to the left atrium (see Fig. 3-2, *C*). Under normal circumstances, the foramen ovale does not allow flow of blood from the left to the right atrium.[242] Defects in this process of atrial septation may result in an ostium secundum atrial septal defect (high in the atrial septum) or in an ostium primum atrial septal defect (low in the atrial septum).

The two endocardial cushions (one each on the anterior and posterior surface of the heart) fuse together. This fusion helps close the central orifice between the atria and ventricles, the atrioventricular (AV) canal. The AV valves are formed from localized proliferations of the mesenchymal tissue and proliferations of the endocardial cushions, which are shaped by the flow of blood. Aberrations occurring during this process can result in a form of endocardial cushion defect (see the discussion of this defect later in this chapter). Tricuspid or mitral valve anomalies may also result from inappropriate endocardial cushion development.

By the end of the fourth week, the ventricles have enlarged and fused together, forming the muscular ventricular septum (Fig. 3-3, *A*). Extension of the truncal conus and development of the membranous ventricular septum will later complete the closure of the ventricular septum (Fig. 3-3, *B*). Inappropriate ventricular septation may cause ventricular septal defects.

The *truncus arteriosus* is a large vessel located in the front of the developing heart (see Fig. 3-1). At approximately the fifth week of development, ridges appear in the trunk; as these ridges grow, they twist, causing a spiral septation of the truncus into the aorta and pulmonary artery (Fig. 3-4, *A*). The truncus arteriosus also shifts to the left so that it is centered over the ventricular septum. During the septation of the truncus arteriosus, additional swellings, conus

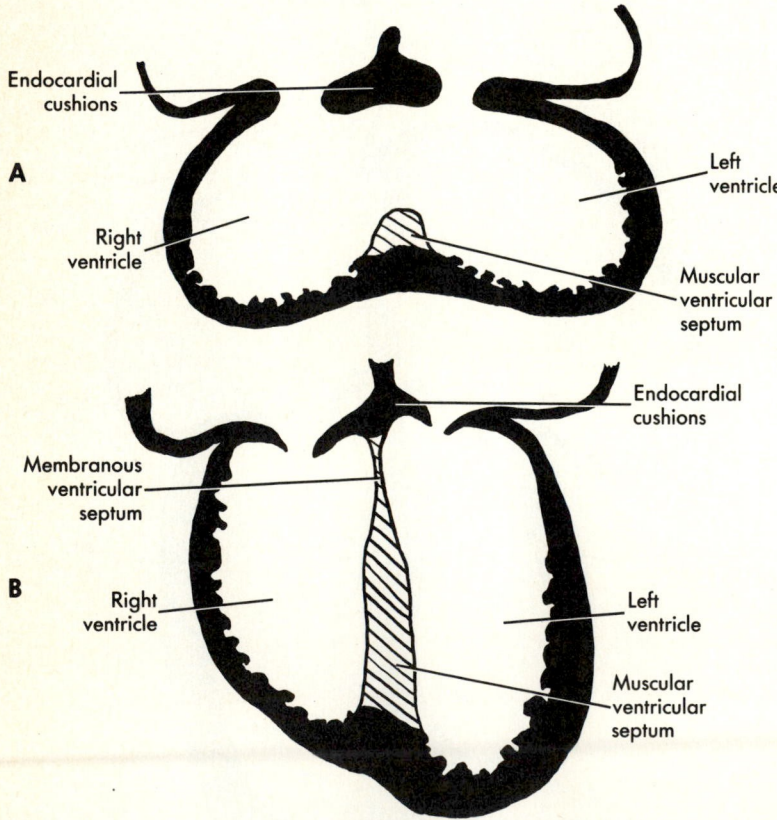

Fig. 3-3　Cardiac embryologic development—ventricular septation. Ventricular septation occurs between the fourth and eighth weeks of fetal life. It is accomplished by the formation of the muscular ventricular septum, growth of the endocardial cushions, extension of the conal septum (from the truncus arteriosus), and formation of the membranous ventricular septum. When the right and left ventricle fuse, the muscular ventricular septum is formed; at approximately the thirty-third to thirty-seventh days of life, the muscular ventricular septum begins to grow toward the endocardial cushions, **A.** Extensions of the endocardial cushions, swelling of conal cushions, and extensions of the conotruncal septum will ultimately fuse with the membranous ventricular septum to form the complete ventricular septum, **B.**

swellings, appear at the base of the truncus. The two conus swellings also fuse, creating the outflow tracts of the right and left ventricles and completing the formation of the ventricular septum[242] (Fig. 3-4, *B*). The semilunar valves form when truncal septation is nearly complete. Tubercles are formed, reabsorbed, and shaped to create the semilunar valve leaflets. Errors that occur during truncal septation, conal formation, or semilunar valve development can cause congenital heart defects, such as persistent truncus arteriosus, tetralogy of Fallot, double outlet right ventricle, pulmonary valve stenosis or atresia, pulmonary infundibular stenosis, or subvalvular, valvular, or supravalvular aortic stenosis. Transposition of the great vessels (known as D-transposition since the heart tube originally still coils to the right during early development) is also thought to result from improper truncal division.

Development of the aortic arch. Two large arteries form at the distal end of the truncus arteriosus during the fourth and fifth week of fetal development. Although these original arteries ultimately disappear, they give rise to six pairs of arteries, the six aortic arches. By the end of the fourth week the first two pairs and the fifth pair of aortic arches have disappeared, and the third, fourth, and sixth pairs of arches are now joined to the pulmonary trunk. Ultimately the third aortic arch will form the common carotid artery, the external carotid artery, and part of the internal carotid artery. The fourth aortic arch forms part of the final aortic arch and the proximal portion of the right subclavian artery. The sixth aortic arch provides the proximal segment of the right pulmonary artery and the ductus arteriosus, and a branch develops with the lung buds to provide pulmonary blood flow. Abnormalities in formation of the aortic arches can result in coarctation of the aorta, inter-

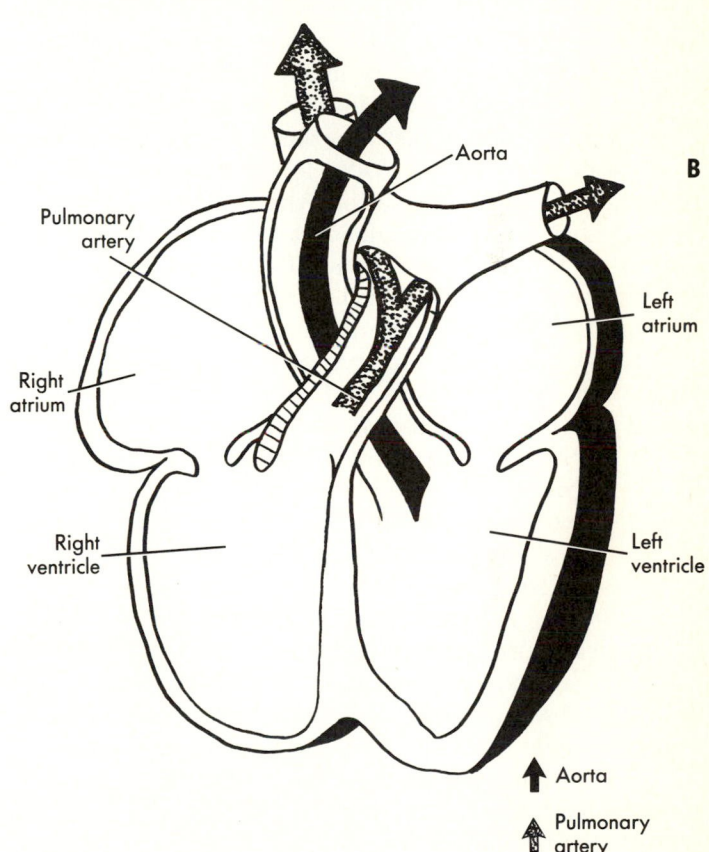

Fig. 3-4 Cardiac embryologic development—division of the truncus arteriosus. The truncus arteriosus begins as a large vessel located at the anterior and superior portion of the coiled cardiac tube by approximately the twenty-eighth day of life. During the next week, this common vessel will be divided into the pulmonary artery and the aorta. Two truncal swellings will begin to form in a spiral fashion, ultimately twisting around one another and fusing together, **A.** Once these swellings have fused, the aorticopulmonary septum (also known as the truncal septum) will form to complete the division of the truncus arteriosus into the pulmonary artery and the aorta. During the development of the truncal swellings, conus swellings develop along the lower anterior and posterior portion of the truncus. These conus swellings ultimately fuse along the plane of the ventricular septum to help close the ventricular septum and to delineate the outflow tracts of the right and the left ventricles, **B.**

rupted aortic arch, aortic atresia, patent ductus arteriosus, vascular rings (including double aortic arches), and aberrant origin of the right subclavian artery.

■ Fetal circulation

Fetal circulation is anatomically and physiologically different than postnatal circulation in several ways. In the fetus, oxygenation of the blood occurs in the placenta not in the lungs. The fetus is not hypoxic, but fetal arterial oxygen tension is much lower than in the infant; the hemoglobin is approximately 60% to 70% saturated, and the fetal arterial oxygen tension is approximately 20 to 30 torr.[189]

The fetal lungs are filled with fluid, and the low arterial oxygen tension produces pulmonary vasoconstriction. As a result pulmonary vascular resistance is high, and the pulmonary circulation receives approximately only 8% of fetal cardiac output.

Fetal systemic vascular resistance is low, and nearly half of the descending aortic blood flow enters the placenta, which provides low resistance to flow.

In the fetal circulation, the highly oxygenated blood comes from the placenta and enters the fetus through the umbilical vein. Fetal blood that has passed through the body is less oxygenated and leaves the fetus through the umbilical artery. Thus the blood with the higher oxygen content is in the umbilical *vein*, and the blood with the lower oxygen content is in the umbilical *artery*.

Three structures provide anatomic shunts in the fetal circulation. These shunts ultimately allow the highly oxygenated blood to be delivered to the fetal brain; they also allow most of fetal cardiac output to bypass the lungs, which are filled with fluid. The *ductus venosus* carries the oxygenated blood from the umbilical vein through the fetal liver to the inferior vena cava. The *foramen ovale* is a flapped opening in the atrial septum that allows this same oxygenated blood to flow from the right atrium to the left atrium. The *ductus arteriosus* provides a route for blood to flow from the main pulmonary artery into the aorta, bypassing the lungs (Fig. 3-5).

Oxygenated blood from the placenta enters the fetus through the umbilical vein and is diverted through the liver to the inferior vena cava by the ductus venosus. When this highly oxygenated blood reaches the right atrium, it streams preferentially toward the atrial septum, through the foramen ovale, and into the left atrium. This oxygenated blood then flows into the left ventricle and into the aorta. Approximately two thirds of the blood from the ascending aorta flows into the fetal brain or the upper extremities (see Fig. 3-5). The remaining third flows into the descending aorta from the ascending aorta.

Venous blood from the head and upper extremities is less oxygenated and has an oxygen tension of 15 to 19 torr and a saturation of approximately 40%. This blood returns to the heart via the superior vena cava, flows through the right atrium into the right ventricle, and enters the pulmonary artery. Since pulmonary vascular resistance is very high and systemic vascular resistance is low, most blood in the main pulmonary artery flows through the ductus arteriosus and into the descending aorta, bypassing the lungs. Thus the lower part of the fetus' body is perfused with a mixture of the well-oxygenated blood from the ascending aorta and poorly oxygenated blood from the ductus arteriosus; as a result the oxygen tension in the descending aorta is approximately 19 to 23 torr with a saturation of 55% to 60%.[190]

■ Normal perinatal circulatory changes

At birth the neonate begins to breathe, and the lungs become filled with air. The umbilical cord is tied, separating the placenta from the circulation. With these events the neonate switches from placental to pulmonary oxygenation of the blood and secondary hemodynamic adaptations are required.

When the umbilical cord is tied and cut, the umbilical arteries and vein constrict. They will eventually undergo fibrous infiltration, becoming the medial umbilical ligament and the ligamentum teres respectively. The ductus venosus constricts within 3 to 7 days of birth; it ultimately undergoes fibrous infiltration and becomes the ligamentum venosum.

When the lungs expand and become filled with air, the fluid from the lung is primarily absorbed into the pulmonary capillaries.[297] Since the lungs provide more efficient oxygenation of the blood than the placenta, the neonate's arterial oxygen tension rises. This is thought to be the most potent stimulus causing constriction of the ductus arteriosus. The rise in the oxygen tension of the blood bathing the ductus (the perivascular oxygen tension) may also contribute to ductal constriction. A fall in endogenous prostaglandin levels and acidosis also promote ductal closure.[190]

Because the foramen ovale is a flapped opening, it opens primarily when right atrial pressure is higher than left atrial pressure, and it allows blood to shunt from the right atrium to the left atrium. After birth, the fall in pulmonary vascular resistance produces a drop in right ventricular and right atrial pressures. At

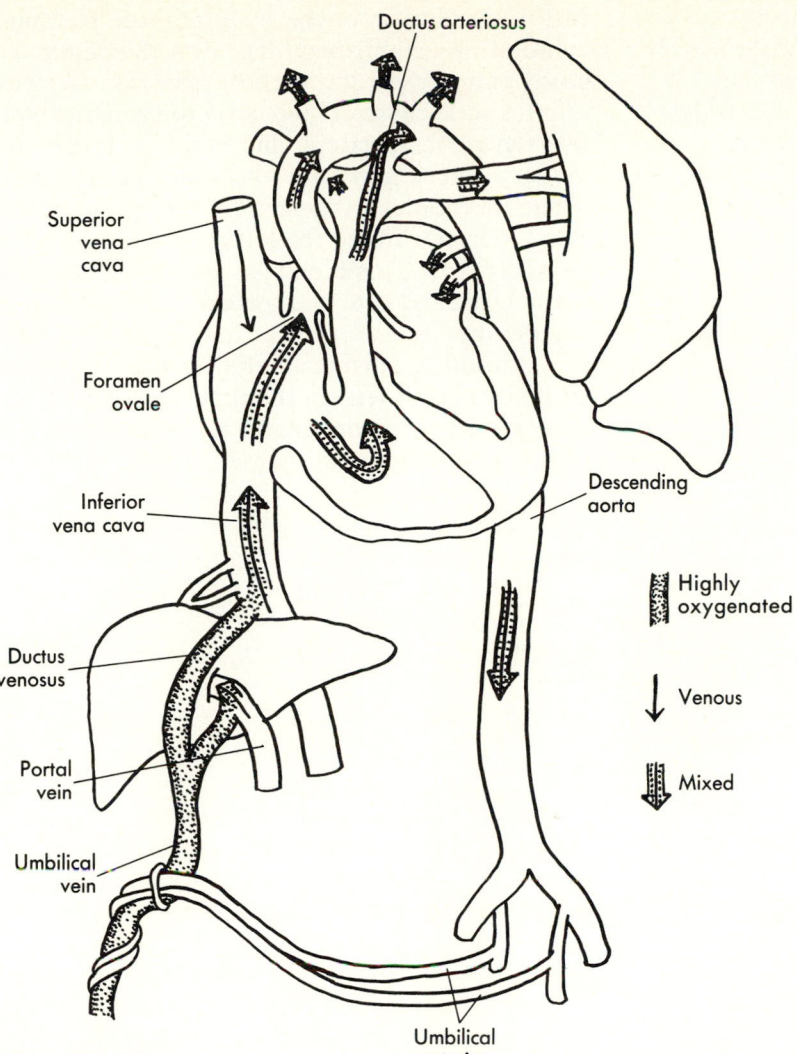

Fig. 3-5 Fetal circulation. In the fetus, the blood is oxygenated in the placenta not in the lungs. The oxygenated blood enters the fetus through the *umbilical vein* and enters the ductus venosus; this allows the blood from the placenta to bypass the hepatic circulation and enter the inferior vena cava. When this blood reaches the right atrium, it is diverted by the *crista dividens,* so that it flows directly toward the atrial septum, through the *foramen ovale,* and into the left atrium. Thus the highly oxygenated blood enters the left atrium and flows through the left ventricle and into the aorta; two thirds of this blood perfuses the brain and the upper extremities. Venous blood from the brain and upper extremities returns to the heart through the superior vena cava. This blood then enters the right ventricle and flows into the pulmonary artery. Since pulmonary vascular resistance is high and systemic vascular resistance is low, most blood from the pulmonary artery flows through the *ductus arteriosus* into the descending aorta. Ultimately, nearly half of the blood from the descending aorta will return to the placenta through the *umbilical arteries.*

the same time, elimination of the placenta causes systemic vascular resistance to rise, causing left ventricular and left atrial pressures to begin to increase. As a result, the foramen ovale usually closes by compression of the two portions of the atrial septum; this form of closure is called *functional* closure of the foramen ovale.[341]

In most individuals the foramen ovale becomes sealed by deposition of fibrin and cell products during the first months of life; this is referred to as *anatomic* closure of the foramen ovale. In approximately 25% of the population, however, the foramen ovale is not anatomically sealed and remains probe-patent beyond adolescence,[322] meaning that a catheter can be passed from the right atrium to the left atrium during cardiac catheterization or that a probe can be passed through the foramen ovale during cardiovascular surgery.

Unless or until the foramen ovale is anatomically sealed, anything that produces a significant increase in right atrial pressure can reopen the foramen ovale so that it becomes patent. Because of the structure of the opening, the shunt through the patent foramen ovale is primarily from the right to the left atrium. However, if both atria become very enlarged, the foramen ovale can be stretched open to allow bidirectional shunting of blood at the atrial level.

The three major fetal shunts, the ductus venosus, foramen ovale, and ductus arteriosus, are normally eliminated within the first days after birth.

Following closure of these shunts, the postnatal circulation is established (Fig. 3-6). Systemic venous blood enters the right atrium from the superior and inferior vena cavae. This poorly oxygenated blood enters the right ventricle, and passes through the pulmonary artery and into the pulmonary circulation where it becomes oxygenated. The pulmonary venous blood then returns to the left atrium through the pulmonary veins. This blood passes through the left side of the heart and into the aorta to supply the systemic circulation.

Although closure of the fetal anatomic shunts normally occurs within the first days of life, there are other qualitative changes in the circulation that occur more slowly.

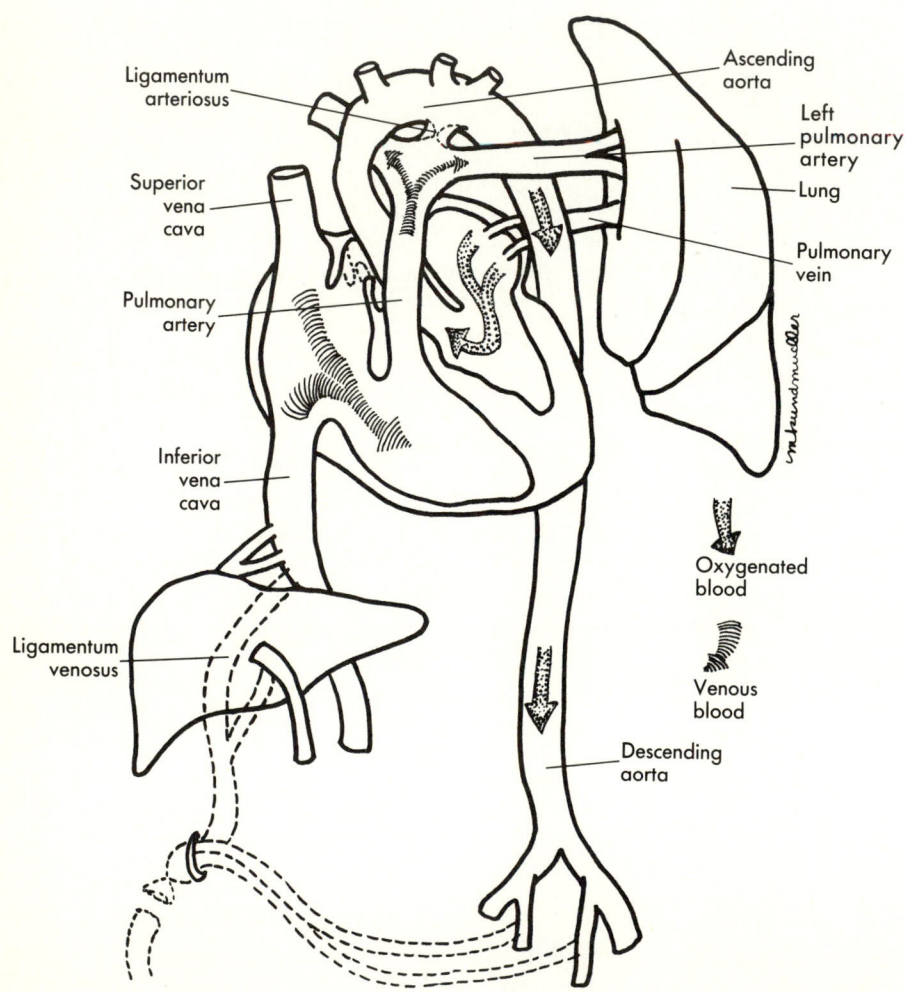

Fig. 3-6 Postnatal circulation. Systemic venous blood returns to the heart through the superior and inferior vena cavae. This blood then flows through the right atrium and right ventricle, into the pulmonary artery, and into the pulmonary circulation. The blood is oxygenated in the lung, and returns to the left atrium through the pulmonary veins. The oxygenated blood then flows through the left atrium and left ventricle, into the aorta, and through the systemic arterial circulation.

■ Perinatal changes in pulmonary vascular anatomy

During the final weeks of gestation there is an increase in the smooth muscle layer of the pulmonary arterioles. After birth the rise in the neonate's arterial oxygen tension and the increase in alveolar oxygenation releases the pulmonary vasoconstriction and may produce pulmonary vasodilation. In addition there is rapid thinning of the medial muscle layer of the pulmonary arterioles. These changes produce a rapid fall in pulmonary vascular resistance and consequently, a fall in pulmonary pressure. Calculated pulmonary vascular resistance falls immediately after birth by approximately 80% and reaches near adult levels by the first weeks after birth. Normal pulmonary vascular resistance is 8-10 U/m² body surface area during the first week of life. By approximately 24 hours after birth, mean pulmonary artery pressure has fallen to approximately one half of mean systemic pressure, if the ductus arteriosus has constricted.[112]

During the first 2 to 9 weeks of life, the medial muscle layer of the pulmonary arterioles continues to thin, and pulmonary vascular resistance decreases further.[189] During this time, the pulmonary arterioles remain very reactive and can constrict if hypoxia, acidosis, or hypothermia develop. By the time the infant is approximately 2 months of age, pulmonary vascular resistance has fallen to approximately normal adult values (1 to 3 U/m² body surface area), and the anatomy of the pulmonary arterioles is the same as in the adult.

If the infant is born prematurely, the medial muscle layer of the pulmonary arterioles may not have thickened completely, so the medial layer may regress in a shorter period of time. This could cause pulmonary vascular resistance to fall within a few days of birth in the premature infant. However, if the premature neonate is hypoxic (as a result of cyanotic heart disease or respiratory distress syndrome, for example), pulmonary vascular resistance may remain high until the hypoxia is corrected. If the hypoxic stimulus remains, the pulmonary arterioles will retain more smooth muscle and a higher pulmonary vascular resistance will be present.

If the infant has a congenital heart defect that is producing increased pulmonary blood flow (such as a patent ductus arteriosus or a ventricular septal defect), pulmonary vascular resistance does not fall normally after birth. These neonates demonstrate a delayed and less marked drop in pulmonary vascular resistance during the first 4 to 12 weeks of life (this drop may occur over a shorter period of time in the premature neonate). Because of this delayed fall in pulmonary vascular resistance, symptoms attributable to increased pulmonary blood flow often do not become apparent until the child is 4 to 12 weeks of age. These symptoms may develop earlier if the neonate was premature.

■ Perinatal changes in systemic vascular pressure

The neonate's systemic vascular resistance gradually rises after birth. Normal systemic vascular resistance is 10 to 15 U/m² body surface area in an infant and 20 to 30 U/m² body surface area in a child. Mean arterial blood pressure also rises from 43 mm Hg in the full-term (3 kg) newborn at 12 hours of life,[430] to 64 mm Hg at 1 year of age.[86]

Low-birthweight neonates tend to have lower mean arterial blood pressure than larger infants, whether or not these neonates are small for gestational age or appropriate for gestational age. Mean arterial blood pressure during the first 12 hours of life is 33 mm Hg (range 24 to 42) in a 750 gm infant and 34.5 mm Hg (range 25 to 44) for a 1000 gm infant.[43]

After birth the neonate's right and left ventricular muscle volumes and ventricular pressures change. These changes will be considered within the brief review of cardiovascular physiology that follows.

■ GROSS ANATOMY
■ The right side of the heart

The systemic venous blood returns to the right atrium via the superior and inferior vena cavae. The *sinoatrial (SA) node* is located near the junction of the superior vena cava and the right atrium, just under the surface of the epicardium. The right atrium lies just under the sternum and forms the right lateral border of the cardiac silhouette on the anteroposterior chest radiograph. Much of the inside of the right atrium has a trabeculated appearance, resulting from the presence of pectinate muscles that compose the anterior and lateral walls.

The atrial septum forms the posterior border of the right atrium, extending from right to left. The fossa ovalis (remnant of the foramen ovale) can usually be visualized high in the septum. The *coronary sinus*, which returns coronary venous blood to the heart, normally lies between the inferior vena cava and the tricuspid valve. The *atrioventricular (AV) node* is located anterior and medial to the coronary sinus and above the tricuspid valve.[209]

Three internodal conduction pathways are thought to provide more rapid conduction between the SA and AV nodes than normal myocardium. Although conduction can occur along any of these three pathways, preferential internodal conduction probably occurs along the anterior internodal pathway, which courses from the sinus node, around the superior vena cava, and along the anterior portion of the atrial septum to the AV node. If these pathways are injured during cardiovascular surgery, AV conduction block can result.

The tricuspid valve is the anterior AV valve. It is positioned so that blood passing through the valve must flow in an anterior, inferior, and leftward direction into the right ventricle. The leaflets of the tricuspid valve are not equal in size, and they are not immediately identifiable as three distinct leaflets. The anterior leaflet extends from the pulmonary infundibulum to the lower anterior portion of the ventricle. The septal (or medial) leaflet attaches to the membranous and muscular portions of the ventricular septum. The posterior leaflet lies along the posterior aspect of the tricuspid ring. Each leaflet is attached to several chordae tendineae, which are, in turn, attached to one of three papillary muscles in the right ventricle.

The right ventricle is normally the most anterior of the four cardiac chambers, and its inferior border forms much of the left inferior cardiac border on an anteroposterior chest radiograph. The right ventricle receives blood from the right atrium and pumps blood into the low-resistance pulmonary circulation. Because the right ventricle normally generates low pressure, it has a thinner wall and a smaller lumen than the left ventricle. The right ventricle contains muscle bundles, called trabeculations, which give the ventricle a flocculated appearance on angiocardiograms. The *moderator band* is a larger muscle bundle that traverses the right ventricle from the posterior portion of the ventricular septum to the anterior right ventricular wall.[209]

The right ventricle is functionally divided into an inflow and an outflow portion by the *crista supraventricularis*, a thick muscle that extends from the lateral wall of the right ventricle to the anterior leaflet of the tricuspid valve and that encircles the pulmonary outflow tract. The pulmonary outflow tract is also called the pulmonary *infundibulum*; blood flows from the right ventricle and is directed posteriorly and superiorly into the pulmonary artery.[209]

The pulmonary valve is a *semilunar valve* that is normally located above, in front of, and to the right of the aortic valve. Its three cusps are labeled the anterior, right, and left cusps.

Beyond the neonatal period, the pulmonary circulation is normally a low-resistance circulatory pathway that carries systemic venous blood to the lungs and then returns pulmonary venous (oxygenated) blood to the heart. The typical pulmonary branch artery has a thinner wall (with thinner medial muscle layer) and larger lumen than a comparable systemic artery.

■ The left side of the heart

Oxygenated blood returns from the lungs via the four pulmonary veins to the left atrium. The left atrium is the most posterior of the four cardiac chambers and normally does not contribute to the definition of the cardiac border on the anteroposterior chest radiograph. The left atrium has a slightly thicker and smoother wall than the right atrium. The left atrial appendage, a trabeculated extension of the left atrium, abuts the pulmonary artery.

Pulmonary venous blood flows from the left atrium through the mitral valve and into the left ventricle. The mitral valve consists of two leaflets: the septal leaflet extends from the muscular ventricular septum to the anterior wall of the left ventricle and the posterior leaflet, the larger of the two leaflets, extends across the remaining portion of the valve annulus. The mitral leaflets attach to several chordae tendineae, which in turn attach to two groups of papillary muscles.

The left ventricle is located behind the right ventricle so that pulmonary venous blood passing through the mitral valve must flow inferiorly and laterally. The left ventricle may not form a distinct part of the cardiac border on the anteroposterior chest radiograph. This ventricle is characterized by a thick wall and a large lumen; it will appear to have smooth walls when seen on angiocardiograms. The septal leaflet of the mitral valve divides the left ventricle into an inflow and an outflow chamber. This division is only present when the mitral valve is open; the ventricle functions as a single chamber during systole.

The aorta has a thicker wall and a smaller lumen than the pulmonary artery. The aortic valve is a semilunar valve. Since the coronary arteries arise immediately above the aortic valve, the valve cusps are labeled in reference to the coronary arteries. The cusp immediately below the left coronary artery is called the left coronary cusp; the cusp immediately below the right coronary artery is called the right coronary cusp; and the cusp that is not related to any coronary artery is called the noncoronary cusp.

There are normally two coronary arteries: the left coronary artery, which branches into the left anterior descending and the left circumflex arteries, and the right coronary artery. After the cardiac tissue is perfused, the coronary venous blood drains into the anterior cardiac veins or the coronary sinus and then into the right atrium.

A systemic artery has a thicker medial muscle layer, a relatively smaller lumen, and more elastic tissue than a pulmonary artery. Systemic arteries normally carry oxygenated blood under relatively high pressure to the tissues.

■ NORMAL CARDIAC FUNCTION
■ The cardiac cycle

The heart receives systemic venous blood, which it pumps to the lungs and blood from the lungs, which it pumps to the body. This serial circulation allows the atria to relax and contract together, and it allows the ventricles to relax and contract together; however, the circulation in the right side of the heart and in the left side of the heart is separated.

Systemic venous return enters the right atrium. During atrial and ventricular diastole, the tricuspid valve is open and systemic venous blood flows passively into the right ventricle. Approximately 70% of ventricular filling occurs during this period. Mean right atrial pressure is equal to right ventricular end-diastolic pressure in the absence of tricuspid valve disease.[171] Mean right atrial pressure in infants (beyond the neonatal period) is approximately 0 to 4 mm Hg; mean right atrial pressure in older children is 2 to 6 mm Hg.[360]

Atrial contraction provides the final 30% of ventricular filling, which is not essential for normal cardiac function. However, this final portion does improve ventricular stroke volume, and loss of atrial systole may further compromise the ventricular performance of a patient with myocardial dysfunction.

The right ventricle fills rapidly at the beginning of ventricular diastole, then ventricular filling is slower until atrial systole. Immediately after atrial contraction, ventricular contraction begins. Initially, ventricular contraction produces only a rise in ventricular pressure (with no movement of blood); this is called the isovolumetric phase of ventricular systole. When right ventricular pressure exceeds right atrial pressure, the tricuspid valve closes and ventricular pressure rises rapidly. Once right ventricular pressure exceeds pulmonary artery pressure, the pulmonary valve opens and blood flows into the pulmonary artery. Right ventricular systolic pressure is normally 15 to 25 mm Hg in older children and adults (it is higher in neonates). Pulmonary artery systolic pressure at birth is approximately 65 to 80 mm Hg (mean 40 to 70 mm Hg); once pulmonary vascular resistance falls, pulmonary artery systolic pressure is approxi-

mately 15 to 25 mm Hg, and diastolic pressure is approximately 8 to 12 mm Hg (mean of 10 to 16 mm Hg).[360]

The blood that enters the pulmonary circulation passes through the alveolar capillary bed, enters the pulmonary veins, and flows into the left atrium. Since there are no valves between the precapillary pulmonary arteriole and the left atrium, pulmonary capillary wedge pressures are assumed to be roughly equivalent to left atrial pressure. During ventricular diastole, left atrial pressure should equal left ventricular end-diastolic pressure, in the absence of mitral valve disease. As a result pulmonary capillary wedge pressure is approximately equal to left ventricular end-diastolic pressure. Left atrial pressure is normally 3 to 6 mm Hg in infants and 5 to 10 mm Hg in older children. The hemoglobin in the left atrium is normally 97% saturated with oxygen.

Left ventricular filling also occurs largely during atrial and ventricular diastole. Left atrial contraction contributes the final 30% of ventricular filling. Immediately after left atrial contraction, the left ventricle begins to contract. When left ventricular pressure exceeds left atrial pressure, the mitral valve closes. When left ventricular pressure exceeds aortic pressure, the aortic valve opens and blood flows into the aorta and systemic circulation. Left ventricular systolic pressure is approximately equal to the child's systemic arterial pressure (Table 3-2) in the absence of aortic valve disease.

Coronary artery perfusion occurs only during diastole. Coronary blood flow uses a very small portion of total cardiac output at rest. With an increased heart rate, diastolic filling time may decrease; if cardiac contractility is improved at the same time (as a result of sympathetic nervous system stimulation), systolic time becomes shorter, so coronary perfusion time is not compromised.

■ Cellular pathology

Membrane and action potentials. The heart contains muscle, connective tissue, and conductive tissue. Both the myocardium and the conductive tissue transmit electrochemical impulses, or *current* (although conduction tissue does so more rapidly). In all tissues of the body, there is a difference between intracellular and extracellular concentrations of each electrolyte. In any excitable tissue, there is also a difference in charge between the inside and the outside of the cell; the inside of the cell is negatively charged, and the outside of the cell is positively charged. This difference in electrical charge across the cell membrane is called a *membrane potential*. The membrane

Table 3-2 Normal pediatric blood pressure ranges*

Age	Systolic (mm Hg)	Diastolic (mm Hg)
Newborns-12 hr (less than 1000 gm)	39-59	16-36
Newborns-12 hr (3 kg)	50-70	25-45
Newborns-96 hr	60-90	20-60
Infants	74-100	50-70
Toddlers	80-112	50-80
Preschoolers	82-110	50-78
School age children	84-120	54-80
Adolescents	94-140	62-88

*The above ranges are taken from the tenth to ninetieth percentile ranges determined by the following studies: de Swiet, M., Fayers, P., and Shinebourne, E.A.: Systolic blood pressure in a population of infants in the first year of life: the Brompton study, Pediatrics 65:1028, May 1980; National Heart, Lung, and Blood Institute's Task Force on Blood Pressure Control in Children, Pediatrics 59(sup. 5):797, 1977; Versmold, H., and others: Aortic blood pressure during the first 12 hours of life in infants with birth weight 610-4220 gms, Pediatrics 67:107, May 1981.

potential of a myocardial cell is approximately −75 to −85 mV. This potential is created by several related factors: (a) the difference in potassium concentration between the inside and the outside of the cell—this is called the potassium concentration gradient; (b) the action of the sodium/potassium pump, which pumps sodium ions out of the cell while allowing potassium ions to enter the cell; (c) the low permeability of the resting membrane to sodium, and (d) the presence of nondiffusable anions—negatively charged proteins—inside the cell (Fig. 3-7). The magnitude of the membrane potential is most closely linked to the potassium gradient.[171]

Potassium concentration is relatively high inside the cell and relatively low outside the cell. These differences result in the development of a *concentration gradient* and an *electrical gradient* across the cell membrane. Since there is a lower potassium concentration outside the cell, there is a tendency for potassium to diffuse out of the cell. However, since the inside of the cell is negatively charged and the outside of the cell is positively charged, potassium is held inside the cell and can only diffuse out if enough other positively charged ions replace it.

There is also a concentration and electrical gradient for sodium across the cell membrane. Since sodium concentration is lower inside the cell, there is a tendency for sodium to diffuse to the inside of the cell. Since the inside of the cell is negatively charged, this also draws the sodium ions into the cell. These tendencies are repelled, however, by the low cell membrane permeability to sodium and by the action of the sodium-potassium pump.

Stimulation of an excitable cell produces a change in the intracellular electrical charge; this charge is called an *action potential*. To create an action potential the cell must have been stimulated sufficiently so that the cell membrane permeability to sodium increases. Once membrane permeability increases, sodium ions rapidly enter the cell. With this influx of sodium ions the inside of the cell transiently becomes *positively* charged; this means the cell has been *depolarized* (Fig. 3-8, *A*). Depolarization takes only a fraction of a second. The cell membrane then becomes impermeable to sodium again so that the sodium influx stops. At the same time potassium

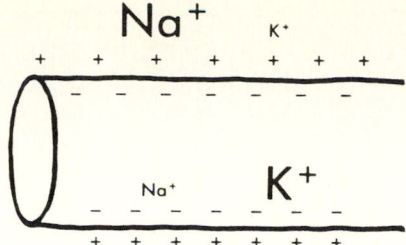

Fig. 3-7 The excitable cell—the membrane potential. The difference in electrical charge across the membrane of an excitable cell is called the membrane potential. This membrane potential exists because there is a difference in the electrical charge between the inside and the outside of the cell; the inside of the cell is negatively charged, and the outside of the cell is positively charged. Potassium ion concentration is higher intracellularly and lower extracellularly; conversely, sodium ion concentration is lower intracellularly, and higher extracellularly. Although the cell membrane is permeable to potassium, the potassium is held inside the cell by the negative intracellular charge. The membrane is normally relatively impermeable to sodium, and a sodium-potassium pump also keeps sodium on the outside of the cell and allows potassium to diffuse inside the cell. The normal membrane potential of myocardial cells is approximately -75 to -85 mV.

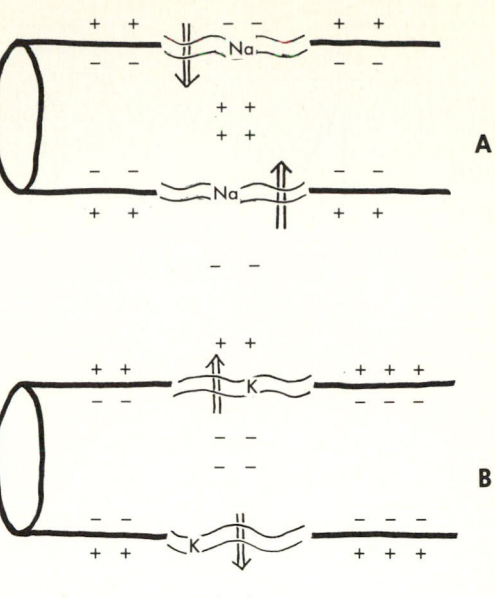

Fig. 3-8 Depolarization and repolarization of an excitable cell. When the excitable cell is stimulated, the membrane permeability to sodium increases, causing sodium ions to rapidly enter the cell (they are drawn by both a concentration gradient and an electrical gradient). This rapid influx of the positively-charged sodium ions temporarily makes the inside of the cell positively charged—it is *depolarized,* **A.** Immediately after depolarization, the cell membrane again becomes impermeable to sodium ion diffusion, so the sodium influx is abruptly terminated. Potassium ions move out of the cell to maintain electrical neutrality (and because the concentration of potassium ion is lower on the outside of the cell). As a result of this rapid potassium ion efflux from the cell, the inside of the cell again becomes negatively-charged—it is *repolarized,* **B.** Ultimately, the action of the sodium-potassium pump will return the ions to their normal positions.

ions move out of the cell. As a result within a fraction of a second the inside of the cell again becomes more negatively charged than the outside of the cell; this means the cell has become *repolarized* (Fig. 3-8, *B*). Ultimately, the sodium-potassium pump returns the ions to their normal positions; sodium is again pumped out of the cell and potassium is allowed to enter the cell.

To create the action potential, the cell must have been stimulated sufficiently so that the electrical changes caused by sodium movement reached a *threshold value*; once threshold is reached, the development of the action potential becomes inevitable (this is referred to as an "all-or-none" phenomenon).[171] Once membrane permeability to sodium increases at one point in the cell membrane and an action potential is generated, membrane permeability to sodium tends to increase along the length of the cell; this causes a propagation of the action potential. As the outside of the cell becomes negative (or depolarized), a *current* is generated. This current can be measured on the surface of a nerve or muscle in the laboratory; at the bedside, depolarization and repolarization of myocardial cells is summated and represented graphically by the electrocardiogram (ECG).

The *action potential* of any excitable cell can be illustrated by graphing the changes in intracellular electrical charge, with electrical charge on the vertical axis and time on the horizontal axis. The action potential of a myocardial cell is unique in several ways; it has a plateau and a prepotential (Fig. 3-9). This action potential typically is described in four phases, according to the appearance of the curve and corresponding electrolyte movement. During phase 0, there is a rapid sodium influx to the cell. This influx peaks and membrane permeability to sodium suddenly decreases, causing a short, sharp drop in intracellular charge, labeled phase 1. The plateau, phase 2 in the action potential, is unique to myocardial cells and is produced by a further reduced sodium ion influx, a slow influx of calcium ions, and only slow potassium efflux. Phase 3 begins with a more rapid

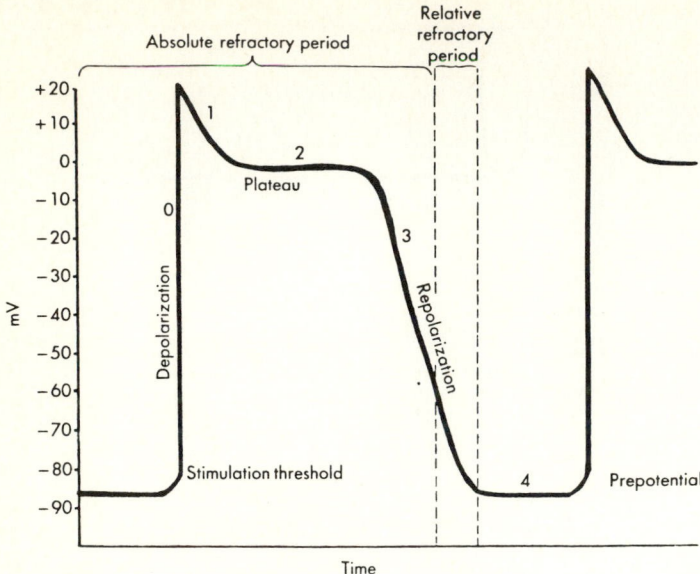

Fig. 3-9 The action potential of a myocardial cell. The action potential of the myocardial cell is described in four phases, according to the electrical charge of the inside of the cell. During *phase 0*, there is a rapid sodium ion influx, causing the inside of the cell quickly to become positively-charged. When the membrane permeability to sodium is abruptly halted, there is a short, sharp drop in the intracellular charge; this short drop is labeled *phase 1*. *Phase 2* is characterized by a plateau in the action potential that is unique to myocardial cells; this phase is caused by a further small influx of sodium ions, a significant influx of calcium ions, and a slow efflux of potassium ions. *Phase 3* is the repolarization phase of the action potential, and it is caused by the rapid efflux of potassium ions from the cell; this quickly returns the intracellular charge to approximately −75 to −85 mV. In *phase 4*, the cell is initially hyperpolarized (the inside is more negatively-charged than usual). Soon, however, a slow leak of sodium ions into the cell creates a gradual *prepotential*. This prepotential will allow the myocardial cell to spontaneously depolarize if it is not stimulated by another cell. Once the myocardial cell has depolarized, it can not be stimulated again until it has partially repolarized—the interval between the onset of depolarization and the time the myocardial cell is absolutely refractory to stimuli is called the *absolute refractory period*. Once the cell is depolarized to a charge of approximately −55 or −60 mV, the cell is still less excitable, so only a very strong stimulus would be capable of depolarizing the cell; during this time the cell is relatively refractory to stimuli, so the interval is known as the *relative refractory period*.

potassium efflux from the cell, which restores the negative intracellular charge and returns the membrane potential to its resting value. Phase 4 is characterized by an initial "hyperpolarization" (the cell initially has a more negative charge than normal). A slow leak of sodium ions into the cell creates a gradual *prepotential*. This prepotential is characteristic of and unique to all myocardial cells and causes the myocardium to be self-excitable. If the cell is not stimulated more rapidly by another cell or by mechanical stimulus, the cell will eventually depolarize because the slow leak of sodium ions will slowly bring the intracellular charge to a threshold value, and the action potential will be created.

Once an excitable cell reaches threshold it is refractory to other stimulation until the membrane potential again becomes negative. The myocardial cell is absolutely refractory until the cellular membrane potential returns nearly to the threshold value. This prevents the heart from responding to rapid stimulation; it cannot be tetanized because it cannot be depolarized in a rapid fashion (each action potential takes a significant amount of time). Once the intracellular charge has fallen to near the threshold value, cell response to further stimulation is reduced; during this period, the cell is relatively refractory to stimuli and would require a larger than normal stimulus to develop an action potential (see Fig. 3-9).

Although all myocardial cells are self-excitable, those with the most rapid rate of spontaneous depolarization are the *pacemaker cells*. These cells have an action potential with a slightly different appearance than the myocardial cell (Fig. 3-10). The resting membrane potential is less negative than the myocardial cell so the pacemaker cell reaches threshold with a smaller net change in intracellular charge. As with all myocardial cells, pacemaker cells have a prepotential, which is produced by a slow influx of so-

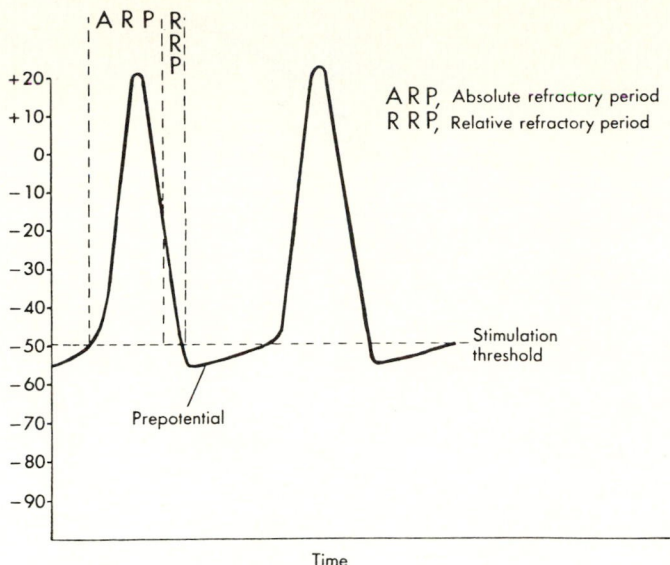

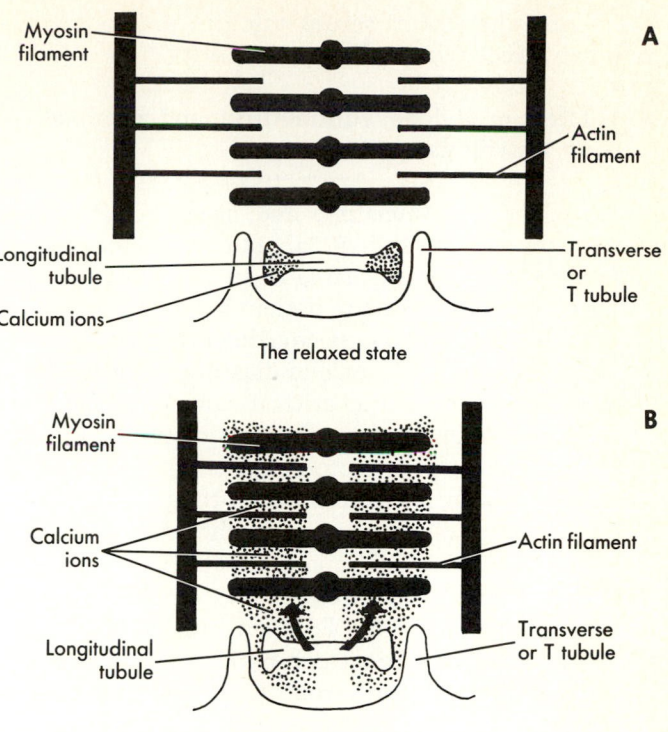

Fig. 3-10 The action potential of a pacemaker cell. The action potential of the pacemaker cell is different from that of other myocardial cells because it has a shorter, sharper prepotential and no plateau. All myocardial cells have the ability to spontaneously depolarize, but the pacemaker cell normally has the most rapid rate of spontaneous depolarization because it is less negatively charged and because its membrane is more permeable to sodium ions. As a result there is a greater influx of sodium ions during the prepotential of the pacemaker cell, and this influx of sodium will bring the pacemaker cell to threshold in a relatively short period of time. Since the pacemaker cell has no plateau, its absolute refractory period is shorter and it can be stimulated more frequently.

Fig. 3-11 The sarcomere. The contractile unit of the myocardial cell is the sarcomere, which consists of overlapping actin and myosin filaments, transverse or T tubules, and longitudinal tubules. In the relaxed state, the actin and myosin filaments overlap slightly, but are not bound to one another, **A.** When the myocardial cell is depolarized, the electrical current flows into the cell through the T tubules and passes through the walls of the longitudinal tubules. When the longitudinal tubules are stimulated, they release calcium ions; the calcium reacts with sites on both the actin and myosin filaments, and aids in the binding of cross-linkages between the actin and myosin filaments. As a result of these cross-linkages, the actin filaments are pulled together between the myosin filaments, and the myocardial fiber shortens, or contracts, **B.**

dium ions before depolarization. However, the prepotential of the pacemaker cell brings the cell to threshold more rapidly than other myocardial cells. Because the action potential of the pacemaker cell also has no plateau, it may be more rapidly stimulated (its absolute refractory period is shorter). Once the pacemaker cell depolarizes, it will in turn stimulate other myocardial cells so they will all depolarize in rapid succession.

Since the electrolyte concentration gradients across the cell membrane determine the magnitude of the membrane potential, alterations in intracellular and extracellular potassium and sodium concentrations can influence the excitability of myocardial cells. Vagal stimulation can alter myocardial membrane permeability and decrease the excitability of the cell. Sympathetic nervous system stimulation increases sodium ion movement so that myocardial cells depolarize more rapidly and the heart rate increases.

Myocardial contraction. The contractile element of a myocardial cell is a sarcomere. The sarcomere contains protein filaments of actin and myosin (Fig. 3-11, *A*). The flow of electrical current (myocardial depolarization) causes the release of calcium ions within the myofibrils. The calcium ions bind the actin and myosin filaments and cause them to slide together; this shortens the myocardial fiber, producing contraction (Fig. 3-11, *B*). It is important to note that myocardial contraction occurs *after* electrical depolarization and that adequate depolarization of the myocardium does not ensure effective contraction. Since calcium ions bind the actin and myosin filaments, changes in serum calcium ion concentration can affect myocardial contractility.

■ Effect of preload, contractility, and afterload on ventricular performance

Preload, contractility, and afterload are three terms from the physiology laboratory that have been applied to the clinical setting in an attempt to understand factors affecting the patient's cardiac output.

Preload and the Frank-Starling law. *Preload* refers to the presystolic or end-diastolic length of the myocardial fiber. In the critical-care unit, the ventricular presystolic volume cannot be measured; instead, the presystolic stretch of the ventricular fibers is estimated from measurement of the patient's right or left atrial pressures since, in the absence of AV valve disease, these are equal to the patient's ventricular end-diastolic pressures.

O. Frank (1895) and E.H. Starling (1914)[323] demonstrated that the strength of myocardial contraction (or ventricular work or stroke volume index) can be increased by increasing the stretch of the myocardial fibers before contraction (Fig. 3-12). The general principle of the Frank-Starling law of the heart is that increasing the left atrial pressure (preload) will increase left ventricular stroke work or stroke volume. In the critical-care unit, it is possible to graph the patient's ventricular function curve using the patient's measured left atrial pressure and cardiac output or stroke volume.

Initially, the Frank-Starling law only appeared to be applicable to normal patients. In 1954, Sarnoff and Berglund[375] demonstrated the presence of a family of ventricular function curves, which are created by varying degrees of myocardial contractility.

Contractility. *Contractility* is commonly used synonymously with strength of contraction. In fact the term refers to the speed of myocardial fiber shortening.[378] If cardiac contractility is increased, systole takes less time (because the fibers shorten rapidly and relax rapidly), so at the same heart rate, diastolic filling time and coronary artery perfusion time are increased; with increased ventricular contractility, stroke volume will increase.

There is no way to readily measure cardiac contractility in the clinical setting. Indirect evaluation of the child's myocardial contractility can be made by monitoring the child's ventricular performance curve. If the child's cardiac output is low, despite high left atrial pressure (or high filling pressure), the child's myocardial function curve is one of decreased contractility or *negative inotropy*. If the child demon-

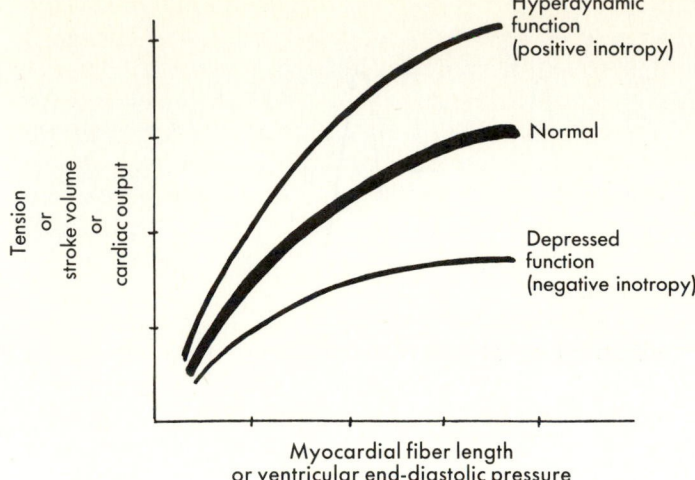

Fig. 3-12 The Frank-Starling curve. In their initial description of this law, Frank and Starling used *isolated normal* myocardial fibers and found that increasing the presystolic length of the fibers improved the tension that those fibers were able to generate when they contracted. In the clinical setting, it is impossible to measure presystolic myocardial fiber length or even presystolic volume; as a result, end-diastolic pressure is used as an indirect indicator of the presystolic length of the myocardial fibers. To a point, increasing the end-diastolic pressure will increase the ventricular stroke volume and, ultimately, the cardiac output (*normal* curve). It is now clear that a family of Frank-Starling curves exist. If myocardial function is depressed, higher end-diastolic pressure will be required to maximize the patient's cardiac output (*depressed* curve). In addition it will be necessary to attempt to improve the patient's myocardial function curve through correction of acid-base or electrolyte imbalance or with administration of inotropic medications. If the patient's myocardial function is hyperdynamic, cardiac output will be high even if end-diastolic pressure is low (*hyperdynamic* curve).

strates a high cardiac output with very low left atrial (or filling) pressure, the myocardial function curve is one of increased contractility or *positive inotropy*.

Contractility is largely independent of presystolic stretch. Decreased cardiac contractility (or negative inotropy) can be caused by acidosis, hypoxemia, hypoglycemia, hypocalcemia, hyperkalemia, hypokalemia, drug toxicity, or infection. Cardiac contractility can be enhanced by correction of these problems. In addition contractility can be further improved by administration of cardiac glycosides or sympathomimetic agents.

Ventricular function will also be influenced by

ventricular *compliance.* Compliance is defined as the ratio of change in ventricular volume to change in ventricular diastolic pressure. If the child's end-diastolic pressure increases sharply with administration of only small amounts of intravenous (IV) fluids, the ventricle has reduced *compliance;* in other words, the ventricle is stiff. If the child's ventricular end-diastolic pressure does not increase despite administration of large amounts of IV fluids, the ventricle is compliant.[378]

Afterload. *Afterload* is the resistance against which the ventricles must pump when ejecting blood. A primary component of right ventricular afterload is pulmonary vascular resistance; a major component of left ventricular afterload is systemic vascular resistance.

If systemic vascular resistance is high, systemic blood flow will decrease unless left ventricular pressure increases since pressure is the product of flow and resistance.

$$Pressure = Flow \times Resistance$$

Since increased systemic vascular resistance (such as that produced by systemic vasoconstriction) increases the afterload of the ventricle, left ventricular work is increased. This increase in work may not create a problem for a normal, healthy ventricle, but it may cause a marked decrease in cardiac output if ventricular function is already compromised.

These same concepts apply to the right ventricle; if the child has high pulmonary vascular resistance (as a result of pulmonary hypertension, hypoxia, acidosis, or hypothermia), the right ventricle must generate a higher pressure to maintain normal pulmonary blood flow. This results in increased right ventricular work and may result in decreased right ventricular stroke volume.[378]

Valvular stenosis or coarctation of the aorta would also increase ventricular work and the pressure the ventricle(s) must generate.

■ **Regulation of cardiac output**

The sympathetic nervous system. The sympathetic nervous system compensatory mechanisms are activated at times of stress. These mechanisms are regulated by the vasomotor center through peripheral sympathetic fibers (from the spinal cord through thoracic nerves to the sympathetic ganglion) and by the secretion of norepinephrine from the adrenal medulla. Sympathetic nervous system stimulation produces the "fight or flight" response; this includes tachycardia, increased cardiac contractility, periph-

eral vasoconstriction (including renal arterial and splanchnic constriction), diaphoresis, and pupil dilation.

Tissues and organs innervated by the sympathetic nervous system contain alpha- or beta-adrenergic receptors (Table 3-3). Sympathomimetic agents may be administered to selectively stimulate only some of the sympathetic receptors (e.g., beta-sympathomimetic agents).

The parasympathetic nervous system. The parasympathetic nervous system fibers are contained in the vagus nerve. Vagal fibers are almost exclusively present in the atria, and vagal stimulation produces a fall in heart rate. Some vagal fibers may be present in the ventricles, and vagal stimulation may produce a slight decrease in cardiac contractility.

The baroreceptor reflexes. The baroreceptors are located in the walls of the carotid sinuses and in the aortic arch. These pressure receptors are stimulated by signals in the patient's arterial blood pressure, and they transmit signals to the patient's vasomotor and vagal centers of the medulla. Stimulation of the baroreceptors by high arterial pressure causes inhibition of the sympathetic portion of the vasomotor center and stimulation of the parasympathetic (vagal) center. This normally results in a decrease in arterial blood pressure.[378]

If systemic blood pressure falls, the baroreceptors become inactive; this removes their inhibitory effect on the sympathetic vasomotor center and results in increased sympathetic stimulation, a rise in

Table 3-3 Adrenergic receptors and effects of stimulation

Receptor	Action
Beta-1	Increased heart rate
	Enhanced atrial and ventricular contractility
	Increased AV conduction
Beta-2	Peripheral vasodilation
	Bronchodilation
Alpha	Peripheral vasoconstriction

Modified from Huss, P., and others: The new inotropic drug, dobutamine, Heart Lung **10:**121, 1981.

heart rate and contractility, peripheral vasoconstriction, and an increase in arterial blood pressure.

■ Common Clinical Conditions

Since the cardiovascular problems most commonly seen in the critical-care unit are congestive heart failure, low cardiac output, hypoxemia, and arrhythmias, these are discussed in detail here. For each problem, the etiology, pathophysiology, clinical signs and symptoms, medical treatment, and nursing care are discussed.

■ CONGESTIVE HEART FAILURE
■ Etiology

Congestive heart failure refers to a set of clinical signs and symptoms that indicate myocardial dysfunction and cardiac output inadequate to meet the metabolic demands of the body. In children it may be caused by congenital heart defects that produce an increase in cardiac preload or afterload, impairment of cardiac contractility, or alterations in the sequence or rate of cardiac contraction (see the following boxed material).

Congestive heart failure in children develops most frequently during the first year of life and is caused most often by congenital cardiovascular anomalies. Defects that cause congestive heart failure in the first weeks of life are those that cause severe left heart or aortic obstruction (such as interrupted aortic arch), large arteriovenous fistula, or combined shunt lesions (see the box on congenital cardiovascular anomalies).[407] Defects that cause high pulmonary blood flow under high pressure, such as a large ventricular septal defect or aortopulmonary window, usually do not cause congestive heart failure until pulmonary vascular resistance falls at approximately 2 to 9 weeks of age.*

*References 3, 113, 134, 179, 208, 226.

CAUSES OF CONGESTIVE HEART FAILURE IN CHILDREN

Problems causing change in cardiac preload or afterload

Congenital heart defects resulting in:
 High pulmonary blood flow under high pressure
 Pulmonary venous, left heart, or aortic obstruction
 AV or semilunar valve atresia, severe stenosis, or regurgitation

Arteriovenous fistula

Surgical repair of congenital heart defects

Severe pulmonary hypertension

Anemia (Hb less than 7 gm%)

Acquired valvular dysfunction

Problems resulting in decreased cardiac contractility

Myocarditis (inflammatory, infectious, metabolic, toxic)

Metabolic disorders (including acid-base, blood gas, calcium, potassium, and glucose imbalances)

Anomalous (congenital) coronary arteries

Endocrine disorders

Fibroelastosis

Disorders of cardiac rate and rhythm

Tachyarrhythmias (ventricular rate greater than 180-200 per minute)

Bradyarrhythmias

Heart block (with slow ventricular rate)

From Hazinski, M.F.: Critical care of the pediatric cardiovascular patient, Nurs. Clin. North Am. **16:**673, 1981.

Surgical correction of congenital heart defects may cause congestive heart failure as a result of intraoperative cardiac manipulation and resection, with subsequent alteration in pressure, flow, and resistance relationships.[16] Surgical repairs of congenital heart defects that require a right or left ventriculotomy approach, conduit insertion, or significant ventricular muscle resection (e.g., repair of severe tetralogy of Fallot, truncus arteriosus, or muscular ventricular septal defect) are those most commonly associated with postoperative heart failure.[336]

■ **Pathophysiology**

When cardiac output becomes insufficient or cardiac dysfunction occurs, sympathetic nervous system compensatory mechanisms are activated, producing the characteristic "fight or flight" response. As part of this response, peripheral vasoconstriction develops to divert blood away from skin, renal, and splanchnic circulations and to direct blood toward the heart and brain. With decreased renal blood flow and reduced renal perfusion, the renin-angiotensin-aldosterone mechanism is activated. This causes renal sodium and water retention and results in an increased circulating blood volume.[28,394] With right ventricular dysfunction and/or volume overload, right ventricular end-diastolic pressure rises, producing systemic venous engorgement. With left ventricular dysfunction or volume overload, left venricular end-diastolic pressure rises, producing pulmonary venous engorgement. The ventricles also dilate and hypertrophy.[412]

An isolated right or left heart volume load or lesion may initially produce signs of right or left ventricular dysfunction and associated systemic or pulmonary venous engorgement. However, signs of biventricular failure are evident most commonly in children, and both systemic and pulmonary venous engorgement are observed.

It is important to note that congestive heart failure does not necessarily cause poor systemic perfusion. Initially, the sympathetic nervous system and renal compensatory mechanisms may be sufficient to maintain cardiac output at a satisfactory level. If the child does not receive medical treatment and decompensates further, low cardiac output may result.

■ **Clinical signs and symptoms**

Sympathetic nervous system stimulation produces tachycardia, peripheral vasoconstriction, and diaphoresis. The child's nail beds often appear pale, the skin appears mottled rather than cyanotic, and extremities are usually cool. Infants may demonstrate significant diaphoresis, particularly over the head and neck. A third or fourth heart sound or a summation gallop may be heard on auscultation.[290]

The renal compensatory mechanisms produce oliguria; the child's urine output will be less than 0.5 to 1.0 ml/kg body weight/hour. If the child has been cared for at home, the mother may note that the infant's diapers are rarely wet or that the child is making fewer trips to the bathroom (see the boxed material on p. 84).

Systemic venous engorgement produces a high

CONGENITAL CARDIOVASCULAR ANOMALIES PRODUCING CONGESTIVE HEART FAILURE IN THE NEONATAL PERIOD

Hypoplastic left heart syndrome

Severe coarctation of the aorta (alone or in combination with other defects)

Severe aortic stenosis

Pulmonary venous obstruction (e.g., mitral stenosis or insufficiency, cor triatriatum, total anomalous pulmonary venous return below the diaphragm)

Tricuspid or pulmonary atresia

Transposition of the great vessels (without pulmonary stenosis)

Combined lesions (e.g., ventricular septal defect with coarctation of the aorta or patent ductus arteriosus)

Single ventricle

Arteriovenous fistula

From Hazinski, M.F.: Critical care of the pediatric cardiovascular patient, Nurs. Clin. North Am. **16**:674, 1981.

SIGNS AND SYMPTOMS OF CONGESTIVE HEART FAILURE IN CHILDREN

Decreased cardiac output—sympathetic nervous system stimulation
   Tachycardia
   Increased cardiac contractility
   Increased vasomotor tone
   Peripheral vasoconstriction
   Diaphoresis

Decreased renal perfusion—renin-angiotensin-aldosterone mechanism
   Sodium and water retention

Systemic venous engorgement
   Hepatomegaly
   Jugular venous distention (difficult to perceive in infants)
   Periorbital and facial edema
   Ascites and dependent edema are rare

Pulmonary venous engorgement
   Tachypnea (and decreased tidal volume)
   Increased respiratory effort (retractions, nasal flaring)
   Grunting (indicates significant distress)
   Rales (may not be perceived)

From Hazinski, M.F.: Critical care of the pediatric cardiovascular patient, Nurs. Clin. North Am. **16:**675, 1981.

---

central venous pressure. Since the hepatic vein is the last large vein to join the inferior vena cava before venous blood enters the heart, high central venous pressure produces liver congestion. As liver sinusoids expand with blood, the liver enlarges and becomes palpable below the child's right costal margin; this is one of the earliest signs of systemic venous engorgement in children. The infant and child may also demonstrate periorbital edema. Because jugular venous distention is difficult to perceive in the short, fat neck of the infant, it is rarely observed until the child is approximately school age. Dependent edema, or ascites, is rarely seen in children unless congestive heart failure is severe and chronic or unless it is associated with other metabolic problems such as hypoalbuminemia or renal failure.

If ascites does develop, it is the result of high central venous pressure, obstruction to hepatic vein flow, severe engorgement of liver sinusoids, and loss of fluid from the surface of the liver. Since liver sinusoids are more permeable than normal capillaries, ascitic fluid contains both fluid and protein. The protein, in turn, may draw even more fluid into the peritoneal cavity, and once it develops the ascites may continue to get worse (see Chapter 8). If ascites is present, the nurse will note an increase in the child's abdominal girth. The child's abdomen will appear full and the skin will be taut and shiny. If two examiners are present, a *fluid wave* may be elicited and areas of

shifting dullness may be noted during percussion (these and other signs and symptoms of ascites are discussed in detail in Chapter 8).[22]

When the child develops *pulmonary venous engorgement*, lung compliance decreases and the work of breathing increases.[3,412] The child demonstrates tachypnea and increased respiratory effort. Infants will demonstrate intercostal, subcostal, sternal, supraclavicular, or suprasternal retractions with nasal flaring. The neonate will demonstrate "head bobbing" with respirations since neck muscles are not strong enough to maintain head control. Older children may demonstrate use of accessory muscles of respiration, such as use of scapular muscles and the sternocleidomastoid. The infant or child with severe respiratory distress will grunt with expiration; this is an instinctive attempt to maintain positive end-expiratory pressure by expiring against a closed glottis, and it is a sign of severe respiratory distress.

Rales are often not observed in infants who develop congestive heart failure. This may be because the child is breathing shallowly and alveolar sounds cannot be heard. Rales may be noted if the child has congestive heart failure that results from left heart or aortic obstruction or if the child has a concurrent respiratory infection.

Subtle signs of congestive heart failure in infants include irritability or lethargy. The infant usually requires prolonged feeding times, sucks poorly,

Table 3-4 Oral digitalizing doses of digoxin for infants and children*

Age	Total digitalizing dose†	Maintenance dose
Preterm neonate	0.025-0.05 mg/kg	0.008-0.012 mg/kg/24 hr
Full-term neonate	0.04-0.08 mg/kg	0.01-0.02 mg/kg/24 hr
2 wk to 2 yr	0.06-0.08 mg/kg	0.015-0.02 mg/kg/24 hr
2 yr to 10 yr	0.04-0.06 mg/kg	0.01-0.015 mg/kg/24 hr
10 yr to adult	Average 0.5-1.0 mg	0.1-0.25 mg/24 hr

Modified from Berman, W.: The relationship of age to the effects and toxicity of digoxin in sheep. In Heymann, M.A., and Rudolph, A.M., co-chairpersons: The ductus arteriosus, Report of the seventy-fifth Ross Conference on Pediatric Research, Columbus, 1978, Ross Laboratories, Inc.; Hazinski, M.F.: Critical care of the pediatric cardiovascular patient, Nurs. Clin. North Am. **16**:675, 1981.
*Intravenous dosage should be calculated at two thirds of these dosages
†Sequence of digitalization: Initial digitalization—one-half of total digitalizing dose initially, one-fourth of total digitalizing dose 6 to 8 hr later, rhythm strip to precede third dose, one-fourth of total digitalizing dose 6 to 8 hr later. Maintenance digitalization—one-eighth of total digitalizing dose given 12 hr later and every 12 hr thereafter

takes only small amounts of fluid, and falls asleep during or immediately after the feeding. This is probably because the effort of sucking and breathing rapidly is exhausting for the infant. The baby may also vomit after feedings, or he may develop gastric distention because of air swallowed with rapid breathing. These children often demonstrate poor weight gain.

■ **Medical treatment and nursing interventions**

Digitalization.   Care of the child with congestive heart failure is aimed at improving cardiac contractility and eliminating excess intravascular fluid. Beyond the neonatal period, the drug of choice for treatment of congestive heart failure is digoxin. During the neonatal period however, use of this drug is controversial since the risk of toxicity is high and therapeutic effects may not be significant.[41,220,240]

When the child is digitalized, several doses of digoxin are administered over a 12 to 24 hour period to provide therapeutic serum digoxin levels; once these levels are achieved, the child is placed on maintenance digoxin, which is administered to replace the child's calculated daily renal excretion of the drug.

The oral digitalizing dose for children is roughly 0.07 mg/kg body weight (Table 3-4). The nurse should always recheck the calculations for the digitalizing and maintenance doses since an error in placement of a decimal point could cause the child to receive a toxic dose. If the child is receiving digoxin intravenously, these doses are calculated at two thirds of the oral dose.

The total digitalizing dose is usually administered in three or four divided doses that are separated by 6 to 8 hours. Usually, the first half of the digitalizing dose is given and then followed by an additional quarter of the digitalizing dose 6 to 8 hours later. The final quarter of the digitalizing dose is usually ordered to be given 6 to 8 hours after the second dose. Before this final dose is administered, the nurse should obtain an ECG rhythm strip to monitor for therapeutic and toxic effects of the drug. Since digoxin slows conduction through the AV node, an increased P-R interval is often present when the child has been digitalized.[178,235,401] Toxic effects of digoxin in children include bradycardia, heart block, and atrial or ventricular premature contractions.[113] Less specific and less common signs of digitalis toxicity in children include anorexia, nausea, vomiting, and diarrhea. If digitalis toxicity is suspected, the physician should be notified, and the medication is usually held, pending results of serum digoxin level testing. A blood specimen is usually drawn for laboratory analysis, but many institutions only perform the analysis a few times each week. Nontoxic serum digoxin levels vary from institution to institution but are in the range of 1.1 to 2.2 ng/ml (nontoxic levels for infants may be up to 3.5 ng/ml). The presence of clinical symptoms compatible with digitalis toxicity is often interpreted more strongly than the serum digoxin level alone.[243,318]

If the child is to be discharged while taking digoxin, the parents must be taught what to do if a dose is omitted or if the child vomits after the medication. It is usually helpful to provide the parents with an approximate schedule of digoxin administration. For example, the nurse may suggest that the digoxin be given at 8 AM and 8 PM daily. If the morning or evening dose is forgotten but remembered by noon or midnight respectively, it may be given; if the drug is forgotten and not remembered until after those hours, that dose should be omitted. If the parents are unsure if a specific dose was administered, it is probably safest to omit it. If the child vomits after receiving the digoxin, I do not advise repeating the dose since it is impossible to determine how much of the drug was absorbed. Vomiting may also be a sign of digoxin toxicity. The parents should notify the physician if more than one dose is omitted or if the child appears ill for any reason since digoxin toxicity may be present.[205] I do not always teach the parents to count the child's pulse because this seems to focus the parents' attention on specific numbers rather than on overall assessment of the child; however, some nurses may prefer to include this teaching. The parents must be aware that digoxin overdose can cause serious illness or even death and that the drug must be kept out of reach of children.[205]

Diuresis. Digitalization alone may improve cardiac output so that renal perfusion is increased and diuresis occurs. However administration of diuretics is frequently necessary (Table 3-5).

Furosemide (Lasix) is the drug of choice for diuresis in the acutely ill child because of the rapid effect of the IV dose (15 to 30 minutes or less). Generally, an IV dose of 1 mg/kg body weight is effective; however, this dose may be doubled in children with severe heart failure who have required chronic diuretic therapy. Furosemide may also be given intramuscularly for rapid action (1 mg/kg body weight/dose). Oral furosemide is given in doses of 1 to 2 mg/kg body weight when less acute diuresis is required (peak action: 2 to 4 hours).

Furosemide inhibits chloride and/or sodium transport in Henle's loop and in the proximal and distal tubules[60,90]; this causes excretion of sodium chloride and water. Since potassium ion is also lost in urine, the child's potassium concentration may fall significantly with diuresis. Since an adequate serum concentration of chloride is required for sodium ex-

cretion, furosemide will be ineffective in the presence of significant hypochloremia. Metabolic alkalosis can develop following furosemide administration because either hypokalemia or hypochloremia will enhance renal hydrogen ion excretion and bicarbonate ion reabsorption. Repeated administration of furosemide is usually contraindicated in the presence of renal failure, particularly in the small infant.[10]

Ethacrynic acid (Edecrin) has a different composition than furosemide, but it has a similar renal action. This drug is prescribed less frequently for children because it is reported to be associated with a higher incidence of gastrointestinal side effects than furosemide; there is also a significant incidence of ototoxicity following administration of this drug.[60,130]

Chlorothiazide (Diuril) may be administered when less acute oral diuresis is required (peak effect: 2 to 4 hours). Chlorothiazide may be given once or twice a day in doses to total 20 to 40 mg/kg/24 hours. It works by blocking sodium and water reabsorption in Henle's loop. It does not produce as profound a potassium loss as furosemide.

Spironolactone (Aldactone) is an aldosterone antagonist that is administered when chronic diuretic therapy will be required since it works more gradually (onset: 1 to 4 days) and results in potassium "sparing." This drug is most effective when administered in conjunction with another diuretic that has a different site of renal action. Since effects of this drug are slow to develop and since they continue days after the drug is discontinued, this drug should be regulated well before the child is discharged.

The combination of *hydrochlorothiazide and spironolactone* (Aldactazide) provides the effects of two oral diuretic drugs with different renal sites of action; this usually produces more significant diuresis than either used alone. The potassium-sparing properties of the spironolactone component may prevent the development of hypokalemia, but serum potassium levels should still be monitored until the child's dosage schedule and fluid balance are stable for several days.

When a child is receiving diuretics, it is important for the nurse to note the exact time of diuretic administration as well as the timing and quantity of the child's diuretic response. It may be helpful to highlight the diuretic response on the nursing flowsheet so that it is easily recognizable. The physician should be notified immediately if the child does not demonstrate a urinary response to the diuretic since the dosage may need to be increased. If the child demonstrates decreased urine response to a previously successful diuretic dose, this may indicate worsening heart failure, low cardiac output, or renal failure.

Table 3-5   Diuretic dosages in children

Drug (trade name)	Peak effect	Action	Dosage	Effect on serum K⁺
Furosemide (Lasix)	Immediate (IV) 2-4 hr (oral)	Inhibits Na⁺ transport in ascending limb of Henle's loop and in proximal and distal tubules	IV: 1-2 mg/kg or Oral: 1-4 mg/kg	↓↓↓
Ethacrynic acid (Edecrin)	Few minutes (IV) ½-8 hr (oral)	Same as furosemide	IV: 1 mg/kg or Oral: 2-3 mg/kg	↓↓↓
Chlorothiazide (Diuril)	2-4 hr	Inhibits tubular reabsorption of Na⁺ primarily in the distal tubule but also in Henle's loop; inhibits H_2O reabsorption in cortical diluting segment of ascending limb of loop	Oral: 20-40 mg/kg/day	↓↓
Spironolactone (Aldactone)	1-4 days; persists for days beyond discontinuation	Aldosterone antagonist (inhibits exchange of Na⁺ for K⁺ in distal tubule)	Oral: 1.5-3.3 mg/kg/day	K⁺ is "saved"
Hydrochlorothiazide and spironolactone (Aldactazide)	2-4 hr (thiazide component); persists for days beyond discontinuation (spironolactone component)	(See above discussion for aldosterone antagonist.) Hydrochlorothiazide inhibits Na⁺ reabsorption in distal tubule and in Henle's loop; inhibits H_2O reabsorption in cortical diluting segment of ascending limb of loop	Oral: 1.65-3.3 mg/kg/day	Remains approximately unchanged

*Modified from Hazinski, M.F.: Critical care of the pediatric cardiovascular patient, Nurs. Clin. North Am. **16:**677, 1981.

With severe congestive heart failure the child's absorption of and response to oral diuretics may not be satisfactory, and it may be necessary to provide parenteral diuretics until systemic venous engorgement is relieved. The nurse should also be aware of any changes in the child's clinical appearance (e.g., decrease in respiratory rate or effort) that may accompany the diuretic response.

Electrolyte balance, particularly serum potassium and chloride ion concentrations, must be monitored while the child is receiving diuretics. Since hypokalemia may augment digitalis toxicity, it should be prevented in these children. Potassium replacement of 1 to 4 mEq/kg/day should be sufficient to maintain serum potassium levels of 3.5 to 4.5 mEq/L in the child with increased urinary loss of potassium. Acid-base balance should also be monitored, and treatment of hypochloremic alkalosis with ammonium chloride may be necessary.

If diuretics are administered late in the evening, the child's sleep will be interrupted for voiding or diaper change unless a Foley catheter is in place. Therefore unless the child's heart failure is severe, some adjustment in scheduling of the evening diuretic dose should be made so that the child experiences diuresis before bedtime.

The parents need to be taught about any medications that the child will be receiving at home. Such information should include the technique of administration, potential effects of drug overdose, flexibility (or lack of it) in the administration schedule, and indications for contacting a physician.

Fluid therapy and nutrition. *Accurate* measurement and recording of the child's daily weight and intake and output is imperative when the child has congestive heart failure. The child should be weighed on the same scale at the same time of day (preferably by the same nurse) so that weight gain or loss can be evaluated. Significant weight changes (greater than 50 gm/24 hours in infants or 200 gm/24 hours in children or 500 gm/24 hours in adolescents) should be verified and reported to a physician.

Normal urine output in children should average 1.0 to 2.0 ml/kg body weight/hour, if fluid intake is adequate. Sources of fluid loss that are not measured, such as increased diaphoresis with fever or increased respiratory rate, should also be considered. If the child does not have a Foley catheter in place and is not "potty-trained," all diapers and drawsheets or pads must be weighed before and after use. One gram of weight increase resulting from urine is counted as 1 ml urine output.

All sources of the child's fluid intake must be totaled to evaluate the child's fluid status and the effectiveness of diuresis. If the child has IV lines in place, total IV and oral fluid intake must be considered. Fluids required to flush IV or arterial lines, to dilute medications, or to obtain cardiac output measurements are often sources of unrecognized fluid intake for the child.

During diuretic therapy the nurse must assess clinical signs of the child's fluid balance. The *hypovolemic* child characteristically demonstrates urine output of less than 0.5 ml/kg body weight/hour and has dry skin and mucous membranes, a flat or sunken fontanelle (in infants under 18 months of age), and decreased or normal tearing; the child may demonstrate weight loss. The child's central venous or pulmonary capillary wedge pressure is usually low when hypovolemia is present, although congestive heart failure or cardiac dysfunction may cause increased systemic and pulmonary venous pressures.

The child with *hypervolemia* will usually demonstrate signs and symptoms of systemic and/or pulmonary venous engorgement. The central venous and/or pulmonary capillary wedge pressure will be elevated, and the child usually gains weight. In addition the child's mucous membranes will be moist, and periorbital edema and hepatomegaly are usually noted. If the child has an endotracheal tube in place, the nurse may notice that she is suctioning the child's airway more frequently as a result of copious pulmonary secretions.

Infants with congestive heart failure often will not tolerate oral feedings. Small, frequent feedings are usually more successful than infrequent, larger ones. If the infant is breathing faster than 60 times per minute or is requiring nearly an hour to ingest 1 to 2 ounces of formula, it may be better to gavage feed the infant until the heart failure has improved; continued attempts at oral feedings may cause the infant to use *more* calories breathing and feeding than he can possibly ingest. The child's daily caloric maintenance requirements should be calculated (Table 3-6), and the nurse should consult with the physician if the child's caloric intake is inadequate.

The child may require fluid restriction if heart failure is severe (see Table 3-7 for calculation of daily fluid requirements). If an infant is vigorously demanding more oral fluids than the amount allowed, the nurse should consult with the physician about increasing the oral fluid allowance and diuretic therapy proportionally.

Excessively salty foods, such as bacon, ham, sausage, potato chips, and some soft drinks, are to be avoided if the child is requiring diuretic therapy. Low-sodium infant formulas (such as Similac PM 60/40) are available, but their increased cost should be considered when deciding if the child requires the formula for home care. If a low-sodium diet is absolutely necessary for an older child, the dietitian must be consulted, and the child's mother (or primary caretaker) must be included in the dietary planning.

Comfort measures and thermoregulation. The child with congestive heart failure usually breathes easier if placed in the semi-Fowler or sitting position so that abdominal contents can drop away from the diaphragm; this allows maximal diaphragmatic excursion and lung expansion. In addition, placement of a small linen roll under the child's shoulders will extend the child's airway and may help the child to breathe with less difficulty.

The child's environment should be kept as quiet as possible to reduce stimulation and to encourage rest. The nurse must decide when and how to consolidate nursing care so that the child is allowed periods of uninterrupted sleep and so that excessive stimulation is avoided.

Premature infants and neonates with little subcutaneous fat have more difficulty maintaining body temperature when environmental temperature is low. In addition, the infant's oxygen requirements are increased when the environmental temperature is excessively warm or cold. The "neutral thermal environment" is that environmental temperature at which the neonate maintains a rectal temperature of 37° C with the lowest oxygen consumption; the neutral thermal environment for infants of various ages and weights have been identified[186,259,381] (see Appendix G). In general, premature infants and neonates will require a higher environmental temperature than older infants.

The nurse is responsible for maintaining an appropriate environmental temperature while the infant is in the unit or during diagnostic tests or transport. Incubators are usually the easiest method of maintaining a warm environment for the infant. However, if the infant must be repeatedly disturbed for vital sign measurement or nursing care activities, it may be better to care for the child on a bed with an overbed warmer so the child will be kept warm yet accessible for treatment. If the child is nursed with an overbed warmer, insensible fluid loss is increased by approximately 40% to 50%.[259]

Evaluation of therapy. The nurse must be aware of the signs and symptoms of increasing heart failure, including continued tachycardia, increased peripheral vasoconstriction, decreased urine output, increased hepatomegaly, and increased respiratory rate and effort. Some of these symptoms may be noted easily in the vital sign sheet and record of intake and output. However, hepatomegaly and respira-

Table 3-6 Calculation of caloric requirements in children

Age	Daily requirements
High-risk neonate	120-150 calories/kg
Normal neonate	100-120 calories/kg
1-2 yr	90-100 calories/kg
2-6 yr	80-90 calories/kg
7-9 yr	70-80 calories/kg
10-12 yr	50-60 calories/kg

NOTE: Ill children (with disease, surgery, fever, or pain) may require extra calories above the maintenance value, and comatose children may require fewer calories (because of lack of exercise).

Table 3-7 Calculation of daily maintenance fluid requirements for children*

Child's weight	Kilogram body weight formula
Newborns (0-72 hr old)	60-100 ml/kg
0-10 kg	100 ml/kg (may increase up to 150 ml/kg if renal and cardiac function adequate)
11-20 kg	1000 ml for the first 10 kg + 50 ml/kg for each kg over 10 kg
21-30 kg	1500 ml for the first 20 kg + 20 ml/kg for each kg over 20 kg

*Administration of 1500 ml/m² body surface area per 24 hours will also provide maintenance fluids.

tory distress may be less specifically described. It is helpful to mark the edge of the liver at the beginning of the day (with another nurse or physician present to validate) so that changes in liver size will be easily recognized throughout the day. Location and severity of any existing retractions should always be recorded with the vital signs so that an increase in respiratory distress will be apparent to even a new nurse caring for the child.

■ **LOW CARDIAC OUTPUT**
■ **Etiology**

Definition. *Cardiac output* is the volume of blood ejected by the left or right ventricle in 1 minute; it is the product of heart rate and stroke volume and is reported in milliliters (or liters) per minute. Since children of different sizes have different normal ranges of cardiac output (Table 3-8), the term "cardiac index" is used for comparison. *Cardiac index* is equal to the child's cardiac output divided by the child's body surface area in square meters (m²). Normal cardiac index in the child is approximately 3.5 to 4.5 L/minute/m².[54]

The term "low cardiac output" is used to refer to a set of clinical signs consistent with poor systemic perfusion, hypotension, and metabolic acidosis, with or without hypoxemia. Occasionally children will demonstrate evidence of low cardiac output and inadequate systemic perfusion with a normal blood pressure; this usually occurs as a result of profound systemic arterial vasoconstriction. The term is also used to apply to children with a measured or calculated cardiac index of less than 2.2 L/minute/m².[228] An excellent review of the etiology, pathophysiology, and treatment of low cardiac output in children has been provided by Perkin and Levin.[328,329]

Causes of low cardiac output in children. Low cardiac output may be caused by an inadequate circulating blood volume or venous return (reduced preload), decreased cardiac function, or increased systemic or pulmonary arterial resistance (afterload). These causes are summarized in the box that follows.

Loss of intravascular fluid volume results in reduced cardiac preload and inadequate circulating blood volume. If the child experiences hemorrhage with an unreplaced volume loss totaling 10% to 15% of the child's circulating blood volume over a short period of time, signs of low cardiac output will result. Severe dehydration (10% or more) will also produce

Table 3-8   Ranges of normal cardiac output in children at different ages

Age	Cardiac output (L/min)	Heart rate	Normal stroke volume
Newborn	0.8-1.0	145	5 ml
6 mo	1.0-1.3	120	10 ml
1 yr	1.3-1.5	115	13 ml
2 yr	1.5-2.0	115	18 ml
4 yr	2.3-2.75	105	27 ml
5 yr	2.5-3.0	95	31 ml
8 yr	3.4-3.6	83	42 ml
10 yr	3.8-4.0	75	50 ml
15 yr	6.0	70	85 ml

Modified from extrapolation of normal postnatal changes in cardiac output, heart rate, and stroke volume from Rudolph, A.M.: Changes in the circulation after birth. In Congenital diseases of the heart, Chicago, 1974, Year Book Medical Publishers, Inc., p. 27.

cardiovascular compromise. Peritonitis, sepsis, or burns can cause "third spacing" of fluid, so that significant amounts of fluid leave the intravascular space, resulting in low cardiac output.

Cardiac dysfunction reduces the heart's ability to pump blood effectively. Acidosis, hypoxemia, electrolyte imbalances, or drug toxicity can alter myocardial electrochemical function and result in decreased excitability or contractility. Untreated congestive heart failure can result in low cardiac output. Myocardial, endocardial, or pericardial inflammation can alter cardiac structure and/or impair cardiac function.

Systemic and pulmonary arterial tone and any existing aortic or pulmonary stenosis provide the resistance against which the ventricles must pump (the afterload). The higher this resistance, the greater the pressure the ventricles must generate to maintain the same amount of flow (pressure = flow × resistance). Increased pulmonary or systemic vascular resistance or pulmonary or aortic outflow tract obstruction cause increased ventricular myocardial work.

■ Pathophysiology

When cardiac output falls, sympathetic nervous system compensatory mechanisms produce tachycardia, peripheral vasoconstriction, decreased urine output, and diaphoresis. Renal arterial constriction causes a fall in the glomerular filtration rate and renal perfusion and activates the renin-angiotensin-aldosterone mechanism; this results in renal sodium and water retention and in an increase in circulating blood volume. With any fall in systemic arterial blood pressure the baroreceptors stimulate the vasomotor center, causing increased heart rate and vasomotor tone. This increase in circulating blood volume and in vasomotor tone may initially be sufficient to maintain the child's systemic arterial blood pressure. If, however, the intravascular volume loss, myocardial dysfunction, or inappropriate ventricular afterload persists, low cardiac output (shock) develops.

With profound systemic vasoconstriction, systemic perfusion is compromised; blood flow to the kidneys, skin, and splanchnic circulation is severely reduced or stopped completely. When cardiac output begins to fall, tissue oxygen extraction can increase up to three times the normal amount. If cardiac output continues to fall, however, tissues will have inadequate oxygen supply to maintain aerobic metabolism, and use of anaerobic metabolic pathways will result in accumulation of lactic acid with the development of metabolic acidosis.[164]

A fall in systemic arterial blood pressure results in decreased coronary perfusion. This compromises the flow of oxygen and nutrients to the myocardium and results in further reduction in cardiac output.

Unless lost intravascular volume is replaced, myocardial function improves, appropriate ventricu-

---

CAUSES OF LOW CARDIAC OUTPUT IN CHILDREN

Sources of inadequate preload (hypovolemia)
  Hemorrhage
  Significant fluid loss (10% or more dehydration or "third spacing" of fluid)
  Sepsis with "capillary leak"
  Peritonitis
  Burns

Causes of cardiac dysfunction
  Acidosis, hypoxemia
  Electrolyte imbalance
  Congestive heart failure
  Arrhythmias
  Inflammatory cardiac diseases
  Drug toxicity

Sources of inadequate or excessive ventricular afterload
  Pulmonary or systemic hypertension
  Aortic stenosis or coarctation of the aorta
  Pulmonary outflow tract obstruction
  Severe systemic vasodilation (e.g., anaphylactic shock, neurogenic shock)

Modified from Hazinski, M.F.: Critical care of the pediatric cardiovascular patient, Nurs. Clin. North Am. **16:**680, 1981.

lar afterload is restored, or metabolic acidosis or electrolyte imbalances are corrected quickly, the child's cardiovascular function will continue to deteriorate and death will result.

■ **Clinical signs and symptoms**

The earliest signs of low cardiac output are usually those of sympathetic nervous system stimulation; these include tachycardia, peripheral vasoconstriction, decreased urine output, and diaphoresis. The child's extremities may be cool, with pale or mottled skin and pale nailbeds and mucous membranes. Urine output will be less than 0.5 ml/kg/hour.

When sympathetic compensatory mechanisms are no longer adequate, the child demonstrates hypotension (refer to Table 3-2 for normal arterial blood pressure ranges). Since the child's normal blood pressure is lower than the adult's, smaller *quantitative* changes in the child's blood pressure may represent significant *qualitative* changes in his clinical condition. If the child has an arterial line in place, the nurse may detect changes in the appearance of the displayed arterial waveform; the waveform may appear to be dampened, and the child's *pulse pressure* is often narrowed. The child's *mean arterial pressure* should be calculated as follows:

$$\frac{(Systolic\ pressure) + (2 \times Diastolic\ pressure)}{3}$$

The mean arterial pressure is usually decreased when low cardiac output develops.

The quality and intensity of the child's peripheral pulses will reflect decreased perfusion. When the child is in shock, the pulses are diminished in intensity and distal pulses may be impossible to feel. If the nurse attempts to obtain a blood pressure measurement by cuff, the Korotkoff sounds may be muffled or impossible to hear. The child's extremities will be cool or cold because of the drastic reduction in skin perfusion. The skin of the child in shock usually develops a gray pallor. The child's nailbeds will be pale or cyanotic, and the capillary filling time (the amount of time blanched skin requires to reperfuse) will be lengthened.

The child's urine volume is initially reduced despite adequate fluid intake. With persistent or profound circulatory compromise, the child becomes anuric.

Since the infant has a large surface area–to–volume ratio, the infant loses a lot of heat to the environment by convection and evaporation. The infant with low cardiac output may not be able to generate heat to replace that lost, and the infant's rectal

(core body) temperature may fall. With significant reduction of skin perfusion, the child is also not able to eliminate heat through the skin; as a result, older children may demonstrate a low skin temperature and a high rectal (core body) temperature.[201]

The child with low cardiac output will be very lethargic or extremely irritable. Although these children still require adequate analgesics if they are in pain, narcotics such as morphine should be given carefully since they may further depress cardiorespiratory function.

If the child's low cardiac output is the result of hemorrhage or other intravascular volume loss, the child will demonstrate signs of *hypovolemia*. Signs of sympathetic nervous system compensation and poor systemic perfusion will be present. In addition, the child will have dry skin and mucous membranes, a flat or sunken fontanelle (in infants younger than 16 months), and decreased or normal tearing. The child's central venous pressure will be below 3 to 5 mm Hg, and the child's pulmonary capillary wedge pressure will be less than 5 to 8 mm Hg.

If low cardiac output is the result of myocardial dysfunction, signs of sympathetic nervous system compensation and poor systemic perfusion will be accompanied by signs of systemic and/or pulmonary venous engorgement (see the boxed material concerning signs and symptoms of congestive heart failure in children). Signs of systemic venous engorgement include hepatomegaly, periorbital edema, and a central venous pressure exceeding approximately 15 mm Hg. Signs of pulmonary venous engorgement include tachypnea, increased respiratory effort (retractions, nasal flaring, possible grunting), and a pulmonary capillary wedge pressure or left atrial pressure above 15 mm Hg.

Because infants have high glucose needs and low glucose stores, the development of low cardiac output may quickly deplete glycogen stores, producing hypoglycemia.[331] Untreated hypoglycemia will further depress myocardial function. Hypocalcemia may also develop in the critically ill infant or child, particularly if frequent transfusions with citrate-phosphate-dextran bank blood have been administered. Since hypocalcemia can depress cardiac contractility, it must be treated promptly.

■ **Calculation of cardiac output**

Fick method. If the child has an arterial as well as a pulmonary artery (Swan-Ganz) line in place, simultaneous arterial and mixed venous blood samples may be obtained to determine the child's arterial-venous oxygen (AV O_2) difference. If the child's AV O_2 difference is low, cardiac output must be high; if the child's AV O_2 difference is high, tissue oxygen extraction is increased and cardiac output must be low. The Fick formula for calculation of the child's cardiac output using AV O_2 difference is as follows*:

$$\text{Cardiac output (L/min)} = \frac{\text{Oxygen consumption (ml/min)}}{\text{Arterial oxygen content (ml/L)} - \text{Mixed venous oxygen content (ml/L)}}$$

To use this formula the child's oxygen consumption must be measured or assumed (normal oxygen consumption is 5 to 8 ml/kg/minute), and the child's hemoglobin concentration must be known (to calculate arterial and venous oxygen content). The following case study is provided to demonstrate use of the Fick calculation and the Grossman formula to calculate cardiac output.[164]

CASE STUDY

A 5 kg, 4-month-old infant has just returned from cardiac surgery. His body surface area is 0.33 m², his hemoglobin concentration is 14 gm/dl, and his oxygen consumption is 25 ml/minute (5 ml/kg/minute). His arterial oxygen saturation is 91%, and his mixed venous (pulmonary artery) oxygen saturation is 64%. What is his cardiac output? What is his cardiac index?

Step 1: Theoretical oxygen-carrying capacity:

$$\text{Hb concentration} \times 1.36 \text{ ml } O_2/\text{gm Hb} \times 10 = \underline{\hspace{1cm}} \text{ ml } O_2/\text{L}$$

$$14 \text{ gm/dl} \times 1.36 \text{ ml } O_2/\text{gm Hb} \times 10 = 190.4 \text{ ml } O_2/\text{L}$$

Step 2: Arterial oxygen content†:

$$\text{Theoretical capacity (step 1)} \times \text{Arterial oxygen saturation} = \underline{\hspace{1cm}} \text{ ml } O_2/\text{L}$$

$$190.4 \text{ ml } O_2/\text{L} \times 0.91 = 173.3 \text{ ml } O_2/\text{L}$$

Step 3: Mixed venous oxygen content:

$$\text{Theoretical capacity (step 1)} \times \text{Mixed venous oxygen saturation} = \underline{\hspace{1cm}} \text{ ml } O_2/\text{L}$$

$$190.4 \text{ ml } O_2/\text{L} \times 0.64 = 121.9 \text{ ml } O_2/\text{L}$$

Step 4: Arterial venous oxygen difference:

$$\text{Arterial oxygen content (step 2)} - \text{Mixed venous oxygen content (step 3)} = \underline{\hspace{1cm}} \text{ ml } O_2/\text{L}$$

$$173.3 \text{ ml } O_2/\text{L} - 121.9 \text{ ml } O_2/\text{L} = 51.4 \text{ ml } O_2/\text{L}$$

Step 5: Fick cardiac output*:

$$\text{Cardiac output} = \frac{\text{Oxygen consumption}}{\text{Arterial venous oxygen difference (step 4)}}$$

$$= \frac{25 \text{ ml/min}}{51.4 \text{ ml/L}} = 0.48 \text{ L/min}$$

Step 6: Cardiac index:

$$\text{Cardiac index} = \frac{\text{Cardiac output (step 5)}}{\text{Body surface area}}$$

$$= \frac{0.48 \text{ L/min}}{0.33 \text{ m}^2} = 1.46 \text{ L/min/m}^2$$

Thermodilution method.   If the child has a pulmonary artery thermistor probe or a balloon-tipped pulmonary artery (Swan-Ganz) catheter with pulmonary artery thermistor, the child's cardiac output may be calculated using a cardiac output computer. IV indicator fluid is injected into the right atrium, and its appearance and concentration in the pulmonary artery are measured. The indicator is usually 5% glucose in water and is usually injected at a temperature different from the patient's body temperature. When the indicator reaches the pulmonary artery, its temperature will have blended with the patient's blood temperature; the cardiac output can be calculated by measuring the temperature change of the blood in the pulmonary artery over time. The injectate may be either 0° to 2° C or room temperature; however, use of cold injectate is thought to provide more accurate calculations. The cardiac output computer has either an external thermometer to measure injectate or an adjustable factor to allow for different injectate temperatures, injectate volumes, or catheter sizes (see Chapter 9).[231,263,365]

The graph of the pulmonary artery time-temperature curve should reveal a logarithm curve that begins at and returns to a consistent baseline.

Three successive measurements are usually performed in children, and any unusually high or low result is discarded. The average of the remaining measurements is presumed to equal the child's cardiac output. Thermodilution cardiac output measurements usually are within 2% to 14% of those obtained using indicator-dilution dye curves.[285]

Since injectate volumes of 3.5 or 10.0 ml are

*For further information, the reader is referred to Rudolph, A.M.: Cardiac output and shunts. In Congenital diseases of the heart, Chicago, 1974, Year Book Medical Publishers, Inc., p. 120.
†For absolute accuracy, the amount of dissolved oxygen should also be added to the amount of oxygen carried by hemoglobin. This is calculated by multiplying the oxygen tension by 0.003.

*For further information see Grossman, W.: Blood flow measurement: the cardiac output, In Cardiac catheterization and angiocardiography, ed. 2, Philadelphia, 1980, Lea & Febiger.

usually required for each cardiac output calculation, the number of injections may have to be restricted to prevent fluid overload in infants.

The nurse must be familiar with the technique of injection required for each computer and catheter. It is essential that manufacturer's recommendations be followed specifically since small variations in technique can result in significant error in calculations.[262]

It is important to note that the thermodilution cardiac output calculates right ventricular output; right ventricular output normally is equal to left ventricular output. If an intracardiac shunt is present, however, adjustments will have to be made in the calculations to allow for the presence of the intracardiac shunt.[365]

■ **Medical treatment and nursing interventions**

Heart rate. Since cardiac output is a product of heart rate and stroke volume, an inappropriate heart rate can produce a fall in the child's cardiac output. If the heart rate is slow, cardiac output will fall unless the child's stroke volume increases proportionally. Children with limited myocardial function must usually maintain an adequate heart rate to maintain a satisfactory cardiac output. Bradycardia in these children should be treated with chronotropic agents or pacemaker therapy.

Extremely high heart rates can also compromise cardiac output, because ventricular diastolic filling time is significantly reduced. Children with extreme tachycardia require treatment with antiarrhythmic agents or pacemaker therapy (see the section on arrhythmias).

Low cardiac output in the critically ill pediatric patient often reflects elements of both inappropriate fluid volume and cardiac failure. The nurse must be able to assess the patient's response to each therapeutic intervention, detect signs of patient deterioration, and respond with appropriate emergency measures.

Volume therapy and diuresis. Any blood loss the child experiences should be considered in terms of the child's total circulating blood volume (Table 3-9). Blood loss should be replaced once it totals 5% to 7% of the child's circulating blood volume. Unreplaced blood loss of 10% to 15% of the child's circulating blood volume constitutes hemorrhage and will compromise systemic perfusion.

Treatment of low cardiac output that results from *hypovolemia* requires insertion of a large bore venous catheter and expansion of intravascular volume. Insertion of a central venous line is preferred but may be very difficult to insert in a critically ill

Table 3-9   Calculation of circulating blood volume in children[364]

Age of the child	Ml/kg body weight
Neonate	85-90
Infant	75-80
Child	70-75
Adult	65-70

neonate; as a result the umbilical, femoral, or subclavian veins may be used. Once the IV lines are inserted, the nurse must secure and protect them carefully since the child depends on them for central fluid therapy.

Once an appropriate venous catheter is in place, a parenteral fluid challenge of approximately 10 ml/kg is provided in the form of glucose and water, saline, colloidal agents, or blood components.[76,328,329] The child's response to fluid challenge must be carefully monitored: venous (central venous, left atrial, or pulmonary capillary wedge) and arterial pressure measurements (and cardiac output, if available), urine output, rectal and skin temperatures, and any changes in blood gas measurements must be noted. If all of these parameters improve with the fluid challenge, hypovolemia probably contributed to the child's low cardiac output and further fluid administration may be required. The cause of the hypovolemia should also be determined and continued fluid losses prevented or replaced immediately. Coagulopathies should be treated with appropriate blood component therapy (Table 3-10). The nurse should note the "filling" (central venous, left atrial, or pulmonary capillary wedge) pressures at which cardiac output seems to be best since these pressures can then be used as a guideline for later fluid administration.

If signs of *hypervolemia* are present (including) signs of systemic and/or pulmonary venous engorgement and increased right or left atrial pressure), diuresis may be required. Intravenous furosemide is the drug of choice for acute diuresis. This drug is given in doses of approximately 1 to 2/ml/kg/dose. The child's potassium concentration must be monitored before and after diuresis since furosemide produces significant potassium loss in the urine (see Table 3-5).

Intravenous mannitol may be administered in

doses of 0.15 to 0.3 gm/kg[48] over 30 to 60 minutes to promote osmotic diuresis in children. However, excessive use of osmotic diuretics may produce an increase in serum osmolality above 350 mOsm/L and may produce renal damage.[173,265]

Correction of electrolyte and acid-base imbalances. If myocardial function is adequate, administration of IV fluid should increase the child's right ventricular end-diastolic pressure and increase the child's stroke volume by increasing ventricular end-diastolic fiber length, according to the Frank-Starling law of the heart (see the discussion of essential anatomy and physiology). If the child's cardiac output does not improve significantly with volume therapy, the cardiac function must be depressed and correction of any acid-base imbalance or electrolyte imbalance must be accomplished since these can all reduce cardiac contractility.

The child with low cardiac output will often require mechanical ventilation to ensure optimal oxygenation and carbon dioxide elimination. If *metabolic acidosis* develops, it should be treated with sodium bicarbonate. A dose of approximately 1 to 3 mEq/kg may be administered and repeated as needed, although the maximum dose should not exceed 8 mEq/kg/24 hours. Since the buffering action of sodium bicarbonate results in the formation of carbon dioxide, it is essential that the child's ventilation is effective and that carbon dioxide elimination is optimal or hypercapnia and its complications can result.[331]

If a laboratory calculation of the child's base excess is available (this is usually part of blood gas results), this value may be used to determine the appropriate sodium bicarbonate dose. For example:

Base excess × Kg body weight × 0.3 =
_____ mEq NaHCO₃

This calculated dose of sodium bicarbonate may be divided into two doses or it may be given slowly in one dose. In neonates the sodium bicarbonate is usually diluted to half strength before administration.

TRIS buffer, tromethamine (Tham), may be administered to buffer combined metabolic and respiratory acidosis. The dosage is usually calculated using the base excess in the following formula:

Base excess × Kg body weight × 0.3 =
_____ ml tromethamine

This calculated dose is administered in divided doses over several hours. The total 24-hour tromethamine dose should not exceed 33 to 40 ml/kg. Side effects include hypoglycemia, hyperkalemia, and osmotic diuresis. This drug is contraindicated for children with renal failure.[48]

If *hypoglycemia* is present, it may be corrected with administration of concentrated glucose solutions. If 50% glucose (D₅₀) is administered, a dose of 0.5 to 1.0 ml/kg is usually required; if 25% glucose (D₂₅) is administered, a dose of 1.0 to 2.0 ml/kg is given.

Hypokalemia may be gradually corrected with a daily supplement totaling 2 to 4 mEq/kg/day in divided doses; the supplement may be administered intravenously or orally. Acute correction of hypokalemia is accomplished with administration of up to 1 mEq/kg. Any IV potassium chloride supplement should be diluted; if the solution is administered in a peripheral IV line, the concentration should be no stronger than the equivalent of 40 to 50 mEq/L or 4 to 5 mEq/dl.[449] Administration of this dilute potassium solution reduces the risk of vasculitis. In addition, the child is protected from inadvertent administration of a potassium chloride bolus if the rate of fluid infusion is suddenly increased during an emergency. Some hospitals advise that IV potassium solutions be given only through central venous lines in small infants and children. Intravenous potassium supplements should not be given by bolus infusion since this may produce arrhythmias. The supplement should be administered over several hours.

Before any potassium supplement is administered the nurse should be sure the child's renal function is adequate since renal failure may produce hyperkalemia, which would only be worsened with further administration of potassium. In addition, the nurse should be familiar with the child's acid-base status. Alkalosis or the correction of acidosis will cause a decrease in the child's intravascular potassium concentration, resulting from hydrogen and potassium ion shifts. As a result, if the child's serum potassium concentration is low in the presence of acidosis, it can be expected to fall further when the acidosis is corrected. Acidosis or the correction of alkalosis will produce a rise in the child's serum potassium concentration; if a potassium supplement is also administered during correction of the alkalosis, the child may become hyperkalemic.

If *hyperkalemia* is present, administration of a concentrated glucose solution alone may increase potassium movement out of the vascular space and into the cells. Fifty percent glucose (D₅₀) is usually given in a dose of 0.5 ml/kg. If necessary, insulin may also be administered in older children in a dose of 1 U/4 gm of glucose or 0.5 U/kg.[275] The effect usually requires approximately 30 minutes. During this time, 50 mg/kg of 10% calcium gluconate is often administered intravenously to counteract the adverse effects of hyperkalemia on myocardial cells.

A cation exchange resin, such as sodium poly-

Table 3-10 Treatment of blood loss or coagulopathies in children[275,352,353,354]

Problem	"Classic" coagulation panel abnormalities	Blood component or medication therapy	Guidelines for quantity
Anemia	Hematocrit <40 (infants) <30 (children)	Whole blood or packed red blood cells	10 ml/kg of packed red blood cells should raise Hct by approximately 10 points
Thrombocytopenia	↓ platelets (isolated) ↑ template bleeding time Clot formation but lack of retraction	Platelets	1 U/5 kg (maximum: 10 units)
Thrombocytopathia	Normal or only slightly decreased platelet count ↑ template bleeding time Clot formation but lack of clot retraction	Platelets	1 U/5 kg (maximum: 10 units)
Lack of coagulation factors in general*	↑ PT, PTT, and thrombin time ↓ fibrinogen Slow clot formation	Fresh frozen plasma (concentrated vitamin K dependent factors may be given)	10 ml/kg
Heparin excess†	↑↑ PTT, thrombin time, and template bleeding time PT may be slightly increased Platelet count normal (initially) Slow clot formation	Protamine sulfate (as titrated, will result in correction of thrombin time)	1 mg/kg (slowly)

Protamine sulfate excess†	↑↑ PTT, thrombin time, and template bleeding time PT may be slightly increased Platelet count normal (initially) Slow clot formation	When protamine sulfate is titrated and thrombin time does not improve, then heparin is administered	Heparin IV load: 50 U/kg Maintenance IV drip: 10-20 U/kg/hr IV bolus: 50-75 U/kg q 4 hr
ASA given in preoperative period	↑ in template bleeding time	Platelets	1 U/5 kg (maximum: 10 units)
Fibrinolysis (primary)	↓ fibrinogen Platelets normal or slightly low ↑ fibrin split products	Aminocaproic acid (Amicar)	200 mg/kg IV, then 150 mg/kg IV q 2 hr for 12 hr
Disseminated intra-vascular coagula-tion (DIC)	↓ fibrinogen and platelets (lower than expected) ↑ PT, PTT ↑ fibrin split products	Heparin or platelets with fresh frozen plasma (see above dosages)	Heparin IV load: 50 U/kg Maintenance IV drip: 10-20 U/kg/hr IV bolus: 50-75 U/kg q 4 hr

From Hazinski, M.F.: Critical care of the pediatric cardiovascular patient, Nurs. Clin. North Am. 16:694, 1981.
*Usually, this results from a complex function of dilution and lack of replacement during surgery, inability of the liver to compensate, and occasionally due to excessive loss of plasma protein via chest tubes.
†The only way to distinguish these two problems is through protamine sulfate titration—see column 3.

styrene sulfonate (Kayexalate) may be administered rectally; such a resin promotes exchange of sodium for potassium in the gut. A dose of 1 gm of resin/kg usually reduces the child's serum potassium concentration by approximately 1 mEq.

Administration of intravenous sodium bicarbonate may also promote potassium movement from the vascular space into the cells. A dose of 2.5 mEq/kg of sodium bicarbonate lowers the child's serum potassium by approximately 2 mEq/L.[250] If the child's serum potassium exceeds 7.0 to 7.5 mEq/L despite the above measures, the child probably requires urgent peritoneal dialysis to prevent ventricular fibrillation and other cardiovascular complications of hyperkalemia.

Hypocalcemia may be treated with either calcium gluconate, calcium chloride 10% IV solution, or calcium gluconate oral solution. IV calcium gluconate is most commonly given in doses of 100 to 200 mg/kg (maximum 2 gm), or calcium chloride may be administered in doses of 20 to 50 mg/kg (maximum 1 gm).

Inotropic support. Correction of hypovolemia and metabolic disorders should improve cardiac contractility and cardiac output. However, if the child's systemic perfusion remains poor despite these measures, use of sympathomimetic agents will be required to improve cardiac contractility and to increase heart rate. These medications are selected and titrated to activate specific (beta$_1$, beta$_2$, or alpha) adrenergic receptors (see Table 3-3). The drugs are administered by continuous IV infusion (Table 3-11).

Dopamine (Intropin) is a norepinephrine precursor that provides "dopaminergic" and direct and indirect beta$_1$- and alpha-adrenergic effects that are dose-dependent. At low infusion doses (1 to 5 μg/kg/minute) the dopaminergic effects dominate, producing selective dilation of the renal, mesenteric, cerebral, and coronary vessels. The renal artery dilation increases renal blood flow and glomerular filtration rate, which causes improved urine output.[97]

At moderate infusion rates (5 to 8 or 10 μg/kg/minute) the dopaminergic effects persist, although beta$_1$-adrenergic effects predominate. These beta$_1$ effects produce increased cardiac contractility, increased heart rate, and increased cardiac output. Dopamine usually does not directly effect systemic vascular resistance, although peripheral vasomotor tone may be reduced if cardiac output increases sufficiently. Pulmonary vascular resistance is not directly lowered with dopamine administration. Therefore when cardiac output (flow) increases without a fall in pulmonary vascular resistance, the child's

pulmonary artery pressure may rise.[196,406] As a result dopamine should be used with caution in children with pulmonary hypertension.

When dopamine is administered at higher rates (those above 8 to 10 μg/kg/minute), alpha-adrenergic effects are thought to predominate. These produce peripheral vasoconstriction, decreased renal blood flow, and decreased urine output[148]; these effects are usually undesirable when the child has low cardiac output.

These dopamine dose-related effects have primarily been determined in full-term neonates, infants, and children.[92,97,241] The effect of dopamine administration in premature neonates has not been elaborated; some evidence indicates that these neonates may require higher doses to achieve an increase in cardiac output.[199] Therefore the titration of dopamine in any child, but particularly in the premature neonate, must be performed while closely monitoring direct and indirect evidence of systemic perfusion and urine output.

Children with low cardiac output following cardiovascular surgery seem to respond more consistently to dopamine administration than those with low cardiac output resulting from sepsis.[97]

Adverse effects of dopamine administration in children include arrhythmias and increased pulmonary artery pressure.[406] The "dopaminergic" effects of dopamine (particularly the increase in renal blood flow and urine output) seem attenuated with concurrent administration of phenothiazines (such as prochlorperazine [Compazine]), apomorphine, butyrophenones (such as haloperidol or Innovar), and bulbocapnine.[135,149] The alpha-adrenergic effects of dopamine (primarily those producing peripheral vasoconstriction) are antagonized by phentolamine (Regitine).[149]

Dobutamine (Dobutrex) is a synthetic sympathetic amine that has beta$_1$-adrenergic cardiovascular effects. Dobutamine does not seem to have any "dopaminergic" effects at lower doses or alpha-adrenergic effects at higher doses. The beta$_1$ effects produce increased cardiac output by increasing myocardial contractility, and they also produce increased heart rate. As a result of the improvement of cardiac output, the child's systemic arterial and mean blood pressures increase. Although systemic vascular resistance is not directly affected by dobutamine, it may fall slightly if cardiac output increases sufficiently.[330] Dobutamine is usually administered at an infusion rate of 2 to 10 μg/kg/minute.[98] Dobutamine may produce pulmonary venoconstriction, elevation in pulmonary capillary wedge pressure, and pulmonary edema (this effect is unusual and has only been re-

Table 3-11 Pediatric inotropic and chronotropic agents for low cardiac output*

Drug (trade name)	Dosage	Effects
Dobutamine (Dobutrex)	2-10 μg/kg/min	Beta$_1$ cardiovascular effects: augments cardiac output by increasing myocardial contractility; less chronotropic effects than isoproterenol (Isuprel); increases systemic arterial and mean blood pressure; slightly decreases systemic vascular resistance (increases cardiac output); no selective renal vasodilation; no alpha peripheral vasoconstriction
Dopamine (Intropin)		Direct and indirect beta-adrenergic agonist: additional alpha-adrenergic properties at higher doses
	Low doses (1-5 μg/kg/min)	Dopaminergic effects dominate: increases renal blood flow, glomerular filtration rate, sodium excretion, and urine output
	Moderate doses (5-10 μg/kg/min)	Dopaminergic effects persist; beta$_1$ effects dominate: increases cardiac contractility, cardiac output, and heart rate; peripheral resistance is unchanged (or slightly decreased); may increase pulmonary artery pressure
	High doses (Above 10 μg/kg/min)	Alpha effects dominate: peripheral vasoconstriction and increased afterload; tachycardia more pronounced
Epinephrine (Adrenelin)	0.05-1 μg/kg/min	Sympathomimetic agent with alpha, beta$_1$ and beta$_2$ effects: systemic vasoconstriction. Increased cardiac rate and contractility NOTE: At lower doses, beta$_2$ effects may promote systemic vasodilation CAUTION: Will increase myocardial oxygen consumption
Isoproterenol (Isuprel)	0.05-0.5 μg/kg/min	Beta$_1$ and beta$_2$ adrenergic effects: increases cardiac rate (chronotropic effects predominate) at lower doses; decreases systemic vascular resistance; less marked increase in renal perfusion than dopamine; bronchodilation CAUTION: Monitor for tachyarrhythmias and venous pooling

Modified from Hazinski, M.F.: Critical care of the pediatric cardiovascular surgical patient, Nurs. Clin. North Am. **16:**683, 1981.
*See references 76, 97, 196, 197, 250, 330, and 406.

ported at dosage rates exceeding 7.0 to 7.5 μg/kg/minute).[330] Dobutamine dosage and effects have not yet been specifically determined for neonates.

Isoproterenol (Isuprel) may be administered to promote an increase in heart rate and/or systemic arterial blood pressure. This drug provides beta$_1$- and beta$_2$-adrenergic effects. It produces a more profound tachycardia than either dopamine or dobutamine.[97,197] At lower infusion rates (0.05 to 0.1 μg/kg/minute) isoproterenol produces an increase in heart rate; at higher doses (0.1 to 0.5 μg/kg/minute) increased car-

diac contractility produces an increase in cardiac output. Since the beta$_2$-adrenergic effects of isoproterenol produce systemic vasodilation, the child's systemic vascular resistance and mean arterial pressure may fall and venous pooling may result. An additional effect of isoproterenol is bronchodilation, which results from beta$_2$ stimulation.

Epinephrine (Adrenaline) administration produces beta$_1$-, beta$_2$-, and alpha-adrenergic cardiovascular effects. This causes increased heart rate, cardiac contractility, and systemic vasoconstriction. Epinephrine may be given in a continuous infusion of 0.05 to 1 μg/kg/minute or it may be given in a bolus of 0.1 ml of 1:10,000 dilution or 0.01 ml of 1:1000 dilution. At extremely low infusion rates, beta$_2$ effects may promote systemic vasodilation. However, epinephrine administration generally increases systemic vascular resistance, so will increase the afterload of the left ventricle and myocardial oxygen consumption. Increased peripheral vasoconstriction produced by epinephrine administration will also reduce renal blood flow and urine output.

Afterload reduction. Systemic vasodilation has been used to treat congestive heart failure and low cardiac output for a long time; it has recently become more popular in the treatment of children. Vasodilator therapy is used to reverse or reduce the pulmonary and/or systemic vasoconstriction that results when cardiac output begins to fall. Since systemic vasoconstriction increases left ventricular work, vasodilation should decrease left ventricular work and improve myocardial performance.[142] In addition, vasodilators produce venodilation, so cardiac preload is also reduced. Continuous vasodilator infusion can produce a fall in left or right atrial pressure and mean arterial pressure while cardiac index rises.[37] The parenteral vasodilators most frequently used in pediatric critical care include nitroglycerine, nitroprusside, and hydralazine. Dobutamine and isoproterenol may also be administered since they have secondary vasodilatory effects.

Nitroglycerin administration produces systemic and pulmonary dilation, so left and right ventricular afterload will be reduced. Venodilatory effects also produce a decrease in venous return to the heart. The net effect of nitroglycerin therapy may be a fall in systemic arterial blood pressure, and an increase in cardiac index.[142] If parenteral fluid administration is titrated during nitroglycerin therapy to maintain an adequate left or right atrial pressure, cardiac index may increase 20% to 30%. Mean arterial pressure and heart rate are not significantly changed with nitroglycerin therapy.[37] IV infusion of the drug may be started at 0.1 μg/kg/minute and increased to 10 μg/kg/minute if necessary. Maximal therapy may be as high as 25 μg/kg/min.

Polyvinyl chloride, the material used in the manufacture of disposable infusion sets, buretrols, and IV tubing, adsorbs nitroglycerin. This adsorption is enhanced when the material is newly exposed to the nitroglycerin (e.g., immediately after the IV tubing has been changed) and when the flow rate of the nitroglycerin is slow.[20,75] As a result, when this drug is administered to small children, the concentration of the drug that the patient receives is far less than

the concentration of the drug originally mixed in the buretrol, and it is impossible to know exactly how much nitroglycerin the patient actually receives. To minimize adsorption of the drug during administration, a large (60 ml) disposable or glass syringe, a syringe pump, and a short length of microbore IV tubing should be used. The disposable syringe is made of polypropylene, which does not appreciably adsorb nitroglycerin, and the microbore tubing has such a small diameter and length that adsorption of nitroglycerin is minimal.[230] Recently, infusion pump tubing made of polyethylene has also become available for IV administration of nitroglycerine by infusion pump. This material does not adsorb significant amounts of nitroglycerin.

Topical nitroglycerin (2% ointment) may also be applied to the chest. A dose of approximately 1 to 1.5 cm may produce effects for ½ to 6 hours. Long-acting nitroglycerin paste discs are also available; these produce vasodilatory effects for up to 12 hours.

Sodium nitroprusside (Nipride) is a smooth muscle relaxant that produces arterial and venous dilation. Sodium nitroprusside administration reduces ventricular afterload by reducing pulmonary and systemic vascular resistance, and it increases venous capacitance reducing venous return and ventricular preload. As a result ventricular end-systolic volume is decreased and ejection fraction is increased. In continuous infusion doses of 0.5 to 8 μg/kg/minute, nitroprusside causes an increase in heart rate and cardiac index and results in a significant decrease in pulmonary and systemic vascular resistance.[406]

Sodium nitroprusside is sensitive to light. It is stored in dark vials before use and must be protected from light after mixing. Since nitroprusside may rapidly lose its potency, the solution is usually mixed in a buretrol and is changed every 24 hours. Some hospitals require that the buretrol and tubing should be covered unless the solution will clear the tubing within a few hours. Sodium nitroprusside can also be administered with a syringe pump.

Since the breakdown of sodium nitroprusside results in the formation of thiocyanate and cyanide, the patient who requires sodium nitroprusside infusion for 48 hours or more should be monitored closely for evidence of thiocyanate or cyanide toxicity. This toxicity will develop more rapidly if renal or hepatic disease is present. Thiocyanate levels should be checked every 2 days (more frequently if the patient has renal or liver disease); toxic serum levels are above 10 mg/dl. Signs of thiocyanate toxicity include anorexia, hypothyroidism, weakness, skin rash, tinnitus, confusion, and fatigue. Signs of cyanide toxicity include agitation, diminished level of consciousness, tachypnea, incontinence, seizures, and cardio-respiratory arrest.[116]

Because sodium nitroprusside also may produce decreased platelet function,[376] the child's platelet count should be monitored. More importantly, the nurse should watch closely for signs of petechiae or ecchymoses, prolonged bleeding from puncture sites, or gastrointestinal bleeding.

Hydralazine (Apresoline) is another vascular smooth muscle relaxant; it has a more pronounced effect in lowering arteriolar resistance. The recommended parenteral dose is 0.15 mg/kg every 4 hours or 1.7 to 3.5 mg/kg/day divided into four to six doses. Hydralazine may also be given orally to total 0.75 mg/kg/day divided into four doses. This oral dose may be gradually increased as much as tenfold over several weeks.[48]

When a child receives vasodilator therapy, the nurse must watch carefully for signs and symptoms of excessive vasodilatory effects, including hypotension, diaphoresis, tachycardia, dizziness, headache, irritability or lethargy, nausea, vomiting, or nasal stuffiness.[116] Since hypotension is more likely to occur when vasodilators are administered in the presence of hypovolemia, the child's fluid status must be evaluated very carefully before vasodilator therapy is initiated. Volume expanders should be available at the bedside, and vasopressors should be on hand for emergency use if the patient develops profound hypotension.

Vasodilators should not be mixed with any other drug. The parenteral lines containing these medications should not be flushed since this delivers a bolus of vasodilator to the patient and can cause acute hypotension. When changing the IV tubing, the nurse must be extremely careful to avoid providing excessive or inadequate vasodilator therapy. The child should not be rapidly elevated to a sitting position during vasodilation therapy since orthostatic hypotension can result.

If possible, the child's systemic vascular resistance and pulmonary vascular resistance should be calculated before the vasodilator therapy is initiated and at frequent intervals thereafter to evaluate the effectiveness of therapy. The following formula is used to calculate systemic vascular resistance.

$$\text{Systemic vascular resistance (U/m}^2 \text{ body surface area)} = \frac{\text{Mean systemic arterial pressure} - \text{Mean right atrial pressure}}{\text{Cardiac index}}$$

Normal systemic vascular resistance is approximately 10 to 15 U/m² body surface area in the neonate, approximately 15 to 20 U/m² body surface area in the older infant (1 to 1½ years), and approximately 15 to 30 U/m² body surface area in the child.[360] To obtain the resistance in dynes-sec/cm², the resistance units are multiplied by 80.

The following formula is used to calculate the child's pulmonary vascular resistance.

$$\text{Pulmonary vascular resistance (U/m}^2 \text{ body surface area)} = \frac{\text{Mean pulmonary arterial pressure} - \text{Mean left atrial pressure}^*}{\text{Cardiac index}}$$

In neonates, pulmonary vascular resistance is normally 8 to 10 U/m² body surface area; by approximately 6 to 8 weeks of life, the infant's pulmonary vascular resistance has fallen to the adult values of 1 to 3 U/m² body surface area.[360] To obtain the resistance in dynes-sec/cm², these resistance units are multiplied by 80.

It is important that these resistance calculations are recorded on the nursing flow sheet near the recorded vasodilator dosage so that the patient's response to changes in these medications can be readily assessed.

It is also important to evaluate any other medications that the patient is receiving since there may be interactions between the effects of the vasodilator and other drugs that produce venodilation or fluid loss (such as morphine sulfate or furosemide).

If the child's dosage of an IV vasodilator is tapered, it may be necessary to simultaneously introduce an oral vasodilator or nitroglycerin ointment to maintain uninterrupted administration of the drug. Prazosin (Minipress), in doses of 25 μg/kg/dose every 6 hours, may be administered to produce systemic vasodilation in children.[89]

Combination therapy. The use of an IV inotropic agent plus an IV vasodilator in children with low cardiac output may produce a more significant increase in cardiac output than that produced by either drug separately. The action of a vasodilator (such as sodium nitroprusside) should reduce systemic and pulmonary vascular resistance sufficiently so that the increased cardiac contractility produced by the inotropic agent (such as dopamine) produces a far more significant increase in the child's cardiac index.[406,411] If two drugs are used for such therapy, it is extremely important that any changes in dosage are made in only one drug at a time so that patient response can be evaluated. Since both inotropic agents and vasodilators can produce tachycardia or tachyarrhythmias, the child's heart rate and rhythm should be monitored closely during therapy.

*NOTE: Pulmonary artery wedge pressure may be substituted for mean left atrial pressure.

Maintenance of continuous infusion medications. Drip concentrations and infusion rates of any medication should always be recalculated by each nurse on every shift to avoid perpetuation of inadvertent calculation errors. Pump infusion rates should be checked every hour with vital sign measurements and more frequently if a change in the patient's condition occurs since flow rate dials may be accidentally bumped and changed or stopcocks turned when many members of the health care team are near the child's bedside. "Piggyback" infusions should be taped securely to prevent accidental dislodgement during movement of the patient for x-ray examinations or linen changes. Any IV line containing continuous infusion of inotropic medication should be labeled prominently near injection sites. This prevents unintentional "bolusing" of the medication or the mixing of incompatible drugs during emergency situations.

The nurse must be aware of the therapeutic and toxic effects of each drug administered and of the compatibility of that drug with other medications (such as antibiotics, potassium or calcium chloride, or sedatives) that the child is receiving.[135,149] The dose of continuous drips should be charted hourly on the vital sign and medication sheets, and fluid and medication quantities should be added to the fluid intake record. The fluids given with continuous infusion medications may be a source of excessive fluid intake for the child. If fluid restriction is necessary, the medication concentration may need to be doubled (and, of course, the administration rate halved). The medication concentration in the buretrol must be clearly labeled.

Whenever the dosage of a continuous drip medication is changed, careful evaluation of patient response (including changes in heart rate, urine output, systemic perfusion, cardiac output, and arterial and venous pressures) must be made.

Mechanical support of ventricular and cardiopulmonary function. The *intraaortic balloon pump* (IABP) is a mechanical circulatory assist device that uses an inflatable balloon positioned in the descending aorta to provide intermittent diastolic counterpulsation to augment diastolic and coronary artery flow. This device has had limited success when used in children. It is most successful when it is used in children with severe cardiac dysfunction of a temporary nature (e.g., during recovery from cardiac surgery or trauma).

The IABP device consists of a long balloon that is attached to a catheter and a pump monitor console. The console monitors the patient's ECG, then provides balloon inflation during ventricular diastole.

The balloon can be inserted percutaneously or through a cutdown in the child's external iliac artery; the balloon catheter is then inserted retrograde in the aorta until it is positioned below the left subclavian artery but above the hepatic and mesenteric arteries. Although initial use of the IABP device yielded only fair results, recent use has provided more consistent improvement in cardiac index and in survival rates.[133,340]

When the child is receiving balloon counterpulsation, the nurse must monitor the child's arterial waveform tracings and ECG to ensure that the IABP device is in fact cycling properly to provide diastolic counterpulsation. The child's arterial *diastolic* pressure will often be greater than the child's arterial *systolic* pressure during counterpulsation. If the child's heart rate exceeds approximately 140 to 150 beats per minute, it may be impossible for the console to cycle rapidly enough to provide balloon inflation during diastole. In this case, some institutions use helium to inflate the balloon[437] since it allows more rapid balloon inflation and deflation. If arrhythmias are present, it may be difficult to synchronize balloon inflation with ventricular diastole. As a result significant arrhythmias should be treated promptly (see the section on arrhythmias in this chapter).

Complications of intraaortic balloon counterpulsation include bleeding, thromboembolic events, infection, leg ischemia, aortic dissection, and decreased mesenteric and renal artery perfusion. The child receives anticoagulants while the balloon is in place to prevent thrombosis formation around the balloon and catheter. As a result the nurse must watch closely for signs of bleeding, and pressure must be applied to any puncture sites. The balloon insertion site must be covered and carefully protected since local infection can progress to endocarditis or sepsis. The color and warmth of the catheterized extremity must be checked constantly since arterial compromise and leg ischemia may result from iliac artery obstruction or thromboembolic phenomenon.

Aortic dissection can occur during retrograde insertion of the balloon. If the balloon is too long, it may occlude the mesenteric and renal arteries, producing bowel ischemia and/or renal failure. It is essential that balloon position be verified frequently and that any evidence of abdominal distention, gastrointestinal bleeding, or decreased renal function be investigated immediately. The child's abdominal girth should be measured and recorded every 2 to 4 hours, and all gastrointestinal secretions should be checked for the presence of blood. Evidence of gastrointestinal bleeding or urine output less than 0.5 to 1.0 ml/kg/hour should be reported to the physician.

Extracorporeal membrane oxygenation provides support of cardiopulmonary function through the use of external (outside of the body) cardiopulmonary bypass with a membrane oxygenator.[396,440] This system can be used to provide cardiopulmonary support for infants and children with potentially short-term and reversible cardiac or respiratory failure.

Initially, extracorporeal membrane oxygenation was used for adults and children with trauma, multisystem failure, infections, or profound primary cardiac or pulmonary failure. Survival rates for those patients treated with this system were approximately 15%, which did not differ significantly from those patients treated with conventional support.[26,456] More recently however, use of this system in neonates with cardiorespiratory failure, particularly that resulting from persistent fetal circulation (often associated with diaphragmatic hernia), has produced survival rates of 25% to 75% in newborns thought to be moribund.[25,140,175]

Indications for use of extracorporeal membrane oxygenation include respiratory failure, cardiogenic shock, hemorrhagic shock, septic shock, or multisystem failure not responsive to conventional management techniques. The problem should also be thought temporary or reversible so that short-term support of cardiopulmonary function will allow time for recovery.

Several methods of extracorporeal membrane oxygenation may be provided. All forms require removing venous blood from the body, warming and oxygenating the blood with a heat coil and a membrane oxygenator, and returning the blood to the body. This requires surgical insertion of cannulae into large vessels and maintenance of these cannulae while the child receives extracorporeal membrane oxygenation.[161]

Complications include bleeding (7% to 34%), mechanical or technical problems (35%), and infection (20%).[24] In addition, intracranial bleeding has been reported in a significant number of neonates requiring this procedure.[25,161]

At least one nurse and one perfusionist must be at the bedside at all times to monitor the patient and equipment function. Because the child will receive paralytic agents, he is totally dependent on the medical team for provision of adequate ventilation. Even though oxygenation is provided, mechanical ventilation is required to maintain lung aeration and to provide oxygenation of any blood that is allowed to enter the lungs. The child also requires adequate analgesia and sedation. The nurse must be able to readily detect changes in the child's condition and to verify appropriate equipment function immediately.

Since cannula dislodgement could result in immediate hemorrhage, the cannulae must be secured and all tubing must be in sight at all times. Emotional support of the child and family is essential.

The *left ventricular assist device* has been used in clinical trials on a limited basis under grants funded by the National Institutes of Health (NIH). The left ventricular assist device is an artificial valved pump that receives and pumps blood in a manner similar to the right or the left ventricle. The pump is powered by a hydraulic generator that is located in a console at the patient's bedside. The pump itself may be located at the bedside or implanted in the patient's chest. The pump receives blood from the child's ventricle via a ventricular apical cannula; it returns blood to the circulation with pulsatile flow via an aortic cannula.

Indications for the use of this device and/or a right ventricular assist device include cardiogenic shock unresponsive to conventional management methods. The cardiac failure must be thought temporary or potentially reversible. Potential complications of this device include bleeding, thromboembolic events, sepsis, or mechanical (pump) failure. The child who is using a left (or right) ventricular assist device requires a nurse at the bedside at all times. The child receives paralytic drugs and still requires adequate sedation and analgesia. Since this device only provides cardiac function, the child also requires mechanical ventilation. Emotional support of the child and family is essential.

Emotional support. The child with low cardiac output requires excellent medical and nursing care. Health care personnel are constantly surrounding the child's bedside to assess the child, to provide treatment, and to adjust and care for all of the equipment used in the child's care. The gravity of the child's clinical condition and the complexity of the child's care can be overwhelming to the staff; it is even more overwhelming for the parents of the child. Too often the child requires such constant attention that the parents are not given as much support as they need. It is essential that physicians and nurses relieve one another at the bedside so that someone is frequently free from patient care responsibilities to talk to and be with the parents. It is also essential that all health care personnel discuss the child's clinical condition, treatment, and prognosis using consistent terms so the parents will not be confused by variations in vocabulary.

The nurse at the bedside is usually the most consistent member of the health care team involved with the parents. She must be aware of their concerns and questions, and she must communicate these to other members of the team. She is also in the best position to support the parents and to comfort them and their child. The nurse can usually best comfort the parents by providing the child with gentle, compassionate care so the parents will know that their child is receiving emotional support not just technical intervention. It is helpful for the parents to be reminded that the child has received appropriate analgesia and sedation and that he is not experiencing any pain. When the parents visit the child, they may need encouragement (when they are ready) to touch the child and speak to the child; they will need to know that the child is still able to hear them and that he knows they are there. Finally, the parents are usually helped far more by a tender gesture or a kind word to them or their child than by lengthy or detailed explanations of the child's treatment plan.

■ ARRHYTHMIAS

Several excellent texts are currently available that provide detailed discussion of interpretation of ECGs[72] and etiology, recognition, and treatment of pediatric cardiac arrhythmias.[348] Therefore the following section will not review interpretation of pediatric ECGs but will focus on etiology, clinical significance, and treatment of those arrhythmias most commonly seen in the pediatric critical-care unit.

Normal components of the ECG are provided in Fig. 3-13, and time and amplitude calculations with ECG grid paper are reviewed in Fig. 3-14. For detailed information of ECG rate, interval, and amplitude standards for children, an excellent series of tables has been published.[81]

■ Etiology

Bradyarrhythmias may result from hypoxia, sinus node dysfunction, heart block, acidosis, hypothermia, increased vagal tone (especially in infants), hyperkalemia, digitalis effects or toxicity, and antiarrhythmic therapy.[160,349]

Supraventricular tachycardias include atrial fibrillation or flutter, sick sinus syndrome, paroxysmal atrial tachycardia, Wolff-Parkinson-White syndrome, or multiple intraatrial conduction pathways; these may be congenital or idiopathic in origin, or they may result from intraatrial cardiovascular surgery, or drug toxicity.[46,144,416] Atrial fibrillation and flutter are almost invariably caused by organic heart disease,[225,343] although they may be seen in otherwise normal neonates.[396]

Ventricular tachycardia may be idiopathic in origin,[39,166,184] but it usually indicates ventricular irrita-

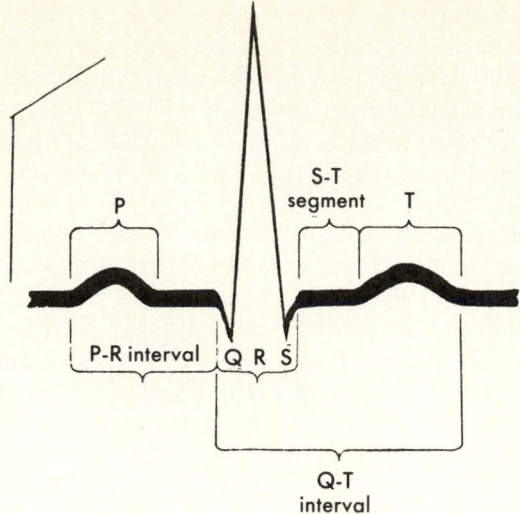

Fig. 3-13 The normal electrocardiogram. Normal depolarization of the atria is indicated by the P wave. The P-R interval indicates the time between sinus node depolarization and ventricular depolarization. Ventricular depolarization is indicated by the QRS complex (the Q deflection may not always be present), and the QRS duration indicates the time of ventricular conduction. The Q-T interval is the time from the onset of ventricular depolarization to the end of ventricular repolarization; this interval normally is shorter when the heart rate is faster.

Modified from Conover, M.B.: Understanding electrocardiography: physiological and interpretive concepts, ed. 4, St. Louis, 1984, The C.V. Mosby Co., p. 59.

bility secondary to hypoxia, acidosis, hyperkalemia, hypokalemia, hypercalcemia, drug toxicity, anomalous AV conduction pathways, creation of an irritable focus during cardiovascular surgery, or the presence of myocarditis or myocardiopathy.[46,167,198,253,295]

Complete heart block may be congenital in origin; it is frequently observed in children with congenital corrected transposition.[11] Heart block may also result from infectious or inflammatory myocardiopathies or from surgical correction of congenital heart defects.[99]

■ Pathophysiology

Effect of electrolyte imbalance. Electrolyte imbalances, especially potassium, calcium, and sodium imbalances, can cause arrhythmias because they alter myocardial electrochemical events. This can affect tissue excitability or the mechanism of cardiac depolarization.

The cell membrane potential is determined predominantly by the difference in potassium concentration (the concentration gradient) between the inside

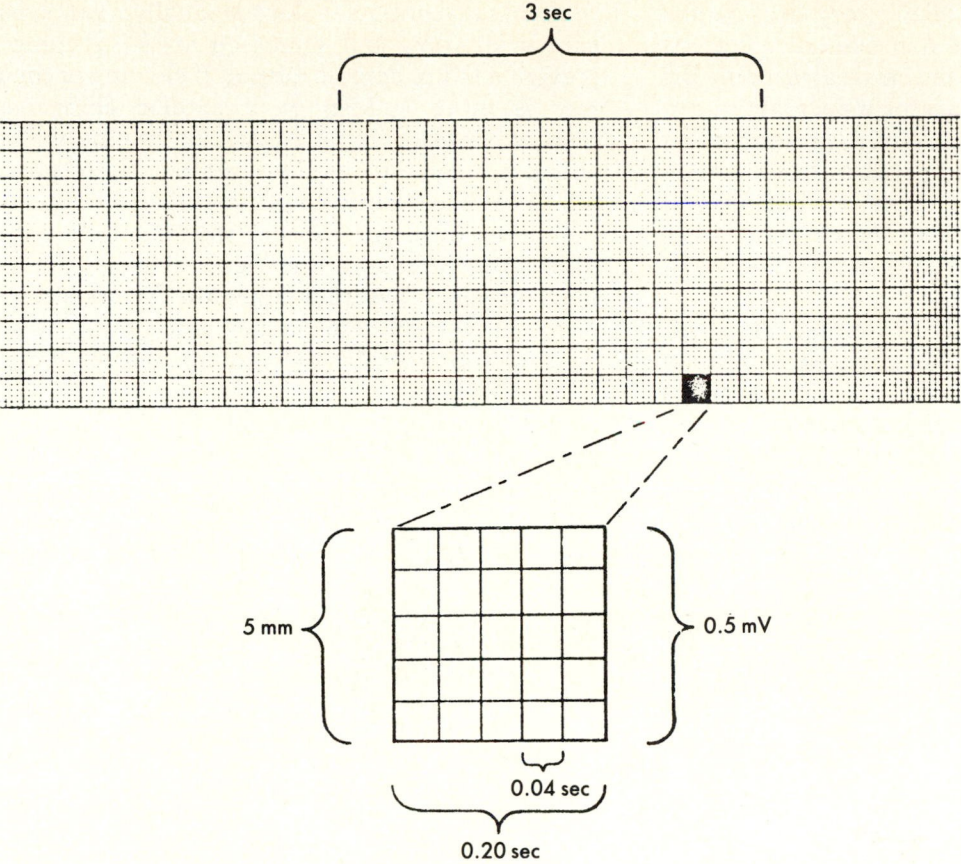

Fig. 3-14 Calculation of time and voltage intervals using electrocardiographic grid paper.

From Conover, M.B.: Understanding electrocardiography: physiological and interpretive concepts, ed. 4, St. Louis, 1984, The C.V. Mosby Co., p. 58.

of the cell and the outside of the cell. The child's serum potassium reflects the extracellular potassium concentration. Any significant changes in the serum potassium concentration can produce arrhythmias. A U wave (a positive deflection in the ECG immediately after the T wave) may be seen in the ECG of the child with hypokalemia.

Hyperkalemia reduces the potassium concentration gradient so the myocardial membrane potential is smaller; a smaller stimulus can excite the myocardium. The ECG of the child with significant hyperkalemia may reflect slow conduction time with an increased Q-T interval or heart block. A peaked T wave may be present. If the child's serum potassium concentration exceeds 7.0 mEq/L, the child is at risk for the development of ventricular fibrillation.[72,390]

Serum hypocalcemia can increase myocardial spontaneous discharge and prolong myocardial repolarization, producing an increase in the child's Q-T interval. Profound hypercalcemia (greater than 15 mg/dl) may produce myocardial rigor.[72]

Hyponatremia enhances calcium myocardial influx, so can increase cardiac contractility. Hypernatremia can, conversely, depress myocardial performance.[390]

Metabolic acidosis also alters myocardial electrochemical events. A fall in extracellular pH can reduce the rate of spontaneous pacemaker firing and the rate of diastolic depolarization. Hypercapnia can produce bigeminy.

Hypoxia reduces the function of the sodium-potassium pump and results in a decrease in the magnitude of the membrane potential. As a result the myocardial conduction time slows, although pacemaker depolarization rate may increase, causing ectopy.[349]

Cardiac surgery. Cardiac surgery can produce arrhythmias because of direct trauma to the conduction tissue at the time of surgery, development of edema of other inflammatory reactions near sutures, or interference with myocardial perfusion. This may produce various forms of heart block and escape rhythms. In addition, myocardial injury or ischemia can produce an irritable focus that causes ectopy.[349]

The arrhythmias that require treatment in the critically ill child are those causing a decrease in cardiac output: bradyarrhythmias (with a ventricular rate less than 70 to 80 beats per minute), tachyarrhythmias (with ventricular rates exceeding 180 to 200 beats per minute), heart block, premature ventricular contractions, or ventricular tachyarrhythmias.

Bradycardia. Bradycardia is defined as a persistent heart rate of less than 100 beats per minute in the infant and less than 80 beats per minute in the child (Fig. 3-15).[429] It is important to note that transient bradycardia can be normal in the neonate, particularly during feeding or sleeping[284,400]; therefore the term "bradycardia" is usually only applied to significant or persistent decreases in an infant's heart rate.

If bradycardia develops gradually, compensatory cardiac dilation and increased stroke volume may prevent a fall in cardiac output. If slowing of the heart rate is more sudden or if cardiac compensatory mechanisms are impaired, stroke volume will probably *not* be able to increase sufficiently to prevent a fall in cardiac output. In addition, a slower heart rate will allow time for "escape" rhythms to be initiated from other areas of the heart (Fig. 3-16). Escape rhythms generated from below the AV node generally result in less efficient cardiac contraction since the ventricles are depolarized through abnormal conduction pathways.

Tachycardia. Tachycardia is defined as a heart rate above 200 beats per minute in an infant and above 140 to 160 beats per minute in a child (Fig. 3-17).[429] Since a transient increase in a neonate's heart rate (up to 200 bearts per minute) can occur with cry-

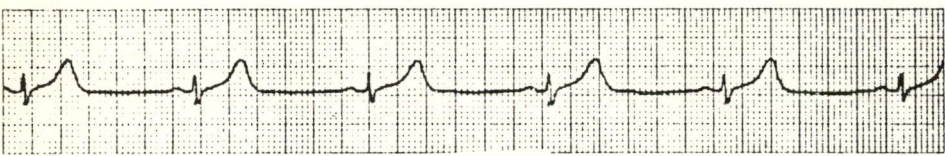

Fig. 3-15 Sinus bradycardia. The heart rate is 48; this is abnormally low for any child. The rhythm is sinus, since all of the P waves are followed by a QRS complex at a regular interval, and each QRS complex is preceded by a P wave of the same configuration. The rhythm is regular. If this rhythm developed in a young patient, the nurse should immediately assess indirect evidence of the child's systemic perfusion to determine if this bradycardia is compromising cardiac output.

From Conover, M.B.: Understanding electrocardiography: physiological and interpretive concepts, ed. 4, St. Louis, 1984, The C.V. Mosby Co., p. 258.

V_1

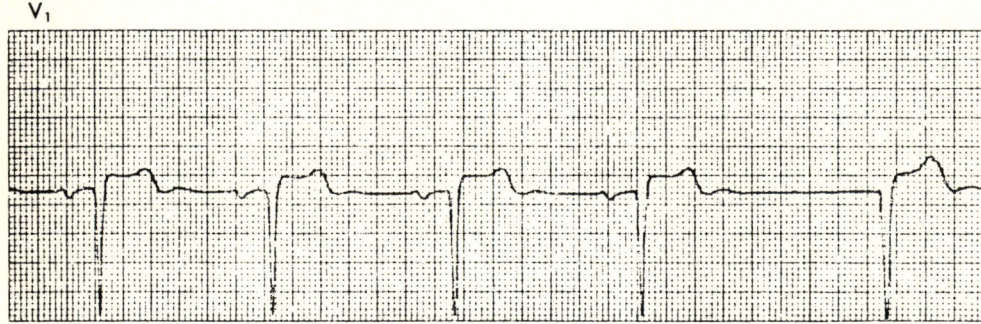

Fig. 3-16 Sinus bradycardia with a junctional escape. The heart rate on this rhythm strip is approximately 48. The first four complexes indicate sinus bradycardia—all of the P waves are of the same configuration, the P-R interval is constant, each P wave is followed by a QRS complex, and each QRS complex is preceded by a P wave. One of the problems with a very slow sinus rhythm is, however, that the long interval between sinus depolarization will allow time for junctional or ventricular escape rhythms to develop. This, in fact, happens in this strip—the fifth complex represents a junctional escape beat. Note that the QRS complex has the same appearance as the previous ones, so the sequence of ventricular depolarization remains unchanged. However, that QRS complex is not preceded by a P wave. It also follows a long pause that is the result of SA node block.

From Conover, M.B.: Understanding electrocardiography: physiological and interpretive concepts, ed. 4, St. Louis, 1984, The C.V. Mosby Co., p. 261.

ing or other activity,[284,400] the term "tachycardia" is usually only applied to significant and persistent increases in an infant's heart rate. Tachycardia normally occurs during periods of increased oxygen requirement, such as exercise. The child's heart rate generally increases 10 beats per minute for each degree centigrade elevation in the child's temperature. In addition, tachycardia will occur if ventricular stroke volume decreases (e.g. with congestive heart failure, tamponade, or low cardiac output).

Although tachycardia may succeed in maintaining cardiac output in the presence of a decrease in stroke volume, it reduces diastolic ventricular filling and coronary perfusion times and increases myocardial oxygen consumption. If the tachyarrhythmia is supraventricular in origin and if some of the impulses are blocked at the AV node, the ventricular rate may not be excessive, and cardiac output may remain adequate (Fig. 3-18). However, if the ventricles depolarize and contract faster than 180 to 200 times per minute,

ventricular diastolic filling time and stroke volume will be seriously impaired, and cardiac output usually falls.[125]

If the tachyarrhythmia is ventricular in origin, cardiac output is usually impaired because the ventricles are depolarized in a less efficient manner and because coronary artery perfusion time is drastically reduced (Fig. 3-19). In addition, because the ventricles do not receive the final filling provided by atrial systole, stroke volume may be critically reduced.

Complete heart block. Complete heart block prevents atrial impulses from being conducted to the ventricles. As a result, the ventricular pacemaker produces ventricular depolarization at a slower rate, independent of atrial activity (Fig. 3-20). Although this may result in increased ventricular diastolic and coronary artery perfusion times, the slow ventricular rate may be inadequate to maintain cardiac output (since cardiac output is the product of heart rate and stroke volume). If ventricular function is impaired,

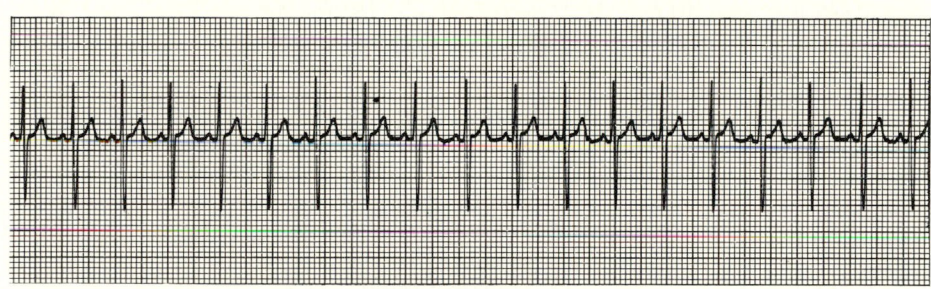

Fig. 3-17 Sinus tachycardia. The heart rate is 168. This represents tachycardia in the 4-year-old child in whom it was observed. The rhythm is very regular. All of the P waves are of the same configuration, and all are followed by a QRS complex. The P-R interval is identical throughout the strip. All of the QRS complexes are of the same configuration, and all are preceded by a P wave.

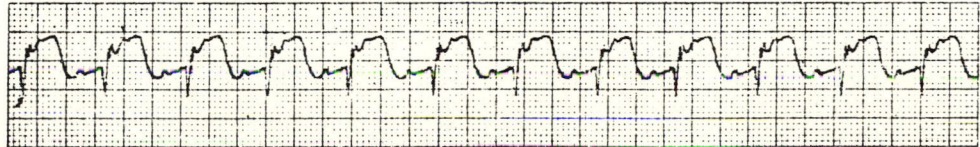

Fig. 3-18 Atrial tachycardia with 2:1 AV conduction. The atrial rate is 200. There are two P waves preceding every QRS complex. One P wave can be seen clearly approximately 0.20 seconds before each QRS complex. The second P wave is actually "buried" or hidden in the S-T segment (it makes the T wave appear biphasic). These P waves all occur at regular intervals, and the QRS complexes appear at regular intervals, with a rate exactly one-half the rate of the atrial complexes—there is 2:1 AV block.

From Conover, M.B.: Understanding electrocardiography: physiological and interpretive concepts, ed. 4, St. Louis, 1984, The C.V. Mosby Co., p. 259.

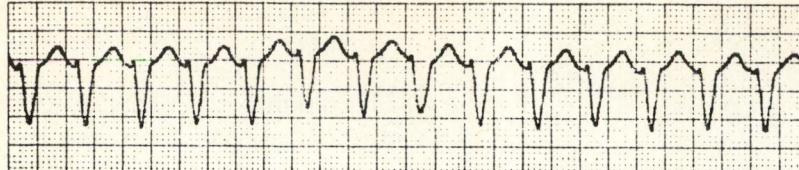

Fig. 3-19 Ventricular tachycardia. The ventricular rate is approximately 135. No P waves are seen. The QRS complexes are wide and regular. This child also demonstrated a significant drop in blood pressure, so required immediate attention.

From Conover, M.B.: Understanding electrocardiography: physiological and interpretive concepts, ed. 4, St. Louis, 1984, The C.V. Mosby Co., p. 103.

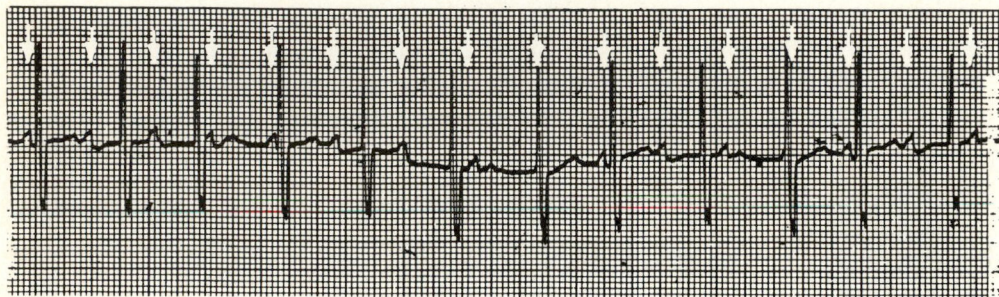

Fig. 3-20 Complete heart block. This infant demonstrated temporary complete heart block following repair of an atrial and ventricular septal defect. The P waves can be seen at very regular intervals throughout the strip *(arrows),* although some of the P waves are "buried" or hidden within the QRS complexes. The atrial rate is approximately 140, and the ventricular rate is approximately 100. The P waves have no consistent temporal relationship to the QRS complexes. The QRS complexes are all narrow and at regular intervals; this indicates that the infant has complete heart block with an idiojunctional rhythm. This patient spontaneously converted to a sinus rhythm 3 days after surgery.

the loss of the extra volume provided by atrial systole (normally 30% of ventricular filling) may reduce stroke volume and result in a further fall in cardiac output. The slow ventricular rate also provides time for ectopic ventricular foci to initiate aberrant rhythms (see the section on premature ventricular contractions that follows).[23]

Premature ventricular contractions (PVCs). Premature ventricular contractions are ectopic depolarizations that originate from the ventricles at a site outside of the normal conduction sequence. Premature ventricular contractions are easily recognized because the ventricular complex is broad, appears earlier than the expected ventricular complex, and has an abnormal T wave that is usually of opposite polarity than the T waves associated with sinus rhythm.

Since premature ventricular contractions represent aberrant cardiac depolarization, the associated cardiac contraction is often less efficient. Premature ventricular contractions are often associated with decreased stroke volume since they abbreviate ventricular diastolic filling and coronary artery perfusion times (Fig. 3-21). Infrequent premature ventricular contractions may be normal.[295]

Frequent or multifocal premature ventricular

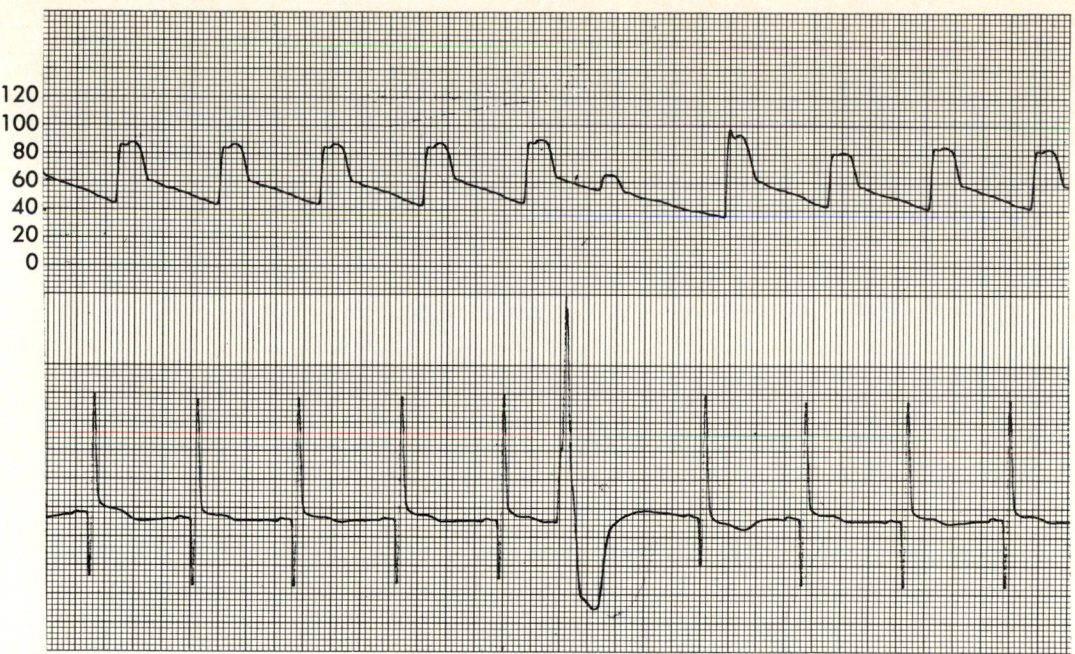

Fig. 3-21 Premature ventricular contraction (PVC). This 3-year-old child demonstrates a sinus rhythm with a heart rate of approximately 85. The arterial pressure tracing is illustrated above the ECG, and some dampening of the waveform is seen. A premature ventricular contraction is seen in approximately the middle of the strip. The QRS complex is early and widened, and the repolarization of the ventricle is aberrant. The effect of the premature ventricular contraction on the child's arterial pressure can be seen immediately above and to the right of the premature ventricular contraction—the child's systolic pressure falls from approximately 84 to 62 mm Hg. There is a compensatory pause following the premature ventricular contraction; the child's normal sinus rhythm then resumes. The systolic pressure associated with the next sinus beat is higher than normal since the ventricles have had a longer time to fill.

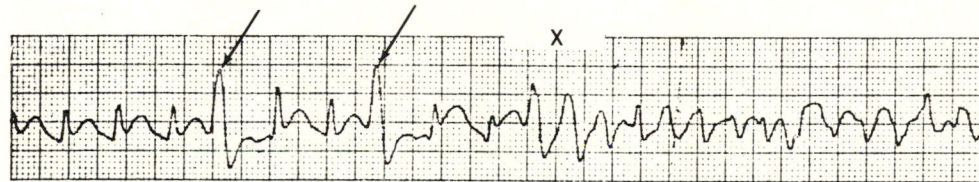

Fig. 3-22 Frequent premature ventricular contractions progressing to ventricular fibrillation. This child has a rapid supraventricular rate of approximately 160 at the beginning of the strip. Two premature ventricular contractions can be seen (*arrows*), which occur early in diastole. When two such premature ventricular contractions occur together (*X*), ventricular fibrillation results. This child required immediate resuscitation.

From Conover, M.B.: Understanding electrocardiography: physiological and interpretive concepts, ed. 4, St. Louis, 1984, The C.V. Mosby Co., p. 267.

contractions may critically reduce cardiac output. In addition, they are worrisome because they indicate the presence of significant ventricular irritability that may progress to ventricular tachycardia or fibrillation (Fig. 3-22).

Ventricular flutter and fibrillation. Ventricular flutter is a very rapid ventricular tachycardia; this rhythm does not allow sufficient time for ventricular filling and results in inadequate cardiac output (Fig. 3-23). Ventricular flutter usually deteriorates rapidly to ventricular fibrillation.

Ventricular fibrillation is characterized by chaotic myocardial electrical activity (see Fig. 3-23). Because myocardial depolarization is not occurring in

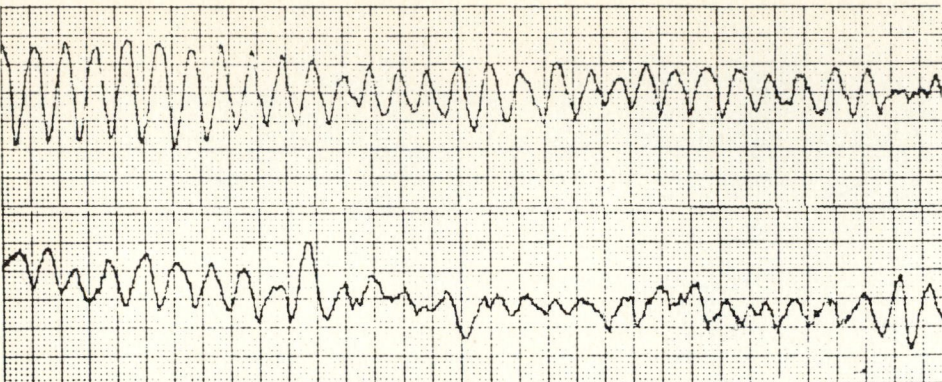

Fig. 3-23 Ventricular fibrillation and flutter. At the top, left corner of the strip, the patient demonstrates a very rapid ventricular tachycardia, which may also be called ventricular flutter. This rapid rhythm soon deteriorates into ventricular fibrillation. This patient required prompt resuscitation and defibrillation.

From Conover, M.B.: Understanding electrocardiography: physiological and interpretive concepts, ed. 4, St. Louis, 1984, The C.V. Mosby Co., p. 105.

any organized fashion, organized cardiac contraction cannot occur. As a result the ventricles quiver and do not pump blood. Ventricular fibrillation is not seen frequently in critically ill children; bradycardia is a more common form of electrocardiographic deterioration.

These rhythms constitute a medical emergency and resuscitation and defibrillation should be instituted promptly. *There is no flow of blood during ventricular flutter or fibrillation unless cardiac massage is performed.*

■ Clinical signs and symptoms

When caring for any critically ill patient, the nurse should ensure that the electrocardiographic monitoring system is functioning properly. Artifacts may be introduced by dry or loose electrodes, damaged electrode cables, or interference from electrical equipment. Too often, physicians are called to see patients with "arrhythmias" that result from such preventable artifacts.

If an arrhythmia is present, the nurse must quickly determine if it interferes with the patient's cardiac output. Appropriate assessment includes vital sign measurement with blood pressure, measurement of urine output, observation of the warmth, color, and capillary filling of the extremities, and comparison of apical cardiac rate with rate and quality of peripheral pulses. If ventricular systole is associated with decreased stroke volume, corresponding peripheral pulses are usually weaker; an arterial pressure tracing may demonstrate such pulse variations (see Fig. 3-21). If ventricular flutter or fibrillation is present, no peripheral pulses will be palpable.

If the cardiac arrhythmia produces persistent inadequate cardiac output so that no peripheral pulses are palpable, cardiopulmonary resuscitation must be initiated immediately. Someone from the resuscitation team should obtain a rhythm strip when possible to document the event.

If the arrhythmia does not produce a life-threatening reduction in systemic perfusion, further assessment and analysis of the patient's rhythm may be performed in a more organized fashion. A representative rhythm strip (including at least a dozen ventricular complexes) should be obtained and a physician should be consulted. Further evaluation of the arrhythmia will require documentation of precipitating or alleviating factors (e.g. suctioning or administration of medications), associated changes in the child's systemic perfusion, timing and dosages of any medications the child is receiving, and documentation of the child's current electrolyte and acid-base balance.

■ Medical treatment and nursing interventions

Arrhythmias that interfere with the child's cardiac output should be treated promptly. When antiarrhythmic therapy is initiated, the nurse must constantly monitor effects of the medication on cardiac rhythm and systemic perfusion. Rhythm strips should be saved and placed in the patient's chart at regular intervals.

If pharmacologic treatment of arrhythmias is required, please note that the dosages of medications provided in this section (Table 3-12) constitute approximate pediatric effective dosage ranges, taken from clinical trials, manufacturers' recommendations, and literature review. These dosages should serve as guidelines only; the correct dose of the drug for the specific patient can only be determined at the bedside. Side and toxic effects of the antiarrhythmic medication should be noted on the child's care plan so they will be detected as soon as they appear. Because some antiarrhythmic medications depress cardiac contractility, it is imperative that careful observation of the child continue throughout therapy.

Bradyarrhythmias may be treated with atropine or isoproterenol; those unresponsive to these medications, including those associated with heart block, will usually require pacemaker therapy. Supraventricular tachyarrhythmias are usually treated with medication, but occasional refractory arrhythmias may require cardioversion, overdrive pacing, or surgical interruption of intracardiac reentrant pathways. Ventricular arrhythmias are initially treated with medications; those arrhythmias unresponsive to medication may also be treated with overdrive pacing. Ventricular fibrillation requires immediate initiation of cardiopulmonary resuscitation and defibrillation.

Pharmacologic treatment of bradycardia. *Atropine* is a belladonna alkaloid that has a vagolytic

Table 3-12 Pediatric antiarrhythmic therapy*

Drug (trade name)	Dose†	Effect	Metabolism/excretion
Atropine	IV: 0.01-0.02 mg/kg/dose Maximum: 0.4 mg	Increases heart rate and AV conduction through anticholinergic effects CAUTION: may also produce decreased heart rate and AV dissociation	Urinary excretion
Digoxin (Lanoxin)	Refer to Table 3-4 for dosage	Decreases SA node rate; decreases atrial automaticity; increases AV nodal conduction time; increases strength of contraction	Renal (60%)
Diphenylhydantoin (Dilantin)	IV: 2-4 mg/kg/dose (over 5 minutes) Oral: 2-8 mg/kg/day Maximum: 500 mg/4 hr	Especially useful in control of digitalis-induced tachyarrhythmias; increases spontaneous depolarization of atria and ventricles; enhances AV nodal conduction; intraventricular conduction usually unchanged CAUTION: may cause bradycardia, decreased myocardial contractility, hypotension, or ventricular fibrillation	Hepatic

Modified from Hazinski, M.F.: Critical care of the pediatric cardiovascular surgical patient, Nurs. Clin. North Am. **16**:688, 1981.
*See references 139, 176, 178, 229, 247, 351, 374, 380, 389, 397, and 414.
†Note: The dosages provided are only approximate ranges taken from literature review. Individual patient problems and response to therapy should always be considered when these drugs are prescribed.

Continued.

Table 3-12 Pediatric antiarrhythmic therapy—cont'd

Drug (trade name)	Dose†	Effect	Metabolism/excretion
Lidocaine (Xylocaine)	IV: bolus: 1 mg/kg/dose Maximum: 5 mg/kg Drip: 10-20 μg/kg/min	Especially useful in treatment of ventricular tachyarrhythmias; depresses spontaneous ventricular depolarization usually does not affect SA or AV node depolarization or conduction rates; may produce seizures in toxic doses	Hepatic
Procainamide (Pronestyl)	IV bolus: 3-10 mg/kg/dose (given over 5 minutes) Maximum bolus: 500 mg IV drip: 20-50 μg/kg/min Oral: 15-50 mg/kg/day	Especially useful in treatment of atrial fibrillation and flutter and premature ventricular contractions; suppresses automaticity in atria and ventricles and depresses AV nodal conduction; does have anticholinergic properties, so moderate doses may cause increased ventricular response to supraventricular tachyarrhythmias CAUTION: may decrease cardiac contractility	Hepatic
Propranolol (Inderal)	IV: 0.01-0.1 mg/kg or 10-100 μg/kg (given over 10 min) Oral: 0.2-8 mg/kg/day	Especially useful in treatment of supraventricular tachycardias; decreases heart rate, conduction, and contractility (beta-adrenergic block); may augment AV block CAUTION: may cause severe bradycardia, AV conduction disturbances, and decreased cardiac contractility (may be contraindicated in patient with severe myocardial dysfunction)	Hepatic

Table 3-12 Pediatric antiarrhythmic therapy—cont'd

Drug (trade name)	Dose†	Effect	Metabolism/ excretion
Quinidine	Oral: 15-60 mg/kg/day	Useful for atrial fibrillation and flutter, as well as for premature ventricular contractions; suppresses automaticity in atria and ventricles and depresses AV nodal conduction; does have anticholinergic properties, so moderate doses may cause increased ventricular response to supraventricular arrhythmias CAUTION: may depress myocardial contractility; may increase serum digoxin levels	Hepatic
Tocainide	No controlled pediatric studies reported; effective adult ranges: 1200-2400 mg/day	An oral amine analog of Lidocaine; suppresses ventricular arrhythmias	Hepatic metabolism and renal excretion
Verapamil (Cordilox)	IV: 0.15-0.25 mg/kg/dose Oral: 20-80 mg/dose every 6-8 hours	Especially useful in treatment of paroxysmal supraventricular tachycardias; blocks slow calcium inward channel (i.e., calcium-mediated slow-channel potential); particularly slows sinus node and AV conduction; may produce hypotension CAUTION: may decrease cardiac contractility; verapamil administration may decrease renal clearance of digoxin, producing increased serum digoxin levels and possible digoxin toxicity in those patients who are concurrently receiving verapamil and digoxin (so digoxin dose may need adjustment); contraindicated in patients with myocardial dysfunction or those receiving beta-blockers	Hepatic (80%)

effect; its administration produces an increase in SA node discharge and increased rate of AV nodal conduction.[380] The IV pediatric dose of atropine is approximately 0.01 to 0.02 mg/kg to a maximum of 0.4 mg (see Table 3-12).

Isoproterenol is a sympathomimetic amine with beta$_1$- and beta$_2$-adrenergic effects. Continuous IV drip doses of 0.05 to 0.1 μg/kg/minute generally produce an increase in the child's heart rate (see Table 3-11).

Pacemaker therapy. Several forms of pacemaker therapy are currently available for use in children. The type of pacemaker used will be determined by the experience and preference of the pediatric cardiologist and surgeon. The following discussion pertains to the more common "demand" external pacemakers most frequently used for temporary pacing in the critical-care unit (see the section on pacemakers in Chapter 9 also).[275]

A demand pacemaker allows the child's intrinsic cardiac rhythm to continue, provided that the child's ventricular rate equals or exceeds the rate at which the pacemaker is set. If the child's ventricular rate falls below the pacemaker rate, the pacemaker will initiate an electrical impulse (Fig. 3-24). A demand pacemaker may initiate an atrial impulse, a ventricular impulse, or both. Simple atrial pacemakers require that the child's AV conduction system be intact, as they only provide an atrial electrical impulse if the child's ventricular rate falls. Because ventricular demand pacemakers provide only ventricular electrical impulses, a paced rate will be generated in the ventricles if the child's ventricular rate falls below the pacemaker rate. With ventricular pacing, ventricular depolarization will proceed regardless of atrial electrical activity; as a result ventricular contraction occurring as a result of ventricular pacing will often occur without the additional ventricular filling provided by atrial systole.

Another type of demand pacemaker is called the AV sequential pacemaker, which can provide both atrial and ventricular impulses in sequence. This pacemaker consists of a ventricular sensing component, an atrial stimulator, and a ventricular stimulator. The stimulators can both be inhibited by patient-initiated ventricular impulses. If the child's *ventricular* rate falls below the pacemaker rate, the pacemaker will provide an atrial impulse (whether or not patient atrial activity is present). Following generation of the atrial impulse, the pacemaker waits a preset interval (this is set by the physician as a "P-R interval" and usually ranges between 0.16 to 0.25 sec-

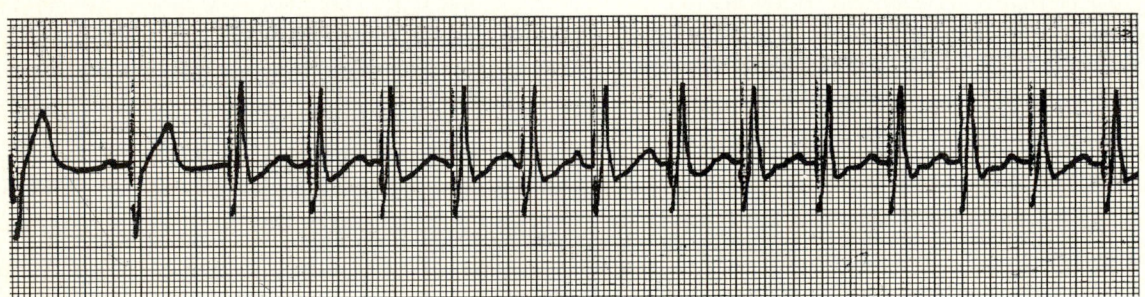

Fig. 3-24 Ventricular demand pacing. This child has temporary pacing wires in place following cardiovascular surgery; these wires were attached to an external ventricular pacer that was set at a demand rate of 130. The first complete complex seen on the strip is sinus rhythm. No pacer firing is seen since the pacemaker is appropriately inhibited by the patient's own ventricular depolarization. Following the sinus beat, a pause is seen; because the ventricular sensing wire did not sense any ventricular depolarization, the pacemaker fires. Pacemaker firing is indicated by the presence of a very narrow spike; if the pacemaker is "capturing" the ventricle appropriately, each narrow pacer spike should be followed by a wider QRS complex, which indicates the ventricular depolarization in response to the pacer. In the remainder of the strip, the pacemaker is "pacing" the ventricle.

onds). If the pacemaker does not sense a patient-initiated ventricular impulse within that "P-R interval," the pacemaker will generate a ventricular electrical impulse (Fig. 3-25). Thus the normal sequence of atrial and ventricular depolarization, including appropriate P-R interval, may be maintained. It is important to note that AV sequential pacemakers will be suppressed if the patient has junctional or ventricular tachycardia since ventricular impulses at a rate faster than the pacemaker rate will inhibit both atrial *and* ventricular pacemaker activity.[246]

A second form of AV sequential pacemaker has recently been developed that has both atrial and ventricular sensors *and* stimulators. With this form of pacemaker, patient atrial impulses can inhibit the atrial stimulator, and ventricular impulses can inhibit the ventricular stimulator.

A "fixed" pacemaker is another type of pace-maker; it is used infrequently in children. This pacemaker fires at a set rate, regardless of patient cardiac electrical activity. Some external pacemakers may be set at either a "demand" or a "fixed" (or "asynchronous") mode; generally the demand mode is preferable since it will not compete with the child's intrinsic cardiac rhythm.

If an external pacemaker is used, the following information should be recorded on the vital sign sheet at least every 8 hours: pacemaker mode (demand or fixed), demand rate, sensitivity (should be set to maximum levels if demand pacing is desired), and pacemaker electrical output (in milliamperes [ma]). The nurse should also note if the pacer is turned "off" or "on," how frequently the patient is "paced," and the child's underlying rhythm. The physician should check the patient's myocardial threshold (the minimum pacemaker electrical stimulus that will consis-

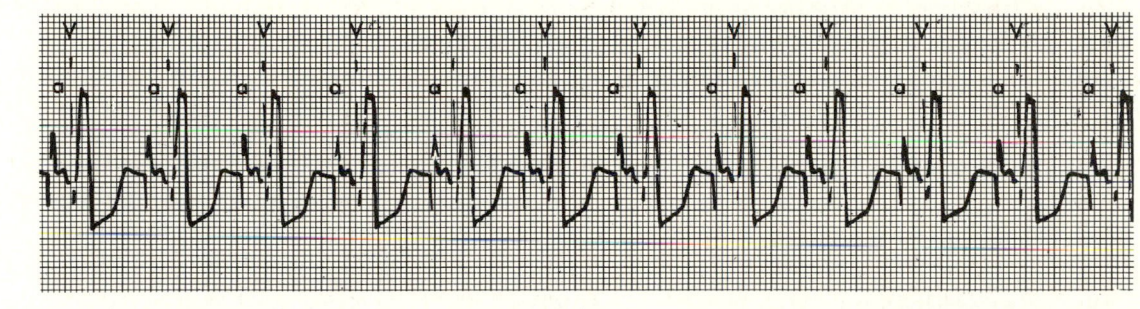

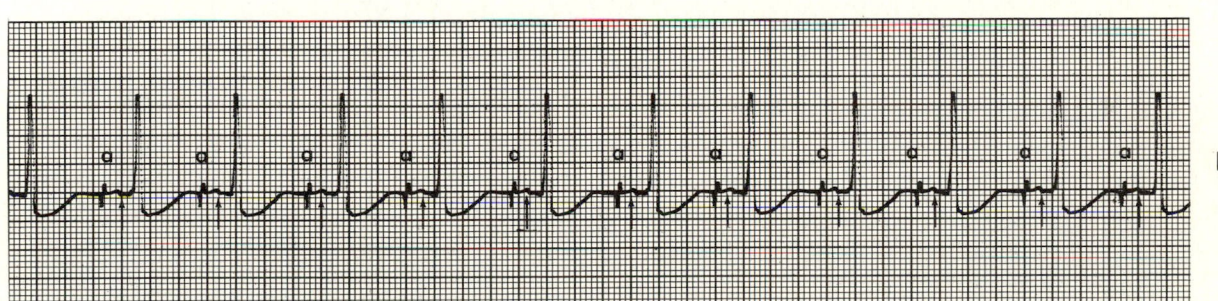

Fig. 3-25 Atrioventricular (AV) sequential pacing. **A,** This strip demonstrates both components of AV sequential pacing. The ventricular demand rate is 90. The AV interval (also called the PR interval) is preset at 0.18 seconds. When the pacemaker does not sense a ventricular depolarization within an adequate interval (consistent with a rate of 90), an *atrial* impulse is generated—this spike appears as a short, narrow biphasic complex *(a)*. Following the atrial impulse, if the pacemaker does not sense a ventricular depolarization within 0.18 seconds, a *ventricular* impulse is generated—this ventricular impulse appears as a taller, narrow spike *(v)*, which is followed immediately by ventricular depolarization. **B,** This strip demonstrates atrial pacing. This patient's AV conduction is intact, so atrial pacing is followed by ventricular depolarization. The pacemaker demand rate is 90 (these pacemakers are accurate to within 10% to 15% of the demand rate set). When the pacemaker does not sense a ventricular depolarization within the appropriate interval, an *atrial* impulse is initiated *(a)*. The pacemaker AV (or PR) interval is 0.20 seconds; because the patient's junctional tissue depolarizes within that interval, the pacemaker does *not* generate a ventricular impulse. This AV sequential pacemaker does not have an atrial sensing component; if it did, even the atrial impulse might be inhibited since the patient demonstrates regular atrial depolarization *(arrow)*.

tently produce a cardiac electrical response) every morning; this threshold should be noted on the vital sign sheet and the pacemaker electrical output set accordingly. All pacemaker wires should be kept covered and dry, and the pacemaker dials *must* be protected with a "childproof" cover.

If the pacemaker is functioning properly, the patient's heart rate should *never* fall below the set pacemaker rate (some pacemakers have an accuracy of ±15% of the set pacemaker rate). In addition, each "paced" electrical impulse on the ECG should be followed by the patient's (atrial or ventricular) cardiac response (see Fig. 3-24). If the child's ventricular rate is consistently faster than the pacemaker rate, no pacemaker spikes (impulses) should be visible because the demand pacemaker should be inhibited by the child's ventricular activity. If pacemaker activity or the child's cardiac response is inappropriate, the pacemaker settings and the integrity of the external wires and connections should be rechecked. The nurse must also obtain patient vital signs and a rhythm strip and note the effect of the apparent pacemaker malfunction on the child's heart rate, blood pressure, and systemic perfusion. A physician should be notified.

Pacemaker malfunction may be caused by internal equipment failure, battery failure, a faulty connection between the pacemaker and pacing wires, increased epicardial or endocardial impedance, or pacing wire fracture or dislodgement.

The nurse must keep in mind that *the presence of a satisfactory heart rate on the cardiac monitor does not ensure effective cardiac contraction and cardiac output.* Frequently, with severe cardiovascular collapse, a pacemaker will continue to provide electrical stimuli (possibly interpreted by older digital cardiac monitors as adequate heart rate), despite inadequate cardiac response. In addition, a ventricular demand pacemaker will continue to fire even if the patient develops ventricular fibrillation—the fibrillation may be difficult to recognize on the ECG because the pacemaker spikes will be superimposed at regular intervals. When the critically ill child requires pacemaker therapy, the nurse must not only ensure the proper functioning of the pacemaker but must continue to monitor the child's cardiovascular function.

Antiarrhythmic medications for supraventricular tachycardia. Supraventricular tachycardia that results in a fall in the child's cardiac output or other significant symptoms requires treatment. Pharmacologic therapy is most often used (see Table 3-12); if this is unsuccessful, cardioversion, overdrive pacing, or surgical interruption of accessory AV conduction pathways may be required. These latter methods will be discussed in the next section.

Digoxin (Lanoxin) is still the drug of choice for initial treatment of supraventricular arrhythmias. Digoxin not only has direct effects on the myocardium, but it interacts with portions of the autonomic nervous system. Digoxin slows the heart rate through vagal effect on the SA node.[414] Because digitalis administration also hypopolarizes atrial cells, a larger stimulus is required to initiate atrial depolarization. Digoxin also slows AV conduction and prolongs the effective refractory period (Table 3-4).[139]

Procainamide (Pronestyl) is useful in the treatment of a wide variety of pediatric dysrhythmias, including atrial fibrillation and flutter and premature ventricular contractions. Procainamide given intravenously is especially effective in controlling reentrant tachycardia.[389] An indirect vagolytic (anticholinergic) effect of procainamide may produce increased sinus node firing and AV node conduction and an increase in ventricular response to atrial tachycardias.[139] Procainamide may be administered intravenously in intermittent doses (3 to 10 mg/kg/dose) or by continuous infusion (20 to 50 μg/kg/minute). Most frequently it is administered orally (15 to 50 mg/kg/day divided into four to six doses). Indirect evidence of the child's systemic perfusion should be monitored carefully since reduced cardiac contractility may result as a side effect of this drug. Another significant and not infrequent complication of chronic procainamide administration in children is the development of a syndrome similar to lupus erythematosis, which usually disappears if procainamide therapy is discontinued.[139]

Propranolol (Inderal) is a beta-adrenergic blocking agent. It depresses impulse formation and membrane responsiveness, slows AV conduction, and increases the refractory period. Propranolol is especially useful in treatment of supraventricular tachycardia that arises from adrenergic stimulation (including anxiety and exercise) or anesthesia. The usual pediatric IV dose of propranolol is 0.01 to 0.1 mg/kg/dose. Since gastrointestinal absorption is variable, oral administration is used infrequently. A significant and potentially harmful effect of this drug is that it may significantly depress cardiac contractility; this may result in reduced cardiac output. As a result use of propranolol is often contraindicated in children immediately following cardiovascular surgery.

Quinidine is also useful in the treatment of a wide variety of pediatric arrhythmias. Its action and effect are very similar to those of procainamide, although quinidine seems to have a more significant depressant effect on the myocardium (negative inotropic effect).[384] Quinidine is administered orally in doses of 15 to 60 mg/kg/day. Gastrointestinal dysfunction, particularly diarrhea, thrombocytopenia, fever, dermatitis, and hepatotoxicity are among the reported side effects.[139]

Verapamil (Cordilox) is a relatively new pediatric antiarrhythmic drug that blocks the slow inward movement of calcium (it does not seem to alter the rapid inward movement of sodium) during depolarization. As a result verapamil is most effective in slowing impulse formation in the sinus node and conduction through the AV node.[110,397] Verapamil is especially effective in treating paroxysmal supraventricular tachycardia, including that caused by Wolff-Parkinson-White syndrome.[373] It is not effective in the treatment of atrial flutter[374] or ventricular arrhythmias. If verapamil is administered intravenously, doses totaling 0.15 to 0.25 mg/kg are administered in increments or as a single dose; effects of this drug are usually apparent within minutes. Oral verapamil may be administered in doses of 20 to 80 mg given every 6 to 8 hours (this requires ingestion of several tablets). Side effects of verapamil therapy in children include hypotension, bradycardia, heart block, and asystole.[139] The development of asystole is more likely if verapamil is administered to the child who is already receiving beta blocking agents. In addition, verapamil administration in adults has been found to produce decreased renal excretion of digoxin. As a result, if the child is concurrently receiving digoxin and verapamil, the digoxin dose may have to be reduced, and the child should be watched closely for signs of digitalis toxicity.[229]

Other treatment for supraventricular tachycardia. Vagal stimulation (by gagging) or unilateral carotid massage may also be attempted to interrupt supraventricular tachycardia.[167] Application of ice or cold water to the infant's face may also terminate episodes of supraventricular tachycardia because the "diving reflex" is stimulated; this primitive reflex produces bradycardia. Administration of ocular pressure is not recommended since it may cause retinal detachment in infants.

Cardioversion is the application of synchronized external electrical current to the heart directly or through the chest wall to depolarize any excitable cardiac fibers and to allow the SA node to reinstitute normal sinus rhythm. A defibrillator with a synchronizer is used to provide the DC electric current. Cardioversion is used to convert children with atrial flutter or fibrillation unresponsive to medical management to a sinus rhythm. Since the incidence of postcardioversion arrhythmias is significantly increased if the child is receiving digitalis, the drug is usually discontinued 24 to 48 hours before cardioversion. The current required for cardioversion is generally 1 to 2 watt-seconds/kg; this dose may be repeated and increased if the child does not respond to the initial current. If the child has received digoxin recently, the initial current is usually reduced.

The child generally receives sedation or general anesthesia during cardioversion. The nurse should monitor for arrhythmias during the cardioversion and immediately after the procedure.

Overdrive pacing for treatment of tachyarrhythmias uses a programmable pacemaker to slowly gain control of the child's rhythm and then slow the heart rate. Transvenous or epicardial pacing wires may be used; these are attached to a programmable pacemaker that provides rapid stimuli at a rate faster than the child's tachyarrhythmia. Once the pacemaker is controlling the child's rhythm, the pacemaker firing rate may be gradually reduced or abruptly terminated. Cessation of pacemaker stimulus should allow the child's sinus node to resume control of the rhythm at an acceptable rate.[127] These programmable pacemakers may also be implanted for patient-activated termination of recurrent tachyarrhythmias.[100,177]

Surgical interruption of multiple intraatrial conduction and reentrant pathways may be required if the child's supraventricular tachycardia is unresponsive to any other treatment and if this tachycardia is producing significant cardiovascular compromise. Surgical treatment requires use of cardiopulmonary bypass and open-heart surgery. Conduction system mapping is performed once the right atrium is opened, and accessory pathways are identified and divided. Postoperative care is similar to that following any open-heart surgery (see the section on postoperative care in this chapter).[145]

Antiarrhythmic medications for ventricular arrhythmias. *Lidocaine* (Xylocaine) is extremely effective in the treatment of ventricular irritability. It slows conduction, abolishes reentrant arrhythmias, and depresses automaticity. An IV bolus of 1 mg/kg/dose may be administered and repeated (maximum total dose: 5 mg/kg), or a continuous drip of 10 to 20 μg/kg/minute may be given. Since lidocaine is metabolized by the liver, a reduction in dose should be considered when the child has hepatic dysfunction. Toxic effects of lidocaine administration include mental confusion or lethargy, slurred speech, seizures, and diplopia. Lidocaine does not seem to depress myocardial function significantly.[139]

Tocainide is an oral amine analog of lidocaine that has been effective in controlling refractory ventricular arrhythmias in children in limited clinical trials. It is especially suitable for children requiring long-term therapy.[247,351] Complications of tocainide therapy include central nervous system symptoms (ataxia, paresthesia, dizziness, anxiety, tremor), nausea, and allergic symptoms (fever, pruritus, rash).

Procainamide may also be effective in the treatment of ventricular arrhythmias. It may be administered in intermittent or continuous IV doses, or it may be administered orally. Dosages and side effects have been discussed previously (see the section on antiarrhythmic medications for supraventricular tachycardia).[155]

Defibrillation and overdrive pacing. Cardiac massage and emergency deliverance of an external AC or DC electric current is required immediately for the child with ventricular fibrillation. It is hoped that application of sufficient current will produce simultaneous depolarization (and, subsequently, repolarization) of all excitable myocardial cells so that an ordered cardiac rhythm can resume. Because defibrillation is less likely to be effective if the child is acidotic and/or hypoxemic, resuscitative efforts must be prompt and thorough before and between defibrillation attempts. DC current is usually more effective than AC current if the child is hypoxic. The American Heart Association recommends use of 2 watt-seconds/kg/attempt but notes that this dose may be doubled if the initial current is ineffective.[63]

Defibrillation can also be accomplished by the use of an implanted defibrillator. This unit has been provided for those patients at high risk for the development of sudden arrhythmias and fibrillation.

Overdrive pacing with an external or an implanted programmable pacemaker may be used to treat refractory ventricular arrhythmias unresponsive to medical management. The principles of overdrive pacing have been discussed previously (see the sections on other treatment of supraventricular tachycardia and overdrive pacing).

■ **HYPOXEMIA (ARTERIAL OXYGEN DESATURATION)**
■ **Etiology**

Definition. Cyanosis is the blue color that may be observed in the mucous membranes, nail beds, skin, and/or sclera of the child with arterial oxygen desaturation. Cyanosis is usually not visible until there are at least 5 gm of reduced hemoglobin (hemoglobin not bound with oxygen) per 100 ml of blood. This usually correlates to an arterial oxygen saturation of 75% to 85%. Since the degree of cyanosis visible is dependent upon both the total amount of hemoglobin present and its saturation, cyanosis itself is not a reliable indicator of the degree of hypoxemia present. An anemic patient may be profoundly hypoxemic before cyanosis is observed, and a polycythemic patient may appear extremely cyanotic at only modest levels of arterial oxygen desaturation. In addition, the detection of cyanosis depends on the

experience of the observer and the ambient lighting conditions. Mildly cyanotic children can appear extremely cyanotic when they are surrounded by blue linen and acyanotic when surrounded by pink linen.

Acrocyanosis, or peripheral cyanosis, is observed in the extremities and around the mouth of the newborn but does not involve the mucous membranes or nailbeds. Acrocyanosis is normal in the newborn and is considered the result of vasomotor instability. It generally disappears when the child is swaddled (to produce increased warmth) or becomes more active.[347]

Causes of hypoxemia in children. Since arterial oxygen desaturation can be caused by either cardiac or respiratory disease, it is important for the nurse to carefully document the distribution and degree of cyanosis, as well as any precipitating or alleviating factors. Cyanosis that *decreases* with cry is generally thought to be *respiratory* in origin and is relieved by the increase in tidal volume during vigorous cry. Cyanosis that *increases* with cry is usually *cardiac* in origin since the expiratory phase of crying tends to increase resistance to pulmonary blood flow and enhance right-to-left intracardiac shunting in the presence of cyanotic heart disease. Cyanosis that is respiratory in origin usually improves with oxygen administration; cyanosis that is cardiac in origin does not (since the intracardiac shunt allows blood to pass into the systemic circulation without ever entering the lungs).[51] The child with cyanosis resulting from respiratory disease will often demonstrate other signs of respiratory distress, including tachypnea and increased respiratory effort (retractions, nasal flaring, and grunting). The child with cyanosis resulting from heart disease may also be tachypneic but will usually not demonstrate signs of increased respiratory effort unless congestive heart failure or acidosis are also present.

To aid in differentiation of respiratory versus cardiac causes of cyanosis, physicians may obtain an arterial blood gas specimen when the child is breathing room air and then obtain an arterial blood gas specimen when the child is receiving 100% oxygen. If the child's arterial oxygen tension increases by more than 20 torr or rises above 200 torr while breathing 100% oxygen, the cyanosis is probably respiratory in origin. If the child's oxygen tension does *not* increase appreciably with administration of oxygen, the cyanosis is probably cardiac in origin.[300] Since the child with cyanotic congenital heart disease has intracardiac shunts, some systemic venous blood bypasses the lungs and that shunted blood is never exposed to the increased alveolar (inspired) oxygen concentration.

When the child has cyanotic heart disease,

venous (deoxygenated) blood is entering the systemic (arterial) circulation. This can occur because of: (1) severe obstruction to right heart or pulmonary flow and shunting of blood from the right to the left side of the heart (or from pulmonary artery to aorta), (2) mixing of arterial and venous blood within the heart or great vessels, or (3) transposition of the great vessels. The specific cardiac defects that cause cyanosis are discussed in the fourth section of this chapter. The following discussion summarizes the potential systemic consequences of arterial oxygen desaturation and medical and nursing interventions.

■ **Pathophysiology**

Chronic arterial oxygen desaturation stimulates erythropoiesis (red blood cell production), resulting in polycythemia. Perinatal polycythemia is normal, and the neonate may have a hematocrit as high as 65% within the first hours of life (particularly if the umbilical cord was "milked" toward the infant before being cut). Within the first weeks of life, however, if the hematocrit does not fall, polycythemia is present.

Digital clubbing (rounding and enlargement of the tips of fingers and toes) occurs after several weeks or months of chronic hypoxemia. The mechanism that causes clubbing is poorly understood but is thought to be related to abnormal peripheral circulation secondary to the hypoxemia and polycythemia.

When polycythemia is present, the viscosity of the blood is increased. The development of microcytic anemia further increases the viscosity of the blood and red blood cells[249]; this increases the child's risk of thromboembolic events. The incidence of spontaneous cerebrovascular accidents among children with cyanotic congenital heart disease is approximately 1.6%. The risk is highest among those patients less than 4 years of age with a mean hematocrit above 60%, a mean hemoglobin concentration of approximately 20 gm/dl, and microcytic anemia (a low mean corpuscular hemoglobin concentration and/or mean corpuscular volume).

Approximately 2% of children with cyanotic congenital heart disease develop brain abscess. The incidence is highest in children over 2 years of age and in those children with tetralogy of Fallot or transposition of the great vessels. The development of a brain abscess is rare in children before the age of 2 years.[126] The pathophysiology of brain abscess formation is not completely understood, but it seems to be related to an episode of bacteremia and some compromise in cerebral microcirculation.[387]

Children with polycythemia and chronic hypoxemia also demonstrate a hemorrhagic diathesis,

which may produce severe postoperative bleeding. They may demonstrate thrombocytopathia with or without thrombocytopenia since platelet survival time is shorter[405,434] and platelet aggregation is significantly reduced.[108] Synthesis of vitamin K-dependent clotting factors in the liver is also impaired, but does not improve with administration of vitamin K.[183]

The risk of bacterial endocarditis is increased for children with congenital heart disease, particularly when the child has a ventricular septal defect, aortic stenosis, or a systemic-to-pulmonary communication. Tetralogy of Fallot is associated with a significant portion of reported cases of bacterial endocarditis in children.[141]

Vascular shear stresses are increased when blood viscosity increases. As a result pulmonary vascular resistance increases as the hematocrit rises, especially when pulmonary blood flow is reduced and the hematocrit approaches 60%.[307] A significant number of children with transposition of the great vessels have been shown to develop increased pulmonary vascular resistance within 1 year, even if pulmonary blood flow is normal. It is thought that these vascular changes are related to the shear stresses and the development of pulmonary microemboli. Thus children with cyanotic heart disease and polycythemia may develop pulmonary hypertension whether their pulmonary blood flow is decreased, normal, or increased.[301,305,306]

Approximately 40% of children with cyanotic heart disease may demonstrate paroxysmal hypercyanotic episodes.[168] These episodes can be very frightening to observe because the child suddenly becomes deeply cyanotic and hyperpneic and may lose consciousness or develop seizures because of acute hypoxemia. In children with tetralogy of Fallot, these episodes are called "tet" spells and are considered the result of a sudden spasm of the child's pulmonary infundibulum with a dramatic fall in pulmonary blood flow and an increase in the right-to-left intracardiac shunt. In children with other forms of cyanotic heart disease, the spells are not readily explained but seem to be related to an acute increase in oxygen requirement; because the child has a fixed right-to-left intracardiac shunt, the child is unable to significantly increase his arterial oxygen content and so may develop an oxygen debt, becoming acutely hypoxemic. Blood gas analysis obtained in children during hypercyanotic episodes has shown arterial oxygen saturations as low as 15% to 33%. The development of spells is not correlated with the degree of cyanosis or the child's hematocrit and is noted most commonly during the first year of life. The spells occur most commonly during the morning and are most frequently precipitated by crying, defecation, or feeding.[289] Since these spells reflect the development of profound hypoxemia and seem to be associated with cerebral hypoxia, the child who develops hypercyanotic spells requires urgent medical attention and is usually scheduled immediately for surgical treatment of the congenital defect.

■ Clinical signs and symptoms

The child with cyanotic heart disease is *hypoxemic* (has a lower arterial oxygen tension than normal) but is not necessarily *hypoxic*. Since polycythemia increases the oxygen-carrying capacity of the blood, the child's arterial *oxygen content* may be adequate. Using the equations discussed in the case study in the second section of this chapter (see Fick cardiac output on p. 93), the reader may wish to calculate a 10 kg child's oxygen content when the child's arterial oxygen saturation is 79% and hemoglobin concentration is 16 gm/dl; the reader should then compare this to the same child's arterial oxygen content when his arterial oxygen saturation is 87% but his hemoglobin concentration is only 10 mg/dl.

The signs of deterioration in the child with cyanotic heart disease include deterioration in clinical appearance (development of pallor, increased respiratory distress, gasping respirations, lethargy, and evidence of decreased systemic perfusion), development of acidosis, and/or a significant fall in the child's arterial oxygen tension (less than normal for that child or to less than 30 torr).[51] The cyanosis will increase with cry and will not disappear with oxygen administration.

The child's hemoglobin and hematocrit should be checked since the development of anemia can significantly reduce the child's arterial oxygen-carrying capacity and oxygen content and can increase the child's risk of thromboembolic events,[249] particularly the development of cerebrovascular accident.[333] Signs of cerebral vascular accident include sudden onset of paralysis, paresthesia, altered speech, seizure, and extreme irritability or lethargy.

Signs and symptoms of brain abscess formation can be extremely vague. Therefore it is necessary for medical personnel to be aware of the risk of brain abscess in these children, particularly during episodes of bacteremia. Signs of brain abscess can include seizures, focal neurologic abnormalities, fever, nausea, vomiting, headache, or signs of increased intracranial pressure.[264]

If significant polycythemia is present, the child's coagulation profile will be abnormal; his clotting time will be prolonged, fibrinogen may be re-duced, and vitamin K-dependent clotting factors will be reduced.[183]

If the cyanotic child develops hypercyanotic episodes, it is important that the nursing staff recognize the spells immediately, notify a physician, and begin treatment immediately, since these spells may produce cerebral hypoxia with resultant brain damage or death. The cyanotic spell will often occur in the morning, following a good night's sleep. The child may become deeply cyanotic following feeding, a bowel movement, or vigorous crying. Often the child is diaphoretic, irritable, and hyperpneic, and he may soon lose consciousness and become limp. Many children sleep deeply following the spells.[289] Treatment of these hypercyanotic episodes is discussed in the following section.

When cyanotic heart disease is suspected in the newborn, a chest x-ray examination (possibly with barium swallow) and a 12-lead ECG will be performed. Careful physical examination may reveal a murmur characteristic of a specific cyanotic defect and will reveal the presence or absence of concurrent congestive heart failure or poor systemic perfusion. A hyperoxygen test may be administered, and an M-mode and 2-dimensional echocardiogram are usually performed immediately. Cardiac catheterization is performed if cyanosis is observed within the first days of life (see the section on diagnostic tests in this chapter).

■ Medical treatment and nursing interventions

The following discussion will focus on supportive measures that maximize the child's arterial oxygen content and minimize the child's risk of systemic consequences of chronic arterial oxygen desaturation and polycythemia. Surgical repair of specific forms of cyanotic congenital heart disease will be discussed in the section on specific diseases in this chapter.

As with any critically ill child, it is important that the nurse be able to immediately recognize changes in the child's condition. As discussed in the previous section, signs of deterioration in the child with cyanotic heart disease include increased severity or distribution of cyanosis, increased respiratory rate or effort (including gasping respirations), irritability or lethargy, a significant fall in the arterial oxygen saturation (from the child's normal level), and the development of acidosis. These changes must be brought to the attention of a physician immediately. Metabolic acidosis, poor systemic perfusion, or respiratory failure must be treated promptly (see the section on low cardiac output in this chapter and the section on respiratory failure in Chapter 4).

If the neonate is dependent upon the ductus arteriosus to provide pulmonary blood flow, prostaglandin E_1 will be administered. When the child with cyanotic heart disease deteriorates despite aggressive medical management, urgent surgical intervention is usually indicated.

If the child develops a hypercyanotic spell, the child should be placed in the knee-chest position immediately. This position often improves pulmonary blood flow and relieves the hypercyanotic episode for reasons that are not clear. This position seems to increase resistance to systemic arterial flow (by kinking the femoral arteries).[336] Oxygen is administered during these episodes to produce pulmonary vasodilation and possibly improve pulmonary blood flow. Intravenous morphine sulfate (0.1 mg/kg/dose) or propranolol (0.15 to 0.25 mg/kg/dose, which is given slowly and which may be repeated once)[48] is often administered with physician order in an attempt to reduce pulmonary infundibular muscle spasm (if tetralogy of Fallot is present).

The child with cyanotic heart disease and polycythemia should not be allowed to become dehydrated, since this can cause hemoconcentration and result in an increase in the child's hematocrit and blood viscosity, increasing the child's risk of spontaneous thromboembolic events. If the cyanotic child is returning home, the parents should be taught to seek medical attention immediately if the child develops a fever, vomiting, or diarrhea since these can rapidly result in dehydration. When the child is hospitalized for diagnostic tests or surgery, the child's level of hydration should be evaluated frequently and carefully. The infant's fontanelle should not be sunken, mucous membranes should be moist, and tearing should be present with cry in infants older than approximately 8 weeks. Skin turgor should be good, and the eyes should not appear sunken. If the infant is placed "NPO" for tests and surgery, the nurse should monitor the length of time the child is without fluid intake. If this period is longer than a few hours, an IV line may be started to provide the child with fluids.

Since the child with cyanotic heart disease has some systemic venous blood directly entering the child's systemic arterial circulation, *absolutely no air can be allowed in the child's IV line* since any air can produce a cerebral air embolus. The entire length of the IV line should be checked frequently for air, and tubing connections should be taped securely. Any air in injection ports or stopcocks must be carefully removed. Even if the child's IV line is regulated by an infusion pump with an "air in line" alarm, this alarm cannot be counted on to detect small amounts of air.

Since anemia reduces the child's arterial oxygen-carrying capacity and since microcytic anemia increases the cyanotic child's risk of cerebrovascular accident, the child's hemoglobin, hematocrit, mean corpuscular volume, and mean corpuscular hemoglobin concentration should be monitored. Iron supplements or blood transfusions (see Table 3-10) should be administered as needed.

If the cyanotic child develops a fever, bacteremia should be suspected. Blood cultures may be ordered, and antibiotic prophylaxis may be administered. If the cyanotic child is returning home, the child's parents and primary physician should both be aware of the necessity of administration of antibiotic prophylaxis surrounding times of risk of bacteremia, including any minor or dental surgery, high fever, or exposure to other ill individuals. Dosages of penicillin antibiotic prophylaxis are listed in Table 3-13. Antibiotic administration for prevention or prompt treatment of bacteremia should reduce the child's risk of bacterial endocarditis and brain abscess formation.

If the cyanotic neonate has a ductus-dependent cyanotic congenital heart defect (so most or all of the child's pulmonary blood flow flows through the ductus arteriosus), prostaglandin E_1 or E_2 will be administered intravenously. Prostaglandins are endogenous lipids with a variety of systemic effects.[317] IV administration of exogenous prostaglandin E_1 (PGE_1 or Prostin VR) has been found to produce vasodilation and smooth muscle relaxation, particularly in the ductus arteriosus and pulmonary and systemic circulations. This not only dilates the ductus arteriosus but enhances effective pulmonary blood flow in these infants. Since nearly 80% of prostaglandin E_1 may be metabolized in one pass through the infant's lungs,[424] the drug must be administered continuously. Some recent successful research has been reported using intermittent oral administration of this drug, although this form of prostaglandin E_2 is not yet readily available in the United States.[68]

Initially, the IV dose of prostaglandin will be 0.05 to 0.1 μg/kg/minute.[188] Some institutions recommend administration of an initial bolus of 0.1 μg/kg when the infusion is begun.[132] PGE_1 may be administered intraarterially or intravenously; peripheral IV administration appears to be as effective as central venous administration. Once the infant has demonstrated a good response to the PGE_1 infusion, the dosage may be tapered to 0.025 μg/kg/minute.[187] Since systemic arterial hypotension can occur as a result of systemic vasodilation, the infant's arterial blood pressure should be monitored throughout the PGE_1 infusion.

Prostaglandin E_1 administration to neonates with cyanotic congenital heart disease generally pro-

Table 3-13   Antibiotic prophylaxis for prevention of bacterial endocarditis in children*

Drug	Dosage
Routine prophylaxis for dental or upper respiratory infections or procedures *No allergies:*	
Penicillin V *plus*	1 gm po 1 hr before procedure
Penicillin V	250 mg q 6 hr × 3 → 8 doses if <27 kg
	500 mg q 6 hr × 3 → 8 doses if >27 kg
Penicillin sensitive:	
Erythromycin *plus*	20 mg/kg po 1 hr before procedure
Erythromycin	10 mg/kg po q 6 hr × 3 → 8 doses
Routine prophylaxis for urologic procedures *No allergies:*	
Ampicillin *plus*	50 mg/kg IM or IV 1 hr before and 12 hr after procedure
Streptomycin *or*	20 mg/kg IM 1 hr before and 12 hr after procedure (NOTE: This dose may be repeated for a total of 8 doses)
Gentamicin	2 mg/kg IM or IV slowly
Penicillin sensitive:	
Vancomycin *plus*	20 mg/kg IV 1 hr before and 12 hr after procedure
Streptomycin	20 mg/kg IM 1 hr before and 12 hr after procedure

*These guidelines are modified from the following sources: Committee on Rheumatic Fever and Bacterial Endocarditis of the Council on Cardiovascular Disease in the Young of the American Heart Association: Prevention of bacterial endocarditis, Circulation **56**:139A, 1977; and Keys, T.F.: Antimicrobial prophylaxis for patients with congenital or valvular heart disease, Mayo Clinic Proceedings **57**:171, 1982.

duces an increase in the infant's arterial oxygen tension by 15 to 40 torr and an increase in arterial oxygen saturation by 25% to 100%.[38,153,188,299] This increase in oxygenation may prevent or eliminate acidosis in these infants and allow them to be stabilized before urgent surgical repair of their congenital heart defect.

Side effects of PGE$_1$ administration include vasodilation or cutaneous flush, hypotension, bradycardia, pyrexia, seizure-like activity, respiratory depression, and infection. The incidence of these complications increases with higher doses of PGE$_1$ administration, longer periods of administration (more than 48 hours), and younger ages of the infants.[188] Fluid administration may be required if hypotension develops during PGE$_1$ administration. If apnea occurs, the infant usually resumes breathing when stimulated, although respiratory support may be indicated if apnea recurs. The seizure-like activity that is occasionally observed does not seem to indicate the presence of neurologic pathology, and the activity usually disappears with reduction in dosage or discontinuation of PGE$_1$ administration.[38,95,153,299,317] Prostaglandin E$_1$ administration can precipitate congestive heart failure in neonates if pulmonary blood flow is significantly increased. As a result the infant's fluid balance should be carefully assessed, and signs of congestive heart failure (tachycardia, hepatomegaly, periorbital edema, tachypnea, and increased respiratory effort) should be reported to a physician immediately (see the section on congestive heart failure in this chapter).

When the child with cyanotic congenital heart disease and polycythemia undergoes surgical repair, postoperative bleeding should be anticipated. Fresh frozen plasma and platelets may be ordered for postoperative administration (see Table 3-10). In some in-

Table 3-13   Antibiotic prophylaxis for prevention of bacterial endocarditis in children—cont'd

Drug	Dosage
High-risk prophylaxis for dental or upper respiratory infections or procedures (for children with valvular or other cardiac prostheses) *No allergies:*	
Procaine penicillin and	600,000 U IM 1 hr before procedure
Aqueous crystallin penicillin G *plus*	30,000 U/kg 1 hr before procedure
Streptomycin	20 mg/kg IM 1 hr before procedure (NOTE: This dose may be repeated for a total of 8 doses)
Penicillin sensitive:	
Vancomycin	20 mg/kg IV 1 hr before procedure (NOTE: Erythromycin may be administered in dosage of 10 mg/kg q 6 hr × 3 → 8 oral doses)
High-risk prophylaxis for urologic procedures (for children with valvular or other cardiac prostheses) *No allergies:*	
Ampicillin *plus*	50 mg/kg IM or IV 1 hr before and 12 hr after procedure
Streptomycin or	20 mg/kg IM 1 hr before and 12 hr after procedure (NOTE: 10 mg/kg is occasionally administered q 6 hr for an additional 3 → 8 doses)
Gentamicin	2 mg/kg IM or IV (slowly)
Penicillin sensitive:	
Vancomycin *plus*	20 mg/kg IV 1 hr before and 12 hr after procedure
Streptomycin	20 mg/kg IM 1 hr before and 12 hr later (NOTE: 10 mg/kg may be administered q 6 hr × 3 → 8 doses)

stitutions, unrefrigerated fresh whole blood is made available for use in the immediate postoperative period, to provide the child with the most active clotting factors and platelets[201,283] (see the section on postoperative care).

If the older child with inoperable cyanotic heart disease and polycythemia becomes symptomatic when his hematocrit approaches or exceeds 60% to 70%, periodic phlebotomies may be performed as a palliative measure. The child should be admitted to the hospital for the phlebotomy since the risk of cerebrovascular accident and bleeding is significant in these children. A central line is inserted, blood is withdrawn in small increments and may be replaced with saline, half-normal saline, or a glucose and saline or glucose and water solution. Although the child's red blood cell production will soon replace any blood withdrawn, the periodic phlebotomy may pro-

vide temporary relief of symptoms such as dyspnea, poor exercise tolerance, headache, and malaise experienced by these terminally ill children. Phlebotomy has been shown to reduce peripheral vascular resistance, improve ventricular stroke volume, increase systemic blood flow, and improve systemic oxygen transport.[355]

■ Postoperative Care for the Pediatric Cardiovascular Surgical Patient

Postoperative care of the pediatric cardiovascular patient is discussed on the following pages and is summarized in the care plan at the end of this section. Although many of the following sections are applicable to the care of the child following closed-heart surgery, this discussion refers primarily to care of the child following open-heart surgery.

General principles of postoperative care are similar for all patients following cardiovascular surgery; however, unique aspects of pediatric care are soon appreciated by members of the medical team. Children generally require cardiovascular surgery because of congenital heart defects. Their surgical repairs tend to involve more intracardiac reconstruction than adult surgery for acquired heart disease. Therefore each child needs a specific perioperative care plan that takes into consideration that child's cardiovascular pathophysiology and clinical condition, surgical repair, and developmental and emotional requirements. In addition care must be taken to provide support to the child's parents or primary caretakers. Such special care necessitates careful selection and preparation of pediatric equipment (see Chapter 9) and personnel.

The purpose of this section is to highlight essential concepts in the care of the child hospitalized for cardiovascular surgery.

■ **PREPARATION OF THE CHILD AND FAMILY**

Preparation of each child and family for cardiovascular surgery must be designed only after consideration of the child's cognitive and social level of development and the child's and family's perception of the child's health. Clearly, a child who considers himself to be well should not be told that the surgeon will "make his heart better" since he will actually feel worse immediately after surgery. Conversely, a child who is acutely conscious of his cyanosis may find the prospect of looking at his (pink) lips and fingernails after surgery to be reassuring and exciting.

Parents may feel in some part responsible for their child's cardiac defect. The nurse may help parents to discuss fears and concerns and may reduce the parents' guilt by emphasizing that the cause of most congenital heart disease is unknown.

Preoperative teaching must always be done at a level appropriate to the child's cognitive abilities and anxiety level. Much information can be obtained from the child during play. For preschool and school age children, it is helpful to make a suitcase including hospital equipment (dressings, tape, syringes, monitor "pasties," IV equipment) and dolls, for use by the child in nonstructured but monitored play. While the nurse ensures that the child will not enter unsupervised into physically or emotionally traumatic activity, she also can observe the child's comments about and use of particular hospital equipment. Since dolls

are also present, the child may choose to use the equipment during doll play, or to completely ignore threatening hospital equipment and pursue doll play only. In either case, he is providing valuable information regarding his coping styles. The same suitcase and equipment may be used later in a structured session to prepare the child for the upcoming surgery. During this structured session, the nurse can tell a story about a doll having the noise in his heart fixed; then the child is free to draw personal comparisons at his own pace. This structured play session also provides an opportunity for the nurse to clarify significant misconceptions the child may have regarding his health care.

Preoperatively it is important that the child and family have time to become familiar with the nurses and physicians who will be caring for the child during the postoperative period. If the same nursing staff is involved throughout the child's hospitalization, continuity of care is fostered. If an entirely new staff will be involved in the child's care immediately after surgery, the family should have the opportunity to meet the new staff before surgery.

The child's preoperative visit to the intensive care unit must be planned and supervised carefully. If the child glimpses a critically ill patient unclothed and covered with tubes, he may be overwhelmed and frightened but unable to verbalize fears or clarify misconceptions. Such a sight can increase the child's anxiety about his own postoperative care. For this reason, too, the staff should be careful in the choice of words used to describe postoperative monitoring equipment. "Chest tubes" may be better called "drains," and monitoring leads can be called "special bandaids." It is best to familiarize the child with only that equipment he will definitely see or feel postoperatively since much of the equipment will be removed or out of sight by the time the child is awake enough to look beyond the horizon of the bed. Parents often cope more effectively with specific definitions of particular tubes once they see their child safely returned from surgery (see Chapter 2).

■ **PREOPERATIVE ASSESSMENT**

To best anticipate postoperative complications the nurse must be aware of the child's preoperative health status, intraoperative cardiovascular function, and the particular postsurgical complications associated with the child's cardiac surgery.

The critical-care nurse should assess the child's cardiac, respiratory, and neurologic function *preoperatively,* so that she is better able to recognize changes in the child's condition *postoperatively.* If congestive heart failure is present preoperatively, it will probably be present to some degree postoperatively. If the child has complex cyanotic heart disease and/or demonstrates significant respiratory distress and pulmonary vascular engorgement preoperatively, respiratory support is usually planned for several hours or days postoperatively. By becoming familiar with the child's preoperative verbal and nonverbal response to requests before surgery the nurse will be better able to assess the child's neurologic status after surgery. It is also important for the nurse to determine the child's unique words or expressions to indicate pain, fear, thirst, and the need to void or have a bowel movement and to record these in the nursing care plan. The nurse should also note any specific objects, people, or behavior the child uses for comfort. The parents may bring a special small toy or blanket to the unit during the child's surgery to be kept on the child's bed, so the child will see a familiar object immediately after surgery.

If the child demonstrates a preoperative coagulopathy, this should be documented, and additional appropriate blood components should be ordered preoperatively to be available for postoperative administration. If the neonate requires surgery in the first days of life, the nurse should ensure that he has received the normal postnatal oral or parenteral dose of vitamin K.[233]

Since the child will require measurement of daily weight after surgery, it is advisable for the child to be weighed the evening before surgery on the critical-care unit scale that will be used postoperatively so that direct comparison of preoperative and postoperative weights may be made.

While the child is in surgery, the child's intensive care bed and bedside area should be prepared for an organized acceptance of the child after surgery. The bed should be prepared with appropriate linen, including a small linen roll to be placed under the child's shoulders (to extend the child's neck and straighten the airway) and cloth restraints for use as needed. IV poles and oxygen supply equipment (including tank, tubing, hand resuscitation bag, adaptor, and mask) should be affixed to the child's bed. All equipment should be turned on and tested to ensure proper working order *before* the child returns from surgery. Proper "warm-up" time should be allowed if needed for transducers and other monitoring equipment. The appropriate mechanical ventilator should be set up at the bedside; the nurse should check the ventilator settings to ensure that appropriate variables (including tidal volume, respiratory rate, minute ventilation, peak inspiratory pressure, alarms, and positive end-expiratory pressure) are used, according

to hospital and nursing procedures. An additional manual resuscitation bag and endotracheal tube of the appropriate size should also be set up at the bedside. Sterile saline for endotracheal tube irrigation should be prepared, and syringes, tubes, and laboratory requisition slips should be assembled for blood sampling. A blood pressure cuff of the appropriate size should also be at the child's bedside.

Two or three suction systems should be prepared at the bedside. Suction is usually applied to the child's chest tube drainage system, and a suction system is also required for endotracheal or pharyngeal suctioning. A third suction system may be required for nasogastric drainage. IV lines including bags, infusion pumps, and extension tubing should be at the bedside and ready for use. One or more hemostats should be taped to the child's bedframe to clamp the child's chest tubes if they inadvertently become disconnected or if a sudden air leak develops in the chest drainage system.

A sign should be taped to the child's bedframe in a prominent position listing the child's length, weight, body surface area (if used for fluid administration or medication dosage calculations), and allergies. It is helpful if a preoperative assessment sheet is made summarizing the child's preoperative clinical condition, results of preoperative laboratory studies (including hemoglobin, hematocrit, serum electrolyte concentrations, and arterial blood gases), and preoperative medications and allergies. Any abnormal cardiopulmonary or neurologic findings should also be recorded. Such a reference sheet is extremely useful postoperatively.

■ ADMISSION OF THE CHILD TO THE CRITICAL-CARE UNIT

Two nurses are usually required to "accept" the child to the critical-care unit after surgery. Before the child returns, the nurses should discuss and divide responsibilities so the child's arrival and admission to the critical-care unit is accomplished smoothly and safely. Unnecessary personnel should be asked to stay away from the area immediately surrounding the child's bed, so stimulation (of the patient and the nurse) and confusion can be kept to a minimum. A sample division of these responsibilities is included in Table 3-14.

■ POSTOPERATIVE CARE
■ Cardiovascular function

The child's cardiovascular function must be monitored closely during the postoperative period. To

Table 3-14   Receiving the postoperative cardiac patient*

Nurse 1	Time	Nurse 2
Assess child—note color and warmth of extremities, strength of pulses, cardiac rhythm per portable monitor, respiratory status	Immediately	Regulate all IV lines to appropriate rate to prevent bolus infusion of fluid or medications or clotting of lines
Obtain vital signs—including arterial and venous pressures—and relay them to surgeon and anesthesiologist; assess lung aeration to ensure proper ventilation and proper tube placement	Within minutes	Attach chest tubes to suction, making sure that water seal chamber has been filled to the 2 cm mark; label pleural drainage systems (#1, #2, etc.), reinforce connections with tape, and secure them to the floor or bed frame
Attach child to cardiac monitor and ensure clear tracing; note any arrhythmias or inappropriate heart rate and discuss with physician; attach any arterial or venous monitoring lines to appropriate monitoring systems—calibrate as needed	After vital signs	Strip chest tubes, and record amount of drainage; notify primary nurse and surgeon if bleeding pronounced; measure and record urine output from operating room
Remain at head of bed for patient needs—suctioning, administration of drugs, repetition of vital signs, etc. Vital signs should be repeated every 5 minutes initially, then at increasing intervals, to *maximum interval of q1hr* (for 24 hr and while child is intubated)	After several minutes	Transfer IVs to infusion control pumps, regulate to proper rate, and label; assist in calibration of arterial and venous monitoring systems
When child is stabilized, you may wish to ask the surgeon about the following: 1. Location of chest tubes (pleural versus mediastinal) 2. Complications or areas of concern during surgery 3. Nature of repair (i.e., direct suture, patch insertion, etc.) 4. Child's fluid and medication requirements during surgery	When area quiet	Assist primary nurse in obtaining supplies or drugs not at bedside and blood samples for laboratory analysis; order chest x-ray examination and ECG

*NOTE: Priority should be given to stabilization of the child's respiratory and cardiovascular function. *If the child is intubated, stabilization of the child on the ventilator is given first priority.*

maintain adequate cardiac output the child must have sufficient cardiac preload or circulating blood volume, adequate myocardial function, and appropriate ventricular afterload (resistance to ventricular ejection). If cardiac preload or myocardial function is inadequate or if ventricular afterload is excessive, cardiac output may fall.

Postoperatively inadequate circulating blood volume can result from hemorrhage, excessive diuresis, or inadequate fluid administration. The child's circulating blood volume should be calculated before the child returns from surgery (see Table 3-9), and all blood losses should be considered as a proportion of the child's circulating blood volume.[364] If the child's chest tube output averages *3 ml/kg/hour* these losses will total 10% to 15% of the child's circulating blood volume within 3 hours. If this blood loss is unreplaced, significant cardiovascular compromise and shock can result. It is usually advisable to replace chest tube output once it totals 5% to 10% of the child's circulating blood volume. If chest tube output is *3 to 5 ml/kg/hour,* this constitutes significant hemorrhage, and the source of the bleeding must be determined. A coagulation panel is drawn, and if abnormalities are present, appropriate blood components should be administered (see Table 3-10).[352,354] If excessive chest tube output continues despite normal clotting function, the child usually requires reoperation (see the section on fluid therapy in this chapter).

The child's hematocrit should be monitored closely postoperatively to assess the need for further blood administration. Whole blood is usually administered to replace whole blood losses, and packed cells may be administered when the child's hematocrit is low and fluid administration must be kept to a minimum. Colloid solutions may be administered to increase the child's intravascular volume when the hematocrit is adequate.

An osmotic diuresis may occur postoperatively, particularly if a glucose-containing solution was used in the bypass pump prime.[201] In some institutions mannitol is added to the pump prime; this also produces a postoperative osmotic diuresis resulting from glycosuria. If postoperative diuresis is excessive, replacement of urine fluid losses may then be required to maintain adequate circulating blood volume; colloid or crystalloid solutions are frequently used.[328,329]

Cardiac contractility may be poor postoperatively because of hypoxemia, acidosis, or electrolyte imbalance, because significant myocardial resection was required intraoperatively, or because surgical repair has significantly altered cardiac pressure, flow, and resistance relationships. If hypercapnia or alveolar hypoxemia are present, ventilatory support must be instituted or adjusted. Acidosis must be treated promptly since it can depress cardiac contractility.

Electrolyte imbalance can be seen frequently after cardiovascular surgery, and these imbalances can depress myocardial function. *Hypokalemia* is often present in the early postoperative period; it can result from an increase in intravascular water,[332] from correction of acidosis, and from increased renal potassium loss resulting from perioperative diuretic therapy. *Hyperkalemia* may occur postoperatively, particularly if renal failure develops. *Hypocalcemia* is more likely to develop postoperatively if the patient is a young infant, or if citrate-phosphate-dextran blood is administered rapidly without calcium infusion.[316] (See Chapter 1). *Hypoglycemia* is also frequently seen postoperatively in infants, particularly during periods of stress and reduced caloric intake,[64] and *hyperglycemia* can develop if glucose-containing solutions are used in the bypass pump prime.

A postoperative cardiac index of less than 2.0 to 2.5 L/min/m² body surface area indicates the presence of low cardiac output, and this is associated with high postoperative mortality in children.[321] Early signs of postoperative low cardiac output include decreased intensity of peripheral pulses, cool and pale (or mottled) extremities, prolonged capillary refill time, decreased urine output, and extreme irritability or lethargy. Later signs of low cardiac output include hypotension, bradycardia, hypoxemia, and metabolic acidosis. Treatment of low cardiac output resulting from decreased cardiac contractility includes correction of metabolic abnormalities, and, if necessary, administration of sympathomimetic inotropic medications (refer to the section on low cardiac output).

Low cardiac output can also result from increased ventricular afterload. If systemic vascular resistance is high—or even normal—in the presence of low cardiac output or if the child demonstrates significant peripheral vasoconstriction with poor systemic perfusion, treatment with IV vasodilators is usually indicated. Vasodilators such as nitroglycerin or sodium nitroprusside are thought to reduce ventricular preload and afterload because they produce venous and arterial dilation (see the section on low cardiac output). During vasodilator therapy, the warmth of the child's extremities, capillary refill, and urine output should be assessed to determine the effectiveness of therapy. In addition, it is helpful to calculate the child's systemic vascular resistance before and throughout therapy as a means of documenting the child's response to treatment.

An increase in the child's pulmonary vascular resistance may also be an acute cause of low cardiac output postoperatively.[442] Those children especially at risk for the development of postoperative pulmonary hypertension are those who had evidence of high pulmonary vascular resistance at preoperative catheterization. In addition, some children with apparently normal pulmonary vascular resistance preoperatively may develop reactive pulmonary hypertension in response to alveolar hypoxia, hypothermia, or acidosis. The child with perioperative pulmonary hypertension must be kept well ventilated and warm. Mechanical ventilatory support is often the most important aspect of the care of these children since alveolar hypoxia, hypoxemia, acidosis, and hypothermia can augment pulmonary vasoconstriction. These children are usually ventilated for several days, and *gradual* weaning is then attempted. During weaning, the child's pulmonary pressure and systemic perfusion should be monitored carefully since hypoventilation will produce alveolar hypoxia and can result in pulmonary vasoconstriction. Prevention or prompt correction of acidosis will also be required (see the section on respiratory function in this chapter).[442]

When pulmonary hypertension is present, pulmonary vasodilation is most frequently accomplished through administration of intravenous nitroglycerin or sodium nitroprusside.[406] Tolazoline may also be administered directly into the pulmonary artery (1 mg/kg) and then administered by continuous infusion of 1 to 2 mg/kg/hour.[201] Prostaglandin E_1 or prostaglandin D (which is available for approved research only) may also be administered to promote pulmonary vasodilation in the newborn. These vasodilators are usually administered in conjunction with a sympathomimetic inotropic agent (see the section on low cardiac output).

If afterload reduction is attempted, it is important that the child's fluid volume status be assessed before vasodilation is begun since hypotension is more likely to occur during therapy if hypovolemia is present. If the child is receiving several medications by continuous infusion, it is advisable that each be administered through a separate IV line so that the infusion rate of each can be adjusted separately. It is also important that the dosage of *only one medication be changed at any one time* so that the patient's response to each change can be determined (see the section on low cardiac output in this chapter).

Congestive heart failure (CHF) can also be present postoperatively, particularly if the child demonstrated it preoperatively or if repair of complex cyanotic heart disease (such as severe tetralogy of Fallot or truncus arteriosus) was performed. The nurse should monitor for signs of congestive heart failure, including signs of systemic and pulmonary venous engorgement (see the boxed material on signs and symptoms of congestive heart failure in children). Signs of systemic venous engorgement in the postoperative patient include a high central venous or right atrial pressure, hepatomegaly, and periorbital edema. Ascites may also be present if systemic venous pressures are high. Signs of pulmonary venous engorgement include a high pulmonary capillary wedge or left atrial pressure. If the child is mechanically ventilated, high-peak inspiratory pressures and decreased lung compliance may be noted. If the child is breathing spontaneously, tachypnea and increased respiratory effort will be present. The size of the heart on the chest radiograph is usually large, and pulmonary vascular markings will be prominent. Congestive heart failure requires treatment with diuretics and possibly with a digitalis derivative (see the discussion of congestive heart failure in the section on common clinical conditions).

Tamponade can be a sudden and fatal cause of decreased systemic perfusion in the postoperative cardiovascular patient. Signs of tamponade may be similar to those of congestive heart failure or low cardiac output, and they may include hypotension and tachycardia, a narrowing of the child's pulse pressure, and a high central venous and left atrial pressure. The child's heart sounds may become muffled, or the QRS complexes on the child's ECG may become smaller, but these are inconsistent and often late findings.[298] The chest radiograph may show increased heart size and pulmonary vascular congestion, although these findings may be difficult to differentiate from those caused by congestive heart failure. Tamponade should be suspected if the child's systemic perfusion becomes poor and if right and left atrial or central venous and pulmonary capillary wedge pressures rise simultaneously and equally. The child may also demonstrate *pulsus paradoxus* (a fall in systolic blood pressure by 8 to 10 mm Hg during inspiration).[2] Clotting of the chest tube and resultant tamponade should be suspected if the child has excessive chest tube output that decreases abruptly as the child's systemic perfusion worsens and right and/or left atrial pressures rise. If clots have formed around the right or left side of the heart alone, signs of isolated right or left heart tamponade (and isolated systemic or pulmonary venous engorgement, respectively) may occasionally be noted.[27] The child with tamponade requires *immediate* evacuation of pericardial fluid, and an emergency thoracotomy (through the median sternotomy) may have to be performed in the critical-care unit.[117]

Arrhythmias that compromise cardiac output or systemic perfusion must be treated promptly. If the child's surgical repair involves manipulation near the intracardiac conduction system, two temporary pacing wires are usually placed at the time of surgery. One wire is hooked into the epicardium of the right ventricle, the other wire lies just under the child's skin and serves as a "ground" wire. Both wires are brought through the child's chest wall and both end with a needle that may be attached to a pacemaker cable. The function of the temporary pacing wires is usually tested in the operating room. If the pacer wires are not attached by cable to an external pacemaker in the operating room, the pacemaker should be tested soon after the child returns to the critical-care unit, and the child's cardiac threshold should be determined and recorded on the nursing flow sheet. If the child has heart block, it is important that the physician determine the appropriate pacemaker demand rate so that the child will receive appropriate pacing support when needed (see the section in this chapter on arrhythmias). If permanent heart block is anticipated postoperatively, the surgeon may implant permanent and temporary pacing wires during surgery. Then, if permanent pacing becomes necessary, a permanent pacing unit can be implanted and joined with the permanent wire that is already in place. This eliminates the need for a second, later thoracotomy procedure when the unit is implanted.

The most common arrhythmias following pediatric cardiovascular surgery include supraventricular tachycardia, various forms of heart block, and right bundle branch block. Significant ventricular arrhythmias, such as ventricular tachycardia or ventricular fibrillation, are relatively uncommon in children following cardiovascular surgery,[349] and the appearance of such arrhythmias usually indicates serious deterioration in the child's cardiovascular function (see the section in this chapter on arrhythmias).

The moment the child returns from surgery the nurse should form an opinion of the child's cardiovascular function. She should be aware of the "filling" (central venous, pulmonary capillary wedge, or left atrial) pressures at which systemic perfusion is best. It is also important that the nurse is aware of the child's fluid balance (total fluid intake less total fluid loss) and the response of the child to volume therapy. If the child demonstrates excessive chest tube output and has poor systemic perfusion despite high left and

right atrial pressures, there is cause for concern. If, on the other hand, the child's chest tube output is minimal and urine output and systemic perfusion are good at low right and left atrial pressures, the child's cardiovascular function is probably very good.

■ **Respiratory function**

If the child is intubated postoperatively, the nurse must frequently assess the effectiveness of the child's ventilatory support. If the child has been sedated or paralyzed, he will not demonstrate restlessness as a sign of hypoxemia or hypercapnia, so it is imperative that the nurse detect early evidence of ventilatory insufficiency and make appropriate adjustments in ventilatory support as ordered.

If the child's endotracheal tube is in the proper position, the tip should be above the child's carina, providing equal aeration of both lungs. This should result in the presence of equal breath sounds bilaterally. In infants the endotracheal tube can easily migrate to the right mainstem bronchus, producing right lung hyperinflation and left lung hypoinflation. If right mainstem bronchus intubation is not corrected, left lung atelectasis can result, producing a large ventilation-perfusion mismatch, profound hypoxemia, increased pulmonary vascular resistance, and sudden clinical deterioration (see Fig. 5-12, *B*). Right mainstem bronchus intubation should be suspected if the breath sounds over the child's right chest are much louder than the breath sounds over the corresponding areas of the child's left chest. If the nurse suspects tube migration to the right mainstem bronchus, she can confirm this by placing *gentle* tension (if hospital policy allows) on the endotracheal tube while listening to breath sounds over the left chest. If left lung breath sounds improve dramatically when the endotracheal tube is pulled *slightly* (withdrawn only approximately 0.5 to 1.0 cm), the tube should be retaped in its new position and the physician should be notified. If breath sounds do not improve with this gentle manipulation, a physician should be consulted, since the child may have a significant left pneumothorax or hemothorax or left lung atelectasis. A chest radiograph should be obtained so position of the endotracheal tube can be confirmed and other lung pathology can be ruled out (see Chapter 5).

When the child requires mechanical ventilation, his clinical appearance, breath sounds, and chest expansion should be checked frequently to be sure that his ventilator variables are adjusted appropriately. While the child requires controlled mechanical ventilation, the child's arterial carbon dioxide tension must be kept low enough to inhibit the child's independent respiratory drive. Most intubated children should be placed on 2 to 4 cm H_2O of positive end-expiratory pressure (PEEP) whether they are requiring controlled ventilation or breathing spontaneously, since this simulates the physiologic PEEP provided by normal coughing or talking.[293]

If the intubated child suddenly becomes restless or combative, endotracheal tube obstruction should be suspected. The child should be hand ventilated, the endotracheal tube should be suctioned, and the child's breath sounds and resistance to hand ventilation should be assessed. If the endotracheal tube is occluded, minimal or absent breath sounds or chest expansion will be noted despite vigorous attempts at hand ventilation.[345] If vigorous suctioning does not remove the obstruction immediately, the tube will have to be removed and the child will require hand ventilation with a bag and mask until a new tube can be placed.

Patient agitation and decreased breath sounds may also be the result of the development of a significant pneumothorax. If pneumothorax is present, hand ventilation may only produce expansion of the unaffected lung and chest, and the child's breath sounds may be diminished over the involved side of the chest. It is important to note, however, that since breath sounds are easily transmitted through the infant's thin chest wall, it may be difficult to appreciate a difference in the intensity of breath sounds between the affected and unaffected lung. With development of a tension pneumothorax, a shift in heart sounds toward the uninvolved side (resulting from a mediastinal shift) may be detected, and *pulsus paradoxus* (a drop in systolic blood pressure by 10 mm Hg or more during inspiration) may be noted. If a large pneumothorax develops suddenly in the infant, the most significant clinical finding may be the development of hypotension and bradycardia resulting from severe hypoxemia. Treatment of a large pneumothorax requires immediate evacuation of the air by needle aspiration or chest tube insertion.

The child's color, peripheral perfusion, and arterial blood gases should be assessed whenever respiratory distress is present. The child's color may not be the most reliable tool to determine the level of oxygenation because cyanosis is not apparent until severe hypoxemia is present and it may not be observed if the child is anemic. The quality of the child's peripheral perfusion will provide indirect evidence of the effectiveness of the child's cardiac and respiratory function.

The child's arterial oxygen and carbon dioxide

tensions can be monitored through use of conventional arterial sampling, skin surface blood gas electrodes, or heel stick blood sampling. However, if the infant is unstable or if he will require prolonged intubation and frequent blood sampling, an arterial line should be inserted to provide a reliable method of obtaining blood gas specimens.

Skin surface (or "transcutaneous") blood gas electrodes may be used to monitor blood gas values continuously without loss of patient blood for sampling. Use of these skin surface monitors can also help the nurse to immediately and continuously evaluate effects of medication adjustments or nursing care measures (such as suctioning and chest physiotherapy) on the child's blood gases.[181]

If an arterial line is not in place, a heelstick blood gas sample may be obtained from the infant to evaluate arterial oxygenation. If the infant's heel is well warmed, the capillary blood is "arterialized." To obtain the sample the infant's heel is punctured, and the blood is massaged—not squeezed—from the heel. The blood sample is collected in a capillary tube; it should not be exposed to air for prolonged periods before collection or analysis. These heelstick blood gas results can approximate the child's arterial blood gas tensions.

The child should not be extubated until his cardiac and respiratory function are good. Ventilatory support should be continued if hemorrhage, severe congestive heart failure, significant arrhythmias, or low cardiac output is present. If right ventricular function is poor, hypoventilation, acidosis, and hypothermia can produce pulmonary vasoconstriction; this will increase right ventricular afterload and can result in right ventricular failure. Therefore children who have had surgical repair of defects such as severe tetralogy of Fallot or truncus arteriosus should receive planned, prolonged mechanical ventilatory support until their cardiac function is stable. They should then be weaned gradually, with careful attention given to both cardiac and respiratory response to weaning.

If the child is extubated, the nurse must carefully assess the child's breath sounds and respiratory effort; tachypnea is often the first sign of cardiorespiratory distress in infants.[339] Respiratory distress may develop as a result of congestive heart failure, low cardiac output, upper airway obstruction, hemothorax, pneumothorax, or atelectasis. If the child demonstrates increased respiratory effort and gasping or grunting accompanied by a deterioration in cardiovascular status, the physician should be notified immediately and the nurse should assemble equipment for reintubation of the child. The appropriate size endotracheal tube should already be at the bedside; if significant subglottic edema is the cause of the reintubation, the child may only tolerate insertion of an endotracheal tube that is one half or one size smaller than the operative endotracheal tube size (see Chapter 4).

Racemic epinephrine nebulizer treatments may be administered to reduce mild or moderate postoperative (postintubation) subglottic edema. Usually, 0.125 to 0.5 ml of 2.25% racemic epinephrine is diluted with 2.0 to 3.0 ml of water or normal saline and is administered by aerosol or intermittent positive pressure breathing (IPPB) treatments. Racemic epinephrine may produce glottic vasoconstriction and reduction of edema, as well as bronchodilation (and decreased airway resistance). The nurse must watch the child closely for development of tachyarrhythmias during treatment.[291] In addition, some children may develop a "rebound" bronchoconstriction.

Once the child is extubated, high humidity oxygen or room air is usually administered by hood, tent, or face mask.[201,282] Chest physical therapy should be administered as soon as the child's cardiovascular function is stable. Postural drainage, percussion, vibration, and "rib-springing" have been shown particularly helpful in prevention of postintubation atelectasis.[121] An excellent review of chest physiotherapy techniques for children has been provided by Jacoby[207] (see Chapter 4 also).

Potential postoperative respiratory complications include atelectasis, pneumothorax, hemothorax, pleural effusion, or chylothorax. Postoperative right upper lobe *atelectasis* develops frequently in infants, although this complication can be prevented by aggressive chest physical therapy.[121] Left lung atelectasis can also develop from inadvertent right mainstem bronchus intubation during mechanical ventilation. Following extubation, left lower lobe atelectasis may develop if significant cardiomegaly causes compression of this lobe or of the left main bronchus. Signs of atelectasis include decreased intensity of breath sounds over the involved area, although this may be difficult to appreciate since breath sounds are easily transmitted from other lung areas. Chest expansion may be decreased on the involved side. The involved lung areas are dull to percussion, and atelectasis produces increased opacification of the involved lung on the chest radiograph. Treatment includes vigorous chest physical therapy. If a mucous plug is thought to be the cause of persistent atelectasis, bronchoscopy and bronchial lavage may be performed by a physician.

A *pneumothorax* can develop postoperatively if the pleural spaces were entered during surgery and if the air is inadequately drained by the chest drainage system. Pneumothorax can also develop spontaneously, or during chest tube removal. Signs of pneumothorax would also include decreased intensity and/or quality of breath sounds over the involved area. If the child with a pneumothorax is receiving mechanical ventilation, peak inspiratory pressures are often elevated and the nurse may note increased resistance to hand ventilation. If the child is breathing spontaneously, he may demonstrate tachypnea and increased respiratory effort. Chest expansion may be decreased on the involved side. If the child develops a tension pneumothorax, he will demonstrate agitation, hypotension, a shift in the mediastinum, and extreme cardiorespiratory distress.

If the pneumothorax is small, treatment may include only chest physical therapy and frequent assessment to ensure that air accumulation has not increased. If a significant pneumothorax is present, a thoracentesis will be performed or a chest tube will be inserted. The development of a tension pneumothorax constitutes a medical emergency and requires prompt aspiration of the air by thoracentesis or chest tube.

A *hemothorax* can develop from bleeding in the mediastinum (if the pleural spaces are entered and communicate with the mediastinum) or from bleeding from the great vessels. Hemothorax can also result from erosion of the aorta by the tip of a thoracic chest tube. If a chest tube is in place, the diagnosis of hemothorax is apparent if a large quantity of blood enters the chest drainage system. If a chest tube is not in place, a hemothorax will cause a decrease in intensity or a change in quality (pitch) of breath sounds over the involved area. If blood accumulation is significant and if the child is mechanically ventilated, his peak inspiratory pressures may rise and there may be resistance to hand ventilation. If the child is breathing spontaneously, tachypnea and increased respiratory effort are usually noted. Chest expansion on the involved side is usually decreased. If significant amounts of blood are lost into the chest, the child may develop hypotension and signs of hypovolemia. The presence of fluid in the chest will create opacification on the chest radiograph. Treatment requires evacuation of the fluid by thoracentesis or chest tube insertion. Surgical exploration of the bleeding site may also be indicated, and administration of whole blood or packed red blood cells may be required.

Pleural effusions may develop as a result of congestive heart failure or postcardiotomy syndrome.[251] Accumulation of thoracic fluid can cause symptoms similar to those observed with a hemothorax. Treatment requires thoracentesis or chest tube insertion. The fluid obtained is sent for culture to rule out the presence of an empyema. If congestive heart failure is present, the child usually receives diuretics to prevent reaccumulation of fluid. If postcardiotomy syndrome is suspected, aspirin or steroids may be ordered (see the section on postcardiotomy syndrome).

Chylothorax is the accumulation of lymph fluid in the chest. It occurs as the result of injury to the thoracic duct or to a large lymphatic vessel during aortic or cardiac surgery. Chylothorax typically occurs as a result of cardiovascular surgery that requires mobilization of the aortic arch (e.g., repair of coarctation of the aorta or patent ductus arteriosus) or following creation of a subclavian-pulmonary artery shunt.[42,191] Chylothorax has less frequently been reported following open-heart surgery using a median sternotomy approach.[217] It may also develop in children with high central venous pressure, such as children with tricuspid atresia (especially following a Fontan procedure) or those children who develop vena caval obstruction following the Mustard procedure for repair of transposition of the great vessels. Chylothorax may also be congenital in origin.[42]

If the surgeon observes lymph in the child's chest at the time of surgery, the health care team should be notified so that the chest tubes will be left in place until the presence of chylothorax is confirmed or ruled out. Since the child does not eat for several hours before and after surgery, there is often very little fat apparent in lymph drainage during the immediate postoperative period; as a result it may not be apparent that there is lymph fluid in the drainage. If the chest tubes are left in place until after the child resumes eating a regular oral diet (one that contains fat), the presence of white or creamy lymphatic drainage from the chest tube will confirm the presence of a chylothorax. If a chest tube is not in place and significant lymphatic drainage is present in the chest, the child can develop severe respiratory distress.

Treatment of chylothorax requires drainage of the lymph fluid by a chest tube or repeat thoracentesis. Many physicians recommend that the child be placed on a medium-chain triglyceride diet,[217,232] because these triglycerides can be absorbed directly in the intestines and passed into portal venous blood rather than into lacteals and into the lymphatic system. Administration of these triglycerides and avoidance of long-chain fatty acids is thought to reduce

thoracic duct lymph flow and promote healing of the chylothorax.[232] During this conservative management the child still requires maintenance fluids and calories, and supplemental administration of fat-soluble vitamins (A, D, and E). Parenteral alimentation may be used to provide supplemental caloric intake. If the chylothorax fails to heal after a prolonged period of chest drainage and medium-chain triglyceride diet, surgical ligation of the thoracic duct may be attempted. The child should resume a regular oral diet before discharge so that chylothorax can be promptly detected and treated in the hospital if it persists.

■ Fluid therapy and renal function

Because the stress of surgery increases antidiuretic hormone secretion and, consequently, sodium and water retention,[332] fluid administration is often restricted during the immediate postoperative period. Generally, 50% to 75% of maintenance fluids are administered during the first 24 hours postoperatively.[2,201,282] Regardless of the policy for fluid administration, the nurse must evaluate each patient's response to fluid therapy. Early in the child's postoperative care, the health care team should identify the central venous pressure and left atrial pressure (or pulmonary artery wedge pressure) at which the child's systemic perfusion is best. This pressure may be maintained through infusion of whole blood, packed red blood cells, fresh frozen plasma, albumin, hetastarch, lactated ringers, saline, or glucose solutions. The appropriate solution is determined by the child's hematocrit, recent blood loss, presence of coagulopathies, electrolyte and acid-base status, and urine output. If the hematocrit is low and if the child is bleeding, packed red blood cells or whole blood are given. If the child's hematocrit is adequate and if cardiac or renal dysfunction is present, a colloidal solution may be administered. If the hypovolemic child has no evidence of congestive heart failure or renal failure, glucose solutions or saline may be given.

As noted earlier, hemorrhage is present if the child's chest tube output is equal to or greater than 3 ml/kg body weight/hour for 3 hours or more. This blood loss must be replaced to prevent low cardiac output as a result of hypovolemia. In addition, the cause of the bleeding must be identified and corrected. A coagulation profile is usually obtained whenever chest tube output is excessive. If clotting factors or fibrinogen are low, they are replaced with fresh whole blood or fresh frozen plasma as needed.

Platelet transfusion will be necessary if thrombocytopenia or thrombocytopathia is present. If there is an excess of heparin, protamine sulfate will be administered slowly—hypotension can follow rapid infusion (approximate dose: 0.25 to 1.0 mg/kg body weight). If inadequate clot formation is observed in the proximal chest tubes when bleeding is present, coagulopathy is strongly suspected. The presence of ecchymotic lesions, petechiae, or diffuse bleeding from puncture sites would also reinforce the diagnosis of coagulopathy (see Table 3-10 for a review of blood component therapy).[352,354]

Bleeding that requires reoperation is called "surgical bleeding" and may be caused by oozing from a suture line, a residual atrial or aortic opening, or a divided collateral vessel. Surgical bleeding should be suspected when the child's chest tube output totals 3 to 5 ml/kg body weight/hour for several hours, despite evidence of good clot formation in the chest tubes. Persistent surgical bleeding requires reoperation, so that the site of bleeding can be sutured or cauterized, and the possibility of tamponade is eliminated.

Children especially at risk for postoperative bleeding include those with cyanotic heart disease since they may develop a coagulopathy related to their polycythemia. Any child who requires repeat operations may also demonstrate postoperative bleeding since scar tissue, which is highly vascular, must be dissected to gain cardiac exposure.

Electrolyte imbalances most commonly observed following pediatric cardiovascular surgery have been discussed previously; these include hypokalemia, hyperglycemia, hypoglycemia, and hypocalcemia.[2,30] These should be treated promptly (see the section on low cardiac output) to avoid depression of cardiac contractility and arrhythmias.

Urine output should remain at 0.5 to 1.0 ml/kg body weight/hour if fluid intake is adequate. Urine specific gravity should also be measured to monitor urine concentration, although osmotic diuresis produced by hypergycemia or mannitol in the pump prime may produce a concentrated urine that does not reflect renal concentrating ability. If urine output is inadequate, it is important to determine whether decreased renal perfusion is the result of congestive heart failure, low cardiac output, or inadequate circulating blood volume. This determination is important since treatment of congestive heart failure or low cardiac output may require elimination of excessive intravascular water (diuresis) or inotropic therapy and the treatment of inadequate circulating blood volume requires fluid administration. The nurse should assess the child's hydration and check for evidence of systemic venous engorgement (hepatomegaly, high central venous pressure, periorbital edema) or pulmonary venous engorgement (tachypnea, decreased lung compliance, increased respiratory effort, high left atrial or pulmonary artery wedge pressure). Occasionally a fluid challenge totaling 5 to 10 ml/kg body weight may be administered; the fluid challenge can then be followed by furosemide (1 mg/kg body weight) if urine output does not improve.

Occasionally, children will develop significant intravascular hemolysis during or immediately following cardiopulmonary bypass. Signs of hemolysis include excretion of a rusty-colored urine that contains cell casts and hemoglobin. In addition, the child may demonstrate bleeding from the gastrointestinal tract, chest tubes, or endotracheal tube as a result of damage to platelets and erythrocytes.[352] If the child demonstrates hemoglobinuria, it is essential that renal blood flow and urine volume be kept at satisfactory levels, so the hemoglobin can be "flushed out" of the kidneys. In addition, the kidneys should not be required to concentrate urine maximally until cell fragments and hemoglobin have been excreted.

If the child's urine output is inadequate despite the presence of adequate systemic perfusion, adequate hydration, and the administration of diuretics, renal failure should be suspected. Too often the assumption is made that the child with decreased urine output requires further fluid administration. It is only after several large boluses of fluid are administered without result, that the diagnosis of renal failure is made; at this point, the child may be hypervolemic. If renal failure is thought to be present, fluid intake should be restricted and potassium administration curtailed. Serum samples are usually sent for analysis of blood urea nitrogen (BUN), creatinine, and potassium. Unless the child is anuric, simultaneous urine sampling for creatinine is also accomplished, so some estimation of urine creatinine clearance can be made. Peritoneal dialysis may be required to eliminate excess intravascular fluid (especially if congestive heart failure or low cardiac output is present) and control the child's serum potassium concentration. Sodium polystyrene sulfonate enemas or administration of glucose and insulin and calcium gluconate may also be required to reduce serum potassium concentrations and cardiac irritability (see Chapter 7).

If the child will not receive oral feedings for several days postoperatively, provision of daily maintenance caloric requirements should be planned immediately. If bowel function is adequate and the gastroesophageal spincter is competent, this may be accomplished through nasogastric feedings. If bowel function is inadequate, IV alimentation is required.

■ Neurologic function

The child's neurologic function should be assessed as soon as the child returns from surgery. The child's pupils should constrict in response to light, the child's movements should be appropriate for his age, and seizures and pathologic posturing should not be present. If abnormalities in postoperative neurologic function are suspected, a neurologic evaluation is usually ordered so that the extent and severity of the child's injury can be immediately evaluated by a specialist. If the neurologic dysfunction is temporary and minimal, the parents often are reassured when such a conclusion is verified by a neurologist. However, if the child has suffered permanent neurologic damage, the early involvement of the neurologist is usually very helpful.

Hemiplegia or coma may result from hypoxia, acidosis, a thromboembolic event, or low cardiac output. Paraplegia may result from the same factors, as well as from local injury to spinal cord circulation during coarctation repair. Seizures may result from perioperative neurologic damage, fever, or electrolyte imbalance. *It is very difficult to evaluate the presence of seizures in the child who is receiving paralyzing agents postoperatively.* Nystagmus, sluggish pupil response, or wide fluctuation in blood pressure may be the only clinical signs of seizures in these patients. In this case an electroencephalogram may be required to determine if seizures are present. Since status epilepticus causes reduced cerebral blood flow and since it can cause brain damage, it must be promptly recognized and vigorously treated.

Hypoxic encephalopathy may occur hours after a significant or prolonged fall in cardiac output. Osmotic diuretics or steroids are often prescribed for the child who has sustained a hemorrhagic or hypotensive episode in an effort to prevent cerebral edema.[201]

It is important to remember that administration of large doses of sympathomimetic medications (such as isoproterenol, dopamine, dobutamine, or epinephrine) or vagolytic drugs (such as atropine) will produce pupillary dilation, and so will affect evaluation of the pupil's constrictive response to light until these medications are reduced in dosage or discontinued.

Horner's syndrome may develop following any surgery that requires dissection around the aortic arch and the sympathetic cervical ganglion. The symptoms of Horner's syndrome include ptosis of the upper eyelid, pupil constriction, narrowing of the palpebral fissure, and decreased perspiration.[73] These signs appear on the same side as the injury, and the ipsilateral pupil constriction may make the contralateral pupil appear to be dilated. Although the signs of Horner's syndrome do not disappear, they often become less obvious over a period of months.

■ Thermoregulation

The neonate is unable to shiver to generate heat when exposed to cold stress.[186] Instead, the infant breaks down brown fat to generate heat; this is an energy-requiring process. As a result cold stress increases the infant's oxygen consumption. Immediately following cardiovascular surgery or during any period of critical illness, it is important to prevent cold stress so that the infant's oxygen requirements will be kept minimal. Scopes[381] has identified the environmental temperatures at which the normal young infant can maintain a rectal temperature of 37° C with the lowest oxygen consumption; this environmental temperature would provide a *neutral thermal environment* for the infant (see Appendix G). It is important that these environmental temperatures be maintained through the use of an Isolette or overbed warmer. Although an Isolette provides the most draft-free environment for the infant, the Isolette structure may reduce the nurse's access to the infant and ability to adjust his support or monitoring equipment. If constant care and manipulation of tubes or equipment are required, it is often best to care for these infants in beds with overbed warmers.

It is important to note that any heating device with a servocontrol is usually designed with a skin probe in the feedback loop. The heat output of the unit is then increased when the child's skin temperature falls and decreased when the child's skin temperature rises. If the child has decreased skin perfusion resulting from low cardiac output, the warmer may continue to generate heat whether the infant's core temperature is high or low. Therefore the nurse should monitor both the infant's rectal and skin temperatures whenever the warmers are used for patients with cardiovascular compromise.

Older children are able to shiver to generate heat. However, they may also require warming if hypothermic bypass was used during cardiovascular surgery.

If the child is hypothermic and peripherally vasoconstricted after surgery, the nurse will have to regulate fluid administration carefully while warming the child. While the child is peripherally vasoconstricted, little fluid administration may be required to maintain adequate cardiac "filling" pressures. Once the child's temperature increases, peripheral vasodilation may produce expansion of the intravascular space, and the child may require additional fluid administration to maintain adequate cardiac "filling" pressures.

■ Infection

Children requiring cardiovascular surgery are at risk for the development of postoperative infection. The infection can occur at the incision, at the site of skin puncture for any vascular catheter, or as a result of endotracheal intubation or genitourinary catheterization. Factors thought to increase the child's risk of postoperative infection include poor nutritional status, lengthy surgical procedure, multiple blood transfusions, and reoperation for bleeding.[91] Lack of handwashing by hospital personnel before and after patient contact can also contribute to the development of nosocomial infections in these critcally ill children. Since studies have documented inconsistent handwashing practices in critical-care units,[4] it is imperative that critical-care nurses practice good handwashing themselves and ensure good handwashing technique by other hospital personnel.

IV administration of broad spectrum staphylocidal antibiotic in the operating room *before the incision is made* has been found to decrease the postoperative incidence of deep and superficial wound infections following thoracic operations.[203,227] Often these prophylactic antibiotics are also administered for 2 to 5 days postoperatively in an attempt to prevent perioperative bacteremia.[201,227] Many children may demonstrate a low-grade fever on the night of surgery[201]; however, the child who develops a fever beyond the first 48 hours postoperatively should be examined carefully for evidence of infection. Blood cultures are usually drawn if the fever exceeds 39° C, and cultures of urine and tracheal aspirate may also be ordered. If the child has required insertion of prosthetic material for intracardiac or great vessel repair, it is especially important to prevent and to promptly treat postoperative bacteremia since the prosthetic material is particularly susceptible to bacterial aggregation. See Table 3-13 for antibiotic prophylaxis dosages.

The nurse should assess the appearance of the child's wound and catheter insertion sites daily and report any evidence of infection (erythema, drainage, etc.) to a physician. Wound drainage should be cultured immediately. Deep wound infections usually require incision and drainage and may require fre-

quent or continuous irrigation with antibiotics. Mediastinitis can cause endocarditis in the child with a cardiac prosthetic valve, patch, or conduit.[91]

■ Postcardiotomy syndrome

Postcardiotomy (or postpericardiotomy) syndrome indicates the association of fever (above 38.5° C), leukocytosis, substernal or pericardial chest pain, pericardial friction rub, pericardial and/or pleural effusion, and serial electrocardiographic evidence of pericarditis.[251] Less specific and less consistent findings include malaise and arthralgia.

The causes of postcardiotomy syndrome have not been identified. Since many patients with the syndrome have an elevated erythrocyte sedimentation rate and antiheart antibodies,[114,245,251] an autoimmune process has been implicated. In addition, a rise in viral titers has also been documented in many of the patients,[114] suggesting that a viral illness may also be involved. The incidence of postcardiotomy syndrome in children following cardiovascular surgery may be as high as 25%.[114,251]

Postcardiotomy syndrome should be suspected in any child who develops unexplained persistent fever and leukocytosis (white blood count more than 12,000/cm³) beyond the first postoperative week. If the child complains of chest or pericardial pain that increases with respiration and radiates to the shoulder, this provides additional support for the diagnosis. A pericardial friction rub is present in approximately half of the patients with postcardiotomy syndrome.[356] If laboratory tests reveal the presence of antiheart antibodies (AHA) and an erythrocyte sedimentation rate (ESR) above 50 mm/hour, the diagnosis is confirmed.[245]

Treatment of postcardiotomy syndrome involves administration of anti-inflammatory agents, observation for and treatment of pleural or pericardial effusions, and general supportive care. Aspirin and/or steroids are usually administered to reduce pericardial inflammation.[245,251] The nurse should monitor for evidence of fluid retention and she should be alert for signs of pleural and pericardial effusion, including signs of cardiac tamponade. The patient must also be protected from exposure to secondary infections while he is receiving anti-inflammatory agents. The aspirin therapy usually reduces the chest pain and arthralgia, and bedrest may be recommended until the symptoms of pericarditis subside.

All of these nursing assessments and interventions are summarized in Table 3-15.

Text continued on p. 165.

Table 3-15 Nursing care of the pediatric cardiovascular surgical patient

Nursing diagnosis	Expected outcomes	Nursing activities

A. Patient and family may demonstrate anxiety related to child's cardiovascular disease, surgery, prognosis, and/or hospitalization	1. Child will not demonstrate loss of control that interferes with medical care
	2. Family members will demonstrate an understanding of child's disease, purpose of hospitalization, goals and potential complications of surgery, planned postoperative management, and child's prognosis, as indicated by their discussion and questions
	3. Child and family (as appropriate) will participate in planning and providing child's care
		1. Provide child and significant family members with an orientation to the nursing care unit (including the preoperative unit and the intensive care unit)
		2. Assess child's preparation for surgery:
		  a. Ascertain what child has been told about his hospitalization and surgery
		  b. Ask parents how they think child can best be prepared for surgery
		  c. Assess child's level of cognitive and psychosocial development
		3. Plan a preoperative teaching approach based on child's prior preparation and individual level of comprehension; collaborate with other members of the health care team
		  a. Most children under 2-3 yr of age do not have sufficient conceptual abilities to grasp details about surgery or postoperative care; they usually benefit most from general information and repeated assurances that their parents will be waiting for them after surgery (if this is true), and that they will be returning home soon
		  b. Children may enjoy and benefit from use of dolls or other play equipment preoperatively and postoperatively; plan unstructured sessions to assess child's understanding of hospital procedure, and his fears and concerns; plan structured sessions for the child older than approximately 2 yr, to teach child about planned treatment or to clarify serious misconceptions; it is important that child not be given more detailed information than he can handle—take cues from child about tolerance and acceptance of information

Table 3-15 Nursing care of the pediatric cardiovascular surgical patient—cont'd

Nursing diagnosis	Expected outcomes	Nursing activities
A. Patient and family may demonstrate anxiety related to child's cardiovascular disease, surgery, prognosis, and/or hospitalization—cont'd		c. Describe the postoperative experience according to child's (and family's) *need to know* and *readiness to learn*; do not overwhelm child with threatening details about events that will occur while he is asleep, or about things that he won't see, hear, or feel; *take cues from child and family* and do not give child more information than he is able to handle; it may be necessary to provide child with small amounts of information at a time, with frequent reinforcement of important points d. School-age child may benefit from use of human figure drawings during explanation of his preoperative and postoperative care (see Chapter 2 and the box on preparations of children and adolescents for procedures and surgery) e. Plan timing of child's teaching carefully; if child does not have a well-developed sense of time intervals, give explanations the evening before surgery, explanations should not be complex; if child has a well-developed concept of time intervals, preparation may be accomplished gradually, focusing on different aspects of postoperative care at different sessions f. Teach child those things that *he* can do that will hasten his recovery (e.g., deep breathing and coughing) g. If child is asymptomatic, avoid telling child that the surgery will "make him feel better" since child will actually feel worse in the early postoperative period; it may be more accurate to tell child that the noise in his heart will be fixed (child may be frightened to hear that he has a "leaky" heart or a "hole" in his heart, so these terms should probably be avoided)

Continued.

Table 3-15   Nursing care of the pediatric cardiovascular surgical patient—cont'd

Nursing diagnosis	Expected outcomes	Nursing activities

A. Patient and family may demonstrate anxiety related to child's cardiovascular disease, surgery, prognosis, and/or hospitalization—cont'd		4. Provide child (as appropriate) and family with the opportunity to visit the critical-care unit and to meet with the nursing staff; very young children, however, may be more frightened by the sight of critically ill children, so a preoperative visit to the critical-care unit should be carefully planned and supervised
		5. Discuss child's general activity schedule (preoperative and postoperative) with child (as appropriate) and family. Review the following information:
		  a. Time of surgery
		  b. Need for preoperative NPO orders
		  c. Approximate length of surgery (overestimations are usually better than underestimations)
		  d. Anticipated length of stay in the critical-care unit (overestimations are usually better than underestimations)
		  e. Anticipated postoperative and posthospitalization activity
		6. Encourage child and family to ask questions and discuss their concerns; it may be helpful to ask child to "name the one scariest thing," to obtain concrete examples of child's fears
		7. Assist in preparing child for diagnostic procedures
		8. Continuously assess child's and family's level of anxiety and be prepared to provide more information or reassurance or comfort as needed; occasionally an anxious parent continues to ask many questions, when, in fact, reassurance or comfort is really needed; in this case, the nurse should avoid providing more and more information and should attempt to determine what the parent is *really* wanting to know

Table 3-15 Nursing care of the pediatric cardiovascular surgical patient—cont'd

Nursing diagnosis	Expected outcomes	Nursing activities
A. Patient and family may demonstrate anxiety related to child's cardiovascular disease, surgery, prognosis, and/or hospitalization—cont'd		9. Record specific teaching information (including specific terminology used to describe procedures or equipment) in child's chart or care plan, so health care team can reinforce the same information consistently 10. Provide further teaching as new problems arise 11. Provide child with postoperative opportunities to discuss the surgical or intensive care experience through play, art, or games 12. Encourage child's expression of feelings and emphasize the acceptability of such expression (e.g., it is "okay to cry" if it hurts); if some of child's expressions of anger are harmful (e.g., if child pulls out an IV line), place consistent limits on this form of expression and discuss this with child 13. Assess and document family strengths and family stresses, since these may influence the family's response to stress 14. Assess family's need for financial assistance or other additional support and refer them to appropriate hospital support personnel, including social worker, hospital financial advisor, or state cr local agencies, as needed
B. Postoperatively, patient may develop inadequate systemic perfusion and low cardiac output related to: 1. Hypovolemia (as a result of hemorrhage, diuresis, or inadequate fluid administration) 2. Tamponade	1. Patient will demonstrate adequate systemic perfusion as demonstrated by: a. Warm extremities b. Pink mucous membranes and nailbeds c. Strong peripheral pulses d. Brisk capillary refill e. Urine output of 0.5-1 ml/kg/hr	1. Assess indirect evidence of child's systemic perfusion, including: a. Temperature of extremities (should be warm) b. Color of mucous membranes and nailbeds (should be pink) c. Quality and intensity of peripheral pulses d. Capillary refill time (should be brisk) Notify physician of signs of poor systemic perfusion

Continued.

Table 3-15 Nursing care of the pediatric cardiovascular surgical patient—cont'd

Nursing diagnosis	Expected outcomes	Nursing activities
B. Postoperatively, patient may develop inadequate systemic perfusion and low cardiac output related to—cont'd 3. Decreased cardiac contractility (related to hypervolemia, electrolyte imbalance, or cardiac dysfunction) 4. Increased systemic or pulmonary vascular resistance 5. Arrhythmias 6. Hypothermia NOTE: Each of these problems will be discussed separately later in the table	2. Patient will demonstrate normal arterial blood pressure ("normal" range for each patient is determined after consideration of normal range for patient's age and patient's preoperative blood pressure) 3. Patient will demonstrate normal arterial blood gases (pH of 7.35-7.45; P_{O_2} 80-100 torr in child or 60-80 in neonate; P_{CO_2} of 35-45 torr)	2. Measure and record hourly urine output; report output of <0.5-1.0 ml/kg/hr to physician; measure urine specific gravity every 4-8 hr and correlate with urine volume; if urine volume is low and if specific gravity is low, renal dysfunction may be present 3. Measure patient's arterial blood pressure; notify physician of arterial hypotension or hypertension (see Table 3-2) 4. If cardiac output thermistor probe is in place, measure child's cardiac output as ordered or as indicated by patient's condition; include amounts of fluid injected as part of patient's fluid intake; convert any cardiac output measurements to *cardiac index*; report a cardiac index of less than 2.5 L/minute/m² body surface area to physicians immediately 5. If a Swan-Ganz catheter is in place, simultaneous arterial and venous oxygen saturation measurements may be made and used to calculate arterial and mixed venous oxygen content; if the difference between child's arterial and mixed venous oxygen content is increasing, the cardiac output is probably falling; if the difference is decreasing, the cardiac output is probably increasing 6. Monitor child's arterial blood gases and report any metabolic acidosis, hypoxemia, or hypercapnia to a physician 7. Total all fluid intake patient is receiving and discuss with physician if total fluid intake greatly exceeds total fluid output

Table 3-15 Nursing care of the pediatric cardiovascular surgical patient—cont'd

Nursing diagnosis	Expected outcomes	Nursing activities

C. Patient may develop postoperative hypovolemia related to hemorrhage, diuresis, or inadequate fluid administration	1. Patient will demonstrate minimal chest tube drainage (<3 ml/kg/hr or <5%-7% of total circulating blood volume during first 3 hr postoperatively); if excessive chest tube drainage is present, physician will be notified immediately and blood loss will be replaced with appropriate blood component
	2. Patient will demonstrate adequate hematocrit (to be specifically determined by health care team—approximate ranges are 40% minimum for infants and 30% minimum for children)
	3. Patient will demonstrate signs of adequate intravascular volume as demonstrated by:
	  a. Adequate central venous or right atrial pressure
	  b. Adequate pulmonary artery wedge or left atrial pressure
	  c. Moist mucous membranes
	  d. Good skin turgor
	  e. Urine output of 0.5-1 ml/kg/hr with appropriate specific gravity
		1. Calculate child's circulating blood volume (see Table 3-9) and consider all blood loss in terms of that blood volume; notify physician if unreplaced blood loss totals 5%-7% of child's circulating blood volume; transfusion may then be ordered
		2. Record running total of unreplaced blood drawn for laboratory analysis for any patient under 1 yr of age; discuss replacement of this blood with physician once it totals 5%-7% of infant's circulating blood volume
		3. Strip chest tubes gently but firmly enough to keep them free of clots. Notify physician if chest tube output totals ≥3 ml/kg/hr for 3 hr or more, or 5 ml/kg/hr in any 1 hour since this is excessive
		NOTE: *Bleeding totaling 3 ml/kg/hr for 3 hr constitutes a 12%-15% hemorrhage*
		4. Draw blood sample for hematocrit determination immediately after surgery (as ordered), and repeat sample as patient condition or physician order indicates; if patient's hematocrit is low or has fallen suddenly, report this to physician immediately
		5. If excessive chest tube output is present, draw blood samples for coagulation studies (as ordered by physician or per unit policy); discuss abnormal results with physician so appropriate blood component therapy may be administered
		6. If excessive chest tube output is present in the absence of any coagulopathy, discuss possibility of surgical bleeding with physician; patient may require reoperation to locate and repair the site of bleeding; surgical bleeding should be suspected when any patient demonstrates excessive chest tube bleeding with evidence of good clot formation in the tube; these patients are most at risk for clot obstruction of chest tubes and resultant tamponade

Continued.

Table 3-15 Nursing care of the pediatric cardiovascular surgical patient—cont'd

Nursing diagnosis	Expected outcomes	Nursing activities

C. Patient may develop postoperative hypovolemia related to hemorrhage, diuresis, or inadequate fluid administration—cont'd		7. Total all fluid intake and output and report patient's fluid balance to physician
		8. Measure patient's central venous and/or right atrial pressure, pulmonary artery wedge and/or left atrial pressure; maintain these cardiac filling pressures at the level where systemic perfusion is best, or as per physician order (see expected outcomes 1 and 2 in nursing diagnosis B)
		  a. Postoperative filling pressures are usually maintained at 5-15 mm Hg, but the specific ideal pressures should be determined by surgeon and other members of the health care team; these filling pressures are usually maintained with infusion of blood components or crystalloid or colloid solutions
		  b. Whole blood or packed cells are usually administered if additional fluid administration is required and if child's hematocrit is low; fresh frozen plasma, albumin, or other colloid or crystalloid solutions are usually administered if additional fluid is required and if child's hematocrit is satisfactory
		  c. If high filling pressures are required to maintain satisfactory systemic perfusion, child's cardiac contractility is probably low, and correction of acid-base or electrolyte balance, or administration of inotropic medications may be required (with physician order); see nursing diagnosis E
		  d. If child's filling pressures rise rapidly with administration of only small volumes of fluid, child's ventricular compliance is reduced, and fluid administration should be accomplished very slowly

Table 3-15 Nursing care of the pediatric cardiovascular surgical patient—cont'd

Nursing diagnosis	Expected outcomes	Nursing activities
C. Patient may develop postoperative hypovolemia related to hemorrhage, diuresis, or inadequate fluid administration—cont'd		9. Assess patient's level of hydration: a. Mucous membranes should be moist b. Infant's fontanelle should be level (not sunken or bulging) c. Tearing should be present with cry beyond 4-8 weeks of age d. Skin turgor should be good (it should not remain "tented" after pinching, and it should not be taut and shiny) e. Urine output should be ≥0.5-1.0 ml/kg/hr if fluid intake is adequate; urine specific gravity should be <1.020 Report signs of inadequate or excessive hydration to physician
D. Patient may develop tamponade and resultant low cardiac output as the result of mediastinal bleeding and inadequate mediastinal drainage	1. Patient will not demonstrate any signs of cardiac tamponade: a. High central venous (or right atrial) and left atrial (or pulmonary artery wedge) pressures with falling systemic arterial pressure and decreasing systemic perfusion b. Pulsus paradoxus c. Decreased intensity of heart sounds (late) 2. Any evidence of cardiac tamponade will be reported to physician immediately, so prompt treatment can be initiated	1. Assess patient continuously for signs of cardiac tamponade: a. Elevated venous and atrial pressures NOTE: Isolated right or left atrial tamponade can produce isolated elevation in right or left atrial pressure b. Poor systemic perfusion c. Pulsus paradoxus (fall in systolic arterial pressure by more than 8-10 mm Hg with spontaneous inspiration) NOTE: Pulsus paradoxus may not be observed if patient is receiving positive pressure assisted ventilation Other *late* signs of tamponade include: a. Distant heart sounds b. Bradycardia c. Hypotension d. Widening of mediastinum on chest radiograph Report any of these findings to physician and be prepared to institute emergency measures as needed

Continued.

Table 3-15 Nursing care of the pediatric cardiovascular surgical patient—cont'd

Nursing diagnosis	Expected outcomes	Nursing activities
D. Patient may develop tamponade and resultant low cardiac output as the result of mediastinal bleeding and inadequate mediastinal drainage—cont'd		2. Keep chest tubes patent with gentle stripping NOTE: Tamponade as the result of clotted chest tubes is especially likely in patient with a history of excessive mediastinal chest tube output and good evidence of clotting, which ceases abruptly with a concurrent deterioration in patient's clinical appearance; "back-stripping" of mediastinal tubes or direct suctioning of mediastinal tubes may be necessary (with physician order) if tamponade is suspected 3. If tamponade develops, prepare thoracotomy tray for emergency thoracotomy (or for patient return to operating room, as hospital policy dictates)

E. Postoperatively, patient may develop decreased cardiac contractility related to hypervolemia, acid-base or electrolyte imbalance, or cardiac dysfunction	1. Patient will demonstrate no persistent signs of systemic or pulmonary venous engorgement (see nursing diagnosis I)
	2. Patient will demonstrate an arterial pH of 7.35-7.45, an arterial oxygen tension of 80-100 torr (60-80 torr in neonates) and an arterial carbon dioxide tension of 35-45 torr
	3. Patient will demonstrate normal serum electrolyte concentrations (particularly glucose, calcium, and potassium)
	4. Patient will demonstrate minimal fluid weight gain:
	  a. ≤50 gm/24 hr in infants
	  b. ≤200 gm/24 hr in children
	  c. ≤500 gm/24 hr in adolescents
		1. Monitor for signs of systemic venous engorgement:
		  a. High measured central venous or right atrial pressure
		  b. Hepatomegaly
		  c. Jugular venous distention (useful only in older children)
		  d. Periorbital edema
		  e. Pleural effusion
		  f. Ascites
		Discuss these findings with physician; patient may require diuresis (per physician order)
		2. Monitor for signs of pulmonary venous engorgement:
		  a. Tachypnea (if patients breathing spontaneously)
		  b. Increased respiratory effort (if patient is breathing spontaneously)
		  c. Increased peak inspiratory pressures or decreased lung compliance (as assessed during hand ventilation with a manual resuscitator when patient is intubated), or increased volume of pulmonary secretions (if patient is intubated and mechanically ventilated)
		  d. Increased pulmonary vascular markings on chest radiograph
		  NOTE: Child's heart size may also be increased, and a pleural effusion may also be present when child has cardiac dysfunction

Table 3-15 Nursing care of the pediatric cardiovascular surgical patient—cont'd

Nursing diagnosis	Expected outcomes	Nursing activities
E. Postoperatively, patient may develop decreased cardiac contractility related to hypervolemia, acid-base or electrolyte imbalance, or cardiac dysfunction—cont'd		3. Monitor patient's arterial blood gas values and report development of acidosis, hypoxemia, or hypercapnia to physician; initiation of, or adjustment in, ventilatory support may be required (see nursing diagnosis J)
		4. Monitor child's serum electrolyte concentration, and report any abnormalities to physician so treatment can be instituted, as indicated below:
		a. If metabolic acidosis is present, sodium bicarbonate may be ordered as follows:
		1. 1-4 mEq/kg/dose, or
		2. Base excess × kg body weight × 0.3 = ____ mEq sodium bicarbonate required
		3. Maximum of 8 mEq/kg/24 hr of sodium bicarbonate is recommended
		NOTE: Since administration of sodium bicarbonate results in the formation of carbon dioxide, it is imperative that ventilatory function and/or ventilatory support be adequate to prevent the development of a secondary hypercapnia and respiratory acidosis
		b. If hypoglycemia is present, administration of hypertonic glucose solution will be ordered as follows:
		1. D_{50}: 0.5-1.0 ml/kg/dose, or
		2. D_{25}: 1-2 ml/kg/dose
		c. If hypocalcemia is present, administer calcium solution as ordered:
		1. 10% calcium chloride (20-50 mg/kg) or calcium gluconate (100-200 mg/kg)
		2. Daily supplement of 200 mg/kg/24 hr of calcium gluconate may be ordered intravenously for neonate
		Administer any calcium infusion through a large-bore venous catheter, and administer slowly to prevent bradycardia (administration rate should not exceed 100 mg/minute)

Continued.

Table 3-15   Nursing care of the pediatric cardiovascular surgical patient—cont'd

Nursing diagnosis	Expected outcomes	Nursing activities

E. Postoperatively, patient may develop decreased cardiac contractility related to hypervolemia, acid-base or electrolyte imbalance, or cardiac dysfunction—cont'd		d. If hypokalemia is present, administer potassium chloride (as ordered) as follows:
		1. Approximately 1 mEq/kg/dose may be given intravenously or
		2. IV or oral daily supplement of 2-4 mEq/kg/dose may be ordered
		Administer IV potassium chloride through a large bore or central venous catheter; if peripheral administration of potassium chloride is required, the solution should be sufficiently diluted so vascular irritation is prevented; inadvertent bolus administration of the drug can be prevented if IV tubing is carefully labeled during potassium chloride infusion
		e. If hyperkalemia is present, physician may order administration of a sodium polystyrene sulfonate enema, glucose ± insulin, or calcium gluconate as follows:
		1. 1 gm resin of sodium polystyrene sulfonate/kg/rectal dose or
		2. Glucose and insulin administration
		   a. 0.5 mg D_{50}/kg and
		   b. 1 unit insulin/4 gm glucose
		3. Calcium gluconate (10%) 50 mg/kg may be ordered to reduce myocardial irritability
		5. NOTE: If poor systemic perfusion persists despite presence of adequate (or even high) cardiac filling pressures and correction of acidosis, hypoxia, or electrolyte imbalances, discuss initiation of inotropic cardiac support or afterload reduction with physician (see also Table 3-11)

Table 3-15 Nursing care of the pediatric cardiovascular surgical patient—cont'd

Nursing diagnosis	Expected outcomes	Nursing activities
E. Postoperatively, patient may develop decreased cardiac contractility related to hypervolemia, acid-base or electrolyte imbalance, or cardiac dysfunction—cont'd		6. Administer dopamine by continuous IV infusion as ordered; desired dose of dopamine will be titrated according to desired clinical effect, as indicated below: a. 1-4 μg/kg/minute will generally provide "dopaminergic" effects, including renal arterial dilation and increased urine output b. 4-8 or 10 μg/kg/minute will usually provide primary beta$_1$-adrenergic effects, including increased heart rate and increased cardiac contractility; the dopaminergic effects should also persist at this dose c. $\geq$8-10 μg/kg/minute will provide primarily alpha-adrenergic effects, including peripheral vasoconstriction NOTE: These effects and dosages are approximate and individual response of patient should always be considered when titrating the dose 7. Administer dobutamine by continuout drip IV infusion as ordered (usually 2-10 μg/kg/minute); dobutamine provides primarily beta$_1$-adrenergic effects, including increased cardiac contractility and increased cardiac output, *dobutamine produces no selective renal artery dilation* 8. If any continuous infusion medication is ordered, administer that medication through a separate IV line so that the infusion will not have to be interrupted for administration of other medications or fluid therapy; verify dosage, concentration, and function of the infusion system hourly and with any change in patient's condition; include fluid administered with infusion in calculation of hourly fluid intake

Continued.

Table 3-15 Nursing care of the pediatric cardiovascular surgical patient—cont'd

Nursing diagnosis	Expected outcomes	Nursing activities

F. Patient may demonstrate decreased cardiac output postoperatively related to an increase in systemic or pulmonary vascular resistance	1. Patient will demonstrate good peripheral perfusion as indicated by:
	  a. Warm extremities
	  b. Pink mucous membranes and nailbeds
	  c. Strong peripheral pulses
	  d. Brisk capillary refill
	  e. Urine output of 0.5-1 ml/kg/hr
	2. Patient will demonstrate normal systemic vascular resistance:
	  a. 10-15 U/m² body surface area in neonate
	  b. 15-20 U/m² body surface area in toddler
	  c. 15-30 U/m² body surface area in child
	3. Patient will demonstrate normal pulmonary vascular resistance:
	  a. 8-10 U/m² body surface area in neonate
	  b. 1-3 U/m² body surface area in infant and child
		1. Assess child's indirect evidence of systemic perfusion (see the nursing activities for nursing diagnosis B) and notify physician if patient demonstrates evidence of poor systemic perfusion
		2. If child's cardiac output is measured and if a central venous or right atrial pressure measurement is available, child's systemic vascular resistance (SVR) can be calculated
		NOTE: Even a "normal" systemic vascular resistance may be too high if child's cardiac contractility is significantly reduced; therefore trends in child's calculated SVR and child's clinical status are usually considered more important than any single SVR measurement
		3. If high systemic vascular resistance is thought to be producing increased left ventricular afterload and decreased cardiac output, afterload reduction may be attempted with any of the following IV medications:
		  a. Nitroglycerin: 0.1-10 μg/kg/minute (an ointment form of the medication may be given instead of the IV form)
		  b. Sodium nitroprusside: 0.5-8.0 μg/kg/minute
		  c. Dobutamine: 2.0-10.0 μg/kg/minute
		  d. Isoproterenol: 0.05-0.1 μg/kg/minute
		NOTE: These drugs are often administered concurrently with a sympathomimetic inotropic drug
		4. If continuous infusion systemic vasodilators are used:
		  a. Administer the vasodilator through a separate IV line, and label the line carefully; prevent interruption in or acceleration of rate of vasodilator infusion, and prevent inadvertent "bolus" administration of medication when IV tubing is changed

Table 3-15 Nursing care of the pediatric cardiovascular surgical patient—cont'd

Nursing diagnosis	Expected outcomes	Nursing activities
F. Patient may demonstrate decreased cardiac output postoperatively related to an increase in systemic or pulmonary vascular resistance—cont'd		b. Keep crystalloid or colloid solution available at bedside for administration if hypotension results from venodilation; fluid administration is often ordered to maintain a stable right or left atrial pressure during vasodilator therapy NOTE: Hypotension is more likely to occur during vasodilator therapy if hypovolemia is present c. Throughout vasodilator therapy, monitor indirect evidence of child's systemic perfusion and notify the physician of signs of inadequate systemic perfusion 5. If child's cardiac output, pulmonary artery, and left atrial pressures are measured, calculate child's pulmonary vascular resistance (PVR), and record on flow sheet 6. If child's calculated pulmonary vascular resistance is high, or if child is known to have increased pulmonary vascular resistance from preoperative catheterization studies: a. Ensure that child's alveolar ventilation is adequate since alveolar hypoxia can produce pulmonary arterial vasoconstriction and increased pulmonary vascular resistance; as a result, child with high pulmonary vascular resistance or reactive pulmonary vascularity should be weaned from ventilatory support *very slowly* b. Prevent hypothermia, since it may contribute to development of pulmonary vasoconstriction and increased pulmonary vascular resistance

Continued.

Table 3-15 Nursing care of the pediatric cardiovascular surgical patient—cont'd

Nursing diagnosis	Expected outcomes	Nursing activities

F. Patient may demonstrate decreased cardiac output postoperatively related to an increase in systemic or pulmonary vascular resistance—cont'd		c. Prevent or ensure prompt treatment of acidosis since acidosis can also produce pulmonary arterial vasoconstriction
		NOTE: Postoperative care of child with pulmonary hypertension requires excellent respiratory support since inadequate ventilation will enhance pulmonary arterial vasoconstriction, and can quickly produce a fall in cardiac output
		7. If pulmonary vascular resistance is high, administration of a systemic vasodilator, particularly nitroglycerin (0.5-10 μg/kg/minute) or sodium nitroprusside (0.5-8.0 μg/kg/minute) is usually ordered; additional pulmonary vasodilators may also be prescribed:
		  a. Tolazoline: 1-2 mg/kg IV push test dose; then, if effective, 1-2 mg/kg/hr will be administered by continuous infusion; NOTE: watch for signs of systemic hypotension
		  b. Isoproterenol: 0.05-0.1 μg/kg/minute
		8. If child receives sodium nitroprusside therapy for 48 hr or more, child's platelet concentration should be checked since sodium nitroprusside administration can produce thrombocytopenia; in addition, child's serum thiocyanate level should be checked since metabolism of nitroprusside produces thiocyanate and cyanide; toxic thiocyanate levels are >10 mg/dl
		9. When patient is being weaned from vasodilator or inotropic support, it is important that *only one medication dose be changed at a time* so that child's response to change can be evaluated

Table 3-15 Nursing care of the pediatric cardiovascular surgical patient—cont'd

Nursing diagnosis	Expected outcomes	Nursing activities

G. Patient may develop a decrease in cardiac output postoperatively, as the result of an arrhythmia	1. Patient will demonstrate normal ECG
	2. If arrhythmia develops, patient will demonstrate no hemodynamic compromise (decreased systemic perfusion) because treatment will be initiated promptly (if needed)
		1. Monitor patient ECG continuously with monitor; ensure the display of a clear tracing with proper lead placement and good skin preparation
		2. If child develops any arrhythmias, immediately assess the effect on child's systemic perfusion
		  a. Assess indirect evidence of child's systemic perfusion (warmth of extremities, color of mucous membranes and nailbeds, strength of peripheral pulses, quantity of urine output)—notify physician of any arrhythmias associated with decreased systemic perfusion immediately
		  b. If arrhythmia causes inadequate systemic perfusion, initiate cardiopulmonary resuscitation as needed
		3. Obtain a rhythm strip to document any arrhythmia (include at least 10-12 ventricular complexes)
		4. Attempt to determine potential contributing factors when any arrhythmia develops:
		  a. Changes in intravascular potassium and calcium concentrations
		  b. Acidosis
		  c. Hypoxemia
		Obtain blood sample for arterial blood gas and/or serum electrolyte concentrations (as ordered or per unit policy); if patient is receiving digoxin therapy, check with physician before administering next digoxin dose, and obtain blood sample for digoxin level as ordered
		5. If temporary pacing wires are in place and connected to an external pacemaker, check the function of the wires and the pacemaker
		  a. If patient becomes bradycardic even though his temporary pacing wires are connected to a demand pacemaker, the pacemaker may not be "capturing" the ventricle, and the pacemaker impulse voltage may require adjustment (it usually should be increased)

Continued.

Table 3-15 Nursing care of the pediatric cardiovascular surgical patient—cont'd

Nursing diagnosis	Expected outcomes	Nursing activities
G. Patient may develop a decrease in cardiac output postoperatively, as the result of an arrhythmia—cont'd		b. If child becomes tachycardic while his pacemaker wires are attached to a demand external pacemaker, check to see if pacemaker is "competing" with child's ventricular rhythm (pacemaker may require adjustment or replacement) c. If pacemaker is not functioning properly, check demand rate, sensitivity level, impulse voltage (or output), and battery level; in addition, check the connections between wires and pacemaker, and make sure that both wires are intact 6. Administer electrolyte supplements, sodium bicarbonate, or antiarrhythmic medications as ordered, and assess patient response
H. During early infancy, patient may develop low cardiac output postoperatively as a result of hypothermia	1. Patient will demonstrate a rectal temperature of approximately 37° C, and a skin temperature of approximately 36-36.5° C 2. Patient will demonstrate evidence of good systemic perfusion (including warm extremities, pink mucous membranes and nailbeds, strong peripheral pulses, good capillary reflill, and urine output of 0.5-1.0 ml/kg/hr)	1. Monitor patient rectal and skin temperature every hour and more often as needed postoperatively 2. Use an overbed warmer or an isolette to provide the infant with a neutral thermal environment (that environmental temperature at which infant can maintain a rectal temperature of 37° C with the lowest oxygen consumption—these temperature ranges can be found in Scope's charts and should be posted in every critical-care unit caring for neonates; see Appendix G) 3. Notify physician if infant has a rectal temperature below 36-36.5°C despite warming measures 4. Notify physician if patient's rectal temperature *exceeds* 37° C in the presence of a low skin temperature or poor systemic perfusion since this may indicate presence of low cardiac output
I. Patient may develop postoperative congestive heart failure as a result of: 1. An uncorrected congenital heart defect (e.g., after palliative surgery)	1. Patient will demonstrate good systemic perfusion. (see nursing diagnosis B) 2. Patient will demonstrate no evidence of systemic venous engorgement, including:	1. Monitor child's heart rate and evidence of systemic perfusion (including the warmth of extremities, color of mucous membranes and nailbeds, strength of peripheral pulses, speed of capillary refill, and urine output); notify physician if evidence of poor systemic perfusion is present

Table 3-15 Nursing care of the pediatric cardiovascular surgical patient—cont'd

Nursing diagnosis	Expected outcomes	Nursing activities
I. Patient may develop postoperative congestive heart failure as a result of—cont'd 2. Correction of a congenital heart defect (and alteration in ventricular preload, contractility, and afterload) 3. Postoperative hypervolemia 4. Electrolyte imbalance 5. Arrhythmia	a. High central venous or right atrial pressure b. Hepatomegaly c. Periorbital edema d. Ascites e. Pleural effusion 3. Patient will demonstrate no evidence of pulmonary venous engorgement, including: a. Tachypnea (if breathing spontaneously) b. Increased respiratory effort, including retractions, nasal flaring, and grunting (if breathing spontaneously) c. Increased left atrial or pulmonary artery wedge pressure d. Increased peak inspiratory pressure or decreased lung compliance (if patient receiving mechanical ventilation) 4. Patient will demonstrate minimal fluid weight gain: a. ≥50 gm/24 hr in infants b. ≥200 gm/24 hr in children c. ≥500 gm/24 hr in adolescents	2. Measure urine output hourly, and notify physician if it totals <0.5-1.0 ml/kg/hr a. If decreased urine output is accompanied by an increased urine specific gravity and if fluid intake is thought to be inadequate, physician may order additional fluid administration b. If child's central venous pressure is high and if periorbital edema, hepatomegaly, or ascites are present, decreased urine output is probably the result of congestive heart failure and diuretic administration will usually be ordered 3. Monitor for evidence of systemic venous engorgement: a. High central venous or right atrial pressure b. Hepatomegaly c. Periorbital edema d. Ascites or pleural effusion Discuss these findings with physician as soon as they are observed 4. Monitor for signs of pulmonary venous engorgement: a. Tachypnea (if patient is breathing spontaneously) b. Increased respiratory effort, as indicated by nasal flaring, retractions, and grunting (if patient is breathing spontaneously) c. Increased left atrial or pulmonary artery wedge pressure d. Increased peak inspiratory pressure or decreased lung compliance (as assessed during hand ventilation of intubated patient), or increased volume of respiratory secretions in patient receiving mechanical ventilatory assistance e. Pleural effusion

Continued.

Table 3-15 Nursing care of the pediatric cardiovascular surgical patient—cont'd

Nursing diagnosis	Expected outcomes	Nursing activities

I. Patient may develop postoperative congestive heart failure as a result of—cont'd		5. Monitor patient fluid intake and output and discuss positive fluid balance with physician
		6. Administer digitalis derivative as ordered; check dosage before administration (see Table 3-4), and monitor for arrhythmias or other signs of toxicity
		7. Administer diuretic therapy as ordered
		  a. Check dosage and possible urinary electrolyte losses
		  b. Assess patient urinary response to diuretic therapy and notify physician if this response is inadequate
		  c. Check patient electrolyte concentration (per physician order or unit policy) and administer electrolyte supplement as ordered
		8. Measure child's weight daily or twice daily on same scale at same time of day; notify physician of significant weight gain:
		  a. ≥50 gm/24 hr in infants
		  b. ≥200 gm/24 hr in children
		  c. ≥500 gm/24 hr in adolescents

J. Patient may develop respiratory distress as a result of:
  a. Atelectasis
  b. Pneumothorax
  c. Hemothorax
  d. Pleural effusion
  e. Chylothorax
  f. Congestive heart failure
  g. Low cardiac output
  h. Pulmonary hypertension
  i. Inadequate ventilatory support
	1. Patient will demonstrate normal respiratory rate (normal range is determined by consideration of normal range for child's age and clinical condition and child's preoperative respiratory rate)
	2. Patient will demonstrate minimal evidence of increased respiratory effort (including nasal flaring, retractions, and grunting)
		1. Assess child's chest expansion, lung aeration, respiratory rate, respiratory effort (if patient breathing spontaneously), lung compliance, and evidence of lung compliance (as evidenced by ease of hand ventilation of intubated patient); report abnormal findings to physician
		2. Monitor for evidence of atelectasis (especially of right upper lobe):
		  a. Decreased breath sounds
		  b. Change in quality or pitch of breath sounds
		  c. Chest dullness to percussion
		  d. Decreased chest movement with inspiration

Table 3-15 Nursing care of the pediatric cardiovascular surgical patient—cont'd

Nursing diagnosis	Expected outcomes	Nursing activities

J. Patient may develop respiratory distress as a result of—cont'd
  j. Malfunctioning pleural drainage system
  k. Pain and "splinting" of incision and resultant hypoventilation
	3. Patient will demonstrate adequate and equal lung aeration bilaterally with no evidence of congestion heard by auscultation
	4. Patient will maintain pH 7.35-7.45, PO_2 80-100 torr (60-80 torr in neonates), Pco_2 35-45 torr
		e. Tachypnea (if patient breathing spontaneously)
		  f. Evidence of atelectasis on chest radiograph
		NOTE: Since breath sounds are easily transmitted through thin chest wall of infant, significant atelectasis can be present without an appreciable decrease in intensity of associated breath sounds; as a result nurse must be alert to the appearance of changes in quality or pitch of breath sounds
		3. Monitor for evidence of pneumothorax:
		  a. Decreased breath sounds
		  b. Change in pitch of breath sounds
		  c. Hyperresonance of chest to percussion
		  d. Decreased chest movement during inspiration
		  e. Increased respiratory rate, effort and dyspnea (if child is breathing spontaneously)
		  f. Increased peak inspiratory pressures and increased resistance to hand ventilation (if patient is intubated and mechanically ventilated)
		  g. Evidence of pneumothorax on chest radiograph
		Notify physician if any of these signs develop, and prepare for chest tube insertion or tap as ordered
		4. Monitor for signs of development of a tension pneumothorax:
		  a. Marked respiratory distress
		  b. Restlessness or agitation with significant respiratory distress
		  c. Mediastinal shift away from side of pneumothorax (heart sounds will be heard better on the side of chest opposite the pneumothorax)
		  d. Hypotension (resulting from decreased venous return and decreased ventricular diastolic filling)

Continued.

Table 3-15   Nursing care of the pediatric cardiovascular surgical patient—cont'd

Nursing diagnosis	Expected outcomes	Nursing activities

J. Patient may develop respiratory distress as a result of—cont'd		e. High peak inspiratory pressures and extreme difficulty in providing hand ventilation (if patient intubated and receiving mechanical ventilatory support)
		f. Decreased arterial oxygen tension and possible cyanosis
		Notify physician of these findings immediately; emergency decompression of the pneumothorax is required or child may die; prepare for emergency needle aspiration of the pneumothorax or for chest tube insertion
		5. Monitor for signs of development of a hemothorax or a pleural effusion:
		  a. Increased respiratory rate and effort (if patient is breathing spontaneously)
		  b. Decreased intensity or change in quality of breath sounds
		  c. Dullness to percussion of chest
		  d. Increased peak inspiratory pressures or resistance to hand ventilation (if patient is intubated and receiving mechanical ventilatory assistance)
		  e. Evidence of free pleural fluid on chest radiograph (this will especially be apparent if a lateral decubitus film is obtained)
		  f. If a significant hemothorax develops, patient may develop signs of circulatory compromise resulting from hypovolemia (see the nursing activities for nursing diagnosis C)
		Notify physician if any of these signs develop and prepare for thoracentesis and/or chest tube insertion.
		6. Check patient chest radiograph as ordered or per unit policy (see Chapter 5)
		7. Observe appearance of chest tube drainage (if pleural tube is in place); if lymph fluid is present or if large amount of serosanguineous fluid is draining continuously, notify physician; chest tube is usually left in place until such drainage ceases; if a chylothorax is present:

Table 3-15 Nursing care of the pediatric cardiovascular surgical patient—cont'd

Nursing diagnosis	Expected outcomes	Nursing activities

J. Patient may develop respiratory distress as a result of—cont'd		a. The chest drainage often becomes milky after patient ingests food or liquid containing fat
		b. A chest tube may be placed to prevent the development of respiratory insufficiency; child may be placed on a special (medium-chain triglyceride) diet to reduce quantity of drainage; child usually also requires administration of supplemental fat-soluble vitamins (A, D, and E)
		8. If congestive heart failure, low cardiac output, or pulmonary hypertension are present, please refer to nursing activities discussed under these specific problems.
		9. If child is intubated, ensure provision of adequate ventilatory support:
		  a. Monitor chest expansion and aeration; child's chest is soft and compliant, and therefore it will move if adequate inspiratory volume is provided—*if child's chest is not expanding with inspiration, ventilatory support is not adequate*
		  b. If child appears restless, irritable, or cyanotic, notify physician and check endotracheal tube patency, position, and effectiveness of ventilation—suction patient's endotracheal tube and provide hand ventilation as necessary
		  c. Provide effective tidal volume (7-20 ml/kg—specific volume is determined by manufacturer's recommendations, ventilator dead space, tubing compliance, and unit policy) and positive end-expiratory pressure (a PEEP of 2-4 cm water is considered physiologic), as ordered
		  d. Verify ventilator settings at least every hour with vital sign measurement and more often if patient's condition changes
		  e. Check the patient's arterial blood gases per hospital policy or physician order; notify physician of abnormal results

Continued.

Table 3-15 Nursing care of the pediatric cardiovascular surgical patient—cont'd

Nursing diagnosis	Expected outcomes	Nursing activities

J. Patient may develop respiratory distress as a result of—cont'd		f. If problems arise, hand ventilate patient while ventilator is checked, assure tube patency and adequate lung aeration, and notify physician if hand-ventilation is difficult or unsuccessful (if tube is obstructed, it may be necessary to remove the tube and hand ventilate child with a bag and mask until tube can be replaced)
		NOTE: If child "fights" the ventilator and hypoxemia is not present, it may be necessary to paralyze the child to enable provision of effective ventilation; if child will be paralyzed, it is important to tell him that he won't be able to move and it is also imperative that child continue to receive analgesics
		10. If child requires mechanical ventilatory support, frequently verify tube patency and proper endotracheal tube position through frequent auscultation of breath sounds and provision of pulmonary toilet
		  a. Hand ventilate patient and suction endotracheal tube as needed to keep endotracheal tube clear and lungs clear to auscultation
		  b. Turn patient frequently (if stable), and provide percussion, vibration, and rib-springing, as needed
		  c. Provide postural drainage as ordered or needed (per patient condition or unit policy)
		  d. See Chapter 4
		11. Monitor child's arterial blood gases (as ordered and per unit policy) and discuss results with physician
		12. When child is extubated, provide bronchial (postural) drainage, chest percussion and vibration, rib-springing, and deep-breathing exercises as needed
		13. Elevate head of child's bed (to allow maximal diaphragmatic excursion) and place a small linen roll under child's shoulders (to extend airway)

Table 3-15 Nursing care of the pediatric cardiovascular surgical patient—cont'd

Nursing diagnosis	Expected outcomes	Nursing activities
J. Patient may develop respiratory distress as a result of—cont'd		14. When child is extubated, monitor for signs of upper airway obstruction (stridor, decreased air movement, increased respiratory effort) as result of subglottic edema; also monitor effectiveness of child's spontaneous ventilation 15. Ensure proper function of pleural drainage system (see Chapter 9) 16. Provide adequate pain medication per physician order; if child is breathing spontaneously, be alert for signs of respiratory depression if narcotics are administered 17. Assist child in splinting chest incision when child attempts to cough or take deep breaths, to minimize child's discomfort and maximize child's inspiratory effort
K. Patient may develop postoperative electrolyte imbalance related to use of cardiopulmonary bypass, use of diuretics, stress response, and fluid and blood component administration	1. Patient will demonstrate normal serum electrolyte concentrations 2. Patient will not demonstrate any secondary signs or complications of electrolyte imbalance	1. Monitor patient serum electrolyte balance; in young infants serum glucose and potassium balance should be monitored closely during periods of illness or stress 2. If metabolic acidosis, hypoglycemia, hypocalcemia, hypokalemia, or hyperkalemia develop, please refer to the nursing activities for nursing diagnosis E for dosages of sodium bicarbonate and electrolyte supplements 3. If serious acid-base or electrolyte imbalances develop, monitor patient closely for evidence of depressed cardiovascular function or arrhythmias, or for other systemic signs of electrolyte imbalance (such as a decrease in muscle tone or neuromuscular irritability)
L. Patient may develop renal dysfunction related to poor systemic perfusion, intravascular hemolysis, thromboembolus, or complications of medications	1. Patient will demonstrate urine output of 0.5-1.0 ml/kg/hr when fluid intake is adequate 2. Patient will demonstrate appropriate urine concentration when urine volume is reduced 3. Patient will maintain a normal serum creatinine and BUN concentration.	1. Measure patient urine output, and discuss with physician if output totals <0.5-1.0 ml/kg/hr 2. If child's urine output is inadequate and if central venous pressure is low, physician may order administration of a fluid bolus totaling 5-10 ml/kg; this bolus will often be followed by administration of a diuretic (such as furosemide: 1 mg/kg/dose)

Continued.

Table 3-15 Nursing care of the pediatric cardiovascular surgical patient—cont'd

Nursing diagnosis	Expected outcomes	Nursing activities
L. Patient may develop renal dysfunction related to poor systemic perfusion, intravascular hemolysis, thromboembolus, or complications of medications—cont'd		3. If urine output remains inadequate despite the presence of an adequate circulating blood volume (a central venous pressure or right or left atrial pressure of 5-10 mm Hg) and administration of diuretics, fluid administration should be curtailed (with physician order)
		4. Urine should be tested for the presence of blood and protein, and specific gravity should be measured every 4 hr postoperatively; if urine is positive for the presence of blood and appears rusty in color, urine sample should be spun down in a centrifuge; if blood precipitates after spinning, this suggests that whole red blood cells are present in urine and that bleeding is probably the result of bleeding from bladder trauma; if, despite centrifuge spinning, urine remains rusty in color, this suggests that urine contains red blood cell fragments as the result of intravascular hemolysis
		NOTE: If intravascular hemolysis is present, it is important that adequate urine flow be maintained to "flush" red blood cell fragments from kidneys (especially glomeruli); adequate urine flow may be maintained through judicious use of fluid and diuretic administration (per physician order)
		5. If acute tubular necrosis or renal failure is suspected, child's fluid intake should be restricted to equal urine output plus child's insensible fluid losses (if this is possible without compromising systemic perfusion)
		6. If renal dysfunction is suspected, child's serum creatinine, BUN, and potassium should be monitored closely; if urine output is present, a simultaneous sample of urine and serum for creatinine measurement will probably be requested, to attempt to determine child's urine creatinine clearance

Table 3-15 Nursing care of the pediatric cardiovascular surgical patient—cont'd

Nursing diagnosis	Expected outcomes	Nursing activities
L. Patient may develop renal dysfunction related to poor systemic perfusion, intravascular hemolysis, thromboembolus, or complications of medications—cont'd		7. Peritoneal or hemodialysis will be considered if child becomes severely hypervolemic, hyperkalemic, uremic, or acidotic; drug dosages will have to be reevaluated for any drug that requires renal excretion; (see Acute renal failure, Peritoneal dialysis, and Hemodialysis, Chapter 7) 8. Sodium polystyrene sulfonate enema may be prescribed (1 gm resin/kg) if hyperkalemia develops 9. Refer to Chapter 7
M. Patient may develop neurologic impairment postoperatively as a result of: 1. Hypoxia 2. Acidosis 3. Poor systemic perfusion 4. Thromboembolism 5. Electrolyte imbalance	1. Patient will demonstrate appropriate movement of extremities with no abnormal posturing, clonus, or flaccidity 2. Patient will respond in an age-appropriate fashion to stimulation and questions 3. Patient will demonstrate brisk, equal pupil constriction in response to light	1. Assess child's neurologic function as soon as possible after child returns from surgery: a. Check pupil size and response to light b. If child is awake, check movement and strength of all extremities c. If child is asleep, note muscle tone and withdrawal from mildly noxious stimuli Report any abnormal findings to a physician immediately NOTE: Pupil dilation is normally present when patient is receiving sympathomimetic agents (such as dopamine) or vagolytic agents (such as atropine) 2. If child requires paralyzing agents postoperatively, the clinical diagnosis of seizure activity becomes very difficult; seizures should be suspected if child demonstrates wide fluctuations in blood pressure in the absence of any cardiovascular problem; an electroencephalogram is often required to determine if seizures are present in these children 3. Assist in the correction of hypotension, hypoxemia, or acidosis (per physician order) as quickly as possible to prevent neurologic sequelae a. Assess child's neurologic status if any of these problems arise b. Suggest that a neurologic consult be obtained (with physician order) if abnormalities are suspected

Continued.

Table 3-15   Nursing care of the pediatric cardiovascular surgical patient—cont'd

Nursing diagnosis	Expected outcomes	Nursing activities
M. Patient may develop neurologic impairment postoperatively as a result of—cont'd		4. If neurologic impairment is suspected, discuss plan of care with physicians immediately, and document *all* information that is given to parents in the nursing care plan so that consistent information can be provided; parents will require extra support.
		5. If neurologic impairment is present, begin to provide passive range-of-motion exercises to prevent development of contractures (when child is stable) 　a. Obtain order for physical therapy or occupational therapy consult 　b. Develop a rehabilitative care plan and share this with all members of health care team
		6. Monitor for evidence of seizure activity: 　a. If seizures develop, notify physician immediately and position patient for maximal safety—*do not stick anything in patient's mouth* 　b. Check blood gas and serum electrolyte concentrations (as ordered or per unit policy), if metabolic imbalance is thought to be a cause of seizures; report any abnormal results to physician 　c. Administer anticonvulsant medications as ordered; check dosage and monitor for therapeutic and side effects 　d. See Seizures, Chapter 6
		7. Provide for periods of rest, and attempt to reduce visual and auditory stimulation
		8. Provide meaningful stimulation between periods of rest; orient child to time and place, and reinforce information that surgery is over, and that child's parents are nearby
		9. Administer pain medications as needed

Table 3-15 Nursing care of the pediatric cardiovascular surgical patient—cont'd

Nursing diagnosis	Expected outcomes	Nursing activities
M. Patient may develop neurologic impairment postoperatively as a result of—cont'd		10. Monitor for signs of increased intracranial pressure if hypoxic encephalopathy is present: a. Increased irritability or lethargy b. Pupillary dilation or constriction and decreased response to light c. Bradycardia d. Changes in respiratory pattern (if patient breathing spontaneously) e. Increased systolic blood pressure with widening of pulse pressure (this is a very *late* sign) Report signs of increased intracranial pressure to physician immediately; attempt to hyperventilate patient since this can produce an immediate reduction in cerebral blood volume and intracranial pressure; see Increased intracranial pressure, Chapter 6 11. If increased intracranial pressure is present, administer osmotic diuretics (e.g., mannitol) or steroids (e.g., dexamethasone) as ordered; in addition, administer antipyretics (with physician order) if rectal temperature exceeds 39°C 12. Refer to Chapter 6
N. Patient may develop postoperative infection or inflammation as a result of: a. Cardiovascular surgery b. Insertion of prosthetic material c. Invasive monitoring techniques d. Compromised nutritional status e. Postcardiotomy syndrome	1. Patient will demonstrate no evidence of overt infection, including: a. Fever above 38.5° C b. Chills c. Leukocytosis d. Local wound infection or inflammation (including erythema, wound exudate, or wound fluctuance) e. Positive wound cultures f. Positive blood cultures 2. Patient will demonstrate no evidence of postcardiotomy syndrome, including: a. Low-grade fever approximately 10 days postoperatively	1. Monitor child's temperature; notify physician if fever >38.5° C develops; physician may order blood cultures (particularly if child's surgical repair required insertion of prosthetic material) NOTE: Neonates may become hypothermic when serious infection develops 2. Keep all incisions and venous and arterial catheter entrance sites clean and dry; observe all skin puncture sites for signs of erythema, drainage, or fluctuance; notify physician of any signs of inflammation 3. Maintain strict aseptic technique when handling invasive equipment; ensure that all staff members wash hands before and after each patient contact

Continued.

Table 3-15 Nursing care of the pediatric cardiovascular surgical patient—cont'd

Nursing diagnosis	Expected outcomes	Nursing activities

N. Patient may develop postoperative infection or inflammation as a result of—cont'd	b. Leukocytosis
	c. Pleural or pericardial effusions
	d. Elevation of erythrocyte sedimentation rate
	e. Serologic evidence of anti-heart antibodies
	f. Rise in viral titers
	If postcardiotomy syndrome develops, cardiovascular compromise will be prevented
		4. Approximately 7-10 days after surgery, monitor for signs of postcardiotomy syndrome, including:
		  a. Fever >38.5° C
		  b. Substernal or pericardial chest pain, which is exacerbated by respiration and may radiate to the shoulder
		  c. Pericardial friction rub
		  d. Pericardial effusion (may be apparent on echocardiogram)
		  e. Pleural effusion (may be evident on clinical examination and chest radiograph)
		  f. Leukocytosis
		  g. Malaise or arthralgia
		  h. Elevation in erythrocyte sedimentation rate
		  i. Serologic evidence of anti-heart antibodies
		  j. Rise in viral titers
		  k. Serial electrocardiographic evidence of pericarditis
		Report these findings to physician
		5. If postcardiotomy syndrome develops, administer aspirin and/or steroids, as ordered
		6. Monitor for evidence of urinary tract infection, including:
		  a. Burning sensation with urination (or other signs of patient discomfort with voiding)
		  b. Cloudy or odorous urine
		  c. Hematuria
		NOTE: Glycosuria may be a sign of infection in children
		7. Calculate child's maintenance caloric requirements; if child is unable to take oral maintenance calories within 24-48 hr after surgery, discuss alternative methods of alimentation with physician (e.g., nasogastric feeding or parenteral alimentation) (see section on total parenteral nutrition through a central venous catheter, Chapter 8)
		8. Administer antibiotics as ordered; check dosage and monitor for side effects

Table 3-15 Nursing care of the pediatric cardiovascular surgical patient—cont'd

Nursing diagnosis	Expected outcomes	Nursing activities
N. Patient may develop postoperative infection or inflammation as a result of—cont'd		9. Change all dressings according to hospital policy; apply occlusive dressings and iodine ointment (per physician order and unit policy) to all central venous lines
O. Patient and family may possess inadequate information for patient home care	1. Patient (as appropriate) and family will demonstrate knowledge of medications and care techniques necessary for child's care at home	1. When patient's condition is stable, begin to provide child (as age-appropriate) and parents with information necessary to provide child's care at home, including: a. Dosage, route, effects, and side effects of all medications that child will receive b. Times and intervals of child's follow-up appointments with physicians c. Indications for contacting a physician d. Telephone numbers of child's primary nurse and physician e. Techniques for special care treatments (e.g., postural drainage) 2. Initiate appropriate referral to supportive services, including: a. Social services b. Visiting nurse or home care nurse c. Outpatient physical therapy d. Outpatient physician contacts 3. Document all teaching in child's care plan so that all information will be reinforced consistently

■ Specific Diseases

In this section, the etiology, pathophysiology, clinical signs and symptoms, and medical treatment and nursing interventions for the child with congenital heart disease are summarized. When common clinical problems such as congestive heart failure or hypoxemia are mentioned, the reader is asked to refer to the detailed discussion of these problems in the section on common clinical conditions in this chapter. When postoperative complications are reviewed it is presumed that the nurse will monitor for signs of low cardiac output, congestive heart failure, bleeding, arrhythmias, and respiratory distress. Those postoperative complications listed here include those *most likely* to occur following the specific procedure discussed; however, the nurse should still assess the patient for signs of other complications.

■ CONGENITAL HEART DEFECTS

Congenital heart defects are present in approximately 8 to 10 of every 1000 newborns.[219] During the first year of life, nearly 25% of infants with heart defects will require treatment (cardiac catheterization or surgery) or die within the first year of life.[134] In addition, nearly one third of infants with congenital heart defects have additional noncardiac anomalies (see Table 3-1) that may require medical or surgical attention.[309,310]

Since all forms of congenital heart defects occur as a result of problems during fetal or perinatal development, the etiology of each defect will not be elaborated (the reader is referred to the embryology section of this chapter). It is important that the nurse remember that the term "congenital" means only that the cardiac defect is present from birth. Most congenital heart disease is thought to be the result of *multifactorial inheritance,* a complex interaction of genetic and environmental factors. Teratogens are associated with only a very small percentage of congenital defects, and very few factors have been shown to *cause* congenital heart disease. The only well-documented teratogens include maternal alcoholism and maternal thalidomide, trimethadione, and hydantoin ingestion.[219,244,288,309,310]

Despite frequent attempts to link maternal illness during pregnancy with increased incidence of congenital malformations in offspring, only a few maternal health factors are associated with an increased risk of congenital heart disease. When the pregnant woman contracts rubella during the first 8 weeks of pregnancy, there is a 50% risk that her baby will have congenital rubella syndrome. This syndrome can include patent ductus arteriosus and/or pulmonary artery branch stenosis.[346] Approximately 10% of offspring of insulin-dependent diabetic mothers have congenital heart disease, most commonly transposition of the great vessels, ventricular septal defect, or hypertrophic cardiomyopathy.[170,450] Nearly 50% of infants with fetal alcohol syndrome have congenital heart disease.[310]

Some congenital heart defects are associated with chromosomal anomalies or syndromes. Most notable among these are Down's syndrome; approximately 30% to 40% of affected children have congenital heart disease. Other associated anomalies are summarized in Table 3-1.

Parents of the child with congenital heart disease often assume that they are in some way responsible for their child's heart defect. These concerns may be reinforced when the mother is questioned in detail about her pregnancy every time a health history is obtained when the child is admitted to the hospital. The health care team can often avert much of the parents' anxiety by providing a few facts about the epidemiology of congenital heart disease when the child is initially diagnosed. If the child's heart defect is thought to be associated with a specific chromosomal anomaly or syndrome, the parents may wish to obtain genetic counseling so that recurrence risks will be known before they conceive another child. Most often, the parents can be assured that there was nothing they could have (or should not have) done to prevent the child's heart disease.

The following section begins with a discussion of acyanotic defects that produce increased pulmonary blood flow. Cyanotic defects that produce increased or decreased pulmonary blood flow are then presented, and the discussion of congenital heart lesions concludes with a summary of defects that produce left heart or aortic obstruction.

■ PATENT DUCTUS ARTERIOSUS (PDA)
■ Etiology

Patent ductus arteriosus results from persistence of the fetal ductus arteriosus beyond the perinatal period (Fig. 3-26). The fetal ductus arteriosus is normally a wide, muscular vessel that allows blood to be diverted from the pulmonary artery into the aorta. Following a normal, full-term birth, the neonate's arterial oxygen tension rises; this produces constriction of the normal ductus arteriosus within days or weeks of life.[118] Ductus closure may be delayed or prevented completely if the neonate is born prematurely or if the arterial oxygen tension does not rise normally after birth. Patent ductus arteriosus can also occur as part of the rubella syndrome, and it may be seen in a small number of otherwise normal, healthy, full-term infants.

Patent ductus arteriosus is responsible for approximately 12% of all congenital heart defects. The incidence of patent ductus arteriosus in infants less than 36 weeks gestation is 32%; in most of these infants over 32 weeks gestation, the ductus will close spontaneously by 6 months of age. The incidence of

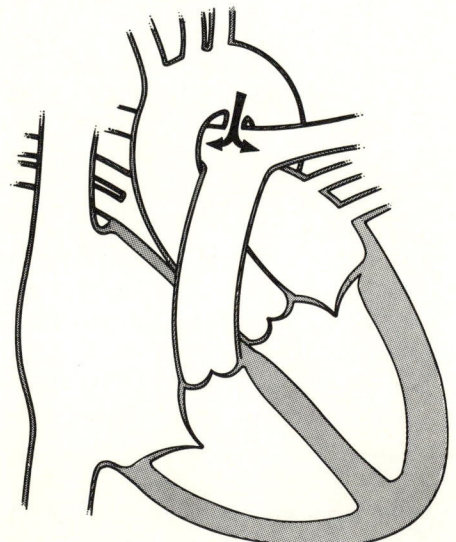

Fig. 3-26 Patent ductus arteriosus.

From Hazinski, M.: The cardiovascular system. In Howe, J., and others, editors: The handbook of nursing, New York, 1984, John Wiley & Sons, Inc.

patent ductus arteriosus is 75% in infants 28 to 30 weeks gestation and in those infants with a birthweight of less than 1200 gm.[111],[206] Approximately 25% of premature infants do become symptomatic from patent ductus arteriosus.[418]

■ **Pathophysiology**

Immediately after birth and for as long as the infant's pulmonary vascular resistance is high, there may be little shunting of blood through the patent ductus. Once the infant's pulmonary vascular resistance begins to fall, however, blood will shunt from the aorta into the pulmonary artery during systole and then during systole and diastole. Characteristically, the premature neonate with lung disease will develop symptoms of patent ductus arteriosus once his lung disease begins to resolve and once pulmonary constriction from alveolar hypoxia decreases.

The amount of blood that flows through the ductus and the extent of the child's symptoms are determined by the difference between systemic and pulmonary vascular resistance, the size of the radius, and the length of the ductus. There is also some evidence that increased fluid administration to premature infants may contribute to the development of symptoms from the ductus arteriosus.[33],[154] If pulmonary vascular resistance is low and if the ductus is wide and short, a large shunt will develop between the aorta and the pulmonary artery. Increased pulmonary blood flow under high pressure can produce increased pulmonary interstitial water, decreased lung compliance, and increased work of breathing. Cardiomegaly will result from a large shunt, and left ventricular dilation and hypertrophy and congestive heart failure can develop. High pulmonary blood flow under high pressure can also produce increased pulmonary vascular resistance. Pulmonary hypertension will cause right ventricular enlargement.

NOTE: The ductus arteriosus may be life saving in infants with cyanotic heart disease and decreased pulmonary blood flow. In these infants, the ductus may provide the major source of pulmonary blood flow.

■ **Clinical signs and symptoms**

Once the infant's pulmonary vascular resistance falls, the patent ductus arteriosus produces a characteristic harsh murmur heard at the second left intercostal space along the mid-clavicular line. Initially the murmur is systolic; it then becomes continuous as pulmonary vascular resistance continues to fall. The murmur may be accompanied by a thrill over the suprasternal notch and along the upper left and right

sternal border. If the shunt is not large, this may be the only sign of a patent ductus arteriosus that the child demonstrates.

With a large patent ductus arteriosus shunt, bounding peripheral pulses and a widened pulse pressure are noted, resulting from the "aortic runoff" into the pulmonary artery. As noted earlier, increased pulmonary blood flow under high pressure produces pulmonary vascular engorgement and increased work of breathing. A large shunt causes a large volume of pulmonary venous return, resulting in enlargement of the left atrium and ventricle. Congestive heart failure can develop.[194]

The premature neonate who becomes symptomatic from a ductus arteriosus often develops signs of respiratory distress, including tachypnea, retractions, hypoxemia, and hypercapnia. One of the most sensitive signs of symptomatic patent ductus arteriosus in these infants may be increased inspired oxygen requirements.

Evidence of left (and possibly right) ventricular hypertrophy may be noted on clinical examination and by electrocardiographic criteria. The echocardiogram usually documents the presence of a large left atrium, and two-dimensional echocardiography may demonstrate the presence of the ductus itself or of abnormal flow patterns in the aorta and pulmonary artery. The chest radiograph may be normal in asymptomatic patients, but it usually demonstrates cardiomegaly and increased pulmonary vascular markings. The main pulmonary artery may be prominent.

If the child's clinical presentation is typical and if no additional abnormality is suspected, a cardiac catheterization may not be ordered since the diagnosis may be made on the basis of clinical examination, chest radiograph, and echocardiogram. If the child's presentation is atypical or if the presence of other cardiac anomalies is suspected, a cardiac catheterization will be performed. The catheterization will reveal an increase in oxygen saturation in the pulmonary artery. Right ventricular and pulmonary artery pressures will be elevated if pulmonary hypertension is present. Aortic contrast injection will demonstrate the shunt into the pulmonary artery.

If pulmonary hypertension develops, the patent ductus arteriosus murmur may decrease in intensity. If pulmonary vascular resistance is approximately equal to systemic vascular resistance, the child may develop bidirectional shunting through the patent ductus arteriosus. This causes arterial oxygen desaturation; the child may demonstrate cyanosis, particularly of the lower extremities and particularly with cry.

If the infant has a ductus-dependent cyanotic congenital heart defect, he may develop profound cyanosis if the ductus begins to constrict.

■ Medical and surgical treatment and nursing interventions

When the premature neonate becomes symptomatic from the ductus arteriosus, medical management will be attempted in order to avoid surgical repair while the neonate is critically ill. Restriction of fluid intake and administration of diuretics should reduce the symptoms of congestive heart failure.[362] The hematocrit is maintained above 45% in these neonates to maximize arterial oxygen-carrying capacity.[418] The use of digoxin in premature neonates is controversial since digoxin serum half-life may be prolonged in these infants and the incidence of digoxin toxicity is high.[41,418] It is also thought that heart failure in neonates is caused more by volume overload and by decreased left ventricular compliance than by myocardial failure.[194] As a result digoxin may not be helpful and may be harmful in these infants.

Administration of a prostaglandin synthetase inhibitor (indomethacin) to premature neonates under 13 days of age has been found to produce ductal constriction in approximately 50% of these neonates.[7,270] If the child has evidence of infection or coagulopathy, indomethacin administration is contraindicated because it is an anti-inflammatory agent and because it may produce bone marrow depression and decreased platelet aggregation. Indomethacin administration is also contraindicated in the presence of renal disease since it decreases renal blood flow and glomerular filtration rate. Since indomethacin binds to albumin, it is not administered to nenonates with hyperbilirubinemia since it may displace the bilirubin from the albumin and increase the risk of kernicterus. Potential side effects of indomethacin include gastrointestinal ulceration, oliguria, increased pulmonary artery pressure, bone marrow depression, and reduced platelet aggregation. If medical management of the symptomatic neonate fails, surgical elimination of the patent ductus arteriosus will be required.

If a patent ductus arteriosus is diagnosed in an older child, surgery is recommended since the turbulent blood flow around and through the ductus may provide a site for development of bacterial endocarditis.[214] If congestive heart failure is present, it is treated with digoxin and diuretic therapy.

Surgical treatment of patent ductus arteriosus requires closed-heart surgery through a left thoracotomy incision. The left lung is retracted to gain access to the ductus arteriosus. The ductus may be ligated (tied) or divided (cut) and oversewn. If the ductus is calcified, hypertensive, and fragile (generally, this only occurs in elderly patients), the procedure is performed with cardiopulmonary bypass on standby.[451] Morbidity and mortality following elimination of the ductus are usually extremely low (less than 2%); surgical risks are highest in critically ill preterm infants,[106,150,420] in children with severe pulmonary hypertension, and in adults. Postoperative complications include those of thoracotomy (bleeding, atelectasis, hemothorax, pneumothorax) and phrenic and recurrent laryngeal nerve injury.

If the child has a ductus-dependent cyanotic heart defect, prostaglandin E₁ may be administered to *maintain* ductal patency (see the section of hypoxemia earlier in the chapter).

■ AORTOPULMONARY WINDOW (AORTOPULMONARY SEPTAL DEFECT)
■ Etiology

An aortopulmonary window results from imperfect septation of the aorta and pulmonary artery during fetal life. It results in a communication between the aorta and pulmonary artery. Aortopulmonary window accounts for less than 1% of all congenital heart defects.

■ Pathophysiology

The hemodynamic consequences of the defect depend on its size and on the magnitude of the shunt produced. Most commonly, the defect is large and unrestrictive, and it provides a large pathway for shunting of blood from the aorta into the pulmonary artery. Increased pulmonary blood flow under high pressure occurs during systole and diastole, resulting in congestive heart failure and an increased risk of pulmonary hypertension.

If the aortopulmonary window is small, the child may have only a mild increase in pulmonary blood flow and minimal symptoms. Rarely, the child has a large aortopulmonary window with persistence of fetal pulmonary hypertension, so the defect does not produce high pulmonary blood flow as a result of high pulmonary vascular resistance.

■ Clinical signs and symptoms

The large aortopulmonary window will produce a harsh murmur heard along the upper left sternal border that is similar to that produced by a patent ductus arteriosus. The murmur is usually continuous, and it may be accompanied by a thrill.

If the defect is large, bounding pulses and widened pulse pressure will occur as a result of "run-off" of aortic flow into the pulmonary artery. Signs of congestive heart failure are often present, and left ventricular hypertrophy may be apparent on the clinical examination, the chest radiograph, and the ECG. Signs of right ventricular hypertrophy will be present if pulmonary hypertension has developed. An echocardiogram may reveal the defect, or it may merely reveal evidence of a large pulmonary shunt. The chest radiograph may demonstrate cardiomegaly and increased pulmonary vascular markings.

Cardiac catheterization is usually necessary to determine the size and specific location of the defect and to allow calculation of pulmonary vascular resistance. The defect will produce an increase in oxygen saturation in the main pulmonary artery, and pulmonary artery pressures will be elevated. Contrast injection in the aorta will reveal the shunt into the pulmonary artery.

Pulmonary hypertension may develop rapidly in those infants with a large aortopulmonary window. They are also at risk for the development of bacterial endocarditis. Other cardiac or great vessel anomalies are frequently present.

■ **Medical and surgical treatment and nursing interventions**

If the aortopulmonary window is small, the infant may respond to medical management of congestive heart failure, with elective surgical intervention planned when the infant is a few months of age. Most commonly, however, the infant has a large defect and severe congestive heart failure that does not respond to medical management alone. Since the risk of pulmonary hypertension is high, early surgical intervention is often advocated.

Surgical treatment of an aortopulmonary window requires a median sternotomy approach. Most commonly, cardiopulmonary bypass (and hypothermia for small infants) is used for surgical repair. The defect is closed with direct visualization by suture or with a patch placed through an aortic incision. Postoperative complications include bleeding, low cardiac output, and congestive heart failure.

■ **ATRIAL SEPTAL DEFECT (ASD)**
■ **Etiology**

An atrial septal defect, a hole in the atrial septum, develops as the result of improper septal formation early in fetal cardiac development. Atrial septal defects are responsible for approximately 12% of all congenital heart defects and can be of three major types: the ostium secundum, the ostium primum, and the sinus venosus. The ostium secundum atrial septal defect is the most common (Fig. 3-27); it is located in the region of the fossa ovalis (the foramen ovale). It may be associated with mitral valve prolapse. The ostium primum atrial septal defect is a form of an endocardial cushion defect. It is located low in the atrial septum and is usually associated with a defect in the amount of ventricular septal tissue as well as with anomalies of one or both AV valves (see the section on endocardial cushion defect). The sinus venosus atrial septal defect is located near the junction of the superior vena cava and the right atrium and is often associated with partial anomalous pulmonary venous return (some of the pulmonary veins empty directly into the right atrium or superior vena cava instead of into the left atrium).

If the child has severe obstruction to right atrial or ventricular outflow, the foramen ovale may be stretched open, and shunting of blood from the right to the left atrium can occur through the patent foramen ovale.

■ **Pathophysiology**

The atrial septal defect usually does not produce a significant shunt during the first weeks of life. Once pulmonary vascular resistance begins to fall, right ventricular end-diastolic and right atrial pressures fall.

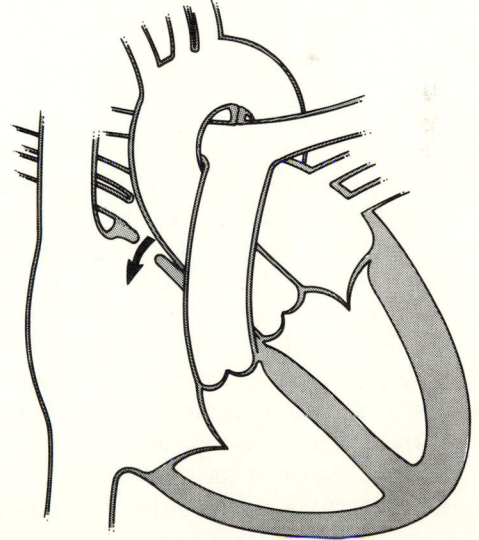

Fig. 3-27 Atrial septal defect (ostium secundum type).

From Hazinski, M.: The cardiovascular system. In Howe, J., and others, editors: The handbook of nursing, New York, 1984, John Wiley & Sons, Inc.

If a defect is present in the atrial septum, left-to-right shunting of blood will occur since the right ventricle is compliant and since the pulmonary circulation is a low resistance circulation. The uncomplicated atrial septal defect produces right ventricular volume overload and increased pulmonary blood flow under low pressure.

This defect is usually well tolerated and often produces no symptoms during childhood. Occasionally, however, an infant will demonstrate significant symptoms, and congestive heart failure may develop; these symptoms are more likely to develop if the infant has a small left ventricle or reduced ventricular compliance.

If an atrial septal defect remains unrepaired into adulthood, significant right atrial and right ventricular hypertrophy can develop, producing atrial arrhythmias, congestive heart failure, and possible paradoxical emboli.

Whereas the risk of developing pulmonary hypertension is low in the child with an uncomplicated atrial septal defect, this complication is reported in 10% to 20% of all adults with unrepaired atrial septal defects, although it usually does not occur before the patient is 20 to 30 years of age.[174,258] The risk of bacterial endocarditis in association with an uncomplicated atrial septal defect is very low.[258]

When the child has cyanotic congenital heart disease, an atrial septal defect may provide an important shunt that allows mixing of oxygenated and venous blood within the atria. In this case, the size of the atrial septal defect can influence the degree of mixing as well as the child's arterial oxygen saturation.

■ Clinical signs and symptoms

Most children with secundum or sinus venosus atrial septal defects are asymptomatic (see the section on endocardial cushion defects for a discussion of ostium primum atrial septal defects). The characteristic heart murmur associated with atrial septal defect is a systolic murmur heard over the second intercostal space at the left sternal border; the murmur may be accompanied by a thrill. The murmur is the result of increased blood flow across an otherwise normal pulmonary valve; this causes a "relative stenosis" since a *normal* valve orifice may not be large enough to allow greatly *increased* blood flow without turbulence. The pathognomonic auscultatory finding is the presence of fixed splitting of the second heart sound; this is the result of prolonged right ventricular ejection, which results from the increased pulmonary blood flow.[319] If a large shunt is present, a diastolic tricuspid rumble may be noted along the lower left or lower right sternal border. This rumble results from increased blood flow across the tricuspid valve into the right ventricle.

Congestive heart failure occurs only rarely in infants; the incidence of this complication does not seem to be related to the size of the atrial septal defect, the magnitude of the shunt, or the pulmonary artery pressure.[402]

Older patients (those in late adolescence or early adulthood) may develop atrial fibrillation or flutter and palpitations as a result of right atrial hypertrophy.[383] Paradoxical embolus can also occur. Congestive heart failure and/or dyspnea is also reported in approximately half of affected adult patients.[174,258]

Right ventricular hypertrophy may produce a sternal lift on the clinical examination and right ventricular hypertrophy may be apparent on the ECG. The echocardiogram will demonstrate right ventricular hypertrophy and abnormal paradoxical septal motion resulting from right ventricular hypertrophy. The atrial septal defect may or may not be visualized.[324,377] The chest radiograph may be normal, or it may show cardiomegaly and increased pulmonary vascular markings. The main pulmonary artery is often prominent on the chest radiograph.

Cardiac catheterization documents the increase in oxygen saturation in the right atrium that results from the left-to-right shunt. Contrast injections are performed only to depict pulmonary venous return (to determine presence of anomalous pulmonary venous drainage) or the size and contractility of the left ventricle.

■ Medical and surgical treatment and nursing interventions

Medical treatment for the child with an atrial septal defect is directed toward alleviation of symptoms of congestive heart failure or treatment of arrhythmias, if these are present.

Surgical closure of an atrial septal defect is recommended during infancy for the child who develops congestive heart failure. When the child is asymptomatic, surgery is usually recommended on an elective basis before the child reaches school age to eliminate the risk of later development of atrial arrhythmias, pulmonary hypertension, or right ventricular dysfunction.

Surgical closure of the atrial septal defect generally requires a median sternotomy incision and use of cardiopulmonary bypass. Recently, closure has been accomplished using a lateral thoracotomy incision and cardiopulmonary bypass. A secundum atrial septal defect is closed primarily (with sutures) or with a pericardial or synthetic patch. If a sinus venosus defect is present, it may also be closed primarily, although pericardial or synthetic patch closure is performed more frequently. Such a patch would be placed so that any anomalous pulmonary veins empty into the left atrium. Mortality of surgical repair during childhood is less than 1%.[238]

Postoperative complications following repair of atrial septal defect include arrhythmias, such as heart block or sick sinus syndrome[238]; these arrhythmias are usually transient. Approximately 2% of patients who have surgical closure of atrial septal defect develop postoperative congestive heart failure.[43] Those patients particularly at risk for the development of heart failure are those with preoperative or intraoperative evidence of a small, noncompliant left ventricle and lower preoperative cardiac index. These patients tend to have a stiff left ventricle, which is unable to accept the total volume of pulmonary venous return following closure of the atrial septal defect. Left ventricular failure can be precipitated by administration of even a small volume challenge postoperatively. Treatment of this congestive heart failure requires strict restriction of fluid intake and aggressive diuresis. If left ventricular failure is refractory to medical management, the atrial septal defect may be surgically reopened to allow resumption of some left-to-right atrial shunting and decompression of the left ventricle.

Surgical closure of the atrial septal defect usually alleviates most symptoms. Occasional patients demonstrate persistent arrhythmias, dyspnea, or poor exercise tolerance. Cardiomegaly may be evident on the chest radiograph or ECG for months or years postoperatively.[453] Residual atrial septal defects may be present in up to 10% of the operated patients, particularly following closure of a sinus venosus defect.[335,453]

Recently, closure of atrial septal defects has been accomplished experimentally using an umbrella patch inserted during cardiac catheterization. This procedure remains under investigation.[276]

■ **VENTRICULAR SEPTAL DEFECT (VSD)**
■ **Etiology**

A ventricular septal defect is a defect or opening in the ventricular septum that results from imperfect ventricular division during early fetal development (Fig. 3-28). There are four major types of ventricular septal defects; these are labeled according to their location. The most common form of ventricular septal defect is located just below the crista supraventricularis and is called an infracristal ventricular septal

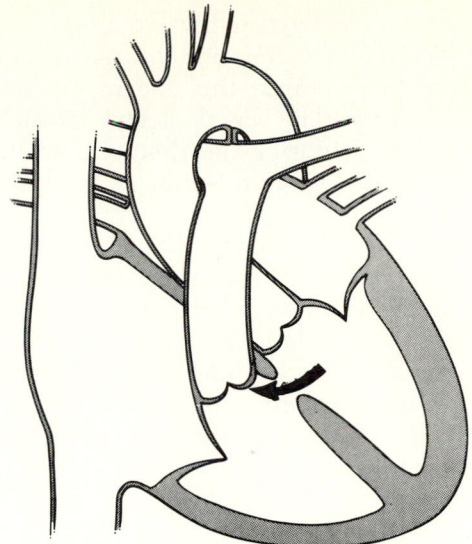

Fig. 3-28   Ventricular septal defect.

From Hazinski, M.: The cardiovascular system. In Howe, J., and others, editors: The handbook of nursing, New York, 1984, John Wiley & Sons, Inc.

defect. Another form of this defect is the supracristal or conal ventricular septal defect, which is located just above the crista supraventricularis and just below the pulmonary valve. The third type of ventricular septal defect is located immediately under the AV valves and occurs as a part of an endocardial cushion defect. Muscular ventricular septal defects are located in the muscular portion of the ventricular septum. These account for approximately one third of all ventricular septal defects, and are often are caused by a single defect on the left ventricular side of the septum that effectively produces many defects on the right ventricular side of the septum, as a result of all the right ventricular trabeculations.[336]

A fifth type of ventricular septal defect allows shunting of blood between the left ventricle and the right atrium. This is a very unusual form of membranous ventricular septal defect, and does not produce classical signs and symptoms of this defect.

■ **Pathophysiology**

The hemodynamic consequences of a ventricular septal defect depend primarily on the size of the defect and on the reactivity of the child's pulmonary vascular bed. To a lesser extent, the location of the defect may also determine its consequences.

Many ventricular septal defects (20% to 60%) are thought to close spontaneously.[9,195,294] The mechanisms of closure are unclear, although it is known that a leaflet of the tricuspid valve may occlude the defect and that proliferation of tissue around the defect may also reduce the size of the defect. Spontaneous ventricular septal defect closure is most likely to occur during the first year of life in children with defects that are small or moderate in size.[50,74,195]

Beyond the neonatal period, the pulmonary circulation normally offers less resistance to blood flow than the systemic circulation. In the presence of an uncomplicated ventricular septal defect, blood will shunt from the left ventricle into the right ventricle and into the pulmonary circulation. As a result pulmonary blood flow is increased and the pulmonary to systemic flow ratio is greater than 1:1 since more blood is passing through the pulmonary circulation than through the systemic circulation. The risk of pulmonary hypertension depends primarily on the size of the defect and to some extent on its location; this is discussed further below.

Since ventricular septal defects frequently occur in association with other congenital heart lesions, it is important to consider the effects of those other lesions on the magnitude and direction of ventricular septal defect shunt flow. In the presence of a simple defect, the shunt will be toward the pulmonary circulation (left-to-right) once pulmonary vascular resistance falls. Anything that increases resistance to aortic flow (such as coarctation of the aorta) would be expected to enhance the left-to-right shunt, and anything producing obstruction to pulmonary blood flow (such as pulmonary stenosis or increased pulmonary vascular resistance) would be expected to reduce the magnitude of the left-to-right shunt. The following discussion pertains to uncomplicated ventricular septal defect.

If the ventricular septal defect is *small*, it allows a small shunt, and the pulmonary to systemic flow ratio is usually no greater than 1.5:1. This means that because of the shunt, 1.5 times as much blood flows through the pulmonary circulation as passes through the systemic circulation. The small radius of the defect itself provides resistance to blood flow and dampens the pressure of blood passing through it. Therefore a small ventricular septal defect produces slightly increased pulmonary blood flow under relatively low pressure. These defects usually produce few symptoms, and approximately one third of them close spontaneously.[74,195]

If the ventricular septal defect is *supracristal* it may be located just under the pulmonary valve. This can allow a jet of blood to flow directly from the left ventricle into the pulmonary artery; even if the defect is moderate in size, this jet can produce increased pulmonary blood flow under high pressure[123]; signs of

congestive heart failure can result.

If the ventricular septal defect is *moderate* in size, it allows a larger shunt, and the pulmonary to systemic flow ratio is 1.5 to 2:1 (up to twice as much blood is passing through the pulmonary circulation as through the systemic circulation). Most often, the size of the defect is still restrictive enough so that the increased pulmonary blood flow still occurs with relatively low pressure. Most of these children are asymptomatic and have a low risk of pulmonary hypertension. Occasionally, their pulmonary vascular resistance is slightly elevated, but it usually does not progress in severity.[50,195]

Children with *large* ventricular septal defects have a large amount of pulmonary blood flow, and their pulmonary to systemic flow ratio is at least 2:1 or greater (twice as much blood flows through the pulmonary circulation as flows through the systemic circulation). Large ventricular septal defects are at least as large as the aortic valve area; the defect and its flow pathway into the pulmonary circulation offer less resistance to flow than the aortic outflow tract and its flow pathway into the systemic circulation. Since the defect is unrestrictive in size, pressure in the right and left ventricles is equalized and blood is shunted from the left ventricle into the pulmonary artery under high pressure; this produces high pulmonary blood flow under high pressure. Many children with large ventricular septal defects become symptomatic at approximately 1 to 2 months of age; this is when their pulmonary vascular resistance has fallen sufficiently to allow a large shunt. The high-pressure pulmonary blood flow and large pulmonary venous return to the left heart produces congestive heart failure. Left atrial and ventricular hypertrophy and dilation develop, and the right ventricle may also enlarge. These infants have the highest risk for the development of pulmonary hypertension, whether or not they have significant symptoms. If pulmonary vascular resistance increases, biventricular hypertrophy will be present.[123,336]

If the child develops pulmonary hypertension and increased pulmonary vascular resistance, left-to-right shunting of blood through the ventricular septal defect is reduced since the pulmonary and systemic circulations offer approximately equal resistance to flow. The child's symptoms may actually improve during this period. As pulmonary vascular resistance increases further, a *right-to-left* shunt will develop, and the child demonstrates cyanosis. This *reversal of the direction of the shunt* as a result of pulmonary vascular disease is called *Eisenmenger syndrome*. Once this develops, pulmonary vascular disease is irreversible[336] and usually progressive.

If the child has a ventricular septal defect that

allows shunting of blood from the left ventricle to the right atrium, the shunt can be large because the right atrium is compliant and offers much less resistance to flow than the aorta and systemic circulation.

Aortic insufficiency develops in approximately 2% to 7% of children with ventricular septal defect.[74,193,221,438] It occurs most commonly with infracristal or supracristal types of ventricular septal defect, and is thought to result from inadequate support of the aortic root as a result of the defect in the ventricular septum. Once it develops, the aortic insufficiency is often progressive.

Approximately 5% of children with ventricular septal defect develop secondary pulmonary infundibular stenosis.[74] This stenosis causes increased resistance to right ventricular outflow and usually reduces the magnitude and pressure of the left-to-right shunt through the ventricular septal defect. If the stenosis becomes severe, symptoms of a right-to-left shunt through the defect may develop (similar to tetralogy of Fallot). The presence of significant pulmonary infundibular stenosis reduces the risk of pulmonary hypertension.

The child with an unrepaired ventricular septal defect has an increased risk of development of bacterial endocarditis. The incidence is approximately 3% to 10% and is highest in patients older than 15 years and in children with aortic insufficiency. The incidence of bacterial endocarditis is lowest in infants.[50,74,193,438]

■ Clinical signs and symptoms

The infant with a ventricular septal defect usually demonstrates no signs or symptoms at birth. Once the infant's pulmonary vascular resistance falls and a shunt develops, a characteristic systolic murmur can be heard along the infant's left lower sternal border. If the defect is small, the murmur is soft, occurs in mid-systole, and may not be accompanied by a thrill. Congestive heart failure usually is not present. Mild left ventricular hypertrophy may be evident on clinical examination (producing a left ventricular heave) and on the ECG or chest radiograph. The chest radiograph will be normal, or it will reveal only slightly increased pulmonary vascular markings. The child is usually asymptomatic.

If the ventricular septal defect produces a larger shunt, the murmur is usually holosystolic and is frequently accompanied by a thrill. A mid-diastolic rumble may be heard at the apex as a result of large pulmonary venous return crossing the mitral valve into the left ventricle. The presence of a mitral diastolic rumble usually indicates the presence of a large shunt, with a pulmonary to systemic flow ratio of 2:1

or greater.[294] A gallop rhythm may also be noted if congestive heart failure is present.

If the ventricular septal defect allows a left ventricle-to-right atrial shunt, a ventricular septal defect murmur is present; it is often accompanied by a tricuspid diastolic rumble heard at the right or left lower sternal border, resulting from the large flow across the tricuspid valve.

The infant with an uncomplicated large ventricular septal defect is asymptomatic until pulmonary vascular resistance begins to fall at approximately 4 to 12 weeks of age. Once a large shunt into the pulmonary circulation develops, the mother often reports that the infant breathes rapidly, feeds poorly, and is diaphoretic; these are classic signs of congestive heart failure. Left and often right ventricular hypertrophy are noted on clinical examination (producing, respectively, a left ventricular heave and a sternal lift) and on the ECG and chest radiograph. Pulmonary vascular markings are increased on the chest radiograph.[294] Hepatomegaly is present, and urine output is decreased.

The M-mode echocardiogram reveals a large left atrium (the result of the large amount of pulmonary venous return) and can help rule out the presence of other defects, such as aortic insufficiency. In addition to demonstrating the defect itself, two-dimensional echocardiography often demonstrates the presence or location of any complicating lesions.

If the child has developed increased pulmonary vascular resistance, the ventricular septal defect murmur may be decreased in intensity. The second heart sound is characteristically increased in intensity because pulmonary valve closure is accentuated. The second heart sound may also appear to be single.[336] The echocardiogram will reveal a shortened right ventricular systolic time interval. Right ventricular hypertrophy is evident on clinical examination and on the ECG and chest radiograph.

If pulmonary vascular resistance equals or exceeds systemic vascular resistance, right-to-left shunting of blood occurs through the ventricular septal defect (Eisenmenger syndrome). Initially this produces exertional cyanosis; as the right-to-left shunt increases, cyanosis at rest is noted. The ventricular septal defect murmur often disappears, and a diastolic murmur of pulmonary valve insufficiency or a systolic murmur of tricuspid insufficiency may develop as pulmonary hypertension and right ventricular dysfunction progress.

If aortic insufficiency develops, a blowing diastolic murmur (possibly accompanied by a thrill) is noted along the right upper sternal border (the aortic area) as well as at the apex. The development and progression of aortic insufficiency will be accompanied by evidence of progressive left ventricular hypertrophy on clinical examination and on the ECG and by signs of left ventricular dilation on chest radiograph.

The development of pulmonary infundibular stenosis produces a systolic pulmonic murmur heard along the left upper sternal border. If the infundibular stenosis is severe, the child may develop right-to-left shunting through the ventricular septal defect, and cyanosis will be noted. The child's symptoms will then be similar to those seen with tetralogy of Fallot.

■ Medical and surgical treatment and nursing interventions

If the child's ventricular septal defect is small and if the child is asymptomatic, the child is often followed on an outpatient basis to allow the ventricular septal defect time to close spontaneously. The child should receive antibiotic prophylaxis surrounding periods of increased risk of bacteremia to prevent endocarditis (see Table 3-13). The defect may be surgically closed on an elective basis if it fails to close spontaneously by the time the child reaches school age.

If the child's ventricular septal defect is moderate in size, the child is usually catheterized so that pulmonary vascular resistance can be calculated. This child should also receive antibiotic prophylaxis during periods of increased risk of bacteremia. If the child is asymptomatic and pulmonary artery pressure and pulmonary vascular resistance are normal, the child is usually followed to allow the ventricular septal defect time to close. If the defect remains moderate in size, it is often closed on an elective basis during the preschool years.

If the child is symptomatic during infancy, a moderate or large ventricular septal defect is usually present. Commonly, the full-term infant develops signs of congestive heart failure at approximately 4 to 12 weeks of age; the premature infant may develop symptoms earlier. These infants require digitalization and diuretic therapy (see the section on congestive heart failure). Cardiac catheterization is necessary to calculate pulmonary vascular resistance, to document the location of the defect, and to rule out the presence of other cardiac anomalies. If the infant's congestive heart failure does not respond to medical treatment, surgical intervention is required. If the child's congestive heart failure resolves with medical management, the child usually receives follow-up care by the cardiologists for several months. If the ventricular septal defect has not closed or become significantly smaller by that time, it is closed surgically at approximately 2 to 4 years of age.

Surgical repair is also indicated if the infant develops high pulmonary artery pressure and increased pulmonary vascular resistance regardless of shunt size, if the infant demonstrates failure to thrive, or if the child develops significant aortic insufficiency.[221] When aortic insufficiency develops, the child will require antibiotic prophylaxis during any period of increased risk of bacteremia.

If the child develops moderate pulmonary infundibular stenosis, the risk of pulmonary vascular disease is almost eliminated. However, surgical repair of the stenosis and closure of the ventricular septal defect will be necessary if the stenosis becomes significant.

Palliative surgery for a ventricular septal defect consists of *banding of the pulmonary artery*. This procedure is performed through a thoracotomy and does not require use of cardiopulmonary bypass. A strip of woven prosthetic material is passed around the main pulmonary artery and used to constrict the artery (Fig. 3-29). This procedure is used to reduce the volume and the pressure of pulmonary blood flow so that symptoms of congestive heart failure are relieved and pulmonary vascular disease is prevented. In the past, pulmonary artery banding was used routinely as the first of two stages in the correction of ventricular septal defect.[385] Currently the procedure is reserved for palliation of complex congenital heart defects that produce high pulmonary blood flow under high pressure, those defects for which surgical repair is unavailable or carries a very high risk, or when the ventricular septal defect is only one of several defects present.[96] Postoperative mortality following pulmo-

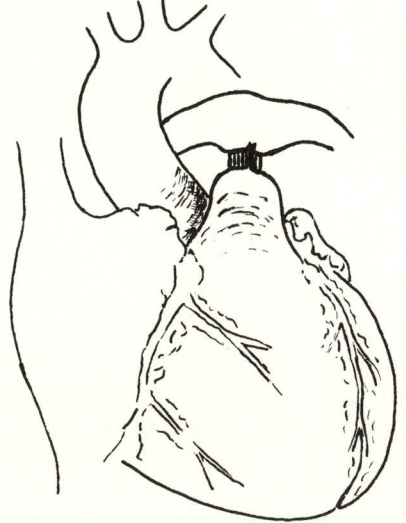

Fig. 3-29 Pulmonary artery banding.

Courtesy Robert J. Szarnicki, MD, Pacific Medical Center, San Francisco, Calif.

nary artery banding is approximately 7% to 40%; it is lowest when a simple ventricular septal defect is present and highest among infants with complex heart defects and/or heart defects that cannot be corrected.[96,255] Early postoperative mortality following a pulmonary artery banding generally results from congestive heart failure and low cardiac output; sudden death has been reported. Late complications of pulmonary artery banding include thickening of one or more pulmonary valve leaflets, stenosis and deformity of the main or right or left pulmonary artery, and abnormalities in regional lung flow and function. Rupture of a pseudoaneurysm at the banding site and development of subaortic stenosis have also been reported.[255,336,366] When the child's ventricular septal defect is closed during later open-heart surgery, the pulmonary artery band is removed, and a patch may be required to enlarge the pulmonary artery at the band site.

Closure of the ventricular septal defect is performed through a median sternotomy with use of cardiopulmonary bypass. Hypothermia may also be used in critically ill infants. If the defect is high in the ventricular septum, an atriotomy cardiac incision may be used, and the defect is repaired from the right atrium through the tricuspid valve. If the defect is difficult to visualize or close through an atriotomy, a right ventriculotomy is performed. Occasionally, an apical *left* ventriculotomy is required to close single or multiple defects located low in the muscular ventricular septum.

The ventricular septal defect may be closed directly with sutures, but a woven prosthetic patch is used most often. If aortic insufficiency is present, a simultaneous aortic valvuloplasty may be performed. If pulmonary infundibular stenosis is present, this is resected before the ventricular septal defect is closed.

Mortality following ventricular septal defect closure is approximately 1% to 33%; mortality is extremely low among children with uncomplicated defects, and it is highest among critically ill infants with severe congestive heart failure, children with preoperative pulmonary hypertension, those with complex heart defects, and those with muscular ventricular septal defect requiring left ventriculotomy.[128,163,336,392] Postoperative complications include congestive heart failure and arrhythmias; right bundle branch block generally occurs if a right ventriculotomy was performed, and heart block may develop. Myocardial damage, left ventricular dysfunction, and low cardiac output may occur following left ventriculotomy for closure of muscular ventricular septal defect.[163] If severe congestive heart failure develops following surgical closure of a ventricular septal defect, the presence of a persistent defect should be suspected, and the child may require reoperation for closure of the defect if the heart failure remains refractory to medical management.

Late results of surgical closure of ventricular septal defects are good. Late complications are largely related to progression of preoperative pulmonary hypertension or aortic regurgitation or to persistence of postoperative arrhythmias.

■ ENDOCARDIAL CUSHION DEFECTS
■ Etiology

Endocardial cushion defects are congenital heart lesions that result from inappropriate fusion of the endocardial cushions during fetal life, producing abnormalities in the atrial septum, ventricular septum, and AV valves. As a result a wide variety of defects, including ostium primum atrial septal defect, ventricular septal defect, and/or AV valve anomalies can result. Several classifications of endocardial cushion defects have been proposed. The variations and contradictions in terminology often tend to confuse rather than define the defects. A description of the more common terms has been provided in Table 3-16. All forms of endocardial cushion defects are characterized by downward displacement of the AV valves as a result of deficiency in ventricular septal tissue; as a result, the left ventricular outflow tract is elongated.

The two terms most frequently used to describe forms of endocardial cushion defects are *partial* and *complete AV canal*. If a *partial* form of AV canal is present, the two AV valve rings are complete and separate. The most common form of partial AV canal is an ostium primum atrial septal defect (located low in the atrial septum) with a cleft in the septal or anterior leaflet of the mitral valve. Other less common forms of partial AV canal include an isolated ostium primum atrial septal defect, a common atrium with AV valve anomalies, an endocardial cushion-type of ventricular septal defect with or without AV valve anomalies, and isolated AV valve anomalies; these defects, however, are better called incompletely displayed forms of AV canal. They do have in common the fact that the mitral and tricuspid valve rings are separate and complete.

When the child has a form of *complete* AV canal, the AV valve rings are incomplete, so there is a common AV valve orifice. In addition, there are defects in both atrial and ventricular septal tissue (Fig. 3-30). The term "canal" is used because the common AV valve orifice and the deficient septal tissue create a large opening in the center of the heart between the atria and the ventricles.[417]

Intermediate forms of AV canal defects have

Table 3-16   Classifications of endocardial cushion defects[47,119,131417]

Defect	Cardiac abnormalities
Partial or incomplete AV canal	In the partial form of AV canal, there are two separate and complete AV valve rings a. In its most common form, an ostium primum atrial septal defect is present with a cleft in the septal leaflet of the mitral (and possibly tricuspid) valve; deficiency in ventricular septal tissue is present with or without a shunt at the ventricular level b. An isolated ostium primum atrial septal defect may also be present c. Rarely, an isolated cleft in the mitral or tricuspid valve may be present with no other abnormality d. Occasionally the child has a common atrium with a cleft in a leaflet of the mitral or tricuspid valve e. A ventricular septal defect may be present alone or in combination with an AV valve deformity (without an associated atrial septal defect)
Complete, common, or persistent common AV canal	One common orifice is located between the atria and ventricles; the mitral and tricuspid valve rings are incomplete
Rastelli classifications of complete AV canal	These classifications are all forms of complete AV canal; classifications are determined by the anatomy of the anterior AV valve leaflet; an atrial and ventricular septal defect are usually present; with any form of AV canal, AV valve tissue can obstruct the left ventricular outflow tract
Type A AV canal (most common)	The anterior common leaflet is roughly divided in half, into tricuspid and mitral components; attachments of the chordae tendineae are normal
Type B AV canal	The anterior common leaflet is roughly divided in half, into tricuspid and mitral components; however, chordae tendineae from the mitral portion of the valve pass through the ventricular septal defect to insert into the right ventricular wall
Type C AV canal	The anterior common leaflet is not divided and has no chordal attachments so it "floats" freely
Intermediate (transitional) form of AV canal	The AV valve rings are incomplete; although adherence of AV valve tissue to the ventricular septum *appears* to close the rings and separate the valve area into the tricuspid and mitral valves; there is no true mitral valve cleft, but there is a deficiency in anterior (and possibly posterior) mitral valve tissue; either right or left ventricular dominance may be present; right ventricular dominance is especially distressing because this means the left ventricle is extremely small (a form of hypoplastic left ventricle is present)

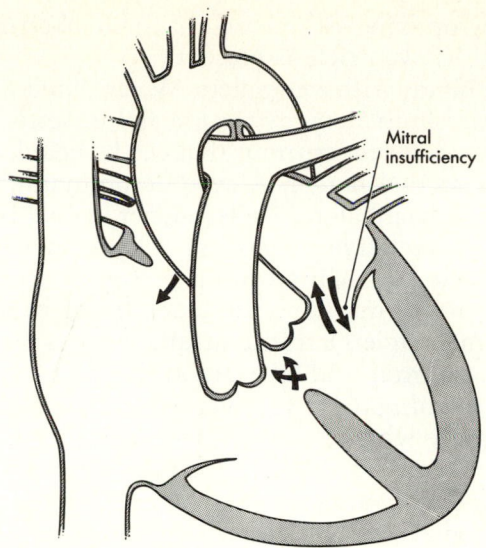

Fig. 3-30 Complete atrioventricular canal.

From Hazinski, M.: The cardiovascular system, In Howe, J., and others, editors: The handbook of nursing, New York, 1984, John Wiley & Sons, Inc.

also been described. In these forms, the tricuspid and mitral valve rings are incomplete, but they both adhere to the rim of the ventricular septal tissue, so they appear to be separate. In this form of AV canal, there is a deficiency in the amount of mitral valve tissue. Either right or left ventricular dominance can be present with an intermediate form of AV canal; if right ventricular dominance is present, the left ventricle is extremely small and may be hypoplastic.[47,131]

Endocardial cushion defects are responsible for approximately 5% of all congenital heart defects.[134] They are the most common form of congenital heart disease seen among children with Down's syndrome (trisomy 21).[336] Endocardial cushion defects are also commonly seen among children with asplenia or polysplenia. Tetralogy of Fallot or double outlet right ventricle may also be associated with the complete forms of AV canal defects.[336]

■ **Pathophysiology**

The direction and magnitude of the intracardiac shunt occurring as the result of an endocardial cushion defect depends on the combination of cardiac anomalies present as well as on the child's pulmonary vascular resistance. Immediately after birth, while the neonate's pulmonary vascular resistance is high, there is minimal shunting of blood through the defect. If the mitral valve is insufficient, a systolic murmur is heard at the apex. The small shunt through the existing septal defect is bidirectional as long as pul-

monary and systemic vascular resistances are approximately equal. At this time, the neonate may demonstrate cyanosis with exertion or vigorous cry since exertion temporarily increases resistance to pulmonary blood flow, enhancing the right-to-left intracardiac shunt and producing arterial oxygen desaturation. Occasionally the infant's pulmonary vascular resistance does not fall normally and the infant remains minimally cyanotic with a bidirectional intracardiac shunt. Most commonly, however, once the infant's pulmonary vascular resistance falls at approximately 4 to 12 weeks of age, a predominantly left-to-right intracardiac shunt develops; as a result, pulmonary blood flow will be increased.

If the child has an uncomplicated ostium primum atrial septal defect, hemodynamic effects are similar to those seen as the result of a secundum atrial septal defect. A cleft mitral valve leaflet produces mitral insufficiency, but this may not be hemodynamically significant because the blood regurgitated from the left ventricle to the left atrium usually passes through the atrial septal defect to the right atrium. An ostium primum atrial septal defect produces right ventricular volume overload. Development of pulmonary vascular disease is rare among children with isolated ostium primum atrial septal defect.[399]

If a ventricular septal defect is present, pulmonary blood flow will be increased once pulmonary vascular resistance falls. The larger the defect, the greater the shunt through the ventricular septal defect, and the higher the pressure of the pulmonary blood flow. An endocardial cushion defect can also produce a left ventricular-to-right atrial shunt, further increasing the volume of blood flow to the right ventricle and pulmonary circulation.

Shunts to the right atrium produce right atrial enlargement and right ventricular volume overload. If pulmonary blood flow is great, pulmonary venous return to the left heart is great. If there is a large left-to-right shunt at the atrial level, left atrial and ventricular hypertrophy will not develop unless significant mitral insufficiency is also present.

High-volume, high-pressure pulmonary blood flow and/or severe mitral insufficiency produce marked signs of congestive heart failure. Pulmonary vascular disease commonly develops during the first year of life if complete AV canal is present.[304]

The defect in ventricular septal tissue that occurs with an endocardial cushion defect causes downward displacement of the AV valves. The abnormal location of the mitral valve produces elongation of the left ventricular outflow tract, resulting in its characteristic "gooseneck" deformity.

The conduction system does not develop normally in infants with endocardial cushion defect because of the deficiency in atrial and ventricular septal tissue. The AV node is displaced posteriorly, producing prolongation of the P-R interval (first degree heart block) on the ECG. The His bundle is also displaced posteriorly, and it courses along the inferior rim of the ventricular septal defect. Left axis deviation is also present.

The incidence of bacterial endocarditis among children with endocardial cushion defects is low preoperatively,[336] but significant after repair.[273]

■ **Clinical signs and symptoms**

Children with an ostium primum atrial septal defect and mild mitral insufficiency are usually asymptomatic during childhood.[399] A systolic pulmonic murmur and fixed splitting of the second heart sound are present. If mitral insufficiency is present, a systolic murmur will be heard at the apex. Signs of right ventricular hypertrophy may be noted on clinical examination and on the ECG or chest radiograph. Increased pulmonary vascular markings may also be seen on the chest radiograph. The ECG will demonstrate prolongation of the P-R interval and left axis deviation; this usually allows differentiation between a primum atrial septal defect and a secundum atrial septal defect. The two-dimensional echocardiogram demonstrates the downward displacement of the AV valves and the "gooseneck" deformity of the left ventricular outflow tract. The atrial septal defect may also be seen.

Cardiac catheterization will reveal an increase in oxygen saturation in the right atrium. Pulmonary hypertension is usually not present during childhood, and the left ventricular angiocardiogram will document the "gooseneck" deformity of the left ventricular outflow tract, the degree of mitral insufficiency, and the presence of any ventricular shunt.

If the infant has a complete AV canal, symptoms depend on the volume and pressure of pulmonary blood flow, the degree of AV valve incompetence, and pulmonary vascular resistance. Cyanosis with exertion may be present during the first weeks of life while pulmonary vascular resistance is high. If a large ventricular septal defect is present, a large left-to-right ventricular shunt will develop when the infant's pulmonary vascular resistance falls at approximately 4 to 12 weeks of age. This will produce high pulmonary blood flow under high pressure, and signs of congestive heart failure will develop (see the section on congestive heart failure). The magnitude of the shunt into the pulmonary circulation and the severity of the

infant's symptoms will increase if aortic obstruction or a small left ventricle is present.

The infant with a complete AV canal and a large ventricular shunt demonstrates a holosystolic ventricular septal defect murmur that can be heard at the left lower sternal border. A systolic pulmonic murmur is often heard along the left upper sternal border as a result of relative pulmonary valve stenosis. If a large shunt to the right atrium is present, a tricuspid diastolic rumble may be heard along the right or left lower sternal border. If mitral insufficiency is present, a systolic murmur will be heard at the apex.

Since pulmonary vascular resistance can increase rapidly when the infant has complete AV canal, the magnitude of the left-to-right intracardiac shunt may begin to decrease as pulmonary vascular resistance increases. If pulmonary vascular resistance is high, cyanosis may be noted during exertion or vigorous cry. This means that some systemic venous blood is shunting into the left heart or systemic circulation. If pulmonary vascular resistance is approximately equal to systemic vascular resistance, cyanosis may be noted even at rest. With the development of pulmonary hypertension, signs of congestive heart failure usually disappear since pulmonary blood flow is reduced. In addition, the second heart sound is often accentuated over the left upper sternal border.

Cyanosis will also be present if the child has tetralogy of Fallot and a complete AV canal. It may also be present as a result of mixing of pulmonary and systemic venous blood in the atria if a common atrium is present.

With complete AV canal, signs of biventricular hypertrophy will be present on clinical examination and on the ECG. The ECG will also demonstrate the long P-R interval and left axis deviation characteristic of endocardial cushion defects. The chest radiograph often reveals gross cardiomegaly with enlargement of all heart chambers. Pulmonary vascular markings will be increased. The two-dimensional echocardiogram will demonstrate the downward displacement of the AV valves and the elongation of the left ventricular outflow tract. The atrial and ventricular septal defects may be visualized, and the common anterior leaflet of the AV valve may be seen.

Cardiac catheterization will reveal an increase in oxygen saturation at the right atrium and/or ventricle, resulting from the left-to-right intracardiac shunt(s). If a right-to-left intracardiac shunt is present, blood in the left side of the heart and aorta will be desaturated. The size of the septal defect(s) and the degree of AV valve insufficiency is often best determined by viewing the angiocardiogram. If the child has atrial and ventricular shunts, calculation of pulmonary blood flow and pulmonary vascular resistance is made more difficult, but the measurements are extremely important. It is not possible to determine the type of complete AV canal that is present from the angiocardiogram, although size of the ventricles and configuration of the AV valves is demonstrated. The left ventricular angiocardiogram will also reveal the characteristic gooseneck deformity of the left ventricular outflow tract. Pressure measurements within the heart and great vessels will also reveal the presence of any areas of stenosis.

■ Medical and surgical treatment and nursing interventions

If the infant with an endocardial cushion defect develops congestive heart failure, medical treatment is the same regardless of the specific type of defect involved (see the section on congestive heart failure). Once an endocardial cushion defect is suspected, cardiac catheterization will be planned to determine the specific type of defect present, to rule out other associated defects, and to determine the presence or degree of pulmonary hypertension.

If the infant has a *primum atrial septal defect* with mild mitral insufficiency and no pulmonary hypertension, surgical repair is usually planned on an elective basis before the child reaches school age. If the left ventricle is small, the infant may require more urgent surgery, as a result of progression of symptoms of congestive heart failure refractory to medical therapy. If pulmonary vascular resistance is high or if significant pulmonary hypertension is present, surgical repair would also be recommended on an urgent basis.

Surgical repair of the ostium primum atrial septal defect requires a median sternotomy incision and use of cardiopulmonary bypass. Hypothermia may be used in infants. The atrial septal defect is most frequently closed with a pericardial or prosthetic patch (rather than with direct closure). A tricuspid or mitral valvuloplasty is performed as needed to reduce AV valve insufficiency; clefts in the valve leaflets are usually closed with sutures. The cleft(s) must be closed carefully so that valvular insufficiency is minimized without producing valvular stenosis. As a result some mitral insufficiency usually remains postoperatively. Perioperative mortality has recently been reported at 10% or less.[252,266,267] Preoperative factors associated with higher operative risk include the presence of significant symptoms, urgent need for surgery, pulmonary hypertension, and increased pulmonary vascular resistance. Low cardiac output is most frequently the cause of early postoperative

death.[252] Postoperative complications include low cardiac output, congestive heart failure, respiratory failure, arrhythmias (especially transient heart block), bleeding, neurologic complications, and postoperative hemolysis. A small number of patients may require permanent cardiac pacing as a result of persistent complete heart block.

Late death following repair of an ostium primum atrial septal defect has been reported in several patients. Late death is related to arrhythmias, residual mitral insufficiency, or (rarely) to progression of pulmonary vascular disease.

If the infant with *complete AV canal* develops severe congestive heart failure and failure to thrive refractory to medical management, palliative or corrective surgery is recommended. Pulmonary artery banding may be performed to reduce the volume and pressure of pulmonary blood flow, thus relieving the signs of congestive heart failure and minimizing the risk of pulmonary hypertension. However, banding of the pulmonary artery previously carried an operative risk as high as 30%.[40,115] When this risk is added to the higher risk of the surgical repair following previous pulmonary artery banding, the total surgical risk for the patient can be very high.[410] In addition, many patients who underwent pulmonary artery banding still developed pulmonary hypertension.[410] Pulmonary artery banding is contraindicated in those patients with severe mitral insufficiency, those with a left ventricular-to-right atrial shunt, or those with primarily an atrial level shunt because the banding significantly increases the magnitude of these shunts.[115] The choice of palliative or corrective surgical treatment of the symptomatic infant with AV canal will depend on the experience and preference of the cardiovascular surgeon.

Total repair of complete AV canal is now often recommended for the symptomatic pediatric patient regardless of age. A median sternotomy incision is required, and cardiopulmonary bypass (with hypothermia in neonates) is used. An incision is made in the right atrium, and the common AV valve leaflet is divided and separated from any abnormal septal or chordal attachments. The septal defects may be closed with a single prosthetic patch or with two separate patches.[287] The AV valve tissue is then mounted to the septal defect patch, and a valvuloplasty is performed to make the AV valve as competent as possible without creating stenosis; the mitral valve may be left with three rather than two leaflets (Fig. 3-31).[410] Perioperative mortality ranges from 4% to 25%.[36,66,273] Operative risks are highest among symptomatic infants, and those patients with significant preoperative symptoms, left ventricular hy-

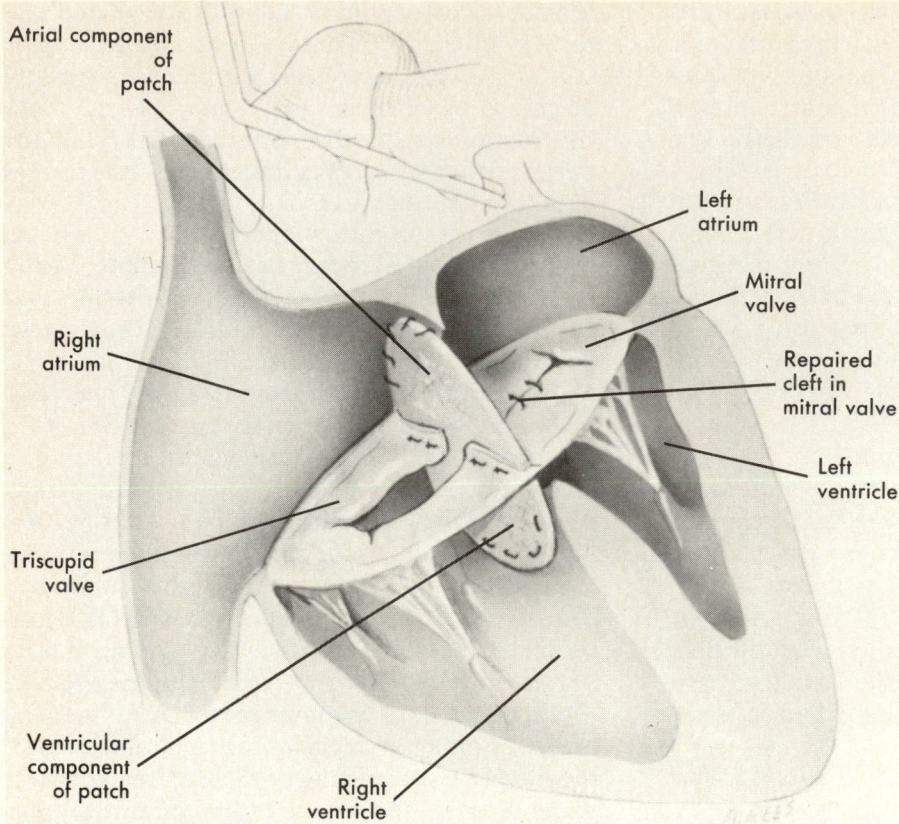

Labels on figure:
Atrial component of patch
Left atrium
Mitral valve
Right atrium
Repaired cleft in mitral valve
Left ventricle
Triscupid valve
Ventricular component of patch
Right ventricle

Fig. 3-31 Repair of complete atrioventricular canal using a single patch. This cut-away view of the heart provides a three-dimensional representation of the repair of a complete atrioventricular canal. The common anterior and posterior leaflets of the AV valve have been divided. A single patch has been used to close both the atrial and ventricular septal defects, and the tricuspid and mitral valve tissues have been remounted to the septal patch. In addition, the cleft in the septal leaflet of the mitral valve has been repaired with sutures. The cleft in the tricuspid valve has not, however, been repaired.

From: Bender, H.W., and others: Repair of atrioventricular canal malformation in the first year of life, J. Thorac. Cardiovasc. Surg. **84:**518, 1982.

poplasia, pulmonary hypertension, previous pulmonary artery banding, additional cardiac defects, or severe mitral regurgitation.

Postoperative complications following repair of complete AV canal include congestive heart failure, low cardiac output, arrhythmias (especially heart block), hemorrhage, and respiratory failure.[119] Occasional reports of hemolysis and coagulopathy thought to be related to dehiscence of the mitral valve repair have been noted; this complication often necessitates reoperation. Many patients require pharmacologic cardiac support in the early postoperative period

(such as sympathomimetic drugs or vasodilators).[273] Persistent postoperative low cardiac output or congestive heart failure is more likely if significant mitral insufficiency or persistant ventricular septal defect is present.[36,66,410] If the child has preoperative pulmonary hypertension, postoperative weaning from mechanical ventilatory support must be done gradually. Hypoventilation and alveolar hypoxia, acidosis, or hypothermia can produce pulmonary arteriolar vasoconstriction. This increases right ventricular afterload and can result in congestive heart failure, low cardiac output, and hypoxemia.

Late postoperative death has been reported in several patients following repair of complete AV canal. Late death most commonly results from bacterial endocarditis,[273] arrhythmias, persistent congestive heart failure, or low cardiac output; late death also results during later mitral valve replacement.[36,66,410] Approximately 1% of postoperative patients per year require mitral valve replacement for persistent mitral regurgitation.[267]

Following surgical repair, patients with endocardial cushion defects still require antibiotic prophylaxis during periods of risk of bacteremia to prevent bacterial endocarditis.[273] (See Table 3-13.)

■ DOUBLE OUTLET RIGHT VENTRICLE (DORV)
■ Etiology

When double outlet right ventricle is present, both great vessels arise from the right ventricle.[336] Double outlet right ventricle is thought to occur as the result of inadequate migration and rotation of the truncus arteriosus during fetal cardiac development. In a normal patient, the pulmonary artery is anterior to the aorta and the pulmonary valve is higher than the aortic valve. When double outlet right ventricle is present, the great vessels lie side-by-side in the same (anteroposterior) plane, and the aortic and pulmonic valves lie at the same level. Because the aorta arises from the right ventricle and has a conus, the normal aortic-mitral valve continuity is absent. There is usually a conus below both the aorta and the pulmonary artery; subpulmonary stenosis is present in nearly one third of the involved patients, and subaortic stenosis may also be present. A ventricular septal defect is nearly always associated with double outlet right ventricle.[403] The great vessels may be normally related or transposed. Double outlet right ventricle is responsible for approximately 0.5% of all congenital heart defects.[336] Additional cardiovascular anomalies, including anomalous coronary arteries, occur in approximately half of the patients with double outlet right ventricle.[403,455]

■ Pathophysiology

Since both vessels rise from the right ventricle, there must be a ventricular septal defect present as an outlet for the left ventricle. There are many forms of double outlet right ventricle; the hemodynamic consequences of each form are determined by the location of the ventricular septal defect, its relationship to the great vessels, the presence and severity of subpulmonic stenosis, and the degree of mixing between systemic and pulmonary venous blood within the right ventricle. In all forms of double outlet right ventricle, right ventricular hypertension and hypertrophy are present since the right ventricle ejects into both the pulmonary artery and aorta. Since three forms of double outlet right ventricle occur most frequently, only these three forms are discussed. These forms include double outlet right ventricle with a subaortic ventricular septal defect, double outlet right ventricle with a subaortic ventricular septal defect and pulmonary stenosis, and double outlet right ventricle with a subpulmonic ventricular septal defect.

In nearly half of the patients with double outlet right ventricle, the great vessels lie side-by-side, there is a *subaortic ventricular septal defect* (the ventricular septal defect is located just below the aorta), and *pulmonary stenosis is absent.* As a result, much of the pulmonary venous blood from the left ventricle will flow through the ventricular septal defect, directly into the aorta. While pulmonary vascular resistance is high during the neonatal period, pulmonary blood flow is not increased. Aortic blood flow comes primarily from the pulmonary venous blood in the left ventricle through the ventricular septal defect, therefore cyanosis is usually *not* present. Once pulmonary vascular resistance falls, at approximately 4 to 12 weeks of age, there is increased blood flow into the pulmonary artery and pulmonary circulation since the pulmonary circulation provides less resistance to flow. Blood flow into the pulmonary artery comes from the right and left ventricles (through the ventricular septal defect) and is under high pressure since both the right and left ventricles are generating high pressure. This high pulmonary blood flow, which is under high pressure, usually produces congestive heart failure and increases the patient's risk of development of pulmonary hypertension. As a result the hemodynamic effect of this form of double outlet right ventricle is similar to that seen with a simple large ventricular septal defect.

If the infant has double outlet right ventricle with a *subaortic ventricular septal defect and pulmonary stenosis,* the hemodynamic effect is similar to that of tetralogy of Fallot. If the stenosis is mild, most of the right ventricular output continues to enter the pulmonary artery, and left ventricular output enters the aorta (through the ventricular septal defect); congestive heart failure is unlikely because the pulmonary stenosis prevents a large shunt into the pulmonary circulation. If the stenosis is moderate or severe, however, pulmonary blood flow is reduced, and systemic venous blood from the right ventricle enters the aorta in an amount proportional to the degree of pulmonary stenosis; the greater the stenosis, the greater the effective right-to-left shunt of blood into the aorta. The infant will be cyanotic.

If the infant has a *subpulmonic ventricular septal defect without pulmonic stenosis*, systemic venous blood from the right ventricle flows preferentially into the aorta, and pulmonary venous blood from the left ventricle flows preferentially into the pulmonary artery through the ventricular septal defect. This form of double outlet right ventricle is referred to as a Taussig-Bing malformation; the result of these anomalies produces hemodynamics similar to those seen with transposition of the great vessels.[336] While pulmonary vascular resistance is high during the neonatal period, the infant is cyanotic with no signs of congestive heart failure. Once pulmonary vascular resistance falls, at approximately 4 to 12 weeks of age, blood from the right and left ventricles will flow preferentially into the pulmonary artery since the pulmonary circulation offers less resistance to flow. These infants usually develop congestive heart failure in addition to their cyanosis at this time. To survive these infants must have another intracardiac shunt (such as an atrial septal defect or a patent ductus arteriosus) to allow oxygenated pulmonary venous blood from the left heart to enter the aorta and systemic circulation.

■ Clinical signs and symptoms

As noted earlier, there are a wide variety of clinical signs and symptoms caused by a double outlet right ventricle. The symptomatology is determined by the location of the ventricular septal defect, its relationship to the great vessels, and the presence of pulmonic stenosis.

If a *subaortic ventricular septal defect is present without pulmonic stenosis*, the infant will have the signs and symptoms similar to those infants seen with a large ventricular septal defect. The neonate is usually asymptomatic while pulmonary vascular resistance is high. Once pulmonary vascular resistance falls, pulmonary blood flow increases, pulmonary hypertension is present, and signs of congestive heart failure develop.[218] A harsh, holosystolic murmur is present at the left lower sternal border as a result of the ventricular septal defect. A systolic pulmonic murmur is noted, and a gallop rhythm may be present as a result of congestive heart failure. If pulmonary blood flow is large, a mitral diastolic rumble may be heard at the apex, resulting from the large flow of pulmonary venous blood from the left atrium to the left ventricle. Because both ventricles are large, a sternal lift and a left ventricular heave may be noted on clinical examination. Biventricular hypertrophy is noted on the ECG and echocardiogram.

The origin of both great vessels from the right ventricle will be seen on the echocardiogram; the lack of continuity between the aorta and the mitral valve and the abnormal relationship of the great vessels will also be apparent. The relationship of the ventricular septal defect to the aorta may not be apparent on the echocardiogram. The chest radiograph will reveal cardiomegaly with biventricular hypertrophy and increased pulmonary vascular markings.

Cardiac catheterization will reveal an increase in oxygen saturation in the right ventricle and pulmonary artery, as a result of the left-to-right shunt through the ventricular septal defect. Right ventricular pressure will equal left ventricular pressure. The right and left ventricular angiocardiograms will reveal the origin of both great vessels from the right ventricle, the relationship of the aorta and aortic valve to the pulmonary artery and pulmonic valve, and the relationship of the ventricular septal defect to the great vessels will be seen. The diagnosis of double outlet right ventricle will be confirmed when aortic-mitral valve discontinuity is observed. Pulmonary pressure and flow and pulmonary vascular resistance will be calculated carefully since the risk of pulmonary hypertension is high in these patients.

If the infant has a *subaortic ventricular septal defect with pulmonic stenosis*, clinical signs and symptoms will be similar to those produced by tetralogy of Fallot.[218] The neonate may be minimally cyanotic at birth. However, as the pulmonic stenosis becomes relatively more severe, more systemic venous blood shunts into the aorta, and the infant becomes progressively more cyanotic. Hypercyanotic spells may be noted (see the section on hypoxemia). These infants have a systolic harsh murmur heard over the left lower sternal border as a result of the ventricular septal defect, and a systolic pulmonic murmur as a result of the pulmonic stenosis. Congestive heart failure does not occur. Biventricular hypertrophy is apparent on the clinical examination, ECG, and chest radiograph (this is one way this form of double outlet right ventricle can be distinguished from tetralogy of Fallot). The chest radiograph also demonstrates decreased pulmonary vascular markings.

The ECG most commonly demonstrates biventricular hypertrophy. In addition, first degree AV block (prolonged P-R interval) and complete right bundle branch block may also be noted. A superior axis is usually present.[409]

Cardiac catheterization reveals an increase in oxygen saturation in the right ventricle, just at the level of the ventricular septal defect, since pulmonary venous blood from the left ventricle must flow through the ventricular septal defect to the right ventricle before passing into the aorta. Arterial oxygen desaturation will also be noted when samples are taken from the aorta. Right and left ventricular pressures are usually equal, and measurement of a pressure gradient between the right ventricle and pulmonary artery will confirm the presence of pulmonic stenosis. Right and left ventricular angiograms will confirm the location and relationship of the great vessels and the location of the ventricular septal defect. In addition, the location and degree of pulmonic stenosis will be documented.

If the infant has double outlet right ventricle with *subpulmonic ventricular septal defect without pulmonic stenosis* (the Taussig-Bing malformation), the infant will have symptoms similar to those produced by transposition and a ventricular septal defect. The infant usually demonstrates mild to moderate cyanosis, and congestive heart failure develops once pulmonary vascular resistance falls, at approximately 4 to 12 weeks of age. The Taussig-Bing malformation is one of the few congenital heart defects in which high pulmonary blood flow and congestive heart failure can be associated with severe cyanosis. A harsh systolic ejection murmur is present at the left lower sternal border, resulting from the ventricular septal defect. A gallop murmur may be noted when congestive heart failure develops.

Signs of right ventricular hypertrophy are present on clinical examination, and on the ECG and chest radiograph. Signs of left ventricular hypertrophy are usually also noted. Conduction abnormalities are rare.[409]

The echocardiogram reveals the dextroposition (rightward displacement) of the aorta and the position of pulmonary artery, which overrides the ventricular septal defect. Certain forms of this defect (so-called "left-sided Taussig-Bing anomaly") may be difficult to differentiate with certainty from transposition of the great vessels with a ventricular septal defect.

The chest radiograph reveals generalized cardiomegaly with right (and often left) ventricular hypertrophy. Pulmonary vascular markings will be increased.

Cardiac catheterization reveals equal right and left ventricular pressures. An increase in arterial oxygen saturation is noted in the right ventricle (and often, again, in the pulmonary artery) as a result of the flow of oxygenated blood from the left ventricle, through the ventricular septal defect, into the right ventricle, and into the pulmonary artery. Blood in the aorta is desaturated since this blood comes primarily from the right ventricle. A right ventricular angiogram reveals the emergence of the pulmonary artery and the aorta from the right ventricle. The aorta is usually located to the right of the pulmonary artery,

and the aortic valve is at the same level as the pulmonic valve. A left ventricular angiogram reveals the location of the ventricular septal defect and the preferential streaming of left ventricular blood into the pulmonary artery.[409] Pulmonary pressure will be high, and pulmonary vascular resistance should be calculated carefully since the risk of pulmonary vascular disease is high.

■ **Medical and surgical treatment and nursing interventions**

When the infant with a double outlet right ventricle and *subaortic ventricular septal defect* develops congestive heart failure, aggressive medical management will be required. Cardiac catheterization will be performed at a young age since surgical repair should be scheduled before pulmonary vascular disease develops. Although pulmonary artery banding may be performed initially as a palliative measure, many surgeons prefer early total correction of this defect unless additional cardiac anomalies are present.

Surgical correction requires a median sternotomy incision and use of cardiopulmonary bypass. Hypothermia is also used in small infants. A right ventriculotomy cardiac incision is made, avoiding any anomalous coronary arteries. The ventricular septal defect is closed with a prosthetic patch so that left ventricular outflow is diverted into the aorta. Postoperative complications include congestive heart failure, low cardiac output, and arrhythmias. Operative risk is especially high if pulmonary hypertension or severe symptoms were present preoperatively.

If the infant has double outlet right ventricle with a *subaortic ventricular septal defect and pulmonic stenosis,* that infant is followed as would be an infant with tetrology of Fallot. During IV therapy, *no air should be allowed in IV lines* since air may flow into the systemic arterial circulation, producing a cerebral air embolus. Nurses caring for the infant with this form of double outlet right ventricle should be alert for the development of hypercyanotic episodes. If these develop, the infant should be placed in a knee-chest position, and oxygen should be administered. Morphine sulfate or propranolol may be administered in an attempt to relieve pulmonary infundibular muscle spasm. These infants should be kept well hydrated to avoid hemoconcentration and resultant increase in the serum hematocrit and blood viscosity. This information should also be taught to the infant's parents (see the section on hypoxemia).

If the infant with double outlet right ventricle of the tetralogy type is extremely hypoxemic or develops hypercyanotic episodes, surgical creation of a systemic-to-pulmonary artery shunt is often recommended. This palliative surgery does not require use of cardiopulmonary bypass and should reduce the infant's hypoxemia (see Table 3-17 and the section on tetralogy of Fallot). Postoperatively, it is still imperative that no air be allowed in any IV lines since systemic venous blood is still entering the systemic arterial circulation, and IV air can produce a cerebral air embolus.

Corrective surgery for the infant with a double outlet right ventricle of the tetralogy type is similar to that performed for repair of tetralogy of Fallot. A median sternotomy incision is used, and cardiopulmonary bypass is required. Hypothermia may also be used in small infants. The surgical repair is usually performed through a right ventriculotomy. The pulmonic stenosis is relieved by excision of the muscular stenotic pulmonary infundibulum, and a pulmonary valvotomy may also be performed. The ventricular septal defect is closed with a prosthetic patch so that left ventricular outflow enters the aorta—the ventricular septal defect patch helps to divert this blood into the aorta. One or two patches may be used to enlarge the right ventricular outflow tract to minimize residual pulmonic stenosis.[218] If an anomalous coronary artery crosses the right ventricular outflow tract where the surgical incision would be made or where the patch would be placed, or if it is difficult to patch the ventricular septal defect without obstructing the flow of blood from right ventricle to pulmonary artery, a valved conduit may be placed between the right ventricle and the pulmonary artery. Postoperative complications include congestive heart failure, low cardiac output, bleeding, arrhythmias, infection, and neurologic complications.[218,408,409]

If the infant has a double outlet right ventricle with a *subpulmonic ventricular septal defect without pulmonic stenosis*, medical management can be difficult. If the infant develops severe symptoms of congestive heart failure at approximately 1 to 3 months of age, treatment with digoxin and diuretics is indicated (see the section on congestive heart failure). However, because the infant is also hypoxemic and polycythemic, aggressive diuresis should be avoided since it may produce hemoconcentration, causing a rise in the infant's hematocrit to unacceptable levels (see the section on hypoxemia). Therefore medical management must strive for a balance between adequate treatment of congestive heart failure and prevention of systemic consequences of polycythemia. Whenever the infant is hospitalized, *no air can be allowed in any IV line* since some systemic venous blood is passing into the systemic arterial circulation, and IV air may cause a cerebral air embolus (stroke).

If the infant's congestive heart failure is refractory to medical management, pulmonary artery banding may be recommended to reduce the quantity and pressure of pulmonary blood flow. Banding should relieve the infant's symptoms of congestive heart failure and reduce the infant's risk of pulmonary vascular disease. However, since the reduction in pulmonary blood flow by banding may worsen the infant's hypoxemia, it may be necessary to create a systemic-to-pulmonary artery shunt at the same time. Both of these procedures are performed through a thoracotomy and neither requires use of cardiopulmonary bypass. (See the sections on management of the child with ventricular septal defect and systemic-to-pulmonary artery shunts—see Table 3-17.)

Surgical correction of the double outlet right ventricle with subpulmonic ventricular septal defect without pulmonic stenosis requires a median sternotomy and use of cardiopulmonary bypass. Hypothermia is also often used for repair during infancy. Surgery may be performed through a right atriotomy or ventriculotomy incision. The ventricular septal defect is closed with a prosthetic patch. If possible, the patch is placed so that left ventricular outflow is diverted to the aorta. This may require placement of a valved conduit between the right ventricle and pulmonary artery. Occasionally, surgical repair must be performed as though the infant had transposition of the great vessels and a ventricular septal defect. In that case, the ventricular septal defect is closed (using a prosthetic patch) so that left ventricular outflow is diverted to the *pulmonary* artery. This effectively creates transposition hemodynamics. Correction of the transposition is then performed through insertion of an intraatrial baffle (see the section on transposition of the great vessels). Operative risk is highest for this form of repair. Postoperative complications include congestive heart failure, low cardiac output, bleeding, arrhythmias, and neurologic complications.[408,409]

If the infant with double outlet right ventricle has preoperative pulmonary hypertension, postoperative weaning from ventilatory support must be done very gradually since hypoventilation and alveolar hypoxia, acidosis, or hypothermia can produce pulmonary arteriolar constriction and increased pulmonary vascular resistance. This increases right ventricular afterload and can produce congestive heart failure, low cardiac output, and hypoxemia.[408,409]

Late complications following surgical repair of double outlet right ventricle include progression of pulmonary vascular disease, persistent arrhythmias, conduit failure, recurrent ventricular septal defect, and development of left ventricular outflow tract obstruction.[62,218,408] A significant incidence of late sudden death has been reported and is probably the result of arrhythmias.[218] If prosthetic material is used for the surgical repair, the child will require antibiotic prophylaxis at times of increased risk of bacteremia since endocarditis can result from bacteremia and since it would be particularly difficult to eliminate if the prosthetic material also became infected (see Table 3-13).

■ PULMONARY VALVE STENOSIS
■ Etiology

Pulmonary valve stenosis results from abnormal formation of pulmonary valve leaflets during fetal cardiac development. Most commonly, valve commissures fail to develop properly and the valve leaflets are thickened and fused. In a small number of patients, the valve leaflets are dysplastic (abnormally shaped) and the pulmonary valve annulus small. Pulmonary valve stenosis results in obstruction to blood flow from the right ventricle to pulmonary artery. Isolated pulmonary valve stenosis is responsible for approximately 6% of all congenital heart defects.[14,134] Pulmonary valve stenosis is frequently present in association with other forms of congenital heart defects, including ventricular septal defects. The following discussion relates primarily to uncomplicated pulmonary valve stenosis.

■ Pathophysiology

Because the radius of the valve orifice is reduced, resistance to flow through the pulmonary valve is increased. To maintain flow through the valve, the right ventricle must generate higher pressure; the greater the pulmonary stenosis, the greater must be the pressure generated by the right ventricle. As a result of the right ventricular hypertension and the valve obstruction, a gradient is present between the right ventricle and the main pulmonary artery that is proportional to the degree of valve stenosis. Mild pulmonary valvular stenosis is present when the valve gradient is approximately 25 to 49 mm Hg. Moderate pulmonary valvular stenosis is present when the valve gradient is approximately 50 to 70 mm Hg. Severe pulmonary valvular stenosis is present when the valve gradient is equal to or greater than 80 mm Hg.[315]

Since right ventricular afterload is high, right ventricular hypertrophy is present. If the valvular obstruction is significant, secondary pulmonary infundibular stenosis or right ventricular fibrosis may develop.[336]

If the pulmonary valve stenosis is mild or mod-erate, moderate right ventricular hypertension is present and pulmonary blood flow is normal. If the valve stenosis is severe, right ventricular pressure may exceed left ventricular pressure. Over time, this can produce right ventricular fibrosis and dysfunction, and increased right ventricular end-diastolic pressure. When this occurs, right atrial pressure increases, and signs of systemic venous engorgement (including hepatomegaly) develop. Right-to-left atrial shunting can then develop through a stretched foramen ovale, producing hypoxemia. Pulmonary blood flow is then reduced.

If a true atrial septal defect or tricuspid insufficiency are present, right-to-left atrial shunting can develop with less significant levels of valve stenosis.[350] Once tricuspid insufficiency develops, the child's symptoms usually progress rapidly.

Occasionally, severe pulmonary valve stenosis is associated with an extremely small right ventricle and tricuspid valve stenosis or atresia. This is known as hypoplastic right heart and produces more severe obstruction to pulmonary blood flow than isolated pulmonary stenosis (see the section on tricuspid atresia).

Adults with congenital pulmonary valve stenosis often have smaller lungs with decreased diffusion capacity and smaller airway dimensions than healthy adults.[87]

■ Clinical signs and symptoms

Most patients with pulmonary valve stenosis are asymptomatic, have a mild or moderate valve gradient, and do not develop an increase in the significance of the valvular stenosis with growth.[315] Those patients who have signs and symptoms of pulmonary valve stenosis during infancy and early childhood usually have more severe valve stenosis, and it is this group of patients that is most likely to develop progression of symptoms and progression in the severity of the stenosis.[315]

Children with *mild* pulmonary valve stenosis usually have a soft systolic murmur heard best over the second intercostal space to the left of the sternum. The second heart sound is normal, but there may be a click heard after the first heart sound as a result of the opening of the stenotic pulmonary valve. The click may disappear during inspiration, and it is often absent in neonates. Mild right ventricular hypertrophy may be evident on clinical examination (causing a sternal lift) or by electrocardiographic voltage criteria. On the chest radiograph, the cardiothoracic ratio is normal, although right ventricular fullness may be noted on the lateral film. The pulmonary artery is often prominent as a result of poststenotic dilation. M-mode and two-dimensional echocardiography may demonstrate mild right ventricular hypertrophy. The two-dimensional echocardiogram will provide the most sensitive indicator of decreased valve leaflet motion and small changes in right ventricular wall thickness.[441]

Cardiac catheterization confirms the presence of right ventricular hypertension and a gradient across the pulmonary valve of approximately 25 to 49 mm Hg. The valve will appear domed on right ventricular angiogram if the leaflets are fused. The main pulmonary artery is usually enlarged as a result of poststenotic dilation.

These children are generally acyanotic and asymptomatic with no signs of congestive heart failure. They usually do not develop progression in the severity of their valve stenosis.

If the infant or child has *moderate* pulmonary valve stenosis, a loud systolic murmur is heard along the left sternal border, at the second intercostal space; it may be accompanied by a thrill. The second heart sound is usually widely split, because the intensity of pulmonic valve closure is diminished. A click may be heard just after (or nearly simultaneous with) the first heart sound and is the result of the opening of the stenotic pulmonary valve; the click usually disappears with inspiration. Signs of right ventricular hypertrophy are evident on clinical examination (causing a sternal lift) as well as on the ECG. The chest radiograph documents prominence of the main pulmonary artery, and right ventricular fullness is usually recognized on a lateral chest film. The cardiothoracic ratio is increased only rarely. The echocardiogram confirms the presence of right ventricular hypertrophy and decreased movement of the pulmonary valve leaflets.

Cardiac catheterization documents the presence of significant right ventricular hypertension; right ventricular pressure is usually equal to one half or two thirds of left ventricular systolic pressure. A gradient across the pulmonary valve of approximately 50 to 70 mm Hg is measured. If right ventricular pressure is equal to left ventricular pressure, the cardiologist may not attempt to enter the pulmonary artery since the catheter can occlude the tiny pulmonary valve orifice, preventing any pulmonary blood flow; this would cause the child to decompensate rapidly. In this case, the valve gradient is calculated assuming a normal pulmonary artery pressure.[361] Systemic arterial oxygen desaturation and left atrial desaturation are noted if a right-to-left shunt is present at the atrial level. The right ventricular angiogram will reveal the presence of a domed pulmonic valve (if the commissures are fused) and possibly of a small valve annulus. The main pulmonary artery is usually enlarged as a result of poststenotic dilation.

Infants with moderate pulmonic stenosis may demonstrate cyanosis as a result of right-to-left atrial shunting through a stretched foramen ovale or a true atrial septal defect. Cyanosis is usually not present in children with moderate pulmonary stenosis over the age of 2 years,[315] and congestive heart failure usually does not occur. Some of these infants and children may develop progression in the severity of their pulmonary valve stenosis, especially before they reach school age.[315]

Infants and children with *severe* pulmonary valve stenosis are often symptomatic. A systolic murmur is heard over the second intercostal space at the left sternal border, and it is usually accompanied by a thrill. The pulmonic component of the second heart sound may be inaudible since the pulmonary valve barely opens and since closure is very delayed. The click may be absent or heard in diastole. A harsh systolic murmur may also be heard at the right or left lower sternal border, resulting from the development of tricuspid insufficiency. Signs of congestive heart failure may be observed, including tachypnea, hepatomegaly, periorbital edema, increased respiratory effort, and decreased exercise tolerance. Cyanosis is often noted, especially when severe pulmonary stenosis is present in young infants.

A sternal lift is palpated as a result of right ventricular hypertrophy. The ECG often shows significant right ventricular hypertrophy by voltage criteria, and right axis deviation. Right ventricular "strain" patterns are often also observed; these include the presence of an upright T wave in lead V_{4R} or V_1 and an R wave in V_1 that is greater than 10 mm in voltage. A Q wave is often also noted in lead V_1.

An echocardiogram documents the presence of severe right atrial and right ventricular hypertrophy, and the presence of reduced pulmonary valve leaflet motion is especially visible on two-dimensional echocardiogram.[441] The infant's chest radiograph will demonstrate cardiomegaly and right atrial hypertrophy. Pulmonary vascular markings are often normal.

Cardiac catheterization confirms the presence of severe right ventricular hypertension. Right ventricular systolic pressure is often greater than left ventricular systolic pressure, and it usually exceeds 100 mm Hg. Right ventricular end-diastolic pressure is often also increased, causing an increase in right atrial pressure. If right-to-left atrial shunting is present, left atrial, left ventricular, and systemic arterial oxygen desaturation will be noted. A pressure gradient across the pulmonary valve exceeding 80 mm Hg will be noted. The cardiologist may calculate the valve gradient by measuring only the right ventricular pressure and assuming normal pulmonary artery pressure since it is extremely dangerous to pass a catheter through a small pulmonary valve orifice—it could totally obliterate the orifice, preventing pulmonary blood flow and resulting in acute cardiovascular decompensation.[361] Subvalvular (infundibular) pulmonary stenosis may also be observed. The right ventricular angiogram may demonstrate the presence of any pulmonary subvalvular stenosis or tricuspid valve regurgitation.

In summary, most children with pulmonary valve stenosis are asymptomatic.[109] Those that do demonstrate symptoms are most frequently infants with moderate or severe valvular stenosis. Cyanosis is observed in approximately one third of involved children under 2 years of age, and these have moderate or severe pulmonic stenosis. Cyanosis is rarely observed in the child older than 2 years, and then it is only present if pulmonary valve stenosis is severe. Congestive heart failure is rarely observed; when it does develop, it is usually seen in infants with severe pulmonic stenosis.

The risk of subacute bacterial endocarditis is low unless additional congenital cardiac anomalies are present.[315]

■ **Medical and surgical treatment and nursing interventions**

Infants and children with mild pulmonic stenosis require no surgical intervention and are given follow-up care to be sure that there are no signs of progression of the stenosis. Progression of pulmonary valve stenosis occurs in approximately 14% of involved children; progression is most likely before the age of 4 years and in those children with valvular gradients exceeding 40 mm Hg at the time of diagnosis. Progression in severity of pulmonary valve stenosis is rare beyond the age of 12 years.[315]

Since it is often difficult to correlate clinical signs and symptoms with the degree of pulmonic stenosis, the child may be catheterized to document the severity of the stenosis once the diagnosis is established. The child may also be catheterized if signs of progression of the pulmonary stenosis develop. In children over the age of 2 years, the most consistent signs of development of severe pulmonic stenosis include electrocardiographic evidence of severe right

ventricular hypertrophy (including voltage criteria and presence of right ventricular "strain" pattern), dyspnea, fatigability, and development of congestive heart failure.[109]

Antibiotic prophylaxis may be prescribed during periods of increased risk of bacteremia (see Table 3-13), although the incidence of bacterial endocarditis associated with pulmonary valvular stenosis is low.

Surgical intervention is recommended for infants and children with pulmonic valvular stenosis whenever significant symptoms, such as congestive heart failure, cyanosis, syncope, or decreased exercise tolerance develop. When the child becomes symptomatic, cardiac catheterization is performed to document the severity and distribution of the stenosis. Surgery is also recommended whenever right ventricular systolic pressure exceeds 50 to 60 mm Hg or two thirds of left ventricular systolic pressure.[162] Surgical relief is recommended because prolonged or severe right ventricular hypertension can produce pathologic ventricular hypertrophy, resulting in eventual fibrosis of the right ventricle. Once this severe hypertrophy and fibrosis develops, it may not regress, even after relief of the pulmonary valve stenosis.[286,444] A significant number of children with significant pulmonic stenosis may also develop secondary pulmonary infundibular stenosis.[162]

Surgical treatment of severe pulmonary valvular stenosis during the neonatal period is performed through a median sternotomy incision; one method of valvulotomy is called *closed transventricular pulmonary valvotomy* (the Brock procedure). The procedure is called "closed" because it does not require use of cardiopulmonary bypass. To perform the valvotomy a curved blade is inserted through a small stab incision in the pulmonary outflow tract that is surrounded by "purse-string" sutures to prevent bleeding. The surgeon quickly incises the valve and withdraws the blade. Although this technique produces a "blind" pulmonary valvotomy, it is quick and it avoids the use of cardiopulmonary bypass; these advantages are very important when the infant is critically ill at the time of surgery. Although these infants may require reoperation later during childhood for residual stenosis, the closed valvotomy is usually effective in reducing severe pulmonary stenosis and right ventricular hypertension during infancy. Perioperative mortality for the closed valvotomy is approximately 20%.[80]

A closed pulmonary valvotomy may also be performed during the neonatal period using cardiac inflow occlusion and an incision in the pulmonary artery. The results of this transarterial valvotomy are approximately the same as for the closed transventricular pulmonary valvotomy.[278]

Open-heart pulmonary valvotomy with hypothermia may also be performed to relieve severe pulmonary valve stenosis during the neonatal period or to relieve moderate or severe pulmonary valvular stenosis during childhood. This procedure uses a median sternotomy and cardiopulmonary bypass. The pulmonary artery is opened, and fused valve leaflets are incised along the valve commissures. The surgeon attempts to open the valve sufficiently to relieve stenosis yet prevent the development of significant pulmonary insufficiency. If the valve is extremely deformed, part or all of the valve may be removed.[436] After the valvotomy, the surgeon palpates the pulmonary infundibulum through the valve. If the infundibulum is extremely small, an incision may be made in the pulmonary outflow tract to allow resection of the infundibular stenosis under direct visualization. Patch enlargement of the right ventricular outflow tract is occasionally necessary if the pulmonary valve annulus is extremely small.[428] After completion of the procedure, pressure measurements are made in the right ventricle and pulmonary artery to ensure that right ventricular hypertension and valvular stenosis are relieved adequately. Some residual right ventricular hypertension may be tolerated since the right ventricular pressure may continue to fall during the immediate postoperative period. If a patent foramen ovale or a true atrial septal defect is present, it is closed during the surgery.

If the right ventricle is extremely small, so small that pulmonary blood flow is reduced despite relief of the pulmonary valve stenosis, a systemic-to-pulmonary artery shunt (such as a subclavian-to-pulmonary artery or Blalock-Taussig shunt) may also be created at the time of the pulmonary valvotomy.[292] The shunt may be taken down later if the right ventricle grows adequately. If the right ventricle and pulmonary outflow tract are extremely small, the surgeon may elect to perform open-heart surgery to place a woven prosthetic patch across the pulmonary valve annulus.[422]

Perioperative mortality following pulmonary valvotomy is low, except in symptomatic neonates, those children with severe right ventricular hypertension, and those with a small right ventricle.[80] Postoperative complications include congestive heart failure, low cardiac output, and arrhythmias.[428] Many patients develop some pulmonary valvular insufficiency following the valvotomy, although most children do not develop symptoms from the insufficiency. Most infants and children demonstrate a relief of symptoms and reduction of signs of right ven-

tricular hypertrophy.[162] They will receive follow-up care, however, to ensure that the pulmonary stenosis does not recur.

■ TETRALOGY OF FALLOT
■ Etiology

Tetralogy of Fallot (Fig. 3-32) refers to the association of four cardiac abnormalities described in detail by Fallot in 1888. The four cardiac anomalies are ventricular septal defect, pulmonic stenosis, dextroposition (displacement toward the right) of the aorta, and right ventricular hypertrophy. If an atrial septal defect is present, this association of five anomalies has been called the "pentalogy of Fallot."[336]

Tetralogy of Fallot is thought to occur as the result of lack of development of the subpulmonary conus during fetal life.[427] This not only produces pulmonary infundibular stenosis but also causes malalignment of the conal septum during fetal cardiac development, resulting in a large ventricular septal

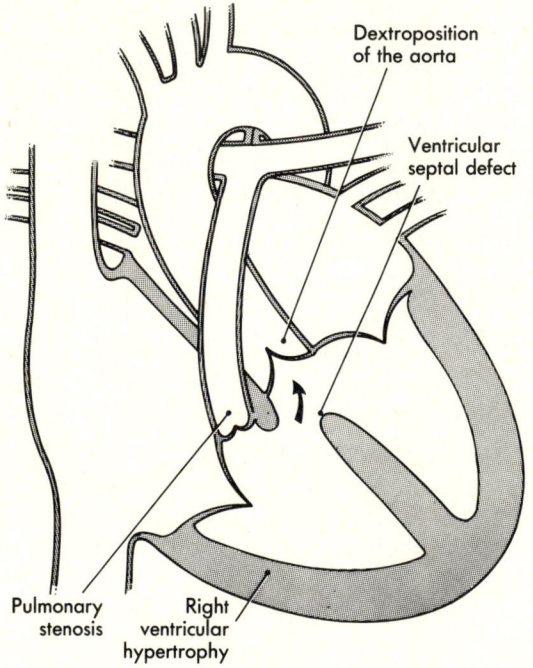

Fig. 3-32 Tetralogy of Fallot. The four components of tetralogy of Fallot are illustrated: pulmonary infundibular (and often valvular) stenosis, a large ventricular septal defect, dextroposition of the aorta (the aorta is shifted to the right so that it overrides the ventricular septal defect), and right ventricular hypertrophy.

From Hazinski, M.: The cardiovascular system, In Howe, J., and others, editors: The handbook of nursing, New York, 1984, John Wiley & Sons, Inc.

defect that is approximately equal to the size of the aorta. Pulmonary valvular stenosis may be present in addition to the infundibular stenosis. The aorta is displaced to the right because of the lack of development of the subpulmonary conus and the pulmonary outflow tract. As a result the aorta sits directly over the ventricular septal defect; this may also be referred to as an "overriding aorta." Right ventricular hypertrophy is merely the result of obstruction to pulmonary flow.

Occasionally, the pulmonary stenosis is so severe that there may be no anatomic connection between the right ventricle and the pulmonary artery. This severe form of tetralogy of Fallot, which may also be referred to as pulmonary atresia or pseudotruncus arteriosus, is discussed briefly here and again in a discussion of truncus arteriosus.

Rarely, tetralogy of Fallot is associated with a rudimentary or totally absent pulmonary valve. This produces valvular insufficiency during the neonatal period. However, the most significant problem caused by tetralogy of Fallot with absent pulmonary valve results from dilation of the main pulmonary artery and its right and left arterial branches.[202] Consequences and management of tetralogy of Fallot and absent pulmonary valve are noted separately in the following discussions.

Tetralogy of Fallot is the most common cyanotic congenital heart defect and is responsible for approximately 9% of all congenital heart defects.[134]

■ Pathophysiology

The hemodynamic changes that occur as the result of tetralogy of Fallot are determined by the severity of obstruction to pulmonary flow. If the pulmonary infundibular and valvular stenosis is mild, the right ventricular pressure will be mildly increased. There is minimal shunting of blood in either direction through the ventricular septal defect because resistance to pulmonary flow is approximately equal to resistance in the systemic circulation. This form of tetralogy may be referred to as "pink" (acyanotic) tetralogy.

During infancy, the pulmonary infundibular muscle may spasm. This produces an acute increase in resistance to pulmonary blood flow; as a result pulmonary blood flow will be severely reduced, and systemic venous blood from the right ventricle will shunt through the ventricular septal defect, almost directly into the aorta. The infant develops acute arterial oxygen desaturation and may become extremely irritable or may lose consciousness. These

spells (called "tet" spells) occur in approximately one third of all patients with cyanotic congenital heart disease and reduced pulmonary blood flow,[168] and they most commonly develop during the first months of life.[289]

If severe pulmonary infundibular or valvular stenosis is present, resistance to pulmonary flow may approach or exceed systemic vascular resistance. Consequently, a large amount of systemic venous blood shunts from the right ventricle into the aorta, producing systemic arterial oxygen desaturation. Initially, this shunt may occur only during periods of exertion (such as during vigorous cry), but when significant pulmonary stenosis develops, cyanosis will be present even at rest. Right ventricular hypertrophy develops as the result of the resistance against which the right ventricle must pump. The extremes of right ventricular hypertension encountered with severe pulmonary valve stenosis without a ventricular septal defect (or pulmonary stenosis with intact ventricular septum) are not seen with tetralogy of Fallot since the ventricular septal defect serves to "vent" the right ventricle. The greater the resistance to pulmonary blood flow, the greater will be the right-to-left shunt through the ventricular septal defect.

The left ventricle may be small, particularly if pulmonary blood flow and pulmonary venous return are reduced or if a large atrial septal defect is also present. When pulmonary blood flow is chronically reduced, collateral circulation to the lungs develops. These collateral vessels consist of branches from the bronchial arteries and the descending aorta, which fuse with pulmonary arteries and arterioles to enhance pulmonary blood flow.

When the infant or child develops chronic arterial oxygen desaturation, polycythemia will result. This increases the child's risk of the development of cerebrovascular accidents; these occur particularly under the age of 4, during episodes of bacteremia, or when microcytic anemia is present.[249,333] The incidence of brain abscesses is also increased in these patients, especially beyond the age of 2 years and during episodes of bacteremia.[126] In addition, infants and children with polycythemia develop coagulopathies and decreased platelet number or function.[183,405] For further discussion of pathophysiology and treatment of potential systemic consequences of polycythemia, see the section in this chapter on hypoxemia.

Approximately 8% of children with tetralogy of Fallot have abnormalities in coronary artery anatomy. In most of these children a single coronary artery rises from the aorta (with later branching into the right and left coronary arteries), or the left anterior descending artery rises from the right coronary artery. As a result of these anomalies, the left anterior descending artery may cross over the right ventricular outflow tract. It is extremely important that this anomalous coronary artery distribution be identified preoperatively so that surgical repair of the tetralogy can be planned to avoid coronary artery injury.[79,271]

Tetralogy of Fallot is one of the congenital heart defects most commonly identified among children with subacute bacterial endocarditis[141]; thus the risk of endocarditis is significant. As a result antibiotic prophylaxis will be prescribed for periods when the child is at risk for the development of bacteremia (see Table 3-13).

It was previously thought that infants and children with decreased pulmonary blood flow (such as occurs with tetralogy of Fallot) did not develop pulmonary hypertension. However, research studies indicate that the presence of a high hematocrit (especially greater than 54%) and low pulmonary blood flow produces an increase in blood viscosity and pulmonary vascular resistance.[307] When tetralogy of Fallot is present, the media of the pulmonary arterioles often is thinner than normal, and thromboses may develop in the smaller arterioles.[342] For discussion of systemic consequences of polycythemia see the section in this chapter on hypoxemia.

If the infant has tetralogy of Fallot with absent pulmonary valve, tracheobronchial obstruction is caused by the dilated pulmonary artery and aortic arch,[274] which produces respiratory distress. In addition, significant pulmonary valve regurgitation can cause severe right ventricular dysfunction.[202] These infants generally develop right-to-left shunting of blood through the ventricular septal defect, and resultant arterial oxygen desaturation. Frequently, as the infant gets older and right ventricular compliance decreases, there is less pulmonary diastolic regurgitation, so the right-to-left shunt through the ventricular septal defect and the child's cyanosis may decrease or disappear.

■ **Clinical signs and symptoms**

The most striking clinical sign of tetralogy of Fallot is cyanosis; the degree of cyanosis is usually directly proportional to the degree of pulmonary stenosis. If the stenosis is mild, there is a minimal right-to-left shunt through the ventricular septal defect, and the infant or child may be cyanotic only with vigorous cry or other exertion. If the pulmonary stenosis is severe, the right-to-left shunt through the ventricular septal defect will be significant, and the infant or child will demonstrate severe cyanosis even at rest (see the section on hypoxemia for discussion of potential systemic consequences of polycythemia).

Typically, the newborn with tetralogy of Fallot demonstrates minimal cyanosis, particularly while the ductus arteriosus is patent and providing additional pulmonary blood flow. After the ductus constricts, the neonate may demonstrate cyanosis with exertion. As the infant grows and becomes more active, the pulmonary stenosis usually becomes relatively more severe. Since the pulmonary stenosis provides a fixed obstruction, it is difficult for the infant to increase pulmonary blood flow during periods of increased oxygen requirement (such as exercise). The infant usually begins to demonstrate more cyanosis and decreased exercise tolerance at approximately 4 to 6 months of age.

If the neonate's main pulmonary artery or right or left pulmonary arteries are extremely small, severe cyanosis is present shortly after birth and becomes profound when the infant's ductus arteriosus begins to constrict since the ductus is the major route of pulmonary blood flow. These neonates become profoundly hypoxemic and acidotic and deteriorate rapidly unless prostaglandin E_1 is administered to maintain ductal patency. Ultimately, a systemic-to-pulmonary artery shunt will be surgically created to provide a permanent source of pulmonary blood flow. It is important to note that the hypoxemia that develops will not improve with the administration of oxygen; the neonate requires some circulatory pathway that allows blood to enter the pulmonary circulation.

Hypercyanotic episodes may develop during the first months of life. They may occur in infants with mild or severe forms of tetralogy of Fallot. The spells occur more commonly in the morning and more often during crying, defecation, or feeding. These activities may precipitate the spells because they all increase the infant's oxygen requirements; in addition, crying and defecation may further increase resistance to pulmonary blood flow (through a mechanism similar to the Valsalva's maneuver).[289] Cardiac catheterization may also precipitate spells.

With the onset of a hypercyanotic spell, the infant becomes acutely cyanotic, hyperpneic, irritable, and diaphoretic. Late in the spell, the infant becomes limp and may lose consciousness. If arterial blood gases are obtained during the spell, hypercapnia, hypoxemia, and acidosis will be noted.

The toddler may instinctively squat during play or assume the knee-chest position in bed. This position seems to increase resistance to systemic arterial blood flow, so that the right-to-left cardiac shunt is decreased and pulmonary blood flow is increased.

The infant with chronic hypoxemia will develop polycythemia. When the hematocrit approaches 60%, the infant may demonstrate a more rapid respiratory rate and increased respiratory effort because polycythemia increases blood viscosity and may decrease the velocity of pulmonary blood flow. Infants with chronic hypoxemia demonstrate clubbing of the tips of the fingers and toes beyond the age of 4 months (see the section on hypoxemia).[336]

If the infant's iron intake is inadequate, a microcytic anemia will develop. The infant may have a normal hemoglobin for his age but be relatively anemic because of the polycythemia. Therefore the mean corpuscular hemoglobin concentration (MCHC) and the mean corpuscular volume (MCV) should be followed to prevent the development of a microcytic anemia since its development will increase the infant's risk of cerebrovascular accident.[249]

The infant or child with tetralogy of Fallot demonstrates a systolic ejection murmur heard best at the second intercostal space along the left sternal border; this murmur is caused by blood flow through the stenotic pulmonary outflow tract. There may be a thrill over the same area. Some attempts have been made to correlate the loudness of the murmur with the degree of pulmonary stenosis, but this is not possible. Bruits may be heard over the child's back if extensive collateral circulation to the lungs has developed.

If moderate or severe pulmonary stenosis is present, a sternal lift will indicate the presence of right ventricular hypertrophy. Right ventricular hypertrophy will also be evident on the ECG and the echocardiogram. The two-dimensional echocardiogram will demonstrate the presence of a large ventricular septal defect, dextroposition of the aorta, and pulmonic stenosis. The size of the main and right and left pulmonary arteries can also be assessed to some extent with the two-dimensional echocardiogram.

A narrow mediastinum is observed on the chest radiograph since the main pulmonary artery segment is small. The classic radiographic cardiac contour in the child with tetralogy resembles the shape of a boot. The apex of the heart is elevated because of right ventricular hypertrophy; as a result the apex resembles the upturned toe of a boot. Pulmonary vascular markings will be decreased once pulmonary stenosis is severe, unless collateral vessels to the lungs have proliferated dramatically (this usually does not occur until adolescence). Approximately one fourth of patients with tetralogy of Fallot have a right aortic arch.

Cardiac catheterization is performed extremely carefully in the critically ill infant or in the infant subject to hypercyanotic spells since risk of catheterization is higher in these infants. Catheterization demonstrates the right ventricular hypertension and the pressure gradient across the pulmonary infundibulum and possibly across the valve. If right ventricular systolic pressure is equal to left ventricular systolic pressure, the cardiologist may not pass the catheter from the right ventricle into the main pulmonary artery since this may produce acute obstruction to pulmonary blood flow and may precipitate a hypercyanotic spell. Arterial oxygen desaturation will be present in a degree proportional to the child's right-to-left intracardiac shunt.

Infants with tetralogy of Fallot and absent pulmonary valve often have mild cyanosis, congestive heart failure, and respiratory distress. These infants have a muffled, single second heart sound since only the aortic valve closure is heard. A harsh, systolic ejection murmur (caused by pulmonary infundibular stenosis) and a prominent, low-frequency diastolic murmur (resulting from pulmonary insufficiency) may be present and accompanied by a thrill.[202] Right ventricular hypertrophy is evident on clinical examination and on the ECG. The echocardiogram reveals right ventricular dilation, and the two-dimensional echocardiogram may document the dilation of the main and right and left pulmonary arteries. The pulmonary valve is absent. The chest radiograph reveals cardiomegaly and dilation of the main pulmonary artery. Pulmonary vascular markings may be normal or increased, and atelectasis, pneumonia, or emphysema may also be noted. Cardiac catheterization data may be difficult to interpret until a right ventricular or pulmonary artery angiocardiogram is performed. The contrast material will reveal the pulmonary insufficiency and the extreme dilation of the main and right and/or left pulmonary arteries.

■ **Medical and surgical treatment and nursing interventions**

If the infant has mild pulmonary stenosis, he receives close follow-up care; medical treatment focuses on prevention of complications until elective surgical repair is performed between 18 months and 5 years of age. The infant should be kept well hydrated to prevent hemoconcentration, and microcytic anemia should be avoided since it increases the child's risk of cerebral thromboembolic events. The parents are taught to notify a physician if the infant develops diarrhea, nausea, vomiting, or fever so dehydration can be prevented and antibiotic prophylaxis can be prescribed if needed. (See the section on hypoxemia also.) The parents are also taught to watch for signs of hypercyanotic episodes. They must know how to place the infant in the knee-chest position and to notify a physician immediately. If spells develop, surgical palliation or correction is usually scheduled on an urgent basis.

Whenever the infant or child with tetralogy of Fallot is admitted to the hospital, it is essential that *no air is allowed to enter any IV line* since systemic venous blood may shunt directly into the aorta and any IV air may cause a cerebral air embolus.

All staff members should be aware that infants with tetralogy of Fallot may develop hypercyanotic spells. If the infant has a history of such spells, the weight-appropriate dose of morphine sulfate (0.1 mg/kg) and propranolol (0.15 to 0.25 mg/kg/IV dose) are usually prepared and kept at the bedside; oxygen should also be at the bedside. The staff should immediately place the infant in a knee-chest position, administer oxygen, and notify a physician if a hypercyanotic spell develops (see the section on hypoxemia).

If the infant with tetralogy of Fallot develops profound cyanosis in the first days of life, it is apparent that a severe form of tetralogy (or pulmonary atresia) is present. Because these neonates usually have a very small pulmonary outflow tract and main pulmonary artery, they are dependent upon the ductus arteriosus to provide pulmonary blood flow. If the neonate begins to develop profound hypoxemia, cyanosis, and acidosis when the ductus begins to close, IV prostaglandin E_1 will be administered to maintain ductal patency and pulmonary blood flow until cardiac catheterization and surgery can be performed. (See the section on hypoxemia for further information.)

If the cyanotic neonate has large main, right, and left pulmonary arteries, total repair of the tetralogy may be performed at this time. Most commonly, however, these neonates have a hypoplastic (extremely small) pulmonary outflow tract and pulmonary arteries, so repair is not feasible and palliative surgery is required. Palliative procedures that are performed to increase pulmonary blood flow in children with cyanotic heart disease are discussed in detail in Table 3-17. The purpose of all of these palliative procedures is to reduce hypoxemia by increasing pulmonary blood flow and to stimulate growth of the small pulmonary arteries. Most of these procedures do not require use of cardiopulmonary bypass and most are accomplished through a thoracotomy incision.

The most popular palliative procedures performed during early infancy use the infant's own subclavian artery or prosthetic material to create a shunt between the aorta and the pulmonary circulation (Fig. 3-33). The small size of the infant's subclavian artery or of the prosthetic tube used will limit the magnitude and the pressure of flow through the shunt so that the volume but not the pressure of pulmonary blood flow is increased; this minimizes the risk of later pulmonary vascular disease.[84,94] If the infant's subclavian artery is used for creation of a Blalock-Taussig shunt, collateral circulation will maintain adequate arterial flow to the arm. During the immediate postoperative period, the arm may feel cool, and it may not be possible to obtain a blood pressure by cuff; however, a *flush blood pressure* should correspond to the infant's mean arterial blood pressure.* To prevent further compromise of the arterial circulation of the arm, arterial punctures of that arm should be avoided preoperatively and postoperatively, and frequent cuff blood pressure measurements should not be performed immediately after surgery.

Although the Waterston-Cooley anastomosis is associated with significant later complications, such as pulmonary vascular disease and deformity of the right pulmonary artery,[19,303,448] this shunt may be created in very ill or very young infants because it is technically the easiest shunt to create (see Fig. 3-33, *C*).

Perioperative mortality for a closed-heart shunt procedure ranges from zero to 18%. Postoperative complications include bleeding and respiratory complications of the thoracotomy. If a large shunt has been created, a wide pulse pressure (resulting from aortic "runoff" into the shunt) and bounding pulses may be noted postoperatively. During the immediate postoperative period, the nurse should report signs of an increase in cyanosis, a worsening of hypoxemia, or the development of acidosis since these signs may indicate occlusion of the shunt. If the shunt does occlude, immediate reoperation may be required. If polytetrafluoroethylene is used for creation of the shunt, the infant's platelet count should be monitored postoperatively since platelets tend to adhere to this material until it becomes endothelialized.[353] Horner's syndrome may be observed after the creation of a Blalock-Taussig or modified Blalock-Taussig shunt (see the discussion on neurologic function in the section on postoperative care).

Congestive heart failure may develop after the Waterston-Cooley anastomosis is created or after the

---

A flush blood pressure is obtained using a standard arm blood pressure cuff of the appropriate size. With the cuff in place, the arm is elevated until it blanches. The cuff is inflated above the infant's known arterial blood pressure. The arm is lowered until it is level with the infant's heart, and the cuff is deflated. The pressure corresponding to the return of pink color to the infant's nailbeds is equal to the infant's mean arterial pressure.

Table 3-17 Palliative procedures to increase pulmonary blood flow in children with cyanotic congenital heart defects*

Palliative procedure	Resultant anatomic change	Circulatory consequences
Blalock-Taussig anastomosis	Subclavian artery is separated from the arm circulation, and the distal end is sewn to the pulmonary artery (see Fig. 3-33, *A*)	Systemic arterial blood from the aorta flows through the subclavian artery to the pulmonary artery; this produces increased pulmonary blood flow under low pressure; this shunt is easy to take down at later surgery
Prosthetic systemic-to-pulmonary artery shunt (modified Blalock-Taussig anastomosis)	Prosthetic material (most commonly polytetrafluoroethylene [Gore-tex or Impra]) is sewn between the aorta or a major systemic artery and the main, right, or left pulmonary artery; most commonly, the shunt is placed between the proximal subclavian artery and the right or left pulmonary artery (called a modified Blalock-Taussig shunt) or between the aorta and the main pulmonary artery (see Fig. 3-33, *B*).	Systemic arterial blood from the aorta flows through the prosthetic graft into the pulmonary artery; this produces increased pulmonary blood flow under low pressure; the shunt must be made large enough to provide adequate flow when the child grows; the flow also must be adequate to prevent thrombosis formation; this shunt is easy to take down at later surgery
Waterston-Cooley anastomosis	The back of ascending aorta is sewn to the front of the right pulmonary artery where they overlap, and an orifice is made between the back wall of the aorta and the front wall of the pulmonary artery (see Fig. 3-33, *C*)	Some blood from the aorta flows into the pulmonary artery; if the shunt is too large, high pulmonary blood flow under high pressure may produce congestive heart failure, and pulmonary hypertension may result; if the shunt is too small, there will be a negligible increase in pulmonary blood flow; with growth, this shunt often produces distortion of the right pulmonary artery, and may result in preferential flow of the shunted blood into the right or the left pulmonary artery; however, this is an easy shunt to construct, so it may be the shunt of choice in a critically ill cyanotic baby; this shunt also can produce growth of hypoplastic pulmonary arteries; the shunt is difficult to take down, however, at later corrective surgery, and patch enlargement of the right pulmonary artery may be necessary

*References 17, 19, 32, 83, 84, 94, 103, 239, 327, 413, 422, 431, 448.

Continued.

Table 3-17 Palliative procedures to increase pulmonary blood flow in children with cyanotic congenital heart defects—cont'd

Palliative procedure	Resultant anatomic change	Circulatory consequences
Glenn anastomosis	The right superior vena cava is ligated at its junction with the right atrium and is sewn to the right pulmonary artery; the right pulmonary artery may also be separated from the main pulmonary artery (see Fig. 3-33, D) NOTE: If a *left* superior vena cava is present, the same procedure may be performed with the *left* pulmonary artery	Systemic venous blood from the head and upper extremities flows directly into the right pulmonary artery; thus superior vena caval blood no longer enters the heart; the Glenn shunt usually increases pulmonary blood flow since approximately half of systemic venous return is flowing directly into the pulmonary circulation; the flow is under low (central venous) pressure; the shunt may also reduce cyanosis since it reduces the quantity of systemic venous blood returning to the heart, and it increases the quantity of pulmonary venous (oxygenated) blood returning to the heart; the Glenn shunt is difficult to take down; however, recently the shunt has become a permanent part of the two-stage correction of tricuspid atresia
Rashkind balloon septostomy	A balloon-tipped catheter is used to tear a hole in the atrial septum during cardiac catheterization NOTE: This procedure is performed during *cardiac catheterization*, not during surgery	This procedure is generally only effective during the neonatal period; it creates an atrial septal defect to allow better mixing of oxygenated and venous blood within the heart; it can also allow right-to-left shunting at the atrial level; the atrial septal defect created by this procedure may contract over time
Blalock-Hanlon septectomy	A large atrial septal defect is created NOTE: Cardiopulmonary bypass is *not* used	The creation of a large atrial septal defect can allow better mixing of oxygenated and venous blood within the heart (especially if the patient has transposition of the great vessels); it can also allow better flow of venous blood from the right to the left atrium; this increases pulmonary blood flow if the patient has transposition of the great vessels
Patch enlargement of the pulmonary outflow tract	A prosthetic patch is placed across the pulmonary outflow tract. NOTE: This procedure requires use of cardiopulmonary bypass	The patch acts as a gusset to enlarge the pulmonary outflow tract; this increases pulmonary blood flow and produces growth of the main and right and left pulmonary arteries; the patch may be left in place (or enlarged) when later correction is performed

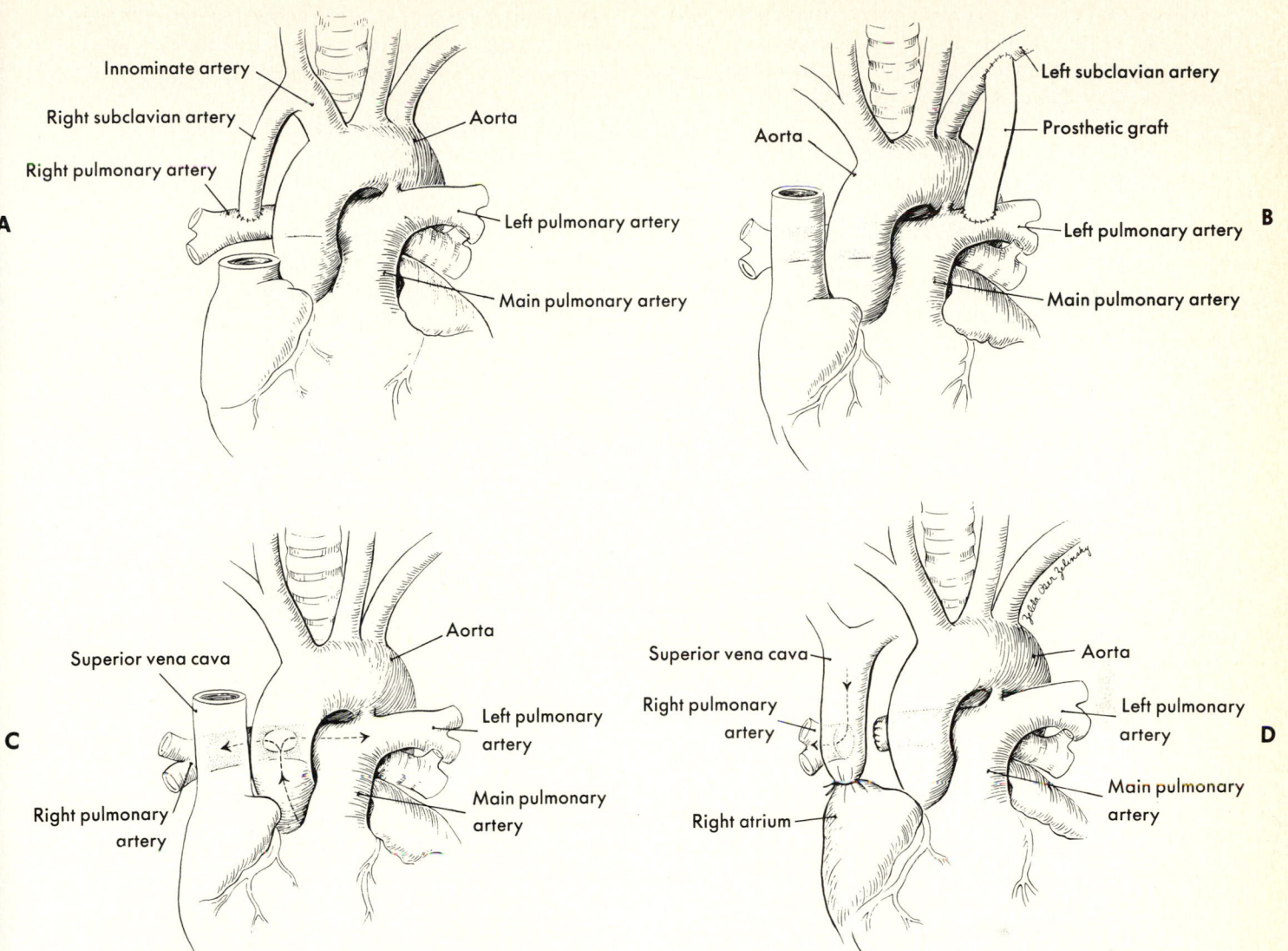

Fig. 3-33 Palliative surgical procedures to improve pulmonary blood flow. **A,** The Blalock-Taussig shunt. The patient's subclavian artery (usually the one arising from the innominate artery) is divided, the proximal portion is brought down, and the end of the subclavian is sewed to the side of the pulmonary artery. **B,** Modified Blalock-Taussig shunt. A prosthetic shunt, usually made of polytetrafluoroethylene (Gore-Tex or Impra), is constructed between the subclavian artery and the pulmonary artery. **C,** Waterston-Cooley shunt. A fistula (hole) is made between the back of the ascending aorta and the front of the right pulmonary artery. **D,** Glenn anastomosis: Ultimately, the superior vena caval flow is directed into the right pulmonary artery. The superior vena cava is often tied off at its junction with the right atrium, so the superior vena caval flow enters only the right pulmonary artery; in addition, the right pulmonary artery is often isolated from the common pulmonary artery.

Courtesy Zelda O. Zelinsky.

creation of any large shunt. If heart failure develops, the physician should be notified immediately, and treatment with a digitalis derivative and diuresis will be required. Rarely, the shunt must be surgically reduced in size to eliminate the congestive heart failure.

Occasionally, the phrenic nerve is injured dur-ing such palliative surgery, and diaphragmatic paralysis results. This paralysis may not be apparent when the infant is receiving positive pressure ventilation, but it should be suspected if the infant has difficulty being weaned from ventilatory support. A chest radiograph obtained while the infant is briefly removed from ventilator support will reveal elevation of the hemidiaphragm. The diaphragmatic paralysis is generally temporary, and frequently diaphragmatic function returns within several weeks. Occasionally, the paralysis is permanent and diaphragmatic plication is later required.

If the young infant with severe tetralogy has a small infundibulum and pulmonary valve annulus, palliative surgery may be performed to enlarge the pulmonary outflow tract.[422] This procedure requires a median sternotomy and use of cardiopulmonary bypass. An incision is made in the pulmonary outflow tract, and some of the hypertrophic infundibular muscle is removed. A patch is placed across the pulmonary outflow tract. This procedure increases blood flow to the main pulmonary artery and thus should enhance growth of both the right and left pulmonary arteries.[422] This pericardial patch may remain in place and later corrective surgery may be performed through the pericardial patch.[422] The disadvantages of this technique include the fact that cardiopulmonary bypass is used and that pulmonary insufficiency is created. Postoperative complications include bleeding, congestive heart failure, low cardiac output, arrhythmias, and neurologic complications of polycythemia.

Indications for corrective surgery for tetralogy of Fallot include the development of severe polycythemia, decreased exercise tolerance, hypercyanotic spells, or severe hypoxemia (an arterial oxygen saturation of less than 80%). The corrective surgery will be performed whenever the pulmonary arteries are of adequate size; it will require a median sternotomy and use of cardiopulmonary bypass. The goals of surgical repair include closure of the ventricular septal defect and reconstruction of the right ventricular outflow tract.[269] Whenever possible, a ventriculotomy is avoided, and the tetrology is repaired through an incision in the right atrium and/or the pulmonary artery. If necessary, however, a right ventriculotomy cardiac incision will be performed The hypertrophic pulmonary infundibular muscle is cut away (resected), and a pulmonary valvotomy is performed if needed. The ventricular septal defect is closed with a woven patch. If the pulmonary outflow tract and main pulmonary artery are small, a patch may be placed across the pulmonary outflow tract and, if necessary, in the main pulmonary artery; one or two patches may be used. An attempt is made to eliminate as much pulmonary obstruction as possible, yet avoid creation of significant pulmonary insufficiency. If severe insufficiency is created, the volume load produced by the insufficiency may produce severe postoperative right ventricular dysfunction.[101]

Occasionally, a conduit (with or without a valve) must be inserted between the right ventricle and the aorta to ensure an adequate, unobstructed flow of blood from the right ventricle to the pulmonary artery.

Perioperative mortality following repair of tetralogy of Fallot is approximately 2% to 8%.[17,269] Postoperative complications include congestive heart failure, low cardiac output, bleeding, arrhythmias, and neurologic complications. Congestive heart failure can result from right ventricular dysfunction and is more likely if residual pulmonary stenosis or pulmonary hypertension is present. Left ventricular dysfunction can result from the sudden increase in pulmonary blood flow and pulmonary venous return, especially if the left ventricle is relatively small. If congestive heart failure is severe and persistent postoperatively, a residual ventricular septal defect may be present; this occurs in approximately 10% of operated patients,[136] and may necessitate reoperation. If low cardiac output develops postoperatively, it requires treatment with a careful balance of fluid administration and diuresis, inotropic support, and possible afterload reduction.[136] Bleeding is more likely if the infant or child had a preoperative coagulopathy related to severe polycythemia.

Many patients develop right bundle branch block following surgical repair, as a result of either right ventriculotomy or closure of the ventricular septal defect.[152] Complete heart block, supraventricular arrhythmias, and premature ventricular contractions may also be noted.[136] Neurologic complications are usually related to thromboembolic events.

Approximately half of those children who undergo correction of tetralogy of Fallot demonstrate excellent cardiovascular function months and years after surgery. Those with a less satisfactory result may demonstrate decreased exercise tolerance,[439] persistent congestive heart failure, or arrhythmias. A poor operative result is most commonly related to persistent right ventricular hypertension (resulting from residual pulmonary stenosis or pulmonary hypertension), a residual ventricular septal defect, or documented coupled or multifocal premature ventricular contractions at rest.[136] The incidence of sudden death late after tetralogy repair is reported at approximately 2% to 7%.[224] The risk of sudden death is extremely low among those patients with an excellent operative result but is significant among those patients with persistent, severe right ventricular hypertension and coupled or multifocal premature ventricular contractions.[136,224,357] For this reason, reoperation is recommended if the patient demonstrates significant residual pulmonary infundibular, valvular, or supravalvular stenosis, pulmonary insufficiency, tricuspid insufficiency, or a significant residual ventricular septal defect.[101] Antiarrhythmic drugs are usually prescribed as needed to reduce the incidence of premature ventricular contractions.[136] The risk of postoperative bacterial endocarditis is low.[224]

If the infant with tetralogy of Fallot and absent pulmonary valve develops signs of respiratory compromise secondary to pulmonary artery compression of the tracheobronchial tree, these infants require careful respiratory care. They usually improve when they are placed in the prone position because the dilated pulmonary artery tends to compress the bronchi when they are supine.[18] Pulmonary toilet must be meticulous, and treatment with bronchodilators is usually helpful. If congestive heart failure is present, treatment with digoxin and diuretics is necessary. If the infant does not respond to medical management, surgical intervention will be necessary.

Surgical repair of tetralogy of Fallot with absent pulmonary valve is most commonly performed

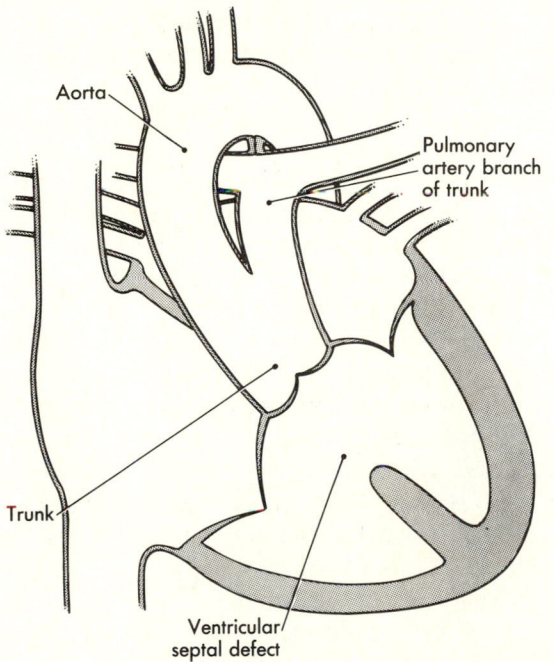

Fig. 3-34 Truncus arteriosus, type I. One single great vessel arises from the ventricles, straddling a large ventricular septal defect; this vessel then gives rise to the systemic, pulmonary, and coronary arterial circulations. In this form of truncus, the main pulmonary artery arises from the lateral aspect of the trunk, and then branches into the right and left pulmonary artery. Pulmonary stenosis may also be present.

From Hazinski, M.: The cardiovascular system, In Howe, J., and others, editors: The handbook of nursing, New York, 1984, John Wiley & Sons, Inc.

through a median sternotomy, and cardiopulmonary bypass is used. The dilated pulmonary artery may be replaced by a prosthetic valved conduit, or portions of the dilated pulmonary artery may be removed (in the form of aneurysmectomy).[18] A prosthetic valve may be inserted initially or as part of a second stage operation.[202] Perioperative mortality is significant, and it is highest among infants with severe symptoms necessitating urgent surgery. Postoperative complications include persistent respiratory failure, congestive heart failure, low cardiac output, and arrhythmias.[202]

■ **TRUNCUS ARTERIOSUS**
■ **Etiology**

Truncus arteriosus results from inadequate division of the common great vessel, the truncus arteriosus, during fetal cardiac development (see the section in this chapter on embryology). As a result a single, large great vessel arises from the ventricles and gives rise to the systemic, pulmonary, and coronary circulations.[57] Since the truncal septum contributes to closure of the conal ventricular septum, failure of truncal division also causes a large ventricular septal defect. The truncus arteriosus usually has a single, large truncal valve with two to four cusps.[44]

There are four major forms of truncus arteriosus; the various types describe the origin of pulmonary arterial circulation from the large trunk. In *type I* truncus arteriosus, the main pulmonary artery rises from the trunk, just above the large truncal valve (Fig. 3-34). In *type II* truncus arteriosus, there is no main pulmonary artery segment, and the right and left pulmonary arteries rise from the back of the truncus at the same level. In *type III* truncus arteriosus, the right and left pulmonary arteries rise separately from the lateral aspect of the truncus, and there is no main pulmonary artery segment.[336] With this type of truncus arteriosus, there may be absence of one pulmonary artery so that the corresponding lung receives blood flow through collateral vessels.[57] Any one of these three forms of truncus arteriosus may be associated with stenosis of the pulmonary artery or arteries.

The fourth type of truncus arteriosus is called *type IV* truncus arteriosus. When this form of truncus arteriosus is present, there is no main pulmonary artery, and pulmonary arterial circulation is supplied from the systemic arterial circulation through collateral vessels of the bronchial arteries (Fig. 3-35). The distribution of the pulmonary arterial circulation is often normal, but it rises from the systemic arterial circulation. Because the hemodynamics that occur as a result of this defect are similar to those resulting

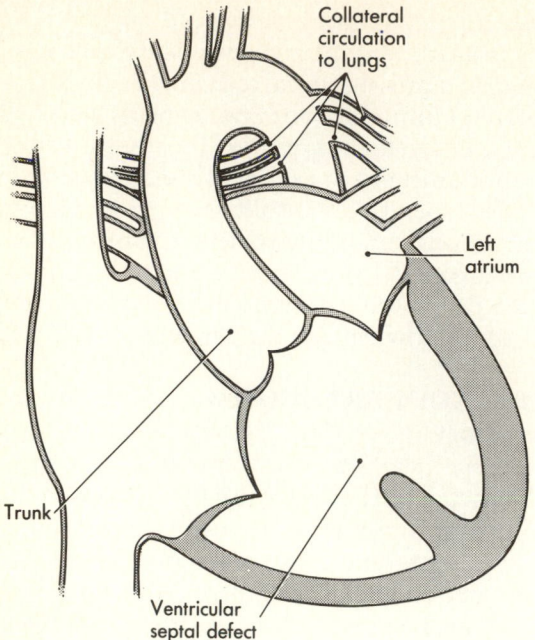

Fig. 3-35 Truncus arteriosus, type IV. The aorta is the single great vessel arising from the ventricles; it straddles a large ventricular septal defect and receives blood from both ventricles. Since there is no main pulmonary artery, pulmonary arterial flow occurs only through collateral vessels arising from the aorta. This blood flow pattern is similar to that occurring with pulmonary artery atresia (pseudotruncus).

From Hazinski, M.: The cardiovascular system, In Howe, J., and others, editors: The handbook of nursing, New York, 1984, John Wiley & Sons, Inc.

from pulmonary artery atresia with a ventricular septal defect, they will be discussed with that defect.

Persistent truncus arteriosus is responsible for approximately 2% of all congenital heart defects.[134]

■ **Pathophysiology**

Since the single great vessel straddles the large ventricular septal defect, it receives the output of both ventricles. The large ventricular septal defect causes equalization of ventricular pressures, and both ventricles share a common outflow tract so that both right and left ventricular pressures will be high.

Since both oxygenated and venous blood from the left and right ventricles is ejected into the common great vessels, both the systemic and pulmonary circulations receive mixed venous blood from both ventricles. However, there is often preferential streaming of systemic venous (desaturated) blood into the pulmonary branches and of pulmonary venous

(oxygenated) blood into the aortic component of the trunk.[57] The level of systemic arterial oxygen saturation usually corresponds to the volume of pulmonary blood flow; the greater the pulmonary blood flow, the larger the proportion of oxygenated pulmonary venous blood that enters the common great vessel from the left ventricle.

If *pulmonary stenosis is absent*, blood flow to both the systemic and pulmonary circulations is approximately equal at birth since both circulations offer approximately equal resistance to flow. Once the neonate's pulmonary vascular resistance falls, the pulmonary circulation provides lower resistance to flow, so there will be a greater tendency for blood from the common great vessel to flow into the pulmonary circulation. Since the main, right, and left pulmonary arteries branch directly from the great vessel, pulmonary blood flow will be under high pressure during both systole and diastole. As a result the infant usually develops signs of congestive heart failure at approximately 4 to 12 weeks of age.[57] Risk of pulmonary vascular disease is high in these infants.[256] If the truncal valve is grossly insufficient, severe congestive heart failure and cardiac decompensation can result.

If *mild pulmonary stenosis* is present, pulmonary blood flow may be sufficient to prevent profound hypoxemia, but it may not be large enough to produce congestive heart failure. If *severe pulmonary stenosis or atresia* of a pulmonary artery is present, pulmonary blood flow may be severely reduced, so little oxygenated blood is returning to the left ventricle and is ejected into the common great vessel; therefore hypoxemia can be severe from birth. In these neonates, the patent ductus arteriosus provides an important source of pulmonary blood flow during the first days of life, and the neonate's hypoxemia can worsen when the ductus begins to close (see the section on hypoxemia in this chapter for a discussion of potential systemic consequences of polycythemia). If there is an absence of one pulmonary artery branch, the lung on the involved side is usually small until collateral circulation to the lung develops.[57]

■ **Clinical signs and symptoms**

Nearly all infants with truncus arteriosus demonstrate signs of congestive heart failure and/or cyanosis in the first months of life. The degree and severity of symptoms is determined by the source and volume of the infant's pulmonary blood flow and by the presence of other intracardiac anomalies.[57,256] The infant with truncus arteriosus without pulmonary stenosis often demonstrates mild or moderate cyanosis within the first days of life; the cyanosis often increases with vigorous cry or exertion. When pulmonary vascular resistance falls, the volume and pressure of pulmonary blood flow increases, and the infant develops signs of severe congestive heart failure. The signs of congestive heart failure are usually more severe than those produced by a simple ventricular septal defect since the shunt into the pulmonary circulation from the trunk occurs during both systole and diastole. These signs and symptoms may develop earlier or be more severe if the truncal valve is grossly insufficient. The infant's cyanosis typically becomes less severe when signs of congestive heart failure develop because the increased pulmonary blood flow improves the proportion of oxygenated blood that is ejected into the trunk and into the aorta.

If the infant has mild pulmonary stenosis, congestive heart failure may not develop unless significant truncal valve insufficiency is present. The infant with mild pulmonary stenosis may be protected from the development of pulmonary vascular disease, yet have enough pulmonary blood flow so that cyanosis is only mild or moderate.

If severe pulmonary stenosis or absence of one pulmonary artery branch is present, the neonate usually has severe cyanosis, particularly once the ductus arteriosus begins to close (see the section on hypoxemia in this chapter).

The infant with truncus arteriosus demonstrates a harsh systolic ejection murmur heard along the left sternal border; the murmur is the result of the ventricular septal defect and is usually accompanied by a thrill. Opening of the truncal valve may produce a click immediately after the first heart sound.[57] The second heart sound is single in half of the patients and split in the remaining patients.[57] It is usually loud, and it will be heard best over the second intercostal space along the right sternal border (the aortic area). A blowing diastolic murmur may be heard along the left lower sternal border if truncal valve insufficiency is present.[57,123] If pulmonary blood flow is large, a diastolic rumble can be heard at the apex as a result of the large flow of the pulmonary venous return from the left atrium across the mitral valve and into the left ventricle.

If pulmonary blood flow is increased, the patient may demonstrate bounding pulses and a widened pulse pressure, as a result of "runoff" of blood from the systemic circulation into the pulmonary circulation.[57]

Biventricular hypertrophy is generally noted on the clinical examination, particularly if pulmonary blood flow is increased. A sternal lift and left ventricular heave are often present. Biventricular hypertrophy is often noted on the ECG, and evidence of left atrial hypertrophy may be noted if pulmonary blood flow is large.[57] The two-dimensional echocardiogram suggests the presence of truncus arteriosus since the large single great vessel will be seen overriding the ventricular septal defect. The diagnosis of truncus arteriosus is confirmed when no pulmonary valve is visualized. The two-dimensional echocardiogram may also reveal the location of the pulmonary artery branch(es) from the trunk.

The chest radiograph will reveal generalized cardiomegaly, particularly if pulmonary blood flow is increased. Pulmonary vascular markings will be increased unless significant pulmonary stenosis is present. Approximately one third of patients with truncus arteriosus have a right aortic arch.[57] The ascending aorta may appear dilated, and the hila of either lung (most commonly the left hilum) may be displaced upward if the corresponding pulmonary artery rises from a point high on the ascending aorta. If significant pulmonary stenosis is present, pulmonary vascular markings will be decreased, and cardiomegaly may not be present.

Cardiac catheterization demonstrates an increase in oxygen saturation in the right ventricle, as a result of the left-to-right shunt through the ventricular septal defect. In most patients, the systemic arterial oxygen saturation will be higher than the pulmonary arterial oxygen saturation because of the preferential streaming of systemic venous blood into the pulmonary circulation and of pulmonary venous blood into the systemic circulation.[57] Right ventricular hypertension is present in all patients. A pressure gradient may be measured across the truncal valve as a result of valvular stenosis. Pulmonary stenosis may also be noted; it occurs most commonly at the origin of the pulmonary artery (or arteries) from the trunk, although peripheral pulmonary artery stenosis has also been noted.[57] The angiocardiogram confirms the presence of a single great vessel and helps differentiate between truncus arteriosus and pulmonary atresia. Both right and left ventricular angiography will demonstrate the location of the ventricular septal defect, the trunk, and the anatomy of the pulmonary arterial circulation. A contrast injection in the common great vessel may demonstrate the presence of truncal valve insufficiency.[57] Pulmonary vascular resistance will be calculated carefully from measurements of pulmonary blood flow and pressure since these infants are at risk for the development of pulmonary vascular disease.

Without surgical intervention, many of these infants die during infancy.[256] As a result the risk of endocarditis in the nonoperated infant is not known. These infants should all receive antibiotic prophylaxis for periods of increased risk of development of bacteremia (see Table 3-13).[336]

■ Medical and surgical treatment and nursing interventions

Medical treatment of the infant with truncus arteriosus is aimed at reducing the signs and symptoms of congestive heart failure and minimizing the risks of systemic consequences of polycythemia.

If the infant has congestive heart failure, treatment with digoxin and diuretics is necessary (see the section in this chapter on congestive heart failure). However, severe diuresis and the resulting hemoconcentration must be avoided since the infant's hematocrit can rise sharply, increasing the risk of thromboembolic events (see the section on hypoxemia). Since infants with truncus arteriosus and high pulmonary blood flow can rapidly develop increased pulmonary vascular resistance, the infant usually receives an echocardiogram and cardiac catheterization as soon as the diagnosis is suspected. Early surgical intervention is also often indicated.

Palliative surgery for the infant with truncus arteriosus and severe congestive heart failure consists of pulmonary artery banding. However, because this procedure is associated with high early and late mortality,[338] many centers now recommend surgical correction of the truncus arteriosus during infancy, providing that the right and left pulmonary artery branches are of adequate size[101] (see the discussion that follows). Pulmonary artery banding is contraindicated in infants with significant truncal valve incompetence.

When the neonate with truncus arteriosus and pulmonary stenosis or absence of a pulmonary artery branch has severe cyanosis at birth, prostaglandin E_1 should be administered intravenously to prevent closure of the ductus arteriosus since the ductus is providing an important route for pulmonary blood flow. An echocardiogram and cardiac catheterization should be performed, and surgical intervention will be necessary. During prostaglandin therapy and diagnostic studies, absolutely *no air can be allowed in the IV lines* since air may enter the systemic circulation, producing a cerebral air embolus (see the section in this chapter on hypoxemia for further nursing interventions).

Palliative surgery for the infant with truncus arteriosus and severe hypoxemia involves creation of a systemic-to-pulmonary artery shunt (see Table 3-17) to improve pulmonary blood flow.[143,422]

If the infant has mild pulmonary stenosis and if congestive heart failure and cyanosis are not severe, that infant may be followed closely and referred for elective surgical repair between 18 months and 4 years of age.[15]

Surgical repair of truncus arteriosus uses a modification of the Rastelli procedure; it requires a median sternotomy incision and use of cardiopulmonary bypass. Hypothermia is often also employed.[336] The pulmonary artery or arteries are separated from the trunk, the ventricular septal defect is closed, and a conduit is placed to join the right ventricle and pulmonary arterial circulation.[336] This procedure was previously reserved for older children because it is not possible to insert a large conduit in small infants. Currently, however, if the pulmonary artery branches are of adequate size, the repair can be performed during early infancy with placement of a small conduit.[102] The small conduit will be replaced with a larger one during the preschool years[101,239]; a third conduit replacement is usually necessary during preteen or early adolescent years.[336] Surgical repair of the truncus arteriosus during infancy should prevent the development of pulmonary vascular disease and systemic consequences of chronic hypoxemia and polycythemia.

To complete the Rastelli repair during openheart surgery, a right ventriculotomy cardiac incision is made. The ventricular septal defect is patched so that left ventricular outflow is directed to the truncal valve; this temporarily isolates the right ventricle and converts the common trunk into the aorta. The pulmonary artery (in type I truncus arteriosus) or arteries (in types II, III, or IV truncus arteriosus) are separated from the aorta and any defect remaining in the aorta is patched. If a pulmonary artery band was placed, it may be removed, and the pulmonary artery is enlarged with a patch if necessary.[336] The band may also be left in place and used to separate the pulmonary artery and the aorta. A prosthetic conduit is then sewn between the right ventricle and the pulmonary artery or arteries.[268] Any palliative shunts are eliminated at the time of repair. Rarely, replacement of a severely insufficient truncal valve with a prosthetic valve is necessary.

Postoperative mortality following repair of truncus arteriosus is approximately 9% to 25%.[101,257,336] Operative risk is highest in small infants, those with severe truncal valve insufficiency, and those with preoperative pulmonary hypertension. Postoperative complications include congestive heart failure, low cardiac output, bleeding, arrhythmias (including heart block), and neurologic complications. Many of these patients require inotropic or vasodilator pharmacologic therapy and assisted ventilation for at least 24 hours postoperatively. If congestive heart failure is severe postoperatively and if it is refractory to medical management, the presence of a residual ventricular septal defect should be suspected and appropriate studies performed. If a large ventricular septal defect is present, reoperation may be necessary to close it.

Late mortality following surgical repair of truncus arteriosus is approximately 9% to 12%.[182,257] This late mortality is the result of valve or conduit failure or obstruction, progression of pulmonary vascular disease, persistent heart failure or low cardiac output, arrhythmias, or reoperation for conduit replacement.[182,257] If a porcine valve is present in the conduit, it may calcify, producing pulmonary valvular stenosis as early as 2 years after placement.[367] When any porcine valve is placed during childhood, it tends to develop obstruction to some degree within 2 to 8 years after initial surgery.[182] If the conduit is placed during infancy, replacement with a larger conduit is planned 1 to 3 years later. Conduit replacement surgery has thus far been associated with a relatively low mortality.[336]

Since calcification of the conduit valve has been frequently reported, repair of truncus arteriosus in the newborn has been attempted using a nonvalved conduit. This procedure has been successful on a limited basis, and it is being investigated further.[325] Use of a nonvalved conduit is contraindicated in infants with significant pulmonary hypertension since this would result in severe pulmonary regurgitation, and can produce right ventricular dysfunction.[101]

Whenever the infant or child has a prosthetic conduit (or any implanted prosthetic material) in place, prevention of bacterial endocarditis is extremely important[101] because the bacteria can lodge in the prosthetic material and be extremely difficult to eliminate. Antibiotic prophylaxis should be administered during periods of increased risk of bacteremia, especially during dental work or infectious illnesses (see Table 3-13). The child's family should be taught to consult a physician whenever the child develops a fever or other signs of infection, and antibiotics will usually be administered. Blood cultures should be drawn whenever the child develops high fever and elevation in white blood cell count, with or without localized signs of infection.

Anticoagulant therapy is not necessary following placement of a porcine or heterograft valved conduit. However, some physicians recommend administration of a small daily dose of aspirin or aspirin and

dipyridamole (Persantine) to reduce platelet adherence to the prosthetic surface.[353]

■ **PULMONARY ATRESIA**
■ **Etiology**

Pulmonary atresia occurs when there is failure of appropriate septation of the truncus arteriosus into both a pulmonary artery and aorta, or failure of pulmonary valve development. The term "atresia" implies that there is a lack of anatomic continuity between the right ventricle and the pulmonary artery. The pulmonary valve annulus may be very small, and the main pulmonary artery may be absent or rudimentary. The right and left pulmonary arteries may be of normal size, or they may be extremely small. A ventricular septal defect may be present.

When pulmonary atresia is present *without* a ventricular septal defect, this defect is called pulmonary atresia with intact ventricular septum. In this case, the right ventricle is usually extremely small and thick-walled, and the tricuspid valve is often stenotic. This association of defects is also known as hypoplastic right heart syndrome. If a ventricular septal defect is present and if no main pulmonary artery is present, the defect is also called "pseudotruncus" and is similar to type IV truncus arteriosus (see Fig. 3-35).

Pulmonary atresia is responsible for approximately 3% of all congenital heart defects.[134]

■ **Pathophysiology**

When there is lack of anatomic continuity between the right ventricle and the pulmonary artery, blood must enter the pulmonary arterial circulation through another shunt or the infant will become profoundly hypoxemic and die. An additional factor is that systemic venous blood which enters the right ventricle must have a way to get out of the right ventricle.

If no ventricular septal defect is present, systemic venous blood that enters the right heart quickly fills the right ventricle but has no outflow path. Right ventricular end-diastolic and right atrial pressures rise, and tricuspid insufficiency often results. The foramen ovale opens, as a result of the increase in right atrial pressure, so systemic venous blood flows from the right to the left atrium and mixes with pulmonary venous blood. The mixed venous blood enters the left ventricle and is ejected into the aorta. There is usually a patent ductus arteriosus or some other form of systemic-to-pulmonary artery shunt present to provide flow from the systemic circulation into the pulmonary arterial circulation.

If a ventricular septal defect is present, blood from the right ventricle is ejected through the ventricular septal defect and into the aorta. Thus the aorta receives both systemic and pulmonary venous blood. There must be a patent ductus arteriosus or some other systemic-to-pulmonary artery shunt present to provide flow from the systemic circulation into the pulmonary arterial circulation. When pseudotruncus arteriosus is present, there is often no common pulmonary artery (which gives rise to the right and left pulmonary arteries), and the distribution of the pulmonary arterial circulation is often abnormal. It is important to determine the presence or absence of a common pulmonary artery since this will affect the type of surgical procedure selected.

The incidence of bacterial endocarditis is not significant in these children preoperatively, and the risk of pulmonary hypertension is low.

■ Clinical signs and symptoms

The neonate with pulmonary atresia usually demonstrates significant cyanosis at birth or within the first days of life and usually develops profound cyanosis once the ductus arteriosus begins to close.

In approximately one fifth of the infants with pulmonary atresia, no murmur is heard.[279] If the infant does not have a ventricular septal defect, a systolic ejection murmur may be heard along the left sternal border; this murmur is caused by the tricuspid insufficiency or a coexistent patent ductus arteriosus. If a ventricular septal defect is present, a systolic ventricular septal defect murmur may be heard along the left lower sternal border.

The neonate's pulses usually are not bounding, even if a significant amount of blood is flowing from the aorta into the ductus arteriosus. This is because the infant is often critically ill so peripheral pulses are often decreased in intensity.

If no ventricular septal defect is present, signs of systemic venous engorgement are usually observed shortly after birth. The neonate demonstrates hepatomegaly and periorbital edema. The enlarged liver will be pulsatile if tricuspid regurgitation is present.[279] Other signs of congestive heart failure may also be noted.

The clinical examination may reveal a left ventricular heave, particularly if no ventricular septal defect is present. If a ventricular septal defect is present, signs of biventricular hypertrophy (including a sternal lift and left ventricular heave) may be noted.

If a ventricular septal defect is not present and if the right ventricle is small, signs of left ventricular hypertrophy are often noted on the ECG, although left axis deviation is uncommon (this helps differentiate pulmonary atresia with intact ventricular septum from tricuspid atresia). If electrocardiographic evidence of left ventricular hypertrophy is pronounced beyond the age of 1 month, the diagnosis of hypoplastic right heart should be strongly considered.[279] Right atrial enlargement is often evident on the ECG, particularly if no ventricular septal defect is present. The echocardiogram demonstrates the presence of an enlarged aorta. It will be impossible to visualize the pulmonary valve, although the tricuspid valve will be seen. If the right ventricle is hypoplastic, this will be evident on the M-mode and two-dimensional echocardiogram. If a ventricular septal defect is present, it may be seen using a two-dimensional echocardiogram.

An increased cardiothoracic ratio is often observed on the chest radiograph; this is the result of enlargement of the right atrium and left ventricle in the infant without a ventricular septal defect, and of the enlargement of both ventricles in the infant with a ventricular septal defect. Pulmonary vascular markings will be diminished. The upper left heart border will be concave because of the absence of the normal main pulmonary artery shadow.

Cardiac catheterization will confirm the absence of anatomic continuity between the pulmonary artery and aorta, and it will document the source, magnitude, and distribution of pulmonary arterial blood flow. It will also be important to determine the presence of a ventricular septal defect and its relationship to the aorta. In addition, the size of the common pulmonary artery or right and left pulmonary artery branches must also be visualized during angiography so that the appropriate surgical intervention can be selected.

■ Medical and surgical treatment and nursing interventions

When the neonate develops cyanosis and when radiographs provide evidence of decreased pulmonary blood flow, prostaglandin E₁ will be administered to maintain patency of the ductus arteriosus. *No air can be allowed in any IV line* since it can enter the systemic arterial circulation, producing an air embolus (see the section in this chapter on hypoxemia). Urgent echocardiography and cardiac catheterization will be performed. If no ventricular septal defect is found, a Rashkind balloon septostomy may be performed during cardiac catheterization to enable better flow of blood from the right to the left atrium. To perform the

Rashkind procedure, a standard venous catheterization is performed, and a balloon-tipped catheter is inserted. The catheter is passed from the right to the left atrium, the balloon is inflated, and it is pulled quickly back into the right atrium. This tears a hole in the atrial septum, and will allow better mixing of systemic and pulmonary venous blood so arterial oxygen saturation will improve. In addition, the septostomy will allow better flow of blood from the right to the left atrium so signs of systemic venous engorgement may be relieved.

Since the neonate must have a permanent route of pulmonary blood flow, surgical intervention is necessary during the neonatal period. If isolated pulmonary valve atresia is present without a ventricular septal defect, a closed transventricular pulmonary valvotomy may be performed. This procedure does not require use of cardiopulmonary bypass. A curved blade is inserted through a small stab wound in the right ventricular outflow tract, which is surrounded by "purse-string" sutures to prevent bleeding, and the valve is incised. A similar procedure may be performed using inflow occlusion and a small incision in the pulmonary artery (see the section on medical and surgical treatment for pulmonary valve stenosis). A valvotomy will decompress the right ventricle and will allow the flow of some blood from the right ventricle to the pulmonary artery. Closed-heart surgical creation of a shunt between the systemic and the pulmonary circulation (see Table 3-17) may also be performed. Most commonly, the neonate's subclavian artery is used to create the shunt, or a prosthetic graft is inserted between the neonate's subclavian artery and pulmonary artery (see the section on medical and surgical treatment for tetralogy of Fallot). Some surgeons recommend that a valvotomy be performed in addition to a shunt in neonates with pulmonary valve atresia.[292]

Open-heart surgery may also be performed during the neonatal period. An open-heart valvotomy may be performed. In addition, a patch may be placed across the outflow tract to enlarge it if the right ventricular outflow is small. This patch procedure seems to allow better growth of the main and distal pulmonary arteries before later surgical correction is attempted.[422]

If the main pulmonary artery is atretic but the right and left pulmonary arteries are of adequate size, total correction of the pulmonary atresia can be performed with the Rastelli procedure. This procedure involves use of a median sternotomy incision and cardiopulmonary bypass. A right ventriculotomy cardiac incision is made. Any existing septal defects are closed. If a ventricular septal defect is present, it is closed with a prosthetic patch so that left ventricular outflow is directed to the aortic valve and the right ventricle is temporarily isolated. Then a valved conduit is placed between the right ventricle and pulmonary artery. Postoperative complications include congestive heart failure, low cardiac output, bleeding, arrhythmias, and neurologic complications. For further discussion of the Rastelli procedure see the section on medical and surgical treatment and nursing interventions for truncus arteriosus.

If the right ventricle is of adequate size to support the pulmonary circulation once the pulmonary valvotomy is performed, the infant will be followed as would be any patient with pulmonary valve stenosis. He should be assessed for signs of development of recurrent pulmonary stenosis, and a repeat valvotomy may be required.

If the right ventricle is too small to support the pulmonary circulation, the long-term surgical intervention planned for the infant may be similar to that planned for the infant with tricuspid atresia. This includes performance of a palliative Glenn procedure and/or correction with oversewing of the tricuspid valve and performance of a Fontan procedure (see the discussion of tricuspid atresia that follows).

■ TRICUSPID ATRESIA/HYPOPLASTIC RIGHT HEART
■ Etiology

Tricuspid atresia results from a complete lack of formation of the tricuspid valve during fetal cardiac development. There is no blood flow between the right atrium and right ventricle. When tricuspid atresia is present, it is generally associated with a hypoplastic (very small) right ventricle and some form of interatrial communication. Usually, a ventricular septal defect is also present (Fig. 3-36).[386]

Tricuspid atresia may be associated with normally related great vessels (this is referred to as type I tricuspid atresia) or with transposition of the great vessels (this is referred to as type II tricuspid atresia). Subcategories of tricuspid atresia have been named according to the presence or absence of associated pulmonary stenosis or atresia.[88,336]

Tricuspid atresia is responsible for approximately 2% of all congenital heart defects.[134]

■ Pathophysiology

Since there is no flow between the right atrium and right ventricle, the only way for blood to leave the right atrium is through an interatrial communication. This often consists of a patent foramen

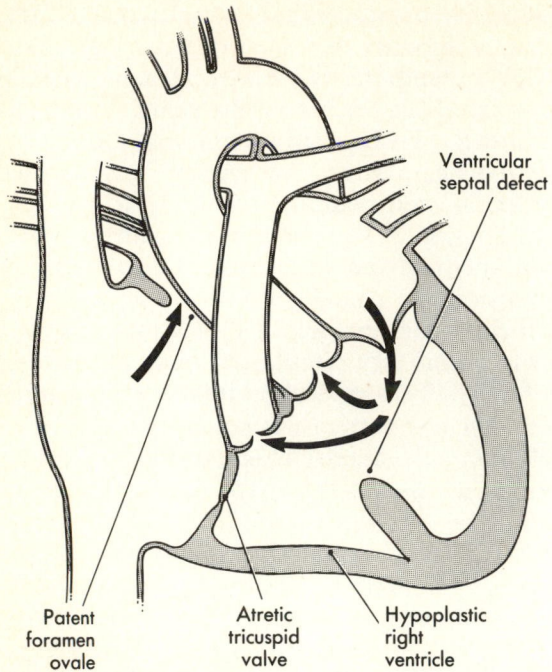

Fig. 3-36 Tricuspid atresia with ventricular septal defect. The tricuspid valve is absent, so there is no anatomic communication between the right atrium and the right ventricle. Systemic venous blood passes through a patent foramen ovale or an atrial septal defect to the left atrium, where it mixes with pulmonary venous blood. If a ventricular septal defect is present (as shown), some of this mixed venous blood will enter the aorta and some will flow through the ventricular septal defect and enter the pulmonary artery. Pulmonary infundibular stenosis and right ventricular hypoplasia may also be present. This illustration depicts normally-related great vessels; transposition of the great vessels may also be present with tricuspid atresia.

From Hazinski, M.: The cardiovascular system, In Howe, J., and others, editors: The handbook of nursing, New York, 1984, John Wiley & Sons, Inc.

ovale.[45] If the interatrial communication is restrictive (too small), right atrial hypertension and signs of systemic venous engorgement will develop.

Systemic venous blood enters the right atrium and passes through the interatrial communication to the left atrium. Thus systemic and pulmonary venous blood mixes in the left atrium and the left ventricle, and arterial oxygen desaturation is present. If a ventricular septal defect is present, the left ventricle ejects blood into both the pulmonary artery and aorta whether or not transposition or malposition of the great vessels is present.

If pulmonary stenosis is present, pulmonary blood flow is decreased, and cyanosis is present and significant. If pulmonary atresia is present, the neo-

nate usually has profound cyanosis, particularly once the ductus arteriosus begins to close since the ductus usually provides the only route of pulmonary blood flow (see the section on hypoxemia for a discussion of systemic consequences of polycythemia).

Over half of all infants with tricuspid atresia have a ventricular septal defect, normally related great vessels, and pulmonary stenosis with decreased pulmonary blood flow.[88] As a result these infants would be expected to develop significant cyanosis but no heart failure.[279] They are at risk for the development of systemic consequences of chronic hypoxemia and resultant polycythemia (see the section on hypoxemia).

If transposition of the great vessels is present with no associated pulmonary stenosis or if the great vessels are normally related with no pulmonary stenosis and with a large ventricular septal defect, pulmonary blood flow will be increased once pulmonary vascular resistance falls at approximately 4 to 12 weeks of age. This pulmonary blood flow will be under high pressure and usually produces symptoms of congestive heart failure. When pulmonary blood flow is increased, there is proportionately more (oxygenated) pulmonary venous blood returning to the left atrium to mix with the (desaturated) systemic venous blood; as a result the infant's cyanosis may decrease as pulmonary blood flow increases. As these infants grow, the ventricular septal defect may become smaller, or the infant may develop pulmonary infundibular stenosis; in either case, pulmonary blood flow is then *reduced*, and the infant will then become more cyanotic. As a result these infants must be followed closely, even if significant cyanosis is not present initially.

Because the incidence of bacterial endocarditis is significant in these children before and after palliative surgery, it is extremely important that antibiotic prophylaxis be administered during periods of increased risk of bacteremia (see Table 3-13).[88] The risk of pulmonary vascular disease is also significant in those patients with tricuspid atresia and with increased pulmonary blood flow who survive infancy.[88]

■ **Clinical signs and symptoms**

Over half of all infants with tricuspid atresia are diagnosed in the first day of life because of the presence of either cyanosis or a heart murmur. Nearly all infants with tricuspid atresia are diagnosed during the first 2 months of life.[88]

If the ventricular septal defect is small with normally related great vessels or if pulmonary stenosis or atresia is present, the neonate will have severe cyanosis at birth. The cyanosis usually becomes profound when the ductus arteriosus begins to close. The infant will develop polycythemia, and clubbing will be observed in infants beyond approximately 4 months of age. These infants may also develop hypercyanotic episodes (paroxysmal hypoxic spells). These episodes may be precipitated by exertion, vigorous cry, feeding, or defecation. The infant who has such a spell can become profoundly cyanotic, irritable, and diaphoretic, and may then lose consciousness (see the section on hypoxemia).

As noted earlier, if a large ventricular septal defect is present, with or without transposition of the great vessels, and if there is no associated pulmonary stenosis, the newborn with tricuspid atresia may demonstrate mild or moderate cyanosis that increases with cry or exertion. Once pulmonary vascular resistance falls at approximately 4 to 12 weeks of age, signs of congestive heart failure develop (see the section on congestive heart failure). At this time, the infant's cyanosis may decrease.

Infants with tricuspid atresia and a patent pulmonary valve may demonstrate a systolic pulmonary murmur at the second intercostal space along the left sternal border. The second heart sound is single (since pulmonary valve closure is decreased in intensity).[123] The precordium is usually quiet, although a left ventricular heave may be palpated. The ECG most often demonstrates left axis deviation and left ventricular, left atrial, and right atrial hypertrophy. The precordial leads show reduced right ventricular forces. The P-R interval is short in approximately half of the patients with tricuspid atresia.[279] The echocardiogram should confirm the presence of tricuspid atresia because the tricuspid valve will not be seen; in addition, the right ventricle is diminutive and the aorta is large.

Right atrial and left ventricular hypertrophy may produce an increased cardiothoracic ratio on the chest radiograph. If a large ventricular septal defect is present without pulmonary stenosis, pulmonary vascular markings will be increased once pulmonary vascular resistance falls. If pulmonary stenosis or atresia is present, pulmonary vascular markings will be decreased.

Cardiac catheterization reveals increased right atrial pressure. The catheter will only pass through an interatrial communication to the left atrium, and left atrial desaturation will confirm the presence of the right-to-left atrial shunt. It may be possible to pass the catheter into the left ventricle, through the ventricular septal defect (if present), and into the small right ventricle. Aortic catheterization will document the presence of arterial oxygen desaturation. Angiocardiograms will confirm the presence of tricuspid

atresia, and they will also help to determine the presence of a ventricular septal defect, the position of the great vessels, and the presence, location, and severity of any pulmonary stenosis.

■ **Medical and surgical treatment and nursing interventions**

Over half of all infants with tricuspid atresia have cyanosis in the first days of life. The cyanosis often progresses as a result of closure of the ductus arteriosus, reduction of the size of the ventricular septal defect, or progression of the pulmonary stenosis. The natural history of the infant with tricuspid atresia is poor. Survival beyond 3 months of age is rare if pulmonary atresia is present. Approximately half of the untreated infants with the defect expire during the first 6 months of life, two thirds by the first year, and 90% by 10 years of age.[58,336] The best natural survival is in infants with associated transposition of the great vessels, an unrestrictive ventricular septal defect, and pulmonary stenosis. Palliative and corrective surgery improves the chance of long-term survival for these infants.[88]

If the neonate with tricuspid atresia develops significant cyanosis in the first days of life, echocardiography and cardiac catheterization are required on an urgent basis. When significant cyanosis is present at this age, the neonate is probably dependent upon the ductus arteriosus to provide a large portion of pulmonary blood flow. Therefore an infusion of prostaglandin E_1 will be administered to maintain ductal patency during the diagnostic studies and possibly until surgery can be performed (see the section on hypoxemia).

During cardiac catheterization, if a large pressure gradient is found between the right and left atria and if systemic venous pressures are high, the interatrial communication is probably restrictive. A Rashkind balloon atrial septostomy will usually then be performed (see the discussion on the medical and surgical treatment and nursing interventions for pulmonary atresia for a description of this procedure.) If angiocardiography confirms that pulmonary blood flow is dependent upon the ductus arteriosus, the prostaglandin E_1 infusion will be continued and the infant will be referred for palliative or corrective surgery.

Throughout the diagnostic and perioperative therapy, it is imperative that *no air be allowed to enter any IV line* since it can enter the systemic arterial circulation, producing an air embolus. The infant should be kept well hydrated to avoid hemoconcentration, although aggressive fluid administration should be avoided since it may cause congestive heart failure. If the infant develops hypercyanotic episodes, he should be placed in the knee-chest position and oxygen should be administered. Since administration of morphine sulfate or propranolol may be required to treat the spell, these medications should be drawn up and kept at the bedside of any infant known to have a history of such spells (see the section on hypoxemia).

The surgical procedure used for the infant with tricuspid atresia and *decreased* pulmonary blood flow will depend on the size of the infant's main pulmonary artery and right and left pulmonary artery branches.[237] If one main pulmonary artery branch is small, a subclavian-to-pulmonary artery shunt (a Blalock-Taussig or modified prosthetic shunt) may be performed to increase flow to that pulmonary artery branch, to stimulate its growth. If the main pulmonary artery is small, a central prosthetic graft may be inserted between the aorta and the main pulmonary artery. These shunt procedures are discussed in greater detail in Table 3-17 and in the section on medical and surgical treatment of tetralogy of Fallot. Reparative surgery will be discussed later. Once the infant is at least 1 year of age, a Glenn shunt may be performed.

If the infant with tricuspid atresia develops congestive heart failure caused by the presence of *increased* pulmonary blood flow under high pressure as the result of a large ventricular septal defect and absence of pulmonary stenosis (with or without transposition of the great vessels), aggressive medical management with diuretics and digoxin is indicated (see the section on congestive heart failure). It is important that the infant not be diuresed too aggressively since hemoconcentration will increase the infant's risk of thromboembolic events, including cerebrovascular accident. Pulmonary artery banding may be performed if congestive heart failure is refractory to medical management or if pulmonary vascular resistance is increasing.[336]

"Corrective" surgery for tricuspid atresia may be accomplished in one or two stages. When Fontan originally described the reparative procedure that carries his name, he used a two-stage correction procedure.[129] Ultimately, as the result of corrective surgery, systemic venous blood will flow directly into the pulmonary circulation or will pass through the right atrium into the pulmonary circulation. If the patient's pulmonary vascular resistance is high, these procedures cannot be performed. In addition, the size of the distal pulmonary arteries must be good, and left ventricular function must be adequate.[336] A previous requirement for the Fontan procedure had been the

presence of a normal sinus rhythm, although recent research has indicated that pulmonary artery perfusion from the right atrium can be adequate even if atrial systole does not occur.[388]

As the first stage of the correction, a Glenn anastomosis is created through a thoracotomy incision without use of cardiopulmonary bypass. In this procedure, the superior vena cava is separated from the right atrium, and the proximal end of the superior vena cava is sewn to the patient's right pulmonary artery. (NOTE: if a left dominant superior vena cava is present, the procedure is performed on the left side.) The right pulmonary artery may be separated from the main pulmonary artery, so it only receives systemic venous blood flow from the superior vena cava through the Glenn shunt. This procedure allows the venous return from the head and upper extremities (approximately 40% of systemic venous return) to flow directly into the right pulmonary circulation (see Fig. 3-33). As a result only venous return from the inferior vena cava will enter the right atrium and flow to the left atrium to mix with (oxygenated) pulmonary venous return. Therefore the infant or child will be less cyanotic following creation of the Glenn anastomosis because the blood ejected by the left ventricle will contain a relatively greater proportion of oxygenated pulmonary venous blood. In addition, the Glenn anastomosis may increase the volume of pulmonary blood flow, and therefore will increase pulmonary venous return to the left heart. Potential early postoperative complications following creation of the Glenn anastomosis include bleeding, chylothorax, pleural effusion, superior vena caval obstruction, and neurologic complications. During the immediate postoperative period, the head of the child's bed should remain elevated approximately 30 degrees; this enhances flow of blood from the superior vena cava into the right pulmonary artery. The child's face often is puffy and looks plethoric for several days after surgery; it is important that the parents be informed about the puffiness in advance. Usually, within several days after surgery, the puffiness recedes, and the child's color returns to normal. A late complication of the Glenn anastomosis is the formation of ipsilateral pulmonary arteriovenous fistulae. These may result in an increase in arterial desaturation (hypoxemia).

The Fontan procedure is the final "corrective" procedure for tricuspid atresia; it requires a median sternotomy incision and use of cardiopulmonary bypass. Hypothermia may also be used. In most patients with tricuspid atresia, the right ventricle is small, so it is bypassed completely. The existing atrial septal defect is closed, and the pulmonary valve may be sewn closed (if severe pulmonary stenosis is present, the valve is not closed because the proximal pulmonary artery flow will not be hemodynamically significant). If a Glenn anastomosis is in place, the right atrium is connected to the *left* pulmonary artery through use of a valved conduit, a valveless conduit, or a portion of the right atrial appendage. If no Glenn anastomosis is in place, the right atrium is connected to the *main* pulmonary artery through use of a valved or valveless conduit, or a portion of the right atrium. Any existing pulmonary artery band, systemic artery-to-pulmonary artery shunt, or ventricular septal defect will also be eliminated at this time. If transposition of the great vessels is present, the ventricular septal defect is *not* closed, and pulmonary venous blood from the left ventricle will continue to flow through the ventricular septal defect into the aorta.

If the right ventricle and pulmonary outflow tract are of adequate size, the Fontan procedure can be modified so that the right atrium is connected to the right ventricle. The ventricular septal defect will be closed with a patch, and the right ventricular outflow tract may be enlarged with a patch.[53,239] In a further modification of these procedures, the right atrium, right ventricle, and pulmonary artery may be joined by a T-shaped conduit so that systemic venous blood from the right atrium can flow into the right ventricle or into the pulmonary artery. It is thought that these modified procedures may encourage growth of the right ventricle. However, since the right ventricle is usually rudimentary, such attempts are possible in only a very few patients. The remainder of the discussion that follows focuses on short- and long-term hemodynamic results and on complications of the more standard Fontan procedure with or without a Glenn anastomosis.

If the Glenn anastomosis is present following the Fontan procedure, systemic venous blood from the head and upper extremities will flow from the superior vena cava directly into the right pulmonary artery (bypassing the heart completely). Systemic venous return from the trunk and lower extremities will return through the inferior vena cava to the right atrium. This blood will be diverted into the left pulmonary artery. Thus the right pulmonary artery receives the venous blood from the head and upper extremities, and the left pulmonary artery receives the venous blood from the trunk and lower extremities. Pulmonary venous blood returns to the left atrium; it flows into the left ventricle and is ejected into the aorta.

If the Glenn anastomosis is not in place following conclusion of the Fontan procedure, all of the systemic venous blood enters the right atrium from both the superior and inferior vena cavae. This blood is diverted to the main pulmonary artery. Pulmonary venous blood return enters the left atrium, flows to the left ventricle, and is ejected into the aorta.

Perioperative mortality associated with the Fontan procedure ranges from zero to 20%.[31,83,234,336] During the immediate postoperative period, patients often demonstrate pronounced signs of systemic venous engorgement, including high central venous pressure, hepatomegaly, pleural effusion, chylothorax, and ascites. Other signs of congestive heart failure or low cardiac output may also be present. There is now some evidence that postoperative mortality and incidence of systemic venous engorgement may be reduced if a Glenn anastomosis is performed as the first stage of the Fontan procedure.[83,327] Bleeding may also occur postoperatively, and it is more likely to occur if the child had a preoperative coagulopathy secondary to polycythemia (see the section on hypoxemia) or if prosthetic polytetrafluoroethylene is used in the repair since this material may produce platelet aggregation along its surface, particularly when it is inserted in low flow areas.[353] Arrhythmias, renal failure, and neurologic complications have also been reported postoperatively.[83,234] Cardiovascular function following the Fontan procedure is most satisfactory for patients with "simple" tricuspid atresia and least satisfactory for patients with complex cyanotic heart disease.

One late complication of the Fontan procedure is conduit obstruction; this may cause sudden death, particularly if a Glenn anastomosis is not in place.[1,34,83] Complete AV block has also been reported and may require pacemaker insertion. Signs of systemic venous engorgement usually subside gradually postoperatively. Many patients are able to resume normal daily activities without difficulty,[83] although others demonstrate persistent signs of cardiovascular dysfunction. If the atrial septal defect patch loosens, intraatrial mixing and cyanosis can result; this usually requires reoperation.[83] If a conduit is inserted during infancy, the child may require placement of a larger conduit during later childhood.

If prosthetic material was used for the corrective surgery, the child will require strict administration of prophylactic antibiotics at times of increased risk of bacteremia to prevent endocarditis (see Table 3-13).

■ **TRANSPOSITION OF THE GREAT VESSELS (TGV)**
■ **Etiology**

Transposition of the great vessels occurs as a result of inappropriate septation and migration of the truncus arteriosus during fetal cardiac development.

When isolated transposition of the great vessels is present, the aorta arises from the anatomic right ventricle and the pulmonary artery arises from the anatomic left ventricle. When dextro-transposition (D-transposition) is present, the aorta lies anterior and to the right of the pulmonary artery (Fig. 3-37). As a result systemic venous blood enters the right atrium, the right ventricle, and is then returned to the systemic circulation through the aorta. Pulmonary venous blood from the lungs enters the left atrium, the left ventricle, and is returned to the lungs via the pulmonary artery. If there is no additional cardiovascular defect to allow mixing of oxygenated and unoxygenated blood, the infant with transposition will die. A patent ductus arteriosus and some form of

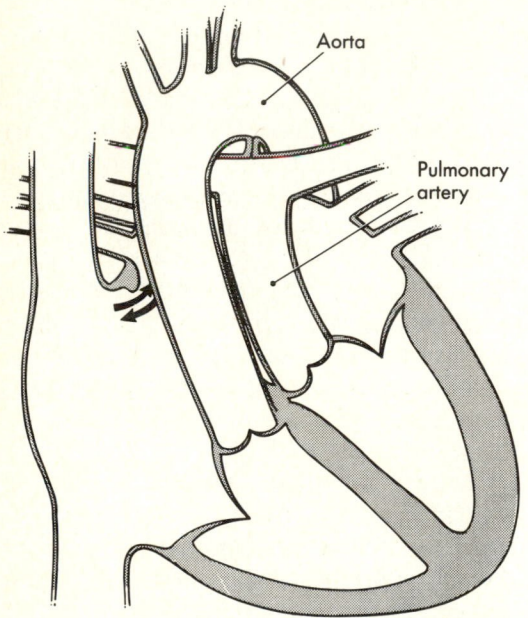

Fig. 3-37 Transposition of the great vessels with an atrial septal defect. The aorta arises from the right ventricle, and the pulmonary artery arises from the left ventricle. As a result systemic venous blood returns to the systemic arterial circulation, and pulmonary venous blood returns to the pulmonary arterial circulation; if there is not an additional defect present to allow mixing of the systemic and pulmonary venous blood, survival is impossible. In this case, an atrial septal defect is present to allow that mixing. This atrial septal defect can occur naturally, can be the result of a Rashkind balloon atrial septostomy performed during cardiac catheterization, or can be the result of an atrial septectomy performed surgically.

From Hazinski, M.: The cardiovascular system, In Howe, J., and others, editors: The handbook of nursing, New York, 1984, John Wiley & Sons, Inc.

interatrial communication are usually present; a ventricular septal defect with or without pulmonary stenosis may also be present.

Transposition of the great vessels is responsible for approximately 9% of all congenital heart defects.[134,279]

■ Pathophysiology

The newborn with transposition of the great vessels usually demonstrates signs of arterial oxygen desaturation at birth. The degree of desaturation present will depend primarily on the amount of mixing between systemic and pulmonary venous blood. If there is no mixing, the aorta receives only desaturated systemic venous blood from the right ventricle; the more mixing between the systemic and pulmonary venous blood that occurs in the heart or great vessels, the more saturated will be the systemic arterial blood.

The degree of arterial oxygen desaturation will also be determined by the amount of *effective* pulmonary blood flow. This refers to the amount of systemic venous blood that enters the pulmonary circulation. It is not helpful if only oxygenated pulmonary venous blood returns to the pulmonary circulation; some systemic venous blood should also enter the pulmonary circulation.

If the neonate has no ventricular septal defect, he will be dependent on the mixing of blood allowed by an interatrial communication and by a patent ductus arteriosus. The most common form of interatrial communication in infants with transposition of the great vessels is a patent foramen ovale.[336] Since a competent foramen ovale is a flapped orifice, it will allow shunting of blood from the right atrium to the left atrium when right atrial pressure is higher than left atrial pressure. If the foramen is incompetent, however, it can allow bidirectional shunting of blood at the atrial level.

The ductus arteriosus also usually remains patent for several days in neonates with transposition of the great vessels because their arterial oxygen tension usually does not increase sufficiently to stimulate ductal constriction. Before pulmonary vascular resistance falls, there may be bidirectional shunting of blood between the pulmonary artery and aorta through the ductus arteriosus.

If adequate mixing of blood is present at the atrial level and through the ductus arteriosus, the neonate may demonstrate an arterial oxygen tension of approximately 30 to 35 mm Hg.[359] If the foramen ovale is competent, however, bidirectional atrial shunting cannot occur. If the ductus arteriosus begins to constrict, the neonate usually develops profound cyanosis, hypoxemia, and acidosis.

If a ventricular septal defect is present, bidirectional shunting of blood will occur at the ventricular level while pulmonary vascular resistance is high. This will produce some mixing of systemic and pulmonary venous blood, and it may improve the neonate's systemic arterial oxygen saturation.[279] Once pulmonary vascular resistance falls, blood will shunt from the right ventricle into the left ventricle and pulmonary artery because the pulmonary circulation will offer less resistance to flow than the systemic circulation. If the ventricular septal defect is large, the high pulmonary blood flow will be under high pressure, and signs of congestive heart failure will result (see the section on congestive heart failure). This shunt at the ventricular level will result in increased pulmonary venous return to the left atrium. If the foramen ovale is incompetent, a greater anatomical left-to-right shunt will occur at the atrial level; this will enhance mixing of systemic and pulmonary venous blood, and it will ultimately increase right ventricular and aortic oxygen saturation. As a result, although the ventricular septal defect may produce congestive heart failure, it may also result in improvement of the infant's arterial oxygen saturation.

If the infant has transposition of the great vessels with a large ventricular septal defect and mild or moderate pulmonary stenosis, a somewhat balanced, bidirectional shunt is present at the ventricular level. The pulmonary stenosis enhances shunting of some pulmonary venous blood from the left ventricle to the right ventricle and aorta. The pulmonary stenosis also prevents excessive, high-pressure pulmonary blood flow, so congestive heart failure does not develop. Systemic venous blood may also shunt into the left heart through a patent foramen ovale or through the ventricular septal defect. As a result these infants have adequate mixing of systemic and pulmonary venous blood, and they demonstrate a higher systemic arterial oxygen saturation than infants with isolated transposition of the great vessels.

If the infant has transposition with a ventricular septal defect and severe subvalvular pulmonary stenosis, the total amount of pulmonary blood flow is reduced. Although the pulmonary stenosis does enhance the shunting of oxygenated blood from the left ventricle into the right ventricle or aorta, the quantity of pulmonary venous return is so small that left-to-right shunting of blood will not greatly improve the infant's arterial oxygen saturation. These infants usually develop profound hypoxemia and acidosis once the ductus arteriosus begins to close since it provides a major source of pulmonary blood flow.

When arterial oxygen saturation is chronically low, polycythemia develops. However, if arterial oxygen saturation is extremely low, tissue hypoxia develops and anaerobic metabolism takes place, producing lactic metabolic acidosis; this is a sign of profound deterioration in the infant with transposition of the great vessels, and it indicates the need for urgent treatment. These infants are also at risk for the development of other systemic consequences of polycythemia, particularly the risk of spontaneous cerebrovascular accident, especially during the period between cardiac catheterization and surgery.[169]

Infants with transposition of the great vessels also have a high risk of development of pulmonary vascular disease within the first years of life. Pulmonary vascular disease can develop in infants less than 1 year of age, with or without a ventricular septal defect.[67,105,305] This pulmonary vascular disease apparently can result from high pulmonary blood flow under high pressure (such as that produced by a large ventricular septal defect or patent ductus arteriosus), but it also seems to occur as the result of development of microthrombi within the pulmonary arterioles.[305] This pulmonary vascular disease may develop or progress even after surgical repair has been performed.[67]

Infants with transposition of the great vessels are at risk for the development of bacterial endocarditis during episodes of bacteremia. As a result they should receive antibiotic prophylaxis whenever they have increased risk of bacteremia (see Table 3-13).

■ **Clinical signs and symptoms**

The infant with transposition of the great vessels is usually cyanotic during the neonatal period. If there is no ventricular septal defect and if there is inadequate mixing of systemic and pulmonary venous blood at the atrial level, the neonate usually demonstrates severe cyanosis at birth. Often the ductus arteriosus provides the main route for mixing of blood, so the neonate's cyanosis becomes profound when the ductus arteriosus begins to constrict, and acidosis can develop quickly.

If a ventricular septal defect is present and if adequate mixing of blood is occurring at the ventricular (and/or atrial) level, the infant may demonstrate only mild or moderate cyanosis that increases with cry or exertion. The infant with transposition of the great vessels and a large ventricular septal defect usually develops signs of congestive heart failure at approximately 3 weeks of age, when pulmonary vascular resistance begins to fall[279] (see the section on congestive heart failure).

If the infant has a ventricular septal defect and if mild or moderate pulmonary stenosis is present, cyanosis may be minimal, although it usually increases with cry or exertion. Congestive heart failure does not often develop in these infants.

If the infant has a ventricular septal defect and severe pulmonary stenosis, cyanosis is severe, particularly once the ductus arteriosus begins to close.

Peripheral pulses are not unusual, and the infant's precordium is usually quiet. Approximately half of infants with transposition of the great vessels have no heart murmur; a systolic murmur of unknown origin may be present in some of the remaining neonates.[279] If a ventricular septal defect is present, a holosystolic murmur may be heard along the left sternal border.[123] If pulmonary stenosis is present, a systolic ejection murmur may be noted along the left or right upper sternal border. The second heart sound is usually single and seems to be the result of the sound of aortic valve closure (since the aorta is anterior in the chest, this is the great vessel nearest the chest wall).

Right ventricular hypertrophy may produce a sternal lift. The ECG may not be helpful during the neonatal period since it usually indicates right ventricular hypertrophy, which is normal during the first days of life. Persistent signs of right ventricular hypertrophy, including upright T waves in V_1 and V_{4R} beyond the first days of life indicate right ventricular hypertension.[336] If a large ventricular septal defect (with or without pulmonary stenosis) is present, clinical and electrocardiographic evidence of biventricular hypertrophy will be noted.

The two-dimensional echocardiogram should confirm the diagnosis of transposition because the pulmonary artery is seen rising from the left ventricle and the aorta is rising from the right ventricle. M-mode echocardiography will also document reversal of normal ventricular systolic ejection times.[336]

Unless a ventricular septal defect is present, the heart size usually appears normal on the chest radiograph, although right atrial and ventricular hypertrophy may be apparent beyond the first days of life. Because the aorta lies in front of the pulmonary artery, the mediastinum often appears to be very narrow, and the cardiac silhouette is said to resemble the appearance of an "egg-on-side."[336] If a large ventricular septal defect is present, generalized cardiomegaly and increased pulmonary vascular markings are usually apparent once pulmonary vascular resistance falls and pulmonary blood flow increases. If severe pulmonary stenosis is present, pulmonary vascular markings will be decreased.

Cardiac catheterization confirms the presence of transposition. The catheter passes from the anterior (right) ventricle into a great vessel with a pressure tracing of the aorta. If the catheter is passed through a patent foramen ovale into the left atrium and posterior (left) ventricle, it will then enter the pulmonary artery. If the catheter is passed retrograde through the aorta, it will enter the anterior (right) ventricle. All of these maneuvers confirm the abnormal relationship between the great vessels and the ventricles before angiocardiography is performed. Arterial oxygen saturation in the aorta will be reduced, and saturation measurements made in the right atrium and ventricle will reveal the presence of any additional intracardiac shunts. Angiocardiography will confirm the presence of transposition and will also demonstrate the presence of additional shunts.

■ Medical and surgical management and nursing interventions

If the neonate demonstrates severe cyanosis during the first days of life, transposition of the great vessels should be suspected. If severe hypoxemia is present, an IV infusion of prostaglandin E_1 is begun, an echocardiogram is obtained on an urgent basis, and plans are made for cardiac catheterization. Throughout the diagnostic testing and hospitalization, it is important that *no air be allowed to enter any IV line* since it may enter the systemic arterial circulation, producing a cerebral air embolus.

The prostaglandin E_1 infusion not only promotes patency of the ductus arteriosus, it also lowers pulmonary and systemic vascular resistance. As a result effective pulmonary blood flow is increased, and the neonate's arterial oxygen saturation usually rises by 25% to 100%. If the neonate has transposition of the great vessels with a ventricular septal defect and no pulmonary stenosis, however, this increased pulmonary blood flow can also produce congestive heart failure.

The diagnosis of transposition of the great vessels should be made using echocardiography. Cardiac catheterization will help determine the presence of other additional cardiac defects, quantify the amount of pulmonary blood flow, measure the arterial oxygen saturation, and enable the performance of a Rashkind balloon septostomy (see the section on medical and surgical treatment of pulmonary atresia). In neonates with transposition of the great vessels, the Rashkind balloon septostomy usually produces a significant increase in the infant's arterial oxygen saturation.[431] Usually, the oxygen saturation rises sharply to above 50% to 60% immediately after the septostomy; it then stabilizes somewhere below 50%.[431] It is extremely important that the infant be watched closely during and immediately following the Rashkind septostomy since arrhythmias, tamponade, and cerebrovascular accident have been reported following this procedure.[279,431] The small amount of blood lost during cardiac catheterization, the manipulation of the septostomy, and the natural fall in arterial oxygen saturation several hours after catheterization may also contribute to a deterioration in the infant's clinical status. For this reason, the prostaglandin E$_1$ infusion begun before catheterization is usually continued for several days after catheterization. The nurse should monitor for evidence of deepening cyanosis, worsening tachypnea, increased respiratory effort, irritability, or lethargy, and these should be reported to a physician immediately. Development of severe hypoxemia (PaO$_2$ less than 30 torr), especially if accompanied by acidosis, should also be reported to a physician immediately. Any blood lost at catheterization or drawn for laboratory studies should be replaced to avoid anemia. If the infant's clinical status deteriorates despite maintenance of a neutral thermal environment, adequate hematocrit and circulating blood volume, and prostaglandin E$_1$ infusion, surgical intervention will be necessary. It is important to note that up to 14% of infants with transposition of the great vessels can die or suffer a cerebrovascular accident between cardiac catheterization and surgery.[169]

If the neonate demonstrates an adequate and sustained increase in arterial oxygen saturation following the Rashkind balloon septostomy, the prostaglandin E$_1$ infusion is usually tapered after several days. During the tapering, the nurse should watch the infant closely for signs of deepening cyanosis, tachypnea, increased respiratory effort, increased irritability or lethargy, or signs of poor systemic perfusion since these can indicate the presence of severe hypoxemia and acidosis. If the infant tolerates the weaning from the prostaglandins, he may be sent home for close observation and return in a few months for elective surgery. The parents should be taught to contact the pediatrician immediately if the infant develops increased cyanosis or respiratory distress or if he feeds poorly. They should also notify the physician if the infant develops a fever, vomiting, or diarrhea since these can produce dehydration and rapid hemoconcentration in these infants. The infant should receive antibiotic prophylaxis during periods of increased risk of bacteremia (see Table 3-13). In addition, supplemental iron is often administered to prevent anemia since the development of microcytic anemia increases the infant's risk of thromboembolic phenomena.[249]

Infants with transposition of the great vessels can demonstrate hypercyanotic episodes during exertion, vigorous cry, feeding, or stooling. These episodes seem to be the result of an increased oxygen demand that the cardiovascular system cannot meet. If the infant has a ventricular septal defect and pulmonary subvalvular stenosis, hypercyanotic episodes can result from a mechanism similar to those producing spells in infants with tetralogy of Fallot.[359] If pulmonary stenosis is present, placement of the infant in the knee-chest position and administration of morphine sulfate or propranolol may help relieve the hypercyanotic episodes (see the section on hypoxemia). Once the infant develops spells, however, surgical intervention is indicated.

If the infant has transposition of the great vessels and a ventricular septal defect without pulmonary stenosis, the infant will be watched closely for the development of congestive heart failure once pulmonary vascular resistance falls. Treatment of heart failure with digoxin and diuretics will be necessary (see the section on congestive heart failure), although vigorous diuresis should be avoided since it may produce hemoconcentration and increase the infant's risk of thromboembolic phenomenon (see the section on hypoxemia).

If the infant demonstrates progressive hypoxemia, acidosis, poor feeding, severe congestive heart failure, or hypercyanotic episodes, surgical intervention is necessary. Palliative procedures performed include the Blalock-Hanlon atrial septectomy (removal of a portion of the atrial septum), pulmonary artery banding, or creation of a systemic-to-pulmonary artery shunt. The selection of palliative surgery will depend on the infant's specific cardiac anatomy, the corrective surgery ultimately planned, and the preference of the surgeon. Reparative surgery may also be performed during infancy. This will be discussed following description of the palliative procedures.

The Blalock-Hanlon septectomy is a less frequently performed palliative procedure; it requires an anterolateral thoracotomy incision and *does not* use cardiopulmonary bypass. The pericardium is entered, and a large clamp is placed on the back of the heart, at the junction of the right and left atrium. The remainder of the procedure is accomplished within the clamp; an atrial incision is made, the atrial septum is withdrawn and excised, and the atrial incision is closed. The clamp is then removed and the thoracotomy incision is closed. Following the atrial septectomy, the infant's systemic and pulmonary venous blood should mix better at the atrial level, producing an improved arterial oxygen saturation.[32]

If the infant with transposition of the great vessels and a ventricular septal defect develops severe congestive heart failure, pulmonary artery banding may be performed (see the discussion of pulmonary artery banding in the section on treatment of ventricular septal defect). The banding will reduce the volume and pressure of pulmonary blood flow; this should ease the symptoms of congestive heart failure and reduce the risk of pulmonary vascular disease in these infants. Since the pulmonary artery banding may produce deformity of the main pulmonary artery, patch enlargement of the main pulmonary artery may be required at the time of later correction of the transposition.

If the infant with transposition of the great vessels demonstrates severe cyanosis as the result of severe pulmonary stenosis, a palliative systemic-to-pulmonary artery shunt may be performed to increase pulmonary blood flow (see Table 3-17). The most popular shunts use the infant's subclavian artery or a prosthetic graft between the subclavian artery and a pulmonary artery (see Fig. 3-33).

Surgical correction of uncomplicated transposition of the great vessels is usually performed during infancy if the infant demonstrates persistent, severe hypoxemia or other symptoms. However, if the infant is relatively asymptomatic, elective repair is usually performed between 6 months and 36 months of age. All corrective forms of surgery use a median sternotomy incision and cardiopulmonary bypass. Hypothermia is usually also used when surgery is performed during infancy.

The most popular procedures for repair of uncomplicated transposition of the great arteries use an intraatrial baffle or portions of the atrial septum to redirect pulmonary and systemic venous blood flow. The Mustard procedure requires complete excision of any remaining atrial septum so that a large, single atrium is temporarily present. A piece of pericardium or of woven prosthetic material (Dacron or Gor-tex) is sewn within the atria as a baffle so that it deflects inferior and superior vena caval (systemic venous) blood to the mitral valve; this venous blood will then flow into the left ventricle and will be ejected into the pulmonary artery. The pulmonary venous blood is deflected by the baffle to the tricuspid valve; this oxygenated pulmonary venous blood then flows into the right ventricle and is ejected into the aorta (Fig. 3-38). The atriotomy cardiac incision is often closed with a patch so that there is more room within the atria.

If the infant also has a simple ventricular septal defect, it is closed with a patch at the beginning of the Mustard procedure, before the intraatrial baffle is placed. The ventricular septal defect is generally closed by manipulation through the tricuspid valve so that an incision is not made in the right ventricle

(since the right ventricle must continue to function as the systemic ventricle postoperatively). Early mortality following the Mustard procedure ranges from zero to 10%.[21,107,138,419,421] Postoperative complications include congestive heart failure, low cardiac output, arrhythmias (including supraventricular arrhythmias and heart block), neurologic complications, and bleeding.

The Senning procedure is another open-heart procedure used to correct transposition of the great vessels. It also results in diversion of systemic and pulmonary venous blood in a manner similar to that accomplished by the Mustard procedure. However, the Senning procedure uses portions of the atrial septal tissue and lateral atrial wall to create the intracardiac baffle. As a result, if the surgeon is planning to perform the Senning procedure to repair transposition, the Blalock-Hanlon septectomy will *not* be performed as a palliative procedure before repair. Perioperative mortality and immediate postoperative complications following the Senning procedure are approximately the same as those following the Mustard procedure.[35]

Both the Mustard and the Senning procedures are associated with some significant late complications. The baffle can obstruct flow from the superior vena cava into the heart; as a result the child can develop a form of superior vena caval syndrome, including edema of the face and head, hydrocephalus, pleural effusion, and chylothorax.[77,393] If the baffle obstructs the flow of blood from the inferior vena cava to the heart, hepatomegaly and ascites can develop. Signs of inferior vena caval obstruction will be difficult to distinguish from signs of congestive heart failure. If the baffle obstructs pulmonary venous return to the heart, pulmonary venous hypertension and pulmonary edema can result.[147] The incidence of postoperative systemic venous obstruction is approximately 10%, and the incidence of pulmonary venous obstruction is approximately 9% following the Mustard procedure.[21,107,147] In some studies, the incidence of venous obstruction following the Senning procedure is lower than that following the Mustard procedure.[35,320]

A significant number of infants and children develop arrhythmias immediately following intraatrial repair of transposition of the great vessels. There is also a disturbing incidence of sudden death that has been reported in approximately 8% of survivors of the Mustard procedure. This sudden death is thought to be the result of an arrhythmia. In some studies, the incidence of sudden death is lower following the Senning procedure.[29,35]

Long-term ability of the right ventricle to func-

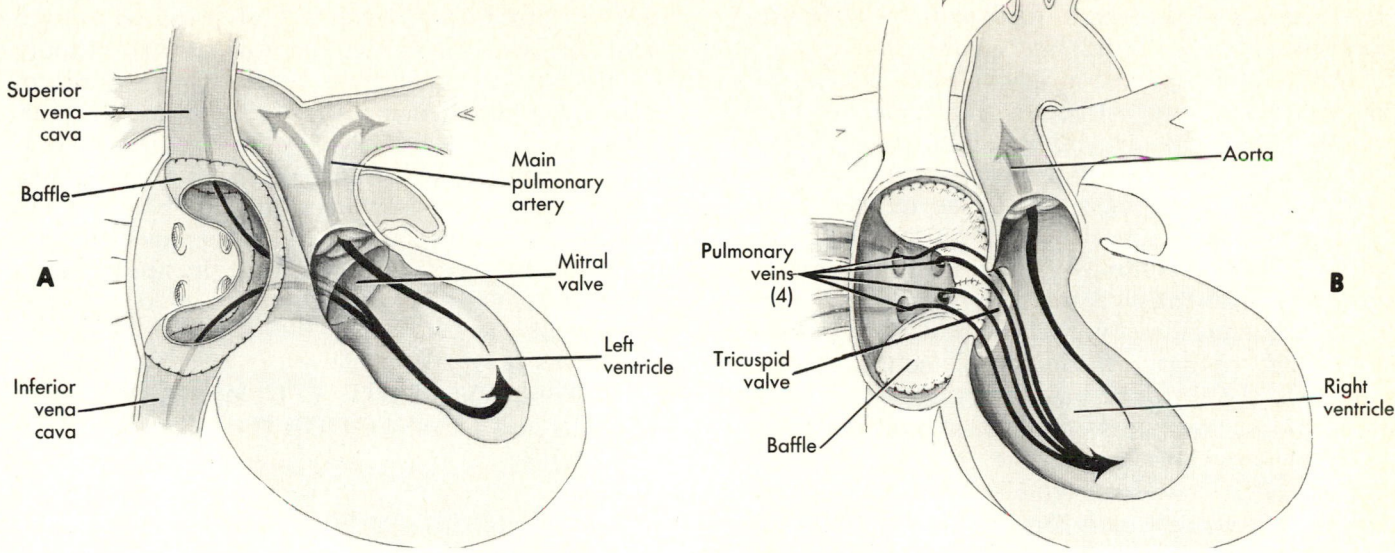

Fig. 3-38 Circulatory pathways following intraatrial repair (Mustard procedure) of transposition of the great vessels. For clarity, two illustrations are utilized to depict separately the paths of systemic and pulmonary venous return. **A,** Systemic venous return from the superior and inferior vena cava enters the heart and is immediately deflected by the baffle to the mitral valve on the left side of the heart. This systemic venous return then enters the *left* ventricle, and is ejected into the pulmonary artery, so it will enter the pulmonary circulation. **B,** Pulmonary venous return enters the heart and is deflected between portions of the baffle to the tricuspid valve on the right side of the heart. This pulmonary venous blood then enters the *right* ventricle and is ejected into the aorta and systemic circulation. As a result of this operation, systemic and pulmonary venous circulations are separated, and systemic venous return (deoxygenated blood) is diverted into the pulmonary circulation, and pulmonary venous blood (oxygenated blood) is diverted into the systemic arterial circulation.

From Paul, M.H.: Transposition of the great arteries. In Adams, F.H., and Emmanouilides, G.C.: Moss' heart disease in infants, children, and adolescents, ed. 3, Baltimore, 1983, The Williams & Wilkins Co.

tion as the systemic ventricle and of the tricuspid valve to remain competent despite right ventricular hypertension is one of the greatest concerns following intraatrial repair of transposition of the great vessels. Right ventricular function is often decreased following repair.[172] If the child develops right ventricular dysfunction or significant tricuspid valve insufficiency, pulmonary venous engorgement and respiratory distress will develop quickly.[419] Since even the earliest survivors of the Mustard and Senning procedures have not yet been followed for 25 years, adequacy of right ventricular function has not yet been sufficiently established.

Because of the potential long-term complications of the intraatrial repairs of transposition of the great vessels, interest has again been directed at anatomic or arterial correction of the transposition; this requires relocation of the great vessels to their appropriate ventricles. This procedure remains technically difficult because the coronary arteries must be removed from the aorta before the switch is accomplished; they must then be reimplanted into the aorta

at its new location. This procedure was first described by Dr. Jatene. Adaptations of this procedure, called the great vessel switch operation, anatomic correction of transposition, or arterial switch procedure, have also been developed. These procedures have recently been accomplished with acceptable operative mortality.[210,447] Since such a procedure is thought to provide a more physiologic correction of the transposition, there is hope that long-term results of the procedure will be better than those of the Mustard or Senning procedure.

If a form of the Jatene procedure is planned for the infant with uncomplicated transposition of the great vessels, the left ventricle must be capable of generating systemic pressure to pump against high systemic arterial resistance. As a result, if pulmonary stenosis is absent, this procedure must be performed during the neonatal period before pulmonary vascular resistance falls or a pulmonary artery banding must be performed during the first month of life as an initial palliative procedure.[452] If the infant has transposition of the great vessels with a ventricular septal defect and no pulmonary stenosis, prior pulmonary artery banding is often performed, and total correction may be scheduled during later infancy.[210]

The Jatene procedure is the most popular procedure for anatomic correction of transposition of the great vessels. It is accomplished through a median sternotomy incision with the use of hypothermia and cardiopulmonary bypass. If any septal defects are present, they are closed at this time, and the pulmonary artery band is removed (if present). If pulmonary stenosis is present, it is resected, and patch enlargement of the pulmonary artery is performed if necessary. The coronary arteries are detached from the aorta, and the aorta and pulmonary arteries are transsected just above the semilunar valves. The aorta is then sewn to the stump of the previous pulmonary artery so that it will receive blood from the left ventricle, and the pulmonary artery is sewn to the stump of the previous aorta so that it will receive blood from the right ventricle. Once the great vessels have been relocated, the coronary arteries are reimplanted in the "new" aorta. Postoperative mortality following the Jatene procedure performed on infants with uncomplicated transposition is approximately 15% to 20%.[210,447] Postoperative complications include low cardiac output, congestive heart failure, bleeding, arrhythmias, and neurologic complications. Long-term follow-up of survivors of this procedure has not been extensive, but long-term complications include aortic insufficiency, supravalvular pulmonary stenosis,[447,452] recurrent ventricular septal defect,[210] and coronary artery stenosis.[151,447] Since the early mortality following the Jatene procedure is still higher than the early mortality following the Mustard or Senning procedures, at the present time, the Jatene procedure is usually reserved for those infants with complex transposition of the great vessels, including those with a ventricular septal defect.

If the infant with transposition of the great vessels has significant pulmonary stenosis or atresia, surgical intervention is very similar to that performed for the child with severe tetralogy, truncus arteriosus with pulmonary stenosis, or pulmonary atresia with a large ventricular septal defect; it is called the Rastelli procedure (see the discussion on treatment of tetralogy of Fallot and truncus arteriosus).

If the infant with transposition of the great vessels demonstrates significant preoperative pulmonary hypertension, postoperative ventilatory support and careful monitoring must be planned regardless of the type of surgical repair performed. The patient should not be allowed to develop hypoxia, acidosis, or hypothermia postoperatively since these may all enhance pulmonary vasoconstriction; weaning from ventilatory support must be performed gradually. Low cardiac output may develop and must be treated promptly (see the section on low cardiac output). These patients may demonstrate progression of pulmonary hypertension even after successful surgical repair.

All patients with transposition of the great vessels should receive antibiotic prophylaxis even following surgical correction. The risk of endocarditis is still present in these children since prosthetic material is often used for the corrective procedure (see Table 3-13).

■ **TOTAL ANOMALOUS PULMONARY VENOUS CONNECTION (TAPVC)**
■ **Etiology**

Total anomalous pulmonary venous connection (also known as total anomalous pulmonary venous *drainage* or total anomalous pulmonary venous *return*) results from failure of the pulmonary veins to join normally to the left atrium during fetal cardiopulmonary development. As a result the pulmonary veins join the systemic venous circulation, and mixed venous blood then returns to the heart. Some of the mixed venous blood then passes from the right atrium through a patent foramen ovale or atrial septal defect to the left atrium.

There are four major types of total anomalous pulmonary venous connection; these types are labeled according to the location of the pulmonary venous connection to the systemic venous circulation. Type I, *supracardiac* total anomalous pulmonary venous connection, is the most common form of this defect and is present in nearly half of all infants with this defect. The pulmonary veins join systemic veins that ultimately enter the superior vena cava or the right atrium. Type II, *cardiac* total anomalous pulmonary venous connection, is the second most common form of the defect; in this case, the pulmonary venous blood drains into the right atrium directly, or through the coronary sinus to the right atrium. When *infradiaphragmatic* total anomalous pulmonary venous connection (type III) is present, the pulmonary veins join to form a common pulmonary vein that descends below the diaphragm and drains into the ductus venosus or portal vein so that pulmonary blood passes through the liver before entering the hepatic vein and returning to the right atrium through the inferior vena cava. When type IV, or *mixed* total anomalous pulmonary venous connection is present, some pulmonary veins join the systemic circulation at one site, and other pulmonary veins enter the systemic circulation at a second site.

This is the least common form of this defect.[137,336]

Total anomalous pulmonary venous connection is responsible for approximately 1% of all congenital heart defects. Approximately half of the involved infants have an associated patent ductus arteriosus.[312]

■ Pathophysiology

With all forms of total anomalous pulmonary venous connection, pulmonary and systemic venous blood mix, and this mixed venous blood ultimately returns to the right atrium. Some mixed venous blood will enter the left atrium through a patent foramen ovale or through a true atrial septal defect. As a result the oxygen saturation of the blood in both the right side of the heart and in the left side of the heart (and, ultimately, in the systemic arterial circulation) will be the same.

In most cases of total anomalous pulmonary vein connection, once pulmonary vascular resistance falls, more of the mixed venous blood returning to the right atrium will flow preferentially into the right ventricle and ultimately into the pulmonary circulation; this produces increased pulmonary blood flow under low pressure, similar to that produced as a result of a large atrial septal defect. When pulmonary blood flow is large, pulmonary venous return is large. If this large pulmonary venous return passes unobstructed into the systemic venous circulation, the mixed venous blood returning to the heart will then have a relatively high-oxygen saturation because a large proportion of the blood is from the pulmonary venous circulation. Some of this highly saturated venous blood will ultimately pass from the right to the left atrium, into the left ventricle, and into the aorta and systemic circulation. As a result the greater the quantity of the infant's pulmonary blood flow, the greater the infant's arterial oxygen saturation.

Obstruction to pulmonary venous drainage is present in approximately one third of all patients with total anomalous pulmonary venous connection; it can occur with any form of the defect, although it is most common when infradiaphragmatic total anomalous pulmonary venous connection is present.[306] When pulmonary venous return is obstructed, pulmonary venous pressure rises, and pulmonary interstitial edema develops. The high pulmonary venous pressure produces an increase in pulmonary vascular resistance and pulmonary arterial pressure. These changes in pulmonary arterial resistance and pressure develop within the first months of life. The risk of development of pulmonary hypertension is high among all infants with this defect, whether pulmonary drainage is obstructed or not. Pulmonary vascular resistance is increased in all infants with obstruction to pulmonary venous return, and histologic evidence of pulmonary arterial hypertension has been observed by 1 to 3 months of age.[306]

■ Clinical signs and symptoms

Over half of all infants with total anomalous pulmonary venous connection are cyanotic during the first month of life. Nearly two thirds of affected patients have developed congestive heart failure by 3 months of age,[85,137,211,336] and over 90% of infants with this defect have congestive heart failure and/or cyanosis during the first year of life. Cyanosis usually increases significantly with exercise or vigorous cry.[312]

If pulmonary hypertension is present as the result of pulmonary venous obstruction, the infant usually becomes critically ill during the first months of life and will usually die within months unless surgical repair is performed. If pulmonary hypertension is absent, the infant usually develops signs of failure to thrive or congestive heart failure in the first year of life, although occasional patients with supracardiac or cardiac total anomalous pulmonary venous connection have survived to adulthood without development of significant symptoms.[137,211,336,423]

Approximately half of infants with total anomalous pulmonary venous connection have a cardiac murmur. It is usually a soft systolic murmur heard best at the lower left sternal border. If pulmonary blood flow is large and unobstructed, mixed venous return to the right atrium is large, and a tricuspid diastolic rumble may be heard at the lower right and left sternal border. If pulmonary hypertension is present, a loud second heart sound will be heard, and if congestive heart failure is present, a gallop may be noted.[124]

If the patient has no pulmonary venous obstruction, cyanosis may be minimal, and physical and electrocardiographic findings will be similar to those observed when a large atrial septal defect is present. Signs of congestive heart failure may not be present. Right ventricular hypertrophy will cause a sternal lift, and right ventricular hypertrophy and right axis deviation will be apparent on the ECG in all patients. Right atrial hypertrophy is also noted beyond 1 month of age. [124,137,336] The echocardiogram will document the presence of right atrial and ventricular enlargement. A two-dimensional echocardiogram will usually reveal the presence of a patent foramen ovale; inability to demonstrate continuity between the pulmonary veins and the left atrium will help confirm the diagnosis.

If obstruction to pulmonary venous flow is present, the infant will be more cyanotic. Once pulmonary edema develops, signs of respiratory distress and congestive heart failure will be observed. There may be no heart murmur noted, although the second heart sound will be loud once pulmonary hypertension develops. Since there is obstruction to pulmonary venous drainage into the systemic circulation, the amount of mixed venous return to the right atrium will not be excessive. Right ventricular hypertrophy will develop once pulmonary vascular resistance is increased so that a sternal lift may be noted, and right ventricular hypertrophy and right axis deviation will be noted on the ECG. Right atrial hypertrophy may or may not be noted. The echocardiogram will reveal right ventricular hypertrophy, and two-dimensional echocardiography will often demonstrate the presence of the patent foramen ovale and no visible continuity between the left atrium and pulmonary veins.

When the infant has total anomalous pulmonary venous connection without obstruction, cardiomegaly is usually apparent on the chest radiograph. In addition, pulmonary vascular markings are increased. If supracardiac total anomalous pulmonary venous connection to the left innominate vein is present, a characteristic bilateral bulge in the superior mediastinum may be noted, giving the entire mediastinum the appearance of a figure eight or of a snowman.[124,336] If pulmonary venous obstruction is present, the heart size is usually normal, and pulmonary interstitial edema will give the lung fields a "ground glass" appearance of passive pulmonary congestion.[137]

Cardiac catheterization is usually performed as soon as the diagnosis of total anomalous pulmonary venous connection is suspected. There will be an increase in arterial oxygen saturation in the systemic venous system at the location of the pulmonary venous connection. Infants with supracardiac total anomalous pulmonary venous connection will have a higher oxygen saturation in the superior vena cava than in the inferior vena cava. Unless obstruction is present, the infant with supracardiac total anomalous pulmonary venous connection will also have a mixed venous oxygen saturation in the right side of the heart that is equal to the oxygen saturation in the left side of the heart and in the systemic arterial circulation. Right atrial and ventricular pressures will be increased, and pulmonary arterial pressure will also be elevated (it may be near systemic pressure if pulmonary hypertension has developed).

If infradiaphragmatic total anomalous pulmonary venous connection is present, pulmonary venous obstruction is usually present. Cardiac catheterization reveals a mixed venous oxygen saturation in the inferior vena cava that is higher than that of the superior vena cava. Since pulmonary blood flow is reduced once pulmonary vascular resistance is high, oxygen desaturation is present in the right and left atria and ventricles and in the systemic arterial circulation. Right atrial and ventricular pressures are usually elevated, and pulmonary artery pressure may equal or exceed systemic arterial pressure.[124,336] The pulmonary arterial wedge pressure will also be elevated.

Injection of contrast material in the main pulmonary artery will opacify the pulmonary arterial circulation and the pulmonary venous circulation, and it should depict the anomalous pulmonary venous connection. Left ventricular angiography will allow evaluation of the size of the left ventricle and will demonstrate the presence of an associated patent ductus arteriosus.[336]

■ Medical and surgical treatment and nursing interventions

The symptomatic infant with total anomalous pulmonary venous connection requires vigorous management of any congestive heart failure and the prevention of pulmonary vascular disease, endocarditis, and systemic consequences of cyanotic heart disease and polycythemia (see the sections on congestive heart failure and hypoxemia). If the infant develops pulmonary venous obstruction, respiratory support and prompt surgical intervention are necessary. Surgical intervention is required on an urgent basis for the symptomatic patient, and it is generally indicated during the first 6 months or year of life if the infant is asymptomatic.

Correction of total anomalous pulmonary venous return is performed through a median sternotomy with use of cardiopulmonary bypass and profound hypothermia. Once the infant is cooled to 18° to 20° C, cardiopulmonary bypass is discontinued and the repair is accomplished during hypothermic circulatory arrest or with only a small cardiopulmonary bypass flow. The surgical correction requires attachment of the anomalous pulmonary veins to the left atrium, elimination of the anomalous pulmonary venous connection, and closure of any interatrial communication. If a patent ductus arteriosus is present, it is also ligated.

Repair of *supracardiac total anomalous pulmonary venous connection* is accomplished by anastomosis of the back of the left atrium and the common pulmonary venous sinus (where the right and left pulmonary veins join). The atrial septal defect is closed with a pericardial or woven patch. When the infant has *cardiac total anomalous pulmonary venous con-*

nection to the coronary sinus, the surgeon joins the ostium of the coronary sinus to the foramen ovale (an incision in the atrial septum is made to join the coronary sinus and foramen ovale and create one large atrial septal defect). A woven patch is then placed over the common orifice so that pulmonary venous return remains on the left atrial side of the patch. When *infradiaphragmatic total anomalous pulmonary venous connection* is present, the descending common pulmonary vein is joined to the left atrium, and the patent foramen ovale is closed.

Perioperative mortality for repair of total anomalous pulmonary venous return is approximately 10% to 15%.[85,223,312,423] A significantly higher mortality is reported for repair of infradiaphragmatic total anomalous pulmonary venous connection, particularly if the infant is acidotic with profound pulmonary edema at the time of surgery.[52] Since many of these infants have pulmonary hypertension at the time of surgery, pulmonary artery pressure is usually high during the immediate postoperative period. Controlled mechanical ventilatory support is then required during the postoperative period, and weaning must be performed slowly and carefully while monitoring the infant's pulmonary pressure. Since acidosis, hypothermia, and alveolar hypoventilation can produce pulmonary arterial constriction, these must be prevented. If the infant demonstrates severe congestive heart failure preoperatively or if the infant has a small left ventricle, severe congestive heart failure or low cardiac output may develop postoperatively. Arrhythmias (particularly supraventricular tachyarrhythmias or heart block) must be treated promptly since they may quickly compromise cardiac output. If a small left atrium is present or if there is some stenosis at the junction of the pulmonary veins and the left atrium, pulmonary interstitial edema may complicate the infant's postoperative course. Postoperative respiratory care must be meticulous.[52,223,312,336,423]

Late mortality varies following repair of total anomalous pulmonary venous connection, but it is significant. The late mortality is most often the result of progressive pulmonary vascular disease caused by pulmonary venous obstruction at the site of anastomosis to the left atrium.[52,306,423]

■ COARCTATION OF THE AORTA
■ Etiology

Coarctation of the aorta is a discrete narrowing in the aortic arch. Most commonly, the narrowing is located just distal to the origin of the left subclavian artery (Fig. 3-39). The coarctation may occur as a

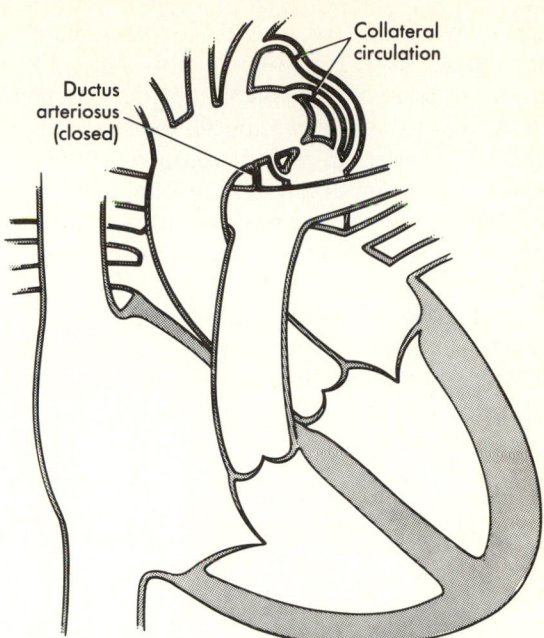

Fig. 3-39 Postductal coarctation of the aorta with schematic representation of collateral circulation. The narrowing in the aorta can be seen just distal to the left subclavian artery and the ligamentum arteriosus. Collateral circulation can develop from the internal mammary arteries and the parascapular arteries; this will maintain flow to the distal aorta.

From Hazinski, M.: The cardiovascular system, In Howe, J., and others, editors: The handbook of nursing, New York, 1984, John Wiley & Sons, Inc.

single lesion, as the result of improper development of the involved area of the aorta, or as the result of constriction of that portion of the aorta when the ductus arteriosus constricts. In addition, coarctation of the aorta is frequently seen in association with defects such as a ventricular septal defect.[248] These patients also often have a small aortic arch (especially a small aortic isthmus). Coarctation does not occur in association with defects that produce severe pulmonary stenosis (such as tetralogy of Fallot).[336,358]

Coarctation of the aorta is responsible for approximately 12% of all congenital heart defects. Approximately 60% of all children with coarctation of the aorta have a bicuspid aortic valve that may later become stenotic.[336]

■ Pathophysiology

Aortic narrowing increases resistance to flow from the proximal to the distal aorta. As a result pressure in the aorta proximal to the narrowing is increased, and pressure in the aorta distal to the narrowing is decreased. Since the renal arteries receive *hypo-*

tensive flow, renin release is stimulated; this produces further hypertension in the ascending aorta proximal to the coarctation, but it does not increase the pressure in the aorta distal to the coarctation.[8] Collateral circulation can develop to maintain adequate flow into the distal descending aorta; this flow is derived from the internal mammary arteries and from the parascapular arteries. These arteries flow into the intercostal arteries that, in turn, carry blood to the descending aorta.

It is important to note that although the *pressure* of blood in the descending aorta is often reduced, the *flow* through the descending aorta is usually adequate once collateral circulation is established so that tissues normally perfused from the descending aorta usually remain adequately perfused.

A coarctation of the aorta was previously classified as an infantile or adult type of coarctation, according to the age at which the patient was expected to develop symptoms. The term "infantile coarctation" was used to describe a narrowing in the aorta proximal to the ductus arteriosus, and the term "adult coarctation" was used to refer to a narrowing in the aorta distal to the ductus arteriosus. Now the terms are used to describe the coarctation according to its location, and the coarctation is classified as preductal, postductal, or periductal.

A *preductal* coarctation is a narrowing in the aorta proximal to the ductus arteriosus. Theoretically, when this form of coarctation develops during fetal life, there is no stimulus for the development of collateral circulation since the normal fetal circulatory pathway is unchanged; right ventricular output continues to flow through the ductus arteriosus into the descending aorta, and left ventricular output continues to flow into the ascending aorta to supply the head and upper extremities (see the section on fetal circulation in this chapter). After birth, this fetal circulatory pathway persists as long as the ductus arteriosus remains patent and as long as pulmonary vascular resistance is high. If the aortic narrowing is severe, there is little antegrade flow from the proximal to the distal aorta so that the infant will develop signs of congestive heart failure and poor systemic perfusion once the ductus arteriosus begins to constrict.

If a *postductal* coarctation is present, the narrowing in the aorta is distal to the ductus arteriosus. As a result, there is obstruction to flow from the ductus into the aorta during fetal life so that theoretically there is stimulus for the development of collateral circulation from the proximal to the distal aorta (see Fig. 3-39). The signs and symptoms demonstrated by the infant with a postductal coarctation will depend

on the severity of the aortic narrowing, as well as on the extent of the collateral circulation.

If a *periductal* coarctation is present, the aortic narrowing is located at the level of the ductus arteriosus. In this case, the ductus arteriosus often fails to constrict, and bidirectional shunting of blood (from the proximal aorta into the ductus, and from the ductus into the distal aorta) often occurs through the ductus.

Regardless of the location of the coarctation, the onset and the extent of the child's symptoms depend on the severity of the aortic narrowing, the presence of associated defects, and the extent and effectiveness of collateral circulation to the distal aorta.

If a large ventricular septal defect is present with a coarctation, signs of congestive heart failure usually develop when pulmonary vascular resistance falls at several days or weeks of age. The ventricular septal defect itself normally produces a left-to-right intracardiac shunt and high pulmonary blood flow under high pressure. The presence of an aortic coarctation further increases the resistance to left ventricular outflow, so flow of blood into the pulmonary circulation is enhanced, producing severe congestive heart failure.[336,358]

Subacute bacterial endocarditis can develop at the coarctation. The incidence of endocarditis is approximately 0.6% to 1.5% per patient a year when the coarctation is unrepaired. Patients with unrepaired coarctation have a shortened lifespan with a mean age at death of 34 years.[59] If aortic coarctation is unrepaired until adulthood, the patient has a higher risk of aortic aneurysm or rupture, cerebral vascular accident, mitral or aortic valve disease, myocardial infarction, or persistent hypertension. Premature death as a result of cardiovascular disease occurs in approximately 10% to 15% of these patients even after repair of the coarctation.[69,248]

■ Clinical signs and symptoms

When severe coarctation is present during infancy, congestive heart failure usually results; approximately half of all children with coarctation of the aorta develop some symptoms of congestive heart failure during the first months of life.[248] Nearly half of these symptomatic infants will have an associated ventricular septal defect.[134] One of the most common causes of congestive heart failure during the first two weeks of life is coarctation of the aorta with or without additional associated congenital heart defects.

Regardless of the location of the coarctation, hypertension is usually present in the aorta and in systemic arterial branches proximal to the coarctation, and hypotension is usually present in the aorta and in systemic arterial branches distal to the coarctation. If the coarctation lies between the innominate artery and the left subclavian artery, the strength of the radial pulse and the arterial blood pressure in the child's right arm will be greater than the intensity of the radial pulse and the arterial pressure in the child's left arm. If the coarctation is located distal to the left subclavian artery, hypertension will usually be present in both upper extremities, and hypotension will be present in both lower extremities.

It is difficult to appreciate a difference in intensity of peripheral pulses or in blood pressure if severe congestive heart failure is present since all pulses may be diminished until the congestive heart failure is treated. In addition, if the child has a preductal coarctation in which the descending aorta is perfused by the right ventricle through the ductus arteriosus, there may be little discrepancy between the upper and lower extremity pulses or blood pressures until the ductus arteriosus begins to constrict. The pulse discrepancy is also less obvious in the older child once collateral circulation has increased to provide flow to the distal aorta.

Most infants with coarctation of the aorta are acyanotic. Theoretically, if a preductal coarctation is present, the upper extremities should be pink and the lower extremities should be cyanotic (since the descending aorta is perfused with systemic venous blood from the right ventricle through the ductus arteriosus). This difference in color between the upper and lower extremities is called *differential cyanosis*; it is infrequently observed because the infant with severe preductal coarctation usually demonstrates severe congestive heart failure and poor peripheral perfusion so that his color is pale and mottled in all extremities.

Children with coarctation who do not develop congestive heart failure in infancy usually remain asymptomatic until adulthood. The child may occasionally complain of dyspnea or exercise intolerance. *Claudication* may develop in the lower extremities because collateral circulation cannot adequately increase flow to the distal aorta during exercise. Of course, hypertension will be present in the upper extremities.

Many children with coarctation have a systolic murmur that is heard best over the child's back near the left side of the upper thoracic vertebrae; this murmur is caused by blood flow through the narrowed aortic segment. If a postductal coarctation is present in the older child, bruits may be heard in the posterior intercostal spaces; these are caused by flow through the large intercostal arteries (which serve as

collateral vessels to provide flow to the distal aorta). If a bicuspid aortic valve is present, a systolic murmur, possibly accompanied by a click, may be heard over the right upper sternal border. If an associated ventricular septal defect is present, a harsh systolic murmur is heard over the left lower sternal border. If a patent ductus arteriosus is present, a systolic or continuous murmur may be heard over the second left intercostal space at the mid-clavicular line.

Left ventricular hypertrophy may produce a left ventricular heave. If the infant has a preductal coarctation, right ventricular hypertrophy is also present and may produce a sternal lift. Right or biventricular hypertrophy are usually noted on the ECG of the symptomatic infant less than 3 months of age. Older children may demonstrate only mild left ventricular hypertrophy on the ECG. A two-dimensional echocardiogram will often document the presence and location of the coarctation, as well as the presence of an associated ventricular septal defect or patent ductus arteriosus. In addition, both M-mode and two-dimensional echocardiography will allow evaluation of aortic valve movement, structure, and function, and left ventricular size and function.[122,336,391]

The chest radiograph of the symptomatic infant with coarctation of the aorta will document the presence of cardiomegaly with prominent pulmonary venous congestion. If an associated ventricular septal defect or patent ductus arteriosus is present, pulmonary vascular engorgement may also be noted. In the older, asymptomatic child with coarctation of the aorta, the heart size is usually normal on the chest radiograph. Occasionally, the aortic silhouette on the radiograph will demonstrate the presence of the aortic narrowing, producing a "letter E" or "number 3" shape to the aorta. When the child has coarctation of the aorta beyond the age of 7 or 8 years, the dilated intercostal arteries, which serve as collateral vessels to provide flow into the distal aorta, can erode the inferior surface of the child's ribs, producing *rib notching* on the chest radiograph. Occasionally, the adolescent with unrepaired coarctation may develop left ventricular dilation.

Cardiac catheterization is usually performed to determine the exact location of the aortic narrowing, to determine the presence of associated defects, and to allow evaluation of the extent of collateral circulation, size of the aorta, severity of aortic valvular stenosis, and the size and function of the left ventricle. When preductal coarctation is present and when the right ventricle is ultimately perfusing the descending aorta through the ductus arteriosus, right ventricular hypertension will be present, and right ventricular pressure will equal descending aortic pressure. Right and left ventricular pressures may be equal. Left ventricular and ascending aortic pressures will both be elevated. If a postductal aortic coarctation is present, left ventricular and ascending aortic hypertension will be noted, and pressure in the descending aorta will be lower and nonpulsatile. If aortic valvular stenosis is also present, a pressure gradient will be measured between the left ventricle and the ascending aorta. If an associated ventricular septal defect is present, it will be confirmed by the increase in oxygen saturation in the right ventricle. Careful left ventricular and aortic angiography will demonstrate the location of the coarctation and associated defects.[358] Since the aortic narrowing is often severe, the cardiologist may not attempt retrograde aortic catheterization through the coarctation of the symptomatic neonate since the catheter may perforate the aorta at the site of the coarctation. The amount of contrast material used for angiography in the symptomatic neonate with coarctation must be limited, because the risk of renal damage is significant in these infants.[358]

■ Medical and surgical treatment and nursing interventions

Any symptomatic infant with coarctation of the aorta requires prompt treatment of congestive heart failure; generally, digoxin and furosemide are the drugs of choice for treatment (see the section on congestive heart failure). If the infant has a simple postductal coarctation, he will generally respond to medical management of the congestive heart failure. These infants generally return for elective repair of coarctation at 1 to 4 years of age. If, however, congestive heart failure persists, surgical repair of the coarctation is required. Until repair is performed, the child requires antibiotic prophylaxis for periods of increased risk of bacteremia (see Table 3-13).

If the neonate has a preductal coarctation of the aorta and if the flow of blood in the descending aorta is entirely dependent on the ductus arteriosus, prostaglandin E_1 (PGE$_1$) is administered to maintain ductal patency (see the section on medical treatment and nursing interventions for hypoxemia in this chapter). The administration of PGE$_1$ produces ductal dilation and maintains adequate perfusion of the tissues supplied by the descending aorta (including the kidneys). Administration of PGE$_1$ in infants with preductal coarctation often prevents the development of acidosis, anuria, and profound circulatory collapse that can accompany ductal constriction.

Occasionally, the infant with severe unrecognized coarctation of the aorta suddenly develops severe congestive heart failure and poor systemic perfusion at several days of age. These infants require careful, thorough, and rapid evaluation, insertion of appropriate venous lines, and treatment of electrolyte and acid-base imbalance (see the section on low cardiac output). Administration of prostaglandin E_1 and intravenous sympathomimetic drugs and mechanical ventilation may be required initially. Echocardiography and cardiac catheterization will be performed on an urgent basis, and the infant is referred for surgery if his clinical condition does not improve.

Surgical repair of coarctation during infancy is generally required for those symptomatic infants unresponsive to vigorous medical management; this group of infants frequently has a severe coarctation, a preductal coarctation (with descending aortic flow dependent upon the ductus arteriosus), or an associated ventricular septal defect or ductus arteriosus. Elective surgical repair between 1 and 4 years of age is recommended for the asymptomatic child with coarctation. If the coarctation is discovered after the child has entered school, repair is usually recommended at that time since the incidence of preoperative and late postoperative cardiovascular complications increases when operative age exceeds 8 to 10 years.[248,260]

Repair of the coarctation is usually accomplished through a left thoracotomy incision and without the use of cardioulmonary bypass. The aorta must be cross-clamped during coarctation repair; if flow to the descending aorta is inadequate during surgery, decreased perfusion of the kidneys and spinal cord can produce renal failure or paralysis postoperatively, therefore the surgeon must ensure adequate distal aortic flow during the repair. If collateral circulation to the aorta does not provide an adequate distal aortic pressure after the aorta is clamped, the surgeon will construct a temporary shunt or tubular graft between the ascending aorta and the descending aorta.

When coarctation repair is performed during infancy or early childhood, special techniques must be used to allow maximal postoperative aortic growth and minimal risk of restenosis. The narrowed aortic segment may be completely excised or the aorta may be opened longitudinally at the area of narrowing. The aorta is then closed, using a patch. The infant's left subclavian artery can be ligated distally, and the subclavian artery can be opened and brought down as a patch on the aorta, or a woven prosthetic material can be used. When this patch enlargement of the aorta is performed at the time of coarctation repair, the incidence of later restenosis is reduced.[71,185,334]

If a patent ductus arteriosus is present, it is divided at the time of coarctation repair. If a significant ventricular septal defect is present, pulmonary artery banding may be performed at the time of coarctation repair (see the discussion of pulmonary artery banding in the summary of treatment of ventricular septal defect). This band will later have to be removed during open-heart closure of the ventricular septal defect.

If coarctation repair is performed in the older child, the narrowed segment is generally excised, and the segments of the aorta are often sewn directly together.

Perioperative mortality for coarctation repair is lowest among asymptomatic young children and highest among symptomatic neonates and those with associated congenital heart defects; the range of perioperative mortality is approximately 4% to 25%.[185,254,326,336] Postoperative complications include congestive heart failure, bleeding, paradoxical hypertension, paralysis or paresis, and mesenteric arteritis.[56] Paradoxical hypertension is thought to be related to high plasma renin activity or to alteration in baroreceptor function as the result of the coarctation.[8] Significant postoperative hypertension can be treated with nitroprusside (continuous infusion of 2 to 8 μg/kg/minute), propranolol (0.1 to 0.25 mg/kg/dose every 6 hours), or reserpine (Serpasil, 0.04-0.07 mg/kg/IM dose every 6 hours).[382,445] This hypertension usually resolves within 1 to 2 weeks after surgery.

If a subclavian flap was used for the coarctation repair, it will not be possible to obtain a cuff pressure from the left arm. Since only collateral vessels are providing the arterial circulation to the left arm, no arterial punctures should be performed postoperatively in that arm.

Postoperative mesenteric vasculitis or arteritis may produce abdominal pain and distention. With progression of the arteritis, bowel ischemia, gastrointestinal bleeding, and bowel necrosis can result.[200] There is some thought that prevention of postoperative hypertension may reduce the risk of mesenteric vasculitis. In addition, frequent and thorough examination for the presence of bowel sounds, abdominal distention, and tenderness must be performed. The infant or child should resume oral feedings slowly, following coarctation repair, and the physician should be notified if the child begins to vomit or develop abdominal distention.

Late results of surgical repair of coarctation of the aorta vary. When the coarctation is repaired during infancy, restenosis may occur, causing hypertension in the aorta (and great vessels) proximal to the narrowing and hypotension in the aorta (and aortic branches) distal to the narrowing. Residual upper extremity hypertension may be present postoperatively,

particularly if the child is over 6 to 10 years of age at the time of repair; the hypertension is often exaggerated during exercise. If significant residual hypertension is the result of restenosis, reoperation may be necessary. If significant hypertension is present that is not related to restenosis, pharmacologic therapy with antihypertensive medications is required.

Children who have coarctation repair should receive follow-up care indefinitely postoperatively since the incidence of residual or secondary cardiovascular problems is significant.[326] If the child has a bicuspid aortic valve, the child will require antibiotic prophylaxis for periods of increased risk of bacteremia (see Table 3-13). In addition, the child should be monitored for the development of calcific aortic stenosis.

■ **INTERRUPTED AORTIC ARCH**
■ **Etiology**

Interrupted aortic arch is a lack of continuity between the aortic arch and the descending aorta that is thought to occur as the result of faulty formation of the aortic arch system during fetal development.

There are three types of interrupted aortic arch and they are labeled according to the site of the interruption. Unless transposition of the great vessels is present, the ascending aorta receives blood from the left ventricle and the descending aorta is perfused from the right ventricle through the ductus arteriosus. In type A interrupted aortic arch, the entire aortic arch is intact and the interruption occurs just beyond the left subclavian artery; approximately 40% of infants with interrupted aortic arch have this type. In type B interrupted aortic arch, the aorta is interrupted between the left carotid and the left subclavian artery; as a result the left subclavian artery arises from the descending aortic segment. This form of interrupted aortic arch is the most common. In type C interrupted aortic arch the aorta is divided between the innominate and the left carotid arteries; as a result the right carotid and subclavian arteries receive flow from the left ventricle through the ascending aorta, and the left carotid and subclavian arteries receive blood from the right ventricle through the ductus arteriosus.[70]

Interrupted aortic arch is responsible for approximately 1% of all congenital heart defects, but it is one of the defects that frequently causes symptoms during the first weeks of life.[134]

Most infants with interrupted aortic arch have additional congenital heart defects, and nearly half of affected infants have additional noncardiac anomalies. There is an association between DiGeorge syndrome and interrupted aortic arch. Since DiGeorge syndrome is associated with congenital absence of the parathyroids (and hypocalcemia) and aplasia of the thymus (and decreased immune response), it is important that the diagnosis of DiGeorge syndrome be considered in the infant with interrupted aortic arch.

■ **Pathophysiology**

Hemodynamic consequences of the interrupted aortic arch are identical to those described for severe preductal coarctation. Since the right ventricle perfuses the distal aorta through the ductus arteriosus, the neonate usually develops severe congestive heart failure and poor systemic perfusion when the ductus arteriosus begins to constrict.

■ **Clinical signs and symptoms**

Clinical signs and symptoms of interrupted aortic arch are identical to those described for a severe preductal coarctation of the aorta. The infant often has no specific cardiac murmur, and he usually develops signs of severe congestive heart failure at a few days of age (see the section on congestive heart failure in this chapter). The infant can develop shock within hours, including decreased systemic perfusion, severe metabolic acidosis, and oliguria or anuria. All peripheral pulses will be decreased in intensity, and the infant will die without prompt and skillful medical, surgical, and nursing care.

In *rare* instances, patients with interrupted aortic arch have survived to adulthood without symptoms, as the result of development of extensive collateral circulation.

The diagnosis of interrupted aortic arch is suspected by the clinical course. It must be differentiated from coarctation of the aorta, aortic atresia, and hypoplastic left heart syndrome. The diagnosis is confirmed by echocardiogram, and the specific anatomy is determined during cardiac catheterization and angiography. If the infant's systemic perfusion improves in the critical-care unit, a difference in blood pressure between the right and left arms or between the upper and lower extremities may be appreciated, although this finding is often obscured when the ductus arteriosus is widely patent during PGE$_1$ therapy. If the infant has a right radial and an umbilical artery line in place, the arterial oxygen saturation should be higher in the sample from the right radial artery than that in the sample obtained from the umbilical artery, since the right radial artery is perfused with blood

from the left ventricle and the decending aorta is perfused with blood from the right ventricle through the ductus arteriosus. However, if a large ventricular septal defect is also present, the difference in oxygen saturations may be minimal. These findings will be altered by the presence of transposition of the great vessels.

■ **Medical and surgical treatment and nursing interventions**

Once the neonate with interrupted aortic arch develops signs of congestive heart failure, medical management must be aggressive and skillful. Appropriate IV lines are inserted, and a continuous infusion of prostaglandin E$_1$ is begun immediately (see the discussion in this chapter on hypoxemia). Correction of existing acid-base and electrolyte imbalances (including acidosis, hypoglycemia, and hypocalcemia) must also be accomplished, and mechanical ventilation is often necessary (see the section on low cardiac output in this chapter). Urine output should be adequate once the prostaglandin infusion is begun, but fluid restriction will be required if oliguria or anuria persists.

Echocardiography should be performed as quickly as possible, and cardiac catheterization is accomplished as soon as the infant is stable. The infant is then referred for surgery on an urgent basis.

Surgical repair of an interrupted aortic arch is usually accomplished through a left thoracotomy incision and without the use of cardiopulmonary bypass. Since the aorta must be clamped above and below the area of interruption, the surgeon must often create a shunt between the ascending and descending aorta to maintain aortic and great vessel flow during the repair. Most commonly, the surgeon joins the two separate portions of the aorta with a woven graft or a patch. The infant's subclavian artery may also be used to enlarge the aorta (see the discussion of coarctation repair during infancy).

A median sternotomy approach and cardiopulmonary bypass may be used occasionally to allow repair of an intracardiac defect and the interrupted aortic arch at the same time.[82] Perioperative mortality for repair of interrupted aortic arch remains high. Postoperative complications are identical to those discussed following repair of severe coarctation of the aorta during infancy. The incidence of postoperative congestive heart failure and low cardiac output is significant, and later restenosis of the site of surgical repair is also frequently reported among survivors.[70,426]

■ AORTIC STENOSIS
■ Etiology

Aortic stenosis results from the obstruction of left ventricular outflow. In the most common form of aortic obstruction, the obstruction is at the level of the aortic valve; this is called *valvular* stenosis. Valvular aortic stenosis can result when the aortic valve is bicuspid instead of tricuspid or when the valve commissures are fused. *Subvalvular* aortic stenosis or *subaortic* stenosis is the second most common form of aortic obstruction. Subaortic stenosis can be caused by a fibrous diaphragm below the aortic valve, from muscular hypertrophy of the ventricular septum (called idiopathic hypertrophic subaortic stenosis), or from fibromuscular tubular narrowing of the left ventricular outflow tract (also called tunnel subaortic stenosis). *Supravalvular* aortic stenosis, or *supraaortic* stenosis is the least common form of aortic obstruction; it is caused by a fibromembranous narrowing of the aorta above the aortic valve and coronary arteries. Children with supravalvular aortic stenosis often have a characteristic facial appearance (including short palpebral fissures and thick lips) and mental retardation; this association has been called the Williams elfin facies syndrome.[215]

Aortic stenosis is responsible for approximately 8% of all congenital heart defects, and it is frequently present in association with other congenital heart defects. Mothers who have a congenital heart defect producing left ventricular outflow tract obstruction may have a significant risk of producing a child with a similar defect.[443]

■ Pathophysiology

Whenever there is obstruction to left ventricular outflow, the left ventricle will generate greater pressure to maintain flow beyond the area of resistance. As a result left ventricular hypertension that is proportional to the degree of aortic obstruction develops. The severity of the obstruction is usually classified according to the gradient across the obstruction when cardiac output is normal. A mild stenosis produces a gradient of 5 to 40 mm Hg; a moderate stenosis produces a gradient that is as high as 50 to 60 mm Hg, and a severe stenosis is thought to produce a gradient exceeding 60 to 80 mm Hg. It is important to note that these classifications vary from institution to institution. In addition, if the cardiac output falls, the gradient across the obstruction falls, even though the severity of the gradient remains unchanged. With exercise, the cardiac output increases, and the gradient

obtained across the area of obstruction increases so the obstruction becomes relatively more severe.

When valvular aortic stenosis is present, valvular insufficiency can also develop. This produces a left ventricular volume load and dilation.

When significant aortic obstruction is present, the left ventricle will hypertrophy. When valvular or subvalvular aortic stenosis is present, the coronary arteries are located *distal* to the area of obstruction, so it may not be possible for the coronary arteries to increase flow during exercise and other periods of increased oxygen requirements. As a result significant subvalvular or valvular aortic stenosis may result in reduced myocardial or subendocardial perfusion, particularly during exercise, and subendocardial fibrosis and ischemia can result. Once left ventricular ischemia is significant and produces angina, syncope, or left ventricular strain patterns on the ECG, the child is at risk of sudden death as a result of ischemia or arrhythmias.

When supravalvular aortic stenosis is present, left ventricular hypertrophy still occurs. However, coronary artery perfusion is usually adequate, because the coronary artery ostia are located proximal to the aortic obstruction. Since the coronary arteries receive hypertensive flow, they often become dilated and tortuous.

Idiopathic hypertrophic subaortic stenosis is an unusual form of dynamic subvalvular aortic stenosis caused by thickening of the left side of the ventricular septum. As the left ventricle hypertrophies, the septum also hypertrophies and the severity of the obstruction increases. This defect is associated with cardiomyopathy, so it is discussed in the section on cardiomyopathies in this chapter.

The child with turbulent aortic blood flow as a result of aortic stenosis is at risk for the development of subacute bacterial endocarditis. The incidence of subacute bacterial endocarditis among patients with aortic stenosis is 4% to 13%, and it is highest among patients with valvular or subvalvular aortic stenosis.[222,372,433] Development of aortic endocarditis is serious since vegetations may embolize to the brain, and valvular inflammation can result in severe aortic insufficiency (see Table 3-13).

■ Clinical signs and symptoms

Most patients with aortic stenosis have a mild or moderate aortic obstruction that does not produce symptoms until late in childhood or during the adult years unless endocarditis or aortic regurgitation develop. Approximately one third of infants and children with mild or moderate aortic stenosis will develop symptoms of dyspnea, exercise intolerance, or fatigability. More rapid progression of stenosis and symptoms can develop as the result of subvalvular aortic stenosis.

If severe valvular aortic stenosis is present during infancy, congestive heart failure will usually develop during the first two months of life. Early signs of decompensation include tachypnea, increased respiratory effort, poor feeding, diaphoresis, and poor weight gain.[336]

Signs of significant aortic stenosis in any patient include the development of angina (this is difficult to evaluate in the child), syncope, poor exercise tolerance, dyspnea, or the appearance of a "strain" pattern on the ECG.

Aortic stenosis produces a systolic murmur that is heard best over the right upper sternal border; during infancy, the murmur may also be heard along the left sternal border. The murmur may be accompanied by a thrill. If valvular aortic stenosis is present, an early ejection systolic click is frequently heard. Approximately one third of the patients with mild or moderate stenosis demonstrate a diastolic murmur as a result of aortic regurgitation.

Peripheral pulses and systemic arterial blood pressure are usually normal when the child has aortic stenosis. If severe aortic stenosis is present, however, the peripheral pulses may be biphasic and the pulse pressure is narrowed. If supravalvular aortic stenosis is present, the right radial pulse may be increased in intensity because of a streaming effect of blood from the left ventricle into the right subclavian artery. If the infant or child develops congestive heart failure as the result of severe aortic stenosis, all pulses will be decreased in intensity.

Left ventricular hypertrophy is often present, although it rarely causes a left ventricular heave.[123] Left ventricular hypertrophy will often be apparent on the ECG. Signs of left ventricular *strain* may develop, including flattening or inversion of the T wave in V_6 and depression or convexity of the ST segment (especially in leads where the QRS complex is predominantly upright); if this strain pattern is not present at rest, it may become apparent with exercise. The development of a left ventricular strain pattern on the ECG indicates the need for urgent surgical attention. Symptomatic infants with valvular aortic stenosis often demonstrate biventricular hypertrophy on the ECG.

M-mode echocardiography can reveal the presence of eccentric aortic valve closure when valvular aortic stenosis is present. In addition, an increased left ventricular shortening fraction (calculated from the M-mode echocardiogram) can identify the presence of a moderate or severe aortic obstruction, and estimates of the gradient can be made after consideration of left ventricular thickness. Two-dimensional echocardiography confirms the location of the aortic obstruction and also allows estimation of the aortic valve gradient. The presence of associated congenital heart defects can also be confirmed through the use of echocardiography.

The chest radiograph of the child with aortic stenosis is often normal since the left ventricular contour will not enlarge unless the left ventricle dilates. If cardiomegaly is present, the child probably has severe aortic stenosis. Often, the ascending aortic silhouette is widened as the result of poststenotic aortic dilation. If congestive heart failure is present, the radiograph will often demonstrate generalized cardiomegaly and prominent pulmonary venous markings with interstitial edema.

Cardiac catheterization is indicated whenever the infant or child with aortic stenosis is symptomatic, whenever significant left ventricular hypertrophy is evident on the ECG, or whenever the valve gradient is thought to be severe. Catheterization will verify the presence of associated defects, and it will document the gradient across the aortic obstruction and the severity of the left ventricular hypertension. In addition, the precise location of the obstruction can be identified, and left ventricular function can be evaluated. Left ventricular and aortic angiography are usually performed to illustrate the obstruction and to document the presence or absence of aortic or mitral regurgitation. The pulmonary artery wedge and right ventricular pressures will only be elevated if congestive heart failure and left ventricular dysfunction are present.

■ **Medical and surgical treatment and nursing interventions**

Because the treatment for each form of aortic stenosis is somewhat different, the medical and surgical treatment of valvular, subvalvular, and supravalvular aortic stenosis is discussed separately in the following section.

Valvular aortic stenosis. If the asymptomatic infant or child has mild *valvular* aortic stenosis, he is followed closely by a physician, and surgical intervention is not indicated. The child will require antibiotic prophylaxis during times of increased risk of bacteremia to prevent endocarditis. The physician will obtain ECGs and echocardiograms at regular intervals, and exercise testing will occasionally be performed to detect any progression in the severity of the child's aortic obstruction.

If the infant with aortic stenosis develops congestive heart failure within the first weeks or months of life, he will require treatment with digoxin and diuretics. Surgical intervention is planned as soon as the diagnosis is established. These infants must be watched closely because they can suddenly develop poor systemic perfusion, acidosis, or an arrhythmia (most commonly ventricular fibrillation) unresponsive to medical management.[104]

Indications for surgery in the infant or child with aortic valvular stenosis include the development of congestive heart failure, the presence of a significant aortic valvular gradient, the development of a left ventricular "strain" pattern on the ECG, narrowing of the pulse pressure, or the development of symptoms such as dyspnea, increased respiratory effort, angina, or syncope.

Once the child develops symptoms or other evidence of *severe* valvular aortic stenosis (particularly evidence of a "strain" pattern on the ECG), surgery is scheduled on an urgent basis. In the time before surgery, the child is placed on *strict* activity restriction since any activities that increase cardiac output requirements will increase left ventricular work and increase the risk of ventricular ischemia, arrhythmias, and sudden death. The risk of sudden death among children with known severe aortic valvular stenosis is approximately 7%,[146] and sudden death has been reported among children with only moderate valvular stenosis.[433]

The goal of surgical intervention for valvular aortic stenosis is relief of the aortic obstruction without creation of significant aortic insufficiency; this is not always possible. When the aortic valvular stenosis produces severe symptoms during early infancy, the aortic valve annulus and the left ventricular chamber may be very small. As a result it may be impossible to completely relieve the aortic obstruction, and the left ventricle may be unable to sustain adequate systemic perfusion postoperatively.[104,236] As a result infants who require surgery for critical aortic valvular stenosis during infancy have a poor prognosis if their left ventricle is also small.

When the child with congenital aortic valvular stenosis requires one or more repeat aortic valvotomies, it may be impossible to relieve the stenosis adequately without producing valvular insufficiency. Ultimately, if the child requires repeat aortic valvotomies during childhood, aortic valve replacement is usually necessary.

Surgical treatment of valvular aortic stenosis is accomplished with the use of a median sternotomy, cardiopulmonary bypass, mild or moderate hypothermia, and cardioplegia. An incision is made in the aorta, just above the coronary arteries, and the valve commissures are incised carefully. As mentioned earlier, valve replacement is performed in the older child if significant aortic insufficiency with or without unrelieved aortic stenosis is present. Peiroperative mortality for aortic valvotomy is approximately 29% to 50% in symptomatic young infants,[93,104,236,372] and up to 4% in children operated on beyond infancy.[12,93,204,216,372] Postoperative complications include congestive heart failure and low cardiac output (particularly if these were present preoperatively), arrhythmias, and sudden death. Most patients will demonstrate a diastolic murmur of aortic insufficiency postoperatively.[204]

Surgical relief of valvular aortic stenosis is considered a palliative operation, since approximately 4% to 33% of the patients will require additional surgery for recurrent or residual aortic stenosis or aortic insufficiency.* In addition, approximately half of the children requiring aortic valvotomy have an unsatisfactory result; and one fourth of the operated patients have major hemodynamic abnormalities within 1 year of surgery.[216] The incidence of late death following aortic valvulotomy is 3.4% to 15%; these late deaths can occur as a result of reoperation, endocarditis, intractable congestive heart failure, and sudden death (probably as a result of arrhythmias).[12,93,104,236,372]

If the child requires aortic valve replacement, further surgery will be necessary as the child grows and requires larger aortic prosthetic valves. If a porcine heterograft valve is used for aortic valve replacement before the child has reached adolescence, calcification, degeneration, and dysfunction can develop within 2 to 8 years after insertion.[371,372,446] If a mechanical valve is inserted, anticoagulation is often required, and this produces a significant risk of thromboembolic or hemorrhagic complications.[49,367] The child and parents will require careful teaching about the importance of the anticoagulation and medical follow-up and about the signs of thromboembolic or hemorrhagic complications. Children with prosthetic valves will still require antibiotic prophylaxis during periods of increased risk of bacteremia, and the incidence of endocarditis among these patients is approximately 2% to 4% per patient-year.[432]

Discrete subvalvular aortic stenosis. Manage-

*References 12, 93, 104, 204, 236, 372.

ment of the asymptomatic infant or child with mild discrete *subvalvular* aortic stenosis is very similar to that of the child with valvular aortic stenosis; the child is followed closely by a physician, and surgical intervention is not immediately indicated. The child will require antibiotic prophylaxis during times of increased risk of bacteremia to prevent endocarditis. The physician will obtain ECGs at regular intervals, and exercise testing will occasionally be performed to detect any progression in the severity of the child's aortic obstruction. Fortunately, however, the incidence of sudden death in children with subvalvular aortic stenosis is lower than that reported as the result of valvular aortic stenosis.[336]

Indications for surgical resection of subvalvular aortic stenosis are similar to those indications for aortic valvotomy; they include the development of a left ventricular "strain" pattern on the ECG, narrowing of the pulse pressure, or development of symptoms such as syncope, dyspnea, increased respiratory effort, angina, or syncope. Once these signs appear, the child is placed on strict activity restriction to minimize the risk of sudden death, and surgery is scheduled. Congestive heart failure does not commonly occur in infants with discrete subvalvular aortic stenosis.

If the subvalvular aortic obstruction is discrete, its severity can increase rapidly.[222,302] In addition, the turbulent blood flow caused by the obstruction can produce secondary deformity of the aortic valve and aortic regurgitation. As a result surgery for discrete subvalvular aortic stenosis is recommended once it produces a 30 to 40 mm Hg gradient.[222,302] If the child has tunnel subvalvular aortic stenosis, the indications for surgery are carefully reviewed since the surgical risk and operative mortality are significant.

Surgical relief of subvalvular aortic stenosis is accomplished through a median sternotomy incision with use of cardiopulmonary bypass, mild or moderate hypothermia, and cardioplegia. The surgeon will make an incision in the aorta, above the aortic valve; he will then open the aortic valve to reach the subvalvular obstruction. If the stenosis is caused by a discrete membrane or fibromuscular ring, the surgeon will cut and remove it. However, if the obstruction is the result of a tunnel narrowing of the left ventricular outflow tract and a small aortic valve annulus, a patch may be required to enlarge the entire left ventricular outflow tract *and* annulus and to allow insertion of an adequate aortic prosthetic valve; this surgical approach is known as the Konno procedure.[277]

The maximum perioperative mortality for relief of subvalvular aortic stenosis is approximately 20%, and it is highest if tunnel aortic stenosis is present.[222,261,277,302] Postoperative complications include congestive heart failure, low cardiac output, arrhythmias (especially complete heart block), and bleeding.

Late results of surgery for subvalvular aortic stenosis vary. Nearly half of operated patients have a residual subvalvular obstruction. In some patients, the obstruction can progress, requiring reoperation.[216,302] Late death following relief of subvalvular aortic stenosis has been reported in approximately 2% to 6% of the patients (the patients at greatest risk are those with a tunnel subvalvular stenosis), and it can occur as the result of endocarditis, sudden death, or severe congestive heart failure.[222,261,277,302] These children should all receive antibiotic prophylaxis indefinitely during periods of increased risk of bacteremia.

Supravalvular aortic stenosis. Infants and children with mild *supravalvular* aortic stenosis are followed closely by a physician, and ECGs and echocardiograms will be obtained at regular intervals to detect an increase in the obstruction. Since relief of supravalvular aortic stenosis can be technically difficult in a small infant, surgery is usually not recommended during infancy unless the obstruction is significant.

Congestive heart failure and other signs of severe aortic stenosis do not commonly occur in infants with supravalvular aortic stenosis.[134] Although the risk of sudden death is present among patients with this form of aortic stenosis, the reported incidence is not as high as that reported with valvular aortic stenosis. These children are at risk for the development of endocarditis, especially during episodes of bacteremia, so antibiotic prophylaxis will be required throughout the child's lifetime.

Indications for surgery for relief of supravalvular aortic stenosis are approximately the same as those for the child with valvular and subvalvular aortic stenosis; they include the presence of a severe aortic gradient, the development of left ventricular "strain" pattern on the ECG, narrowing of the pulse pressure, or the development of symptoms such as dyspnea, increased respiratory effort, angina, or syncope.

Surgical relief of supravalvular aortic stenosis is accomplished through a median sternotomy incision with the use of mild or moderate hypothermia and cardioplegia. If the aorta will require extensive reconstruction, specific perfusion of the individual coronary arteries may be provided during the procedure. A longitudinal incision is made in the aorta across the narrowed segment. If a discrete membrane is present, it is simply excised. If, however, an extensive area of narrowing is present, the aorta will be enlarged with a prosthetic patch.

Perioperative mortality and results following repair of supravalvular aortic stenosis are variable, and they depend primarily on the size of the ascending aorta; the lowest mortality and best results are obtained when a discrete membrane is removed from a large aorta. The highest risk is present when the ascending aorta is small and requires a large patch. Postoperative complications include low cardiac output, bleeding, and arrhythmias. Late complications of surgery include endocarditis, sudden death, residual stenosis, and later aortic valvular dysfunction requiring aortic valve replacement.[65,344]

■ HYPOPLASTIC LEFT HEART SYNDROME
■ Etiology

This congenital cardiac anomaly consists of a diminutive left ventricle, aortic and/or mitral valve stenosis or atresia, normally related great vessels, and an intact ventricular septum. The most serious form of the defect includes aortic atresia. This anomaly occurs as the result of inadequate left ventricular, aortic, and/or mitral valve development during fetal life.

Hypoplastic left heart syndrome is responsible for approximately 2% of all congenital heart defects, but it is the leading cause of death from cardiovascular disease during the first 2 weeks of life[134]; death occurs because the left ventricle is inadequate to maintain systemic perfusion.

■ Pathophysiology

Since there is a small left ventricular chamber with or without aortic or mitral valve obstruction, there is resistance to flow into the aorta and inadequate perfusion of the systemic circulation. As a result the neonate is dependent upon the flow of blood from the pulmonary artery through the ductus arteriosus to supply the descending aorta (with antegrade flow) as well as the aortic arch and coronary circulation (with retrograde flow). When severe mitral or aortic obstruction is present, some blood will shunt from the left to the right atrium through a stretched foramen ovale; this produces increased pulmonary blood flow. In addition, the left atrial pressure will rise, and pulmonary venous engorgement and edema will develop.

■ Clinical signs and symptoms

At birth the neonate may appear to be normal. However, as the ductus arteriosus begins to close, cyanosis or pallor and signs of poor systemic perfusion develop rapidly. In addition, the development of pulmonary venous engorgement will produce respiratory distress. The neonate progressively deteriorates despite aggressive medical management.

There is no specific murmur associated with this defect. Peripheral pulses are not unusual initially, but they become diminished in intensity once systemic perfusion is compromised. Right ventricular hypertrophy is present, and it may produce a sternal lift. The ECG will reveal prominent right ventricular forces and right axis deviation with diminished left ventricular forces. Echocardiography will confirm the presence of an extremely small left ventricle and any associated aortic or mitral atresia. The neonate's chest radiograph will usually reveal cardiomegaly; and pulmonary vascular markings may be increased with evidence of interstitial edema.[370]

A cardiac catheterization is only performed if surgical intervention is planned or if echocardiographic findings are somewhat equivocal.

■ Medical and surgical treatment and nursing interventions

Many neonates with hypoplastic left heart syndrome die before they can be transferred to a tertiary care center or before diagnostic studies are completed. In many centers, this defect is considered inoperable, and the neonate is allowed to die without vigorous intervention. Prostaglandin E_1 may be administered intravenously to keep the ductus arteriosus open until the diagnosis is established (see the section on hypoxemia).

During the past several years, several palliative and corrective procedures for infants with hypoplastic left heart syndrome have been proposed. Each proposed procedure would require that the infant undergo several operations before "correction" could be achieved, and long-term results of such procedures are not yet available.[313,314] If such a procedure is to be attempted, the neonate will receive prostaglandin E_1 preoperatively. The short- and long-term risks and the palliative nature of the procedure will be explained to the infant's parents. At this time, such procedures are still considered to be experimental; it is not clear if these infants will be able to survive for any length of time after the first (or second, or third) palliative operation, and it is not clear if such children will ever be able to lead an active life should such survival occur. As a result some physicians recommend against such a procedure, and some parents request that the surgery not be performed.

If the newborn with hypoplastic left heart syndrome is allowed to die, the nurse's skills and support must be focused on the parents. They should be allowed to be with their infant as much as possible, if that is their wish. Occasionally, the parents are not able to remain constantly at the bedside; in this case it can be very comforting for them to know that a nurse will be holding the baby and keeping the baby comfortable.

■ MYOCARDITIS
■ Etiology

Myocarditis is an inflammatory process that involves the cardiac muscle. It can be caused by almost any pathogen, including bacteria, virus, rickettsia, fungus, protozoa, or parasites, although most known cases of myocarditis in the United States are associated with a viral illness, a systemic infection, or active infective endocarditis. Noninfectious myocarditis may be caused by systemic diseases such as systemic lupus erythematosis, or polyarteritis nodosa. The incidence of myocarditis in pediatric patients is unknown since it is thought that many milder cases remain undiagnosed. Severe cases of myocarditis, however, can produce severe cardiac dysfunction and have been associated with sudden death in children.

■ Pathophysiology

Once the pathogen invades the myocardium, it produces either temporary or permanent damage to the myocardial structure; it can interfere with normal myocardial cell function, resulting in necrosis of some myocardial tissue. In addition, an inflammatory response results in infiltration of the involved area with white blood cells, predominantly polymorphonuclear leukocytes, and the possible formation of antigen-antibody complexes. Over time, necrotic muscle is reabsorbed as infiltration with leukocytes continues. Ultimately, the necrotic area of muscle is replaced with scar tissue. Focal hemorrhage, edema, fatty infiltration of the muscle, and fibrosis may also result.

Although most patients with myocarditis appear to recover from an acute episode with little or no sequelae, some patients develop progressive cardiac dilation with decreased ventricular function and AV valve insufficiency. In other patients, the primary manifestations of the disease are arrhythmias, including those producing sudden death; these patients may demonstrate no signs of myocardial dysfunction.

■ Clinical signs and symptoms

Most children with myocarditis will have a history of bacterial or viral illness or of systemic disease known to be associated with the development of myocarditis. Typically, the child will have fever, tachycardia disproportionate to the degree of fever present, arrhythmias, and signs of congestive heart failure, including a gallop rhythm, tachypnea, and signs of systemic and pulmonary venous engorgement (see the section on clinical signs and symptoms of congestive heart failure in this chapter). The child's parents may note that the child seems lethargic, and the child may complain of chest pain, weakness, myalgia, or constant fatigue.

If significant myocardial dysfunction is present, the child may have signs of poor systemic perfusion or low cardiac output (see the section on clinical signs and symptoms of low cardiac output in this chapter). A systolic tricuspid or mitral murmur may be noted that is consistent with the development of AV valvular insufficiency as the result of progressive ventricular dilation. Pulsus alternans may be noted as the result of decreased ventricular contractility, and a pericardial or pleural friction rub may also be present.

The ECG is occasionally normal, although it frequently reveals nonspecific S-T segment changes consistent with myocardial injury. Diffuse myocarditis characteristically produces a decrease in the QRS and T-wave voltage. Arrhythmias, including premature atrial or ventricular contractions, supraventricular or ventricular tachycardia, heart block, or bundle branch block may be noted. The echocardiogram is necessary to rule out the presence of structural heart disease, and it will enable evaluation of heart size, ventricular contractility, and AV valve function. The echocardiogram will also confirm the presence of any significant pericardial effusion. Radionuclide imaging may be used to assess ventricular function. The chest radiograph of the symptomatic child will reveal cardiomegaly, although this may be difficult to separate from the increase in the size of the cardiac silhouette produced by a pericardial effusion. Pleural effusions may also be noted on the radiograph.

If there is any question about the presence of structural heart disease, pulmonary hypertension, or severe ventricular dysfunction with AV valve disease, a cardiac catheterization may be performed. It usually confirms the presence of elevated ventricular end-diastolic pressures; the presence of poor ventricular contractility and tricuspid or mitral valve insufficiency can then be confirmed with angiography. During the catheterization, the cardiologist may perform an endomyocardial biopsy to allow histologic grading of the myocarditis and possible delineation of the causative organism.

The child with myocarditis typically has an elevated erythrocyte sedimentation rate and a rise in serum myocardial enzymes. Bacterial or viral cultures may identify the causative organism in infectious myocarditis, but such cultures are often negative. Myocarditis must be differentiated from acute rheumatic fever and symptoms resulting from systemic arteriovenous fistula.

■ **Medical treatment and nursing interventions**

Treatment of the child with myocarditis includes treatment of the underlying infection or disease (if identified), maximization of ventricular function, and prevention, early detection, and treatment of possible complications of the myocarditis (including congestive heart failure, low cardiac output, and arrhythmias). Since the symptomatic child with myocarditis is at risk for the development of serious arrhythmias and sudden death, he is often admitted to the critical-care unit for continuous electrocardiographic monitoring and observation.

If an infectious agent is identified, the child may require isolation or treatment with antimicrobial agents. The physician may recommend that the child be maintained on bedrest to reduce cardiac output requirements. Fever should be treated with antipyretics once the appropriate cultures have been obtained since fever will increase oxygen consumption and myocardial work.

Use of corticosteroids in the treatment of myocarditis is controversial since the steroids can suppress the child's immune response, resulting in a progression of the initial infectious process. Occasionally, however, if the myocarditis produces severe complications, including malignant arrhythmias refractory to medical management, corticosteroids may be administered in an attempt to reduce myocardial inflammation.

Treatment of congestive heart failure requires fluid restriction, administration of diuretics, possible digitalization, and the use of inotropic support or vasodilator therapy as necessary (see the section on medical treatment and nursing interventions for congestive heart failure in this chapter). Treatment of low cardiac output requires maintenance of an adequate circulating blood volume, correction of electrolyte or acid-base imbalances, and use of inotropic

and vasodilator therapy (this management is discussed in the section on medical treatment and nursing interventions for low cardiac output in this chapter). Treatment of arrhythmias requires administration of antiarrhythmic drugs, although these medications should be used with caution since many of them also depress myocardial contractility. Therefore, if antiarrhythmic therapy is prescribed, the nurse must assess the child carefully for signs of decreased systemic perfusion and notify a physician immediately if these occur. If arrhythmias remain unresponsive to pharmacologic therapy, esophageal or transvenous pacing wires may be inserted to allow overdrive pacing (see the section on medical treatment and nursing interventions for arrhythmias in this chapter).

If the child with myocarditis has a significant pericardial effusion, he should be watched closely for signs of cardiac tamponade, including a rise in central venous pressure, poor systemic perfusion, and pulsus paradoxus. Pericardiocentesis or pericardial drainage may be required to decompress the pericardium (pericardiocentesis is discussed in more detail in Appendix A).

Throughout the child's care, both the child and family will require sensitive support and provision of clear, concise, and consistent information. If the child is admitted with signs of low cardiac output or malignant arrhythmias, the prognosis is usually guarded, and the possibility of sudden death is a real and frightening one for the child, the parents, and the nursing staff. The parents should be allowed to remain with the child as often as is feasible; this will probably reduce their anxiety and the child's fear of his surroundings. The nurse must be able to recognize early signs of deterioration in the child's cardiovascular function, and she must be able to respond quickly and begin cardiopulmonary resuscitation if arrhythmias result in a fall in systemic arterial pressure to inadequate levels (e.g., a systolic blood pressure less than approximately 40 mm Hg in the infant, 50 mm Hg in the child, or 60 mm Hg in the adolescent—the child's previous systolic blood pressure, mean arterial pressure, and systemic perfusion must also be taken into consideration).

■ **CARDIOMYOPATHY**
■ **Etiology**

A cardiomyopathy, in its broadest sense, is any abnormality of the ventricular myocardium; most commonly, the term is used to indicate myocardial disease unrelated to congenital heart disease, pulmonary or systemic hypertension, or coronary artery or valvular heart disease. It may be idiopathic in origin, or it may be secondary to a systemic disease, to a viral infection, or to exposure to chemicals or drugs. Some forms of cardiomyopathy are thought to be genetically transmitted. In most patients, the cause of the cardiomyopathy is never known.

■ Pathophysiology

Three forms of cardiomyopathies are commonly identified: dilated congestive cardiomyopathy, hypertrophic cardiomyopathy, and restrictive/obliterative cardiomyopathy. A discussion of each of these follows. All forms of cardiomyopathy are associated with ventricular dysfunction, decreased ventricular ejection fraction, and an increase in myocardial mass.

In *dilated congestive cardiomyopathy* (also known as idiopathic dilated cardiomyopathy or congestive cardiomyopathy), the ventricles dilate and contract poorly. As a result the ejection fraction is reduced, and the ventricular end-systolic volume and end-diastolic pressure are increased. Thus the right and left atrial pressures are increased, and atrial dilation develops. The child usually demonstrates signs of congestive heart failure with systemic and pulmonary venous engorgement. Since the ejection fraction is low, there may be stasis of blood in the apices of the heart, resulting in the formation of intraventricular thrombi that can embolize into the pulmonary or systemic circulations. Histologic examination reveals the presence of either hypertrophied or atrophied myocardial cells without the evidence of inflammation and leukocytosis typical of myocarditis.

Hypertrophic cardiomyopathy is also described as *idiopathic hypertrophic subaortic stenosis* (IHSS), or hypertrophic obstructive cardiomyopathy. Although this disease generally appears in the second or third decade of life, it does occasionally produce symptoms during childhood and may be a rapidly progressive and fatal disease. The characteristic feature of this form of cardiomyopathy is the progressive and assymmetrical thickening of the myocardium, especially in the area of the ventricular septum. The thickened myocardium encroaches on the ventricular cavity so that the cavity size is dramatically diminished; left and right ventricular outflow tract obstruction may develop. Histologic examination of the myocardium demonstrates an abnormal and disorganized arrangement of myocardial cells, myofibrils, and myofilaments. Approximately half of involved patients have an abnormally large number of thickened intramural coronary arteries. Hypertrophic cardiomyopathy usually produces a decrease in ventricu-

lar compliance and ejection fraction, and it can result in the development of mitral regurgitation, arrhythmias, congestive heart failure, or low cardiac output. Many children with this form of cardiomyopathy have first-degree relatives with similar heart disease, and sudden death is frequently reported in involved family members. Sudden death is presumably the result of a ventricular arrhythmia or progressive and critical left ventricular outflow tract obstruction.

Restrictive/obliterative cardiomyopathy is the least common form of cardiomyopathy reported in children in the United States; it occurs more commonly in equatorial countries and is thought to be related to repeated tropical infections. With this form of cardiomyopathy, endocardial, subendocardial, or myocardial lesions are present that prevent adequate ventricular diastolic expansion. If endocardial fibrosis is present, it may be noted as a distinct disease entity (called *endomyocardial fibrosis* [EMF] or Leffler's disease), or it may be noted in association with bacterial endocarditis or eosinophilic leukemia. As the endocardial or myocardial lesions progress, ventricular expansion during diastole is restricted so that ventricular end-diastolic pressures are increased, and stroke volume may begin to fall. Eventually, the ventricular lumen may be obstructed by fibrotic tissue and thrombus formation. These ventricular thrombi can also embolize into the pulmonary or systemic circulation. Signs of systemic and pulmonary venous engorgement develop, and mitral regurgitation and low cardiac output may be present.

■ Clinical signs and symptoms

Some children with cardiomyopathy remain asymptomatic during childhood, with only minimal evidence of ventricular dysfunction. However, once the disease progresses to the point where symptoms develop, significant myocardial involvement is usually present, and the child often demonstrates signs of congestive heart failure, low cardiac output, or serious arrhythmias. The child may be extremely lethargic with decreased exercise tolerance. He may also complain of chest pain. Occasional patients are asymptomatic except during times that arrhythmias are present; sudden death may be the first sign of disease in these children.

A systolic murmur is often noted along the left sternal border in children with cardiomyopathy; this may be caused by progressive left ventricular outflow tract obstruction (in the child with hypertrophic cardiomyopathy) or by mitral regurgitation. Other signs of left ventricular outflow tract obstruction, including chest pain and syncope, may be noted (see the section on clinical signs and symptoms of aortic stenosis). If ventricular dysfunction is present, peripheral pulses may vary in intensity, and a diffuse apical impulse will be present. The ECG is usually abnormal, although no specific criteria are diagnostic for cardiomyopathy. Usually, evidence of left (and possible right) ventricular hypertrophy, S-T segment changes consistent with myocardial injury, or arrhythmias are noted. Evidence of atrial hypertrophy may also be present. The echocardiogram demonstrates the presence of ventricular dilation, disproportionate ventricular septal thickening, or possible obstruction of the left and/or right ventricular outflow tracts. The chest radiograph may reveal a normal or increased cardiothoracic ratio; if significant left ventricular dysfunction is present, pulmonary venous engorgement and interstitial edema may also be noted.

Cardiac catheterization is often performed to rule out structural heart disease (such as congenital mitral insufficiency or a septal defect). In addition, the study may be performed to assess AV valve competence or degree of left ventricular outflow tract obstruction or to enable performance of an endomyocardial biopsy.

■ Medical and surgical treatment and nursing interventions

The child with cardiomyopathy requires treatment of any reversible cause of the myopathy (such as drug intoxication) and careful management of congestive heart failure, low cardiac output, and arrhythmias.

Management of the congestive heart failure or low cardiac output usually requires fluid restriction and careful diuresis; however, serious intravascular volume depletion and electrolyte imbalance must be prevented since these may depress cardiac output further. Use of beta-adrenergic agonists may be useful in the treatment of dilated congestive cardiomyopathy but is contraindicated if the child has hypertrophic cardiomyopathy since they may contribute to the development of further ventricular hypertrophy and increased left ventricular outflow tract obstruction. Vasodilator therapy is also often successful in improving systemic perfusion in the presence of low cardiac output; this therapy is also often successful in the treatment of dilated congestive cardiomyopathy but is contraindicated in the child with hypertrophic cardiomyopathy since it may critically reduce cardiac output. Propranolol is often prescribed for the child with hypertrophic cardiomyopathy (0.15 to 0.25 mg/kg/IV dose, then 1 to 2 mg/kg/oral dose every 6 hours)

since it seems to reduce the progressive left ventricular outflow tract obstruction. This drug has also had limited success in the treatment of dilated congestive cardiomyopathy. Use of corticosteroids is controversial in these patients and appears to be most successful in the management of endomyocardial fibrosis. Use of digitalis derivatives is also controversial; if this drug is administered, smaller doses are usually prescribed, and the patient must be watched closely for signs of digitalis toxicity (see the section on medical treatment and nursing interventions for congestive heart failure). This drug is contraindicated in patients with hypertrophic cardiomyopathy.

Prevention or treatment of arrhythmias (particularly those that produce sudden death) can be extremely difficult in these patients since antiarrhythmic drugs usually produce myocardial depression. The child is usually placed on 24-hour electrocardiographic monitoring, and a physician should be notified of any arrhythmias (see the section on medical treatment and nursing interventions for arrhythmias in this chapter). If the child with severe and irreversible cardiac dysfunction is thought to be at risk for the development of sudden malignant arrhythmias, the medical team and the family should discuss the plan for resuscitation before any arrest, and any restrictions in resuscitation that are desired should be written clearly by a physician in the form of an order. This prevents unwanted and vigorous resuscitation in the child with irreversible cardiomyopathy, and it protects the child, the family, and the medical team from any confusion. Regardless of the child's prognosis, it will be extremely difficult, but necessary, to avoid focusing constant attention on the child's ECG. Each member of the health care team should make an effort to express an interest in the child before immediately beginning examination of the child or the ECG.

If the child has developed intraventricular or intraatrial thrombi, anticoagulant therapy will be required.

If aggressive medical management of low cardiac output fails to control the child's symptoms, palliative surgical intervention is occasionally performed. If the child has severe and symptomatic AV valve insufficiency, the tricuspid or the mitral valves may be replaced. If hypertrophic cardiomyopathy is producing severe left ventricular outflow tract obstruction, a cardiomyectomy (removal of some of this muscle) may be attempted (see the section on medical and surgical treatment and nursing interventions for aortic stenosis). If the child has severe endomyocardial fibrosis, surgical resection of the fibrotic endocardial tissue may be attempted. The mortality rate for all of the procedures is high; postoperative complications include low cardiac output, arrhythmias, and bleeding.

Both medical and surgical treatment of symptomatic children with cardiomyopathy have poor results. A significant number of these children develop progressive debilitation from low cardiac output or arrhythmias, and many die suddenly. It is important to note, however, that some children *do* demonstrate significant improvement in exercise tolerance and ventricular performance as a result of medical therapy or regression of the disease. In any event, the child will usually be hospitalized for a long period of time and will require careful attention to nutrition, physical therapy, and emotional support. The medical team should meet regularly with the child and family so that communication remains consistent and clear and so that the family can receive regular reports of the child's progress. The child (as appropriate) should be allowed to participate in decisions about his health care.

■ Common Diagnostic Tests

■ ECHOCARDIOGRAPHY
■ Definition

Echocardiography is a painless, noninvasive diagnostic test. It involves the transmission of high-frequency, pulsed-sound waves into the chest and the reception and recording of those sound waves as they are reflected back to a receiver. Since very high-frequency sound waves are used, the term *ultrasound* has also been used to describe the technique. Since all of the tissues in the body will impede or absorb high-frequency sound waves in a different way, the sound waves reflected back to the receiver will be of differing strengths. When these reflected sound waves are amplified and displayed on an oscilloscope or on photosensitive paper, an image of the tissues will be created. Echocardiography uses the high-frequency pulsed-sound waves to generate an image of the heart, great vessels, and pericardium.[13,120,308] These reflected sound waves and resultant images can be used to evaluate the dimensions of the cardiac chambers and great vessels, the location and motion of cardiac valves, the size and location of septal defects, and (to some degree) ventricular function.

Two forms of echocardiography are currently used. *M-mode* (or motion-mode) echocardiography uses a single crystal to obtain an image of the heart at one point; the only axis that is evaluated is depth, so only structures located directly under the transducer

are visualized. Spatial orientation of objects can only be achieved by moving or angling the transducer. *Two-dimensional* or *cross-sectional* echocardiography uses many crystals to pass a planar beam of ultrasound through the heart to obtain an image of a cardiac plane. Because this form of echocardiography can provide a spatially correct image of the heart and great vessels,[120] it is more useful for determination of anatomic relationships of structures within the heart (Fig. 3-40).

■ Procedure

Echocardiography can be performed at the bedside or in the echocardiography laboratory, and it does not require any specific preparation. The infant or child is placed in a reclining or semireclining position at the start of the procedure, and it may be necessary to turn the patient occasionally during the procedure. Since the images produced during the echocardiogram will be blurred by motion artifact, it is very important that the infant or child be motionless during the procedure. Usually, the infant will be quieted with use of a pacifier or during feeding with a bottle. If all attempts at holding and quieting the infant fail, however, the physician may elect to prescribe a mild (non-narcotic) sedative for the infant. The cooperation of the older child must be won, and it may be useful to allow the child to see his heart working on the oscilloscope. The room or bedside must be somewhat darkened during the recording of the echo so that the images on the oscilloscope can be seen easily.[280]

A single, flat-tipped transducer that is approximately 6 inches in length, is used to obtain the echocardiogram; this transducer sends and receives the sound waves. To minimize artifact and maximize sound transmission, small amounts of electrocardiographic gel or paste are applied to the child's chest, where the transducer will be placed. During the procedure, the infant or child merely feels the touch of the transducer and gel. This procedure is painless.

Occasionally, bubbled saline, dextrose water, or blood is injected into one of the child's veins as the echocardiogram is recorded; this is called *contrast echocardiography*. As the injected fluid enters the child's heart, better visualization of anatomic relationships and better evaluation of intracardiac shunts and blood flow patterns can be made.[6] If an IV line is already in place, the contrast material is simply injected through the existing catheter. However, if no IV catheter is in place, a venipuncture will be required to perform the procedure. If a venipuncture and contrast studies are planned, the nurse must

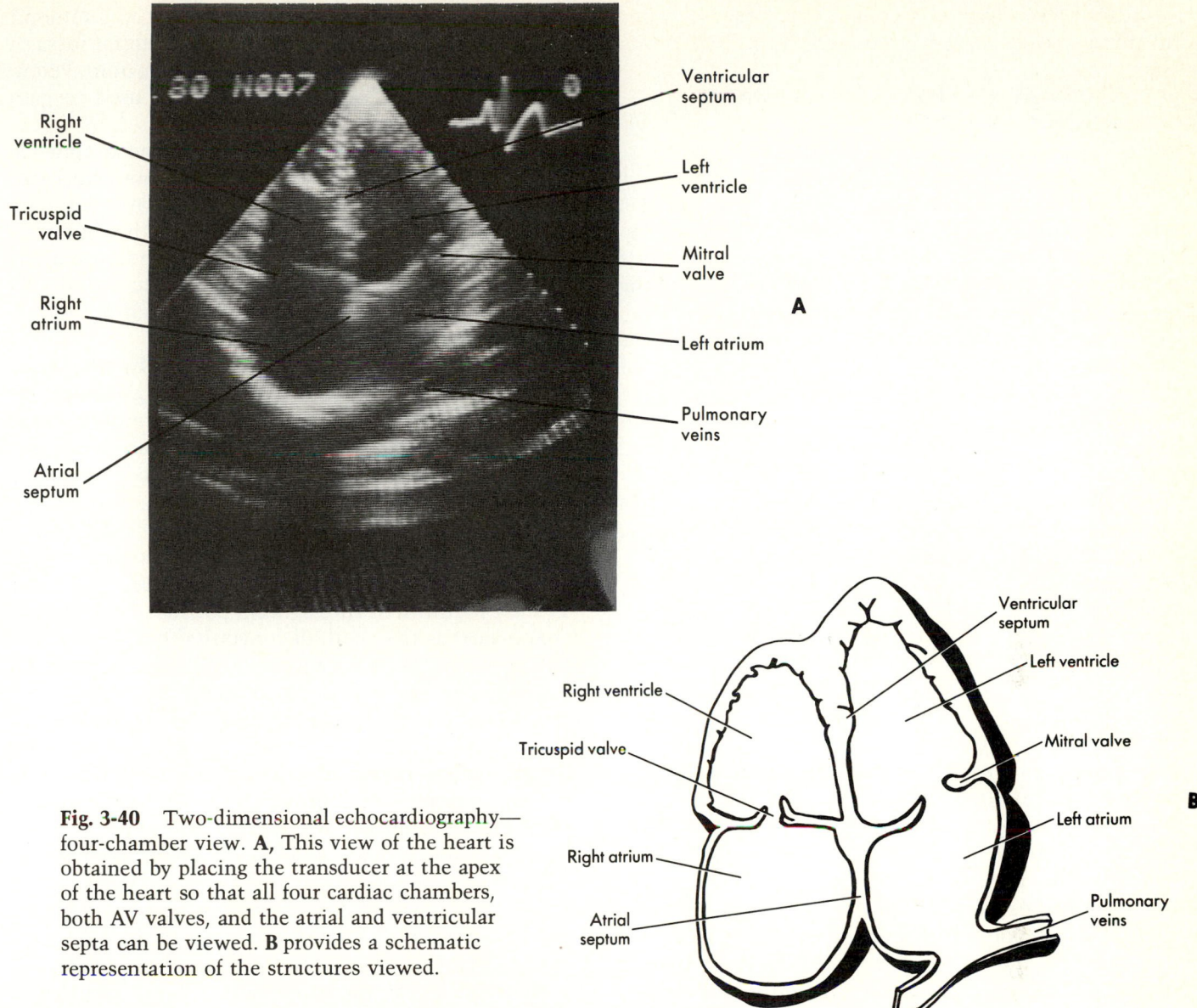

Fig. 3-40 Two-dimensional echocardiography—four-chamber view. **A,** This view of the heart is obtained by placing the transducer at the apex of the heart so that all four cardiac chambers, both AV valves, and the atrial and ventricular septa can be viewed. **B** provides a schematic representation of the structures viewed.

modify her preparation of the child for echocardiography since a simple "echo" will not be painful, but a contrast echo may require a painful venipuncture.

■ **Potential complications**

There are no known complications of simple echocardiography.[272] However, adequate care must be taken to keep the critically ill infant or child warm and comfortable during the procedure. If contrast echocardiography is performed when the child has an intracardiac right-to-left shunt, there is the possibility that an air embolus can result; for this reason, contrast studies are usually avoided in children with cyanotic heart disease.

■ **Nursing interventions**

There is no specific nursing care required before, during, or after simple echocardiography. It is important that the nurse observe the patient carefully throughout the procedure, and keep him warm. The study will progress more quickly if the nurse is able to help keep the infant or child quiet, content, and motionless. Often, this requires creativity and a lot of patience. The nurse should keep a bottle (unless the infant can have nothing by mouth) and pacifier nearby during echocardiography of the infant, and several toys available during echocardiography of the child. Children often enjoy watching their heart "on TV."

Several excellent reviews of pediatric echocardiography have been written, and the nurse is referred to these sources for further information.[368,369,398]

■ **CARDIAC CATHETERIZATION AND ANGIOCARDIOGRAPHY**
■ **Definition**

Cardiac catheterization involves insertion of a radiopaque catheter through an artery and/or vein into the heart. The procedure is performed under fluoroscopy so that the location and movement of the catheter can be seen. Throughout the catheterization, pressure measurements are made and blood samples are drawn via the catheter to provide information about pressures and oxygen saturations within the heart chambers and great vessels. Pressure measurements can demonstrate the presence and severity of obstruction to blood flow (such as that caused by valvular disease), and abnormal oxygen saturations confirm the presence and magnitude of intracardiac or intrapulmonary shunting.

Specific structures, such as cardiac chambers, valves, or great vessels, can be visualized through injection of a radiopaque contrast agent. If such an injection is made, rapid, sequential radiographs, called *angiograms*, are made to record the flow of contrast through the heart. Two excellent references are currently available[165,360] that provide excellent reviews of the technique of cardiac catheterization and analysis of the data gathered.

■ **Procedure***

Cardiac catheterization is performed in a catheterization laboratory where appropriate catheters and radiographic equipment are located. As a result the patient must be transported to and from the catheterization laboratory; if the patient is critically ill, a critical-care nurse usually remains with the patient throughout the study.

The infant or child usually receives nothing by mouth before the catheterization to minimize the possibility of vomiting and aspiration during the procedure. Some form of sedation is usually prescribed for the patient before the catheterization, and additional sedation may be administered during the procedure.

When catheterization is performed during infancy, the patient's right femoral artery and vein are used for the procedure; the umbilical vessels may be

*NOTE: In the interest of simplicity, the description of the catheterization procedure assumes that there are normally related atria, ventricles, and great vessels.

used in the neonate. In the older child, the femoral artery and vein, or vessels in the antecubital fossa or axilla may be used for the catheterization. Percutaneous puncture or cutdown may be used to gain access to the artery or vein.

Right heart catheterization is accomplished through insertion of a catheter into a vein; this catheter is then passed into the superior or inferior vena cava and into the right atrium and then the right ventricle and pulmonary artery. Pressure measurements and oxygen saturation analyses are made initially to detect the presence and location of abnormal chamber hypertension or intracardiac shunts.

The left heart can often be entered by passage of the catheter from the right atrium through the patent foramen ovale to the left atrium. If the cardiologist is not able to enter the left atrium from the right atrium, a catheter can be inserted into a systemic artery, retrograde into the aorta and then into the left ventricle.

When all necessary pressure and oxygen saturation measurements have been recorded, an angiogram is then performed. Angiograms portray the shunting that occurs as the result of congenital heart defects or valvular dysfunction, and will document areas of narrowing or dilation in blood flow pathways.

Associated procedures may be accomplished during cardiac catheterization. His bundle mapping can be performed using an electrically sensitive catheter within the ventricles. Transvenous intracardiac pacing wires may also be inserted during catheterization and fluoroscopy, and overdrive pacing may be performed for refractory arrhythmias. Atrial septal defects may be created (through use of a balloon-tipped catheter) or closed (using an umbrella-tipped catheter).[276,431] Patients may be exercised during the catheterization to monitor effects of exercise on cardiac output, intracardiac shunts, or aortic stenosis. The child may also be asked to breathe from a bag containing hydrogen or nitrogen gas, and the rapidity of the hydrogen or nitrogen circulation will be measured and recorded to detect intracardiac shunts. Medication may also be administered during the catheterization to allow detailed assessment of the patient's hemodynamic response. Recently, percutaneous transluminal angioplasty has been used to successfully dilate a restenotic area of coarctation repair during cardiac catheterization.[218a]

At the end of the catheterization procedure, the catheters are removed, and pressure is applied to the puncture site or the cutdown is sutured. The infant or child is returned to the unit for close observation. If the child is normally ambulatory, the physician will usually request that the child remain in bed for several hours after the catheterization.

■ Potential complications

If cardiac catheterization is performed electively on a stable child, the mortality is less than 1%, and morbidity is low. If, however, the procedure is performed on an emergency basis on a critically ill patient, the morbidity and mortality will be higher. The risks of catheterization are also increased for infants and children with pulmonary hypertension, arrhythmias, or hypoxemia, and for those children with tetralogy of Fallot who have a history of hypercyanotic episodes (see the section on tetralogy of Fallot in this chapter).

Complications following catheterization in infants and children include arrhythmias, bleeding, cardiac perforation, tamponade, cerebrovascular accident, contrast agent reactions, and local vascular complications (e.g., thrombosis within the femoral artery or hematoma).[192,296,379,404]

■ Nursing interventions

If the infant requires cardiac catheterization, the nurse must ensure that the parents understand the purpose of the procedure. It is also important to emphasize that the infant will receive sedation as well as analgesics so that the infant will not be uncomfortable during the procedure, and that he may sleep deeply for several hours after the procedure.

When the child requires cardiac catheterization, explanations should be given according to the level of the child's interest and comprehension. The young child should not be prepared too far in advance or with extensive detail since this can cause more anxiety than it alleviates. In addition, it is important for the child to be prepared for what he will *see, hear,* and *feel.* Older children, on the other hand, may appreciate more detailed explanations of the purpose of the catheterization and the procedures involved. It is important that the child know that he will probably receive some medicine that will help to keep him sleepy during the catheterization, and that the cardiologist can administer additional medication during the procedure itself to minimize pain. Most children benefit from a precatheterization visit to the catheterization laboratory if it is at all possible. Excellent articles have been written regarding preparation of the child for cardiac catheterization, and the reader is referred to these sources[415,425,454] and to Chapter 2 for further information.

During transport of the critically ill infant or child to and from the catheterization laboratory, it is the nurse's responsibility to ensure continuation of all mechanical and pharmacologic support. This means that the nurse should constantly assess the patient's cardiorespiratory function, the adequacy of the oxygen supply, and the accuracy and function of any IV pumps. Any IV lines should be taped securely to prevent dislodgement during patient movement. If an ET tube is in place, it must also be taped securely, and provisions must be made to provide supplemental oxygen and to perform endotracheal suctioning and hand ventilation in the catheterization laboratory. If the patient requires ventilatory assistance, this must be provided without interruption during the transport to and from the catheterization laboratory and throughout the procedure itself.

During the catheterization, the critical-care nurse should frequently assess the patient's cardiorespiratory function and notify the cardiologist of any problems. The nurse is often best able to comfort the infant or child since she may be the most familiar person near the patient. The nurse can keep the child informed of the progress of the test, and often prepare the child for any unexpected procedures. Since many older children feel warm or short of breath during an angiogram (as the result of the contrast injection), it is good to remind the child that he might feel warm just before the angiogram is performed so that the child will not be alarmed by unexpected sensations.

Throughout the catheterization procedure the nurse should be prepared to assist with emergency resuscitation measures. Such measures are rarely necessary, but if they are needed, they must be performed quickly and expertly. As a result the nurse should also ensure that there is appropriate emergency equipment available in the catheterization laboratory.

During and following catheterization, the nurse should monitor the infant or child very closely for any evidence of arrhythmias, bleeding from the catheterization site, cardiac perforation, tamponade, neurologic complications, contrast agent reactions, and vascular complications. These are discussed in the care plan in Table 3-18.[180]

■ Conclusions

This chapter has reviewed the normal structure and function of the cardiovascular system, common cardiovascular problems that require critical care, postoperative care of the child requiring cardiovas-

Text continued on p. 240.

Table 3-18 Care of the child requiring cardiac catheterization

Nursing diagnosis	Expected outcomes	Nursing activities

A. Patient and family anxiety related to patient health status and anticipated catheterization	1. Patient and family will demonstrate comprehension of preparation for procedure, catheterization itself, and post-catheterization care
	2. Patient and family anxiety will not interfere with appropriate activity
		1. Orient patient and family to nursing care unit, policies, personnel, and catheterization laboratory (as appropriate)
		2. Orient patient and family to precatheterization preparation:
		  a. Chest x-ray examination
		  b. Blood tests
		  c. Appropriate medications (including withholding of anticoagulants before catheterization, as needed)
		  d. Need for NPO before catheterization
		  e. Premedication (include possible side effects such as dry mouth, possible blurred vision, as appropriate)
		3. Instruct patient (as appropriate) and family on procedure itself—especially on those aspects that patient will see, hear, or feel—the length of the procedure, and the postcatheterization appearance of catheterization site
		4. Discuss postcatheterization care with patient (as appropriate) and family:
		  a. Need for bedrest
		  b. Postcatheterization feeding orders
		  c. Required care of catheterization site (include need for immobility, ice packs, etc.)
		  d. Frequency of vital sign measurement
		5. If patient is a child over the age of 2, toys or puppets may be used to demonstrate the experiences the child will remember; in preparing any child for catheterization, the nurse must be sensitive to the cues of the child and only prepare the child with information he can handle; if the child has little concept of time intervals, preparation just before injections and separation from parents may be appropriate
		6. During and following the catheterization procedure, provide support and simple explanations of catheterization results; orient patient to time and place frequently while patient is recovering from sedation

B. Possible decrease in cardiac output related to arrhythmia, reaction to sedation or contrast medium, hemorrhage or cardiac perforation	1. Patient will demonstrate stable cardiac output as measured by: a. Adequate blood pressure	1. Note occurrence of any arrhythmias during catheterization procedure 2. Monitor patient vital signs, level of consciousness, and signs of perfusion frequently; note tachycardia, bradycardia, and effect on cardiac output; notify physician

Modified from Hazinski, M.F.: Cardiac catheterization. In Johanson, B.C., and others, editors: Standards for critical care, ed. 2, St. Louis, 1984, The C.V. Mosby Co.

Table 3-18 Care of the child requiring cardiac catheterization—cont'd

Nursing diagnosis	Expected outcomes	Nursing activities
B. Possible decrease in cardiac output related to arrhythmia, reaction to sedation or contrast medium, hemorrhage or cardiac perforation—cont'd	b. Good peripheral perfusion c. Regular cardiac rhythm and rate d. Minimal bleeding from catheterization site e. Good urine output (0.5-1.0 ml/kg/hr)	a. Normal adult heart rate range: 50-75 (note precatheterization range) b. Normal pediatric heart rate ranges: Newborn: 120-160 Toddler: 90-140 Preschooler: 80-110 School-age child: 75-100 Adolescent: 60-90 (note precatheterization ranges) 3. Notify physician of any episodes of hypotension a. Newborn (systolic): 60-90 b. Toddler (systolic): 80-112 c. Preschooler (systolic): 82-110 d. School-age (systolic): 84-120 e. Adolescent (systolic): 94-140 (see Table 3-2 for further information) 4. Notify physician of any arrhythmias (obtain rhythm strip during episodes and monitor blood pressure—have emergency equipment ready) 5. Monitor catheterization site and dressing for evidence of bleeding (dressing saturated with blood or formation of hematoma); if bleeding is excessive, notify physician, obtain hematocrit and carefully monitor blood pressure 6. Monitor for indirect evidence of low cardiac output (cool, clammy extremities, decreased urine output, altered level of consciousness); notify physician if it is observed 7. Monitor for signs of cardiac tamponade (pallor, tachycardia, hepatomegaly, jugular venous distention, decreased blood pressure, decreased pulse pressure, decreased heart sounds, restlessness, cool extremities); notify physician if present (and be prepared for emergency measures) 8. Infants must be kept *warm* during and following cardiac catheterization, especially if they have low cardiac output; their oxygen requirements increase dramatically if a neutral thermal environment is not provided (see Appendix G)

Continued.

Table 3-18 Care of the child requiring cardiac catheterization—cont'd

Nursing diagnosis	Expected outcomes	Nursing activities

C. Possible compromise of circulation to catheterized extremity	1. Perfusion of catheterized extremity is good as measured by:
	a. Warmth
	b. Pink nail beds
	c. Good pulses
	d. Brisk capillary refill
	e. Adequate movement and sensation (use opposite limb for comparison)
		1. If arterial catheterization was performed:
		a. Monitor pulses of extremity distal to catheterization site—notify physician *immediately* of *any* decrease in intensity of pulses; if spasm or thrombus occurs in artery, distal artery can rapidly become clotted, and ischemia of extremity will result; in severe cases, this may ultimately require amputation of extremity, so *prompt* attention must be given
		b. Monitor color and warmth of extremity for reasons noted above
		  NOTE: When arterial circulation is compromised, extremity usually will become "mottled" rather than cyanotic and will become cool; notify physician immediately if either occurs; application of heat to the *contralateral* extremity may help maintain circulation to the catheterized extremity (by producing reflex vasodilation), but heat should *never* be applied to involved extremity, as it merely increases oxygen requirements of already compromised tissue
		c. If thrombus is present, it will require surgical removal; a heparin drip may be ordered to prevent further thrombosis
		d. Attempt to prevent flexion of extremity at catheterization site (this may require frequent repositioning of patient's extremity and gentle reminders)
		e. Maintain bedrest for 6-12 hr postcatheterization (as ordered)
		f. Administer pain medication as ordered (and per patient need)
		g. Apply ice to catheterization site, if ordered
		h. Monitor for evidence of excessive edema or bleeding at catheterization site—notify physician if bleeding is not stopped by application of pressure
		2. If venous catheterization was performed:
		a. Monitor pulses of extremity distal to catheter site
		  NOTE: Often the vein used for the catheterization is tied off or becomes obstructed at the end of the procedure, especially in small infants; in this case, the extremity distal to the catheterization site will become edematous and slightly cyanotic, as venous blood is trapped in that extremity; collateral veins will quickly provide venous drainage, but initial discomfort should be expected

Table 3-18 Care of the child requiring cardiac catheterization—cont'd

Nursing diagnosis	Expected outcomes	Nursing activities
C. Possible compromise of circulation to catheterized extremity—cont'd		b. If edema is present, elevate extremity to facilitate venous return; *notify physician immediately if edema causes a decrease in intensity of pulses;* this may indicate compromise of arterial circulation c. Monitor for evidence of bleeding at catheterization site and notify physician if it is not relieved by pressure d. Maintain bedrest for 4-6 hr following catheterization as ordered

D. Possible infection of catheterization site or intracardiac structures	1. Patient will remain free of symptoms of infection
	  a. Fever
	  b. Leukocytosis
	  c. Erythema or drainage at catheterization site
	  d. Evidence of endocarditis
		1. Monitor catheterization site for edema, erythema, heat, and discharge; notify physician if present
		2. Monitor patient temperature; blood cultures are usually recommended if fever >38.5° C occurs
		3. Monitor white blood cell count if infection is suspected
		4. Monitor for evidence of endocarditis (high fever, appearance of new heart murmur, hematuria) and pericarditis (cardiac friction rub, loss of heart tones, ECG changes)
		5. Administer prophylactic antibiotics as ordered

E. Possible compromise in renal function related to response to contrast medium (the very concentrated contrast medium can cause hematuria or oliguria, which should soon be followed by an osmotic diuresis; rarely, anuria may develop)	1. Patient will demonstrate adequate urine output (0.5-1.0 ml/kg/hr)	1. Monitor urine output—notify physician if urine output is inadequate *despite* sufficient fluid intake NOTE: A small child may become rapidly dehydrated when kept NPO for hours while awaiting catheterization—the nurse must ensure that parenteral and/or oral fluid intake is adequate during the period preceding and following the catheterization 2. If patient is anuric despite sufficient fluid intake, fluid intake will then have to be restricted to prevent overload 3. Monitor for evidence of dehydration (depressed fontanelle in infants, dry mucous membranes, decreased urine output with high specific gravity, poor skin turgor) 4. Hematest all urine after the catheterization and report hematuria to a physician

F. Possible respiratory distress related to sedation	1. Patient will demonstrate adequate respiratory function
	  a. Appropriate rate
	  b. Adequate and equal lung aeration bilaterally
		1. Check precatheterization order against recommended dosage for your patient's age and weight before administering; notify physician if sedation ordered is excessive
		2. Monitor respiratory rate and effort and notify physician if either is insufficient or excessive; normal respiratory rates for children:
		  a. Infant: 30-60
		  b. Toddler: 24-40
		  c. Preschooler: 22-34

Continued.

Table 3-18 Care of the child requiring cardiac catheterization—cont'd

Nursing diagnosis	Expected outcomes	Nursing activities
F. Possible respiratory distress related to sedation—cont'd		d. School-age child: 18-30 e. Adolescent: 12-16 3. Auscultate lungs and encourage patient to change position frequently and to cough and breathe deeply; rib-springing exercises or other forms of chest physical therapy may be necessary if aeration is insufficient; notify physician immediately if respiratory effort is insufficient, and begin emergency resuscitative measures as needed
G. Discharge planning	1. Patient and family will receive adequate information to comply with postcatheterization care regime and general health maintenance	1. Provide patient and family with appropriate instruction regarding wound care, physician follow-up appointments, signs of infection, activity restrictions (if any), and medications 2. Discuss implications of catheterization results with patient and family to obtain their perceptions of physician recommendations and to clarify any misconceptions they may have 3. Provide patient and family with aproppriate telephone numbers and locations of health-team members (primary nurse, cardiologist, cardiac surgeon, etc.)

cular surgery, congenital heart defects, inflammatory diseases of the heart, and common diagnostic tests used to assess cardiovascular function. An extensive reference list has been used in the preparation of this material, and the reader is referred to these articles for further information.

REFERENCES

1. Agarwal, K.C., and others: Clinicopathological correlates of obstructed right-sided porcine valved extracardiac conduits, J. Thoracic. Cardiovasc. Surg. **81:**591, 1981.
2. Agarwala, B.N.: Postoperative management of open heart surgery in infants and children, Hosp. Pract. **17:**40c, Feb. 1982.
3. Agarwala, B.N., and Baffes T.: Congestive heart failure in the infant, Heart Lung **5:**62, 1976.
4. Albert, R.K., and Condie, F.: Hand-washing patterns in medical intensive care units. N. Engl. J. Med. **304:**1465, 1981.
5. Alford, C.A., Neva, F.A., and Weller, T.H.: Virologic and serologic studies on human products of conception after maternal rubella, N. Engl. J. Med. **271:**1275, 1964.
6. Allen, H.D., and others: Ultrasound cardiac diagnosis, Pediatr. Clin. North Am. **25:**677, 1978.
7. Alpert, B.S., and others: Plasma indomethacin levels in preterm newborn infants with symptomatic patent ductus arteriosus—clinical and echocardiographic assessments of response, J. Pediatr. **95:**578, 1979.
8. Alpert, B.S., and others: Role of the renin-angiotensin-aldosterone system in hypertensive children with coarctation of the aorta, Am. J. Cardiol. **43:**828, 1979.
9. Alpert, B.S., and others: Spontaneous closure of small ventricular septal defects: 10 year follow up, Pediatrics **63:**204, 1979.
10. Anand, S.K.: Acute renal failure in the neonate, Pediatr. Clin. North Am. **29:**791, 1982.
11. Anderson, R.H., and others: Congenitally complete heart block, Circulation **56:**90, 1977.
12. Ankeney, J.L., Tzeng, T.S., and Liebman, J.: Surgical therapy for congenital aortic valvular stenosis: a 23 year experience, J. Thorac. Cardiovasc. Surg. **85:**41, 1983.
13. Anthony, C.L., Arnon, R.G., and Fitch, C.W.: Pediatric cardiology, New York, 1979, Medical Examination Publishing Company, Inc.
14. Anthony, C.L., Arnon, R.G., and Fitch, C.W.: Pulmonary stenosis. In Pediatric cardiology, New York, 1979, Medical Examination Publishing Company, Inc.

15. Appelbaum, A., and others: Surgical treatment of truncus arteriosus, with emphasis on infants and small children, J. Thorac. Cardiovasc. Surg. **71**:436, 1976.

16. Appelbaum, A., and others: Afterload reduction and cardiac output in infants early after intracardiac surgery, Am. J. Cardiol. **39**:445, 1977.

17. Arciniegas, E., and others: Classic shunting operations for congenital cyanotic heart defects, J. Thorac. Cardiovasc. Surg. **84**:88, 1982.

18. Arensman, F.W., and others: Early medical and surgical intervention for tetralogy of Fallot with absence of pulmonic valve, J. Thorac. Cardiovasc. Surg. **84**:430, 1982.

19. Azzolina, G., and others: Waterston anastomosis in two-stage correction of severe tetralogy of Fallot: ten years experience, Ann. Thorac. Surg. **34**:413, 1982.

20. Baaske, D.M., and others: Nitroglycerin compatability with intravenous fluid filters, containers, and administration sets, Am. J. Hosp. Pharm. **37**:201, 1980.

21. Bailey, L.L., and others: Mustard operation in the first month of life, Am. J. Cardiol. **49**:766, 1982.

22. Barness, L.A.: Manual of pediatric physical diagnosis, ed. 5, Chicago, 1981, Year Book Medical Publishers, Inc.

23. Barold, S., and Friedberg, D.: Second degree atrioventricular block, Am. J. Cardiol. **33**:311, 1974.

24. Bartlett, R.H., and Gazzaniga, A.B.: Extracorporeal circulation for cardiopulmonary failure, Curr. Probl. Surg. **15**(5):1, May 1978, Year Book Medical Publishers, Inc.

25. Bartlett, R.H., and others: Extracorporeal circulation (ECMO) in neonatal respiratory failure, J. Thorac. Cardiovasc. Surg. **74**:826, 1977.

26. Bartlett, R.H., and others: Extracorporeal membrane oxygenator support for cardiopulmonary failure: experience in 28 patients, J. Thorac. Cardiovasc. Surg. **73**:375, 1977.

27. Bateman, T., and others: Right atrial tamponade complicating cardiac operation, J. Thorac. Cardiovasc. Surg. **84**:413, 1982.

28. Baylen, B.G., and others: The occurrence of hyperaldosteronism in infants with congestive heart failure, Am. J. Cardiol. **45**:305, 1980.

29. Behrendt, D.M.: Current results of the Mustard operation for simple dextrotransposition (editorial), Ann. Thorac. Surg. **31**:201, 1981.

30. Behrendt, D.M., and Austen, W.G.: Patient care in cardiac surgery, ed. 2, Boston, 1976, Little, Brown & Co.

31. Behrendt, D.M., and Rosenthal, A.: Cardiovascular status after repair by the Fontan procedure, Ann. Thorac. Surg. **29**:322, 1979.

32. Behrendt, D.M., and others: The Blalock-Hanlon procedure; a new look at an old operation, Ann. Thorac. Surg. **20**:424, 1975.

33. Bell, E.F., and others: Effect of fluid administration on the development of symptomatic patent ductus arteriosus and congestive heart failure in premature infants, N. Engl. J. Med. **302**:598, 1980.

34. Ben-Shachar, G., and others: Separation of neointima from dacron graft causing obstruction: case following Fontan procedure for tricuspid atresia, J. Thorac. Cardiovasc. Surg. **82**:268, 1981.

35. Bender, H.W., and others: Comparative operative results of the Senning and Mustard procedures for transposition of the great arteries, Circulation **62**(suppl. 1): 197, 1980.

36. Bender, H.W., and others: Repair of atrioventricular canal malformation in the first year of life, J. Thorac. Cardiovasc. Surg. **84**:515, 1982.

37. Benson, L.N., and others: Nitroglycerin therapy in children with low cardiac index, Cardiovasc. Med. **4**: 207, 1979.

38. Benson, L.N., and others: Role of prostaglandin E_1 infusion in the management of transposition of the great arteries, Am. J. Cardiol. **44**:691, 1979.

39. Bergdahl, D.M., and others: Prognosis in primary ventricular tachycardia in the pediatric patient, Circulation **62**:897, 1980.

40. Berger, T.J., and others: Primary repair of complete atrioventricular canal in patients less than two years old, Am. J. Cardiol. **41**:906, 1978.

41. Berman, W., Jr.: The relationship of age to the effects and toxicity of digoxin in sheep. In Heymann, M.A., and Rudolph, A.M., co-chairpersons: The ductus arteriosus, Report of the seventy-fifth Ross Conference on Pediatric Research, Columbus, Ohio, 1978, Ross Laboratories, Inc.

42. Bessone, L.N., Ferguson, T.B., and Burford, T.H.: Chylothorax: a collective review, Ann. Thorac. Surg. **12**:527, 1971.

43. Beyer, J.: Atrial septal defect: acute left heart failure after surgical closure, Ann. Thorac. Surg. **25**:36, 1978.

44. Bharati, S., and others: The surgical anatomy of truncus arteriosus communis, J. Thorac. Cardiovasc. Surg. **67**:501, 1974.

45. Bharati, S., and others: Anatomic variations in underdeveloped right ventricle related to tricuspid atresia and stenosis, J. Thorac. Cardiovasc. Surg. **72**:383, 1976.

46. Bharati, S., and others: The anatomic substrate for pre-excitation in corrected transposition, Circulation **62**: 831, 1980.

47. Bharati, S., and others: Surgical anatomy of the atrioventricular valve in the intermediate type of common atrioventricular orifice, J. Thorac. Cardiovasc. Surg. **79**:884, 1980.

48. Biller, J.A., and Yeager, A.M.: The Harriet Lane handbook, ed. 9, Chicago, 1981, Year Book Medical Publishers, Inc.

49. Bjork, V.O., and Henze, A.: Ten years' experience with the Bjork-Shiley tilting disc valve, J. Thorac. Cardiovasc. Surg. **78**:331, 1979.

50. Bloomfield, D.K.: The natural history of ventricular septal defect in patients surviving infancy, Circulation **29**:914, 1964.

51. Blount, S.G.: Cyanosis: pathophysiology and differential diagnosis, Prog. Cardiovasc. Dis. **13**:595, 1971.

52. Bove, E.L., and others: Infradiaphragmatic total anomalous pulmonary venous drainage: surgical treatment and long-term results, Ann. Thorac. Surg. **31:** 544, 1980.

53. Bowman, F.O., and others: Physiological approach to surgery for tricuspid atresia, Circulation **58**(suppl. 1): 83, 1977.

54. Brandfonbrener, M., Landowne, M., and Shock, N.W.: Changes in cardiac output with age, Circulation **12:** 556, 1955.

55. Braunwald, E., and Swan, H.J.C.: Cooperative study on cardiac catheterization, Circulation **37**(suppl. 3):1, 1968.

56. Brewer, L.A., and others: Spinal cord complications following surgery for coarctation of the aorta: a study of 66 cases, J. Thorac. Cardiovasc. Surg. **64:**368, 1972.

57. Calder, L., and others: Truncus arteriosus communis: clinical, angiocardiographic, and pathologic findings in 100 patients, Am. Heart J. **92:**23, 1976.

58. Campbell, M.: Tricuspid atresia and its prognosis with and without surgical treatment, Br. Heart J. **23:**699, 1961.

59. Campbell, M.: Natural history of coarctation of the aorta, Br. Heart J. **32:**633, 1970.

60. Cannon, P.J., and Kilcoyne, M.M.: Ethacrynic acid and furosemide: renal pharmacology and clinical use, Prog. Cardiovasc. Dis. **12:**99, 1969.

61. Carter, C.O.: The effect of successful treatment on the future birth frequency of congenital heart disease, Eur. J. Cardiol. **213:**374, 1975.

62. Chaitman, B.R,., and others: Late development of left ventricular outflow tract obstruction after repair of double outlet right ventricle, J. Thorac. Cardiovasc. Surg. **72:**265, 1978.

63. Chameides, L., and others: Guidelines for defibrillation in infants and children, Report of the American Heart Association target activity group: cardiopulmonary resuscitation in the young, Circulation **56:**502A, 1977.

64. Chesney, R.W., and others: Acute renal failure: an important complication of cardiac surgery in infants, J. Pediatr. **87:**381, 1975.

65. Chiariello, L., and others: Congenital aortic stenosis: experience with 43 patients, J. Thorac. Cardiovasc. Surg. **72:**182, 1976.

66. Chin, A.J., and others: Repair of complete common atrioventricular canal in infancy, J. Thorac. Cardiovasc. Surg. **84:**437, 1982.

67. Clarkson, P.M., and others: The pulmonary vascular bed in patients with complete transposition of the great arteries, Circulation **53:**539, 1976.

68. Coe, J.W., Radley-Smith, R., and Yacoub, M.: Management of tricuspid atresia with orally administered prostaglandin E₂, J. Pediatr. **100:**496, 1982.

69. Cokkinos, D.V., Leachman, R.D., and Cooley, D.A.: Increased mortality rate from coronary artery disease following operation for coarctation of the aorta at a late age, J. Thorac. Cardiovasc. Surg. **77:**315, 1979.

70. Collins-Nakai, R.L., and others: Interrupted aortic arch in infancy, J. Pediatr. **88:**959, 1976.

71. Connor, T.M., and Baker, W.P.: A comparison of coarctation resection and patch angioplasty using postexercise blood pressure measurements, Circulation **64:** 567, 1981.

72. Conover, M.B.: Understanding electrocardiography: physiological and interpretive concepts, ed. 3, St. Louis, 1980, The C.V. Mosby Co.

73. Conway-Rutkowski, B.L.: Autonomic nervous system. In: Carini and Owen's neurological and neurosurgical nursing, ed. 8, St. Louis, 1982, The C.V. Mosby Co.

74. Corone, P., and others: Natural history of ventricular septal defect: a study involving 790 cases, Circulation **55:**908, 1977.

75. Cossum, P.A., and others: Loss of nitroglycerin from intravenous infusion sets, Lancet **2:**349, 1978.

76. Crone, R.K.: Acute circulatory failure in children, Pediatr. Clin. North Am. **27:**525, 1980.

77. Cumming, G.R., and Ferguson, C.C.: Obstruction of superior vena cava after the Mustard operation for transposition of the great arteries: conservative management of chylothorax, J. Thorac. Cardiovasc. Surg. **70:**242, 1975.

78. Curtis, J.J.: Clinical experience with permanent atrioventricular sequential pacing, Ann. Thorac. Surg. **32:** 179, 1981.

79. Dabizzi, R.P., and others: Distribution and anomalies of coronary arteries in tetralogy of Fallot, Circulation **61:**95, 1980.

80. Daskalopoulos, D.A., and others: Closed transventricular pulmonary valvotomy in infants, J. Thorac. Cardiovasc. Surg. **84:**187, 1982.

81. Davignon, A., and others: ECG standards for children: percentile charts, Pediatr. Cardiol. **1:**133, 1979.

82. DeLeon, S.Y., and others: Transmediastinal repair of complex coarctation and interrupted aortic arch, J. Thorac. Cardiovasc. Surg. **82:**98, 1981.

83. DeLeon, S.Y., and others: The role of the Glenn shunt in patients undergoing the Fontan operation, J. Thorac. Cardiovasc. Surg. **85:**669, 1983.

84. deLeval, M.R., and others: Modified Blalock-Taussig shunt: use of subclavian artery orifice as flow regulator in prosthetic systemic-pulmonary artery shunts, J. Thorac. Cardiovasc. Surg. **81:**112, 1981.

85. Delisle, G. and others: Total anomalous pulmonary venous connection: report of 93 autopsied cases with emphasis on diagnostic and surgical considerations, Am. Heart J. **91:**99, 1976.

86. deSwiet, M., Fayers, P., and Shinebourne, E.A.: Systolic blood pressure in a population of infants in the first year of life: the Brompton study, Pediatrics **65:** 1028, 1980.

87. DeTroyer, A., Yerreault, J.C., and Englert, M.: Lung hypoplasia in congenital pulmonary valve stenosis, Circulation **56:**647, 1977.

88. Dick, M., Fyler, D.C., and Nadas, A.S.: Tricuspid atresia: clinical course in 101 patients, Am. J. Cardiol. **36:**327, 1975.

89. Dillon, T.R., and others: Vasodilator therapy for congestive heart failure, J. Pediatr. **96:**623, 1980.

90. Dirks, J.H.: Mechanisms of action and clinical uses of diuretics, Hosp. Pract. **15**:99, 1979.
91. Disch, J.M.: Wound integrity in the patient undergoing cardiac surgery, Nurs. Clin. North Am. **14**:743, 1979.
92. DiSessa, T.G., and others: The cardiovascular effects of dopamine in the severely asphyxiated neonate, J. Pediatr. **99**:772, 1981.
93. Dobell, A.R.C., and others: Congenital valvular aortic stenosis: surgical management and long-term results, J. Thorac. Cardiovasc. Surg. **81**:916, 1981.
94. Donahoo, J.S., and others: Systemic-pulmonary shunts in neonates and infants using microporous expanded polytetrafluoroethylene: immediate and late results, Ann. Thorac. Surg. **30**:146, 1980.
95. Donahoo, J.S., and others: Prostaglandin E₁ as an adjunct to emergency cardiac operation in neonates, J. Thorac. Cardiovasc. Surg. **81**:227, 1981.
96. Dooley, K.J., and others: Results of pulmonary artery banding in infancy, Am. J. Cardiol. **36**:484, 1975.
97. Driscoll, D.J., Gillette, P.C., and McNamara, D.G.: The use of dopamine in children, J. Pediatr. **92**:309, 1978.
98. Driscoll, D.J., and others: Hemodynamic effects of dobutamine in children, Am. J. Cardiol. **43**:581, 1979.
99. Driscoll, D.J., and others: Management of surgical complete atrioventricular block in children, Am. J. Cardiol. **43**:1175, 1979.
100. Dunnigan, A., and others: A patient-activated radio frequency pacemaker system: therapy for recurrent ventricular tachycardia, J. Pediatr. **101**:403, 1982.
101. Ebert, P.A.: Management of patients with right ventricle to pulmonary artery discontinuity. In Engle, M.A., editor: Pediatric cardiovascular disease, Cardiovascular Clinics, vol. 11, no. 2, Philadelphia, 1981, F.A. Davis Co.
102. Ebert, P.A., and others: Pulmonary artery conduits in infants younger than six months of age, J. Thorac. Cardiovasc. Surg. **72**:351, 1976.
103. Edmunds, L.H., Stephenson, L.W., and Gadzik, J.P.: The Blalock-Taussig anastomosis in infants younger than 1 week of age, Circulation **62**:597, 1980.
104. Edmunds, L.H., Wagner, H.R., and Heymann, M.A.: Aortic valvulotomy in neonates, Circulation **61**:421, 1980.
105. Edwards, W.D., and Edwards, J.E.: Hypertensive pulmonary vascular disease in d-transposition of the great arteries, Am. J. Cardiol. **41**:921, 1978.
106. Eggert, L.D., and others: Surgical treatment of the patent ductus arteriosus in preterm infants, Pediatr. Cardiol. **2**:15, 1982.
107. Egloff, L.P., and others: Early and late results with the Mustard operation in infancy, Ann. Thorac. Surg. **26**:474, 1978.
108. Ekert, H., and Sheers, M.: Preoperative and postoperative platelet function in cyanotic congenital heart disease, J. Thorac. Cardiovasc. Surg. **67**:184, 1974.
109. Ellison, R.C., and others: Indirect assessment of severity of pulmonary stenosis, Circulation **56**(suppl. 1):14, 1977.
110. Ellrodt, G., Chew, C.Y., and Singh, B.N.: Therapeutic implications of slow-channel blockade in cardiocirculatory disorders, Circulation **62**:669, 1980.
111. Emmanouilides, G.C.: Incidence, perinatal factors, and natural history. In Heymann, M.A., and Rudolph, A.M., co-chairpersons: The ductus arteriosus, Report of the seventy-fifth Ross Conference on Pediatric Research, Columbus, Ohio, 1978, Ross Laboratories, Inc.
112. Emmanouilides, G.C., and others: Pulmonary arterial pressure changes in human newborn infants from birth to 3 days of age, J. Pediatr. **65**:327, 1964.
113. Engle, M.A.: When the child's heart fails: recognition, treatment, prognosis, Prog. Cardiovasc. Dis. **12**:601, 1970.
114. Engle, M.A.: Immunologic and virologic studies in the postpericardiotomy syndrome, J. Pediatr. **87**:1103, 1975.
115. Epstein, M.L., and others: Pulmonary artery banding in infants with complete atrioventricular canal, J. Thorac. Cardiovasc. Surg. **78**:28, 1979.
116. Erickson, S.: Administration of sodium nitroprusside (Nipride) independently and in conjunction with dopamine. In Hirsch, J., and Hannock, L., editors: Mosby's manual of clinical nursing procedures, St. Louis, 1981, The C.V. Mosby Co.
117. Fairman, R.M., and Edmunds, L.H.: Emergency thoracotomy in the surgical intensive care unit after open cardiac operation, Ann. Thorac. Surg. **32**:386, 1980.
118. Fay, S.: Mechanism of oxygen-induced contraction of ductus arteriosus. In Heymann, M.A., and Rudolph, A.M., co-chairpersons: The ductus arteriosus, Report of the seventy-fifth Ross Conference on Pediatric Research, Columbus, Ohio, 1978, Ross Laboratories, Inc.
119. Feldt, R.H., editor: Atrioventricular canal defects, Philadelphia, 1976, W.B. Saunders Co.
120. Felner, J.M.: Techniques of echocardiography. In Hurst, J.W., editor: The heart, arteries, and veins, ed. 5, New York, 1982, McGraw-Hill Book Co.
121. Finer, N.N., and others: Postextubation atelectasis: a retrospective controlled study, J. Pediatr. **94**:110, 1979.
122. Fink, B.W.: Aortic stenosis and other lesions. In Congenital heart disease; a deductive approach to its diagnosis, Chicago, 1975, Year Book Medical Publishers, Inc.
123. Fink, B.W.: Congenital heart disease: a deductive approach to its diagnosis, Chicago, 1975, Year Book Medical Publishers, Inc.
124. Fink, B.W.: Total anomalous pulmonary venous connection. In Congenital heart disease: a deductive approach to its diagnosis, Chicago, 1975, Year Book Medical Publishers, Inc.
125. Fink, B.W., and Mandel, W.J.: Supraventricular arrhythmias. In Roberts, N.K., and Gelband, H., editors: Cardiac arrhythmias in the neonate, infant, and child, New York, 1977, Appleton-Century-Crofts.
126. Fischbein, C.A., and others: Risk factors for brain abscess in patients with congenital heart disease, Am. J. Cardiol. **34**:97, 1974.

127. Fisher, J.D., Mehra, R., and Furman, S.: Termination of ventricular tachycardia with bursts of rapid-ventricular pacing, Am. J. Cardiol. 41:94, 1978.

128. Fisher, R.D., and others: Operative closure of isolated defects of the ventricular septum: planned delay, Ann. Thorac. Surg. 26:351, 1978.

129. Fontan, F., and Baudet, E.: Surgical repair of tricuspid atresia, Thorax 26:240, 1971.

130. Freed, M.D.: Cardiac disorders. In Graef, J.W., and Cone, T.E., editors: Manual of pediatric therapeutics, ed. 2, Boston, 1980, Little, Brown, & Co.

131. Freedom, R.M., Bini, M., and Rowe, R.D.: Endocardial cushion defect and significant hypoplasia of the left ventricle: a distinct clinical and pathological entity, Eur. J. Cardiol. 7:263, 1978.

132. Fryer, A.D.: The use of prostaglandins in congenital heart disease. Unpublished protocol, San Francisco, 1981, Presbyterian Hospital of Pacific Medical Center.

133. Fukumasu, H., and others: Intraaortic balloon-pumping device for infants, Clin. Cardiol. 2:348, 1979.

134. Fyler, D.C., editor: Report of the New England Regional Infant Cardiac Program, Pediatrics 65(Feb. suppl.):377, 1980.

135. Gardella, L.A., and others: Intropin (dopamine hydrochloride) intravenous admixture compatability, Am. J. Hosp. Pharm. 33:537, 1976.

136. Garson, A., and McNamara, D.G.: Postoperative tetralogy of Fallot. In Engle, M.A., editor: Pediatric cardiovascular disease, Cardiovascular Clinics, vol. 11, no. 2, Philadelphia, 1981, F.A. Davis Co.

137. Gathman, G.E., and Nadas, A.S.: Total anomalous pulmonary venous connection: clinical and physiologic observations of 75 pediatric patients, Circulation 42:143, 1970.

138. Gay, W.A., and others: The surgical treatment of transposition of the great arteries. In Engle, M.A., editor: Pediatric cardiovascular disease, Cardiovascular Clinics, vol. 11, no. 2, Philadelphia, 1981, F.A. Davis Co.

139. Gelband, H., Myerburg, R.J., and Bassett, A.L.: Management of cardiac arrhythmias. In Roberts, N.K., and Gelband, H., editors: Cardiac arrhythmias in the neonate, infant, and child, New York, 1977, Appleton-Century-Crofts.

140. German, J.C., and others: Management of pulmonary insufficiency in diaphragmatic hernia using extracorporeal circulation with a membrane oxygenator (ECMO), J. Pediatr. Surg. 12:905, 1977.

141. Gersony, W.M., and Hordof, A.J.: Infective endocarditis and diseases of the pericardium, Pediatr. Clin. North Am. 25:831, 1978.

142. Giles, T.D.: Principles of vasodilator therapy for left ventricular congestive heart failure, Heart Lung 9:271, 1980.

143. Gill, C.C., Moodie, D.S., and McGoon, D.C.: Staged surgical management of pulmonary atresia with diminutive pulmonary arteries, J. Thorac. Cardiovasc. Surg. 73:436, 1977.

144. Gillette, P.C., and others: Mechanisms of cardiac arrhythmia after the Mustard operation for transposition of the great arteries, Am. J. Cardiol. 45:1225, 1980.

145. Gillette, P.C., and others: Surgical treatment of supraventricular tachycardia in infants and children, Am. J. Cardiol. 46:281, 1980.

146. Glew, R.H., and others: Sudden death in congenital aortic stenosis: a review of eight cases with an evaluation of premonitory clinical features, Am. Heart J. 78:615, 1969.

147. Godman, M.J., and others: Hemodynamic studies in children four to ten years after the Mustard operation for transposition of the great arteries, Circulation 53:532, 1976.

148. Goldberg, L.: Cardiovascular and renal actions of dopamine: potential clinical applications, Pharmacol. Rev. 24:1, 1972.

149. Goldberg, L.: Dopamine: clinical uses of an endogenous catecholamine, N. Engl. J. Med. 291:707, 1974.

150. Gomez, R., and others: Management of patent ductus arteriosus in preterm babies, Ann. Thorac. Surg. 29:459, 1978.

151. Goor, D.A., Shem-Tov, A., and Neufeld, H.N.: Impeded coronary flow in anatomic correction of transposition of the great arteries, J. Thorac. Cardiovasc. Surg. 83:747, 1982.

152. Goor, D.A., and others: Correction of tetrad of Fallot with reduced incidence of right bundle branch block, Am. J. Cardiol. 48:892, 1981.

153. Graham, T.P., Atwood, G.F., and Boucek, R.J.: Pharmacologic dilatation of the ductus arteriosus with prostaglandin E_1 in infants with congenital heart disease, South. Med. J. 71:1238, 1980.

154. Green, T.P., and others: Fluid administration and the development of patent ductus arteriosus: correspondence, N. Engl. J. Med. 303:337, 1980.

155. Greenspan, A.M., and others: Large dose procainamide therapy for ventricular tachycardia, Am. J. Cardiol. 46:453, 1980.

156. Greenwood, R.D., and Rosenthal, A.: Cardiovascular malformations associated with tracheoesophageal fistula and esophageal atresia, Pediatrics 57:87, 1976.

157. Greenwood, R.D., Rosenthal, A., and Nadas, A.S.: Cardiovascular abnormalities associated with congenital diaphragmatic hernia, Pediatrics 57:92, 1976.

158. Greenwood, R.D., Rosenthal, A., and Nadas, A.S.: Cardiovascular malformations associated with congenital anomalies of the urinary system, Clin. Pediatr. 15:1101, 1976.

159. Greenwood, R.D., and others: Extracardiac anomalies in children with congenital heart disease, Pediatrics 55:485, 1975.

160. Greenwood, R.D., and others: Sick sinus syndrome after surgery for congenital heart disease, Circulation 52:208, 1975.

161. Griffith, B.P., and others: Arteriovenous ECMO for neonatal respiratory support: a study in pregestational lambs, J. Thorac. Cardiovasc. Surg. 77:595, 1979.

162. Griffith, B.P., and others: Pulmonary valvulotomy alone for pulmonary stenosis: results in children with and without muscular infundibular hypertrophy, J. Thorac. Cardiovasc. Surg. **83**:577, 1982.

163. Griffiths, S.P., and others: Muscular ventricular septal defects repaired with left ventriculotomy, Am. J. Cardiol. **48**:877, 1981.

164. Grossman, W.: Blood flow measurement: the cardiac output. In Cardiac catheterization and angiography, ed. 2, Philadelphia, 1980, Lea & Febiger.

165. Grossman, W.: Cardiac catheterization and angiography, ed. 2, Philadelphia, 1980, Lea & Febiger.

166. Guam, W.E., Schwartz, D.C., and Kaplan, S.: Ventricular tachycardia in infancy: evidence for a reentrant mechanism, Circulation **62**:401, 1980.

167. Guntheroth, W.G.: Disorders of heart rate and rhythm, Pediatr. Clin. North Am. **25**:869, 1978.

168. Guntheroth, W.G., Morgan, B.C., and Mullins, G.L.: Physiologic studies of paroxysmal hyperpnea in cyanotic congenital heart disease, Circulation **31**:70, 1965.

169. Gutgesell, H.P., Garson, A., and McNamara, D.G.: Prognosis of the newborn with transposition of the great arteries, Am. J. Cardiol. **44**:96, 1979.

170. Gutgesell, H.P., Speer, M.E., and Rosenberg, H.S.: Characterization of the cardiomyopathy in infants of diabetic mothers, Circulation **61**:441, 1980.

171. Guyton, A.C.: Excitable tissue: muscle. In Textbook of medical physiology, ed. 6, Philadelphia, 1981, W.B. Saunders Co.

172. Hagler, D.J., and others: Right and left ventricular function after the Mustard procedure in transposition of the great arteries, Am. J. Cardiol. **44**:276, 1979.

173. Hahn, J.F.: Cerebral edema and neurointensive care, Pediatr. Clin. North Am. **27**:587, 1980.

174. Hanlon, C.R., and others: Atrial septal defect: results of repair in adults, Arch. Surg. **99**:275, 1969.

175. Hardesty, R.L., and others: Extracorporeal membrane oxygenation: successful treatment of persistent fetal circulation following repair of congenital diaphragmatic hernia, J. Thorac. Cardiovasc. Surg. **81**:556, 1981.

176. Harrison, D.C., Sprouse, J.H., and Morrow, A.G.: The antiarrhythmic properties of lidocaine and procainamide, Circulation **28**:486, 1963.

177. Hartzler, G.O.: Treatment of recurrent ventricular tachycardia by patient-activated radio-frequency ventricular stimulation, Mayo Clin. Proc. **54**:75, 1979.

178. Hayes, A.H.: The pharmacology of cardio-active agents. In Engle, M.A., editor: Pediatric cardiology, Cardiovascular Clinics **4**:104, 1972.

179. Hazinski, M.F.: Congenital heart lesions: pathophysiology, surgery, and postoperative care, parts I and II, Life Support Nurs. **3**:8, Jan. and March 1980.

180. Hazinski, M.F.: Cardiac catheterization. In Johanson, B.C., and others, editors: Standards for critical care, ed. 2, St. Louis, 1984, The C.V. Mosby Co.

181. Hazinski, T.A., and Severinghaus, J.W.: Transcutaneous analysis of arterial PCO_2, Med. Instrum. **16**:150, 1982.

182. Heck, H.A., and others: Conduit repair for complex congenital heart disease, J. Thorac. Cardiovasc. Surg. **75**:806, 1978.

183. Henriksson, P., Varendh, G., and Lundstrom, N.R.: Haemostatic defects in cyanotic congenital heart disease, Br. Heart J. **41**:23, 1979.

184. Hernandez, A., and others: Idiopathic paroxysmal ventricular tachycardia in infants and children, J. Pediatr. **86**:182, 1975.

185. Hesslein, P.S., and others: Comparison of resection versus patch aortoplasty for repair of coarctation in infants and children, Circulation **64**:164, 1981.

186. Hey, E.N., and Katz, G.: The optimum thermal environment for naked babies, Arch. Dis. Child. **45**:328, 1970.

187. Heymann, M.A.: Protocol for PGE_1 infusion during transport to UCSF for diagnostic evaluation and/or surgery. Unpublished protocol, San Francisco, 1980, University of California at San Francisco.

188. Heymann, M.A.: Pharmacologic use of prostaglandin E_1 in infants with congenital heart disease, Am. Heart J. **101**:837, 1981.

189. Heymann, M.A., and Rudolph, A.M.: Effects of congenital heart disease on fetal and neonatal circulations, Prog. Cardiovasc. Dis. **15**:115, 1972.

190. Heymann, M.A., and Rudolph, A.M., co-chairpersons: The ductus arteriosus, Report of the seventy-fifth Ross Conference on Pediatric Research, Columbus, Ohio, 1978, Ross Laboratories, Inc.

191. Higgins, C.B., and Mulder, D.G.: Chylothorax after heart surgery for congenital heart disease, J. Thorac. Cardiovasc. Surg. **61**:411, 1971.

192. Ho, C.S., Krovetz, L.J., and Rowe, R.D.: Major complications of cardiac catheterization and angiography in infants and children, Johns Hopkins Med. J. **131**:247, 1972.

193. Hoffman, J.I.E.: Natural history of congenital heart diseases: problems in its assessment with special reference to ventricular septal defects, Circulation **37**:97, 1968.

194. Hoffman, J.I.E.: Factors affecting shunting and the development of heart failure. In Heymann, M.A., and Rudolph, A.M., co-chairpersons: The ductus arteriosus, Report of the seventy-fifth Ross Conference on Pediatric Research, Columbus, Ohio, 1978, Ross Laboratories, Inc.

195. Hoffman, J.I.E., and Rudolph, A.M.: The natural history of ventricular septal defects in infancy, Am. J. Cardiol. **16**:634, 1965.

196. Holloway, E.L., Polumbo, R.A., and Harrison, D.C.: Acute circulatory effects of dopamine in patients with pulmonary hypertension, Br. Heart J. **37**:482, 1975.

197. Holloway, E.L., and others: Action of drugs in patients early after cardiac surgery: comparison of isoproterenol and dopamine, Am. J. Cardiol. **35**:656, 1975.

198. Horowitz, L.N., and others: Electrophysiologic characteristics of sustained ventricular tachycardia occurring after repair of tetralogy of Fallot, Am. J. Cardiol. **46**:446, 1980.

199. Hoshino, K.: Clinical usefulness of dopamine in the shock state of neonates, Jpn. J. Anesth. **25:**11, 1976.

200. Ibarra-Perez, C., and Lillehei, C.W.: Treatment of mesenteric arteritis following resection of coarctation of the aorta, J. Thorac. Cardiovasc. Surg. **58:**135, 1969.

201. Idriss, F.S., and others: Postoperative management of the pediatric cardiac surgical patient. In Beal, J.M., editor: Critical care for surgical patients, New York, 1982, Macmillan Publishing Co., Inc.

202. Ilbawi, M.N., and others: Tetralogy of Fallot with absent pulmonary valve, J. Thorac. Cardiovasc. Surg. **81:**906, 1981.

203. Ilves, R., and others: Prospective, randomized, double-blind study using prophylactic cephalothin for major, general thoracic operations, J. Thorac. Cardiovasc. Surg. **81:**813, 1981.

204. Jack, W.D., and Kelly, D.T.: Long-term follow-up of valvulotomy for congenital aortic stenosis, Am. J. Cardiol. **38:**231, 1976.

205. Jackson, P.L.: Digoxin therapy at home: keeping the child safe, MCN: Am. J. Matern. Child Nurs. **4:**105, 1979.

206. Jacob, J., and others: The contribution of PDA in the neonate with severe RDS, J. Pediatr. **96:**79, 1980.

207. Jacoby, J.: Performance of chest physiotherapy. In Hirsch, J., and Hannock, L., editors: Mosby's manual of clinical nursing procedures, St. Louis, 1981, The C.V. Mosby Co.

208. James, F.W., and Love, E.: Congestive heart failure in infants and children, Heart Lung **3:**396, 1974.

209. James, T.N., and others: Anatomy of the heart. In Hurst, J.W., editor: The heart, arteries, and veins, ed. 5, New York, 1982, McGraw-Hill Book Co.

210. Jatene, A.D., and others: Anatomic correction of transposition of the great arteries, J. Thorac. Cardiovasc. Surg. **83:**20, 1982.

211. Jensen, J.B., and Blount, S.G.: Total anomalous pulmonary venous return: a review and report of the oldest surviving patient, Am. Heart J. **82:**387, 1971.

212. Jick, H., and others: First trimester drug use and congenital disorders, JAMA **246:**343, 1981.

213. Johanson, B.C., and others, editors: Cardiac surgery. In Standards for critical care, St. Louis, 1981, The C.V. Mosby Co.

214. Johnson, C.M., and Rhodes, K.H.: Pediatric endocarditis, Mayo Clin. Proc. **57:**86, 1982.

215. Jones, K.L., and Smith, D.W.: The William's elfin facies syndrome, J. Pediatr. **86:**718, 1975.

216. Jones, M., Barnhart, G.R., and Morrow, A.G.: Late results after operations for left ventricular outflow tract obstruction, Am. J. Cardiol. **50:**569, 1982.

217. Joyce, L.D., Lindsay, W.G., and Nicoloff, D.M.: Chylothorax after median sternotomy for intrapericardial cardiac surgery, J. Thorac. Cardiovasc. Surg. **71:**476, 1976.

218. Judson, J.P., and others: Double-outlet right ventricle: surgical results, 1970-1980, J. Thorac. Cardiovasc. Surg. **85:**32, 1983.

218a.Kan, J.S., and others: Treatment of restenosis of coarctation by percutaneous transluminal angioplasty, Circulation **68:**1087, 1983.

219. Kannel, W.B.: Incidence, prevalence, and mortality of cardiovascular disease. In Hurst, J.W., editor: The heart, arteries, and veins, ed. 5, New York, 1982, McGraw-Hill Book Co.

220. Kaplan, S., and others: Therapeutic advances in pediatric cardiology, Pediatr. Clin. North Am. **25:**891, 1978.

221. Karpawich, P.P., and others: Ventricular septal defect with associated aortic valve insufficiency, J. Thorac. Cardiovasc. Surg. **82:**182, 1981.

222. Katz, N.M., Buckley, M.J., and Liberthson, R.R.: Discrete membranous subaortic stenosis, Circulation **56:**1034, 1977.

223. Katz, N.M., Kirklin, J.W., and Pacifico, A.D.: Concepts and practices in surgery for total anomalous pulmonary venous connection, Ann. Thorac. Surg. **25:**479, 1978.

224. Katz, N.M., and others: Late survival and symptoms after repair of tetralogy of Fallot, Circulation **65:**403, 1982.

225. Kavey, R.W., Sondheimer, H.M., and Blackman, M.S.: Detection of dysrhythmia in pediatric patients with mitral valve prolapse, Circulation **62:**582, 1980.

226. Kawabori, I.: Cyanotic congenital heart defects with increased pulmonary blood flow, Pediatr. Clin. North Am. **25:**777, 1978.

227. Keys, T.F.: Antimicrobial prophylaxis for patients with congenital or valvular heart disease, Mayo Clin. Proc. **57:**171, 1982.

228. Kirklin, J.W., and Rastelli, G.C.: Low cardiac output after open intracardiac operations, Prog. Cardiovasc. Dis. **10:**117, 1967.

229. Klein, H.O., and others: The influence of verapamil on serum digoxin concentrations, Circulation **65:**998, 1982.

230. Klotz, R., and others: The use of intravenous nitroglycerin in children: clinical applications and method of administration. Unpublished paper, Chicago, 1982, Children's Memorial Hospital.

231. Kohama, F.H., and Cunningham, J.N.: Monitoring of cadiac output by thermodilution after open heart surgery, J. Thorac. Cardiovasc. Surg. **73:**451, 1977.

232. Kosloske, A.M., Martin, L.W., and Schubert, W.K.: Management of chylothorax in children by thoracentesis and medium-chain triglyceride feedings, J. Pediatr. Surg. **9:**365, 1974.

233. Kraybill, E.N.: Needs of the term infant. In Avery, G.B., editor: Neonatology: pathophysiology and management of the newborn, ed. 2, Philadelphia, 1981, J.B. Lippincott Co.

234. Kreutzer, G.O., and others: Atriopulmonary anastomosis, J. Thorac. Cardiovasc. Surg. **83:**427, 1982.

235. Kugler, J.D., Garson, A., and Gillette, P.C.: Electrophysiologic effects of digitalis on sino-atrial nodal function in children, Am. J. Cardiol. **44:**1344, 1979.

236. Kugler, J.D., and others: Results of aortic valvotomy in infants with isolated aortic valvular stenosis, J. Thorac. Cardiovasc. Surg. **78:**553, 1979.

237. Kyger, E.R., and others: Surgical palliation of tricuspid atresia, Circulation **52:**685, 1975.

238. Kyger, E.R., and others: Sinus venosus atrial septal defect: early and late results following closure in 109 patients, Ann. Thorac. Surg. **25:**44, 1978.

239. Laks, H.: Advances in the repair of complex congenital heart disease, Pediatr. Ann. **11:**926, 1982.

240. Lang, D., and von Bernuth, G.: Serum concentration and serum half-life of digoxin in premature and mature newborns, Pediatrics **59:**902, 1977.

241. Lang, P., and others: The hemodynamic effects of dopamine in infants after corrective surgery, J. Pediatr. **96:**630, 1980.

242. Langman, J.: Cardiovascular system. In: Medical embryology, ed. 4, Baltimore, 1981, The Williams & Wilkins Co.

243. Lasagna, L.: How useful are serum digitalis measurements? N. Engl. J. Med. **294:**898, 1976.

244. Lenz, W.: Malformations caused by drugs in pregnancy, Am. J. Dis. of Child. **112:**99, 1966.

245. Lessof, M.H.: Postcardiotomy syndrome: pathogenesis and management, Hosp. Pract. **11:**81, 1976.

246. Levy, S., and others: Long-term results of permanent atrio-ventricular sequential demand pacing, PACE **2:**175, 1979.

247. LeWinter, M.M., Engler, R.L., and Karliner, J.S.: Tocainide therapy for treatment of ventricular arrhythmias: assessment with ambulatory electrocardiographic monitoring and treadmill exercise, Am. J. Cardiol. **45:**1045, 1980.

248. Liberthson, R.R., and others: Coarctation of the aorta: review of 234 patients and clarification of management problems, Am. J. Cardiol. **43:**835, 1979.

249. Linderkamp, O., and others: Increased blood viscosity in patients with cyanotic congenital heart disease and iron deficiency, J. Pediatr. **95:**567, 1979.

250. Link, D.A.: Fluid and electrolytes. In Graef, J.W., and Cone, T.E., editors: Manual of pediatric therapeutics, Boston, 1980, Little, Brown, & Co.

251. Logue, R.B.: Etiology, recognition, and management of pericardial disease. In Hurst, J.W., editor: The heart, arteries, and veins, New York, 1982, McGraw-Hill Book Co.

252. Losay, J., and others: Repair of atrial septal defect primum: results, course, prognosis, J. Thorac. Cardiovasc. Surg. **75:**248, 1978.

253. Lown, B., Temte, J.V., and Arter, W.J.: Ventricular tachyarrhythmias: clinical aspects, Circulation **47:**1364, 1973.

254. Macmanus, Q., and others: Correction of aortic coarctation in neonates: mortality and late results, Ann. Thorac. Surg. **24:**544, 1977.

255. Mahle, S., and others: Pulmonary artery banding: long-term results in 63 patients, Ann. Thorac. Surg. **27:**216, 1978.

256. Marcelletti, C., McGoon, D.C., and Mair, D.D.: The natural history of truncus arteriosus, Circulation **54:**108, 1976.

257. Marcelletti, C., and others: Early and late results of surgical repair of truncus arteriosus, Circulation **55:**636, 1977.

258. Mark, H.: Natural history of atrial septal defect with criteria for selection for surgery, Am. J. Cardiol. **12:**66, 1963.

259. Marks, K.H., and others: Oxygen consumption and insensible water loss in premature infants under radiant heaters, Pediatrics **66:**228, 1980.

260. Maron, B.J., and others: Prognosis of surgically corrected coarctation of the aorta, Circulation **47:**119, 1973.

261. Maron, B.J., and others: Tunnel subaortic stenosis, Circulation **54:**404, 1976.

262. Maruschak, G.F., and others: Overestimation of pediatric cardiac output by thermal indicator loss, Circulation **65:**380, 1982.

263. Mathur, M., and others: Measurement of cardiac output by thermodilution in infants and children after open-heart operations, J. Thorac. Cardiovasc. Surg. **72:**221, 1976.

264. Matson, D.D., and Salam, M.: Brain abscess in congenital heart disease, Pediatrics **27:**772, 1961.

265. Mattar, J.A., and others: A study of the hyperosmolar state in critically ill patients, Crit. Care Med. **1:**293, 1973.

266. McCabe, J., and others: Surgical treatment of endocardial cushion defects, Am. J. Cardiol. **39:**72, 1977.

267. McGoon, D.C., and Puga, F.J.: Atrioventricular canal. In Engle, M.A., editor: Pediatric cardiovascular disease, vol. 11, no. 2, Cardiovascular Clinics, Philadelphia, 1981, F.A. Davis Co.

268. McGoon, D.C., Wallace, R.B., and Danielson, G.K.: The Rastelli operation: its indications and results, J. Thorac. Cardiovasc. Surg. **65:**65, 1973.

269. McNicholas, K.W., and Malm, J.R.: Tetralogy of Fallot. In Engle, M.A., editor: Pediatric cardiovascular disease, vol. 11, no. 2, Cardiovascular Clinics, Philadelphia, 1981, F.A. Davis Co.

270. Merritt, T.A., and other: Patent ductus arteriosus treated with ligation or indomethacin: a follow-up study, J. Pediatr. **95:**588, 1979.

271. Meyer, J., and others: Coronary artery anomalies in patients with tetralogy of Fallot, J. Thorac. Cardiovasc. Surg. **69:**373, 1975.

272. Meyer, R.A.: Echocardiography. In Adams, F.H., and Emmanouilides, G.C., editors: Moss' heart disease in infants, children, and adolescents, ed. 3, Baltimore, 1983, The Williams & Wilkins Co.

273. Midgley, F.M., and others: Experience with repair of complete atrioventricular canal, Ann. Thorac. Surg. **30:**151, 1980.

274. Miller, R.A., Lev, M., and Paul, M.H.: Congenital absence of the pulmonary valve: the clinical syndrome of tetralogy of Fallot with pulmonary regurgitation, Circulation **26:**266, 1962.

275. Mills, L.J., and others: Cardiothoracic surgery: perioperative principles. In Levin, D.L., Morriss, F.C., and Moore, G.C., editors: A practical guide to pediatric intensive care, ed. 2, St. Louis, 1983, The C.V. Mosby Co.

276. Mills, N.L., and others: Transvenous closure of ASD's with a double umbrella device: 7 year minimum follow-up (abstract), Circulation 66(suppl. 2):317, 1982.

277. Misbach, G.A., and others: Left ventricular outflow enlargement by the Konno procedure. J. Thorac. Cardiovasc. Surg. 84:696, 1982.

278. Mistrot, J., and others: Pulmonary valvotomy under inflow stasis for isolated pulmonary stenosis, Ann. Thorac. Surg. 21:30, 1976.

279. Moller, J.H., and Neal, W.A.: Cyanosis and decreased pulmonary blood flow. In Heart disease in infancy, New York, 1981, Appleton-Century-Crofts.

280. Moller, J.H., and Neal, W.A.: Other diagnostic studies. In Heart disease in infancy, New York, 1981, Appleton-Century-Crofts.

281. Moller, J.H., and others: Congenital cardiac disease associated with polysplenia, Circulation 36:789, 1967.

282. Monson, D.O., Hazinski, M.F., and Weinberg, M., Jr.: Management of the pediatric cardiac surgical patient. In Goldin, M.D., editor: Intensive care of the surgical patient, ed. 2, Chicago, 1981, Year Book Medical Publishers, Inc.

283. Monson, D.O., Taylor, W., and Weinberg, M.: The use of fresh unrefrigerated whole blood in cyanotic patients undergoing open heart surgery. Unpublished research findings, Chicago, 1979, Rush Presbyterian St. Luke's Medical Center.

284. Montague, T.J., and others: The spectrum of cardiac rate and rhythm in normal newborns, Pediatr. Cardiol. 2:33, 1982.

285. Moodie, D.S.: Measurement of cardiac output by thermodilution in pediatric patients, Pediatr. Clin. North Am. 27:513, 1980.

286. Morady, F., Laks, M.M., and Parmley, W.W.: Comparison of sarcomere lengths from normal and hypertrophied inner and middle canine right ventricle, Am. J. Physiol. 225:1259, 1979.

287. Moreno-Cabral, R.J., and Shumway, N.E.: Double-patch technique for correction of complete atrioventricular canal, Ann. Thorac. Surg. 33:88, 1980.

288. Morgan, B.C.: Incidence, etiology, and classification of congenital heart disease, Pediatr. Clin. North Am. 25:721, 1978.

289. Morgan, B.C., and others: A clinical profile of paroxysmal hyperpnea in cyanotic congenital heart disease, Circulation 31:66, 1965.

290. Morgan, C.L., and Nadas, A.S.: Sweating and congestive heart failure, N. Engl. J. Med. 268:580, 1963.

291. Morriss, F.C.: Postintubation sequelae. In Levin, D.L., Morriss, F.C., and Moore, G.C., editors: A practical guide to pediatric intensive care, ed. 2, St. Louis, 1983, The C.V. Mosby Co.

292. Moulton, A.L., and others: Pulmonary atresia with intact ventricular septum, J. Thorac. Cardiovasc. Surg. 78:527, 1979.

293. Mushin, W.W., and others: Clinical aspects of controlled ventilation. In: Automatic ventilation of the lungs, Oxford, 1980, Blackwell Scientific Publications.

294. Nadas, A.S., and Fyler, D.C.: Ventricular septal defect: a review of current thought, Arch. Dis. Child. 42:268, 1968.

295. Nadas, A.S., and Fyler, D.C., editors: Electrocardiography. In Pediatric cardiology, Philadelphia, 1972, W.B. Saunders Co.

296. Neches, W.H.: Cardiac catheterization in the newborn, Perinatol. Neonatol. 5:37, 1981.

297. Nelson, N.M.: The onset of respiration. In Avery, G.B., editor: Neonatology: pathophysiology and management of the newborn, ed. 2, Philadelphia, 1981, J.B. Lippincott, Co.

298. Nelson, R.M., Jenson, C.B., and Smoot, W.M., III: Pericardial tamponade following open-heart surgery, J. Thorac. Cardiovasc. Surg. 58:510, 1969.

299. Neutze, J.M., and others: Palliation of cyanotic congenital heart disease in infancy with E-type prostaglandins, Circulation 55:238, 1977.

300. Newfeld, E.A.: Cyanotic congenital heart disease. In Levin, D.L., Morriss, F.C., and Moore, G.C., editors: A practical guide to pediatric intensive care, ed. 2, St. Louis, 1983, The C.V. Mosby Co.

301. Newfeld, E.A., and others: Pulmonary vascular disease in complete transposition of the great arteries: a study of 200 patients, Am. J. Cardiol. 34:75, 1974.

302. Newfeld, E.A., and others: Discrete subvalvular aortic stenosis in childhood: study of 51 patients, Am. J. Cardiol. 38:53, 1976.

303. Newfeld, E.A., and others: Pulmonary vascular disease after systemic-pulmonary arterial shunt operations, Am. J. Cardiol. 39:715, 1977.

304. Newfeld, E.A., and others: Pulmonary vascular disease in complete atrioventricular canal defect, Am. J. Cardiol. 39:721, 1977.

305. Newfeld, E.A., and others: Pulmonary vascular disease in transposition of the great vessels and intact ventricular septum, Circulation 59:525, 1979.

306. Newfeld, E.A., and others: Pulmonary vascular disease in total anomalous pulmonary venous drainage, Circulation 61:103, 1980.

307. Nihill, M.R., McNamara, D.G., and Vick, R.L.: The effects of increased blood viscosity on pulmonary vascular resistance, Am. Heart J. 92:65, 1976.

308. Noble, R.J., and Steinmetz, E.F.: Noninvasive techniques and cardiac catheterization. In Wenger, N.K., Hurst, J.W., and McIntyre, M.C., editors: Cardiology for nurses, New York, 1982, McGraw-Hill Book Co.

309. Noonan, J.A.: Association of congenital heart disease with syndromes or other defects, Pediatr. Clin. North Am. 25:797, 1978.

310. Noonan, J.A.: Syndromes associated with cardiac defects. In Engle, M.A., editor: Pediatric cardiovascular disease, Cardiovascular Clinics vol. 11, no. 2, Philadelphia, 1981, F.A. Davis Co.

311. Nora, J.J., and Nora, A.H.: Recurrence risks in children having one parent with a congenital heart disease, Circulation 53:701, 1976.

312. Norwood, W.I., Hougen, T.J., and Castaneda, A.R.: Total anomalous pulmonary venous connection: surgical considerations. In Engle, M.A., editor: Pediatric cardiovascular disease, Cardiovascular Clinics, vol. 2, no. 2, Philadelphia, 1981, F.A. Davis Co.

313. Norwood, W.I., Lang, P., and Hansen, D.D.: Physiologic repair of aortic atresia: hypoplastic left heart syndrome, N. Engl. J. Med. **308**:23, 1983.

314. Norwood, W.I., and others: Experience with operations for hypoplastic left heart syndrome, J. Thorac. Cardiovasc. Surg. **82**:511, 1981.

315. Nugent, E.W., and others: Clinical course in pulmonary stenosis, Circulation **56**(suppl. 1):38, 1977.

316. Olinger, G.N., and others: Acute clinical hypocalcemic myocardial depression during rapid blood transfusion and postoperative hemodialysis, J. Thorac. Cardiovasc. Surg. **73**:503, 1977.

317. Olley, P.M., and Coceani, F.: The prostaglandins, Am. J. Dis. Child. **134**:688, 1980.

318. O'Malley, K., and others: Plasma digoxin levels in infants, Arch. Dis. Child. **48**:55, 1973.

319. O'Toole, J.D., and others: The mechanism of splitting of the second heart sound in atrial septal defect, Circulation **56**:1047, 1977.

320. Parenzan, L., and others: The Senning operation for transposition of the great arteries, J. Thorac. Cardiovasc. Surg. **76**:305, 1978.

321. Parr, G.V.S., Blackstone, E.H., and Kirklin, J.W.: Cardiac performance and mortality early after intracardiac surgery in infants and young children, Circulation **51**:867, 1975.

322. Patten, B.M.: The development of the heart. In Gould, S.E., editor: Pathology of the heart, Springfield, Illinois, 1953, Charles C Thomas, Publisher.

323. Patterson, S.W., and Starling, E.H.: On the mechanical factors which determine the output of the ventricles, J. Physiol. **48**:357, 1914.

324. Pearlman, A.S., and others: Abnormal right ventricular size and ventricular septal motion after atrial septal defect closure, Am. J. Cardiol. **41**:295, 1978.

325. Peetz, D.J., and others: Correction of truncus arteriosus in the neonate using a nonvalved conduit, J. Thorac. Cardiovasc. Surg. **83**:743, 1982.

326. Pennington, D.G., and others: Critical review of experience with surgical repair of coarctation of the aorta, J. Thorac. and Cardiovasc. Surg. **77**:221, 1979.

327. Pennington, D.G., and others: Glenn shunt: long-term results and current role in congenital heart operations, Ann. Thorac. Surg. **31**:532, 1981.

328. Perkin, R.M., and Levin, D.L.: Shock in the pediatric patient. I., J. Pediatr. **101**:163, 1982.

329. Perkin, R.M., and Levin, D.L.: Shock in the pediatric patient. II. Therapy, J. Pediatr. **101**:319, 1982.

330. Perkin, R.M., and others: Dobutamine: a hemodynamic evaluation in children with shock, J. Pediatr. **100**:977, 1982.

331. Phibbs, R.H.: Resuscitation of the asphyxiated infant. In Avery, G.B., editor: Neonatology: pathophysiology and management of the newborn, ed. 2, Philadelphia, 1981, J.B. Lippincott Co.

332. Philbin, D.M., and others: Antidiuretic hormone levels during cardiopulmonary bypass, J. Thorac. Cardiovasc. Surg. **73**:145, 1977.

333. Phornphutkul, C., and others: Cerebrovascular accidents in infants and children with cyanotic congenital heart disease, Am. J. Cardiol. **32**:329, 1973.

334. Pierce, W.S., and others: Late results of the subclavian flap procedure in infants with coarctation of the thoracic aorta, Circulation **58**(suppl. 1):78, 1978.

335. Pieroni, D.R., and others: Postoperative assessment of residual defects following cardiac surgery in infants and children. III. Atrial septal defects, Johns Hopkins Med. J. **133**:287, 1973.

336. Plauth, W.H., and others: The pathology, abnormal physiology, clinical recognition, and medical and surgical treatment of congenital heart disease. In Hurst, J.W., editor: The heart, arteries, and veins, ed. 5, New York, 1982, McGraw-Hill Book Co.

337. Plumb, V.J., and James, T.N.: Clinical hazards of powerful diuretics, Mod. Concepts Cardiovasc. Dis. **47**:91, 1978.

338. Poirier, R.A., Berman, M.A., and Stansel, H.C.: Current status of the surgical treatment of truncus arteriosus. J. Thorac. Cardiovasc. Surg. **69**:169, 1975.

339. Polgar, G.: Practical pulmonary physiology: a functional analysis of symptoms and therapeutic measures in respiratory disorders of newborn infants, Pediatr. Clin. North Am. **20**:303, 1972.

340. Pollock, J.C., and others: Intraaortic balloon pumping in children, Ann. Thorac. Surg. **29**:522, 1979.

341. Prec, K.J., and Cassels, D.E.: Oximeter studies in newborn infants during crying, Pediatrics **9**:756, 1952.

342. Rabinovitch, M., and others: Growth and development of the pulmonary vascular bed in patients with tetralogy of Fallot with or without pulmonary atresia, Circulation **64**:1234, 1981.

343. Radford, D.J., and Izukawa, T.: Atrial fibrillation in children, Pediatrics **59**:250, 1977.

344. Rastelli, G.C., and others: Surgical treatment of supravalvular aortic stenosis, J. Thorac. Cardiovasc. Surg. **51**:873, 1966.

345. Redding, G.J., and others: Partial obstruction of endotracheal tubes in children, Crit. Care Med. **7**:227, 1979.

346. Reynolds, D.W., Stagno, S., and Alford, C.A.: Chronic congenital and perinatal infections. In Avery, G.B., editor: Neonatology: pathophysiology and management of the newborn, ed. 2, Philadelphia, 1981, J.B. Lippincott Co.

347. Riemenschneider, T.A.: Evaluation of cyanosis in the newborn, J. Fam. Pract. **3**:201, 1976.

348. Roberts, N.K., and Gelband, H., editors: Cardiac arrhythmias in the neonate, infant, and child, New York, 1977, Appleton-Century-Crofts.

349. Roberts, N.K., and Yabek, S.: Arrhythmias following atrial and ventricular surgery. In Roberts, N.K., and Gelband, H., editors: Cardiac arrhythmias in the neonate, infant, and child, New York, 1977, Appleton-Century-Crofts.

350. Roberts, W.C., Shemin, R.J., and Kent, K.M.: Frequency and direction of interatrial shunting in valvular pulmonic stenosis with intact ventricular septum and without left ventricular inflow or outflow obstruction, Am. Heart J. **99**:142, 1980.

351. Roden, D.M., and others: Tocainide therapy for refractory ventricular arrhythmias, Am. Heart J. **100**:15, 1980.

352. Rodvien, R.: Non-surgical hemorrhage associated with cardiopulmonary bypass, J. Extracorporeal Tech. **9**:6, 1977.

353. Rodvien, R.: Personal communication, San Francisco, June, 1982, Presbyterian Hospital of Pacific Medical Center.

354. Rodvien, R., and Hill, J.D.: Coagulation and anticoagulation in the critically ill cardiac patient. In Donoso, E., and Cohen, S.I., editors: Current cardiovascular topics, vol. 5, New York, 1979, Stratton Intercontinental Medical Book Corp.

355. Rosenthal, A., and others: Acute hemodynamic effects of red cell volume reduction in polycythemia of cyanotic congenital heart disease, Circulation **42**:297, 1970.

356. Roses, D.F., Rose, M.R., and Rapaport F.T.: Febrile responses associated with cardiac surgery: relationships to the postpericardiotomy syndrome and to altered host immunologic reactivity, J. Thorac. Cardiovasc. Surg. **67**:251, 1974.

357. Rosing, D.R., and others: Long-term hemodynamic and electrocardiographic assessment following operative repair of tetralogy of Fallot, Circulation 58(suppl. 1):209, 1977.

358. Rudolph, A.M.: Aortic coarctation and isthmus narrowing. In Congenital diseases of the heart, Chicago, 1974, Year Book Medical Publishers, Inc.

359. Rudolph, A.M.: Aortopulmonary transposition. In Congenital diseases of the heart, Chicago, 1974, Year Book Medical Publishers, Inc.

360. Rudolph, A.M.: Cardiac catheterization and angiocardiography. In Congenital diseases of the heart, Chicago, 1974, Year Book Medical Publishers, Inc.

361. Rudolph, A.M.: Pulmonary stenosis with intact ventricular septum. In Congenital diseases of the heart, Chicago, 1974, Year Book Medical Publishers, Inc.

362. Rudolph, A.M., and Heymann, M.A.: Medical treatment of the ductus arteriosus, Hosp. Pract. **13**:57, 1977.

363. Ruttenberg, H.D., and others: Syndrome of congenital cardiac disease with asplenia, Am. J. Cardiol. **16**:387, 1964.

364. Sade, R.M., Cosgrove, D.M., and Castaneda, A.R.: Infant and child care in heart surgery, Chicago, 1977, Year Book Medical Publishers, Inc.

365. Sade, R.M., Richi, A.A., and Dearing, J.P.: Calculation of systemic blood flow with pulmonary artery thermistor probe, J. Thorac. Cardiovasc. Surg. **78**:576, 1979.

366. Sade, R.M., and others: Abnormalities of regional lung function associated with ventricular septal defect and pulmonary artery band, J. Thorac. Cardiovasc. Surg. **71**:572, 1976.

367. Sade, R.M., and others: Cardiac valve replacement in children, J. Thorac. Cardiovasc. Surg. **78**:123, 1979.

368. Sahn, D.J.: Medical progress: real-time two-dimensional echocardiography, J. Pediatr. **99**:175, 1981.

369. Sahn, D.J., and others: Pediatric echocardiography: a review of its clinical utility, J. Pediatr. **87**:335, 1975.

370. Saied, A., and Folger, G.M.: Hypoplastic left heart syndrome: clinicopathologic and hemodynamic correlation, Am. J. Cardiol. **29**:190, 1972.

371. Sanders, S.P., and others: Use of Hancock porcine homografts in children and adolescents, Am. J. Cardiol. **46**:429, 1980.

372. Sandor, G.G.S., and others: Long-term follow-up of patients after valvotomy for congenital valvular aortic stenosis in children, J. Thorac. and Cardiovasc. Surg. **80**:171, 1976.

373. Sapire, D.W., Mongkolsmai, C., and O'Riordan, A.C.: Control of chronic ectopic supraventricular tachycardia with verapamil, J. Pediatr. **94**:312, 1979.

374. Sapire, D.W., O'Riordan, A.C., and Black, I.F.: Safety and efficacy of short- and long-term verapamil therapy in children with tachycardia, Am. J. Cardiol. **48**:1091, 1981.

375. Sarnoff, S.J., and Berglund, E.: Ventricular function. I. Starling's law of the heart studied by means of simultaneous right and left ventricular function curves in the dog, Circulation **9**:706, 1954.

376. Saxon, A.: Inhibition of platelet function by nitroprusside, N. Engl. J. Med. **295**:281, 1976.

377. Schapira, J.N., and others: Single- and two-dimensional echocardiographic features of the interatrial septum in normal subjects and patients with an atrial septal defect, Am. J. Cardiol. **43**:816, 1979.

378. Schlant, R.C., Sonnenblick, E.H., and Gorlin, R.: Normal physiology of the cardiovascular system. In Hurst, J.W., editor: The heart, arteries, and veins, ed. 5, New York, 1982, McGraw-Hill Book Co.

379. Schwartz, D.C., and West, T.D.: Cardiac catheterization in infants and children, Heart Lung **3**:407, 1974.

380. Schweitzer, P., and Mark, H.: The effect of atropine on cardiac arrhythmias and conduction, part I, Am. Heart J. **100**:119, 1980.

381. Scopes, J.W., and Ahmed, I.: Range of critical temperatures in sick and premature newborn babies, Am. J. Dis. Child. **41**:417, 1966.

382. Sealy, W.C., and others: Paradoxical hypertension following resection of coarctation of the aorta, Surgery **42**:135, 1957.

383. Sealy, W.C., and others: Atrial dysrhythmia and atrial secundum defects, J. Thorac. Cardiovasc. Surg. **57**:245, 1969.

384. Selzer, A.: Quinidine in perspective: the rise and fall of quinidine, Heart Lung **11**:20, 1982.

385. Seybold-Epting, W., and others: Repair of ventricular septal defect after pulmonary artery banding, J. Thorac. Cardiovasc. Surg. **71**:392, 1976.

386. Shariatzadeh, A.N., and others: Tricuspid atresia: a review of 68 cases, Chest **71**:538, 1977.

387. Shaw, G.: Pediatric aspects of cyanotic heart disease, Q. Pediatr. Bull. Lutheran General Hospital **6**:37, 1979.

388. Shemin, R.J., and others: Evaluation of right atrial-pulmonary artery conduits for tricuspid atresia: an experimental study, J. Thorac. Cardiovasc. Surg. **77**:685, 1979.

389. Shenasa, M., and others: Procainamide and retrograde atrioventricular nodal conduction in man, Circulation **65**:355, 1982.

390. Shine, K.I.: Ionic basis of excitation and of excitation-contraction coupling. In Roberts, N.K., and Gelband, H., editors: Cardiac arrhythmias in the neonate, infant, and child, New York, 1979, Appleton-Century-Crofts.

391. Shumacker, H.B., and others: Coarctation of the aorta, Curr. Probl. Surg. **15**(1):2, 1978.

392. Sigmann, J.M., and others: Ventricular septal defect: results after repair in infancy, Am. J. Cardiol. **39**:66, 1977.

393. Silverman, N.H., and others: Superior vena caval obstruction after Mustard's operation: detection by two-dimensional contrast echocardiography, Circulation **64**:392, 1981.

394. Skorecki, K.L., and Brenner, B.M.: Body fluid homeostasis in congestive heart failure and cirrhosis with ascites, AJM **72**:323, 1982.

395. Slota, M.C.: Extracorporeal membrane oxygenator support of the infant, Dimen. Crit. Care Nurs. **1**:70, 1982.

396. Slota, M.C.: Pediatric electrocardiography overview, Heart Lung **11**:69, 1982.

397. Soler-Soler, J., and others: Effect of verapamil in infants with paroxysmal supraventricular tachycardia, Circulation **59**:876, 1979.

398. Solinger, R., Elbl, F., and Minhas, K.: Echocardiography: its role in the severely ill infant, Pediatrics **57**:543, 1976.

399. Somerville, J.: Ostium primum defect: factors causing deterioration in the natural history, Br. Heart J. **27**:413, 1965.

400. Southall, D.P., and others: Study of cardiac rhythm in healthy newborn infants, Br. Heart J. **43**:14, 1980.

401. Soyka, L.F.: Clinical pharmacology of digoxin, Pediatr. Clin. North Am. **19**:241, 1977.

402. Spangler, J.G., Feldt, R.H., and Danielson, G.K.: Secundum atrial septal defect encountered in infancy, J. Thorac. Cardiovasc. Surg. **71**:398, 1976.

403. Sridaromont, S., and others: Double outlet right ventricle: hemodynamic and anatomic correlations, Am. J. Cardiol. **38**:85, 1976.

404. Stanger, P., and others: Complications of cardiac catheterization of neonates, infants, and children, Circulation **50**:595, 1974.

405. Steele, P., and others: Platelet survival time in patients with hypoxemia and pulmonary hypertension, Circulation **55**:660, 1977.

406. Stephenson, L.W., and others: Effects of nitroprusside and dopamine on pulmonary arterial vasculature in children after cardiac surgery, Circulation **60**:(suppl. 1):104, 1979.

407. Stevenson, J.G.: Acyanotic lesions with increased pulmonary blood flow, Pediatr. Clin. North Am. **25**:743, 1978.

408. Stewart, R.W., and others: Repair of double outlet right ventricle: an analysis of 62 cases, J. Thorac. Cardiovasc. Surg. **78**:502, 1979.

409. Stewart, S.: Double outlet right ventricle: a collective review with a surgical viewpoint, J. Thorac. Cardiovasc. Surg. **71**:355, 1976.

410. Studer, M., and others: Determinants of early and late results of repair of atrioventricular septal (canal) defects, J. Thorac. Cardiovasc. Surg. **84**:523, 1982.

411. Sturm, J.T., and others: Combined use of dopamine and nitroprusside therapy in conjunction with intra-aortic balloon pumping for the treatment of postcardiotomy low-output syndrome, J. Thorac. Cardiovasc. Surg. **82**:13, 1981.

412. Talner, N.S.: The pathophysiology of congestive heart failure in infancy. In Engle, M.A., editor: Pediatric cardiology, Cardiovasc. Clin. **4**:120, 1972.

413. Taussig, H.B., and others: Long-time observations on the Blalock-Taussig operation. VII. 20 to 28 year follow-up on patients with a tetralogy of Fallot, Johns Hopkins Med. J. **137**:13, 1975.

414. Ten Eick, R.E., and Hoffman, B.F.: Chronotropic effect of cardiac glycosides in dogs, cats, and rabbits, Circ. Res. **25**:305, 1969.

415. Tesler, M., and Hardgrove, C.: Cardiac catheterization: preparing the child, Am. J. Nurs. **73**:80, 1973.

416. Thapar, M.K., and Gillette, P.C.: Dual atrioventricular nodal pathways: a common electrophysiologic response in children, Circulation **60**:1369, 1979.

417. Titus, J.L., and Rastelli, G.C.: Anatomic features of persistent common atrioventricular canal. In Feldt, R.H., editor: Atrioventricular canal defects, Philadelphia, 1976, W.B. Saunders Co.

418. Tooley, W.H.: Clinical considerations. In Heymann, M.A., and Rudolph, A.M., co-chairpersons: The ductus arteriosus, Report of the seventy-fifth Ross Conference on Pediatric Research, Columbus, Ohio, 1978, Ross Laboratories, Inc.

419. Trusler, G.A., and others: Current results with the Mustard operation in isolated transposition of the great arteries, J. Thorac. Cardiovasc. Surg. **80**:381, 1980.

420. Tucker, B.L., Hurvitz, R.J., and Wells, W.J.: PDA: portal to cardiac surgery, Contemp. Surg. **15**:26, 1979.

421. Turley, K., and Ebert, P.A.: Total correction of transposition of the great arteries: conduction disturbances in infants younger than three months of age, J. Thorac. Cardiovasc. Surg. **76**:312, 1978.

422. Turley, K., Tucker, W.Y., and Ebert, P.A.: The changing role of palliative procedures for the treatment of infants with congenital heart disease, J. Thorac. Cardiovasc. Surg. **79**:194, 1980.

423. Turley, K., and others: Total anomalous pulmonary venous connection in infancy: influence of age and type of lesion, Am. J. Cardiol. 45:92, 1980.

424. The Upjohn Company, Prostin VR Pediatric: physician's prescribing information, Kalamazoo, Michigan, 1981. The Upjohn Company.

425. Uzark, K.: A child's cardiac catheterization: avoiding the potential risks, MCN: Am. J. Matern. Child Nurs. 3:158, 1978.

426. van der Horst, R., and others: Interrupted aortic arch operation in the first week of life: hemodynamic and angiographic evaluation one year later, Ann. Thorac. Surg. 27:112, 1979.

427. Van Praagh, R., and others: Tetralogy of Fallot: underdevelopment of the pulmonary infundibulum and its sequelae, Am. J. Cardiol. 26:25, 1970.

428. Vancini, M., and others: Surgical treatment of congenital pulmonary stenosis due to dysplastic leaflets and small valve annulus, J. Thorac. Cardiovasc. Surg. 79:464, 1980.

429. Varghese, P.J.: Sinus node disorders. In Roberts, N.K., and Gelband, H., editors: Cardiac arrhythmias in the neonate, infant, and child, New York, 1977, Appleton-Century-Crofts.

430. Versmold, H., and others: Aortic blood pressure during the first 12 hours of life in infants with birthweight 610-4220 gms, Pediatrics 67:607, 1981.

431. Vlad, P., and Lambert, E.C.: Late results of Rashkind's balloon atrial septostomy. In Kirklin, J.W., editor: Advances in cardiovascular surgery, New York, 1973, Grune & Stratton, Inc.

432. Wada, J., and others: Long-term follow-up of artificial valves in patients under 15 years old, Ann. Thorac. Surg. 29:519, 1979.

433. Wagner, H.R., and others: Clinical course in aortic stenosis, Circulation 56(suppl. 1):47, 1977.

434. Waldman, J.D., and others: Shortened platelet survival in cyanotic heart disease, J. Pediatr. 87:77, 1975.

435. Wallgren, E.I., Landtman, B., and Rapola, J.: Extracardiac malformations associated with congenital heart disease, Eur. J. Cardiol. 7:15, 1978.

436. Watkins, L., and others: Surgical management of congenital pulmonary valve dysplasia, Ann. Thorac. Surg. 24:498, 1977.

437. Weeks, H.: Personal communication, Salt Lake City, Utah, October, 1982, Pediatric Intensive Care Unit, Primary Children's Hospital.

438. Weidman, W.H., and others: Clinical course in ventricular septal defect, Circulation 56(suppl. 1):1, 1977.

439. Wessel, H.U., and others: Lung function in tetralogy of Fallot after intracardiac repair, J. Thorac. Cardiovasc. Surg. 82:616, 1981.

440. Wetmore, N.E., and others: Extracorporeal membrane oxygenation (ECMO): a team approach in critical care and life support research, Heart Lung 8:288, 1979.

441. Weyman, A.E., and others: Cross-sectional echocardiographic visualization of the stenotic pulmonary valve, Circulation 56:769, 1977.

442. Wheedon, D., Shore, D.F., and Lincoln, C.: Continuous monitoring of pulmonary artery pressure after cardiac surgery in infants and children, J. Cardiovasc. Surg. 22:307, 1981.

443. Whittemore, R., Hobbins, J.C., and Engle, M.A.: Pregnancy and its outcome in women with and without surgical treatment of congenital heart disease, Am. J. Cardiol. 50:641, 1982.

444. Wilkman-Coffelt, J., Parmley, W.W., and Mason, D.T.: The cardiac hypertrophy process, Circ. Res. 69:51, 1980.

445. Will, R.J., and others: Sodium nitroprusside and propranolol therapy for management of postcoarctectomy hypertension, J. Thorac. Cardiovasc. Surg. 75:722, 1978.

446. Williams, D.B., and others: Porcine heterograft valve replacement in children, J. Thorac. Cardiovasc. Surg. 84:446, 1982.

447. Williams, W.G., and others: Early experience with arterial repair of transposition, Ann. Thorac. Surg. 32:8, 1981.

448. Wilson, J.M., and others: Persistent stenosis and deformity of the right pulmonary artery after correction of the Waterston anastomosis, J. Thorac. Cardiovasc. Surg. 82:169, 1981.

449. Winters, R.W.: Principles of pediatric fluid therapy, ed. 2, Boston, 1982, Little, Brown & Co.

450. Wolfe, R.R., and Way, G.L.: Cardiomyopathies in infants of diabetic mothers, Johns Hopkins Med. J. 140:177, 1977.

451. Wright, J.S., and Newman, D.C.: Ligation of the patent ductus: technical considerations at different ages, J. Thorac. Cardiovasc. Surg. 75:695, 1978.

452. Yacoub, M., and others: Clinical and hemodynamic results of the two-stage anatomic correction of simple transposition of the great arteries, Circulation 62:(suppl. 1):190, 1980.

453. Young, D.: Later results of closure of secundum atrial septal defects in children, Am. J. Cardiol. 31:14, 1973.

454. Youssef, M.M.S.: Self-control behavior of school-age children who are hospitalized for cardiac diagnostic procedures, Matern. Child Nurs. J. 10:219, 1981.

455. Zamora, R., Moller, J.H., and Edwards, J.E.: Double outlet right ventricle: anatomic types and associated anomalies, Chest 68:672, 1975.

456. Zapol, W.M., Snider, M.T., and Schneider, R.C.: Extracorporeal membrane oxygenation for acute respiratory failure, Anesthesiology 46:272, 1977.

Pulmonary Disorders

JANET SNOW

Acute disease of the respiratory tract is by far the most common cause of illness in infancy and childhood, accounting for approximately 50% of all illness in children under 5 years of age and 30% in children between 5 and 12 years of age.[2] Although these youngsters usually have mild and self-limited problems, some may be severely affected. As a result respiratory disease is commonly seen in the critical-care unit, either as a primary clinical problem or as a secondary complication. The purpose of this chapter is to discuss pediatric respiratory problems and to emphasize developmental factors that may influence the nursing care provided for these patients.

■ Essential Anatomy and Physiology

The primary function of the respiratory system is to move oxygen from air to blood, and carbon dioxide from blood to air; this process of gas exchange is known as *ventilation*. Ventilation is the product of breathing frequency (f) and tidal volume (V_T). Ventilation is adequate if arterial oxygen tension (Pa_{O_2}) and arterial carbon dioxide tension (Pa_{CO_2}) are maintained in the normal range; it is either inadequate or excessive if these blood gases are abnormal.

Oxygen and carbon dioxide move between air and blood in the lung by simple diffusion; that is, gases move from an area of high partial pressure to an area of low partial pressure. Oxygen-rich, carbon dioxide–poor air is brought to the alveolar air spaces by the respiratory muscles through branching airway tubes. Oxygen-poor, carbon dioxide–rich systemic venous blood is pumped by the right ventricle through branching pulmonary arteries to lung capillaries. These capillaries are located within the walls of the alveoli. Because the whole of cardiac output enters the lungs, each blood cell spends about 1 sec-

ond in contact with alveolar air. This brief time is more than sufficient for complete equilibration of oxygen and carbon dioxide between gas and blood.

■ EMBRYOLOGY OF THE LUNG

The rudiment of the respiratory system appears by the fourth week of gestation. A lung bud branches from the primitive esophagus to form the airways and alveolar spaces. The pulmonary arteries form near the branching airways; their growth matches the growth of the airways. Although virtually all other body systems are physiologically ready for extrauterine life as early as 25 weeks of gestation, the lung requires a longer time for complete maturation. Thus lung maturity is the single most important factor that determines whether or not a prematurely born infant can survive.

Table 4-1 summarizes the development of the respiratory system. Although the number of airway branches is fixed at birth, airway dimensions and alveolar number both increase until the child is about 8 years of age.[8,16,19,39]

■ ANATOMY OF THE LUNG

The thoracic cavity is formed by the ribs, intercostal muscles, and diaphragm. It contains both lungs and the mediastinum; within the mediastinum, the heart, great vessels, nerves, trachea, and esophagus are located. Pleural tissue covers each lung and adheres to the surface of the diaphragm and inner surface of the chest wall.

The diaphragm is the principal muscle of inspiration. If the chest wall is sufficiently stiff, contraction of the diaphragm during inspiration decreases the pressure within the thoracic cavity and increases thoracic volume in both its longitudinal and transverse dimensions. The diaphragm is inner-

Table 4-1 Fetal development of the respiratory system[8,16,19,39]

Period of gestation	Development
26 days	Lower respiratory system begins to develop until separation of the respiratory tract from the foregut is achieved
Week 5	Lung buds form and begin to differentiate into the bronchi
Weeks 7-10	Development of the larynx
Weeks 5-16	24 orders of airway branches are formed
Weeks 13-25	Canalicular period; bronchi enlarge and lung tissue becomes highly vascular
Weeks 26-28	Lungs are capable of gas exchange; Type II alveolar cells secrete surfactant
Week 24-birth	Capillary network proliferates around the alveoli. Only about 8%-10% of cardiac output flows through the lung; pulmonary vascular resistance is very high

vated on each side by the phrenic nerve, which is formed by the third, fourth, and fifth cervical spinal nerves. Thus the diaphragm continues to function even when a high thoracic spinal cord injury results in complete paralysis of the arms and legs.

In the older child and adult the angle of rib attachments to the sternum and vertebrae allows the thorax to increase its volume during inspiration. By contrast, in the newborn, the ribs are attached to the spine and sternum almost horizontally, so that chest size is not increased and it may actually decrease during normal breathing. In the infant the diaphragm is inserted horizontally, tending to draw the lower ribs inward during spontaneous inspiration, particularly when the infant is supine.[22] For these reasons the chest of the infant and young child is likely to retract when respiratory distress develops, resulting in "seesaw" respirations. Finally, the accessory muscles of respiration are poorly developed in infants and young children.

The airways distribute gas to all parts of the lung. As air passes through the nose and mouth, it is warmed, humidified, and filtered. The upper airway thus serves as an "air conditioner"; when air reaches the trachea, it has been warmed to body temperature, is fully saturated with water, and is freed of small particles. The amount of water vapor a volume of gas can contain depends on the temperature of the gas. The higher the temperature of the inspired gas, the greater is the amount of water vapor contained in the gas. For example, alveolar air is 100% humidified at body temperature and contains about 44 mg of water per liter of gas; room air at 21° C has a water content of 10 mg or less.

Heat is transmitted to inspired air by convection, while water is added by evaporation from the airway surface. Therefore there may be a loss of heat and water from the body during breathing. The healthy child copes well with this loss, but the small infant with lung disease may lose heat and water when tachypnea occurs. Moreover, as water is lost from the airway surface, ciliary activity is impaired. This impairment of mucociliary clearance may result in the formation of mucous plugs, atelectasis, air-trapping, or infection. Thus great care must be taken with children in whom the upper airway has been bypassed with an endotrachel (ET), or tracheostomy tube. Warm, moist air must be provided to these patients in order to avoid damage to the airway surface.

■ **THE UPPER AIRWAY**

The infant, up to approximately 4 weeks of age, is an obligatory nose-breather and does not adapt well to mouth breathing. Thus any obstruction in the nose or nasopharynx may increase upper airway resistance and increase the work of breathing. For example, respiratory failure has occurred in newborn infants whose eye patches (used to prevent possible eye damage from phototherapy lights) have slipped over the nose and caused obstruction.

Because the upper airway is smaller in diameter in the young child, it may significantly contribute to airflow resistance. In addition, the upper airway is fairly pliable in the young infant, and it may narrow during inspiration. Upper airway patency is maintained by the active contraction of muscles in the pharynx and the larynx. Airway obstruction can occur if these muscles do not function properly or when the neck of an infant is flexed or extended.

The glottis of an infant is located more cephalad than in an older child, and the epiglottis is longer. This may make intubation of the airway more difficult in the small infant, especially when the neck is hyperextended. The narrowest portion of the airway in a baby is at the level of the cricoid, while the glottic area is the narrowest portion of the airway in the adult. Small amounts of edema or obstruction in the cricoid (subglottic) area will produce an increase in airway resistance and may lead to respiratory failure.

The airways continue to increase in length and diameter postnatally. Major changes occur in the terminal respiratory units as the number and size of the alveoli increase after birth.[8,16,39] Alveolar and bronchiolar pathways for collateral ventilation (pores) also develop by middle childhood. These pores allow trapped gas in an obstructed lung unit to be eventually absorbed.

■ COMPLIANCE AND RESISTANCE

From the time of the first breath, the lungs have a tendency to recoil from the chest wall because of the elastic fibers within lung tissue. This tendency is balanced by the propensity of the chest wall to spring outward. The net effect of these two opposing tendencies is to create a subatmospheric pressure in the intrathoracic space at the end of a normal breath. During inspiration the volume of the thoracic cavity is enlarged and intrathoracic pressure becomes more negative; air moves from the mouth to the alveolar spaces. At the end of inspiration the elastic recoil of the lungs and chest wall causes alveolar pressure to rise above atmospheric pressure, thus producing expiratory flow. In a person with normal lungs, expiration requires no muscular work.[39]

The relationship between transpulmonary pressure and volume is called compliance. *Compliance* is a measure of the distensibility of the lungs and is defined as the volume change produced by a trans-

pulmonary pressure change. If the volume change produced by a given pressure change is small, the lungs are stiff, or they have a decreased compliance. Conversely, compliance is increased when the volume change produced by a given pressure change is large. Compliance is decreased by pulmonary edema, pneumothorax, atelectasis, and pulmonary fibrosis. Compliance is increased in diseases such as lobar emphysema, and asthma. Compliance is difficult to measure, but effective compliance or dynamic compliance of the lung and chest wall can be measured in the child who is mechanically ventilated. This is discussed later in this chapter.

Lung compliance is determined primarily by two factors: surfactant and the elasticity of lung tissue. Surfactant is a lipid material that spreads on the alveolar surface and prevents alveolar collapse as the alveoli get smaller during expiration. (See the section on respiratory distress syndrome for further discussion of surfactant.)

Just as compliance is determined by lung tissue factors, resistance depends mostly on the airways. Airway resistance is defined as the driving pressure divided by the airflow rate. In the lung the driving pressure for flow is the transairway pressure, which is equal to mouth pressure minus alveolar pressure during inspiration; and alveolar pressure minus mouth pressure during expiration. Airway resistance is directly proportional to three variables: flow rate, the length of the airway, and the viscosity of the gas. Airway resistance is inversely proportional to the fourth power of the airway radius (Poiseuille's law). Any decrease in the infant's airway radius will significantly increase airway resistance and will increase the work of breathing. For example, if the tracheal radius of an infant is reduced by 1 mm of circumferential swelling or mucus (from 4 mm to 3 mm) the airway diameter is decreased by 25% and airway resistance is increased by $4^4/3^4$, or fivefold. In the adult airway, however, accumulation of 1 mm of mucus would result in a decrease of airway radius by only 15% and only a twofold increase in airway resistance. This difference in airway caliber predisposes the small infant to airway obstruction.

Airway resistance is highest in the nasopharynx and lowest in the small bronchioles. Airway resistance is greatly increased in diseases such as asthma, bronchiolitis, tracheal stenosis, and conditions associated with increased respiratory secretions. High airway resistance increases the work of breathing and is manifested by respiratory distress. If respiratory muscle fatigue develops in a child with increased airway resistance, respiratory failure may develop.

■ VENTILATION

The process of gas movement in and out of the lungs is defined as ventilation. *Minute ventilation* ($\dot{V}$) (volume per minute) is the product of tidal volume (V_T) and respiratory frequency (f) or:

$$\dot{V} = f \times V_T$$

For example, a patient breathing 30 times per minute with a tidal volume of 100 cc has a minute ventilation of 30×100, or 3000 cc per minute. Normally, about 70% of tidal volume reaches the alveolar space and 30% fills the conducting airways. This latter volume is called the *anatomic dead space* V_D and is approximately 2 to 3 cc/kg body weight. The remaining 70% of the volume that actually reaches the alveolar space is referred to as *alveolar ventilation* ($\dot{V}_A$). Alveolar ventilation can be estimated by subtracting the anatomic dead space from the tidal volume (V_T):

$$\dot{V}_A = f \times (V_T - V_D)$$

For example, if the tidal volume is 100 cc, the breathing rate 30 per minute, and the anatomic dead space 20 cc, then alveolar ventilation would equal $30 \times (100 - 20)$ or 2400 cc/minute. Thus alveolar ventilation is always less than minute ventilation.

The rate of removal of carbon dioxide from alveoli and the rate of oxygen delivery to the alveoli are directly dependent on alveolar ventilation. Normal alveolar ventilation is defined as that level of ventilation that results in normal partial pressures of arterial oxygen and carbon dioxide in arterial blood.

Anatomic dead space is just one part of the total dead space ventilation. A more clinically significant portion of dead space is the *physiologic dead space.* This represents the volume of ventilated lung that does not receive any pulmonary blood flow and thus does not participate in gas exchange. Ventilation of this portion of the lung is thus "wasted." This concept is illustrated in Fig. 4-1, *B.* In normal individuals, physiologic and anatomic dead-space measurements are similar, but in patients with lung disease, physiologic dead space is much greater than the anatomic dead space.

■ LUNG VOLUMES

The total volume of the gas contained in the lung at maximum inspiration is the *total lung capacity.* The volume that can be expired following a maximum inspiratory effort is the *vital capacity.* This is an important and useful measurement of lung function and is discussed in detail later in this chapter. Vital capacity may be reduced by any acute or chronic lung disease that increases lung stiffness or

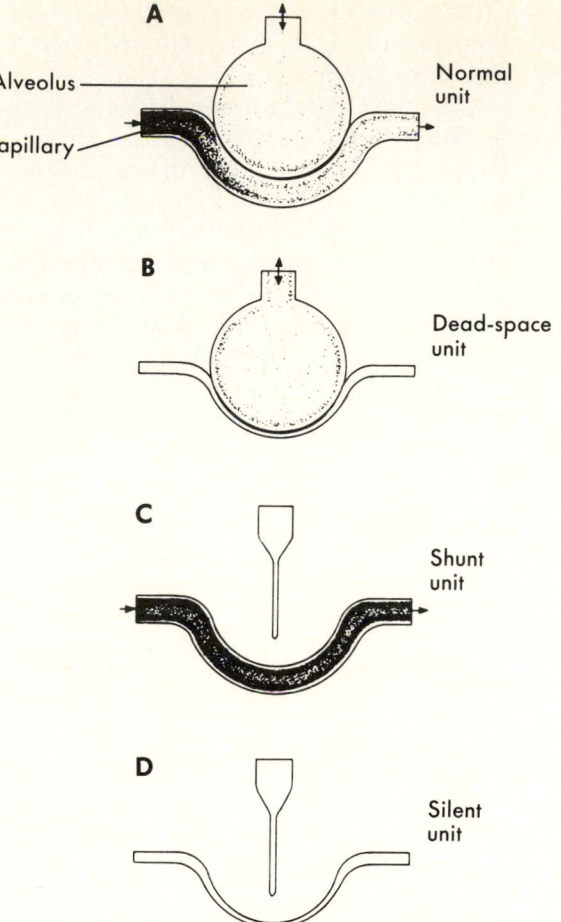

Fig. 4-1 The theoretical respiratory unit with graphic representation of the relationship between ventilation and perfusion in different clinical conditions. **A,** Normal ventilation; normal perfusion. **B,** Normal ventilation; no perfusion. **C,** No ventilation; normal perfusion. **D,** No ventilation; no perfusion.

Reproduced with permission from Shapiro, B.A., Harrison, R.A., and Walton, J.R.: Clinical application of blood gases, 3rd edition. Copyright © 1982 by Year Book Medical Publishers, Inc., Chicago.

by conditions that limit available intrathoracic space (scoliosis, pneumonia, or pleural effusion). These lung volume measurements are extremely dependent on the patient's effort. They are difficult or impossible to obtain in children who are uncooperative or who are less than 5 years of age.

The volume of gas remaining in the lungs at the end of a normal expiration is the *functional residual capacity.* An increase in functional residual capacity usually indicates hyperinflation of the lung, which is found in lobar emphysema, bronchopulmonary dysplasia, cystic fibrosis, or asthma. A decrease in functional residual capacity may be seen in patients with pulmonary fibrosis or scoliosis. Fig. 4-2 shows the subdivisions of lung volume.

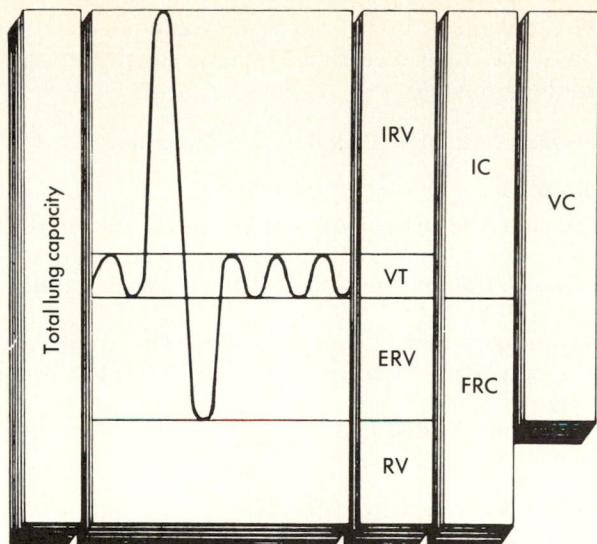

Fig. 4-2 Divisions of total lung capacity. Total lung capacity (TLC) is the maximum amount of air the lungs can hold. The total lung capacity is divided into four primary volumes: inspiratory reserve volume (IRV), tidal volume (V_T), expiratory reserve volume (ERV), and residual volume (RV). Capacities are combinations of two or more lung volumes. These include the inspiratory capacity (IC), functional residual capacity (FRC), and vital capacity (VC).

Reproduced with permission from Shapiro, B.A., Harrison, R.A., and Walton, J.R.: Clinical application of blood gases, 3rd edition. Copyright © 1982 by Year Book Medical Publishers, Inc., Chicago.

■ VENTILATION-PERFUSION RELATIONSHIPS

As atmospheric air reaches the lungs, it comes into contact with pulmonary capillary blood. The distribution of perfusion and ventilation is not uniform in the normal lung. Because of the effects of gravity, blood flow is greatest in the dependent portions of the lung; thus when the patient is lying supine, blood flow is greatest in the posterior portions of the lungs. When the patient is standing or sitting, blood flow is greatest in the inferior portions of the lung.

Because pleural pressure is not uniform, the upper airways receive more ventilation than the lower airways. As a result of these relationships, some portion of pulmonary blood flow does not reach ventilated alveoli. This volume of blood is known as the *physiologic shunt*. Diagram *C* in Fig. 4-1 illustrates this concept. The physiologic shunt can occur either because of an absolute fall in pulmonary blood flow or as the result of an increase in pulmonary blood flow to unventilated portions of the lung. In the

Table 4-2   Normal arterial blood gas values

	Neonate	Child
pH	7.32-7.42	7.35-7.45
P_{CO_2}	30-40 mm Hg	35-45 mm Hg
HCO_3	20-26 mEq/L	22-28 mEq/L
P_{O_2}	60-80 mm Hg	80-100 mm Hg

The neonatal values represent normals for neonates between a few hours after birth and 4 weeks of age. Values for the child are the same as for the adult.

normal person approximately 2% to 5% of right ventricular cardiac output is returned to the left ventricle without entering pulmonary capillaries. This small portion of right ventricular output flows into bronchial, pleural, or thebesian veins and represents obligatory shunt pathways. However, abnormal intrapulmonary shunts may occur as a result of congenital or acquired lung diseases. This increase in physiologic shunt is the basis of most respiratory disorders and is the most common cause of hypoxemia. However, hypercapnia usually does not occur. Carbon dioxide elimination continues at a much greater rate in lung units whose ventilation and perfusion are better matched. The clinical measurement of intrapulmonary shunt is discussed later in this chapter.

The normal neonate, especially the premature infant, has a larger amount of intrapulmonary shunting. This is a result of the presence of either nonventilated or poorly ventilated but perfused areas in the lungs, which causes a decreased Pa_{O_2} in the newborn infant. In these infants a Pa_{O_2} of 60 to 80 mm Hg may be normal in the first day of life but should be greater than 80 mm Hg within 2 or 3 days after birth (Table 4-2).

■ GAS TRANSPORT

The exchange of oxygen and carbon dioxide occurs in the alveolus. Carbon dioxide and oxygen diffuse through the alveolar capillary membranes. The pressure gradient for carbon dioxide causes carbon dioxide to diffuse from the blood into the alveolus, while the pressure gradient for oxygen causes oxygen to diffuse from alveolar air to blood. The amount of oxygen that diffuses through the alveolar-capillary membrane depends on the pressure gradient and on the amount of functional alveolar membrane.

Oxygen is carried in the blood in two ways. A large portion (97.5%) is carried in combination with hemoglobin inside red blood cells. A small portion (2.5%) is carried in the dissolved state in plasma. The normal individual, breathing room air, has approximately 20 ml oxygen per deciliter of arterial blood (or 20 vol%); approximately 19.5 ml of the oxygen is combined with hemoglobin, and approximately 0.5 ml of oxygen is dissolved in the blood. If the patient receives a high inspired oxygen concentration, the amount of blood carried by the hemoglobin will not change; instead the amount of dissolved oxygen will increase. Approximately 0.003 ml O_2 are dissolved per deciliter of blood for every mm Hg rise in oxygen tension (0.003 ml O_2/dl blood/mm Hg Pa_{O_2}).[42]

Whenever the nurse attempts to evaluate the patient's arterial oxygenation, the patient's hemoglobin concentration, arterial oxygen saturation, and Pa_{O_2} must be known. From these values the nurse will be able to calculate the patient's *arterial oxygen content,* that is, the *actual amount of oxygen carried by the blood.* This is equal to the sum of the oxygen carried by the hemoglobin and the oxygen dissolved in the blood. Each gram of hemoglobin (Hb) can carry approximately 1.34 ml oxygen. As already noted, 0.003 ml oxygen is dissolved in each deciliter of blood for every mm Hg in Pa_{O_2}.

Total oxygen content = O_2 bound to Hb + dissolved O_2

The oxygen bound to hemoglobin is calculated by determining the *theoretical oxygen capacity of the blood,* or the amount of oxygen carried by the hemoglobin if the hemoglobin is fully saturated:

Oxygen capacity = Hb concentration (mg/dl) ×   (1)

1.34 ml O_2/gm Hb

Once the patient's arterial oxygen saturation is known, the amount of oxygen bound to the hemoglobin is multiplied by the theoretical oxygen capacity:

O_2 bound to Hb = (O_2 capacity) × Arterial O_2 saturation (2)

To calculate the amount of dissolved oxygen present in the blood, the child's Pa_{O_2} is multiplied by 0.003 ml O_2/dl:

Dissolved oxygen = 0.003 ml O_2/dl × Pa_{O_2} (3)

Finally, the total arterial oxygen content is equal to the sum of the oxygen carried by the hemoglobin and the dissolved oxygen:

Oxygen content = (Equation 2) + (Equation 3)

EXAMPLE 1

Calculate the oxygen content (in ml O_2/dl) for the child with a hemoglobin concentration of 15 gm/dl, a Pa_{O_2} of 100 mm Hg, and an arterial oxygen saturation of 97%:
Oxygen content = O_2 carried by Hb + Dissolved O_2
= (15 gm/dl × 1.34 ml/gm × 0.97) + (.003 ml O_2/mm Hg × 100 mm Hg)
= 19.50 ml O_2/dl + 0.30 ml O_2/dl
= 19.80 ml O_2/dl

EXAMPLE 2

Calculate the oxygen content (in ml O_2/dl) for the child with a hemoglobin concentration of 8 gm/dl, a Pa_{O_2} of 100 mm Hg, and an arterial oxygen saturation of 97%:
Oxygen content = O_2 carried by Hb + Dissolved O_2
= (8 gm/dl × 1.34 ml/gm × 0.97) + (.003 ml O_2/mm Hg × 100 mm Hg)
= 10.40 ml O_2/dl + 0.30 ml O_2/dl
= 10.70 ml O_2/dl

These two examples demonstrate the dramatic fall in oxygen content that occurs with a fall in the hemoglobin. Although both patients have exactly the same Pa_{O_2} and oxygen saturation, the second patient must almost double his cardiac output to maintain the same oxygen delivery as the first patient.

EXAMPLE 3

Calculate the arterial oxygen content (in ml O_2/dl) for the child with a hemoglobin concentration of 15 gm/dl, a Pa_{O_2} of 50 mm Hg, and an arterial oxygen saturation of 85%:
Oxygen content = O_2 carried by Hb + Dissolved O_2
= (15 gm/dl × 1.34 ml O_2/gm × 0.85) + (.003 ml O_2/mm Hg × 50 mm Hg)
= 17.09 ml O_2/dl + 0.15 ml O_2/dl
= 17.24 ml O_2/dl

This example demonstrates the effect of mild hypoxemia on the patient's arterial oxygen content. Most patients tolerate such mild hypoxemia because they are able to maintain oxygen delivery by compensatory increases in cardiac output. It is interesting to note that the arterial oxygen content of the patient in example 3 is still significantly higher than the arterial oxygen content of the patient in example 2, even though the patient in example 2 has a higher Pa_{O_2} and fully saturated hemoglobin. This is explained by the higher hemoglobin concentration of the patient in example 3.

These examples confirm the importance of using hemoglobin concentration, PaO_2, and arterial oxygen saturation to evaluate blood gas results.

The relationship between the PaO_2 and the hemoglobin saturation is expressed by the oxyhemoglobin dissociation curve, as shown in Fig. 4-3. The curve is not linear; instead, it is **S** shaped, with a large plateau at the higher levels of PaO_2.[42] There are several important parts of the oxyhemoglobin dissociation curve. The curve flattens when the PaO_2 exceeds 80 to 100 mm Hg. This means that although the PaO_2 continues to rise, the hemoglobin is fully saturated; it cannot carry any more oxygen. Thus any further rise in the PaO_2 will only reflect an increase in the amount of dissolved oxygen in the blood (which contributes only 0.003 ml O_2/mm Hg PaO_2). Therefore a rise in PaO_2 from 100 to 700 torr does *not* mean that seven times more oxygen is carried in the blood; in fact this rise is associated with only approximately a 10% increase in oxygen content. Since the hemoglobin is fully saturated once the PaO_2 reaches 100 mm Hg, there is usually no advantage to maintaining the patient's PaO_2 any higher.

The slope of the oxyhemoglobin dissociation curve becomes very steep once the PaO_2 is less than 60 mm Hg. Thus when the patient's PaO_2 falls below 60 mm Hg, even small decreases represent a large fall in the arterial oxygen saturation (and thus in the arterial oxygen content). Therefore, if at all possible, the patient's PaO_2 should be maintained above 60 mm Hg.

The shape of the oxyhemoglobin curve may be altered by several factors. If the curve is shifted to the right, this means that hemoglobin binds less oxygen at any partial pressure. Conversely, if the curve is shifted to the left, hemoglobin binds more oxygen at any given PaO_2. Factors that shift the curve to the right include acidosis, hypercapnia, and hyperthermia. Under these conditions, less oxygen is bound at any given PO_2, but within the normal range, oxygen release to tissues is enhanced.[42]

In contrast, the oxyhemoglobin dissociation curve may be shifted to the left by alkalosis, hypocapnia, and hypothermia. While these factors increase hemoglobin saturation with oxygen at any given partial pressure of oxygen, hemoglobin release to tissues may be impaired.[42]

The hemoglobin dissociation curve for fetal hemoglobin is shifted to the left of the adult hemoglobin curve. Thus at a given PO_2 and hematocrit, fetal blood contains more oxygen than adult blood. This ensures that an adequate amount of oxygen will be transferred from maternal blood to fetal blood by the placenta. After birth, fetal hemoglobin usually disappears within 4 to 6 weeks and adult hemoglobin is formed by the infant.

Carbon dioxide is also carried in the blood in several ways. Like oxygen it may be either dissolved in plasma or carried by hemoglobin. In addition, however, carbon dioxide may react with water to form carbonic acid (H_2CO_3), or it may combine with other proteins to form carbamino compounds. In any event, the important thing to remember about carbon dioxide is that the relationship between $PaCO_2$ and arterial CO_2 content is linear. Furthermore, arterial carbon dioxide tension ($PaCO_2$) is directly proportional to the metabolic production of carbon dioxide but inversely proportional to alveolar ventilation. Thus a decrease in alveolar ventilation will result in an increase in $PaCO_2$. For example, an individual whose $PaCO_2$ falls from 40 mm Hg to 20 mm Hg must have doubled his alveolar ventilation. Similarly, if the $PaCO_2$ increases from 40 mm Hg to 60 mm Hg, alveolar ventilation must have decreased by 50%.

If the $PaCO_2$ increases, carbon dioxide combines

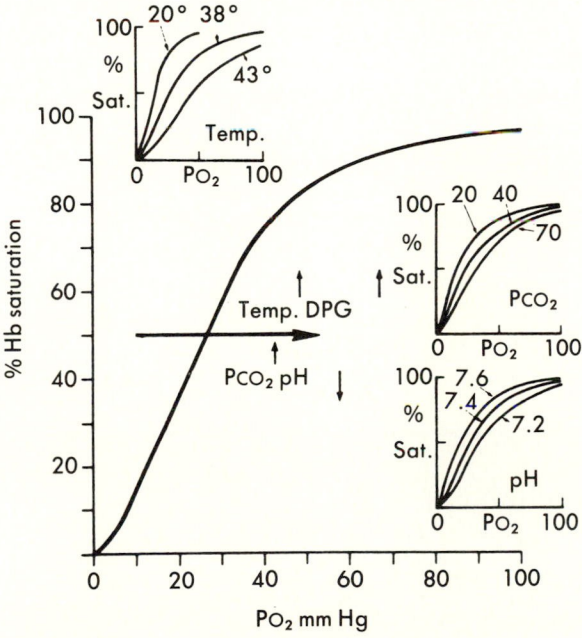

Fig. 4-3 The oxyhemoglobin dissociation curve. The inset curves demonstrate shifts in the dissociation curve which result from changes in temperature, PCO_2, and pH. In addition, a decrease in 2,3,-DPG (which is present in the neonate with large amounts of fetal hemoglobin) shifts the dissociation to left and an increase in 2,3,-DPG shifts the curve to the right.

From West, J.B.: Gas transport to the periphery. In Respiratory physiology—the essentials, ed. 2, Baltimore, © 1979, Williams & Wilkins.

with water to form carbonic acid (H_2CO_3); carbonic acid then dissociates into bicarbonate and hydrogen ion:

$$CO_2 + H_2O \leftrightharpoons H_2CO_3 \leftrightharpoons H^+ + HCO_3^-$$

The net result of these reactions is a rise in hydrogen ion concentration and a fall in pH, that is, respiratory acidosis. If this condition persists for several hours, the kidney will respond with excretion of more hydrogen ion and reabsorption of more bicarbonate. This renal compensation can restore the arterial pH to nearly normal levels (see discussion of renal disorders in Chapter 7).

Alveolar ventilation may either increase or decrease as compensation for primary metabolic disorders. When metabolic acidosis develops, excess hydrogen ions are present. This results in the formation of more carbonic acid, which then dissociates to carbon dioxide and water. Total ventilation is increased, which eliminates additional carbon dioxide, and the carbon dioxide tension (or partial pressure—Pa_{CO_2}) will fall. Thus the arterial pH may increase toward normal levels since hydrogen ions are eliminated as carbon dioxide is excreted by the lungs.

Alveolar ventilation will decrease when metabolic alkalosis is present. Carbon dioxide may be retained until the Pa_{CO_2} is extremely high. This carbon dioxide will combine with water to form carbonic acid, which will dissociate to form hydrogen ion and bicarbonate ion. As a result of the carbon dioxide retention, hydrogen ions accumulate and the arterial pH rises.

Table 4-3 summarizes changes in the arterial pH, P_{CO_2}, and serum bicarbonate (HCO_3) that occur with respiratory and metabolic acidosis and alkalosis.

■ REGULATION OF RESPIRATION

Alveolar ventilation is controlled by both neural and chemical factors. Spontaneous respiration depends on a rhythmic discharge from the respiratory center; this respiratory center is known to be located primarily in the brainstem, but no one specific center has ever been isolated. The respiratory center contains both voluntary and involuntary nerves, so that the pulmonary system participates in functions other than gas exchange (e.g., coughing, swallowing, talking, and vomiting).

The chemical control of breathing is modulated at two respiratory centers—the carbon dioxide sensor and the oxygen sensor. The sensor for carbon dioxide is located in the brainstem and is primarily influenced by the hydrogen ion concentration of the cerebrospinal fluid. Carbon dioxide freely diffuses from blood into cerebrospinal fluid so that an increase in Pa_{CO_2} will quickly increase the hydrogen ion concentration in the cerebrospinal fluid near these sensor cells. The electrical output of these chemosensitive cells results in an increase in ventilation that restores Pa_{CO_2} to normal levels.

The oxygen sensor consists of chemoreceptors located in the carotid body (near the common carotid artery). These peripheral chemoreceptors detect changes in arterial oxygen *tension* and not oxygen *content*. A fall in Pa_{O_2} below 50 to 60 mm Hg results in a progressive increase in the electrical activity of the carotid body, which is transmitted to the respiratory centers in the brainstem. The result is an increase in alveolar ventilation. The carotid body sensors are also responsive to the development of acidosis and, to a lesser extent, hypotension.

Table 4-3 Changes in arterial blood gases with acid-base imbalances

	pH	P_{CO_2}	HCO_3
Respiratory acidosis	↓ or N*	↑	N or ↑*
Respiratory alkalosis	↑ or N*	↓	N or ↓*
Metabolic acidosis	↓ or N*	N or ↓*	↓
Metabolic alkalosis	↑ or N*	N or ↑*	↑

*Complete compensation.
↓, Decreased; ↑, increased; N, normal.

■ **NEURAL CONTROL OF AIRWAY CALIBER**

The walls of the airways are lined with smooth muscle, and constriction of this smooth muscle will cause narrowing of the airway, that is, bronchoconstriction. On the other hand, relaxation of the smooth muscle lining the airways will cause an increase in airway diameter, or bronchodilation. This muscle is innervated by branches of the vagus nerve (cholinergic nerves) and by branches of the sympathetic nervous system (adrenergic nerves). Thus acetylcholine and related compounds cause bronchoconstriction, while acetylcholine antagonists like atropine cause bronchodilation. Adrenergic stimulation of smooth muscle by epinephrine (and related compounds) causes bronchodilation.

Mucous glands in the lung also have a dual cholinergic and adrenergic innervation. Cholinergic stimulation increases mucous secretion, while adrenergic stimulation decreases it.

The neural control of pulmonary blood vessel diameter is less well understood.

■ **Common Clinical Conditions**

■ **AIRWAY OBSTRUCTION**

The nurse is primarily responsible for airway care in the critical-care unit. Therefore the importance of a thorough understanding of airway obstruction in children is extremely important. Every nurse working in the intensive care unit (ICU) must learn how to assess for signs of airway obstruction, when to anticipate it, and how to manage it.

■ **Etiology**

There are several important developmental factors that increase the risk of airway obstruction in infants and children. These factors, discussed at the beginning of this chapter, include small airway size, increased airway resistance, and a pliable chest wall. The accessory muscles of respiration are immature in infants and young children. In addition, since the ribs of the infants are horizontally placed, elevation of the ribs does not increase intrathoracic volume significantly. Since diaphragmatic placement is more horizontal in infants and small children, diaphragmatic contraction tends to draw the lower ribs inward. All of these factors increase the young child's risk of respiratory muscle fatigue if respiratory distress develops.[22]

The infant or child has an increased likelihood of development of sudden airway obstruction for any of the following reasons[7,34]:

1. Recent history of intubation, bronchoscopy, or surgery near the upper airway
2. Presence of an artificial airway or tracheostomy. In these patients, collection of secretions may cause airway obstruction.
3. History of ingestion or inhalation of a foreign body or volatile chemical. In these patients, bronchoconstriction or laryngospasm may result in airway obstruction.
4. Acute inflammation of the airway, including croup, epiglottitis, peritonsillar abscess, and anaphylaxis
5. Recent history of general anesthesia. Bronchospasm may result after anesthesia or mucous plugging, and atelectasis may occur during mechanical ventilation
6. Trauma or congenital malformation of the head, neck, or chest
7. Any disease that results in dehydration. In these patients, the mucociliary system may not function properly, leading to an increased amount of thick secretions.

■ **Pathophysiology**

Airway obstruction can be either partial or complete and may be acute or chronic. Any form of obstruction may cause death from hypoxia and hypercapnia. Complete obstruction can result from occlusion of an ET tube because of mucus. Acute partial obstruction usually results from the inhalation of foreign material or from acute inflammation of the airway such as occurs with croup, epiglottitis, or bronchiolitis. Chronic airway obstruction, on the other hand, results from persistent or recurrent conditions such as cystic fibrosis or asthma.

■ **Clinical signs and symptoms**

The child who has a partial airway obstruction may be restless and tachypneic and may use the accessory muscles of respiration. The child with upper airway obstruction is generally more comfortable sitting forward, and respiratory distress increases when the child is supine. The pitch of the infant's cry may be altered, or the pitch or intensity of the child's voice may be diminished; the patient may appear anxious and cyanotic. Breath sounds are diminished, and there is a tachycardia. As the child's condition deteriorates, bradycardia may develop.[11]

The site of an airway obstruction can sometimes be determined by the patient's signs and symptoms.

For example, inspiratory stridor and hoarseness indicate upper airway obstruction, such as a lesion in the larynx, while expiratory wheezing and prolonged expiratory time indicate lower airway obstruction.

Regardless of the site of airway obstruction, the hallmark of acute airway diseases is a respiratory acidosis. Arterial blood gas analysis will reveal acidosis, an increased P_{CO_2}, and a normal or decreased P_{O_2} (see discussion of respiratory failure later in this chapter).

■ **Medical treatment and nursing interventions**

Airway obstruction can often be anticipated and therefore prevented in young children by proper positioning of the head and neck. All infants with respiratory distress who are breathing spontaneously should be positioned in the upright or prone position, especially after feedings. An infant seat may also be used to keep the infant upright. Care must be taken to avoid complete flexion or hyperextension of the neck, since these positions may cause tracheal compression. For the older child the side-lying position is preferred immediately after surgery, since the tongue and other upper airway muscles may be hypotonic, and they may occlude the upper airway if the patient is supine. Occasionally, children with large tonsils or adenoids may manifest signs of airway obstruction if they are allowed to sleep in the supine position.

Toddlers and older children with upper airway obstruction seem to instinctively assume a posture that maximizes airway caliber. Thus it may be best to avoid manipulating the child's position until personnel experienced in airway management are present. (For management of intubated patients, see the discussion later in this chapter.)

Stimulation of cough. A cough is the normal mechanism for clearing the tracheobronchial tree of foreign particles and secretions. After the patient inspires deeply, the epiglottis and vocal cords close and expiration is attempted against a closed glottis. The glottis then opens suddenly and air is exhaled at a high velocity. Secretions and other particles are propelled toward the larger airways and pharynx, where they are either swallowed or expectorated. An effective cough requires a deep inspiration; a small inspiration will produce an ineffective cough.

Since stimulation of a cough in a young child is often difficult (often the child does not understand what is meant by the word "cough"), intervention may be required. Providing a demonstration for the child may encourage a natural cough. Alternatively insertion of a sterile suction catheter into the back of the orophraynx (without application of suction) can

provoke a cough. However, this will be ineffective if the child bites the catheter, vomits, or gags. In addition, it can increase upper airway irritation and obstruction and thus is contraindicated in children with croup or epiglottitis (unless they are intubated). Sometimes light finger pressure against the trachea just above the sternal notch may stimulate a cough, but excessive pressure on the notch may produce vomiting. In a child old enough to follow directions, a deep inspiration may also stimulate a cough.

Suctioning of the nonintubated patient. If secretions collect in the child's nose or mouth, the work of breathing is increased. For the child who is unable to mobilize these secretions, their removal by suctioning of the upper airway is often dramatically effective in eliminating or reducing respiratory distress. If the infant or child becomes combative during the suctioning, or if the unstable child develops bradycardia, two nurses will be required to suction the child. A sterile glove and sterile catheter should be used. The catheter should be lubricated with a water-soluble lubricant before introduction into the nostril. Table 4-4 contains a list of appropriate catheter sizes.

The child's head is held securely, and the catheter is introduced carefully into the nose. The presence of a deviated nasal septum or nasal polyp may prevent further passage of the catheter. A catheter that does not easily pass into the nasopharynx should not be forced but withdrawn and an attempt made to pass it through the other nostril. Once the catheter does pass freely, it should be inserted further until coughing is

Table 4-4 Catheter sizes for nasopharyngeal and oropharyngeal suctioning of the nonintubated patient

Age	Size of catheter
Newborn	5-6½
6 mo	8
1 yr	8-10
2 yr	10
5 yr	12
≥10 yr	12-14

stimulated. At this point, suction is applied, and the catheter is rotated and withdrawn from the nostril. Suction is applied as the catheter is withdrawn (Table 4-5 indicates appropriate amounts of negative pressure). If deeper suctioning is desired, the catheter may be passed further into the larynx. If repeat suctioning is required, the child should be allowed to rest between each suctioning event. The patient's heart rate and general appearance must be monitored very closely during the suctioning procedure. Prolonged suctioning can result in hypoxemia and bradycardia. If these symptoms occur, the catheter should be withdrawn and the child immediately ventilated with a bag and mask.

Since introduction of a catheter decreases air flow and may produce hypoxemia, it is often advisable that the patient receive supplemental oxygen or ventilation by hand ventilator (ventilator bag) and mask before and after suctioning.[37] A pressure gauge should be attached to the ventilating bag. Since excessive inflation pressure may produce a pneumothorax, inflating pressures of less than 30 cm of water are generally used in the intubated patient.

Any secretions removed by suctioning should be inspected by the nurse and their color, consistency, amount, and odor recorded on the bedside flow sheet. If purulent or bright, bloody secretions are obtained, a physician should be notified. A culture of the secretions may be ordered. (Suctioning of intubated patients is discussed later in this chapter.)

Humidity. Infants and children with acute disease of the upper airway may benefit from humidification of inspired air. Inadequate humidification will cause drying of the upper respiratory mucosa and further injury to the airway. This can result in impairment of ciliary activity with retention of secretions. In addition, atelectasis and infection may develop. Generally, if the inspiratory air is bubbled through

distilled water at or near 37° C, the appropriate amount of humidity will be present in the air.

■ **ACID-BASE DISORDERS**
■ **Etiology**

Acid-base disorders may result from both respiratory and nonrespiratory causes. The pediatric critical-care nurse must be able to recognize signs and symptoms of acid-base disorders, to interpret arterial blood gas results, and to be prepared to initiate appropriate treatment (a brief discussion of normal acid-base balance was presented at the beginning of the chapter). This section deals with acid-base disorders, their causes, clinical presentations, and treatment. Table 4-6 summarizes the characteristics of common acid-base disorders, and the following definitions should be kept in mind:

Acidosis: a condition in which the arterial pH is below 7.35

Alkalosis: a condition in which the arterial pH is above 7.45

Hypoxemia: a PaO_2 of less than 80 torr when the patient is breathing room air at sea level

Hypercapnia: a $PaCO_2$ greater than 45 torr

Torr: a unit of gas tension, which is the same as millimeters of mercury (mm Hg)

The four physiologic causes of hypoxemia are (1) hypoventilation (which can result from central nervous system diseases, depressant drugs, or airway obstruction), (2) anatomic right-to-left shunt (caused by cyanotic congenital heart disease), (3) ventilation-perfusion mismatch (such as occurs with asthma, cystic fibrosis, or pneumonia), and (4) diffusion limitation (which can occur with pneumonia or pulmonary fibrosis).

Acid-base disorders can affect the function of several organs. For example, moderate acidosis (pH of less than 7.3) may cause pulmonary vasoconstriction and decreased pulmonary blood flow. Severe pulmonary vasoconstriction may precipitate right ventricular failure. In addition, with acidosis the oxyhemoglobin dissociation curve (see earlier discussion) is shifted to the right so that, at a given PaO_2 the hemoglobin saturation (and thus the arterial oxygen content) will be less than normal. Alkalosis may cause pulmonary vasodilation and an increase in pulmonary blood flow, and it will shift the hemoglobin dissociation to the left.

Acidosis and alkalosis may also affect cerebral blood vessel diameter. Hypercapnia produces dilation of the cerebral vessels; hypocapnia causes constriction. Patients with increased intracranial pressure are generally hyperventilated to maintain a $PaCO_2$ be-

Table 4-5 Maximum negative pressure for airway suctioning

Age	Amount of negative pressure (cm H_2O pressure)
Infant	60-90
Child	90-110
Older child	110-150

Table 4-6 Common acid-base disorders

Classification	Arterial blood gas criteria
Alveolar hyper-ventilation (acute)	P_{CO_2} <30 mm Hg pH >7.50
Alveolar hyper-ventilation (chronic)	P_{CO_2} <30 mm Hg pH WNL*
Alveolar hypoven-ventilation (acute)	P_{CO_2} >50 mm Hg pH <7.30 May be accompanied by a P_{O_2} <80 mm Hg
Alveolar hypoven-tilation (chronic)	P_{CO_2} >50 mm Hg pH WNL May be accompanied by a P_{O_2} <80 mm Hg
Metabolic acidosis	P_{CO_2} WNL pH <7.30 HCO_3 <22 mEq/L
Compensated metabolic acidosis	P_{CO_2} <30 mm Hg pH WNL HCO_3 <22 mEq/L
Metabolic alkalosis	P_{CO_2} WNL pH >7.50 HCO_3 >28 mEq/L
Compensated metabolic alkalosis	P_{CO_2} >50 mm Hg pH WNL HCO_3 > 28 mEq/L

*Within normal limits

tween 23 and 28 torr. This mild hypocapnia produces a reduction in cerebral blood volume and may reduce intracranial pressure. Severe hypocapnia is to be avoided, however, since it may result in such severe vasoconstriction that cerebral ischemia occurs be-

cause of reduction in oxygen delivery to the brain (see the discussion of increased intracranial pressure in Chapter 6).

An alteration in arterial pH may result from electrolyte abnormalities. For example, diuretic therapy may cause a loss of sodium, potassium, and chloride in the urine. This produces a metabolic alkalosis since the kidneys excrete hydrogen ions in an effort to conserve sodium and potassium. Some infants and children with chronic metabolic alkalosis hypoventilate and develop hypercapnia to maintain their pH at near-normal levels (see Chapter 7).

■ **Pathophysiology**

As previously noted, the Pa_{CO_2} reflects the effectiveness of alveolar ventilation. Thus if metabolic CO_2 production is nearly constant, an increase in alveolar ventilation will lower the Pa_{CO_2} and raise the pH, and a decrease in alveolar ventilation will raise the Pa_{CO_2} and lower the pH. These alterations in alveolar ventilation are mediated by peripheral and central chemoreceptors in three ways: (1) they can occur automatically as a response to a change in extracellular pH, (2) they can occur by voluntary increases or decreases in minute ventilation, and (3) they can occur as a result of drugs that increase or decrease ventilatory drive. For example, theophylline may stimulate breathing, while narcotic drugs may result in respiratory depression.

Respiratory alkalosis. Primary respiratory alkalosis is not often seen in pediatric critical-care units. When respiratory alkalosis develops, a primary increase in alveolar ventilation lowers the Pa_{CO_2} and raises the arterial pH. Chronic alveolar hyperventilation may be caused by central nervous system (CNS) injury or by salicylate intoxication, head injury, Reye's syndrome, brainstem lesions, and hepatic encephalopathy. More commonly, acute respiratory alkalosis in children results from crying, anxiety, or acute hyperventilation due to severe hypoxemia. For example, a child's anticipation of an arterial puncture or the pain of the puncture itself will often cause an acute hyperventilation while the blood sample is drawn; consequently, the analysis will reflect an apparent respiratory alkalosis.

If hyperventilation is sustained beyond 6 to 8 hours, the kidneys will begin to restore pH to near normal by increasing hydrogen-ion reabsorption and increasing the excretion of bicarbonate. This produces a fall in bicarbonate levels and a fall in the pH—both toward normal. Thus when there is a secondary (renal) compensation for primary respiratory alkalosis, arterial blood gas analysis will show a slight increase in the pH, a decrease in the Pa_{CO_2}, a decrease in the bicarbonate ion concentration, and a positive base excess (greater than +2).

CASE STUDY 1

A 3-year-old child is admitted with a fractured femur. She is very frightened and breathing 55 times per minute. Arterial blood gas analysis shows the following:

pH	7.50
Pa_{CO_2}	29 mm Hg
HCO_3	26 mEq/L (normal: 24-28)
Pa_{O_2}	104 mm Hg
Base excess	+1

Interpretation. This child has acute respiratory alkalosis caused by the pain and anxiety of the leg injury and resultant hyperventilation. The bicarbonate level is normal, confirming that the alkalosis is of respiratory origin and that renal compensation has not yet begun.

CASE STUDY 2

A 16-year-old with leukemia in remission is admitted because of tachypnea and fever. Chest radiographs show a bilateral interstitial infiltrate; arterial blood gases are obtained with the patient breathing room air.

pH	7.48
Pa_{CO_2}	29 mm Hg
HCO_3	23 mEq/L
Pa_{O_2}	50 mm Hg
Respiratory rate	60/min
Base excess	+1

Interpretation. This patient has acute respiratory alkalosis because of severe hypoxia. In this case severe hypoxia results in an increased respiratory drive. Oxygen therapy is indicated; if the hypoxia is corrected, the pH may fall to normal levels.

Respiratory acidosis. A primary decrease in alveolar ventilation will raise the arterial P_{CO_2}, lower the arterial pH, and produce respiratory acidosis. Common causes of respiratory acidosis in children are (1) airway obstruction from any cause, (2) central depression of the respiratory drive by such things as drugs and head trauma, and (3) respiratory muscle weakness resulting from muscle disease or chest wall abnormalities. The appropriate compensatory re-

sponse to an increase in the Pa_{CO_2} is an increase in respiratory rate and depth in an effort to eliminate carbon dioxide. However, if it is not possible for the patient to increase ventilation, hypercapnia will persist. The renal response to hypercapnia includes increased excretion of hydrogen ions and potassium, and increased reabsorption of bicarbonate. Thus serum bicarbonate concentration increases, serum potassium concentration decreases, urine pH falls, and arterial pH increases to near normal levels. Since this renal compensation appears slowly and takes several days to occur, acute respiratory acidosis is manifested by a decrease in the pH and an increase in the Pa_{CO_2}, while the serum bicarbonate and base excess remain normal. When respiratory acidosis is chronic, however, the pH is increased toward normal, although both the Pa_{CO_2} and bicarbonate concentration are increased. The two following examples illustrate the differences between acute and chronic respiratory acidosis.

CASE STUDY 1

A 16-month-old boy with bronchopulmonary dysplasia is admitted with a right upper lobe infiltrate and fever. Arterial blood gases were obtained while the infant was breathing room air. They showed the following:

pH	7.36
P_{CO_2}	72 mm Hg
HCO_3	38 mEq/L
Pa_{O_2}	52 mm Hg
Base excess	+9

Interpretation. This child has a primary respiratory acidosis because of chronic respiratory insufficiency. This respiratory acidosis is evidenced by a low pH and an elevated Pa_{CO_2}. Hypoxemia is present as a result of chronic pulmonary disease. Renal compensation has occured, as evidenced by the elevated bicarbonate level. Normally, a person with a Pa_{CO_2} over 70 would require mechanical ventilation; however, in this child, carbon dioxide retention is chronic. As a result, the pH is near normal. Thus mechanical ventilation is probably not necessary. Unless the pH falls further or respiratory muscle fatigue occurs, only antibiotics, chest physical therapy, and oxygen would be required.

CASE STUDY 2

A 7-year-old child is hospitalized for removal of her appendix. Four hours after the surgery, the child is asleep and cannot be awakened. As she breathes room air, her arterial blood gases are:

pH	7.25
Pa_{CO_2}	64 mm Hg
HCO_3	25 mEq/L
Pa_{O_2}	73 mm Hg
Respiratory rate	15/min

Interpretation. This child exhibits acute respiratory acidosis caused by alveolar hypoventilation. The alveolar-arterial oxygen gradient is normal (see later discussion of this A-a gradient). Notice that the 25 mm Hg rise in Pa_{CO_2} (from a normal of 40, to the present 64) is approximately matched by the 22 mm Hg fall in Pa_{O_2} (from a normal of 95 to the present 73). Renal compensation has not occurred since the bicarbonate level is normal. This disturbance is most likely a result of respiratory depression because of anesthesia. In such a patient, administration of narcotic analgesics may prolong or worsen the respiratory depression.

Metabolic alkalosis. Metabolic alkalosis can result from the loss of a strong acid from the extracellular fluid (such as occurs with persistent vomiting and potassium depletion), or it can result from a gain in base (as occurs following infusion of excess bicarbonate). The initial response to metabolic alkalosis is a buffer reaction to lessen the effect on the blood pH of the loss of acid or the gain in base.

As the serum pH rises, stimulus to ventilation is reduced. As a result, alveolar ventilation falls and the Pa_{CO_2} rises. This rise helps offset the gain in base. However, the respiratory response to acute metabolic alkalosis is slow because the pH in the brain increases slowly, even though the plasma pH is high. In addition, respiratory compensation for metabolic alkalosis can never completely restore the pH to normal because once the pH approaches normal, the respiratory inhibition disappears and the child's respiratory rate will increase. Thus acute metabolic alkalosis results in normal Pa_{CO_2} with an elevation in the pH and the bicarbonate ion concentration.

Metabolic acidosis. Metabolic acidosis is caused by a primary gain of strong acid (as in diabetic ketoacidosis) or by a loss of bicarbonate ion from the extracellular fluid (as in diarrhea or renal tubular acidosis).

The initial response to acidosis occurs almost immediately. A buffer reaction lessens the effect on blood pH of an acid load or a bicarbonate ion loss. Over a period of several hours of sustained metabolic acidosis, respiratory compensation will begin. This is a gradual process that can occur over several hours or even a day. Compensation in this case occurs as alveolar ventilation increases in order to increase the

serum pH toward normal. When partial respiratory compensation for metabolic acidosis has occurred, the serum pH, bicarbonate ion concentration, and the Pa_{CO_2} are all decreased. Once respiratory compensation for metabolic acidosis is complete, the pH returns toward normal, but the Pa_{CO_2} and bicarbonate ion concentration remain decreased. The following two case studies involving two infants will illustrate the difference between metabolic alkalosis and metabolic acidosis.

CASE STUDY 1

An 8-month-old infant with bronchopulmonary dysplasia has been admitted to the ICU with a history of low-grade fever and increasing respiratory distress. On initial examination the infant appears irritable but is active and alert. The skin and mucous membranes are dry, and the anterior fontanelle is flat. The infant's respiratory rate is 45 per minute, and retractions are present. The infant has been receiving oral furosemide (Lasix), 15 mg twice daily; the mother states that she "ran out" of potassium chloride supplements several weeks ago. Arterial blood gases obtained while the infant is breathing room air are:

pH	7.50
Pa_{CO_2}	59 mm Hg
HCO_3	34 mEq/L
Pa_{O_2}	60 mm Hg
Base excess	+18

Interpretation. This infant has chronic respiratory disease, which produces respiratory acidosis. Renal compensation can increase the serum pH to near normal but not to normal levels. The fact that this infant has a pH that is *above* normal suggests that an additional element is affecting acid-base balance. Since the infant is receiving diuretic therapy known to increase potassium and chloride excretion and has not received potassium chloride for several days, presumably a furosemide-induced metabolic alkalosis has developed. The diagnosis will be confirmed if hypokalemia and hypochloremia are present.

CASE STUDY 2

A 6-month-old infant is admitted with 10% dehydration as the result of a week-long episode of gastroenteritis. On initial examination the infant looks extremely ill and is lethargic and pale. Tachycardia and tachypnea are both present. The skin is cool to touch, extremities are clammy, and peripheral pulses are decreased in intensity. Initial blood gases obtained while the infant is breathing room air are:

pH	7.20
P_{CO_2}	22 mm Hg
HCO_3	22 mEq/L
Pa_{O_2}	98 mm Hg
Base excess	−18

Interpretation. This infant demonstrates metabolic acidosis as the result of dehydration and decreased systemic perfusion. The metabolic acidosis may be the result of loss of bicarbonate ions through diarrhea, but it now may also be perpetuated by poor systemic perfusion and lactic acidosis. Partial respiratory compensation for the metabolic acidosis is demonstrated by the fact that the child's $PaCO_2$ is low. The low bicarbonate ion concentration confirms the fact that the acidosis was metabolic in origin.

■ **Clinical signs and symptoms**

Acid-base disturbances are usually best identified through analysis of blood-gas results. It is often clinically difficult to access acid-base abnormalities, since so many body systems are involved. Most commonly, the signs and symptoms demonstrated by the child are related to the underlying pathologic condition. Therefore the following discussion separates those clinical signs and symptoms observed as the result of hypoxemia from those that occur in the child with primary acidosis or alkalosis.

Hypoxemia. The term "hypoxia" indicates that there is inadequate tissue oxygenation, while the term "hypoxemia" implies that the child's Pa_{O_2} is less than 80 mm Hg. The initial cardiopulmonary response to acute hypoxemia is an increase in cardiac output, respiratory rate, and tidal volume. The child with hypoxemia demonstrates tachycardia, tachypnea, restlessness, possible drowsiness, disorientation, and headache. With severe hypoxemia, bradycardia, hypotension, and cardiac arrhythmias develop. Pulmonary arteriolar vasoconstriction occurs as the result of hypoxemia, and this produces pulmonary hypertension. If pulmonary hypertension is severe, right ventricular failure can result. Low cardiac output and cardiac arrest may ensue if hypoxemia is not promptly and adequately treated.

Cyanosis is a very late sign of hypoxemia, and its presence is usually a sign that arterial oxygen content is markedly reduced. Cyanosis is defined as a diffuse blue discoloration of the skin and mucous membranes. It develops as a result of an increased amount of unoxygenated (reduced) hemoglobin in the capillaries. Normally, there are approximately 2 gm of reduced hemoglobin per dl of blood in the capil-

laries. Cyanosis is not perceptible until the concentration of unoxygenated hemoglobin increases to 4 to 5 gm per dl of blood. It is important to note that the appearance of cyanosis is related to the absolute amount of unoxygenated hemoglobin, not to desaturation of a certain percent of total hemoglobin. Thus a patient who has polycythemia and whose hemoglobin is greater than 20 gm/dl may appear cyanotic (despite nearly normal hemoglobin saturation) because quantitatively more reduced hemoglobin will be present. By contrast a child with anemia may be severely hypoxemic, yet cyanosis will not be present because the total amount of unoxygenated hemoglobin does not total 4 to 5 gm/dl of blood. Thus the interpretation of the appearance or absence of cyanosis depends on the child's hemoglobin concentration.

In individuals who are not anemic or polycythemic, cyanosis develops when the arterial oxygen saturation falls below approximately 75% to 80% or the Pa_{O_2} is less than 50 mm Hg. Cyanosis is best detected by assessing the color of the mucous membranes and nail beds of the infant and child. The inside of the mouth is usually the most reliable place to observe cyanosis. In addition, the lips, eyelids, and soles of the feet can be good places to observe cyanosis in children.

Acidosis. The signs and symptoms of acidosis are nonspecific and are related to the underlying cause of the acidosis. Primary metabolic acidosis usually results in tachypnea, pallor, and lethargy. The infant or child with acute respiratory acidosis may have respiratory distress if the underlying cause is an airway obstruction; alternatively, the patient may demonstrate periodic breathing or extreme lethargy if the respiratory acidosis results from respiratory depression of the central nervous system.

Alkalosis. Primary respiratory alkalosis is usually caused by an increase in respiratory rate and depth. This may progress to actual dyspnea. The child may be dizzy and may complain of numbness and tingling in the extremities. With progression of the alkalosis, the child's muscles become weak, and twitching of the facial muscles may be noted. *Carpopedal spasm* is a classic sign of severe alkalosis and consists of palmar flexion of the hands and plantar flexion of the feet.

■ **Medical treatment and nursing interventions**

Nursing care of the child with an acid-base disorder requires immediate and continual assessment of the general status of the child. Frequent blood gas analyses are useful, but once a baseline has been established, the nurse should use them basically to confirm clinical impressions of changes or trends in the patient's condition. The accurate and sterile collection of the blood specimen for blood gas analysis is essential (for review of this procedure, see the section of this chapter on common diagnostic tests).

■ RESPIRATORY FAILURE
■ Etiology

Almost any respiratory disorder can ultimately cause respiratory failure. The following discussion focuses on those factors that place the child at risk for the development of respiratory failure and indicates common pathophysiologic mechanisms, clinical signs and symptoms, and appropriate nursing care.

■ Pathophysiology

As noted previously, children are more likely to develop respiratory failure for many reasons: their airways are small in absolute diameter, accessory muscles of respiration are poorly developed, respiratory muscle fatigue may more quickly appear, upper airway resistance is high, and the chest wall of the infant is extremely compliant.

The diagnosis of impending respiratory failure is usually made on the basis of blood gas analysis; it is defined as a Pa_{CO_2} of more than 60 mm Hg or a pH of less than 7.30. Virtually all of these patients are hypoxemic in room air, but oxygen therapy usually can result in a normal Pa_{O_2}.[23]

The Pa_{CO_2} directly reflects the adequacy of alveolar ventilation and thus lung function. As the Pa_{CO_2} rises, the blood pH drops, and respiratory acidosis results. In addition, minute ventilation, cardiac output, and pulmonary vascular resistance increase. In the presence of respiratory acidosis lasting for several days, the kidneys will excrete more acid and reabsorb more bicarbonate in an effort to increase the arterial pH. Once respiratory failure develops, however, these compensatory mechanisms are inadequate to maintain a normal arterial pH in the face of an elevation in the Pa_{CO_2}. If respiratory failure is severe, the Pa_{O_2} is also low, despite oxygen therapy. Hypoxemia results in inadequate tissue oxygenation (hypoxia) and lactic acidosis. Cardiac output and pulmonary blood flow increase initially in response to hypoxemia. In addition, the hemoglobin affinity for oxygen is decreased (the oxyhemoglobin dissociation curve shifts to the right) so that oxygen is more easily released to the tissues.[44] With progressive hypoxemia, cardiac output falls and pulmonary vasoconstriction occurs.

Common causes of respiratory failure in children include[23,27]:

1. Upper airway obstruction: croup, epiglottitis, foreign body aspiration, vascular ring
2. Lower airway obstruction: asthma, bronchiolitis, cystic fibrosis, aspiration pneumonia, and bronchopulmonary dysplasia
3. Decreased oxygen or carbon dioxide diffusion at the alveolar surface: severe interstitial pneumonia, pulmonary edema, oxygen toxicity, respiratory distress syndrome, near-drowning
4. Acute decrease in pulmonary blood flow: pulmonary embolus
5. Respiratory muscle failure: Guillain-Barré syndrome, muscular dystrophy, myasthenia gravis, or drug ingestion (such as narcotics, barbiturates, and sedatives)
6. Other causes: pneumothorax, severe kyphoscoliosis, severe abdominal distention, flail chest caused by trauma, increased intracranial pressure (cerebral trauma, tumors, meningitis, encephalitis, Reye's syndrome)

The single most important factor contributing to respiratory failure in children is alveolar hypoventilation. Any condition in which the alveolar ventilation is severely compromised and compensatory mechanisms are inadequate may result in respiratory failure. The patient who is diagnosed as having impending respiratory failure should be watched carefully, since mechanical ventilatory support may be necessary at any moment.

■ Clinical signs and symptoms

Most patients with respiratory distress do not develop respiratory failure, and those who do usually respond to simple oxygen therapy. There are a few specific signs of impending respiratory failure, including the general signs of respiratory distress such as wheezing, expiratory grunting, decreased or absent breath sounds, flaring of the alae nasi, retractions of the chest wall, tachypnea, bradycardia, or apnea. Progression of these signs strongly suggests the development of respiratory failure. In addition, respiratory failure should be suspected if the child develops sudden unexplained restlessness, irritability, or mental confusion. Note that hypoxemia and cyanosis indicate only a decrease in arterial oxygen content, and they do not confirm a diagnosis of respiratory failure of and by themselves.

■ Medical treatment and nursing interventions

The child with respiratory failure may require mechanical ventilation with oxygen. Vital signs and arterial blood gas measurements must be frequently monitored whenever the child develops respiratory failure. Oxygen therapy should be provided exactly as ordered, and the child's airway patency must be strictly maintained. The child's response to any therapeutic measures should be carefully assessed, as should the child's cardiac output and indirect evidence of systemic perfusion. A planned program of airway management and careful nursing assessment and care will provide the child with the greatest opportunity for full recovery. If specific treatments are ordered, such as chest physical therapy, the nurse should refer to further discussions of these treatment modalities in other sections of this chapter.

Oxygen administration. Oxygen is administered to most critically ill children at some time during their ICU stay. Oxygen should be considered a medication; thus appropriate flow rate and concentration should be checked frequently. While oxygen therapy is potentially very helpful, too much or too little oxygen has obvious hazards.

The most common method to deliver oxygen to infants is via a head hood. An air-oxygen humidified mixture with a flow rate of at least 7 L per minute is administered to prevent carbon dioxide accumulation inside the hood. The oxygen concentration can be continuously monitored to ensure delivery of the appropriate oxygen concentration. Several hood sizes are available.

An oxygen tent is used primarily for older infants and children. Tents can provide humidified air or oxygen in inspired oxygen concentrations up to 0.5. However, oxygen tents have several disadvantages that limit their usefulness in the pediatric critical-care unit. First, they make observation of the patient difficult, especially when the air is highly humidified. Second, whenever the tent is opened, the oxygen concentration within the tent falls quickly, and it returns slowly to previous levels after the tent is securely closed.

Face tents are frequently used for older children and adolescents, although they are not specifically made in pediatric sizes. The soft, plastic, mask-like tent fits around the patient's chin and is held in place around the jaw by elastic straps. Gas flow through the mask should be at a minimum of 7 L per minute to ensure adequate carbon dioxide removal.

Several kinds of oxygen masks are available for pediatric use. To select the appropriate size mask, the nurse should make sure that the mask is just large enough to cover the child's nose and mouth; too large a mask may cause the patient to reinhale his own exhaled gas, and too small a mask can prevent adequate gas flow. Most oxygen masks deliver inspired oxygen concentrations up to approximately 0.55. A mask with a reservoir bag or special blender (Puritan)

can provide inspired oxygen concentrations up to 1.00. Venturi masks are designed to provide more predictable oxygen concentrations; they are particularly effective at delivering inspired oxygen concentrations between 0.24 and 0.5. The Venturi mask differs from the conventional mask because it can successfully deliver specific inspired-oxygen concentrations, since its total liter flow usually exceeds the patient's inspiratory flow. Therefore, all the gas inhaled by the patient is of the same, premeasured oxygen concentration (FIO_2, or inspired oxygen concentration), and no ambient air is entrained. Table 4-7 provides a summary of the advantages and disadvantages of various oxygen delivery systems (see also Table 9-5 and the discussion of principles and techniques of instrumentation in Chapter 9).

Manual ventilator bags. A simple method of delivering positive pressure to the patient is through a bag and mask setup. This unit may be utilized for resuscitation as well as for intermittent ventilatory support. Mechanical ventilation with a bag and mask can be accomplished with or without an artificial airway in place. In the critical-care unit, every patient-care area should be equipped with a manual ventilator bag and mask appropriate for the patient's size.

Two forms of manual ventilator bag setups are currently utilized in pediatric critical-care settings. One type consists of a flow-inflating or "anesthesia" Ambu bag and the second is the self-inflating manual ventilator bag. Both of these bags come in a variety of sizes so that the appropriate tidal volume may be delivered to the patient. However, there are several differences between these two forms of manual ventilator bags that are important to know. The self-inflating bag does not require a souce of gas flow; therefore, it can be used away from oxygen sources. This self-inflating bag usually has a one-way pop-off valve that vents pressure from the bag system when the pressure reaches 40 cm of water, ensuring that inflation pressures delivered to the patient do not exceed the maximum level. Concentrations of oxygen vary greatly (between 0.30 and 0.60) when this bag is used, a result of the elastic recoil of the bag and entrainment of room air. In addition, there is no way to monitor the pressure or volume of inspired air delivered to the patient when this manual bag is used, and the user tends to lose the "feel" of the lungs while providing hand ventilation. Table 4-8 provides information about self-inflating bags currently being used in the care of critically ill children.

The flow-inflating bag does require a continuous gas flow to inflate, but it is able to accurately deliver concentrations of oxygen up to 1.00. Flow through the bag is adjusted by either changing the flow of gas

Table 4-7   Advantages and disadvantages of various oxygen-delivery systems

System	Advantages	Disadvantages
Oxygen masks	Various sizes available Ability to provide a predictible concentration of oxygen (with Venturi mask)	Skin irritation Fear of suffocation Accumulation of moisture on face Possibility of aspiration of vomitus Difficulty in controlling oxygen concentrations
Nasal cannula	Provision of constant oxygen flow even while the child eats and talks Possibility of more complete observation of child because nose and mouth remain unobstructed	Discomfort for the child Possibility of causing abdominal distention and intestinal rupture Difficulty of controlling oxygen concentrations Inability to provide mist if desired
Oxygen tent	Achievement of lower concentrations of oxygen (FIo_2 of 0.3-0.5)	Necessity for tight fit around bed to prevent leakage of gas Probability of cool and wet tent environment Poor access to patient—inspired oxygen levels will fall whenever tent is entered
Oxygen hood	Achievement of high concentrations of oxygen (FIo_2 up to 1.00) Free access to patient's chest for assessment	High humidity environment Need to remove patient for feeding and care

at the wall flowmeter or by changing a screw clamp (or valve) attached to the tail of the bag. Since this manual ventilator system has no pop-off valve, the inflating pressures provided to the patient should be continuously measured with a needle-gauge manometer attached to the bag outlet. Since oxygen flow is continuous through this system, and no one-way valve is present, the child who breathes spontaneously can receive oxygen flow between manual inflations. Since the bag is extremely compliant, the user gets a very good "feel" for the compliance of the child's lungs during manual ventilation. However, the flow-inflating bag has no pop-off valve; thus high inflation pressures may be inadvertently administered to the patient, which may cause, among other things, a pneumothorax.

It is extremely important that the nurse be familiar with each of these two ventilating systems so that appropriate and safe inspiratory pressures are provided during manual ventilation. It should be noted that positive end-expiratory pressure (PEEP) may be delivered with either bag setup. A discussion of hand ventilation techniques is presented later in this chapter (see discussion and care of the child who requires mechanical ventilatory support; see also Chapter 9 on resuscitation bags for hand ventilation and Fig. 9-33).

The artificial airway. Placement of an oropharyngeal or nasopharyngeal airway may be necessary in a child for control of secretions or prevention of airway obstruction. These airways are appropriate for short-term use only, and they must be replaced by ET intubation if the child's ability to maintain a patent airway is doubtful.

Table 4-8 Adult and pediatric resuscitator bags

	Ohio Hope II		Air Shields Ambu		Laerdal			Anesthesia bag	
	Adult	Pediatric	Adult	Pediatric	Adult	Pediatric	Infant	Adult	Pediatric
Desired liter flow	15	15	10-15	10-15	15	15 (1½-10 yr)	15 (up to 2 yr)	$1.5 \times \dot{V}_E$	$3 \times \dot{V}_E$
F_{IO_2} delivery (approximate)									
With resistance	80-90	80-90	80-90	80-90	100	100	100	100	100
Without resistance	35-40	35-40	35-40	35-40	35-40	35-40	35-40	100	100
Bag capacity (approximate)	2 L	0.5 L	2 L	0.5 L	2 L	0.5 L	0.24 L	3 L	1 L
Stroke volume (approximate)	1 L	0.3-0.4 L	1 L	0.3-0.4 L	1 L	0.3-0.4 L	0.2 L	1 L	0.5 L
Type of valve	Spring ball	Spring ball	One-way leaf	One-way leaf	Diaphragm and duck bill			Variable orifice	
Pressure relief	Optional	Optional	Expansion of rubber bag		None	Spring-loaded valve approximately 35 cm H_2O		Variable orifice	
PEEP	Boerhinger valve	Boerhinger valve	Boerhinger valve or Orange spring-loaded valve					Variable orifice	

Developed by R. Wong, Department of Respiratory Therapy, Presbyterian Hospital of Pacific Medical Center, San Francisco, Calif.

Airways come in a variety of sizes; oral sizes begin as small as 000, and nasopharyngeal sizes range from 26 to 34 French. Oral airways are most useful in a comatose patient. A properly placed oral airway prevents the tongue from moving posteriorly, and it allows the patient to breathe both through and around the airway.

Placement of an ET or a tracheostomy tube may be necessary to maintain an open airway. In the adult the smallest part of the upper airway is near the glottis, while in children the narrowest portion of the airway is at the level of the cricoid cartilage. This structural difference means that children can be effectively ventilated, without much air leak, through use of an *uncuffed* ET tube. The narrowness of the cricoid area may, however, cause problems. If an excessively large ET tube is placed, pressure on the child's airway and cricoid cartilage by the tube may result in severe postextubation edema or subglottic stenosis, which may make reintubation necessary. If an excessively small ET tube is placed, a large air leak can develop around the tube, resulting in a loss of inspiratory volume. If the child is breathing spontaneously, a small ET tube diameter will increase the resistance to airflow and therefore increase the work of spontaneous breathing. If the ET tube is of appropriate diameter, once the child is intubated and hand ventilated, a small air leak should develop when the child's inspiratory pressure reaches 40 cm H_2O.

Whenever a child is critically ill or is at risk for the development of respiratory failure or airway obstruction, an ET tube of proper size should be ready and at the bedside. Infants and small children require shorter ET tubes. As a result, before these tubes are placed, they may require cutting to make them the appropriate size. Table 4-9 provides a list of appropriate ET tube sizes and lengths for various ages of infants and children. When the nurse is preparing to cut an ET tube to its proper length, she should measure the length recommended on the chart and then add an additional 1 to 2 cm to that measured length to allow room for attachment of the ET adapter. It is also extremely important that the cutting be done from the nonbeveled edge, that is, at the end of the ET tube that will be attached to the ET adapter. In some units, the ET tube is placed, and *then* the distal end is trimmed after a chest radiograph has confirmed proper tube placement.

The most popular ET tube for use in children has the same internal diameter through the entire length of the tube. This type of tube has a side hole near the tip, which allows for air flow in the event the distal end of the tube becomes plugged. The Cole tube has a tapered internal diameter along its entire

Table 4-9   Endotracheal and tracheostomy tube sizes[32]

Age	Internal diameter (mm)	Oral length (cm)	Nasal length (cm)	Tracheostomy (internal diameter in mm)	Suction catheter (in French sizes)
Premature	3.0-3.5	8	11	4-5	5½-6
Newborn	3.5	8.5	13	4-5	6-8
6 months	3.5-4.0	10	15	5.5	6-8
18 months	4.0-4.5	12	16	6.0	8-10
24 months	5.0-5.5	14	17	6-7	10
2-4 years	5.5-6.0	15	18	6-7	10-12
4-7 years	6.0-6.5	16	19	7.0	12
7-10 years	6.5-7.0	17	21	8.0	12-14
10-12 years	7.0-7.5	20	22-25	9.0	14

length; this tube is rarely used today in children because it often results in problems with postextubation laryngeal dilation.

Intubation of the critically ill child should be attempted only by an experienced individual. Before the intubation is begun, all appropriate equipment must be assembled at the bedside. This equipment includes various sizes of laryngoscope blades and handles, lidocaine (Xylocaine) jelly, McGill forceps, a stylet, a tonsillar suction, suction catheters for oropharyngeal suction, appropriate suction catheters for ET suction, a manual resuscitator bag with a tight-fitting mask and an ET adapter, and a cardiac monitor. The manual resuscitator bag available should be one capable of providing a high inspiratory-oxygen content.

Tracheal intubation can be performed either through the mouth or the nostril. Oral tubes are often easier to place during an emergency situation, but they are more difficult to immobilize when the child is alert and moving, since they stimulate salivation, gagging, or sucking. If an oral tube is placed, its position should be changed from one side of the mouth to the other at least every 48 hours in an at-

tempt to avoid pressure injury to the hard palate and to the lips. An older child may bite an oral tube and occlude the lumen unless a bite block is in place. Nasotracheal tubes may be more difficult to place initially, but they are usually more comfortable for the child and easier for the nurse to immobilize. Disadvantages of the nasal tube include potential development of pressure sores on the nares and possible blockage of the sinus drainage or the eustachian tube.

Once the ET tube is in place, it must be secured immediately. Movement of the ET tube is thought to be one of the most frequent and preventable factors associated with the development of subglottic edema and scarring. Securing of the ET tube is a nursing responsibility; undetected dislodgment of this tube can be fatal.

There are various techniques for securing a nasotracheal tube (one method is illustrated in Fig. 4-4). Regardless of the technique used, it is often advisable to use regular adhesive tape or umbilical tape rather than clear plastic waterproof tape, which may slip. The most common method of securing a nasotracheal tube involves wrapping it with pieces of tape attached to both cheeks. To begin this procedure, the

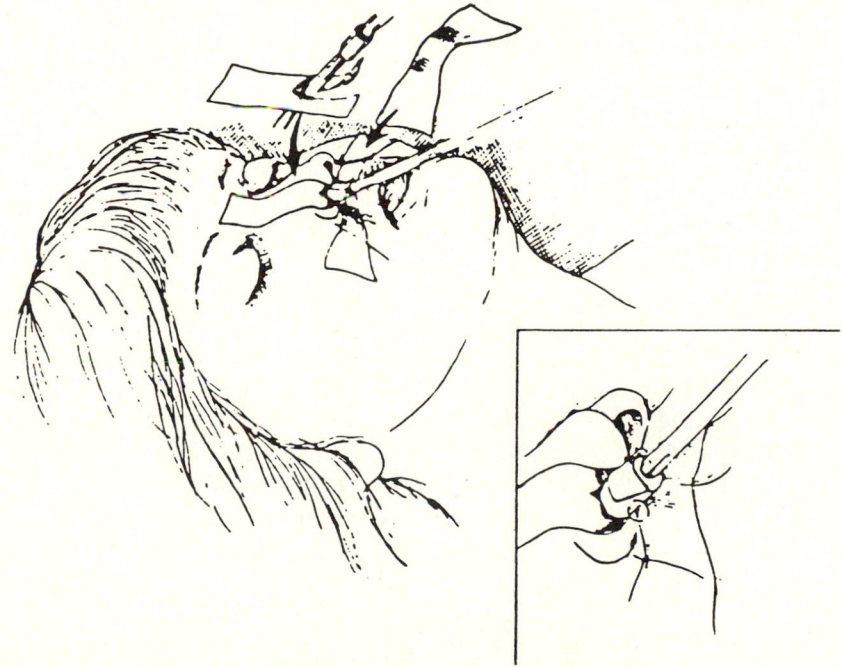

Fig. 4-4 Method of securing the nasotracheal tube with tape reinforced by suture. The tape on the nose is necessary to prevent the tube from slipping out of the nose superiorly. Inset shows position of suture connecting tape on the tube with tape on the upper lip.

From Levin D.L., Morriss, F.C., and Moore, G.C.: A practical guide to pediatric intensive care, ed. 2, St. Louis, 1984, The C.V. Mosby Co.

upper lip and cheeks are lightly painted with tincture of benzoin to ensure tape adhesiveness. When the benzoin is sticky, ½-inch adhesive tape is applied first to the right cheek, drawn across the lip, and wrapped around the tube at least two or three times. The left cheek is then taped, extending the tape around the tube for two or three revolutions. Either piece of tape can then be brought back to the ipsilateral or contralateral cheek to reinforce the taping. If too much tape is used, secretions from the nose and mouth can seep between the layers of tape and result in slipping of the tube or accidental extubation before tube slippage is recognized. It is essential that the breath sounds be auscultated carefully as soon as the ET tube is retaped to be sure that the tube is still in appropriate position. The nurse should auscultate breath sounds bilaterally and compare their loudness as well as their pitch. Bronchial intubation (especially intubation of the right main-stem bronchus) can usually be avoided if the nurse carefully assesses breath sounds and chest expansion before and after ET tube taping. Bronchial intubation should be suspected whenever breath sounds are unequal and when arterial blood gases reveal progressive hypoxemia but normocapnia. A chest radiograph should be performed immediately following intubation and the tube placement adjusted on the basis of radiograph results. The tip of the ET tube should be no lower than 1 to 2 cm above the carina and no higher than the first rib (see Fig. 5-12 for examples of the determination of appropriate ET tube placement).

Great care should be exercised when positioning the intubated child because the position of the tube changes when the neck is moved. When the neck is flexed, the tube moves toward the carina; when the neck is extended, the tube moves toward the larynx (see Fig. 5-11). It is important to rotate the head, neck, and shoulders as one unit rather than allowing the head to remain stationary as the child's torso is rotated. When a chest radiograph is obtained, the nurse should note the child's head and neck position as the film is taken so that the ET tube position can be better evaluated.

Communication with the intubated child is an important aspect of nursing care. The nurse should find some way for the child to communicate. The older child can write using a ''magic slate'' or a paper and pencil. The younger child may wish to point to objects or facial expressions collected on a poster. A circle containing such facial expressions or objects can be attached to a windowed cover so that the child can uncover the desired objects or the facial expression representative of his feelings (see Fig. 2-6 for directions about creation of such a wheel).

The intubated infant or child requires some stimulation and gentle touch. A music box or mobile, especially one from home, may be especially soothing for an infant or a toddler. A tape recording of family voices or favorite music may be comforting for an older child. The child may enjoy hearing stories or having his forehead stroked. It is important that the nurse keep a list on the nursing-care plan of the people, objects, and gestures that are most soothing to the infant or child for use by all nurses involved in the child's care. If possible, arrangements should be made for the mother or nurse to hold the child, even though the youngster is intubated.

■ Nursing Care of the Child Requiring Mechanical Ventilatory Support

■ **VENTILATORY SUPPORT**
■ **Indications for ventilatory support**

Most children with acute lung disease have mild hypoxemia but a normal or low Pa_{CO_2}. For these children oxygen therapy is all that is necessary. However, if the child becomes unable to maintain adequate ventilation, mechanical ventilation with PEEP must be instituted. Mechanical ventilation of the infant and child is an art involving highly specialized technology and skills. The use of assisted ventilation in neonatal and pediatric ICUs has been instrumental in reducing the number of deaths caused by acute lung injury. However, as mortality from these diseases decreases, the group of children who subsequently require long-term ventilatory support increases. Although the long-term nursing care of these ventilator-dependent children is not discussed in this chapter, it can be expected that these patients will be prepared to return home with intermittent or continuous ventilatory support.

There are many indications for mechanical ventilatory support. Obviously, any child with absence of spontaneous ventilation for whatever cause requires such mechanical support. This includes children with drug overdoses, apnea, acute central nervous system abnormalities, or respiratory muscle weakness.

Inadequate alveolar ventilation reflects the failure of the lungs to adequately remove carbon dioxide from the body. Ventilatory failure also leads to hypoxemia (Pa_{O_2} less than 50 mm Hg in 100% oxygen). As the Pa_{CO_2} increases (above 60 mm Hg with serial blood gases) and the pH decreases (below 7.25), there is a direct threat to cardiopulmonary homeostasis. Because some disorders may result in sudden respiratory failure without warning, prophylactic mechanical ventilatory support is sometimes initiated before respiratory failure is documented by blood gases.[4,23]

Infants and children with chronic lung disease may have chronic respiratory insufficiency with hypoxemia and hypercapnia but yet have a nearly normal serum pH. These patients have metabolic compensation for chronic respiratory acidosis and usually do *not* require ventilation when they become ill. In these patients the indication for ventilatory support is a falling pH, usually to less than 7.2 to 7.25.[23]

In addition to arterial blood gases and pH, there are other objective measurements that are used to assess the initial severity and evolution of lung injury. One of these measurements is called the alveolar-to-arterial oxygen pressure gradient or difference—A-aO_2. As the term implies, this is the difference between alveolar and arterial P_{O_2}. It is measured in the following way: a patient breathes a known concentration of oxygen for 15 to 20 minutes, and then an arterial blood sample is obtained. The *inspired oxygen tension* (PI_{O_2}) is calculated by multiplying the fractional inspired oxygen concentration by the difference between the barometric pressure and the water vapor pressure at body temperature (this water vapor pressure at body temperature is 47 mm Hg). The *alveolar oxygen tension* (PA_{O_2}) is equal to the PI_{O_2} less the Pa_{CO_2} as shown below:

$$PA_{O_2} = FI_{O_2} \times (760 - 47) - Pa_{CO_2}$$

$$PA_{O_2} = \underbrace{\phantom{FI_{O_2} \times (760 - 47)}}_{PI_{O_2}} - Pa_{CO_2}$$

The alveolar-arterial oxygen difference or gradient (A-a O_2 difference) is the difference between the calculated PA_{O_2} and the Pa_{O_2}, as follows:

$$\text{A-a } O_2 \text{ difference} = PA_{O_2} - Pa_{O_2}$$

CASE STUDY

If a child has a Pa_{O_2} of 250 mm Hg, a Pa_{CO_2} of 35 mm Hg, and is breathing 100% oxygen ($FI_{O_2} = 1.00$) at sea level (barometric pressure = 760 torr), then to calculate the A-a O_2 difference:

$$PA_{O_2} = 1.00 \times (760 - 47) - 35 = 678$$

So therefore:

$$PA_{O_2} - Pa_{O_2} = 678 - 250 = 428$$

The normal A-a O_2 gradient is less than 50 torr. In this example the A-a O_2 gradient is abnormally elevated and indicates a marked maldistribution of ventilation and perfusion.

There are many ways to artificially support ventilation and oxygenation in a child whose lungs are not working effectively. Ventilatory support can be intermittent or continuous, short or long-term, using positive or negative pressure, with or without patient effort or cooperation.

The topic of ventilatory support can be better understood following consideration of the normal respiratory cycle. Normal mechanics of breathing are dependent on pressure gradients within the pulmonary system (Fig. 4-5). Air flows only when a pressure difference exists between the two areas. Gas always flows from an area of greater pressure to one of lesser

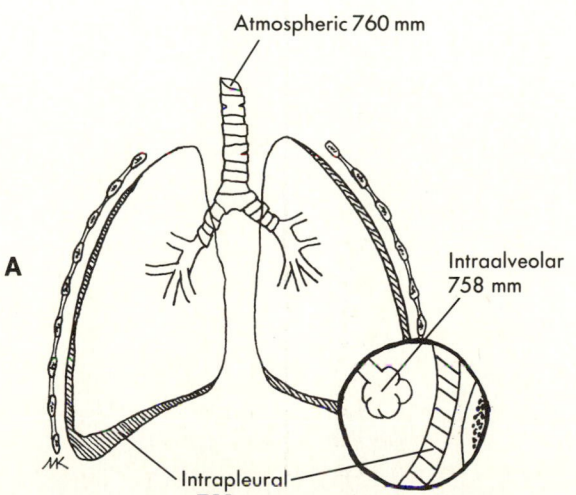

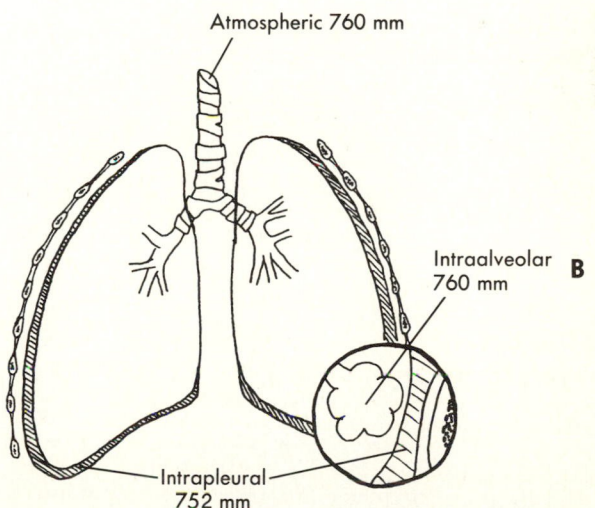

Fig. 4-5 Typical pressures during inspiration. **A,** Represents the beginning of inspiration. The pressure in the intrapleural space decreases, causing a fall in intraalveolar pressure; this creates a pressure gradient between the atmosphere and the intraalveolar space. Since gas always flows from

greater pressure to lesser pressure, air flows into the alveoli. **B,** Depicts the approximate pressures at the end of a normal inspiration. Note that the pressure in the alveoli is equal to the pressure in the atmosphere.

pressure; thus the intraalveolar pressure must be less than the pressure at the airway opening (atmospheric pressure) for inspiratory flow to occur. At end-expiration, intraalveolar and atmospheric pressures are approximately equal. As the diaphragm contracts, the thoracic cavity is enlarged, and the intrapleural pressures become negative with respect to atmospheric pressure. The lung tissue is pulled outward (enlarged) and the alveolar pressure decreases. This pressure change creates a pressure difference between the atmosphere and the alveolus, and gas flows into the lungs until pressures in the atmosphere are again equal to those within the alveoli. The passive elastic recoil of the lung and thorax tend to return the lung volume to its resting state during expiration.

■ Positive- and negative-pressure ventilators

Positive-pressure ventilators. Positive-pressure ventilators can be broadly classified according to the way in which the inspiratory cycle is ended. A ventilator may be time-, pressure-, volume-, or flow-cycled. Many of the ventilators operate by a combination of two or three cycles.

If a ventilator is time-cycled, inspiration ends when a preset inspiratory time is reached. In this case the tidal volume depends on the flow and pressure characteristics of the ventilator, the ET tube, and the patient.

If a ventilator is pressure-cycled, inspiration ceases when the preset inspiratory pressure is reached. In this case the tidal volume delivered is dependent on the compliance of the patient's lung as well as the patient's airway resistance.

Volume-cycled machines terminate inspiration after a predetermined volume is delivered. The pressure necessary to deliver the volume depends on the compliance of both the ventilator and the patient's lung. Most volume-cycled ventilators also have a high-pressure limit at which inspiration will end (see Table 4-10 for classification of mechanical ventilators and a listing of their flow characteristics; Table 9-8 also reviews ventilator specifications).

Positive-pressure ventilators create a pressure at the airway opening greater than the intraalveolar pressure; as a result, gas is forced from the ventilator unit into the lungs. Positive-pressure ventilation results in increased airway pressures and increased intrathoracic pressures. This increase in intrathoracic pressure may cause a decrease in both systemic and pulmonary venous return to the heart and a consequent fall in cardiac output. In addition, positive-pressure ventilation may increase antidiuretic hormone (ADH) secretion; this may promote water retention and also affect cardiovascular function (see Chapter 7 for further information).[26]

Negative-pressure ventilators. Negative-pressure ventilators are occasionally used for the long-

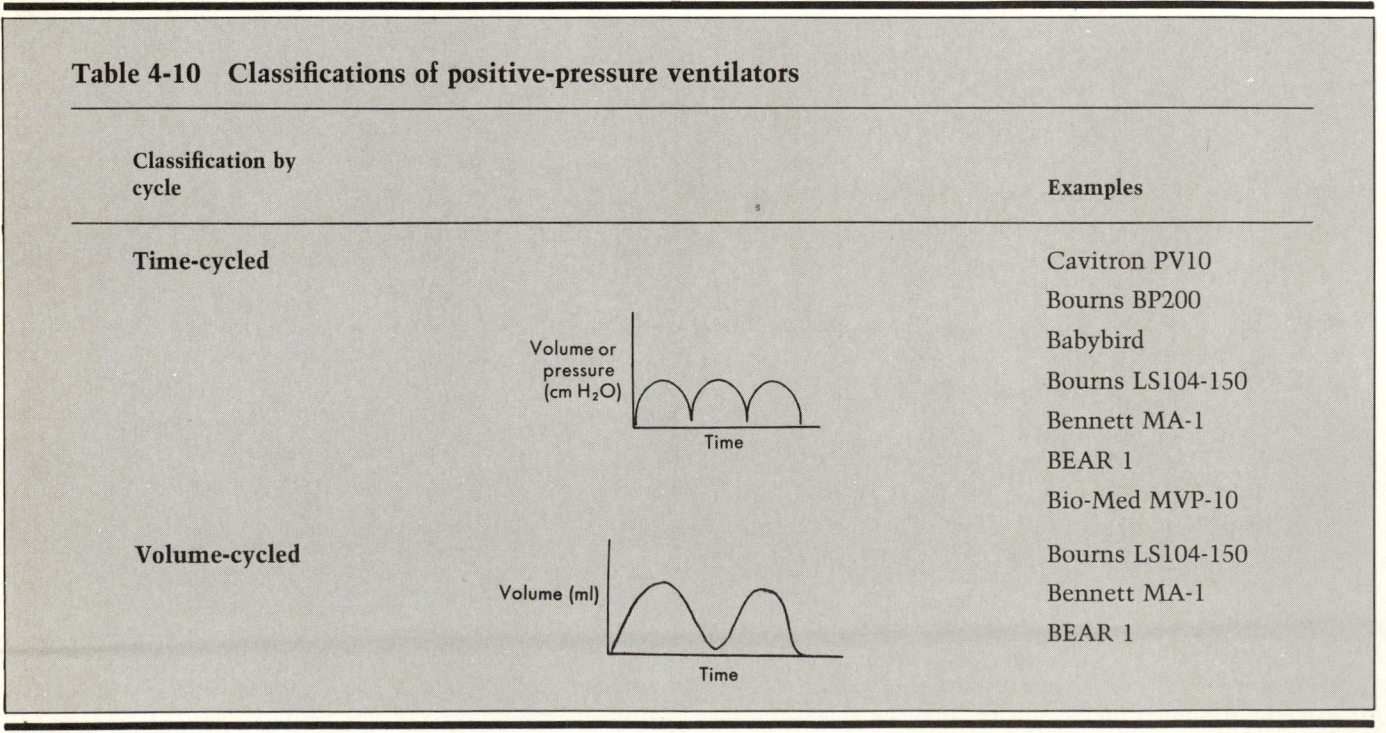

Table 4-10 Classifications of positive-pressure ventilators

Classification by cycle		Examples
Time-cycled	Volume or pressure (cm H₂O) / Time	Cavitron PV10
		Bourns BP200
		Babybird
		Bourns LS104-150
		Bennett MA-1
		BEAR 1
		Bio-Med MVP-10
Volume-cycled	Volume (ml) / Time	Bourns LS104-150
		Bennett MA-1
		BEAR 1

term ventilation of patients with neuromuscular disease. The tank ventilator (so-called iron lung) and the cuirass ventilator are the primary units available. These units create intermittent negative pressure or partial vacuum around the chest and upper abdomen; this results in a pressure gradient that causes expansion of the chest and inspiration. These devices must cover the child's thorax; as a result, the machines are large and limit activity and accessibility of the child. The chief advantage of such a system is the fact that an artificial airway is unnecessary.

■ Ventilatory modes

Mechanical ventilation can be delivered in several *modes*. The selection of the appropriate ventilatory mode is dependent on such factors as the presence of spontaneous breathing, the reason for institution of mechanical ventilation, and the severity of the child's cardiopulmonary disease.

The two major categories of ventilatory support are *control* and *augmented ventilation*. Total control of ventilation implies that the patient cannot contribute any spontaneous breaths during ventilation. The use of this mode has gradually decreased since the development of more sophisticated assist modes, but unstable patients generally require some initial time in the control mode. Children with impaired central nervous system function (coma, apnea, or neuromuscular weakness) or severe cardiovascular instability will often require ventilatory support with the control mode. Children who have recently undergone major surgery may conserve energy and more quickly stabilize if they are placed on mechanical ventilatory support in the control mode. Those children who are able to make sufficient breathing efforts and who may "fight" the ventilator, however, would not be good candidates for the control mode, unless they are sufficiently sedated. Since there is not a constant flow of air to the patient during the expiratory phase of the control mode, it is impossible for the child to breathe spontaneously between machine-delivered breaths. This can be stressful and frustrating for the alert child. The control mode usually requires faster ventilator rates and deeper breaths (totaling 10 to 20 ml/kg tidal volume) than augmented modes, since maintenance of a mild hypocapnia (Pa_{CO_2} between 30 to 40 mm Hg) will eliminate most of the child's stimulus to breathe and enable better ventilatory control of the patient.

With an *augmented mode*, the patient can initiate whatever spontaneous breathing he is capable of, and the machine is used to augment further ventilation as needed. Fresh gas flows through the system continuously so that the patient does not rebreathe expired air.

The *assist* setting available on most ventilators allows the patient to determine ventilatory rate but not tidal volume. Inspiratory flow will begin when the patient creates a subatmospheric pressure or, in the case of ventilation with PEEP, reduces pressure to a preset level, which triggers the ventilator and causes it to cycle. The ease of the patient "triggering" is dependent on the sensitivity setting on the machine. Once triggered, the machine cycles and delivers a full preset tidal volume. One advantage of the assist setting is that, since the patient is allowed to regulate his ventilatory rate, aggressive pharmacologic intervention such as paralysis is avoided. A disadvantage of the assist mode is that the child may be unable to regulate his own tidal volume and may be likely to hyperventilate if he is anxious.

Intermittent mandatory ventilation (IMV) or *intermittent demand ventilation* (IDV) implies that positive-pressure ventilation is delivered at mandatory intervals. With IMV, the patient may breathe spontaneously between each mandatory positive-pressure breath. Synchronized IMV (intermittent mandatory ventilation) also allows the patient to breathe spontaneously between mandatory breaths, but the mandatory breaths are delivered in synchronization with the spontaneous pattern. With IMV and IDV the patient receives ventilatory breaths of preset tidal volumes at predetermined intervals, but the breaths taken by the patient between ventilatory breaths are at his own tidal volume.[43]

Since its introduction in 1973, IMV/IDV has proved to be a real advance in mechanical ventilatory support. IMV with PEEP is currently the ventilatory assistance method of choice for most critically ill infants and children. The chief disadvantage of the IMV mode is that it may be used in a patient who is not ready to resume spontaneous breathing. In this case the patient will be unable to breathe independently between the mandatory positive-pressure breaths; this will result in retention of carbon dioxide.

■ Positive end-expiratory pressure (PEEP)

The use of either *PEEP* or *continuous positive airway pressure (CPAP)* maintains alveolar pressure at a level above atmospheric pressure at the end of expiration. PEEP is used for ventilated patients, while CPAP is reserved for patients who are breathing spontaneously. The physiologic effects of CPAP and PEEP are the same: alveolar volume increases, ventilation and perfusion are better matched, arterial oxygen content increases (shunt fraction decreases), and Pa_{O_2}

rises. In addition, if pulmonary edema is present, the excess lung water may be moved to areas of the lungs that do not interfere with gas exchange. Moreover, the work of breathing is reduced with both PEEP and CPAP, since lung compliance is increased.[4] CPAP was initially used to prevent atelectasis in infants suffering with respiratory distress syndrome, but now CPAP or PEEP is routinely used in the management of all intubated patients. Once it is instituted, it is important that the level of CPAP or PEEP is monitored and continuously maintained at a constant value. Manual ventilator bags can be equipped with a valve and manometer to maintain this positive airway pressure. CPAP can be administered with nasal prongs, face mask, or head hood, or through an ET tube (Fig. 4-6). Most mechanical ventilators can provide PEEP and CPAP. Positive-airway pressures in the range of +2 to +12 cm H_2O are used for children[27]; however, PEEP as high as +40 cm H_2O has been used in adult patients with severe respiratory failure.

CPAP/PEEP pressure is increased or decreased according to the results of blood gas analysis as well as clinical assessment of the patient, including measurement of vital signs, observation of color, and evaluation of the chest radiograph. The CPAP or PEEP can be increased as long as the child's Pa_{O_2} does not fall and the Pa_{CO_2} does not rise above approximately 60 mm Hg. If the child is hypoxemic and the hypoxemia persists after PEEP is initiated, the PEEP may be increased to a maximum pressure of approximately 12 cm H_2O (or according to physician order or unit policy). Once the Pa_{O_2} levels increase to about 50 to 70 mm Hg for the infant or to 70 to 90 mm Hg for the older child, the PEEP does not need to be increased further. If the child remains stable on an existing PEEP for several hours, that PEEP may be slowly decreased by 1 to 2 cm at a time, until a PEEP of approximately +4 cm H_2O is provided. CPAP/PEEP should never be reduced below +2 cm H_2O while the ET tube is still in place because pressures below that level may encourage alveolar collapse or atelectasis and thus result in hypoxia.

Many complications may occur as a result of either CPAP or PEEP therapy. The two most important complications are air leaks (pneumothorax, bilateral emphysema, and pneumopericardium) and low cardiac output. Reduction in cardiac output can be manifested by hypotension, decreased urinary output, increasing acidosis, a decreasing Pa_{O_2}, or a widening of the arteriovenous oxygen difference. In some patients, for example, PEEP may improve Pa_{O_2} but reduce cardiac output, so that the ultimate result of PEEP is a reduction in oxygen delivery.[26,32] Table 4-11 contains a list of some commercially available venti-

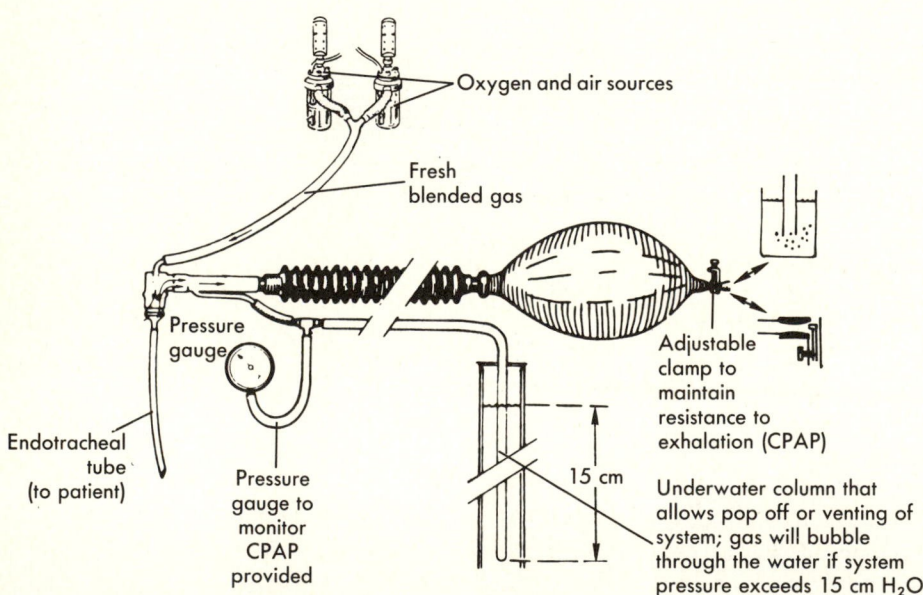

Oxygen and air sources

Fresh blended gas

Pressure gauge

Endotracheal tube (to patient)

Pressure gauge to monitor CPAP provided

Adjustable clamp to maintain resistance to exhalation (CPAP)

15 cm

Underwater column that allows pop off or venting of system; gas will bubble through the water if system pressure exceeds 15 cm H_2O

Fig. 4-6 System for applying CPAP through an ET tube during spontaneous breathing.

Table 4-11 Specifications of commercially available pediatric ventilators

Commercial name	Rate capacity	Flow (L/min)	Tidal volume or pressure range	Size of patient
Bourns LS104-150	5-80	25-200 ml/sec	5-150 ml	Infants
Bourns BP200	1-60	0-20 L/min	0-80 cm of H_2O pressure (variable volume)	Infants
Babybird	0-100	0-30 L/min	0-88 cm H_2O pressure (variable volume)	Infants
Bio-Med MVP-10	1-150	0-12 L/min	0-400 cc	Infants
Bennett MA-1	6-60	10-100 L/min	100-2200 cc	Adults and children, provided small bore tubing is used
Siemens Servo	6-60	0.5-30 L/min	Calculated by dividing minute volume by breaths per minute (ranges from 0.5 L to over 30 L)	Designed for all patients including neonates
Ohio Neonatal		50-200 ml/sec	5-50 ml	Infants

For a more complete listing of ventilator specifications, see Table 9-8.

Table 4-12 Comparison of various modes of positive-pressure ventilation

Mode	Physiologic action	Indications
Controlled PPV*	Provides total ventilation	Apnea Respiratory failure Oxygenation deficit
Augmented PPV (IMV/IDV)	Provides extra support to the spontaneously breathing patient	Same as above except for apnea
Controlled PPV (PPV + PEEP)	Same as above with addition of PEEP to increase functional residual capacity	Intubated patient with central nervous system problems or for control of a patient with oxygenation problems (e.g., after cardiac surgery)
Augmented PPV (IMV/IDV + PEEP)	Same	Useful for the intubated, spontaneously breathing patient with oxygenation problems
CPAP	Used to improve oxygenation by increasing functional residual capacity	Patient who can assume all work of breathing but who has a decreased P_{O_2}

*Positive-pressure ventilation

lators for use with pediatric patients; these ventilators are also reviewed in Table 9-8. Table 4-12 summarizes the physiologic action and indications for each method of ventilation.

The following list presents ideal components of a pediatric ventilator:

Volume- or time-cycled with control, assist-control, and IMV modes
Respiratory rate between 1-100 breaths/min
Tidal volume range from 5-2000 ml
Inspiratory flow rate from 0-100 L/min
Variable I:E ratio 3:1-1:10
PEEP or CPAP capability to 20 cm H_2O
Size: small, portable
Capable of use as a transport ventilator
Capable of remote recording of pressure, flow, and volume waveform

The pediatric ventilator should have alarms (audible and visible) for:

Apnea
Loss of CPAP or PEEP
High and low-pressure
Electrical failure
Overheating of humidifier
Low or high oxygen concentrations
Failure to cycle

The pediatric ventilator should also be equipped with visible readouts for:

Airway pressure (proximal) and temperature
Inspiratory oxygen concentration
I:E ratio
Respiratory rate
Tidal volume
Inspiratory and expiratory time
Flow rate

■ NURSING CARE OF THE CHILD ON A VENTILATOR
■ Humidification

Because the upper airway is bypassed when the patient is intubated, inspired air must be humidified before it is delivered to the patient. Inadequate humidification can cause life-threatening airway obstruction, since drying of secretions and a decrease in ciliary function may cause mucous plugs to develop. Increased viscosity of secretions or significant decrease in secretion quantity should cause the nurse to suspect inadequate ventilatory humidification. Too much humidity, on the other hand, can cause accumulation of water in the ventilator tubing; this can reduce the inspired oxygen concentration, the inspired ventilatory pressure, or the volume of gas delivered to the patient. In very young children, fluid overload may occur as the excess water droplets are absorbed from the air spaces.

The humidification provided by the ventilator is a function of the heat applied to the water in the system. Humidity should be delivered at approximately body temperature, since air is 100% saturated with water vapor at body temperature. A thermometer should always be attached to the inspiratory line to be sure that the desired air temperature is maintained. Excessive heat in the tubing will not only increase humidity within the circuit but may stimulate bronchospasm and raise the patient's body temperature. Inadequate heat in the tubing may result in condensation of water within the ventilator tubing and inadequate delivery of humidification in the inspired air.

■ Suctioning and hand ventilation technique

Sick patients cannot move secretions effectively; thus these secretions must often be removed by suction, which is extremely unpleasant for the conscious patient. Gentle stimulation of the upper airway surface may possibly elicit spontaneous coughs that are highly effective in moving secretions toward the large airways. If such cough stimulation is ineffective, suctioning will be required.

Suctioning of the ET tube and airway must always be performed in a sterile manner. The child should be prepared with an appropriate explanation before the suctioning process.

Since mechanical ventilation is interrupted during suctioning, the duration of suctioning must be as short as possible to prevent hypoxia. Preoxygenation and hyperventilation should nearly always be performed immediately before the introduction of the suction catheter into the ET tube. If the nurse thinks that a plug is present in a larger airway, suctioning should occur before hyperventilation in order to avoid propelling the plug into a distal airway. When normal hyperventilation is performed, approximately 8 to 10 manual breaths are provided at an inspired oxygen concentration that is approximately 10% greater than the child's maintenance inspired oxygen requirements. Some physicians request the use of 100% oxygen during manual hyperventilation before suctioning.[37] The peak inspiratory pressure provided during manual ventilation should be approximately equal to that pressure provided by the mechanical ventilator. It is important to note that the peak inspiratory pressure measured with a hand ventilator system reflects the true peak inspiratory pressure at the proximal airway, while the peak inspiratory pressure measured by a manometer in the ventilator system often is falscly elevated because of internal resistance within the mechanical ventilator circuit. Therefore if hand ventilation is provided at the same pressure reflected by the mechanical ventilator manometer, the patient is often receiving much higher pressures during hand ventilation than he was receiving by mechanical ventilation. As a result, barotrauma and pneumothoraxes can result. In any event, a pressure manometer should be attached to the manual ventilator bag system to help ensure that high inspiratory pressures are avoided.

The use of normal saline instillation into the artificial airway before suctioning is controversial. The rationale for such saline instillation is that it is thought to facilitate removal of fixed secretions and prevent formation of mucous crust within the artificial airway and proximal patient airways. However, since the instilled saline droplets are large in diameter, it will be virtually impossible for those droplets to move beyond the area of the carina. Generally, 0.5 ml is instilled in the airway of an infant and 1 to 3 ml in the airway of an older child. Some physicians also advocate the use of bicarbonate solutions before airway suctioning to facilitate removal of secretions.

The nurse should know the appropriate French size of the suction catheter to use for a specific ET tube (see Table 4-9)—usually obtained by multiplying the child's ET tube size by 2. If the suction catheter has a flared tip, it will be necessary to use a suction cathether that is one size smaller than that calculated to fit into the ET tube. In an effort to maximize secretion removal, the child's head should be rotated if possible during suctioning. However, it is not possible to ensure entrance into the patient's right or left main-stem bronchus through turning of the head.

Throughout the suctioning procedure, the child's heart rate, blood pressure, and skin color should be observed closely. Some centers utilize transcutaneous oxygen electrodes to assess the effect of suctioning on the patient's oxygenation. It has been shown that the use of this device can be a valuable aid in teaching good suction technique. In general, suctioning should be as brief as possible to prevent vagal stimulation and hypoxia. If the child becomes bradycardic, hypotensive, or develops cyanosis, mottling, or pallor during suctioning, the suction procedure should be terminated and the child should be manually ventilated until stable.

To minimize possible microatelectasis produced by suctioning and to reverse any hypoxia or hypercapnia that may have developed, the child should be manually ventilated immediately after any suction procedure. The lungs should be auscultated carefully for adequacy of ventilation and presence of conges-

tion immediately after each suctioning episode. In addition, the nurse should be alert to the possibility that the ET tube may have migrated into a main-stem bronchus during hand ventilation.

The amount of suctioning required for any specific patient is variable. Frequency of suctioning depends on the type of lung injury the patient has sustained. For example, patients with bacterial tracheitis may require suctioning every 15 minutes during their illness, while comatose patients with normal lungs may be suctioned every 1 to 2 hours. Suctioning should be performed, however, whenever there is any evidence that secretions have accumulated or a mucous plug has developed. Suctioning that is unnecessary or haphazardly performed will cause mucosal damage and stimulate more mucus production.[26]

■ **Initial ventilatory variables**

Once the patient is intubated, the specific appropriate ventilator variables must be quickly determined to initiate mechanical ventilatory support. Nursing assessment skills are most vital at this time. Although specific ventilatory variables are determined by the anesthesiologist, intensive-care specialist, or respiratory therapist, the nurse must be able to monitor the patient's response to mechanical ventilation to help evaluate appropriateness of the ventilator variables (Table 4-13).

The most important consideration to be made concerning mechanical ventilation in the pediatric patient is the type of ventilator to be used. A child with extremely noncompliant lungs, for example, would probably be best ventilated through use of a volume-cycled (rather than pressure-cycled) ventilator. In addition, if an "adult" ventilator is used, such as an MA-1 or MA-2, appropriate adaptations must be made in both the ventilator tubing and the ventilator variables before its use for a child. It should be emphasized that while there are many kinds of ventilators and many styles of ventilation, the goals of mechanical ventilation are always the same: to maintain normal gas exchange, to avoid air leaks and oxygen injury, and to maintain oxygen delivery until the lung injury resolves. The following variables should be checked by the nurse at least every hour with vital sign measurements, or any time the patient's condition changes.

1. *Respiratory rate.* The respiratory rate depends on the child's respiratory disease and level of consciousness. If the child is breathing spontaneously, for example, the IMV mode may be used; however, the comatose child will require controlled ven-

Table 4-13 Suggested ventilator variables* for initiation of mechanical ventilation[4]

| Age | Respiratory rate | Tidal volume† | Peak inspiratory pressure† | | I:E ratio |
			Normal lungs	Diseased lungs	
Newborn	30-40	10-20 cc/kg	15-20 cm H_2O	20-30+ cm H_2O	1:2 (1.5:1 or 1:1 may be needed if interstitial lung disease is present)
Infant	20-30	10-20 cc/kg	15-30 cm H_2O	30-40+ cm H_2O	
Child	18-25	10-20 cc/kg	20-30 cm H_2O	30-40+ cm H_2O	
Older child	12-22	10-15 cc/kg	25-35 cm H_2O	30-40+ cm H_2O	

*These variables should always be modified according to the patient's clinical condition. Once mechanical ventilation is begun, the nurse should continuously monitor the child's response to the ventilatory support.
†These variables should be adjusted after consideration of the resistance (or compliance) within the ventilator circuit (including tubing).

tilation. When the nurse is assessing the child's respiratory rate, she should not only count the breaths delivered by the ventilator but also any additional breaths taken entirely by the child. If the child is receiving assisted ventilation, the nurse should record how frequently the child triggers the ventilator.

2. *Tidal volume.* A typical setting for initial ventilation on a volume ventilator is usually 10 to 15 cc/kg body weight. The tidal volume provided will need to be increased if extremely compliant ventilator tubing is utilized or if there is a leak around the ET tube. Higher volumes (15 to 20 cc/kg) are required by the child with significant respiratory disease. If a pressure-limit ventilator is used, a peak inspiratory pressure of between 15 to 30 cm H_2O will deliver the appropriate tidal volume. *It is important to note that a child's chest must expand during each inspiration provided by a mechanical ventilator; if the chest does not move, the tidal volume delivered by the ventilator is inadequate, regardless of the numbers displayed by the ventilator gauges.*

3. *Minute ventilation.* The total inspiratory gas delivered by the ventilator in liters per minute is the minute ventilation. If the child is receiving controlled ventilatory support, the minute ventilation can be calculated by multiplying the child's respiratory rate by the tidal volume delivered. Some mechanical ventilators display the minute ventilation; others do not.

4. *Pressure limit control.* The pressure limit should be determined after considering the child's physiologic condition and the amount of pressure required to achieve adequate chest expansion or deliver

adequate tidal volume. This pressure limit will be the maximum peak inspiratory pressure delivered by either a volume-cycled or a pressure-cycled ventilator. If the child has a volume-cycled ventilator, the peak inspiratory pressure should be watched closely. This pressure will increase when secretions form in the child's airways or when a kink or water buildup is present in the tubing. If the child develops a pneumothorax, the peak inspiratory pressure may increase suddenly; if the patient becomes extubated or disconnected from the ventilator, the peak pressure will decrease suddenly. The amount of pressure required to deliver a given tidal volume depends on the compliance of the ventilator tubing and the compliance of the patient's lungs and chest wall. The child with lung disease or decreased lung compliance will develop higher airway pressures when a given volume is delivered than a child with normal lung compliance. As the disease and compliance improve, however, the inspiratory pressures will usually decrease.

5. *Inspired oxygen concentration (FIO₂).* The amount of oxygen delivered by the ventilator system is the FIO_2. The oxygen concentration delivered should be analyzed continuously or at least every hour.

6. *Positive end-expiratory pressure.* If the child is receiving PEEP, the nurse must remember to continue the PEEP mode at all times. When the child is manually ventilated with a bag, a valve can be added to the manual ventilator system to "hold" the PEEP during manual ventilation. If the child is receiving both PEEP and assist-controlled ventilation, it is im-

portant that the assist trigger be adjusted so that the child can initiate an inspiration from the ventilator without having to override the PEEP.

■ Assessment of the child receiving ventilatory support

The most important nursing responsibility in the care of the child receiving mechanical ventilation is assessment of the adequacy of the ventilatory support. *The fact that the child is being ventilated does not mean that he is being ventilated appropriately.* This nursing assessment is especially important during the first few hours of ventilatory support and whenever a change in ventilatory variables is made. The primary methods of assessment include physical examination and vital sign measurement, arterial blood gas analysis, chest radiograph interpretation, and measurement of pulmonary function variables.

The most reliable method of assessment is the physical examination performed by a skilled practitioner. The objective impression that a child "looks good" or "looks bad" is as important (if not more so) than any other assessment the skilled nurse can make. The vital signs, especially the heart rate and blood pressure, must also be noted. It may be helpful if the nurse asks herself the following questions.

1. Is the child "fighting" the ventilator? If so, remove him from the ventilator, manually ventilate him, and assess lung aeration and chest expansion for evidence of pneumothorax, a misplaced ET tube, or ET tracheal tube obstruction.
2. Is the child's heart rate too fast or too slow for his clinical condition? If the child is extremely tachycardic or bradycardic, it may be an indication of hypoxemia.
3. Is the blood pressure appropriate for the child's clinical condition? The child who is hypertensive may be in pain or may be stressed because of hypoxia. If the child is hypotensive, extreme hypoxemia or acidosis may be present because of inadequate ventilation.
4. Is the child's color and perfusion acceptable? The child's mucous membranes and nail beds should be pink, extremities should be warm, and capillary filling time should be brisk. Urine output should average 1 ml/kg body weight per hour if fluid intake is adequate. If the child's color or systemic perfusion are deteriorating, these could be early signs of hypoxemia because of respiratory insufficiency.

5. Is the chest rising symmetrically with each cycle of positive pressure? Significant atelectasis or pneumothorax can prevent adequate lung expansion on the involved side and thus prevent chest expansion on that side also.
6. Are the breath sounds equal and adequate bilaterally? If the ET tube is in the right bronchus, breath sounds heard over the right chest will be significantly louder than those heard over the left chest. It is important to note, however, that since the chest wall of infants and young children is so thin and transmits breath sounds so easily, the child may appear to have adequate breath sounds even over areas of atelectasis or pneumothorax.
7. What is the pitch of the breath sounds bilaterally? Since breath sounds can be referred so easily from other areas of the lung, the nurse must listen for a change in pitch of the breath sounds over involved areas, which may be the first sign of atelectasis, pneumothorax, or consolidation.
8. Is the child's level of consciousness appropriate for his clinical condition? Extreme irritability followed by lethargy may be signs of severe hypoxemia or hypercapnia.

The presence of any of these abnormalities may reflect abnormal gas exchange. It should be emphasized that when the condition of a ventilated patient suddenly worsens, he should be disconnected from the ventilator and manual ventilation should be performed. The ventilator should be quickly checked for malfunction, and the nurse should assess breath sounds to be sure that the ET tube is not obstructed. If there is no malfunction in the mechanical ventilator, the patient can be returned to the ventilator, and a search should be made for other causes of deterioration. The most common causes of sudden deterioration in a ventilated child can include development of a significant pneumothorax or development of ET tube obstruction or migration.

Laboratory assessment of the ventilated patient should be utilized only to reinforce the clinical impression. Blood gases and a chest radiograph are often ordered once the child is placed on mechanical ventilation or when any change is made in ventilatory variables. Analysis of arterial or capillary blood gases are of fundamental importance, since the pH, Pa_{O_2}, and Pa_{CO_2} ultimately reflect the effectiveness of the child's gas exchange. Blood gas analyses are also useful for calculation of both the A-a O_2 difference and the physiologic shunt.

Chest radiographs are typically performed daily

while the child is intubated in order to assess placement of the ET tube and progression of the child's disease state.

Special care must be provided to the child who has received a neuromuscular blocking agent, such as pancuronium. These children become completely dependent on the health-care team for provision of adequate ventilation and are not able to signal in any way distress or development of hypoxemia. Paralysis and loss of muscle tone also place the child at risk for accidental injury; as a result, whenever the child is turned or moved, the head and extremities must be supported carefully to prevent bone dislocation or other injury. Venous pooling can also occur with loss of muscle tone. The recovery of diaphragmatic muscle tone may be gauged by recovery of the rectus muscle, since both recover at approximately the same rate from pharmacologic paralysis.

Muscle-relaxant drugs are *not* sedatives or analgesics; thus pain and other sensations are still experienced by the paralyzed child. Sedatives or analgesic drugs should be used in conjunction with muscle relaxants to ensure that the child is free of pain and comfortable during treatment. Since the child can still hear, he requires continual explanations (appropriate to his age) and reassurances. It may be useful to provide a tape recording of the voices of parents and siblings or familiar music that can be played through a portable battery-operated recorder at the child's bedside.

■ Weaning

Weaning can be a smooth process or a long difficult one. It should be considered whenever the child's underlying disease process resolves, the blood gases improve, and the cardiopulmonary system stabilizes. The following are specific criteria for beginning the weaning process from ventilatory support[45]:

1. Resolution of the condition that necessitated intubation and mechanical support
2. Blood gases near normal range
3. Central nervous system and cardiovascular stabilization
4. Spontaneous tidal volume greater than 5 ml/kg body weight
5. Vital capacity (measured by a Wright Respirometer) greater than 10 ml/kg body weight

The child should first be assessed for any factors that might hinder the weaning process. These factors include problems with fluid balance, cardiac abnormalities such as arrhythmias, anemia, pain, drug-induced respiratory depression, fever, sleep deprivation, and extreme apprehension. The child's nutritional status and general muscle strength should also be considered, since poor nutrition or poor muscle strength make weaning a difficult or an impossible task.[4] The type of weaning process to be initiated will vary with physician preference and patient needs. The most widely used method of weaning today is a form of IMV. In this mode the ventilator is set to provide continuous fresh gas flow, and the mandatory ventilatory rate is slowly decreased as the patient's independent respiratory effort increases. Eventually, the patient receives only oxygen flow with CPAP.

Another method of weaning involves use of a T piece, without end-expiratory pressure. As the child is stabilized and ready to breathe on his own, the ventilator is discontinued for specific periods of time. The intervals are initially short, totaling perhaps only 5 to 15 minutes at a time. Between these intervals, the child is returned to mechanical ventilatory support. If the child can breathe without difficulty and if arterial blood gases remain stable, the periods on the T piece are gradually lengthened. This method of ventilatory weaning is not recommended for infants and children, since it does not provide even physiologic (+2-+4 cm H_2O) amounts of PEEP.

CPAP may be added to either of the methods just discussed, particularly when the child is breathing spontaneously. CPAP increases the child's resting lung volume or functional residual capacity (FRC) and may change the mechanical properties of the respiratory system and make the patient's inspiratory efforts more effective. In addition, CPAP prevents atelectasis.

Regardless of the weaning protocol selected, the weaning should be performed in an organized manner. It is usually inappropriate to make multiple variable changes at the same time. For example, it is not appropriate to expect to decrease the inspired oxygen concentration, the respiratory rate, and the inspiratory pressure or tidal volume all at once. The cumulative effect of all these changes may be too great for the child to tolerate. A gradual decrease or change in the variables (one at a time) provides the smoothest transition for the child and, in the long run, often the shortest weaning process.[4]

Frequent blood gas analyses may be required to determine the child's tolerance of weaning. If a device is available to analyze the child's end-tidal P_{CO_2}, these values may be utilized to reflect Pa_{CO_2} values. If transcutaneous oxygen or carbon dioxide monitoring is available, this could be utilized in place of frequent blood gas analyses. Transcutaneous carbon dioxide monitoring may be particularly useful if it eliminates the need for intermittent arterial puncture. In awake infants and children, the P_{CO_2} obtained from arterial puncture may be misleading.

■ Extubation

The decision to extubate the patient is obviously made when neither mechanical ventilation nor CPAP is necessary. The overall assessment is based on a number of different factors including satisfactory Pa_{CO_2}; chest radiograph and hematocrit; good cardiac, respiratory, neurologic, and renal function; and the ability of the child to cough effectively. Before actual extubation, reintubation equipment must be placed nearby in case reintubation is necessary on an urgent basis. A high humidity tent, head hood, or face mask should be ready to provide the child with humidified oxygen immediately on extubation. An individual skilled at intubation should be at the bedside before extubation and available for 4 to 6 hours following extubation.

The airway is usually suctioned immediately before extubation. Deep suctioning should be avoided after extubation because it may traumatize glottic and supraglottic tissues, producing edema and upper airway obstruction. The child should be monitored for changes in heart rate and apnea during and after the removal of the tube. Some physicians recommend that corticosteroids such as dexamethasone (Decadron) be given before and after extubation in an effort to reduce airway edema; however, the effectiveness of steroid administration has never been demonstrated in a controlled clinical trial.

The inhalation of an aerosol mist containing epinephrine may be used to enhance bronchodilation and to reduce edema immediately after extubation (see Appendix B for further information about racemic epinephrine).

Oral fluids and chest physiotherapy should usually be withheld for 2 to 4 hours following extubation in order to avoid compromising the airway with swallowing maneuvers or coughing. Arterial blood gases may be useful after extubation to assess respiratory function. A chest radiograph is also usually obtained within the first 2 to 4 hours following extubation to assess lung expansion and to identify lung segments that may benefit from chest physiotherapy.

The child must be observed closely for at least 24 hours following extubation. Changes in respiratory status such as an increase in hoarseness, wheezing, stridor, chest retractions, or decreased air movement, accompanied by tachycardia and anxiety, usually indicate that the child has developed upper airway obstruction caused by postextubation edema. In this case intensive aerosol therapy may be necessary, and reintubation may ultimately be required.

■ COMPLICATIONS
■ Complications from intubation

Complications that arise from intubation range in severity from major to minor. Mild side effects, such as sore throat and hoarseness, usually disappear within several days without therapy. The administration of humidified air may be useful following extubation to relieve these symptoms.

Although the intubated airway can become edematous in different places, the most frequent site of postextubation edema is in the subglottic area. As the laryngeal and subglottic tissues swell, the airway gradually decreases in diameter. The presence of an inspiratory stridor accompanied by increased hoarseness, anxiety, chest retractions, and tachycardia indicate increasing obstruction of the airway.

Prevention of postextubation edema begins while the patient is intubated. Tracheal irritation can be minimized if the appropriate size of uncuffed ET tube has been used. In addition, the ET tube must be secured effectively throughout intubation to prevent tube movement. Adequate airway humidification and skilled pulmonary hygiene must also be provided. Finally, prompt extubation should be performed as soon as it is clinically indicated.

Other potential problems following extubation include ulceration of the tracheal mucosa, vocal cord injury, granuloma or polyp formation, and vocal cord paralysis.

Several factors seem to increase the risk of postintubation sequelae in children. They include young age, long duration of intubation, frequent movement of the tube during intubation, use of high-pressure cuffed tubes, and presence of a respiratory infection.[24] Children exhibiting postextubation sequelae should be placed in humidified air with or without oxygen. Oxygen therapy may be necessary to keep the Pa_{O_2} between 85 and 100 torr. The head of the child's bed should be elevated, and deep suctioning should be avoided to prevent further trauma to the airway. The child should be disturbed as infrequently as possible and allowed to rest so that vigorous crying is avoided. Administration of racemic epinephrine by aerosol may be ordered (see Appendix B for dosages and effects).

■ Pulmonary oxygen toxicity

Prolonged oxygen breathing can produce pulmonary edema and pulmonary fibrosis. In the newborn, high oxygen tensions have caused injury to the blood vessels of the retina (retrolental fibroplasia). The dose and duration of exposure leading to oxygen injury in children is unknown because it is impossible to separate the toxic effects of oxygen from the lung disease that necessitated oxygen therapy. The growing lung is particularly sensitive to oxygen. The addition of positive pressure ventilation (PPV) may increase the likelihood of oxygen injury. Inspired oxygen levels below 0.40 rarely produce acute pulmonary oxygen toxicity in research animals. It should be kept in mind, however, that oxygen must never be denied to a patient who needs it for fear of development of toxicity. Like any drug, the lowest effective amount of oxygen should be used.

■ General complications of mechanical ventilation

Complications of mechanical ventilation are related primarily to physiologic effects of positive pressure. Compression of the great vessels results in low cardiac output, venous pooling, arrhythmias, and possible pulmonary emboli. Barotrauma (pneumothorax, pneumopericardium, and pneumomediastinum) can result from the positive pressure. Atelectasis may occur because of secretion stasis and because of non-uniform ventilation.[10,24] Gastric distention with possible ileus may develop from the increased pressure exerted on the abdominal contents and the swallowing of air associated with mechanical ventilation. Abdominal distention is also caused by use of muscle relaxants. Gastric ulcers may result from the increased acidity of stomach contents, which can occur during periods of generalized stress.[26]

Other complications of mechanical ventilation include problems with immobility (contractures, constipation, and skin breakdown) and psychologic trauma. These complications, their clinical signs and symptoms, and appropriate nursing interventions are summarized in Table 4-14.

Text continued on p. 293.

Table 4-14 Complications of mechanical ventilation

Complication	Cause	Signs/symptoms	Intervention
Pulmonary system			
Atelectasis	Monotonous ventilatory pattern	Decreased breath sounds	Ventilate with hand resuscitator q 1-2 hr
	Decreased ability to cough	Increased A-a O_2 difference	Increase mobility
	Decreased mobility	Decreased Pao_2	Change body position q 1-2 hr
	Decreased stimulation of surfactant	Increased peak pressure	Chest physiotherapy q 2-4 hr in Trendelenburg position; treat specific areas
	Displaced endotracheal tube	Increased body temperature	
	Increased secretions		Auscultate breath sounds
	Pain—causing splinting		Take chest x-ray to identify proper tube placement, areas of infiltration and consolidation
			Suction tracheobronchial tree

Modified from Morrison, M.L.: The mechanically ventilated patient. In Bushnell, S.S., editor: Respiratory intensive care nursing, ed. 3, Boston, © 1980, Little, Brown & Co.

Table 4-14 Complications of mechanical ventilation—cont'd

Complication	Cause	Signs/symptoms	Intervention
Atelectasis—cont'd			Instill NS prior to chest physiotherapy and suctioning
			Provide adequate humidification
			Use in-line bronchodilator or ultrasonic nebulizer treatments
			Hydration
Oxygen toxicity	FIO_2 >50% for longer than 24 hr	Decreased compliance involving:	Chest physiotherapy to improve A-a O_2 difference
		Atelectasis	PEEP to increase functional residual capacity
		Pulmonary edema	
		Fibrosis	
		Intraalveolar hemorrhage	
Trauma to upper airway, vocal cords, or trachea	ET tube, nasotracheal tube, tracheostomy tube	Oral/nasal pressure sore	Provide meticulous mouth care q 2-4 hr
	Unstable positioning in trachea; "riding" tube	Bleeding	Rotate oral ET tube side-to-side q 8 hr
	Decreased humidity to upper airway	Increased air requirement in cuff	Change tape on nasal ET tube prn; note signs of ischemia at nasal tip
			Mark ET tube at lip or nasal line
			Secure ET tube well
			Use Mörch swivel to decrease movement of ET tube
Barotrauma Subcutaneous emphysema	Misplaced tracheostomy cannula	Crepitus over face, thorax, abdomen	Reposition tracheostomy cannula
	Gas leak around tracheostomy cannula		
	Tear in parietal pleura		
Pneumothorax Pneumopericardium Pneumomediastinum Pneumoperitoneum	Increased positive pressure, especially in combination with noncompliant lung tissue	Cyanosis	Chest x-ray
		Decreased PaO_2	Placement of CT
	Increased increments of PEEP	Decreased breath sounds on affected side	Ventilate with hand resuscitator
	Thoracic surgery or injury	Increased peak pressure, usually sudden onset	

Continued.

Table 4-14 Complications of mechanical ventilation—cont'd

Complication	Cause	Signs/symptoms	Intervention
Barotrauma—cont'd		Absence of movement of thorax on affected side	
		Tracheal deviation	
		Hypotension	
		Arrhythmias	
		Cardiac arrest	
Cardiovascular system			
Hypotension	Compression of great vessels	Cyanosis (central or peripheral)	Arterial monitoring
	Interruption of thoracic pump causing decreased venous return, decreased cardiac output	Agitation	ECG monitoring
		Diaphoresis	Ensure proper I/E ratio
	Decreased cardiac filling time	Cardiac arrhythmias	ABG measurements (ensuring normal acid-balance)
	Decreased pulmonary blood flow	Decreased Pao_2	Plasma volume/fluid replacement, i.e., blood, colloid, IV fluid
	Large increments of PEEP		Vasopressor support
	Malfunction of ventilator, i.e., improper I/E ratio		Monitor central venous pressure, pulmonary artery pressure, pulmonary capillary wedge pressure and cardiac output
	Acidosis (metabolic or ventilator induced)		
	Decreased oxygen consumption from a decrease in work of breathing		
Arrhythmias	Hypoxemia	Presence of arrhythmia on ECG	Continuous ECG monitoring
	Hypercarbia	Hypotension	Monitor ABG; ensure and maintain normal acid-base
	Metabolic acidosis/alkalosis		Antiarrhythmic drugs
	Compression of the heart		

Table 4-14 Complications of mechanical ventilation—cont'd

Complication	Cause	Signs/symptoms	Intervention
Emboli (pulmonary)	Decreased mobility Venous stasis	Decreased Pa_{O_2}; increased A-a O_2 difference Hypotension Blood-tinged sputum ECG changes Pain in thoracic region	Range of motion exercise q 2 hr Change position q 2 hr External boot compression to legs to improve venous return and decrease venous stasis Anticoagulation agents (as ordered)
Central nervous system			
Restlessness and disorientation	Hypoxemia CO_2 retention Hypotension Cerebral edema from hypoxia Lack of sleep Cerebral damage	Restlessness and disorientation	Maintain adequate ABG Monitor and maintain arterial blood pressure Neurologic vital signs q 1-2 hr Sedatives for lack of sleep Osmotic diuretics for cerebral edema (as ordered)
Peripheral nerve damage (i.e., popliteal, radial, brachial, and facial nerve plexuses)	Poor positioning and body alignment Improper positioning of IV lines, ET tube, tubes and connections	Decubiti Loss of sensation of body part affected Excoriated areas	Proper body alignment Position monitoring equipment, ET tube, and other tubes to prevent pressure sores Air mattress/egg crate foam mattress Range of motion exercise Change position q 2 hr

Continued.

Table 4-14 Complications of mechanical ventilation—cont'd

Complication	Cause	Signs/symptoms	Intervention
Retinal/conjunctival damage	Lack of meticulous care	Scleral edema, irritation	Eye care q 4 hr with NS and methylcellulose eye drops
			Tape eyelashes to cheek to keep eyelid shut
			Prevent eyes from coming in contact with linens, IV lines, etc., especially when patient positioned on side
Gastrointestinal system			
Gastric distention; ileus	Increased pressure exerted on abdominal contents	Abdominal distention	Nasogastric tube placement
	Temporary decreased gut motility	Decreased bowel sounds	Aspirate, guaiac, and pH test stomach contents q 2-4 hr
	Air swallowing around ET tube	Nausea/vomiting	Nasogastric suction until bowel sounds return
	Use of muscle relaxants		Check for impaction
	Abdominal surgery		Aspirate stomach prior to each feeding; note residual; if residual is equal to the amount of feeding, feedings should be held until residual decreases
	Initiation of gastric feedings without assessment of bowel sounds		
Gastric bleeding	Stress of illess, PICU atmosphere, lack of sleep/wake periods	Guaiac-positive nasogastric aspirate	Nasogastric tube placement
	Increased acidity of stomach contents due to stress	Decreased hematocrit	Aspirate, guaiac, and pH test stomach contents q 2-4 hr
	Lack of nutrition	Hypotension	Antacid therapy
	Drug therapy	Tachycardia	Start GI feedings ASAP
		Nausea/vomiting	

Table 4-14 Complications of mechanical ventilation—cont'd

Complication	Cause	Signs/symptoms	Intervention
Starvation	Lack of nutrient intake	Electrolyte imbalance Muscle wasting/lethargy Negative nitrogen balance Weight loss	Feeding tube placement Check bowel sounds Initiate gastric feeding Watch daily calorie count Hyperalimentation if GI tract unavailable or not tolerating feedings
Constipation	Lack of motility and tone due to decreased mobility and increased pressure applied to abdomen during mechanical ventilation	Absence of bowel movement Diarrhea	Monitor bowel function Place on appropriate medication regimen
Other complications			
Positive water balance	Increased secretion of antidiuretic hormone Increased H_2O intake through respiratory tract due to humidification of delivered air	Increased A-a O_2 difference Increased body weight Electrolyte imbalance Decreased urine output Pulmonary edema Peripheral edema	Strict I&O Daily weights Use of diuretic therapy Swan-Ganz catheter monitoring
Infection (pulmonary, renal, systemic)	Multiple invasive procedures Increased susceptibility due to environment Decreased resistance to infection (compromised host) Antibiotic therapy with subsequent superinfection Steroid therapy	Increased body temperature Diaphoresis Tachycardia Hypertension/hypotension Increased cardiac output	Meticulous handwashing by all personnel Sputum culture and sensitivity daily Provide for safe environment: 1. Aseptic technique for all invasive procedures, i.e., insertion of IV lines, suctioning, dressing changes 2. Individual respiratory equipment 3. Change vent tubing daily 4. Access to clean and dirty utility rooms 5. Isolate patient if necessary

Continued.

Table 4-14 Complications of mechanical ventilation—cont'd

Complication	Cause	Signs/symptoms	Intervention
Infection—cont'd			Aggressive chest physiotherapy for adequate removal of secretions
			Closed urinary drainage systems with meticulous catheter care every 8 hr
			Change IV tubing and transducer lines daily
			Culture and sensitivity of any draining wound
			Take blood culture for temperature spike >101° F
Failure to wean	Decreased muscle strength	Retention CO_2	Provide psychologic support
	Acid-base imbalance	Decreased Pao_2 and increased A-a O_2 difference	Involve patient and explain procedure of weaning (as age-appropriate)
	Drug induced respiratory depression	Hematocrit less than 30%	Prepare for wean as soon as patient is intubated
	Unstable arrhythmias	Inadequate pulmonary mechanics: V_T, VC, IF	Correct anemia
	Anemia	Increased agitation/anxiety	Treat arrhythmias
	Sleep deprivation	Tachycardia, hypertension	Allow for rest periods, wean during day hours, medicate for pain
	Discoordinated breathing	Bradycardia, hypotension	Use intermittent mandatory ventilation method of weaning
	Fear		Increase nutrition
	Pain		
Psychologic trauma	Fear of death/illness	Fear and apprehension communicated by patient, i.e., written notes, facial expression, lip talking	Talk to, *not at* patient
	Lack of ability to communicate verbally		Involve patient
	Threat to self-image and dignity	Communication by family and significant others of the patient's life style, fears, concerns	Explain procedures, introduce health team
	Total dependency on machine and strangers		Provide safe environment, i.e., side rails, equipment alarms
	Decreased access to family members or close support systems		Provide a humane environment

Table 4-14 Complications of mechanical ventilation—cont'd

Complication	Cause	Signs/symptoms	Intervention
Psychologic trauma—cont'd	ICU environment Lack of time sequence Lack of privacy Sleep deprivation Multiple invasive procedures Drug therapy	Stress response: hypertension, tachycardia, diaphoresis, agitation	Provide adequate pain and/or sedation medication Provide primary nurse and psychiatric and/or social work consult

■ **RESPIRATORY PHYSICAL THERAPY TECHNIQUES**
■ **Chest physiotherapy**

An integral part of treatment of both acute and chronic respiratory disorders is administration of chest physical therapy to improve pulmonary hygiene and to maintain normal airway function. These techniques promote deep breathing, effective coughing, and removal of airway secretions. It may be necessary to administer oxygen during the treatment.

Chest physiotherapy requires the use of a series of four techniques: positioning of the patient, percussion, vibration, and coughing by the patient. These maneuvers can be performed on most critically ill patients as long as the patient's tolerance to physical therapy is monitored carefully throughout the procedure. Absolute contraindications to chest physiotherapy include the presence of displaced or fractured ribs, hemoptysis, or pulmonary hemorrhage. The performance of chest physiotherapy should be tailored to each patient. Some patients require treatment every 2 hours, while some do not need treatment more than a few times a day. Some patients can tolerate placement in a Trendelenburg's position, while some will not. Some patients will be able to tolerate therapy on only one side at a time.

Physiotherapy itself requires time and patience on the part of the nurse or therapist. The procedure should be explained to the child and parent. It should be emphasized to both the child and parent that the nurse is not "hitting" the child as percussion is performed. Infants can be positioned in the nurse's lap or in the crib. Older children usually receive the treatment in bed.

Postural drainage utilizes gravity to promote drainage of the tracheobronchial tree. If the patient is positioned so that each major bronchus drains downward, mucus collected in the bronchus is forced by gravity toward the trachea, where it can be expelled by cough or removed by suction. For example, drainage of the bases of the lungs is facilitated by placement of the child in a Trendelenburg's position, while drainage of the apical segment of the upper lobe of either lung is best facilitated with the child in a sitting position (Figs. 4-7 and 4-8). The use of any of these positions may have to be modified in unstable patients. For example, the head-down position would be inappropriate for the child with increased intracranial pressure or the child with significant respiratory distress or severe abdominal distention. Use of the side-lying, prone, or Trendelenburg's positions may need to be modified depending on patient condition and tolerance, and the time spent in these positions will also have to be adjusted according to patient needs.

During postural drainage, *percussion or clapping* is performed over the draining bronchopulmonary segment for 1 to 2 minutes. Percussion is best performed with a cupped hand or a soft mask that has been removed from a resuscitation bag. If a mask is used, tape should be placed over the connection port to create a seal within the mask. The air pocket under the hand or mask cushions the blow of the percussion and is transmitted inward to the chest wall. Percussion is not performed over bony prominences or the abdomen, and treatment is best performed if there is a light layer of clothing over the child's chest to prevent stinging as the percussion is performed. For an

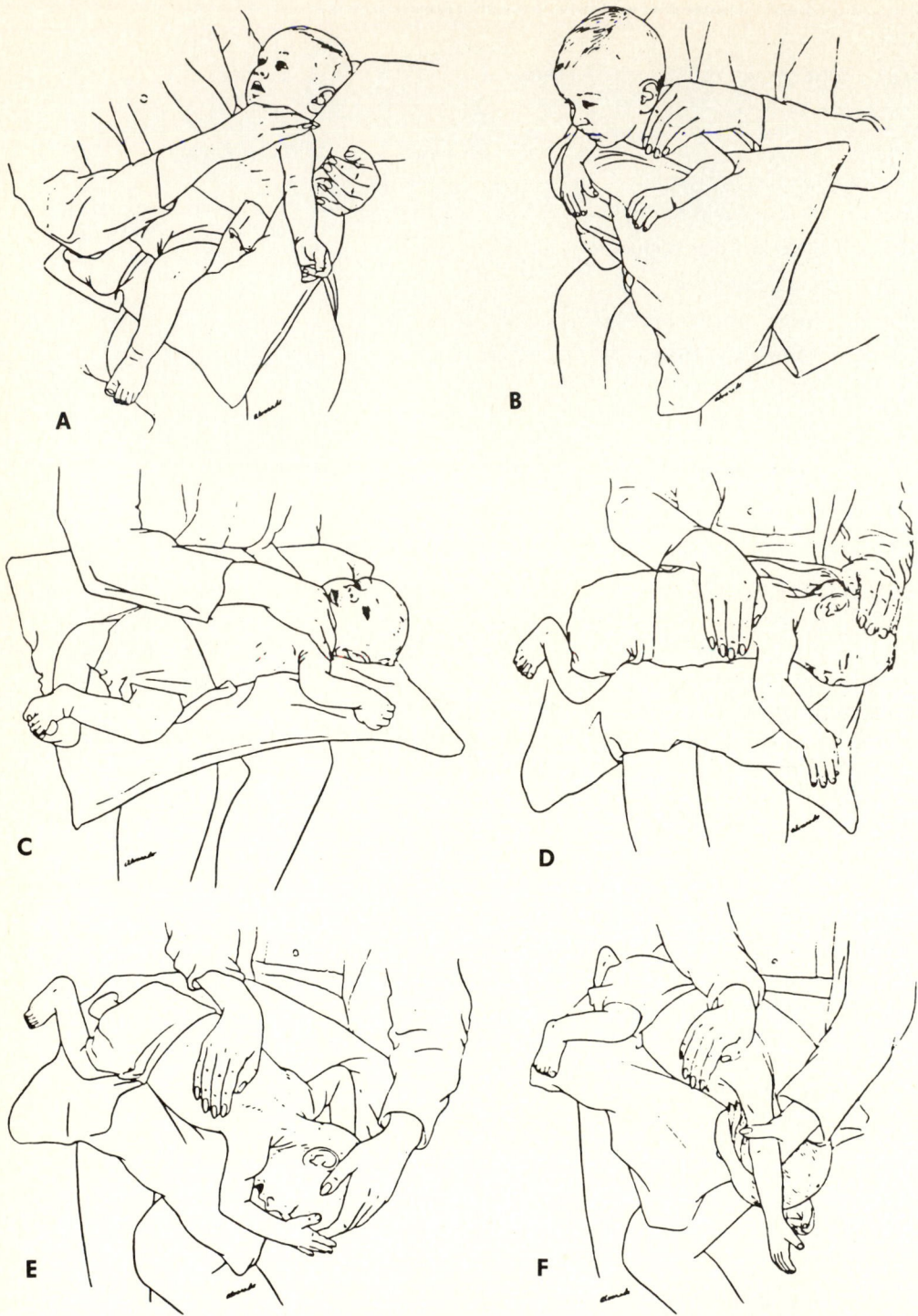

A

B

C

D

E

F

Fig. 4-7 Bronchial drainage positions for the major segments of all lobes in an infant. The procedure is most easily carried out in the therapist's lap. The therapist's hand on the chest indicates the area to be "cupped" or vibrated. **A,** Apical segment of the left upper lobe. **B,** Posterior segment of the left upper lobe. **C,** Anterior segment of the left upper lobe. **D,** Superior segment of the right lower lobe. **E,** Posterior segment of the right lower lobe. **F,** Lateral segment of the right lower lobe.

From Waring, W.: Diagnostic and therapeutic procedures. In Kendig, E., editor: Disorders of the respiratory tract in children, ed. 4, Philadelphia, 1983, W.B. Saunders Co.

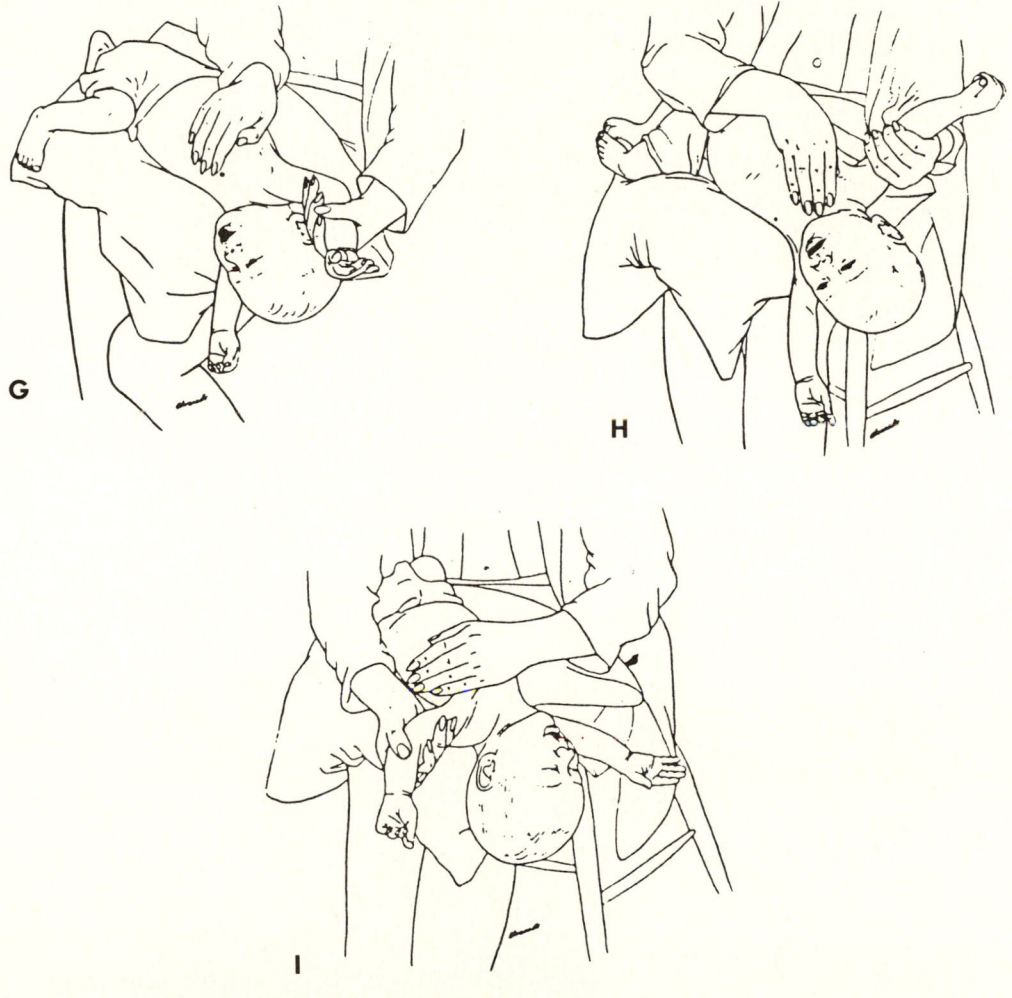

Fig. 4-7, cont'd   G, Anterior basal segment of the
lower lobe. **H,** Right middle lobe. **I,** Lingular
segments of the left upper lobe.

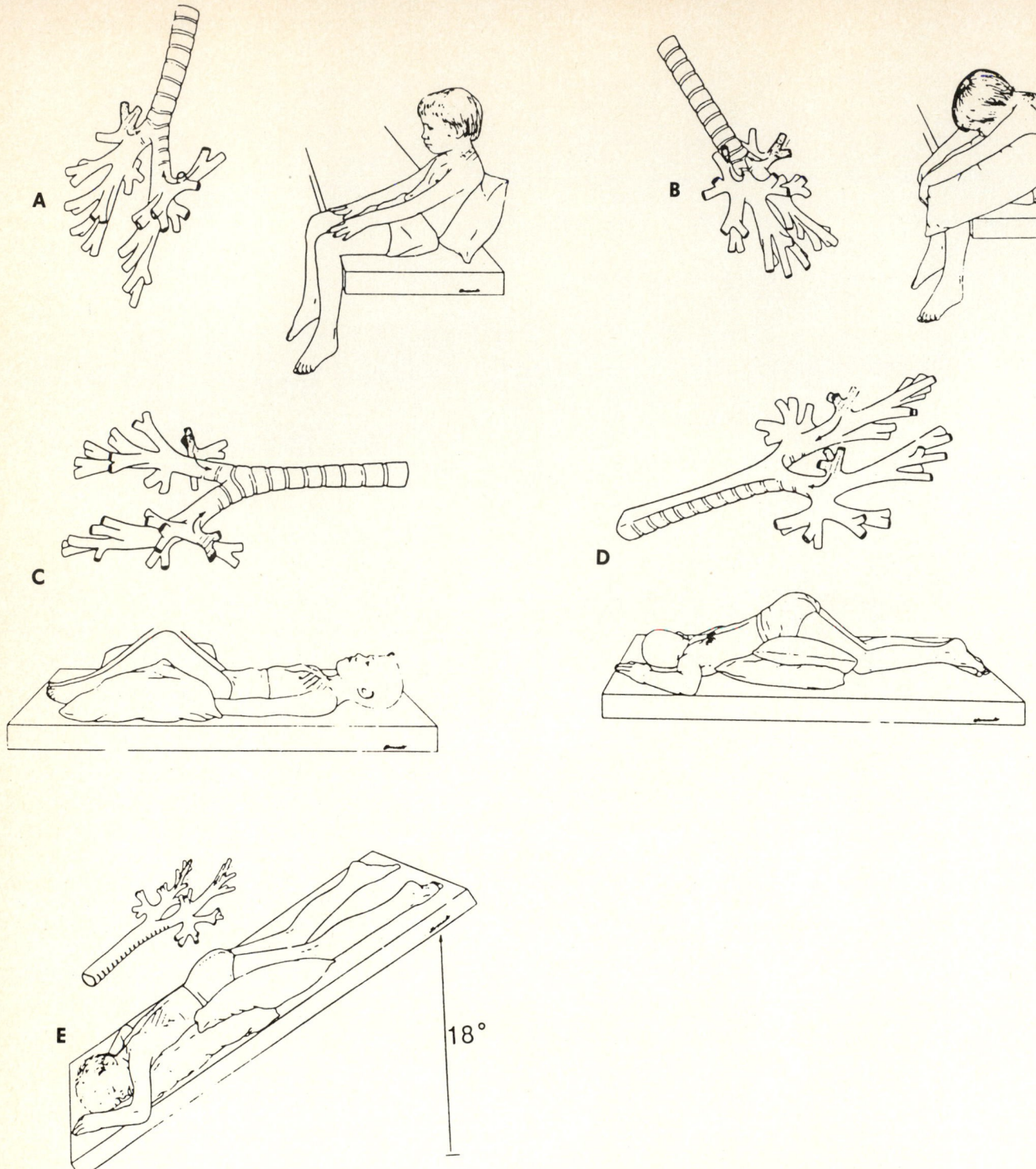

Fig. 4-8 Bronchial drainage positions for the major segments of all lobes on a child. In each position a model of the tracheobronchial tree is projected beside the child in order to show the segmental bronchus being drained (stippled) and the flow of secretions out of the segmental bronchus (arrow). The drainage platform is padded but firm, and pillows are liberally used to maintain each position with comfort. The platform is horizontal unless otherwise noted. A stippled area on the child's chest indicates the area to be "cupped" or vibrated by the therapist. **A,** Apical segment of the right upper lobe and apical subsegment of apical-posterior segment of left upper lobe. Drainage moves secretions into main bronchi from which they can be more easily expelled *(curved arrows)*. **B,** Posterior segment of right upper lobe and posterior subsegment of apical-posterior segment of left upper lobe. Drainage moves secretions into main bronchi from which they can be more easily expelled *(curved arrows)*. **C,** Anterior segments of both upper lobes. The child should be rotated slightly away from the side being drained. **D,** Superior segments of both lower lobes. Although the platform is flat, pillows are used to raise the buttocks moderately. **E,** Posterior basal segments of both lower lobes. The platform is tilted as shown.

Waring, W.: Diagnostic and therapeutic procedures. In Kendig, E.L.: Disorders of the respiratory tract in children, ed. 4, Philadelphia, 1983, W.B. Saunders Co.

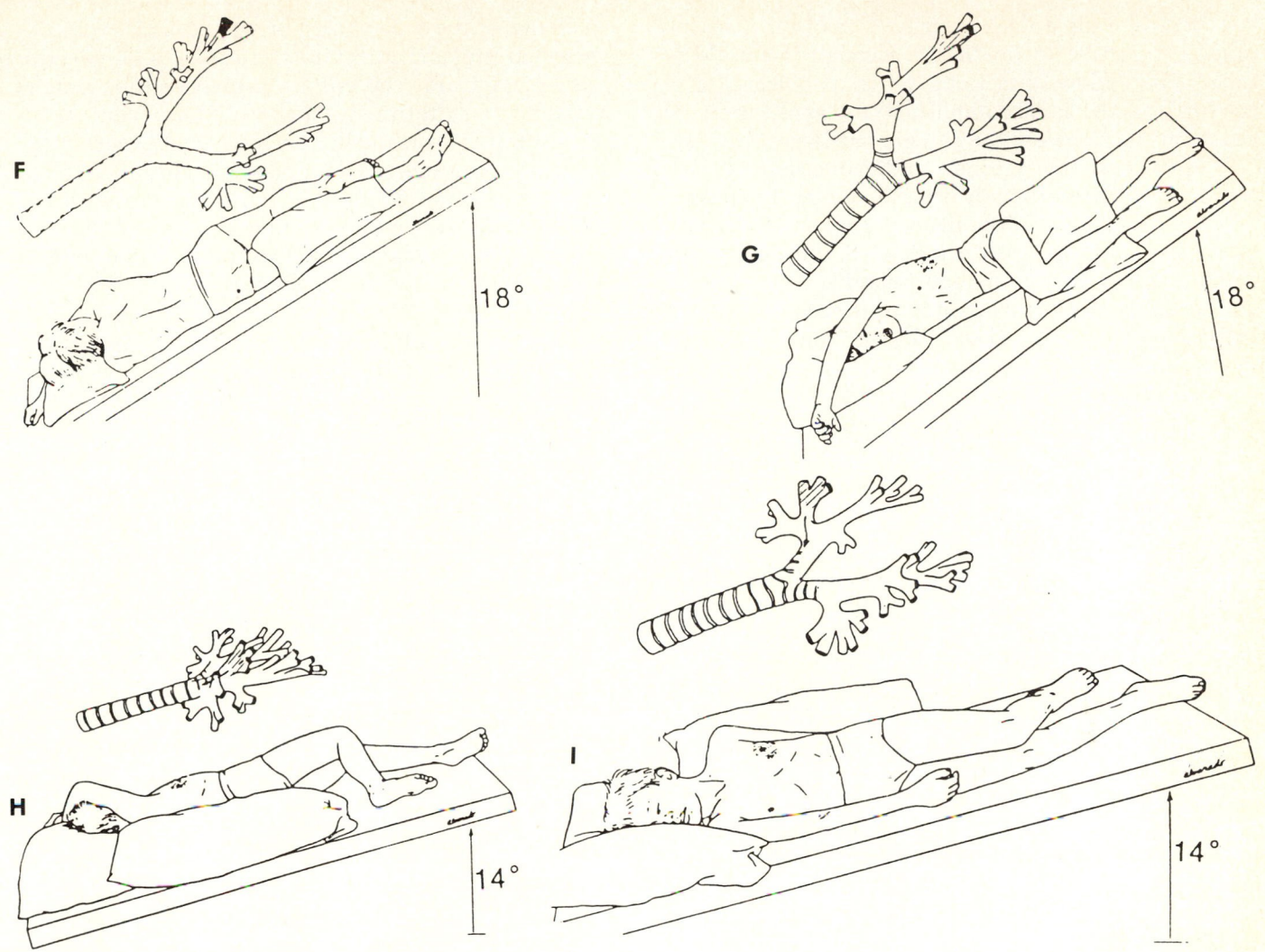

Fig. 4-8, cont'd **F,** Lateral basal segment of the
right lower lobe. The platform is tilted as shown.
Drainage of the lateral basal segment of the left
lower lobe would be accomplished by a mirror
image of this position (right side down). **G,** Anterior
basal segment of the left lower lobe. The platform is
tilted as shown. **H,** Right middle lobe. The platform
is tilted as shown. **I,** Lingular segments (superior
and inferior) of left upper lobe (homologue of right
middle lobe).

infant it may be necessary to use only two or three
fingers to provide the percussion.

The third component of chest physiotherapy is
vibration. The purpose of vibration is to help move
secretions further toward the trachea. Vibration is
best achieved by applying a shaking motion to the
draining bronchopulmonary segment immediately
after percussion, while the patient is exhaling. An
electric toothbrush with foam wrapped around the
bristles may also be used for vibration in small neo-

nates. If the patient is old enough to follow directions,
he should be asked to exhale through pursed lips with
the glottis partially closed; this will help keep the
airways open and will mimic the CPAP technique.

Coughing should always follow percussion and
vibration and is most effective if the child is sitting
up so that diaphragmatic excursion is maximal. Before the child begins to cough, the nurse should demonstrate appropriate coughing technique; the child
should take several deep breaths and then follow the

last breath with a deep cough. A tracheal "tickle" may be effective in producing a cough if a child is unable to follow directions or to cooperate; this tracheal tickle is accomplished by application of gentle pressure below the thyroid cartilage.

If the child has recently undergone thoracic surgery, chest physiotherapy should not be performed directly over the incision; instead, the incisional area should be splinted with a pillow. If the child is in pain, analgesics should be administered 1 hour before the chest physiotherapy treatment to reduce pain and increase cooperation. This will make the physiotherapy treatment most effective.

Chest physiotherapy should not be scheduled any sooner than 1 hour before feedings and should never be performed immediately after meals, since aspiration may occur. If the child is receiving continuous nasogastric feedings by pump, the feedings should be discontinued during therapy, and to prevent aspiration, the Trendelenburg's position should be avoided. The child with a history of gastric reflux will require close monitoring throughout the chest physiotherapy and may require more time between feedings and chest physiotherapy treatments.

■ Incentive spirometry

Incentive spirometry is a relatively new technique intended to augment chest physiotherapy. It is used both to treat and to prevent atelectasis. A device is used that allows the child to inspire maximally and thus optimize lung inflation. This device can only be used in the older, cooperative child who will enjoy the challenge of the incentive. The devices have been designed to provide entertainment as well as positive reinforcement for the child. A small bedside unit is available that illuminates a clown's nose when a preset inspiratory volume has been reached. Another device lifts a colored ball in a plastic column when appropriate inspiratory flow is achieved, and with another, colored water may be moved from one bottle to another during maximum expiration. Each device has a method of increasing the flow required to reach the goal.

Before incentive spirometry is attempted, the technique is first carefully explained to the child and parents (if present). If surgery is planned, the device should be demonstrated to the child before the operation. The initial inspiratory goal should be approximately twice the child's measured tidal volume if the child is able to tolerate this. In an upright position the child is instructed to perform five or six maneuvers every 1 or 2 hours, and the performance should be evaluated at least once daily. The therapy should not be allowed to exhaust or frustrate the child. Often a parent is best able to encourage the child and assist in the treatment.

Less mechanical forms of incentive spirometry include blowing bubbles or blowing paper cups across the bedside table. While these are less scientific methods of encouraging deep breathing, they are often very successful and entertaining for the child.

Table 4-15 provides a nursing care plan that summarizes the care of the child requiring mechanical ventilatory support.

Text continued on p. 305.

Table 4-15 Nursing care of the child requiring mechanical ventilatory support

Nursing diagnosis	Expected outcomes	Nursing actions
A. Possible airway obstruction related to 1. Thick secretions 2. Inappropriate position of ET tube 3. Bronchospasm 4. Accidental extubation	1. Artificial airway will remain in appropriate position and will remain patent	1. Monitor for evidence of airway obstruction a. Chest retractions b. Stridor c. Nasal flaring d. Decreased chest expansion and aeration e. Cyanosis (pallor if patient is anemic or an infant) f. Excessive respiratory secretions

Table 4-15 Nursing care of the child requiring mechanical ventilatory support—cont'd

Nursing diagnosis	Expected outcomes	Nursing actions
A. Possible airway obstruction—cont'd		• If the aforementioned occur, immediately ventilate with a hand resuscitation bag before and after suctioning the airway. If no improvement, call a physician immediately, and begin emergency resuscitation measures, as needed 2. Keep suction, resuscitator bag, oxygen, and appropriate sizes of ET tubes at the bedside (tube will need to be cut to appropriate length for infant; allow extra length to accommodate the adapter) 3. Ensure adequate humidity in the environment, and maintain general state of hydration 4. Keep child's head in straight alignment to avoid tube dislodgment; prevent neck flexion or hyperextension 5. Provide chest physiotherapy with postural drainage every 2-4 hr as tolerated 6. Instill small amounts of sterile normal saline into the artificial airway before suctioning when secretions are thick or crusting 7. If necessary, administer sedation, muscle relaxants, or paralyzing agents to ensure adequate ventilatory control of child
B. Possible restlessness because of 1. Hypoxia 2. Hypercapnia 3. Lack of sleep 4. Inability to "breathe" with ventilator	1. Adequate ventilation as measured by a. Satisfactory arterial blood gas levels b. Pink lips and mucous membranes c. Equal and adequate lung aeration d. Ability to "breathe" with ventilator	1. Monitor for signs of hypoxemia a. Increased heart rate b. Increased respiratory rate (cannot be monitored while maintained on "control" mode of ventilation) c. Peripheral vasoconstriction d. Decreased arterial P_{O_2}, pH (respiratory center is stimulated so hypocapnia may occur initially) e. Cyanosis or pallor 2. Monitor for signs of increased respiratory distress a. Signs noted above b. Decreased lung aeration c. Increased pulmonary congestion d. Arterial oxygen desaturation or hypercapnia

Continued.

Table 4-15 Nursing care of the child requiring mechanical ventilatory support—cont'd

Nursing diagnosis	Expected outcomes	Nursing actions
B. Possible restlessness—cont'd		3. ET tube may be obstructed; hand ventilate and suction patient immediately • If much resistance is felt during manual ventilation and if chest expansion and breath sounds are inadequate bilaterally, the tube is probably blocked and should be removed and the child ventilated by mask until reintubation can be accomplished. A physician should be notified 4. Monitor for signs of pneumothorax a. If the tube is patent but the child is progressively more distressed, the physician should be notified immediately. Hand ventilation should be attempted and a chest radiograph obtained (per unit policy or physician order) b. Chest tube insertion equipment should be available in the room for placement of chest tube and decompression of the pneumothorax NOTE: The pneumothorax can appear suddenly and without warning and can cause severe cardiopulmonary compromise. Action must be taken immediately to relieve the pneumothorax Breath sounds in young infants are usually easily transmitted through the thin chest wall; thus adequate breath sounds may be heard bilaterally even in the presence of a pneumothorax. 5. Monitor ventilator settings at least q hr; check the following (as applicable to the particular machine in use): a. Inspiratory pressure b. Respiratory rate c. Tidal volume d. FIO_2 e. Level of PEEP/CPAP 6. Maintain mechanical ventilation as ordered 7. Monitor blood gas levels and make ventilatory changes as ordered (hypercapnia, hypoxemia, and acidosis indicate increased respiratory failure)

Table 4-15 Nursing care of the child requiring mechanical ventilatory support—cont'd

Nursing diagnosis	Expected outcomes	Nursing actions
B. Possible restless-ness—cont'd		8. Wean the patient from the ventilator in an organized manner: a. Child should be able to generate a satisfactory vital capacity before weaning, and blood gases should be in a near-normal range. The disease process or reason for initial ventilation should be resolving b. Initially, inspiratory or PEEP pressures are decreased. If the child tolerates this, then either the rate or V_T is decreased c. Monitor child clinically for signs of hypoxemia d. Monitor arterial blood gases • Arterial hypocapnia during weaning may indicate the child is hyperventilating; arterial hypercapnia or falling Pa_{O_2} indicates respiratory insufficiency and intolerance of weaning e. Monitor $A\text{-}a_{O_2}$ difference; increased gradient suggests increased intrapulmonary shunting and decreased alveolar ventilation 9. Promote an environment conductive to sleep a. Change position of child every 1-2 hr b. Allow for planned periods of sleep during which no invasive procedures are performed c. Decrease overhead lighting and environmental noise d. Provide psychologic support
C. Potential hypotension caused by 1. Decreased venous return and decreased cardiac output resulting from positive pressure ventilation 2. Hypoxemia	1. Cardiac output will remain stable as measured by a. Effective cardiac rhythm b. Adequate blood pressure c. Pink mucous membranes and nailbeds d. Adequate urine output (1 ml/kg/hr) e. Adequate cerebral perfusion f. Warm extremities with strong peripheral pulses	1. Monitor for evidence of decreased cardiac output • Critical blood pressure in children: systolic less than 80-90 mm Hg; critical blood pressure in infants: systolic less than 60-80 mm Hg (consider patients normal range)

Continued.

Table 4-15 Nursing care of the child requiring mechanical ventilatory support—cont'd

Nursing diagnosis	Expected outcomes	Nursing actions
C. Potential hypotension—cont'd		2. Tachycardia 3. Arrhythmias (document any abnormalities in rhythm; note blood pressure during the arrhythmia and any electrolyte imbalances) 4. Pallor or cyanosis 5. Decreased peripheral perfusion (cold clammy extremities, decreased peripheral pulses, slow capillary refill) 6. Decreased urine output with specific gravity >1.015

D. Possible atelectasis caused by
  1. Monotonous ventilatory pattern
  2. Decreased cough
  3. Increased secretions
  4. Decreased mobility
  5. Inappropriate mechanical ventilation with inadequate PEEP
	1. Aeration of the lungs will remain normal and chest radiograph will show no signs of atelectasis	1. Monitor for signs of hypoxemia and increased respiratory distress (see nursing diagnosis *B*)
		2. Monitor chest radiograph and arterial blood gases
		3. Hand ventilate with bag before and after each suctioning procedure
		4. Change body position q 1-2 hr
		5. Provide chest physiotherapy q 2-4 hr
		6. Check level of PEEP/CPAP (inadequate levels may be present)

E. Possible blood gas abnormalities caused by
  1. Inappropriate support
	1. Pa_{CO_2} level will remain within range of 35-45 mm Hg
	2. Pa_{O_2} will remain 80-100 mm Hg (60-80 mm Hg in neonates)
	3. Arterial pH will remain 7.35-7.45
		1. Monitor for signs of hypoxemia or change in level of consciousness (lethargy)
		2. Obtain arterial sample for analysis of blood gases if aforementioned occurs; check P_{CO_2} and P_{O_2} levels
		3. Check ventilator settings:
		  a. Is V_T at appropriate level (about 10 ml/kg body weight)?
		  b. Is rate appropriate for level of consciousness?
		  c. Is ventilator tubing of appropriate size? (a small size tubing will increase resistance in the system; large compliant tubing may increase volume lost within the ventilator circuit)
		  d. Is flow rate (if applicable) at appropriate level?
		4. Check chest radiograph for increase in disease process
		5. Monitor activity level (increased restlessness may accompany hyperventilation)
		6. Note signs of carpopedal spasm. If so, obtain arterial blood gases and notify physician

Table 4-15 Nursing care of the child requiring mechanical ventilatory support—cont'd

Nursing diagnosis	Expected outcomes	Nursing actions
F. Possible infection of respiratory tract caused by 1. Repeated traumatic suctioning 2. Underlying pulmonary disease 3. Inadequate handwashing or compromise of sterile suctioning technique by nursing or medical staff 4. Compromised nutritional status	1. Absence of local signs of infection a. Fever (or hypothermia in the infant) b. Leukocytosis c. Redness, heat, or discharge at the wound site (tracheostomy site or site of other wounds) d. Copious, cloudy, foul-smelling secretions from respiratory tract	1. Monitor for evidence of pulmonary infection a. Increased pulmonary congestion as evidenced on auscultation or chest radiograph b. Increased respiratory distress c. Change in characteristics of sputum: odor, presence of purulent material, color, thickness; obtain a specimen for culture and sensitivity and Gram's stain 2. Monitor for tracheostomy or other wound infection a. Erythema at wound edges b. Wound drainage c. Odor 3. Maintain meticulous handwashing techniques 4. Maintain aseptic technique with suctioning procedures
G. Possible patient/family anxiety related to 1. Inability to verbally communicate 2. Discomfort 3. Disease process and prognosis 4. Mechanical ventilation	1. Child and family anxiety will remain at manageable levels	1. Provide a means of communication for child (e.g., sign language, paper and pen) 2. Explain all procedures 3. Provide pain and sedation medications as necessary 4. Provide a safe environment (e.g., side rails, equipment alarms on) 5. Involve family in the child's care when appropriate 6. Make appropriate referrals to social services/chaplain
H. Possible trauma to airway caused by 1. Pressure of ET or tracheostomy tube on tracheal wall 2. Frequent ET tube movement (inadequate securing of tube)	1. ET or tracheostomy tube will remain stable, and pressure on the tracheal wall will be prevented	1. Carefully reposition the patient every 1-2 hr 2. Use a swivel adapter between the ET tube and ventilator tubing to decrease movement of the tube 3. Secure ET tube firmly a. Before tape application, apply tincture of benzoin to skin to ensure adhesion of the tape. Apply a double layer of tape from behind the head (do not apply tape directly to hair in back) or from both cheeks b. Attach each piece of tape in front around the ET tube. To avoid skin irritation, use a slightly different area on the face each time the tube is retaped

Continued.

Table 4-15 **Nursing care of the child requiring mechanical ventilatory support—cont'd**

Nursing diagnosis	Expected outcomes	Nursing actions
H. Possible trauma to airway—cont'd		c. Change tape when necessary. Taping of the tube should be performed with two nurses present—one to stabilize the tube throughout the procedure and one to do the taping 4. Monitor position of the tube q hr. The tape may begin to loosen and release the tube. Avoid multiple layering of tape around the tube.
I. Probable nutritional compromise related to 1. Prolonged nasotracheal intubation 2. Bed rest 3. Stress	1. Adequate nutritional status as measured by a. Appropriate weight gain b. Moist mucous membranes c. Good skin turgor d. Normal Hb	1. Calculate child's caloric needs daily, and if child is unable to take oral feedings, ensure caloric intake via gavage feedings or parenteral alimentation 2. Monitor urine and blood glucose levels to determine presence of hypoglycemia 3. Weigh child daily and notify physician of any significant weight gain or loss a. >200 g/24 hr in children b. >50 g/24 hr in infants 4. Monitor intake and urine and stool output. Calculate daily fluid and caloric requirements. Notify physician if the child is not receiving the minimal requirements 5. Monitor for signs of dehydration 6. Rotate child's position in bed q 1-2 hr
J. Possible fluid overload caused by: 1. Increased levels of ADH 2. Water taken into the respiratory system via the ventilator 3. Extremely high PEEP levels	1. Intake and output and serum-electrolyte and concentrations will remain in appropriate balance, and the child will not demonstrate excessive weight because of fluid retention	1. Calculate child's daily fluid requirements. Notify physician if fluid requirements are not being met 2. Monitor urine output. Adequate output should be 1 ml/kg/hr in children if fluid intake is adequate 3. Obtain daily weights (see nutritional problem for significant weight gains and losses) 4. Assess electrolyte levels, specifically Na, K, and Cl levels 5. Monitor specific gravity of urine. An increased loss of sodium in the urine and decreased serum sodium concentration, accompanied by a decreased urine volume with high urine specific gravity (>1.015) may indicate inappropriate ADH secretion (Chapter 7) 6. Monitor levels of PEEP delivered via the ventilator 7. Prevent accumulation of fluid in the ventilator tubing, empty tubing prn to minimize fluid that may reach child's airway; adjust inspired airway temperature as needed

■ Specific Diseases

■ CROUP
■ Etiology

Croup is a general term which refers to the clinical syndrome of laryngitis and laryngotracheobronchitis (LTB). The vocal cords, subglottic tissue, trachea, bronchi, and bronchioles can be involved. Croup may be infectious or noninfectious. The infectious croup can be either viral or bacterial in origin. Viral croup (85% of reported cases) occurs mostly in children between the ages of 3 months and 4 years. Bacterial croup occurs in children aged 2 to 7 years. Noninfectious croup may result from asthma or allergic reactions, or it may follow ET intubation or foreign body aspiration. There often appears to be a positive family history for croup.

■ Pathophysiology

Once mechanical irritation or infection of the laryngeal area develops, the tissues become inflammed and edematous. Secretions from these tissues increase, and partial obstruction of the airway results. Children under 2 years of age are especially susceptible to the development of partial airway obstruction with croup because the glottic opening is small and the mucous membrane of the laryngeal airway is highly vascular and apt to become rapidly edematous in response to inflammation.

■ Clinical signs and symptoms

The child who develops croup may have a history of rhinitis, fever, malaise, and anorexia for 2 to 3 days before the development of specific respiratory signs. The onset of croup is heralded by the development of a hoarse, barking cough. The child, appearing restless and anxious, may demonstrate symptoms ranging from inspiratory stridor to inflammation and obstruction of the laryngeal area. Since the airway obstruction increases resistance to airflow, chest retractions, a sign of increased respiratory effort, will be present. On auscultation, diminished breath sounds can be heard, and rales and rhonchi may also be noted. As the child's condition deteriorates, intermittent cyanosis may be observed during coughing. Hypercapnia, hypoxemia, and tachycardia may develop with progressive airway obstruction and respiratory acidosis may occur.[36]

The differential diagnosis of croup includes epiglottitis and foreign body aspiration. The most important diagnostic test for croup is a lateral radiograph of the neck, which can be expected to show a normal epiglottis and an area of density below the larynx caused by swelling of the tracheal soft tissues. Viral cultures may be positive for parainfluenza and adenovirus.

Direct examination of the oropharynx should be performed only by a skilled physician (see the discussion of epiglottitis in the next section).

■ Medical treatment and nursing interventions

With croup the most important aspect of nursing care is minimization of the child's anxiety and maximization of the child's rest. The patient should be kept as quiet and comfortable as possible. Painful procedures should not be performed until the diagnosis is confirmed and more severe causes of upper airway obstruction (such as epiglottitis) are excluded.

Respiratory distress can be minimized by providing a comfortable environment, which is free from stress and rich in humidity. The nurse should monitor the child's respiratory rate, depth, and pattern and should note the presence of retractions and nasal flaring. Observations should be made for the development of hoarseness, stridor, and cough. The child's heart rate and rhythm are important to monitor; as hypoxia increases, tachycardia will be evident and may be accompanied by arrhythmias such as bradycardia or a premature ventricular contraction. Blood samples for blood gas analysis may be obtained if the child's condition warrants. Equipment for intubation and possible tracheostomy should be readily available.

The nurse should monitor the child's body temperature and administer antipyretics for fever above 38.5° C. If respiratory distress is severe, the child should receive nothing by mouth to avoid the possibility of aspiration. Intravenous fluids should be administered if oral intake is impossible or if dehydration is present. The urine specific gravity is a good indicator of the child's level of hydration, so it should be monitored and a physician should be notified if urine specific gravity above 1.030 is measured (see Chapter 7).

Chest physiotherapy is usually avoided during the acute phase of croup because the child's respiratory distress may increase when he is placed flat in bed; however, chest physiotherapy may be instituted once the child shows signs of improvement.

The inhalation of racemic epinephrine may reduce airway edema, and it has been recommended for use in children with croup; sometimes hourly treatments are necessary (see Appendix B for dosages and effects). If the child receives racemic epinephrine treatments, the nurse must monitor for tachycardia or other signs of intolerance of the treatment. Although antibiotics are usually not prescribed, they may be administered if a bacterial cause of the croup is suspected. Corticosteroids are also advocated for these patients, although there is little clinical or research data to support their use.

Croup is usually a self-limited disease, but occasionally intubation is necessary either because of the development of airway obstruction or respiratory muscle fatigue.

■ EPIGLOTTITIS
■ Etiology

Epiglottitis is a medical emergency characterized by inflammation and swelling of the epiglottis, false cords, and aryepiglottic folds. The bacterial agent most responsible is *Haemophilus influenzae* B. The disorder occurs most commonly in children 3 to 7 years of age, with the peak at ages 3 to 4.

■ Pathophysiology

The epiglottis is a long, narrow structure that closes off the glottis during swallowing. Edema of this area can completely occlude the airway in a matter of minutes or hours. Complete occlusion of the airway can occur in the child with epiglottitis immediately after the gag reflex has been stimulated by examination of the upper airway or by suctioning.[36]

■ Clinical signs and symptoms

Epiglottitis is frequently associated with bacteremia. Signs of distress are usually sudden in onset and accompanied by high fever. The child may develop symptoms over a period of a few hours, and the fever may be above 39° C. The child often has a muffled voice, but rarely is the disorder accompanied by the characteristic "barking" cough of croup. The child may begin to complain of a sore throat. As the epiglottis increases in size, the child exhibits signs of airway obstruction. These signs include a characteristic inspiratory stridor, chest retractions (particularly in the sternal notch area), tachycardia, and decreased breath sounds. The child may appear anxious. Dysphagia and drooling occur if the child is unable or afraid to swallow. Late signs of hypoxia include listlessness, cyanosis, and cardiac arrhythmias, including bradycardia and PVCs[36] (see the earlier discussion in this chapter on airway obstruction).

The most important test for diagnosis of epiglottitis is the lateral radiograph of the neck, which shows the epiglottis as a large, rounded, soft tissue mass below the base of the tongue. With well-penetrated films, the enlarged epiglottis can be seen ob-

structing the upper airway (see Fig. 5-18). Examination of the upper airway reveals a cherry-red and swollen epiglottis. *It is extremely important that inspection or manipulation of the upper airway be performed only if a person skilled in intubation is present at the bedside* and if all equipment necessary for an urgent intubation is readily available. The visualization should take place quickly and with the least amount of manipulation of the patient. Any induction of gagging (such as occurs when the tongue blade is forced down the child's throat or when suctioning is performed) may induce laryngospasm or cause increased swelling of the area and result in acute airway obstruction. Occasionally, intubation is not possible once laryngospasm has occurred, and placement of a tracheostomy may be required.

■ Medical treatment and nursing interventions

Children who are suspected of having epiglottitis should be carefully monitored at all times. The nurse should expect that the child will be anxious and restless. The most important nursing intervention is keeping the child quiet and undisturbed; the nurse must minimize the child's anxiety and episodes of crying. This usually means that the patient is most comfortable in the parent's arms. Older children with severe epiglottis swelling may prefer to sit upright, with the hands out in front of the trunk and the neck thrust out. They should not be forced into the supine position, since this may compromise diaphragmatic excursion and air movement.

Before intubation, care of these children involves careful monitoring of respiratory status, including assessment of the rate and depth of respiration and the presence of retractions, nasal flaring, and stridor. Supportive care should be provided to minimize the child's energy expenditure and to maximize respiratory efficiency. The child should be placed in a humidified oxygen-enriched environment with the head of the bed elevated at all times. Antibiotics are started immediately. Ampicillin remains the drug of choice, but with increased resistance to ampicillin, chloramphenicol or moxalactam may be used (see Appendix B for drug dosages and side effects).

Intubation and tracheostomy equipment (including laryngoscope blades with working bulbs, tube, lidocaine [Xylocaine] jelly, and tracheostomy tray) of the proper size should be placed at the bedside. If the lateral neck radiograph suggests epiglottitis and if direct visualization confirms it, immediate ET intubation is performed. The ET tube inserted may be a size smaller than that normal for the child's age, since reduction in the child's airway size may result from swelling. Mechanical ventilation is or-

CHAPTER 4 *Pulmonary Disorders* ■ **307**

dinarily not necessary, and the ET tube can usually be removed within 48 to 72 hours.

Other important nursing interventions include provision of reassurance for the child and parents, assessment for possible respiratory complications such as ET-tube obstruction or accidental extubation, assessment of body temperature, and provision of adequate fluid and caloric intake. The child with severe respiratory distress should receive nothing by mouth, and intravenous fluids should be administered to ensure adequate hydration. Immediately after the child is extubated, he should receive nothing by mouth for at least 4 hours until the health team is sure that reintubation will not be necessary. Once the child has demonstrated tolerance of extubation, oral fluids may again be provided. Chest physiotherapy is usually not necessary for the child with epiglottitis.

■ FOREIGN BODY ASPIRATION
■ Etiology

Toddlers are particularly prone to aspiration of objects and food. The severity and timing of respiratory distress and the appropriate treatment depend on the type of object aspirated, the location of the object, and the degree of airway obstruction produced. Aspirated objects commonly lodge in the laryngotracheal area because it is narrow, but these objects can also pass into a main-stem bronchus or further down into a segmental bronchus. A small object such as a bead may produce no acute symptoms; aspiration of vegetable material (such as carrots and peanuts) may cause symptoms similar to those produced by croup, asthma, or lobar pneumonia.[5,28]

■ Pathophysiology

The history of aspiration often includes a report that the child has "swallowed" something. A sudden onset of coughing is often noted. Discovery of an open container holding small objects may lead the caretaker to bring the child to the hospital. However, many children who aspirate a foreign body have no history to suggest the diagnosis. Thus when an afebrile child has sudden respiratory distress, foreign body aspiration must be strongly considered.[5,28]

■ Clinical signs and symptoms

Immediate signs of aspiration include the sudden onset of coughing, choking, and gagging. The child's cough may be associated with hemoptysis, and aphonia would suggest that the obstruction is in the larynx. Later signs of airway obstruction include the development of hoarse, muffled voice, and further signs of respiratory distress are dyspnea, wheezing, chest retractions, and cyanosis.

The diagnostic test of choice includes an anteroposterior and lateral chest radiograph. Metallic objects will be visible on the chest radiograph; however, objects such as peanuts or plastics are usually not seen. *A negative chest radiograph does not exclude the possibility of foreign body.*[5]

If foreign body aspiration is suspected, a direct laryngoscopy or bronchoscopy should be performed to allow direct visualization of the airway. Removal of the foreign body can take place simultaneously.

■ Medical treatment and nursing interventions

Whenever the child is in danger of development of acute airway obstruction, the nurse's efforts focus on careful clinical assessment and relief of respiratory distress. A quiet environment should be provided for the child, and the parents should be present to minimize the child's anxieties. The child's vital signs and degree of respiratory distress must be watched carefully. Signs of deterioration in the child's clinical status include an increase in heart rate, an increase and then a decrease in respiratory rate, increased severity and distribution of chest retractions, deterioration in color, loss of ability to speak, and drooling. Emergency equipment for intubation should be kept close at hand.

The most effective intervention for acute aspiration of a foreign body is immediate removal of the object. Following removal, nursing care again requires strict monitoring of the child's heart rate and respiratory rate and effort. The child should be watched carefully for signs of upper airway obstruction that can occur as a result of edema formation at the site of the foreign body removal. If upper airway obstruction occurs, an increase in respiratory distress will be seen. After removal of the foreign body, chest physiotherapy may be helpful for several days, particularly if the object was lodged beyond the main-stem bronchus and signs of infection are present.

It would be most helpful if foreign body aspiration could be prevented through careful teaching of the parents of young toddlers. Whenever possible, parents should be instructed that young children should not be given beans, beads, small toys, or nuts to eat or play with.

■ DIAPHRAGMATIC HERNIA
■ Etiology

Diaphragmatic hernia is a congenital defect in the diaphragm, which results in a free communication between the thoracic and abdominal cavities.

Abdominal organs enter the chest in utero and may interfere with the growth and development of both lungs, even though the defect is unilateral. This condition is most often diagnosed immediately after birth, affecting approximately one in every 2000 to 3500 births. If untreated, approximately 75% of children with diaphragmatic hernia die within 1 month of age.[18] Most children develop severe respiratory distress, which requires surgical intervention during the first days of life.

■ Pathophysiology

The diaphragmatic hernia is on the left side in approximately 80% of all cases. The involved lung is small and hypoplastic, with decreased pulmonary vascularity and increased pulmonary vascular resistance. The mediastinal structures are shifted to the contralateral side of the chest in utero; therefore the heart is most commonly shifted into the right chest. As a result of pulmonary hypertension, there is right-to-left shunting of blood through the patent ductus arteriosus (see the discussion in Chapter 3 on patent ductus arteriosus). The contralateral lung is often partially compressed, and it may also be hypoplastic. Respiration is further compromised by distention of the stomach and intestines with swallowed air as a result of crying.

Once the diagnosis of diaphragmatic hernia is made, surgical intervention should take place immediately, since the neonate usually deteriorates quickly. The defect is generally closed primarily; however, if the defect is large, a synthetic patch may be necessary to close it.

■ Clinical signs and symptoms

The child with diaphragmatic hernia has a large barrel chest and a suspiciously flat abdomen. Tachypnea, with a respiratory rate exceeding 120 breaths per minute, is commonly seen. Other signs of respiratory distress include nasal flaring, severe chest retractions, cyanosis, absent breath sounds, and severe respiratory acidosis. The newborn may exhibit extreme respiratory distress when fed. Once the infant is intubated and mechanically ventilated, the nurse will note extreme resistance to hand ventilation, and the neonate will require high inspiratory pressures.

The diagnostic test of choice is the chest radiograph, which shows that air-filled loops of bowel are located in the chest. Blood gas analysis will demonstrate the presence of respiratory acidosis and hypoxemia.

An echocardiogram may be obtained to measure right ventricular systolic time intervals (STI), which may provide an indirect indication of the degree of the child's pulmonary hypertension.

■ Medical treatment and nursing interventions

It is extremely important that the neonate with diaphragmatic hernia receive excellent ventilatory support. The neonate is usually paralyzed with muscle relaxant and placed in a semi-Fowler's position to help alleviate pressure of the abdominal contents on the thorax. A nasogastric tube is used to decompress the stomach, and the child should receive nothing by mouth. The involved side of the chest may be placed in a dependent position to increase aeration of the uninvolved lung. It is usually necessary to insert one or more chest tubes during preoperative management, since pneumothoraxes may develop; no suction is applied to these tubes. The infant's arterial blood gases should be monitored frequently, and the serum glucose and serum calcium levels should be checked because stress may rapidly produce hypoglycemia and hypocalcemia in neonates. Since the neonate will receive nothing by mouth preoperatively or for many days postoperatively, long-term plans should be made to provide parenteral nutrition.

As soon as the diagnosis is established and the infant's respiratory status is reasonably stable, the infant should be transported to a tertiary care center where surgery is performed immediately.

Postoperatively, the infant should be monitored closely for evidence of respiratory insufficiency, shock, or bleeding. These neonates have highly reactive pulmonary vascular beds, and pulmonary hypertension can produce hypoxemia, right ventricular failure, and low cardiac output in the immediate postoperative period. Tolazoline (Priscoline) is sometimes administered intravenously during the postoperative period to promote pulmonary vasodilation. More recently, intravenous nitroglycerine has been administered in doses of 0.5 to 25 μ/kg/minute in a continuous drip to promote pulmonary vasodilation. Acidosis, hypothermia, and hypoxia must be prevented since they all enhance pulmonary vasoconstriction.

Since these neonates have small, noncompliant lungs, they are especially at risk for the development of pneumothorax and tension pneumothorax during the postoperative period. In addition, they will require extremely high inspiratory pressures to maintain adequate alveolar oxygenation. Tension pneumothorax is particularly life-threatening in these infants because of the "check valve" obstruction that can develop, permitting air into the intrapleural space on inspiration but preventing its exit on expiration.

Signs of tension pneumothorax in the infant include hypertension, tachycardia, sudden decrease in the Pa_{O_2}, asymmetry of chest expansion during inspiration, decreased or absent unilateral breath sounds, and tracheal deviation detected by chest radiograph or palpation. Hypotension and cardiac arrest are late signs of tension pneumothorax in the neonate. Tension pneumothorax is treated, of course, through immediate insertion of a chest tube and evacuation of the chest air. These neonates often require several chest tubes during the course of their critical-care management.

Recently, a few medical centers have successfully treated severe respiratory failure in infants by use of extracorporeal membrane oxygenation (ECMO). However, in some infants, the lungs are still too small, and despite ECMO, postnatal lung growth does not occur and the infants die (see the discussion in Chapter 3 on the treatment of low cardiac output).

The child with diaphragmatic hernia often requires long-term hospitalization following the initial surgery. Throughout this hospitalization, it is imperative that the child receive adequate nutrition (see the section on total parenteral alimentation in Chapter 8). Lung development will usually continue until the involved lung achieves normal or near-normal size. Occasionally, the child will require a second operation for release of abdominal adhesions.

∎ RESPIRATORY DISTRESS SYNDROME (RDS)
∎ Etiology

Respiratory distress syndrome, a syndrome in premature neonates, is characterized by progressive alveolar collapse, atelectasis, hypoxemia, and respiratory insufficiency. RDS occurs in approximately 1 out of every 6000 births. Although premature infants who weigh less than 1500 gm at birth are most frequently affected, even term infants have developed RDS. Other infants at risk include those of diabetic mothers and those delivered by cesarean section. Deficiency or absence of surfactant seems to be largely responsible for the development of RDS.

∎ Pathophysiology

Surfactant is a complex mixture consisting of lipids and proteins. Surfactant is formed by Type II alveolar cells in the lung, and it decreases surface tension at the air-fluid interface in the alveolus. The small alveolar size in the premature infant coupled with the lack of surfactant encourages alveolar collapse and the development of progressive atelectasis. As a result the lungs are stiff and have low compliance; this means that at a given inspiratory pressure,

the alveolar volume is smaller. Once lung compliance is reduced, a much greater negative intrathoracic pressure is required to inflate the alveoli. However, the premature neonate's chest is extremely compliant so that it tends to be drawn inward with each inspiration. Thus the net result is that work of breathing is increased and the infant is unable to maintain adequate ventilation.

As the infant with RDS develops progressive atelectasis and hypoxemia, pulmonary vascular resistance is increased. If the neonate's ductus arteriosus is patent, bidirectional shunting of blood may occur through the ductus arteriosus so that systemic venous blood is able to shunt away from the lungs and into the descending aorta (see the discussion of patent ductus arteriosus in Chapter 3). In addition, right-to-left shunting of blood may occur within the lung as the result of increased pulmonary vascular resistance; as much as 80% of right ventricular output may not perfuse ventilated alveoli. Prolonged hypoxemia produces a metabolic acidosis, which can enhance pulmonary vasoconstriction.[20]

∎ Clinical signs and symptoms

The infant with RDS usually exhibits moderate to severe respiratory distress shortly after birth. There is obvious tachypnea (respiratory rate of 60 to 120 breaths per minute), flaring of the nares, intercostal retractions, and cyanosis in room air. An expiratory grunt can be heard as the infant attempts to exhale against a partially closed glottis to maintain alveolar volume (a natural form of CPAP). Metabolic and respiratory acidosis may occur, and as the infant deteriorates, hypotension and signs of poor systemic perfusion develop.[20]

Arterial blood gas analyses usually provide a good indication of the severity of the infant's distress; as the disease progresses, acidosis, hypoxemia, and hypercapnia develop. A chest radiograph obtained immediately after birth may be normal, but the radiograph usually reveals the characteristic ground-glass appearance of the lung fields with air bronchograms occurring as a result of atelectasis.[20]

∎ Medical treatment and nursing interventions

Most of these infants respond favorably to the application of CPAP because it serves to stabilize the alveoli and to increase the FRC and Pa_{O_2}. Infants with severe respiratory insufficiency require intubation and provision of PPV with PEEP.[20] Oxygen therapy is beneficial for these infants; however, the complications of oxygen therapy can include pulmonary hemorrhage, bronchopulmonary dysplasia (BPD), and retrolental fibroplasia (RLF). Pao_2 is usually maintained between 50 to 70 mm Hg in the premature infant. Retrolental fibroplasia most commonly affects premature infants under 28 weeks' gestational age and those who receive excessive oxygen therapy.

Since these infants have very stiff lungs, they require high inspiratory pressures to maintain adequate ventilation; thus they are at risk for the development of pneumothorax, pneumomediastinum, and pneumopericardium. These air leaks occur most frequently in the infants with severe lung disease and are usually the result of mechanical ventilation or resuscitation. Pneumothorax in the neonate with RDS is usually manifested by the sudden onset of severe hypoxemia or by cardiac arrest. Signs of pneumomediastinum include mediastinal displacement on chest radiograph, hypoxemia, and hypercapnia. A crunch may be heard on auscultation over the mediastinum, or it may be palpated above the sternum.

The premature infant with RDS is also at risk for the development of intracranial or intraventricular hemorrhage (IVH). Whenever the infant deteriorates acutely during the first days of life, the development of an intracranial hemorrhage should be suspected. Its presence may be confirmed by ultrasonography or computed tomography.

Since the premature infant often requires insertion of multiple monitoring lines, intravenous catheters, and an ET tube, he is at risk for the development of severe infections. As a result the nurse must demonstrate meticulous aseptic technique when suctioning the ET tube, and she should wash her hands well before and after every patient contact.

Since cold stress increases the young infant's oxygen consumption, the nurse must make every effort to maintain a neutral thermal environment for the infant at all times. The appropriate neutral thermal environment for a specific baby varies with that baby's weight and age; therefore the nurse should always refer to the neutral thermal environment charts posted in the ICU (see Appendix G).

■ BRONCHOPULMONARY DYSPLASIA (BPD)
■ Etiology

Bronchopulmonary dysplasia typically occurs in infants who survive severe RDS.

■ Pathophysiology

Infants and young children with bronchopulmonary dysplasia demonstrate chronic respiratory insufficiency with chronic respiratory acidosis. Airway resistance is increased and lung compliance is re-

duced. In addition, pulmonary vascular resistance is increased and pulmonary hypertension may be present. Though the pulmonary damage associated with bronchopulmonary dysplasia is usually reversible, complete resolution of the disease often takes months or years. In addition, infection is poorly tolerated in these children and may result in repeated hospitalizations.[38,40,41]

■ Clinical signs and symptoms

Bronchopulmonary dysplasia is usually diagnosed in a young child with a known history of RDS. Such a child usually demonstrates signs of respiratory distress with increased work of breathing. Air trapping and small airway obstruction produces carbon dioxide retention and the development of a barrel-shaped chest. The child is usually tachypneic with chronic hypoxemia and hypercapnia and possible clubbing of the fingers and toes. High pulmonary vascular resistance increases right ventricular afterload and may produce right ventricular hypertrophy (RVH), which is asymptomatic but may be diagnosed by an ECG. If right heart failure develops, tachycardia, tachypnea, hepatomegaly, periorbital edema, and a gallop rhythm may be noted.

The chest radiograph of the child with bronchopulmonary dysplasia characteristically shows scattered linear infiltrates and patchy areas of hyperinflation. Arterial blood gases usually reveal hypercapnia, mild acidosis, and mild hypoxemia.[38,40,41]

■ Medical treatment and nursing interventions

The first priority of medical and nursing care of the child with bronchopulmonary dysplasia is the maintenance of adequate oxygenation. Bronchodilator therapy may be effective in reducing airway obstruction in those patients who also have reactive airway disease. In addition, administration of antibiotics, diuretics, and corticosteroids has been recommended by some physicians, although use of the latter two drugs is controversial.[38,40,41]

Throughout the child's hospitalization, the nurse must monitor for signs of development of respiratory failure, including an increase in hypercapnia or the development of hypoxia. If respiratory failure develops, the child will require mechanical ventilation until the acute phase of the disease is past. The nurse must also monitor for signs of congestive heart failure including tachycardia, tachypnea, hepatomegaly, periorbital edema, and signs of decreased urine output and decreased systemic perfusion. Whenever medications are administered, the nurse must carefully assess the child's response. Since metabolic alkalosis can result from excessive diuretic therapy and metabolic alkalosis can produce hypoventilation, the child's pH must be monitored closely when diuretics are administered (see the case study on metabolic acidosis and alkalosis earlier in this chapter).

Discharge planning should begin as soon as the child's condition improves. In an effort to prevent the development of pulmonary hypertension, home oxygen therapy may be recommended if hypoxemia is present. The parents will require knowledge of home care, oxygen therapy, chest physiotherapy, prevention of respiratory infections, and signs of respiratory distress. The family will often require a great deal of support, since the child's condition is a chronic one and it may not resolve until the child is 3 or 4 years old. It is imperative that the child and family receive good follow-up care and evaluation of respiratory status—these are essential to maximize the child's pulmonary function and to allow the child to grow and develop normally.

■ BRONCHIAL ASTHMA
■ Etiology

Asthma is a recurrent, reversible, generalized obstruction of both large and small airways and is characterized by dyspnea and wheezing. It is a complex disorder involving biochemical, immunologic, allergic, infectious, and psychologic factors.

■ Pathophysiology

Some attacks of asthma begin with an antigen-antibody reaction that causes the release of histamine and the slow-reacting substance of antiphylaxis. This results in dilation of blood vessels, excessive production of mucus, accumulation of secretions, development of bronchial edema, and constriction of small muscles in the airways. The lungs become hyperinflated and air trapping results.[6,35] As hypoxemia increases, alveolar ventilation increases and Pa_{CO_2} decreases.

Children with bronchial asthma do not usually require intensive care unless severe *status asthmaticus* develops. With status asthmaticus, little air exchange occurs, and carbon dioxide retention, respiratory acidosis, hypoxemia, and hypoxia develop. Severe hypoxemia and acidemia produce pulmonary vasoconstriction with severe intrapulmonary shunting; up to 40% to 50% of right ventricular output can bypass ventilated areas of the lung, resulting in a right-to-left intrapulmonary shunt. With extreme pulmonary vasoconstriction, right ventricular failure

(cor pulmonale) can result. The more hypoxic and acidotic the child becomes, the more pulmonary vasoconstriction and right ventricular failure develop.[6]

■ Clinical signs and symptoms

The child in acute asthmatic distress usually exhibits a productive cough, wheezing, low-grade fever, and tachypnea. As the attack progresses, there is increased wheezing, the production of thick mucus, use of accessory muscles of respiration, decreased air movement, cyanosis, and respiratory fatigue.

Analysis of arterial blood gases can indicate the severity of the child's impairment; it may be used to determine the appropriate form of therapy and to evaluate the patient's response. As the child with asthma develops air trapping, hypoxemia occurs, which may produce respiratory stimulation and result in initial hypocapnia and respiratory alkalosis. If inadequate tissue oxygenation develops, lactic acid production will produce a metabolic acidosis. As respiratory failure worsens, carbon dioxide retention occurs and the pH may fall from alkalotic to a normal range, indicating the development of respiratory acidosis. Should respiratory failure progress, severe hypoxemia and hypocapnia occur; thus in the most severe stage of asthma, both respiratory acidosis and metabolic acidosis are present.[6]

Decreased air movement can be detected with careful auscultation of the lung fields. It should be emphasized that as airway obstruction worsens, wheezing may disappear.

The chest radiograph is useful primarily to rule out pneumothorax, foreign body aspiration, or other acute respiratory diseases that cause wheezing. Generalized hyperinflation of the lungs is present on the chest film.

The white blood cell (WBC) differential may demonstrate an increase in eosinophils, and leukocytosis may be present either because of epinephrine therapy, stress, or infection; thus the WBC count is of little value in evaluation of the child with acute asthma.

■ Medical treatment and nursing interventions

The immediate goal of medical and nursing care of the child with asthma is relief of respiratory distress. Tachypnea, prolonged expiratory time, and wheezing are often the early signs of an asthma attack. Wheezing may be audible or heard on auscultation. The quality of the breath sounds should be noted, and assessment of air movement should be made at least hourly or more often if the asthma attack is severe. Other signs of respiratory distress include the development of intercostal retractions and restlessness. With severe hypoxemia and hypercapnia, the child may become lethargic and unresponsive; these are ominous signs and suggest that complete respiratory failure is imminent.[6] As the child's condition worsens, air exchange will become severely diminished and rales may appear, indicating the development of pulmonary edema.

Respiratory failure is present when the pH falls below 7.25, the $Paco_2$ increases above 65 to 75 mm Hg, Pao_2 falls below 50 mm Hg despite oxygen therapy; cyanosis develops, and breath sounds become diminished or absent.[6] Persistent hypoventilation with severe hypoxemia will further reduce the arterial pH and produce a mixed acidosis. Sodium bicarbonate should be administered with caution, since the buffering action of the bicarbonate results in carbon dioxide formation; this may worsen existing hypercapnia.

Administration of oxygen is one of the most important forms of treatment of asthma.[6] Oxygen should be administered by mask or by nasal cannula. If a tight-fitting mask makes the child more anxious, use of a face tent may be appropriate. The oxygen should be administered with a cool mist rather than a warm mist since a cool mist is thought to reduce bronchial swelling.

Intravenous fluids are indicated for correction of dehydration; however, the amount of fluid required for hydration of the child with asthma is somewhat controversial. Previously, overhydration of these children was recommended; however, most physicians discourage this practice, since administration of excessive amounts of intravenous fluids may result in the development of pulmonary edema.[21] It is essential that the nurse maintain an accurate record of total fluid intake and output for any child with status asthmaticus.

Chest physiotherapy is contraindicated during the acute phases of an asthmatic attack because it often worsens the child's condition. However, as the child's respiratory status improves, vigorous chest physiotherapy is indicated to help remove secretions.

Relief of bronchospasm is usually produced through administration of sympathomimetic and methylxanthine drugs (see Appendix B for further information about dosages and side effects).[1] Severe attacks of status asthmaticus are usually treated initially with several doses of subcutaneous epinephrine in a concentration of 1:1000 in dosages of 0.1 to 0.3 ml every 20 minutes.[3] A bolus intravenous amino-phylline dose (5 to 6 mg/kg up to a total of 300 mg) may be administered over a 30-minute period every 6 hours. Aminophylline may also be administered by constant infusion (0.7 to 1.1 mg/kg/hour) after a loading dose is administered. It is important that the child's serum theophylline level is checked frequently so that drug dosages can be adjusted appropriately. The therapeutic range of theophylline is 10 to 20 μg/ml, and theophylline toxicity may occur when the serum level exceeds 20 μg/ml. In some centers, inhaled beta$_2$-agonists, such as metaproterenol, isoetharine, or albuterol are used in addition to intravenous aminophylline.

Steroids, particularly methylprednisolone sodium succinate (Solu-Medrol), may also be given when the child is hospitalized. The antiinflammatory effect of the steroid decreases the airway obstruction and may augment the effect of bronchodilators.[1,3,6,21] Antibiotics may be employed if an underlying infection is suspected.

If oxygen, epinephrine, and intravenous aminophylline do not succeed in improving the child's condition, an isoproterenol IV infusion may be attempted before intubation and ventilation. The isoproterenol infusion is prepared by mixing 0.5 mg of isoproterenol (Isuprel) with 50 ml of intravenous fluid or 1 mg of isoproterenol in 100 ml of intravenous fluid. The mixture is then flushed through the intravenous tubing and placed on a continuous infusion pump. The initial dose of isoproterenol should provide 0.05 to 0.1 μg/kg/minute; this dosage may be increased by 0.05 μg/kg/minute every 15 minutes if the $Paco_2$ does not fall.[3,6] The maximum dose of isoproterenol is determined by the child's heart rate and rhythm and by his clinical improvement.[6] If the child has a heart rate greater than 200 beats per minute and still does not demonstrate improvement in respiratory status, intubation is indicated. The patient should be gradually weaned from the isoproterenol if clinical improvement occurs or if the child is mechanically ventilated.

Since anxiety can contribute to the child's bronchospasm and the severity of the asthma attack, it is important that the nurse provide reassurance to the child and maintain a calm atmosphere around the bedside. The parents can often be effective in reducing the patient's anxiety.[35]

It is extremely important that the child and family receive the information necessary to maintain care when discharge is planned. Both the child and the parents must be aware of the importance of adherence to drug therapy, and additional teaching of chest physiotherapy may be required if the child continues to demonstrate persistent pulmonary infiltrates. The youngster (if age appropriate) and the parents should be familiar with the names of all drugs currently prescribed and with their dosages and side effects. Since asthma may be a chronic disease, the child will require frequent evaluations and follow-up.

■ NEAR-DROWNING
■ Etiology

Near-drowning is the third most common cause of death in infants and children[31,32]; in childhood drowning and near-drowning, approximately 40% of the victims are less than 4 years of age.[25] Drowning is defined as submersion resulting in asphyxia and death within 24 hours. Near-drowning, on the other hand, is defined as submersion of sufficient gravity to require hospitalization but not severe enough to result in death within the first 24 hours.

Drownings occur in private swimming pools, lakes, ponds, canals, and bathtubs. The factors that most commonly contribute to immersion accidents with children are lack of proper adult supervision and lack of adequate barriers around bodies of water.

■ Pathophysiology

Drowning may occur in either fresh water or salt water. Theoretically, when fresh-water drowning occurs, hypotonic fluid enters the alveolar space and can quickly be absorbed into the vascular space, resulting in hemodilution and low serum electrolyte and hemoglobin concentrations. Fresh-water drowning may also produce dilution of surfactant and so can result in atelectasis.

If the child was submerged in salt water, the alveolar space will be filled with hypertonic fluid. This hypertonic fluid can pull free water from the vascular space into the alveoli, resulting in pulmonary edema and hemoconcentration, with resulting increase in hemoglobin and serum electrolyte concentrations. Despite these theoretic considerations, however, clinical experience has shown little difference between fresh- and salt-water drowning, probably because only a small amount of water is necessary to produce asphyxia.[13] Furthermore, approximately 10% of near-drowning victims do not aspirate any water. In these patients laryngospasm probably occurs.

Inhalation of fluid may occur during active gasping. With loss of consciousness, airway reflexes are abolished and fluid can be aspirated into the airways, leading to inflammation, airway obstruction and collapse of small airways, and destruction of alveolar and capillary membranes. Hypercapnia and hypoxemia

with combined metabolic and respiratory acidosis may develop quickly, particularly if pulmonary edema and atelectasis are present.

Other complications of near-drowning include the development of a secondary pneumonia, shock lung or adult RDS, seizures, and disseminated intravascular coagulation (DIC). If a child is comatose on admission to the hospital, with a pH of less than 7.00 and an absence of spontaneous respiration and cranial nerve reflexes, the neurologic prognosis is extremely poor. A better neurologic prognosis may be present if drowning has occurred in cold water, presumably because hypothermia reduces oxygen consumption.[2]

■ Clinical signs and symptoms

When the child is admitted following a near-drowning episode, it is extremely important to obtain a good history of the event, including the duration of submersion, the water temperature, the condition of the patient on recovery from the water, the presence of spontaneous respirations, and duration and quality of any cardiopulmonary resuscitation attempted. Analysis of blood gases should be performed immediately. Most commonly the child has moderate hypoxemia accompanied initially by hypocapnia. Hypercapnia may be present if ventilation/perfusion abnormalities are severe, and metabolic acidosis will develop if hypoxemia is severe. Pulmonary edema, atelectasis, and chemical pneumonitis may also be present.

If the child is breathing spontaneously, pulmonary congestion or airway obstruction will produce signs and symptoms of respiratory distress. The child will be tachycardic and tachypneic and will demonstrate stridor, retractions, nasal flaring, and use of accessory muscles for respiration; excessive respiratory secretions will be present. Auscultation may reveal pulmonary congestion and decreased lung aeration bilaterally. As the child's respiratory distress increases, rales may be heard on auscultation.

If the child's hypoxic episode was severe or prolonged, his level of consciousness may be altered, and he may be lethargic or extremely irritable. In addition there may be changes in pupillary response to light (specifically, a decrease or inequality in response), pathologic posturing, or seizure activity. With severe central nervous system injury, inappropriate antidiuretic hormone (ADH) secretion or diabetes insipidus may occur. With inappropriate ADH secretion, sodium is lost in the urine, hyponatremia develops, and urine specific gravity increases. With diabetes insipidus, the child loses large amounts of very dilute urine, hypernatremia develops, and urine specific gravity decreases (see the discussion of inappropriate ADH secretion and diabetes insipidus in Chapter 7).

The child with near-drowning may develop electrolyte imbalance related to acidosis, fluid shifts, hemodilution, or hemoconcentration. With acidosis the serum potassium will rise as potassium shifts out of the cells into the vascular space; conversely, the serum potassium will fall with correction of acidosis or the development of alkalosis. The serum potassium concentration may also rise if intravascular hemolysis is present (see the discussion of potassium regulation in Chapter 7).

Hemodilution results in a fall in the serum electrolyte concentrations, the hematocrit, and the hemoglobin concentration. Likewise, hemoconcentration will result in a rise in serum electrolyte concentrations and hematocrit and a rise in the hemoglobin concentration.

The chest radiograph of the child with near-drowning reveals infiltrates and diffuse pulmonary edema. Fractured ribs or air leaks may also be seen as the result of resuscitation.

■ Medical treatment and nursing intervention

As soon as the child arrives in the ICU, nursing interventions are focused on continuation of cardiopulmonary resuscitation and assessment of central nervous system functions. Signs of respiratory distress such as stridor, chest retractions, cyanosis, and decreased lung aeration should be reported immediately to a physician since they may indicate that the child requires ventilatory assistance. If the child is intubated and mechanically ventilated, the nurse must ensure that the tube remains patent and that adequate ventilation is provided.

If the child with near-drowning is mechanically ventilated, higher ventilatory and PEEP pressures are usually required. As the child requires high inspiratory pressures, his risk of developing a pneumothorax increases. It is imperative that the nurse assess the child's breath sounds frequently and monitor peak inspiratory pressures closely, especially if the youngster is ventilated with a volume-cycled ventilator. Signs of development of a pneumothorax include unilateral decrease in breath sounds, decrease in chest expansion with ventilation, and resistance to hand ventilation. If the child is ventilated with a volume ventilator, the nurse may notice a sudden and dramatic increase in peak inspiratory pressures. Since the development of a pneumothorax can produce tension pneumothorax and result in severe compromise of cardiorespiratory function, emergency equipment for chest tube insertion should be kept nearby (see Appendix A).

Occasionally, it is difficult to distinguish between the signs and symptoms produced by pneumothorax and those produced by tube obstruction. In both, the child's breath sounds are dramatically reduced and there is resistance to hand ventilation. If a pneumothorax is present, the treatment of choice is to maintain ventilation through the ET tube and to insert a chest tube. If the ET tube is blocked, however, the appropriate intervention is removal of that ET tube, ventilation of the child with a bag and mask, and reinsertion of an ET tube. Therefore whenever the child demonstrates a deterioration in clinical status, the nurse should notify the physician immediately. Sedation and muscle relaxants may be required to ensure ventilatory control of the patient, but these drugs preclude effective neurologic assessment and so they are often avoided if at all possible. As long as the child is ventilated, the ventilatory variables should be checked by the nurse at least every hour when vital signs are assessed.

Analysis of arterial blood gases will help the health-care team to assess the child's ventilatory status and to evaluate his response to therapy. In addition, it is important to monitor the patient's A-a O_2 difference since this difference will increase with the amount of intrapulmonary shunting that is present (see the discussion of A-a O_2 difference earlier in this chapter). As already noted, it is imperative that the nurse auscultate the child's breath sounds frequently; she may note the presence of adventitious sounds such as rhonchi and wheezing. If rales are noted, they may indicate the development of pulmonary edema or infection and so should be reported to a physician.

Throughout the child's care it is important that the nurse assess the indirect evidence of cardiac output and systemic perfusion. Signs of poor systemic perfusion include tachycardia, decreased intensity of peripheral pulses, cool extremities, and decreased urine output—with the excretion of a very concentrated urine. In addition, capillary filling time will be slow (greater than several seconds). The development of hepatomegaly and periorbital edema may indicate the presence of right ventricular failure secondary to pulmonary hypertension. The child with near-drowning may demonstrate cardiac arrhythmias, particularly if electrolyte imbalance is present.

The nurse is responsible for maintaining careful records of the child's total fluid intake and output. Overzealous fluid administration should be avoided in these children, since the risk of pulmonary edema is significant. Urine output should average 0.5 to 1 ml/kg/hour if fluid intake is adequate, and an increase in urine specific gravity and a decrease in urine volume may indicate the development of poor systemic perfusion or ischemia. The type and volume of intravenous solutions should be adjusted frequently according to the results of evaluation of the serum electrolyte concentrations and the child's hematocrit.

Increased intracranial pressure may result from hypoxia. Signs of increased intracranial pressure include a deterioration in the child's level of consciousness; an alteration in pupillary response to light, including pupillary dilation or inequality; change in the child's respiratory pattern; a rise in the child's systolic arterial blood pressure; a widening of the pulse pressure; bradycardia; or apnea (late). The presence of anisocoria, posturing of the extremities, and seizures may also be noted. Neurologic assessment should be performed at least every hour or more often if the patient's condition warrants (see the discussion of clinical signs and symptoms of increased intracranial pressure in Chapter 6). Direct measurement of the child's intracranial pressure may be accomplished through insertion of an indwelling monitor catheter. If such a monitoring line is inserted, the nurse must ensure that the line remains patent and must monitor for signs of local infection. Acute and temporary reduction of high intracranial pressure may be accomplished through hyperventilation of the child and reduction in the child's $Paco_2$, since this results in constriction of cerebral arteries and may cause reduction of intracranial volume. The child with an increase in intracranial pressure may also require mannitol administration. Hypothermia and use of barbiturates may also be indicated (see Chapter 6 for the treatment of increased intracranial pressure).[2]

Since the child with near-drowning requires insertion of multiple monitoring and IV lines, an ET tube, and possibly many chest tubes, he is at risk for the development of infection. Throughout his care the nurse should assess all of the patient's skin-puncture sites and wounds for evidence of inflammation or drainage and should report these to a physician immediately. The nurse should also assess the color, odor, and thickness of any respiratory secretions. Signs of systemic infection include the development of leukocytosis and fever. Antibiotics will be administered if infection is suspected.

The child's body temperature should be controlled carefully, since fever and hypothermia may increase the child's oxygen requirements. If the child is allowed to remain normothermic, a physician should be notified if a fever develops, and administration of antipyretics or use of a cooling blanket is usu-

ally indicated. If the child requires hypothermia to treat increased intracranial pressure, his body temperature should be maintained within very strict limits.

The child is at risk for the development of nutritional compromise as the result of prolonged intubation, stress, and bedrest. The medical team is responsible for ensuring adequate caloric intake, since this is necessary for lung and wound healing. The child should be weighed daily, and the daily weight should be recorded on a bedside growth chart. A significant weight change is one that totals 50 gm or more per 24 hours in an infant, 200 gm or more per 24 hours in a child, or 500 gm or more per 24 hours in an adolescent; this amount of weight change should be discussed with a physician. The nurse should calculate the child's daily fluid and caloric intake, and if inadequate intake is occurring, she should discuss this immediately with the physician. To prevent skin breakdown, the child's skin should be kept dry and the sheets smooth. An egg-crate mattress may be used to decrease the risk of skin breakdown over bony prominences. If the child is comatose or sedated, a physical therapy consultation should probably be obtained so that range of motion exercises can be initiated to prevent the development of contractures.

Finally, psychologic support of the child and family should be provided at all times. Since near-drowning is accidental and often preventable, the family may feel a great deal of guilt for the child's condition. Throughout the youngster's illness and recovery, it is imperative that the health-care team use the same terms so that the family is provided with consistent information and a consistent prognosis. As soon as the child begins to recover, discharge planning should begin. The parents need complete information about any medications or therapy the child will require at home, and they should be given adequate time to learn home-care techniques.

■ **CHEST TRAUMA**
■ **Etiology**

Trauma to the chest may involve damage to the chest wall, lungs, esophagus, diaphragm, or tracheobronchial tree. Penetrating injuries are usually caused by high velocity missiles or sharp objects. Nonpenetrating injuries are caused by forceful contact with a blunt object. Children with chest injuries most frequently have nonpenetrating injuries resulting from automobile accidents. Nonpenetrating chest trauma is a serious problem because of its frequency and because potentially fatal internal injury can occur with few superficial signs of injury.

■ Pathophysiology

The most common traumatic chest wall injury is rib fracture. Rib fractures may be uncomplicated, or they may result in development of hemothorax, pneumothorax, or flail chest. A flail chest occurs with fracture of four or more ribs or fracture of the sternum at the rib junction that renders the chest wall floppy instead of rigid. Ribs 3 to 10 are the most commonly fractured, since the upper ribs are more protected and the lower ribs are more mobile.

Other forms of chest trauma include pericardial tamponade, fracture of the sternum, rupture of the larynx, and lacerations of the trachea, bronchi, and heart. Penetrating wounds of the chest are most often produced by knives, ice picks, or bullets.

Cardiac tamponade can result from accumulation of as little as 30 ml of blood within the pericardial sac, which can cause severe compromise of cardiac output.

Traumatic rupture of the diaphragm is rare. If it occurs, the lacerated diaphragm allows the abdominal contents to enter the pleural cavity. During inspiration the decreased intrathoracic pressure draws the abdominal contents into the chest; during expiration, however, the involved lung becomes partially filled with expelled gas from the contralateral lung. If the mediastinum shifts to the side opposite the injury, the great vessels can be compressed and cardiac output reduced. The child with a ruptured diaphragm often has other major organ injuries. These children require immediate surgical repair.

Rupture of the trachea or bronchi may occur with severe blunt trauma to the upper chest, as the result of shear stresses. Ribs may be fractured, and they may lacerate the airway. With such rupture of a large airway, air leaks from the airway into the chest during both inspiration and expiration. This produces a constant and significant pneumothorax, which may result in insufficient delivery of air to the alveoli.

Contusion of the lung causes hemorrhage with fluid transudation and extravasation into the lung parenchyma and alveoli. As fluid accumulates in both interstitial and intraalveolar spaces, lung compliance decreases and work of breathing increases. Severe hypoxemia can develop as the result of large intrapulmonary right-to-left shunt.

■ Clinical signs and symptoms

Signs and symptoms of rib fractures include tachypnea with shallow breathing and pain during inspiration. Tenderness, crepitus, and swelling may be present over the fracture site. If multiple rib fractures are present, the chest wall may become unstable and retract during inspiration; this is termed *paradoxic respiration* (Fig. 4-9). Such instability of the chest wall can produce alveolar hypoventilation, hypoxia, and hypercapnia. Atelectasis and the increased work of breathing can develop rapidly and ultimately produce respiratory failure.

The presence of a pneumothorax is best diagnosed through careful auscultation of breath sounds and examination of the chest radiograph. Since the chest wall of the infant and young child is so thin, breath sounds are easily referred from other areas of the lung. As a result decreased breath sounds may not

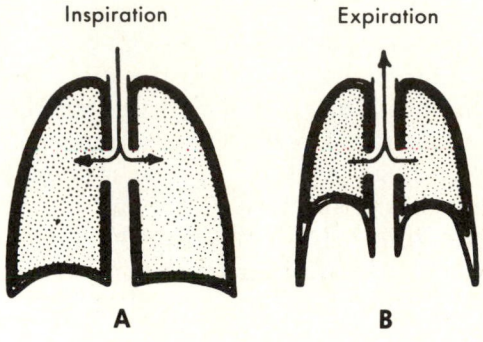

Normal respiration

Inspiration   Expiration

A   B

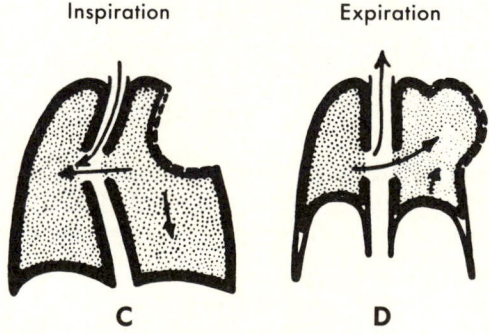

Paradoxical motion

Inspiration   Expiration

C   D

Fig. 4-9 Effects of flail chest and resultant paradoxic motion. **A,** Normal inspiration. **B,** Normal expiration. **C,** During inspiration in the patient with flail chest, the involved lung and mediastinal structures are drawn toward the noninvolved lung. **D,** During expiration in the patient with flail chest, the involved lung expands outward with the nonrigid (flail) chest, and the noninvolved lung is drawn toward the side of injury.

From Salzberg, A.M., and Brooks, J.W.: Disorders of the respiratory tract due to trauma. In Kendig, E., editor: Disorders of the respiratory tract in children, ed. 4, Philadelphia, 1983, W.B. Saunders Co.

necessarily be heard over involved areas of the lung; instead the nurse may note a difference in the quality or pitch of the breath sounds over an area of pneumothorax. Pneumothorax should be suspected in any child who demonstrates tachypnea and increased respiratory effort following chest trauma.

If a large pneumothorax is present (so that the pleural space fills with air), the trapped air will push the mediastinal contents to the side opposite the area of pneumothorax. If this occurs, a *tension pneumothorax* is present; this situation may produce severe hypoxemia and a drastic reduction in cardiac output. Development of a tension pneumothorax should be suspected in any child who demonstrates extreme respiratory distress following chest trauma with signs of systemic venous engorgement (as the result of decreased systemic venous return), poor systemic perfusion, a shifting in the location of heart sounds away from the side of injury, and decreased breath sounds on the side of injury.

The diagnosis of rib fractures with or without pneumothorax can be confirmed through careful examination of the chest radiograph (see Fig. 5-2 for an example of a chest radiograph demonstrating both rib fracture and pneumothorax; see also Fig. 4-10).

Another potential complication of rib fracture is the development of a hemothorax. Bleeding from lung vessels or from the chest wall vessels collects in the pleural cavity. This will produce a decrease in breath sounds over involved areas and a dullness to percussion. However, since the chest wall of the infant and young child is thin and breath sounds can easily be referred from other areas of the lung, the nurse may note only a decrease in the quality or the pitch of breath sounds over the area of hemothorax. The appearance of a hemothorax resembles that of a pleural effusion on the chest radiograph. A lateral decubitus film is often obtained to allow the collection of the hemothorax in dependent areas of the lung so that air-fluid interface may be seen on the radiograph (see Chapter 5). A small hemothorax that resolves spontaneously may produce no compromise in respiratory function; however, accumulation of large amounts of blood in the pleural cavity may compromise ventilation and produce signs of increased respiratory effort and cyanosis.

Signs of cardiac tamponade include those associated with extreme respiratory distress and critical reduction in cardiac output. These signs include tachycardia, tachypnea, increased respiratory effort,

Normal respiration   Open pneumothorax

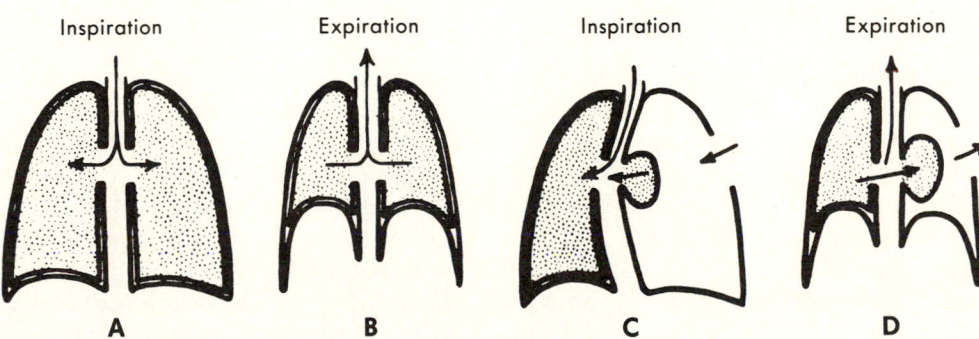

Inspiration   Expiration   Inspiration   Expiration

A   B   C   D

Fig. 4-10 Changes in normal respiratory pattern brought about by the presence of an open, sucking thoracic wall injury. **A,** Normal inspiration. **B,** Normal expiration. **C,** During inspiration in the patient with an open pneumothorax, air is drawn into the involved chest, so that the involved lung and mediastinal structures are shifted toward the noninvolved lung. **D,** During expiration in the patient with an open chest wound, some air is pushed out of the open wound, but the involved lung tends to fill with expired air from the noninvolved lung.

From Salzberg, A.M., and Brooks, J.W.: Disorders of the respiratory tract due to trauma. In Kendig, E., editor: Disorders of the respiratory tract in children, ed. 4. Philadelphia, 1983, W.B. Saunders Co.

hepatomegaly, high central venous pressure, cool, clammy extremities, decreased intensity of peripheral pulses, decreased urine output, and prolonged capillary refill time. The child with cardiac tamponade may also demonstrate a *pulsus paradoxus*; this condition is present when the child's systolic arterial blood pressure falls more than 8-10 mm Hg during spontaneous inspiration. Pulsus paradoxus may be detected during routine measurement of arterial blood pressure by cuff or, if the child has an arterial line in place, through examination of the arterial wave form on the oscilloscope during spontaneous respirations. The chest radiograph of the child with cardiac tamponade may reveal enlargement of the cardiac silhouette or evidence of pulmonary venous engorgement. The diagnosis of cardiac tamponade is confirmed by ultrasonography (echocardiogram).

Traumatic rupture of the diaphragm should be suspected if the child demonstrates severe respiratory distress and evidence of decreased cardiac output and systemic perfusion. In addition, the child with ruptured diaphragm will demonstrate shifting of heart sounds to the side opposite that of injury. The diagnosis may be confirmed through examination of the chest radiograph, which will reveal the presence of abdominal contents in the chest on the side of injury.

Rupture of the trachea or bronchi should be suspected in any child who has severe respiratory distress and evidence of a large pneumothorax. These children will demonstrate hemoptysis and a continuous large air leak during both inspiration and expiration after a chest tube is inserted. The child with tracheal rupture may also have upper airway obstruction if the torn flaps of the trachea obstruct the lumen of the airway (see the section on upper airway obstruction earlier in this chapter).

The child with pulmonary contusion will demonstrate signs of respiratory distress, and evidence of hypoxemia and respiratory acidosis may be evident on examination of arterial blood gas. The chest radiograph will reveal the accumulation of interstitial fluid.

■ Medical and surgical treatment and nursing interventions

Medical and surgical care of the child with chest trauma requires rapid assessment of the extent of the child's injury and maximization of cardiopulmonary function. While, obviously, life-threatening injuries should be treated immediately, the following discussion is organized so that the injuries are discussed in the same order in which they appeared in the section on clinical signs and symptoms. Whenever a child is admitted with chest trauma, a large-bore venous catheter should be inserted to ensure venous access. A chest radiograph should also be obtained, and careful physical assessment must be performed.

Treatment of a simple rib fracture includes relief of pain and bed rest. Uncomplicated rib fractures heal within several weeks. If severe pain is present, an intercostal nerve block may be provided. Restrictive bandaging is seldom useful. The most frequent complication of rib fracture is atelectasis, which occurs as the result of splinting of the affected area, hypoventilation, and inadequate coughing. This splinting can also result in retained secretions and the development of pneumonia.

The child with flail chest requires immediate stabilization of the chest wall. The youngster should be positioned so that the injured side is down, and gentle pressure is placed over the area—for example, through use of a pillow. The child with an acute flail chest requires ET intubation and institution of controlled ventilation with PEEP to maintain adequate oxygenation and carbon dioxide removal. If the child is young and healthy, 7 to 10 days of mechanical ventilation should be sufficient. Weaning from mechanical ventilation should not be attempted, however, until paradoxical chest movement has ceased and the pulmonary parenchyma has recovered from the trauma.

A small pneumothorax may require only observation or a simple needle aspiration. If needle aspiration is planned, this is usually accomplished through insertion of a 14 to 18 gauge needle attached by stopcock to a 20 to 50 ml syringe. Through this setup, air can be aspirated from the chest, the stopcock port to the chest can be turned off, and the air can be flushed from the syringe out of the stopcock. The procedure is carried out under local anesthesia (1%-2% lidocaine [Xylocaine]). The nurse should always record the amount of air removed, and a small dressing should be applied over the needle site after completion of the needle aspiration. Of course, the child will require adequate explanation and support before, during, and after the procedure.

If the pneumothorax is greater than 10%, or if it is accompanied by significant respiratory distress, insertion of a chest tube to underwater seal and suction is often necessary. Whenever insertion of a chest tube is planned, the nurse should assemble all of the appropriate equipment at the bedside and have it prepared for immediate use. This equipment includes a chest bottle or disposable pleural drainage system with both the water-seal and suction chambers filled to the appropriate levels, adequate lighting, sterile gloves, gown, mask, tape, suture material, and the appropriate size of chest tube. Most physicians request a thoracotomy tray so that surgical instruments are available during chest-tube insertion. The child will require adequate preparation and possible sedation or administration of analgesia before the procedure.

To insert the chest tube, lidocaine is infused subcutaneously into the intercostal space. A small incision is made just above the second or third rib. Blunt dissection into the pleural space is performed with a hemostat. The chest tube is then inserted and secured to the skin with suture material and adhesive tape. A gauze dressing is applied over the chest-tube site. Some physicians request use of a petroleum jelly (Vaseline) gauze dressing, which can be changed every 24 to 48 hours or more often if necessary. It is extremely important that after insertion of the chest tube, care is taken not to dislodge it. Whenever the chest-tube dressing is changed, the area should be assessed for evidence of erythema or the presence of any drainage or subcutaneous emphysema (see Appendix A for further information about chest tube insertion and Chapter 9 for information about pleural drainage systems). A chest radiograph should be obtained after a chest tube is inserted to confirm its appropriate placement and to verify that the pneumothorax has been evacuated. The chest tube may be removed once evidence of the air leak has disappeared. Following chest tube removal, a chest radiograph should also be obtained to ensure that a pneumothorax has not occurred during tube removal.

If the child develops a tension pneumothorax, this constitutes a medical emergency and requires immediate decompression of the air collection. Initially, a large-bore needle is inserted into the pleural cavity, and aspiration of the extrapulmonary air is accomplished. Then a chest tube is inserted to permit continuous removal of any further air. A repeat chest radiograph should show that the mediastinal structures have returned to the midline.

The appropriate treatment of a hemothorax is dependent on the size of the blood accumulation and the degree of respiratory distress it produces. Small collections of blood do not require removal, and the child needs only to be observed for the development of respiratory distress. If respiratory distress is present or a significant amount of blood has accumulated in the chest, chest-tube drainage and blood transfusion may be necessary. Surgical exploration is indicated if the hemothorax is significant and continuous or if damage to mediastinal structures is suspected.

If the child has penetrating wounds of the chest, these wounds must be treated immediately. The wound should be covered with an air-tight dressing consisting of gauze bandage and petroleum jelly. Insertion of a chest tube is usually indicated. Cardiac tamponade is a life-threatening condition and must be treated immediately to prevent severe compromise of cardiac output and death. Treatment of cardiac tamponade consists of pericardial aspiration, which is usually performed in the ICU during electrocardiographic monitoring. A large-bore needle attached to a syringe is inserted into the pericardial space, and the pericardial fluid is aspirated. Throughout the procedure the nurse should monitor the child's electrocardiogram (ECG) and evidence of systemic perfusion, and a physician should be informed of any cardiac arrhythmias or evidence of S-T segment changes.

The child with traumatic rupture of the diaphragm or rupture of the tracheobronchial tree usually requires immediate intubation and surgical intervention. Surgery is usually performed immediately when traumatic rupture of the diaphragm is present. If rupture of the tracheobronchial tree is suspected, a bronchoscopy confirms the presence and location of the rupture before surgery is performed. Occasionally, tracheal rupture produces obstruction of the airway with tracheal flap; this makes ET intubation impossible and requires performance of a tracheostomy.

The child with pulmonary contusion tends to rapidly develop evidence of intrapulmonary and parenchymal fluid accumulation. These children require mechanical ventilatory support to maintain adequate oxygenation. Most commonly, lung compliance is reduced, and high levels of PEEP are also required. These high inspiratory pressures place the child at risk for the development of spontaneous pneumothorax and tension pneumothorax so that careful assessment must be made of the child's breath sounds and adequacy of lung expansion. Chest physiotherapy is usually required, and pulmonary hygiene must be meticulous. This condition is usually self-limiting, and resolution occurs within several days.

In summary, nursing care of children with chest trauma requires careful and continuous nursing assessment and rapid response to deterioration in the child's clinical status. The first priority in nursing care is maintenance of adequate cardiopulmonary function and early identification of respiratory failure or low cardiac output (for further information about caring for the child with trauma, see Appendix A).

■ RESPIRATORY INFECTIONS
■ Etiology

Respiratory infection is a major cause of respiratory disease in children. For purposes of this chapter, discussion is limited to pneumonia, the most common form of respiratory infection in critically ill patients.

Children most at risk for the development of pneumonia are those with the following conditions:

1. Congenital immune deficiency
2. Acquired immune deficiency
   a. Treatment with immunosuppressive drugs
   b. Malignancy
3. Preexisting lung injury
4. Congenital malformations of the trachea or esophagus
5. Frequent aspiration episodes
6. Congenital defect of cilia formation

■ **Pathophysiology**

The term "pneumonia" covers a multitude of disorders that differ widely in terms of causative agents, course of disease, pathology, and prognosis. A common feature of all pneumonias is that each involves an inflammatory response. The causative agent is most often infectious, and it is introduced into the lungs through inhalation or through the blood stream. Table 4-16 includes classification of the three major bacterial pneumonias based on their etiologic agents.

Table 4-16 Comparison of the pneumonias based on etiologic agent

Bacterial	Nonbacterial
1. *Diplococcus pneumoniae*	1. Syncytial virus
2. *Staphylococcus aureus*	2. Parainfluenza virus
3. *Haemophilus influenzae*	3. Influenza viruses
4. *Streptococcus pyogenes*	4. Adenoviruses
5. *Mycobacterium tuberculosis*	5. *Mycoplasma species*
6. Miscellaneous	6. Fungi
a. *Escherichia coli*	a. *Histoplasma capsulatum*
b. *Klebsiella pneumoniae*	b. *Aspergillus species*
c. *Salmonella species*	

Pneumonia can be classified as lobar, bronchopneumonia, and interstitial pneumonia on the basis of clinical and radiographic evidence. In a lobar form of pneumonia, one or more lobes are involved; when bronchopneumonia is present, the terminal bronchioles are inflamed. With interstitial pneumonia the inflammatory processes are found within the alveolar walls. The pneumonia can also be described as hemorrhagic, fibrinous, or necrotizing.

Bacterial pneumonia. Most patients with primary bacterial pneumonia require neither hospitalization nor intensive care. However, when an already sick patient acquires a secondary pneumonia, it may be particularly severe. The three major causes of bacterial pneumonia in children are *Streptococcus pneumoniae* (pneumococci), *Haemophilus* species, and Group A *Streptococcus*. Occasional bacterial pathogens are *Staphylococcus* species, *Pseudomonas* species, and anaerobes. In general, bacterial pneumonia affects children younger than 3 years of age. It occurs most frequently during the winter and early spring, and the organisms are transmitted by droplet infection. Pneumococcal pneumonia tends to be lobar with exudative filling of the alveoli. Streptococcal pneumonia most commonly is lobar, with interstitial involvement. Table 4-17 compares the etiology, pathophysiology, diagnostic findings, and signs and symptoms of three common bacterial forms of pneumonia.

Viral pneumonia. Viral pneumonia occurs much more frequently than bacterial pneumonia and often causes interstitial pneumonitis. Respiratory syncytial virus (RSV), adenoviruses, and parainfluenzae usually account for the greatest number of cases. Pathologic changes include interstitial pneumonitis, inflammation of the mucosa and walls of the bronchi and bronchioles, and at times secondary bacterial infections.

Pneumonia in immunosuppressed patients. In patients with congenital or acquired deficiency in immune function, certain rare pathogens must be considered as the cause of pneumonia, since these pathogens must be treated differently. For example, in patients with leukemia, *Pneumocystis carinii* infection may occur, causing a severe interstitial pneumonia. Similarly, fungal infections with *Candida* species or *Aspergillus* species should be suspected in these patients.

■ **Clinical signs and symptoms**

Generally, younger children, especially those between 6 months and 3 years of age, tend to have more severe symptoms than older children when re-

Table 4-17   Comparison of three common bacterial pneumonias

	Pneumococcal pneumonia	Staphylococcal pneumonia	Streptococcal pneumonia
Etiologic agent and epidemiology	Most common agent in lobar pneumonia (approximately 90% of all pneumonias) Occurs most often in late winter and early spring Organisms transmitted by droplet infection Highest attack rate during the first 4 years and declines with increasing age Uncommon in infants less than age 1 year	Most common agent in bronchopneumonia Greatest incidence in first 2 years of life; 30% of all cases occur in children less than 3 months of age; 70% before 1 year of age Occurs most often in winter months Usually contracted as primary infection Cross-contamination common in hospitals	Usually lobar Less common than other bacterial pneumonias Usually occurs as complication of influenza or measles
Pathophysiology	Usually lobar Progresses through four stages: (1) engorgement—lobe is congested, heavy, and dark with effusion of blood and serum into alveoli; (2) red heparinization—lobe is solid, dark red, and airless; alveoli contain fibrin, serum, red blood cells, neutrophils, and pneumococci; (3) gray heparinization—lobe is larger than normal, firm, gray, and pleural surface appears dull; fibrin present in alveoli but decreased cellular elements and bacteria; (4) resolution	Localized abcesses in older children; more diffuse in infants Exotoxin causes necrosis and sloughing of bronchial mucous membranes Formation of peribronchial abcesses Pneumatocele formation—frequently, abscesses erode bronchial wall, abscess material is discharged into lumen; air enters abscess cavity and becomes trapped to form pneumatoceles visible on roentgenograms (pathognomonic of staphylococcus pneumonia), which usually develop during the first 10 days of illness; most disappear within a few weeks	Interstitial pneumonia Spreads via lymphatics
Roentgenographic findings	Areas of consolidation, usually patchy in children in one or more lobes; may involve entire lung	Patchy clouding in one or more lobes Pneumatoceles of varying sizes appear as thin-walled translucencies	Disseminated infiltration

Modified from Whaley, L., and Wong, D.: Nursing care of infants and children, ed. 2, St. Louis, 1983, The C.V. Mosby Co.

Continued.

Table 4-17   Comparison of three common bacterial pneumonias—cont'd

	Pneumococcal pneumonia	Staphylococcal pneumonia	Streptococcal pneumonia
Laboratory findings	Elevated white blood cell count—15,000-40,000/mm³ Positive sputum culture Positive blood culture in 30% of cases	Leukocytosis of 20,000/mm³ or more in older children; WBC count may be normal in infants Positive sputum culture Bacteremia in 10% of cases	Polymorphonuclear leukocytosis Blood cultures positive Elevated antistreptolysin O titer
Complications	Fibrinous pleurisy Pleural effusion Empyema Occasionally postpneumatic pneumatocele formation	Empyema Tension pneumothorax Pyopneumothorax	Pleural effusion Empyema in approximately 20% Streptococcal foci may appear in other areas, for example, bones
Clinical manifestations	Infants: Usually preceded by upper respiratory tract infection Fretfulness and diminished appetite followed by abrupt onset of fever, 39°-40.5° C (102°-105° F) May be accompanied by convulsions Restlessness Apprehension Respiratory distress Appears acutely ill Moderate to severe air hunger Flushed cheeks Circumoral cyanosis Physical—may be decreased breath sounds and crackling rales; exaggerated breath sounds on uninvolved side; pleural friction rub may be heard Older children: Usually follows an upper respiratory tract infection	Usually in infants less than age 1 year, often with history of staphylococcal skin lesion and preceded by upper respiratory tract manifestations Abrupt onset of fever, listlessness and lethargy when undisturbed, irritability on arousal, anorexia, nasal discharge, cough, grunting respirations, progressive and severe dyspnea that may include subcostal and sternal retractions and cyanosis Poor systemic perfusion may be present Symptoms of complications may appear, including pneumothorax, empyema, and septicemia Some infants have gastrointestinal disturbances, for example, vomiting, diarrhea, and sometimes abdominal distention	May appear without evidence of illness May follow streptococcal infection of upper respiratory tract or as complication of contagious disease Symptoms similar to those of pneumococcal pneumonia Onset sudden High temperature Chills Signs of respiratory distress At times, extreme prostration Occasionally, only mild symptoms Tachypnea usually mild Rales generally unilateral and exaggerated by deep inspiration

Table 4-17   Comparison of three common bacterial pneumonias—cont'd

	Pneumococcal pneumonia	Staphylococcal pneumonia	Streptococcal pneumonia
Clinical manifestations—cont'd	Shaking chills followed by high fever, 40°-40.5° C (104°-105° F) Chest pain Drowsiness with intermittent periods of restlessness Tachypnea Hacking, unproductive cough (initially) Anxiety Occasional delirium Circumoral cyanosis Splinting of side caused by pleurisy pain Physical—dullness; diminished breath sounds, tactile and vocal fremitus; consolidation on second or third day evidenced by dullness, increased fremitus, tubular breath sounds, and disappearance of rales With resolution—moist rales; productive cough with large amounts of blood-tinged mucus	Rapid progression of characteristic symptoms Physical findings—early, diminished breath sounds, rales, and rhonchi with effusion or pneumothorax; dullness on percussion; breath sounds diminished; respiratory lag on affected side; exaggerated excursion on opposite side; tubular breathing above fluid level and on unaffected side	

Antibiotic therapy	Pneumococcus highly susceptible to penicillin G:
	
	   Administered intravenously, intramuscularly, or orally
	   Continued 4-5 days after temperature returns to normal
	
	Alternate drugs—ampicillin, tetracycline, chloramphenicol, erythromycin, and sulfonamides
	
	Resolution begins about 24 hours after initiation of therapy
		Methicillin, parenterally
		
		Equally effective are oxacillin, cloxacillin, dicloxacillin, or nafcillin
		
		For penicillin-sensitive organisms, penicillin G may be given
		
		Duration of treatment usually 3 weeks
		
		If empyema—aspiration of empyema fluid and instillation of penicillin
		
		May require closed chest drainage
			Penicillin G (intravenous or intramuscular) is highly effective

Continued.

Table 4-17 Comparison of three common bacterial pneumonias—cont'd

	Pneumococcal pneumonia	Staphylococcal pneumonia	Streptococcal pneumonia
Prognosis	Good when recognized and treated early Mortality less than 1%; higher in debilitated children Rapid recovery with treatment	Prognosis ranges from 5% to 40% mortality and varies with length of illness before treatment Course is usually prolonged, often 6-10 weeks Early recognition and treatment usually effective	Variable in duration Roentgenographic findings may be seen for 3 or 4 weeks, with spontaneous resolution

spiratory infection develops. Children exhibit the following signs and symptoms as the result of a respiratory infection[2]:

1. *Fever.* The temperature can range between 39.4° and 40.6° C with mild infection when the child is 6 months to 3 years of age. Premature infants and newborns, however, may demonstrate a subnormal temperature or temperature instability that suggests the presence of an infection. A sudden increase in temperature to greater than 39° C may be associated with generalized seizure in a young child.
2. *Respiratory distress.* The child with respiratory infection usually demonstrates tachypnea, rapid shallow breathing, rales, rhonchi, and wheezing. The child with viral pneumonia may demonstrate hemoptysis and a productive cough.
3. *Behavior.* The child with respiratory infection usually demonstrates unusual irritability or lethargy; most sick children are irritable, but lethargy is an ominous symptom and warrants immediate evaluation.
4. *Gastrointestinal symptoms.* The child with respiratory infection frequently demonstrates anorexia, vomiting, and diarrhea. These symptoms may also accompany the onset of any infection in the young child. In addition, the child may develop abdominal pain as the result of vomiting or the presence of a pleural effusion.

The chest radiograph confirms the clinical impression of pneumonia and may suggest a specific pathogen. The child with lobar pneumonia may demonstrate a characteristic lobar infiltrate, while the child with viral pneumonia usually has diffuse infiltrates in one or both hilar regions. *Pneumocystis carinii* pneumonia produces a characteristic granular appearance over the lung fields bilaterally (see Fig. 5-15).

All attempts should be made to identify a specific pathogen when a child with respiratory infection is critically ill in order to institute appropriate antimicrobial therapy. Sputum, tracheal aspirate, pleural fluid, and tissue obtained by lung biopsy can all be examined with special stains and cultured for pathogens. Bacterial pathogens may be obtained from routine blood cultures.

■ **Medical treatment and nursing interventions**

When the nurse cares for the child with pneumonia, careful assessment of respiratory function and general supportive care should be performed. This assessment should include evaluation of respiratory rate and effort; it is important to note that a normal respiratory rate is not always appropriate for the child with pneumonia, since tachypnea is expected. Auscultation should be performed over all areas of the lung as part of the hourly assessment of the child; the nurse should pay particular attention to the presence of rales, rhonchi, or wheezing. Once any area of consolidation or congestion is identified, this area should be monitored carefully for evidence of clearing or worsening of the condition, and respiratory therapy should be directed specifically at these areas. Throughout the child's care, the nurse should carefully evaluate the child's color and amount of respiratory effort, and she should notify a physician if signs of deterioration appear.

The child whose respiratory distress is severe should receive nothing by mouth; intravenous and possibly arterial catheters may be inserted. Respiratory secretions from both the nose and mouth should be removed by suctioning if the child is unable to generate an effective cough. Vigorous chest physiotherapy with postural drainage may be needed if the child has difficulty expelling secretions; this physiotherapy should be performed at least every 4 hours. The child may be placed in a cold mist tent to aid in secretion removal if this therapy does not limit direct observation of the child's respiratory status. The child with unilateral pneumonia is positioned with the involved lobe on top to provide postural drainage; thus, too, the uninvolved lung is better perfused in the dependent position. The child with pneumonia may not be able to tolerate a head-down or side-lying position; therefore he may be propped up on pillows in bed or placed in an infant seat to maximize diaphragmatic excursion.

The child's body temperature should be monitored frequently so that excessive rises in temperature, which can increase oxygen requirements, can be treated with antipyretics. In addition, high fevers, which may produce a febrile seizure, should be avoided. The child with fever and tachypnea has a greater insensible water loss and may develop dehydration; consequently, fluid administration should be evaluated several times daily. The child's urine output and specific gravity must be measured carefully, and the urine output should average approximately 1 ml/kg/hour if fluid intake is adequate.

Often antimicrobial therapy is begun before pathogen isolation if the child is critically ill. In these cases three or four antibiotics may be used until the culture and sensitivity tests demonstrate the specific etiologic agent of the infection. Once the specific organism is identified, appropriate antibiotics are administered. Children with bacterial pneumonia are usually isolated until they have received 24 hours of antibiotic therapy. These children should not be placed in a critical-care unit among children recovering from major surgery. Viral pneumonias are usually not treated with antibiotics unless secondary bacterial infection results, and thus they do not require isolation.

Some complications of pneumonia (especially staphylococcal pneumonia) include the development of empyema, pleural effusion, pyopneumothorax, and tension pneumothorax. If fluid has accumulated in the chest as detected by auscultation and chest radiograph, a thoracentesis is performed and the fluid obtained is cultured. Continuous chest drainage may be necessary when purulent fluid is aspirated.[30]

Once the child's respiratory status is stable, nu-tritious oral fluids can be offered, and the IV fluid administration rate should be reduced accordingly. As the child continues to improve, he can receive a diet appropriate for his age.

Whenever the child develops an acute respiratory infection, both the child and family will probably be extremely anxious. The anxiety of the child can be increased by the presence of hypoxemia or hypercapnia. Throughout the child's care, it is necessary that the nurse provide consistent information and support. Once the child is more stable, quiet diversional activities appropriate for the youngster's age should be planned. As the patient becomes more active, the nurse should assess his activity tolerance and report any evidence of increased respiratory distress to a physician.

■ **ASPIRATION PNEUMONIA**
■ **Etiology**

Aspiration pneumonia occurs when food, secretions, or volatile compounds enter the lung and cause inflammation or a chemical pneumonitis. Most cases of aspiration pneumonia occur when there is impaired consciousness or impaired neuromuscular control of swallowing.

■ **Pathophysiology**

Aspiration pneumonia may appear in any lung segment, and it may be acute or chronic. Usually, it is clinically impossible to distinguish between infection and inflammation, since respiratory distress, pulmonary infiltrates, and pulmonary symptoms are identical.

■ **Clinical signs and symptoms**

Aspiration of gastric contents can cause severe distress as a result of the volume of material aspirated, its acidity, the distribution of the aspirated material, and the presence or absence of bacteria. In the critical-care unit, the substance most commonly aspirated is gastric content.

The severity of the lung injury increases as the pH of the aspirated material decreases.[5] Coughing and vomiting usually occur immediately after aspiration. This may be accompanied by tachypnea, dyspnea, and cyanosis. More severe aspiration may produce pulmonary hemorrhage, necrosis, surfactant impairment, and pulmonary edema. If spontaneous ventilation becomes insufficient, intubation and provision of ventilatory support may be necessary.

The chest radiograph may not be a useful diagnostic tool immediately following the aspiration event. The presence of a normal chest radiograph and normal breath sounds do not rule out the possibility of aspiration pneumonia; within 2 to 4 hours after the suspected aspiration, the chest radiograph may begin to show evidence of diffuse alveolar or interstitial pulmonary infiltrates.

■ Medical treatment and nursing interventions

Many episodes of aspiration occur when lethargic or tachypneic patients are carelessly or inappropriately fed or when critically ill infants are overfed. Thus prevention of aspiration pneumonia is most important. Infants and debilitated children should be positioned on their abdomen or with their right side down following feedings to minimize the possibility of aspiration and to promote stomach emptying. The head of the child's bed should be elevated during and after every feeding. When nasogastric feedings are administered with an infusion pump, the child needs to be monitored carefully, since an infusion pump will continue to infuse the feeding material even when the child is vomiting. If it is necessary to administer feedings through an infusion pump, a Y system should be constructed so that there is a vent in the event the child vomits. The feeding should be administered slowly and the child monitored carefully after the feeding is completed. To promote expulsion of air from the stomach and to allow a vent in case vomiting does occur, the nasogastric tube should remain vented to air after the feedings. Before the next feeding the nasogastric tube should be aspirated so that residual undigested feedings can be measured. If the child continues to have significant amounts of residual formula between each feeding, the volume or the concentration of the formula may need to be reduced.

Treatment of aspiration pneumonia is largely supportive, and it includes administration of chest physiotherapy, suctioning, and oxygen. Since there are no reliable guidelines for antibiotic therapy for such patients, the use of these drugs is determined by clinical judgment.[6]

■ Common Diagnostic Tests

There are many pulmonary function tests that are clinically useful. However, most are impractical for use in the critical-care setting because they require maximum efforts from cooperative patients. This section focuses only on those tests performed on critically ill children.

■ PHYSICAL EXAMINATION

The most important diagnostic tool for assessment of respiratory function is the physical examination. A great deal of information can be gained by merely watching the child's behavior and noting his position of comfort. The nurse must know the physical findings normal for the child's age as well as typical physical signs of the patient's disease.

■ CHEST RADIOGRAPH

The chest radiograph is utilized frequently to evaluate pulmonary status in the critically ill child (see Chapter 5 for a detailed discussion of the radiologic examination).

■ BRONCHOSCOPY

Bronchoscopy allows direct visualization of the larynx and larger airways. Emergency bronchoscopy is usually indicated when epiglottitis or foreign-body aspiration is suspected. Bronchoscopy may also be used to evaluate chronically intubated patients for the presence of subglottic stenosis. In addition, the procedure provides an excellent opportunity for obtaining tracheal secretions for culture, although upper airway contamination can occur. Lavage of the tracheobronchial tree may also be performed during bronchoscopy.

A bronchoscopy is generally performed in the operating room after induction of general anesthesia. However, since flexible fiberoptic bronchoscopes are now available, bedside bronchoscopy may also be performed. The typical fiberscope for bronchoscopy cannot be used in children under approximately 11 years of age because it is too large to fit in the child's small airways. Fiberoptic bronchoscopes are smaller in size and thus do not occlude the small child's airways; they can also be used to view the airway of a critically ill child without interruption of the child's ventilation. The fiberoptic bronchoscope, generally more flexible, can be introduced either nasally or orally. When the child receives mechanical ventilation, the bronchoscopy may be performed through use of a special T adaptor so that an airtight seal may be maintained at the attachment to the ventilator during the procedure.

Before bronchoscopy the child (if age appropriate) and the family will require an explanation of the procedure. Since the procedure requires general anesthesia, the youngster will receive nothing by mouth for 4 to 6 hours before bronchoscopy. If the child is critically ill, dehydrated, or has cyanotic heart disease, an IV line may be inserted to maintain hydration preoperatively.

The critically ill child undergoing a bronchoscopy should be carefully monitored throughout the procedure. Cardiovascular status and pulmonary function must be carefully assessed, and supplemental oxygen and humidity should be provided both during and after the procedure for any child with hypoxemia.

Complications of bronchoscopy are rare, and they include laryngospasm, hemoptysis, and vocal cord injury. In addition, since bronchoscopy may traumatize the larynx, it may produce edema and upper airway obstruction. Therefore, it is important that the child be assessed for development of bronchospasm as indicated by the presence of a cough, hoarseness, and cyanosis. If the child is not intubated, the physician may order a mist tent or extra humidity by face mask in an effort to minimize the development of laryngeal edema.

Children often complain of a sore throat immediately following the procedure and may initially have difficulty in swallowing. As soon as the child is able to swallow, clear liquids may be provided. If the youngster demonstrates drooling or persistent coughing, oral fluids may be withheld until these respiratory symptoms disappear. Once the child has completely recovered from general anesthesia and has demonstrated tolerance of a clear liquid diet, he may resume a regular diet. Chest physiotherapy is usually appropriate following the procedure.

■ **EVALUATION OF PULMONARY FUNCTION**
■ **Direct and indirect assessment of arterial blood gases**

The adequacy of gas exchange is best evaluated by measuring the pH, P_{O_2}, and P_{CO_2} of arterial blood. It is also possible to assess "arterialized" capillary samples, but the analysis of Pa_{O_2} by this method is not as reliable, since it is greatly influenced by the perfusion of the sampled capillary bed.

The vessels most frequently used for blood gas analysis include the temporal artery in neonates and the brachial, radial, and femoral arteries in infants and children. The brachial and radial arteries are preferred sites for arterial blood sampling, since arterial spasm occurs more commonly if the femoral artery is used. Since an arterial puncture may produce pain and cause anxiety, the blood gas measurements obtained by intermittent sampling in this manner can be unreliable. As a result, arterial catheters should be placed in those children with severe cardiorespiratory disease that require close observation.

Placement of an indwelling arterial cannula is necessary when the child requires serial blood gas determinations. However, complications such as ischemia, bleeding, infection, and air emboli can occur (see Chapter 9 for additional information about arterial catheterization).

Arterial blood gas analysis. An arterial blood sample can be collected in either a plastic or glass syringe. Since the development of the "micro-method" of blood gas analysis, as little as 0.2 ml of blood may be adequate for blood gas analysis. If the blood gas specimen will be obtained by arterial puncture, a small-gauge needle or a "butterfly" needle can be used for the puncture. The syringe and the needle should always be rinsed with a small amount of sodium heparin (1000 U/ml), although only a drop of heparin should be left at the syringe tip. Even this amount of liquid can lower the pH and the P_{CO_2} of the sample, so that in some centers syringes containing heparin powder are used for blood gas measurements. A local anesthetic (1% to 2% lidocaine) can be administered immediately over the artery to minimize the child's discomfort during the arterial puncture; however, only small volumes of lidocaine are administered, since large volumes can produce arterial spasm.

The arterial puncture is made at an angle of approximately 45 degrees, and the artery is entered with the bevel of the needle pointed downward. As the artery is entered, blood will appear in the syringe. As already noted, a quantity of 0.2 to 0.5 ml should be sufficient for blood gas analysis by the "micro-method." The arterial puncture site should be covered with dry gauze immediately after removal of the needle, and pressure should be applied for at least 5 minutes to ensure that all bleeding has ceased. If a femoral arterial puncture is performed, pressure should be applied for approximately 5 to 15 minutes.

When the arterial sample is obtained, the tube and syringe should contain absolutely no air bubbles, since the room air will equilibrate with the blood specimen and produce errors in the P_{O_2} and P_{CO_2}. As soon as the needle is removed from the vessel, the syringe should be sealed by placing a rubber stopper over the tip to prevent air from entering the tube or syringe. The syringe is rotated to mix the blood with the heparin so that the specimen is uniformly heparinized. Some centers use small pieces of metal called "fleas" in the "micro-tubes." The fleas are put into the tube after the specimen is obtained but before sealing the tube. A magnet is then run over the length of the tube and the heparin is thus mixed with the blood by the metal flea. The metal flea is then removed and the tube sealed.

The blood gas sample should be placed on ice for transport to the blood gas laboratory; because ice slows blood metabolism, the blood gases will be more accurate. Any blood specimen should be analyzed immediately for the most accurate results. If the specimen is not sent to the laboratory within a few minutes, it probably should be redrawn.

Complications of arterial puncture include arterial spasm or hematoma formation; these can produce subsequent occlusion of the artery and compromise of perfusion to the distal extremity.

Capillary sampling for blood gas analysis. Because arterial punctures are sometimes difficult to obtain in infants, capillary samples are often taken. Although an accurate P_{CO_2} and pH can be obtained with a capillary sample, the P_{O_2} will usually be lower than the child's Pa_{O_2}. When the youngster has decreased perfusion of the extremities because of hypothermia or shock, the capillary P_{O_2} will probably not accurately reflect the Pa_{O_2}.

The best area for the capillary stick is one that is highly vascularized. The infant's heel, earlobe, or a large finger or toe is usually tapped. The area must be prewarmed with a warm towel, heat lamp, or warm moist pack for 10 minutes before the tap to encourage blood flow to the area, thus "arterializing" the capillary blood. A puncture wound is made with a lance or scalpel blade so that blood flows freely from the puncture site. Squeezing of the sample area is to be avoided since it will encourage venous blood to mix with the capillary blood. Fig. 4-11 illustrates the circulation of the infant's heel. The best blood gas speci-

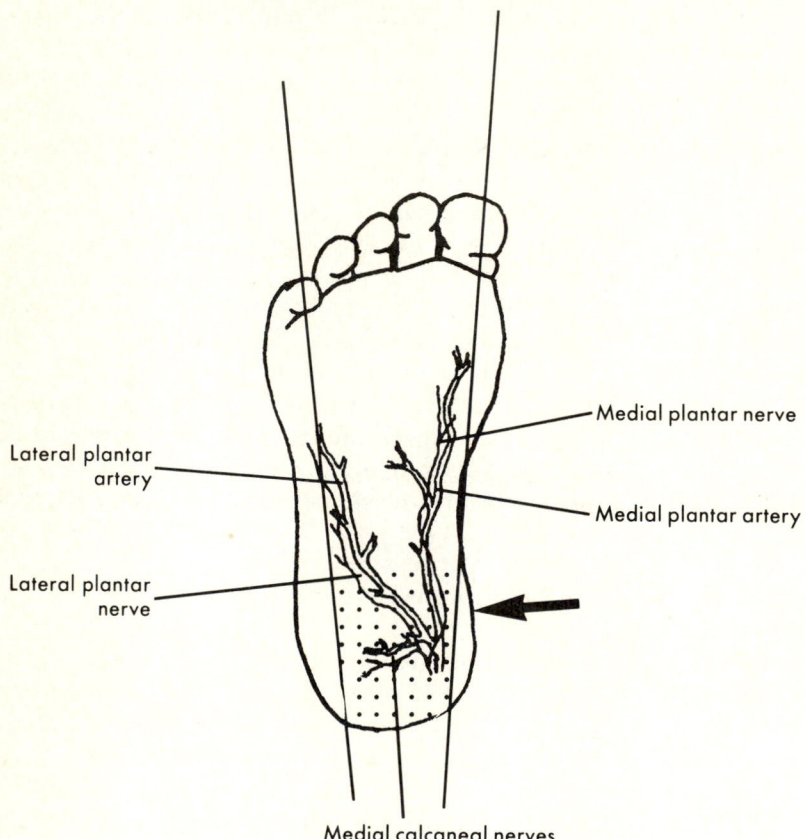

Lateral plantar artery

Lateral plantar nerve

Medial plantar nerve

Medial plantar artery

Medial calcaneal nerves

Fig. 4-11 Vascular anatomy of the infant foot. Heel-stick blood samples for blood gas analysis are best obtained from the medial aspect of the heel *(arrow)*, since this area is highly vascular. To avoid direct injury to the calcaneous or the medial calcaneal nerves, the bottom of the heel should be avoided *(shaded area).* This area can be identified by drawing imaginary vertical lines along the length of the infant's foot—from the middle of the first and fifth toes; the area of the heel between these two lines must be avoided.

mens are obtained by tapping the medial portion of the heel because this area is more highly vascular. Heel-stick capillary blood specimens should not be obtained after the infant has begun walking since calluses have formed on the heel, making the puncture more difficult; in addition, the child may develop an infection once he again begins to walk on the foot.

To obtain the specimen, a preheparinized 0.2 ml capillary tube is used. Once the free-flowing blood has been collected in the tube, the tube is sealed and placed on ice.

Complications from repeated capillary sticks are rare; however, infection may occur if the area is not cleansed properly before the puncture. Osteomyelitis has been reported in neonates after only one or two heel punctures.

Venous samples. Venous blood may be used for blood gas analysis, but interpretation of the P_{O_2} and P_{CO_2} is very difficult. The venous pH may sometimes be helpful, although it is usually significantly lower than arterial pH in critically ill patients.

Pulmonary artery samples. Pulmonary artery blood obtained through a pulmonary artery catheter provides a true mixed venous blood sample. If arterial blood and pulmonary artery blood are obtained and analyzed simultaneously, the arterial-venous oxygen (a-vO_2) content difference can be calculated using the Fick equation (see the discussion on assessment of low cardiac output in Chapter 3). The difference between these two numbers is inversely proportional to the cardiac output; that is, if the a-vO_2 difference is small, the cardiac output is high. Conversely, if the a-vO_2 difference is large or is increasing, cardiac output is low or falling. The normal a-vO_2 content difference ranges from 4.5 to 6.0 volumes percent. A critically ill child with excellent cardiovascular reserves will have an a-vO_2 difference in the range of 2.5 to 4.5 volumes percent. However, a critically ill child with low cardiac output from whatever cause will have an a-vO_2 difference greater than 6.0 volumes percent.

Skin surface (transcutaneous) P_{O_2} and P_{CO_2}. The most reliable method for assessment of the partial pressure of oxygen and carbon dioxide in the body is through analysis of an arterial blood sample; however, in recent years, a new technique has been introduced that is almost as reliable as blood gas analysis. The skin P_{O_2} and P_{CO_2} monitor can be used to estimate, continuously and noninvasively, changes in Pa_{O_2} and Pa_{CO_2}. These devices are modifications of conventional blood gas electrodes that are used to measure arterial blood gases.[10,17] This technique operates on the principle that small amounts of oxygen and carbon dioxide diffuse through the skin. The device warms the skin beneath the electrode membrane

to a temperature of 44° to 45° C; lower temperatures are sometimes used in premature infants. As a result of the warming, the capillaries located beneath the electrode dilate and the arteriovenous connections within the capillary bed open so that the oxygen and carbon dioxide tensions of the heated blood beneath the membrane reach arterial levels. In general, the skin surface P_{O_2} is less than the Pa_{O_2}, particularly in older patients. The skin surface P_{CO_2} is usually 40% to 60% higher than the Pa_{CO_2} in all patients and is not dependent on age or sampling site.[10,14]

The basic requirements for a reliable skin surface oxygen and carbon dioxide sensor system include the following: (1) measurement of specific gases, with no interference from other gases, (2) uniform heat transfer across the sensing area, (3) drift of less than ±5 mm Hg for 24 hours, (4) a machine with mechanical and electrical integrity, and (5) ability to eliminate discrepancies between the transcutaneous and arterial P_{O_2} and P_{CO_2} resulting from hypoperfusion or other factors.

The skin electrodes must be calibrated before each use and applied to skin that is clean, dry, and hairless, such as the abdomen or ventral forearm. The skin should be prepared before application of the electrode. The electrode must be removed at least every 3 to 6 hours and reapplied in another location; the machine must also be recalibrated at these intervals.

Thus far, several instruments are available for simultaneous measurement of P_{O_2} and P_{CO_2}. Since the cost of these instruments is now reasonable, they are standard equipment in most critical-care units (see the discussion of skin-surface monitoring in Chapter 9).

■ **End-tidal carbon dioxide ($P_{et}CO_2$)**

The amount of carbon dioxide in the exhaled air can be measured continuously with a variety of devices. The P_{CO_2} at the end of expiration is approximately equal to the alveolar P_{CO_2}; in patients with normal lungs the alveolar P_{CO_2} is the same as the Pa_{CO_2}. As a result, measurement of $P_{et}CO_2$ may be utilized in lieu of repeated Pa_{CO_2} measurements during weaning of patients from ventilators and during care of children with chronic lung disease.

To measure $P_{et}CO_2$ in intubated patients, a sampling catheter is inserted into the expiratory ventilator tubing, near its junction with the ET tube. Then a small sample of exhaled air is analyzed continuously, using an infrared carbon dioxide sensor or a mass spectrometer. If the patient is breathing spontaneously, the sampling catheter can be placed just inside the nostril or tracheostomy stoma.

While it is relatively simple to measure P_{CO_2}, it is extremely difficult to obtain a true alveolar gas sample (uncontaminated by dead-space gas or ambient air). If measurements of $P_{et}CO_2$ is to be utilized, a simultaneous measurement of the Pa_{CO_2} and the $P_{et}CO_2$ is usually obtained in order initially to assess the relationship between these two measurements.

Although many devices can measure the peak P_{CO_2} of exhaled air, the result may or may not be representative of the alveolar (and arterial) P_{CO_2}. If the patient has severe lung disease, the $P_{et}CO_2$ does not plateau but varies widely during expiration; as a result, it will be difficult to determine which measurement to use.

In general, changes in the $P_{et}CO_2$ accurately reflect trends in the child's Pa_{CO_2}, even if a significant lung disease is present. However, if the patient has severe pulmonary interstitial disease, the $P_{et}CO_2$ correlates poorly with the Pa_{CO_2}.[45]

■ Assessment of lung volumes and flows

Tidal volume. Simple measurements of various lung volumes and capacities can be performed at the bedside to provide an objective estimate of the child's respiratory status (see the beginning of this chapter). The measurement of tidal volume is an easy procedure and can be done by the nurse at the bedside. This measurement, together with assessment of respiratory rate on a serial basis, can provide an indication of inspiratory effort and tidal volume.

To measure tidal volume at the bedside, a hand-held spirometer may be used. A mouthpiece is applied to the spirometer, and the child is asked to breathe normally through the mouthpiece. A needle indicator then instantly records the inspiratory tidal volume. The child should breathe for a full minute. Then to obtain the average inspiratory tidal volume, the total volume recorded is divided by the respiratory rate. If the child is intubated, the spirometer can be easily attached to the ET tube or to the ventilator tubing. A normal predicted tidal volume is 6 to 7 cc/kg. A tidal volume of less than 4 to 5 cc/kg may indicate an inadequate inspiratory effort to sustain spontaneous ventilation, or it may indicate the presence of upper airway obstruction or a decreased lung compliance. It is extremely important to note that the measurement of a normal tidal volume does not exclude the presence of severe restrictive lung disease. As a result, this test is not clinically useful as a predictor of severity of pulmonary symptoms.

Several devices are available for spirometry measurement; one of the most widely used is the Wright Respirometer. The Dräger Volumeter and the Bourns LS-75 Ventilation Monitor are also available. If the child refuses to cooperate, assessment of the tidal volume may be difficult or impossible. Since these bedside tests (even when they are accurately performed) require a great deal of patient effort, the results can be highly misleading.

Vital capacity. The vital capacity is the maximum amount of air that can be exhaled after a maximum inspiratory effort. Predicted values related to the child's sex and height are available. This forced expiratory volume measurement is best evaluated in a cooperative patient.

A hand-held spirometer attached to a mouthpiece or the child's ET tube or a mask can be used to measure the child's vital capacity. The child is instructed to take the deepest inspiration possible and then, with spirometer attached, to exhale the air as quickly, forcefully, and completely as possible.

Normal vital capacity is approximately 65 to 75 cc/kg. Children with significant respiratory disease usually have a vital capacity of approximately 15 to 30 cc/kg; those children with a vital capacity of less than 15 cc/kg usually require assisted ventilation.[45] If the measured vital capacity is low, this may result from inadequate effort on the part of the child or from loss of exhaled air as a result of loose seal around the airway or the patient's mask. These errors in measurement can result in underestimation of the child's vital capacity.[12]

Inspiratory occlusion pressure. A measurement of inspiratory force is occasionally made in patients with neuromuscular disease or in patients who are to be weaned from ventilatory support. The measurement can be made while the child is mechanically ventilated or while he is breathing through a mask. Inspiration is then prevented through either occlusion of the inspiratory tubing of the ventilator or occlusion of the inspiratory port on the mask; then the maximum negative inspiratory pressure generated by the child is measured through use of a standard pressure transducer. Normal inspiratory force is a negative pressure of approximately 75 to 100 cm H_2O. The child with significant respiratory disease can often only generate a negative inspiratory force totaling approximately 25 to 50 cm H_2O. The child usually requires assisted ventilation if the negative inspiratory force totals less than 20 cm H_2O.[45] Since this measurement also requires patient cooperation, it is subject to error.

Static and dynamic lung compliance. Lung compliance is defined as the change in lung volume per unit change in transpulmonary pressure when the lungs are motionless. In the pulmonary function laboratory, volume is measured by a spirometer, and transpulmonary pressure is measured through use of an esophageal catheter. The units of compliance are ml/cm H_2O.[12]

Clinically, the compliance of the lung and the chest wall are often measured together. The best way to measure total compliance in a ventilated patient is as follows. Inspiratory hold is applied after a known volume is delivered by the ventilator (this can be done by occluding the exhalation tubing). The pressure measured at that volume is recorded and then the tidal volume is divided by the measured pressure. This reflects the static lung compliance.

Dynamic compliance is defined as the tidal volume divided by the peak inspiratory pressure. This represents the ratio of change in volume to change in pressure between the points of zero flow at the end of inspiration and expiration. In healthy children the values for static and dynamic compliance are similar. Measurement of dynamic lung compliance can be useful in detecting pneumothorax when the patient is ventilated with a volume-cycled ventilator. In these patients, higher pressures than normal are needed to deliver the desired tidal volume because their lung compliance is decreased.

■ Conclusion

While all of these diagnostic tests may be clinically useful, it should be reemphasized that *physical examination and arterial blood gas analysis provide the most rapid, complete, and objective estimate of pulmonary function.* The nurse should learn to correctly obtain and handle the arterial blood gas specimens and to accurately interpret the results.

REFERENCES

1. American Academy of Pediatrics, Section on Allergy and Immunology: Management of asthma, Pediatrics **68:**874, 1981.
2. Conn, A.W., Edmonds, J.F., and Barker, G.H.: Cerebral resuscitation in near-drowning, Pediatr. Clin. North Am. **26:**691, 1979.
3. Cotton, E., and Parry, W.: Treatment of status asthmaticus and respiratory failure, Pediatr. Clin. North Am. **22:**163, 1975.
4. Crone, R.K.: Assisted ventilation in children. In Gregory, G.A., editor: Respiratory failure in the child, New York, 1981, Churchill Livingstone.
5. Dobrin, R.S.: Perspectives in the management of the child with aspiration and pneumonia. In Gregory, G.A., editor: Respiratory failure in the child, New York, 1981, Churchill Livingstone.
6. Downes, J.J., and Heiser, M.S.: Status asthmaticus in children. In Gregory, G.A., editor: Respiratory failure in the child, New York, 1981, Churchill Livingstone.
7. Duncun, P.G.: Management of upper airway disease in children. In Gregory, G.A., editor: Respiratory failure in the child, New York, 1981, Churchill Livingstone.
8. Farrell, P.M., and Perelman, R.H.: The developmental biology of the lung. In Fanaroff, A.A., and Martin, R.J., editors: Behrman's neonatal-perinatal medicine: diseases of the fetus and infant, ed. 3, St. Louis, 1983, The C.V. Mosby Co.
9. Finer, N.N., and Stewart, A.R.: Continuous transcutaneous oxygen monitoring in the critically ill neonate, Crit. Care Med. **8:**319, 1980.
10. Finer, N.N., and others: Post-extubation atelectasis: a retrospective review and a prospective controlled study, J. Pediatr. **94:**110, 1979.
11. Fox, W.W., and Shaffer, T.H.: Assessment of pulmonary function. In Fanaroff, A.A., and Martin, R.J., editors, Behrman's neonatal-perinatal medicine: diseases of the fetus and infant, ed. 3, St. Louis, 1983, The C.V. Mosby Co.
12. Froese, A.B.: Preoperative evaluation of pulmonary function, Pediatr. Clin. North Am. **26:**645, 1979.
13. Hazinski, M.F.: Near-drowning. In Johanson, B.C., and others, editors: Standards for critical care, ed. 2, St. Louis, 1984, The C.V. Mosby Co.
14. Hazinski, T.A., and Severinghaus, J.W.: Transcutaneous analysis of arterial P_{CO_2}, J. Med. Instrumentation **16:**150, 1982.
15. Hughes, J., editor: Synopsis of pediatrics, ed. 5, St. Louis, 1980, The C.V. Mosby Co.
16. Inselman, L.S., and Mellins, R.B.: Growth and development of the lung, J. Pediatr. **98:**1, 1981.
17. Kendig, E., editor: Disorders of the respiratory tract in children, ed. 4, Philadelphia, 1983, W.B. Saunders Co.
18. Levin, R.: Pediatric respiratory intensive care handbook, New York, 1976, Medical Examination Publishing Co.
19. Loper-Hunter, D.: The beginnings of the respiratory system, Neonatal Network **1:**19, Oct. 1982.
20. Martin, R.J., Fanaroff, A.A., and Skalina, M.E.L.: The respiratory distress syndrome and its management. In Fanaroff, A.A., and Martin, R.J., editors: Behrman's neonatal-perinatal medicine: disease of the fetus and infant, ed. 3, St. Louis, 1983, The C.V. Mosby Co.
21. Milner, A.D.: Changing concepts in asthma, Arch. Dis. Child. **53:**525, 1978.
22. Muller, N.L., and Bryan, A.C.: Chest wall mechanics and respiratory muscles in infants, Pediatr. Clin. North Am. **26:**503, 1979.
23. Newth, C.J.L.: Recognition and management of respiratory failure, Pediatr. Clin. North Am. **26:**617, 1979.
24. Orlowski, J.P., and others: Complications of airway intrusion in 100 consecutive cases in a pediatric ICU, Crit. Care Med. **8:**324, 1980.
25. Pearn, J.: Drowning in Australia: a national appraisal with particular reference to children, Med. J. Aust. **2:**770, 1977.
26. Perkin, R.M., and Levin, D.L.: Adverse effects of positive-pressure ventilation in children. In Gregory, G.A., editor: Respiratory failure in the child, New York, 1981, Churchill Livingstone.

27. Pfenninger, J., and others: Adult respiratory distress syndrome in children, J. Pediatr. **101**:352, 1979.
28. Pinney, M.: Foreign body aspiration, Am. J. Nurs. **81**:521, 1981.
29. Pinney, M.: Pneumonia, Am. J. Nurs. **81**:517, 1981.
30. Raffensperger, J.G., and others: Mini-thoracotomy and chest tube insertion for children with empyema, J. Thorac. Cardiovasc. Surg. **84**:497, 1982.
31. Rowe, M., Arango, A., and Allington, G.: Profile of pediatric drowning victims in a water-oriented society, J. Trauma **17**:587, 1977.
32. Scarpelli, E.M., Auld, P., and Goldman, H.S.: Pulmonary disease of the fetus, newborn, and child, Philadelphia, 1978, Lea & Febiger.
33. Shapiro, B., Harrison, R., and Walton, J.R.: Clinical application of respiratory care, ed. 3, Chicago, 1982, Year Book Medical Publishers, Inc.
34. Shugar, J.M.A., Biller, H.F., and Som, P.M.: Pediatric airway obstruction, Surgical Rounds **11**:56, Aug. 1980.
35. Simkins, R.: Asthma and reactive airways disease, Am. J. Nurs. **81**:523, 1981.
36. Simkins, R.: Croup and epiglottitis, Am. J. Nurs. **81**:519, 1981.
37. Skelley, B.F., Deeren, S.M., and Powaser, M.M.: The effectiveness of two preoxygenation methods to prevent endotracheal suction-induced hypoxemia, Heart Lung **9**:313, 1980.
38. Stahlman, M.T.: Clinical description of bronchopulmonary dysplasia, J. Pediatr. **8**:829, 1979.
39. Tooley, W.H.: Lung disease and lung development. In Hodson, W.A., editor: Development of the lung, New York, 1977, Marcel Dekker, Inc.
40. Tooley, W.H.: Epidemiology of bronchopulmonary dysplasia, J. Pediatr. **85**:851, 1979.
41. Voyles, J.B.: Bronchopulmonary dysplasia, Am. J. Nurs. **81**:510, 1981.
42. West, J.B.: Gas transport to the periphery. In Respiratory physiology: the essentials, ed. 2, Baltimore, 1979, Williams & Wilkins.
43. West, J.B.: Mechanical ventilation. In Pulmonary pathophysiology—the essentials, ed. 2, Baltimore, 1982, Williams & Wilkins.
44. West, J.B.: Respiratory failure. In Pulmonary pathophysiology: the essentials, ed. 2, Baltimore, 1982, Williams & Wilkins.
45. Yeh, T.S., and Holbrook, P.R.: Monitoring during assisted ventilation of children. In Gregory, G.A., editor: Respiratory failure in the child, New York, 1981, Churchill Livingstone.

BIBLIOGRAPHY

Embryology, anatomy, and physiology

Burton, G., Gee, G., and Hodgkins, J.: Respiratory care: guide to clinical practice, Philadelphia, 1977, J.B. Lippincott Co.
Comroe, J., and others: The lung, Chicago, 1962, Year Book Medical Publishers, Inc.

Doershuk, C., Fisher, B., and Matthews, L.: Pulmonary physiology of the fetus, infant and child, Philadelphia, 1975, Lea & Febiger.
Ganong, W.F.: Review of medical physiology, ed. 4, Los Altos, Calif., 1982, Lange Medical Publishers, Inc.
Harper, R.: A guide to respiratory care: physiology and clinical application, Philadelphia, 1981, J.B. Lippincott Co.
Moore, K.: Before we are born, Philadelphia, 1977, W.B. Saunders Co.
Nunn, J.F.: Applied respiratory physiology, Boston, 1977, Butterworth Co.
Shapiro, B.: Clinical application of blood gases, Chicago, 1979, Year Book Medical Publishers, Inc.
Shapiro, B., Harrison, R., and Trout, C.: Clinical application of respiratory care, ed. 3, Chicago, 1982, Year Book Medical Publishers, Inc.
West, J.B.: Respiratory physiology: the essentials, ed. 2, Baltimore, 1979, Williams & Wilkins.

Diagnostic tests

Bone, R.: Compliance and dynamic characteristic curves in acute respiratory failure, Crit. Care. Med. **4**:84, July-Aug. 1976.
Bone, R.: Thoracic pressure: volume curves in respiratory failure, Crit. Care Med. **4**:84, July-Aug. 1976.
Fink, R., Doershuk, C., and Orenstein, D.: Significance of pulmonary function and exercise tests. In Lough, M., editor: Pediatric respiratory therapy, Chicago, 1979, Year Book Medical Publishers, Inc.
MacDonnell, K., and Segal, M.: Current respiratory care, Boston, 1977, Little, Brown & Co.
McBride, J., and Wohl, M.: Pulmonary function tests, Pediatr. Clin. North Am. **26**:3, Aug. 1979.
Polgar, G., and Promadhat, V.: Pulmonary function testing in children, Philadelphia, 1971, W.B. Saunders Co.
Waring, W.: Diagnostic and therapeutic procedures. In Kendig, E., editor: Diseases of the respiratory tract in children, ed. 4, Philadelphia, 1983, W.B. Saunders Co.

Diseases

Barker, G.: Current management of croup and epiglottitis, Pediatr. Clin. North Am. **26**:3, Aug. 1979.
Dunsky, E.: Bronchiolitis differentiated from infantile asthma, Pediatr. Ann. **6**:7, July 1977.
Eigen, H.: Croup or epiglottitis: differential diagnosis and treatment, Respir. Care **20**:12, Dec. 1975.
Gregory, G.: Respiratory care of the child, Crit. Care Med. **8**:10, Oct. 1980.
Holsclaw, D.: Early recognition of acute respiratory failure in children, Pediatr. Ann. **6**:7, July 1977.
Holsclaw, D.: Pediatric pulmonary disease: an overview, Pediatr. Ann. **6**:27, July 1977.
Kattan, M.: Long-term sequelae of respiratory illness in infants and childhood, Pediatr. Clin. North Am. **26**:3, Aug. 1979.
Kendig, E.L., and Chernick, V., editors: Diseases of the respiratory tract in children, ed. 4, Philadelphia, 1983, W.B. Saunders Co.

Landau, L.: Outpatient evaluation and management of asthma, Pediatr. Clin. North Am. **26:**3, Aug. 1979.

Laraga, K., and Causay, L.: Pulmonary sequelae of acute respiratory viral infections, Pediatr. Ann. **7:**42, 1978.

Lochart, C., and Battaglia, J.: Croup and epiglottitis, Pediatr. Ann. **6:**77, April 1977.

Moore, G.: Acute respiratory failure. In Levin, D., Morriss, F.C., and Moore, G.C., editors: A practical guide to pediatric intensive care, ed. 2, St. Louis, 1984, The C.V. Mosby Co.

Moore, G.: Near drowning. In Levin, D., Morriss, F.C., and Moore, G.C., editors: A practical guide to pediatric intensive care, ed. 2, St. Louis, 1984, The C.V. Mosby Co.

Report of Workshop of Bronchopulmonary Dysplasia, Washington, D.C., 1978, U.S. Government Printing Office.

Scarpelli, E.M., Auld, P., and Goldman, H.S.: Pulmonary diseases of the fetus, newborn, and child, Philadelphia, 1978, Lea & Febiger.

Scoggin, C., Sahn, S., and Petty, T.: Status asthmaticus, JAMA **238:**11, Sept. 1977.

Shaw, L., and Mansmann, H.: Decisions in the evaluation and treatment of acute viral croup, Pediatr. Ann. **6:**7, July 1977.

Stalcup, S., and Mellens, R.: Mechanical tones produced pulmonary edema in acute asthma, N. Engl. J. Med. **297:**592, 1977.

Todd, J.: Pneumonia in children, Postgrad. Med. J. **61:**251, 1977.

Voyles, J., and others: Pulmonary problems in infants and children, Am. J. Nurs., March 1981.

Waring, W.: Respiratory diseases in chidren: an overview, Respir. Care **20:**12, Dec. 1975.

Respiratory therapy

Frownfelter, D., editor: Chest physical therapy and pulmonary rehabilitation: an interdisciplinary approach, Chicago, 1978, Year Book Medical Publishers, Inc.

Levison, H., editor: The chest, Pediatr. Clin. North Am. **26:**3, Aug. 1979.

Lough, M., Williams, T., and Rawsen, J.: Newborn respiratory care, Chicago, 1979, Year Book Medical Publishers, Inc.

Lough, M., Doershuk, C., and Stern, R.: Pediatric respiratory therapy, Chicago, 1979, Year Book Medical Publishers, Inc.

Keens, T.: Exercise training programs for pediatric patients with chronic lung disease, Pediatr. Clin. North Am. **26:**3, Aug. 1979.

Walters, P.: Chest physiotherapy. In Levin, D., Morriss, F.C., and Moore, G.C., editors: A practical guide to pediatric intensive care, ed. 2, St. Louis, 1984, The C.V. Mosby Co.

Buyer Information

Babybird ventilator, Bird Corp., Palm Springs, Calif.

Bourns infant ventilator, Bourns Life Systems, Riverside, Calif.

MVP-10 Pediatric Ventilator, Bio-Med Division, Stamford, Conn.

Ventilation

Boros, S.: Mechanical ventilation of newborn infants: an overview. In Lough, M., editor: Newborn respiratory care, Chicago, 1979, Year Book Medical Pubishers, Inc.

Heironimus, T.W., and Bageant, R.: Mechanical artificial ventilation, Springfield, Ill., 1977, Charles C Thomas, Publisher.

Inselman, L., and others: Mechanical ventilation in the neonate, Pediatr. Ann. **7:**4, April 1978.

Jones, M., and Murton, L.: Mechanical ventilation in newborn infants with hyaline membrane disease, Pediatr. Ann. **6:**3, April 1977.

Lough, M., and Schuchardt, B.: Mechanical ventilation. In Lough, M., editor: Pediatric respiratory therapy, Chicago, 1979, Year Book Medical Publishers, Inc.

Mushin, W., and others: Automatic ventilation of the lungs, ed. 3, Oxford, 1980, Blackwell Scientific Publications, Ltd.

Snow, J.: Ventilatory management of the infant, Life Support Nursing, July-Aug. 1979.

CHAPTER FIVE

Chest X-ray Interpretation

MARY FRAN HAZINSKI

JANET SNOW

Assessment skills are essential for any nurse working in a critical-care unit. A basic understanding of the chest radiograph can aid in the assessment and care of critically ill patients. Since the nurse may be the first person to see a patient's chest film, her ability to interpret changes in the radiograph can assist in prevention or early detection of pulmonary disorders and complications of treatment. Nurses can check the location of tubes in the airway, lungs, heart or stomach; the placement of pacemaker wires; and the identification of pulmonary infiltrates to be treated. In addition, they can assess the progress in treatment and assist in determination of changes in treatment. Thus the purpose of this chapter is to present some of the basic concepts used in the interpretation of chest radiographs and the application of these concepts in the care of the critically ill child.

It is extremely important that the chest films be used only in conjunction with careful physical assessment. Often the radiograph simply confirms findings of the physical examination. In any event, the child's clinical condition often dictates the acuity of the treatment required. As a result, no attempt is made in this chapter to discuss treatment of the problems evident on the radiograph. Instead, the focus is on skills needed for careful interpretation of the radiograph itself. For specific discussion of the pathophysiology, clinical signs and symptoms, and treatment of the disorders mentioned, the reader is referred to the appropriate chapters elsewhere in the book.

Since chest radiographs, taken so frequently in the critical-care unit, use radiant energy, it is extremely important that the nurse avoid becoming lax in shielding herself and her patient from stray radiation exposure. The nurse should always wear a lead shield if she remains at the bedside during x-ray examinations and should always be certain the child has a gonadal shield in place.

■ DEFINITION OF TERMS

X-ray films or radiographs are a form of short wavelength radiant energy. They are produced when an electronic (x-ray) beam is directed through an object to a film cassette. The image produced on the film is determined by the composition, or density, of the object through which the beam passes. If the object is very dense, it will block most of the beam and prevent it from reaching and reacting with the film; this creates a gray or white shadow on the film. The object that is not very dense does not block a significant amount of the x-ray beam and thus most of the beam reacts with the film; the resultant image on the film will be dark gray or black. The more x-ray beam an object blocks or absorbs, the more *radiopaque* that object is. If the object does not block or absorb very much of the x-ray beam, it is *radiolucent*.[15]

Most complex objects are not of uniform density; they contain a variety of substances of varying densities, which produce a variety of shadows on a radiograph. Four major categories of densities are used in interpretation of x-ray films; in order of decreasing density these are metal, water, fat, and gas (or air).[4] Metal is extremely dense, and it is the most radiopaque of materials. Pure metals block or absorb all of the x-ray beam and produce a white shadow on the radiograph. Since bones contain a large amount of calcium, they are nearly as dense and radiopaque as metal and also produce white images on the radiograph. Water and other fluids block a significant amount of the x-ray beam so that they too are radiopaque. Body tissues or cavities containing water or fluid (such as the heart) will produce a very light or white image on the radiograph. However, since water and fluids are not as dense as bones, bones and metals will still create a lighter image than water. Because fat is not as dense as water, it does not block as much of the x-ray beam and consequently is less radiopaque or more radiolucent than bone or fluid. As a result the radiograph shadow that fat produces is darker in intensity than bone or water. Fat is contained in subcutaneous tissue and in some muscle; the x-ray image produced by these fat-containing tissues will be dark gray. Gas or air is the least dense of substances visible on the chest radiograph. Since gas does not absorb much of the x-ray beam, it is radiolucent and produces a black image on the radiograph. Gas or air density is normally seen in the lung fields and in the air-filled stomach.

All parts of the body contain one or more of the four densities discussed above (metal/bone, fluid, fat, or gas). The combination of densities in the body will create contrasts on the radiograph. When objects of varying densities are in contact, their borders will be apparent because of the contrasts in their radiographic images; the difference in their images creates a *silhouette.* When structures are visible on a radiograph, their size, shape, and position can easily be evaluated. In addition, if a characteristic density is observed in an abnormal location, it may create an abnormal contrast or obliterate an expected silhouette. This observation of abnormal density can often confirm a diagnosis of inappropriate tissue, fluid, or air accumulation.

An x-ray film creates a two-dimensional image of three-dimensional objects as it compresses the image into one plane. As a result depth of structures often cannot be appreciated by evaluation of only one x-ray view. Many times, studies must be taken from two or more views so that the images can be compared and so that the relative position of objects can be better evaluated.

The standard chest film is an upright *posteroanterior (PA)* film. This film is obtained in the radiology department. The patient stands facing the radiographic film cassette, and the x-ray beam is directed from the back of the patient, through the patient, to the film. Thus the patient's back (posterior aspect) is closest to the x-ray tube. An *anteroposterior (AP)* chest film is often obtained in the critical-care unit because it can be taken with a portable x-ray machine. When an AP view is obtained, the film cassette is placed under or behind the child and the child faces

the x-ray tube. The x-ray beam is then directed from the front of the child, through the child to the film. Thus the front of the child (anterior aspect) is nearest the x-ray tube when the film is taken. The AP film tends to magnify anterior chest structures, including the heart. Whenever heart size is being evaluated, it is important to know if the film was taken with a PA or an AP approach, although the difference is not as significant in infants and small children as it is in older children and adults.[11] Changes in heart size (or in the size of any organ) can best be made by comparing two x-rays obtained using the same approach. Characteristically, chest films obtained in the radiology department under very controlled conditions are clearer and of better quality than those obtained with a portable machine. Therefore, whenever practical, the films should be obtained in the radiology department.

When PA or AP chest films are obtained, evaluation of lateral relationships of structures is possible, but assessment of AP relationships is not possible because of the compression of the image onto a single plane. If determination of depth is necessary or if localization of a density is required, a *lateral* film is taken. Lateral chest films are usually obtained as part of a complete radiographic study of the heart and lungs. To obtain a lateral film, the patient is *upright*, the film cassette is placed on the side of the patient, and the beam is directed from the other side of the patient. The lateral film is labeled according to the side of the patient that is *nearest* the x-ray tube. If the patient's left side is against the film cassette and *right* side is nearest the x-ray tube, the film is a *right lateral* film. Conversely, if the patient's right side is nearest the film cassette and *left* side is nearest the x-ray tube, the film is a *left lateral* film.

Lateral views allow evaluation of the AP relationships of body structures, but they do not allow determination of their lateral relationships. Therefore the comparison and evaluation of both a PA and a lateral film provide much more information than either film does separately. An additional advantage of obtaining radiographs from two views is that thin structures (such as lung septa or fissures) will only be visible on a single film if the x-ray beam strikes the structure parallel to its long axis.[4] As a result, when films of the same object are obtained using two different views, there is a greater chance that small structures will be apparent on one of the views.

A *decubitus* view is obtained with the patient recumbent on one side or the other. The film cassette is placed at the patient's back, and the x-ray beam is then aimed horizontally, or parallel to the floor.[4] A decubitus view can easily be obtained in the critical-care unit, and it is often helpful in determining the presence of air-fluid levels in the lung.

In most x-ray views, the x-ray beam is directed perpendicular to the plane of the film (and the patient). Occasionally, however, a more oblique view of structures is desirable, and a *lordotic* view is obtained. To obtain the lordotic view in an AP projection (the patient is facing the x-ray tube), the tube is elevated slightly above the midline so that the beam must be directed *down* at the patient. Another method of obtaining the AP lordotic view is for the x-ray beam to be directed normally at the film, but the patient leans backward into the film in an exaggerated lordosis.[15] In the lordotic view the clavicles are directed upward so that the apexes of the lungs are more easily seen. In addition, the anterior and posterior segments of the same ribs are superimposed so that the lung tissue may be seen more clearly between the ribs. The lordotic view is less frequently obtained in radiologic evaluation of children since their ribs are more horizontal than adults' and therefore frequently superimposed with a normal AP film. An additional disadvantage of the lordotic view is that it tends to foreshorten the lung fields.

■ INTERPRETATION OF FILM TECHNIQUE

The evaluation of a chest radiograph must include knowledge of the exposure conditions of the film, the angle of the x-ray beam, and the alignment and position of the patient. If the x-ray tube is positioned close to the film (and the patient) the x-ray image of the patient will be very large and blurred. Conversely, if the x-ray tube is farther away from the film and the patient, the image of the patient will be smaller but sharper. To standardize the size of images obtained, the *distance* between the x-ray tube and the film is measured and recorded on the film. The *magnification* of the film should also be noted on the film and should remain constant since changes in magnification will alter the size of the images produced.

The x-ray tube should generally be positioned so that the x-ray beam is exactly perpendicular to the plane of the film. If the patient is positioned properly, the x-ray beam will also be perpendicular to the horizontal or verticle axis of the patient. If the x-ray beam is not perpendicular, a lordotic view will be obtained. A lordotic view is undesirable if it is obtained unintentionally because it foreshortens the lung fields.[18] If the apexes of the lungs are not visible above the clavicles on an AP or a PA chest film, a lordotic view has been obtained, and this must be considered when evaluation of lung size and chest expansion is made.

The alignment and the position of the patient at the time the film is taken must also be considered. If the patient is rotated slightly, the radiographic image of the chest will be oblique; this changes the heart shape and enlarges the cardiac image. To evaluate patient alignment, the position and appearance of the patient's clavicles are assessed. If the clavicles both appear horizontal and of equal size and length, a true AP or PA view was obtained. If, on the other hand, one clavicle appears to be smaller than the other (because it is farther away from the x-ray tube at the time the film was taken) or if one clavicle is at a different angle than the other, the patient was probably rotated, and a more oblique view of chest structures was obtained on the radiograph. This should be noted when any observations about heart size are made.

When the chest film is obtained, the technician and the nurse must be sure to note if the patient was *upright* (sitting or standing) or *supine*. This is important because gravity will affect the position or location of any free air or fluid in the chest. *Free pleural fluid* (such as that accumulating as a result of a hemothorax, chylothorax, or pleural effusion) will assume a *dependent position*. On the other hand, *free* pleural *air* (such as occurs with a pneumothorax) *rises* to the most superior position of the chest. If the child is upright, free fluid tends to accumulate along the bases of the lungs and the diaphragm, and free air will rise toward the apexes of the lung. If the film is taken with the child supine, free pleural fluid will accumulate in the back of the child's pleural cavity, behind the lung(s). This fluid may be difficult to distinguish on an AP film from intrapulmonary congestion. To determine the presence, quantity, and location of free intrapleural fluid, the child should be placed upright before and while the radiograph is taken; if this is impossible or inconclusive, a lateral decubitus film will often be obtained. When the child is supine, free pleural air is usually seen along the diaphragm or the sides of the lung fields on an AP film.[4]

It is generally desirable (unless specifically ordered otherwise) for chest films to be obtained with the child in the upright position so that air and fluid levels can more easily be recognized. In addition, when the child is upright, diaphragmatic excursion is usually better, enabling the child to inspire more deeply, thus producing a better inspiratory film. A supine chest film may be necessary if the child is extremely unstable or if it is not possible to immobilize the child in the upright position while the radiograph is obtained.

The *exposure* of the chest film will also affect the intensity of the images on the chest radiograph. If the film is *underpenetrated* (underexposed), all of the images on the radiograph will appear lighter. The results are hazier images and difficulty in differentiating among images. In addition, pulmonary vascular markings will appear to be more prominent, with less distinct borders; thus they may be mistakenly interpreted to be increased or hazy because of interstitial edema. If a chest radiograph is *overpenetrated* (overexposed), all of the images on the radiograph will be darker. This can obliterate images and may make pulmonary vascular markings appear to be reduced. If the radiograph is appropriately penetrated, the vertebral bodies will be clear and well-delineated behind the heart. In addition, some pulmonary vascular mark-

ings will be visible within the heart shadow because they are present behind the heart.

Unless other orders are specifically given, chest films should be obtained during inspiration. This maximizes the size of the lung fields and makes the cardiac image sharp. If the film is obtained during expiration, the heart will appear larger and less well-defined. The lung fields will appear to be hazier and the pulmonary vascular markings more prominent. Fig. 5-1 illustrates these differences since it includes two views obtained from a normal child during in-

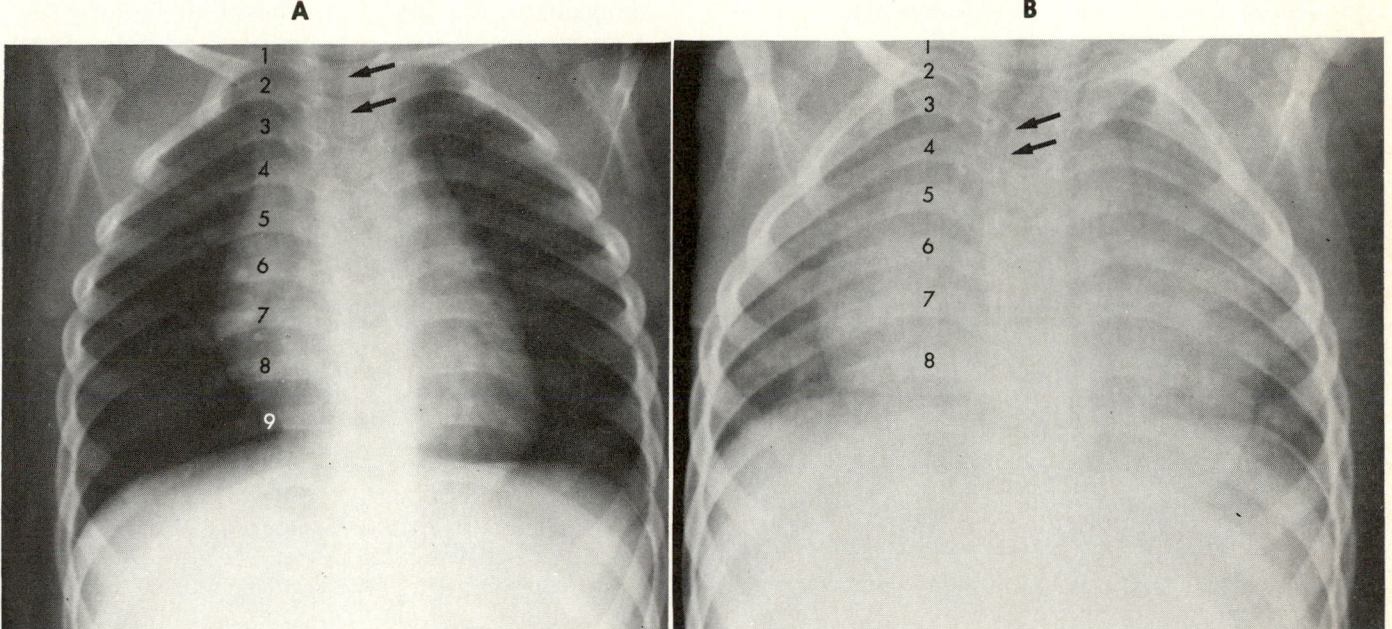

A

B

Fig. 5-1 Normal chest films obtained from the same child during inspiration and expiration. **A,** *Inspiratory phase.* Note that 9 ribs can be counted above the diaphragm (refer to numbering on ribs); this indicates good lung expansion (inspiration). The child is in good alignment since the clavicles are approximately of the same size and appearance. The penetration of the film is good since the outline of the vertebral bodies can be seen, and some pulmonary vascular markings can be seen behind the heart. The intercostal spaces are equal and adequate. Both sides of the diaphragm are clearly visible. The mediastinum is also well defined, but not widened, and the trachea is straight *(arrows).* The heart borders are sharply defined against the air density of the lungs, and the heart size is normal (cardiothoracic ratio is 0.52). The pulmonary vascular markings are normal since they are visible in the proximal two thirds of the lung fields but not prominent in the peripheral lung fields. **B,** *Expiratory phase.* Only 8 ribs are visible above the diaphragm (refer to numbering on ribs); this indicates inadequate expansion of lungs caused

by insufficient inspiration (or expiration) while the film was taken. The clavicles are of approximately the same size and configuration so the child is in good alignment. The penetration of the film is good since the outline of the vertebral bodies is clear. The intercostal spaces are very small since expiration is occurring. Both sides of the diaphragm are hazy; in fact, the patient's left hemidiaphragm is not readily identifiable. The mediastinum appears to be wide, and the trachea seems to buckle to the right *(arrows).* The heart appears to be much larger, although its absolute size has not increased, and the heart borders are obliterated. The silhouette sign seems to be present, suggesting the presence of pulmonary infiltrates. If a cardiothoracic ratio were calculated from this view, it would be 0.71; this is why cardiothoracic ratios *should not be calculated from expiratory chest radiographs.* Pulmonary vascular markings appear to be very prominent; this appearance mimics pulmonary edema.

Chest radiographs courtesy Dr. H. Rex Gardner, Rush Presbyterian-St. Luke's Medical Center, Chicago, Ill.

spiration and expiration. To determine if the chest film was obtained during maximal inspiration, the nurse should count the ribs visible above the diaphragm. With good inspiration and chest expansion, nine to ten ribs should be visible. In addition, the normal trachea should appear to be straight. If fewer than nine ribs are visible above the diaphragm, the child was probably exhaling while the film was taken. Furthermore the trachea will appear to buckle to the right on an expiratory film.[11]

It is imperative that the child be prevented from moving while the film is taken since motion can blur cardiothoracic structures. Blurring of the diaphragm can mimic the appearance of pulmonary infiltrates.[11] If motion is suspected when the film is taken, this should be noted for consideration when the film is interpreted. If excessive motion artifact is present, another film should be taken.

Finally, whenever a chest film is obtained, any metal objects that can cause artifacts on the radiograph should be removed. Occasionally, long hair, wrinkles in clothing, or skin folds can produce artifacts that resemble pulmonary infiltrates or air-fluid interface.

■ INTERPRETATION OF THE CHEST FILM

It is good practice to develop a routine for reviewing chest films. If the nurse always uses an organized approach, she will be less likely to overlook significant abnormalities. It is often advisable to initially ignore the most striking or obvious features of a radiograph in order not to miss other equally important features. The following box provides one method of organizing the review of a chest film. Because there is no one correct way, the nurse must develop a style that is convenient for her. The most important thing about any approach is that all aspects of the film must be reviewed.

Current films should not be reviewed in isolation. They are most valuable when compared with the patient's previous films so that changes are more

CHEST X-RAY INTERPRETATION

1. Check the child's alignment; look at the size and configuration of the clavicles; if the child is rotated, keep this in mind when assessing heart size.
2. Determine if the film was taken during inspiration or expiration; nine or ten ribs should be visible above the diaphragm if the film was taken during inspiration.
3. Look at the *soft tissues of the chest wall* and at extrathoracic structures; check for subcutaneous emphysema.
4. Look at the *soft tissues of the neck;* check for the presence of subcutaneous emphysema.
5. Examine the *bony thorax,* including the clavicles, scapula, ribs, humeri, and the cervical and thoracic spine; check for fractures.
6. Examine the width of the *intercostal spaces.*
7. Examine the *diaphragm* and the *area below the diaphragm;* Note the presence and location of the gastric bubble; note the clarity of the diaphragm and its location (note if one side is elevated).
8. Examine the *pleura and the costophrenic angle;* note if the pleura reach the edge of the bony thorax or if there is a collection of pleural air or fluid; the costophrenic angle should be sharp.
9. Look at the *mediastinum* in both the frontal and lateral projections.
10. Look at the *trachea;* the trachea may appear to buckle to the right on an expiratory film.
11. Look at the *heart and the great vessels;* the borders of the heart and aortic knob should be distinct; the obliteration of these borders (called the silhouette sign) usually indicates atelectasis, pleural congestion, or accumulation of pleural fluid; the cardiothoracic ratio should be approximately 0.5.
12. Look at the *lung fields,* being sure to compare both sides; note the presence of opacities, and attempt to determine if these are caused by atelectasis or congestion; look for fluid lines.
13. Look at the *hili* of the lungs; pulmonary vascularity should be prominent but not enormous.
14. Look at the *peripheral pulmonary vascularity;* pulmonary vascular markings are usually visible in the proximal two thirds of the lung fields; increased or decreased pulmonary vascular markings may be caused by congenital heart disease (and the resultant intracardiac shunt); prominent but hazy pulmonary vascular markings may result from pulmonary edema or pulmonary venous congestion.
15. Check the location or placement of all tubes, wires, and lines.
16. Compare the film to previous films.

Modified from Martz, K.: Chest x-ray interpretation: normal. In Proceedings of the Seventh Annual NTI, Irvine, Calif., 1980, The American Association of Critical-Care Nurses.

readily appreciated. For this reason, the two most recent chest films for each patient are often kept in the
critical-care unit.

Once the technical aspects of the chest film
have been reviewed, the nurse can begin examination
of the structures outlined by the radiograph. Please
note that in the following discussion, emphasis is
placed on examination of the AP chest film since this
is the projection most frequently obtained in the critical-care unit.

The *soft tissues of the chest wall* should be examined for evidence of subcutaneous emphysema (air
density between the skin and bony thorax), which can
result from an air leak around the chest tube or from a
penetrating chest wound. In addition, tissue swelling
may indicate the presence of an injury.

The *soft tissues of the neck* should also be
checked for subcutaneous emphysema. In addition, if
the child is intubated, the position of the child's head
should be noted since flexion or extension of the head
can change the position of the tip of the endotracheal
(ET) tube (this is discussed in more detail later in the
chapter).

The *bony thorax* and the shape of the chest
should be examined. Infants and young children normally have round chests with a horizontal orientation of their ribs (see Fig. 5-1, if necessary). However,
older children and adults have chests that are wider
than they are deep, and their ribs angle downward from
back to front. A round chest in an older child or adult
is abnormal and may be the result of chronic respiratory disease and air trapping. Again, nine to ten ribs
should appear above the diaphragm if a good inspiratory film has been obtained.

The continuity of vertebrae, ribs, and clavicles
should be checked. A fracture will often create a dark
line in the bone because of the presence of air or
tissue between the bone fragments. The vertebral
bodies, particularly the cervical vertebrae, should be
checked very closely for fractures if the child has been
admitted following trauma (Fig. 5-2). Rib notching, or
erosion of the underside of ribs caused by enlargement of the intercostal arteries, can be seen in older
children with coarctation of the aorta (the intercostal
arteries provide collateral circulation around the coarctation).

If the child has had previous cardiothoracic surgery, sternal wires or clips may be noted or the appearance of the ribs may be altered. Significant deformities of the chest wall may alter the location and
appearance of the cardiac silhouette.

The *width of the intercostal spaces* should be
noted. When the child has a thoracotomy, muscle
spasm or sutures can reduce the width of the inter-

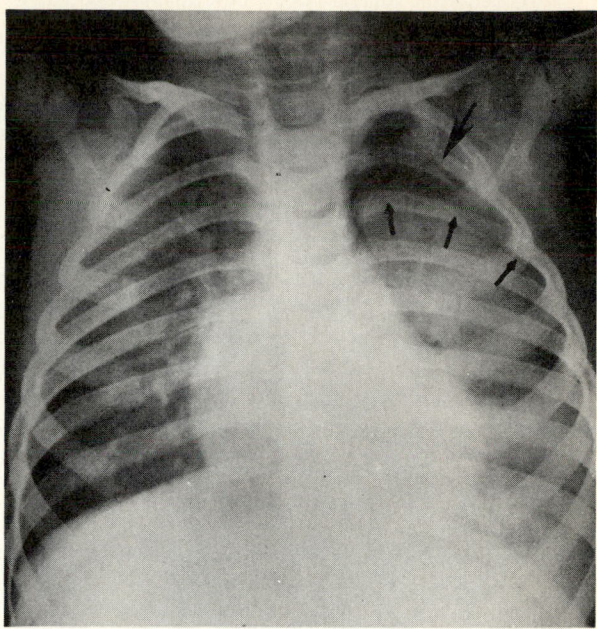

Fig. 5-2 This chest radiograph of a 3½-year-old boy
was taken after he was admitted to the pediatric
critical-care unit for observation following an
automobile accident. On admission the child was
tachypneic (respiratory rate of 40 to 50) and
complained of "tummy" pain, pointing to his left
chest. The nurse observed that the child's breath
sounds were decreased over the left upper chest, and
a chest x-ray examination was ordered. The child
had a *fractured left third rib (wide arrow)*, which
has caused a *left pneumothorax* (see the border
between the pneumothorax and the left lung
indicated by the small arrows). Since the film was
obtained with the child in the upright position, the
free pleural air has accumulated along the apex of
the left lung.

Chest radiograph courtesy Dr. Andrew K. Poznanski, Children's
Memorial Hospital, Chicago, Ill.

costal space at the site of surgery. In addition, significant atelectasis can cause narrowing of the intercostal spaces on the involved side and widening of the
spaces on the noninvolved side.[4]

The *position and appearance of the diaphragm*
should be given particular attention. The patient's
right hemidiaphragm is usually lower than the left
hemidiaphragm since the stomach lies under the left
lung. Unilateral elevation of either side of the diaphragm may be caused by diaphragmatic paralysis;
this may be seen with congenital diaphragmatic
paralysis or after injury to the phrenic nerve during
thoracic surgery (Fig. 5-3). Atelectasis and abdominal
organ distention can also cause unilateral elevation of
the diaphragm. Bilateral elevation of the diaphragm

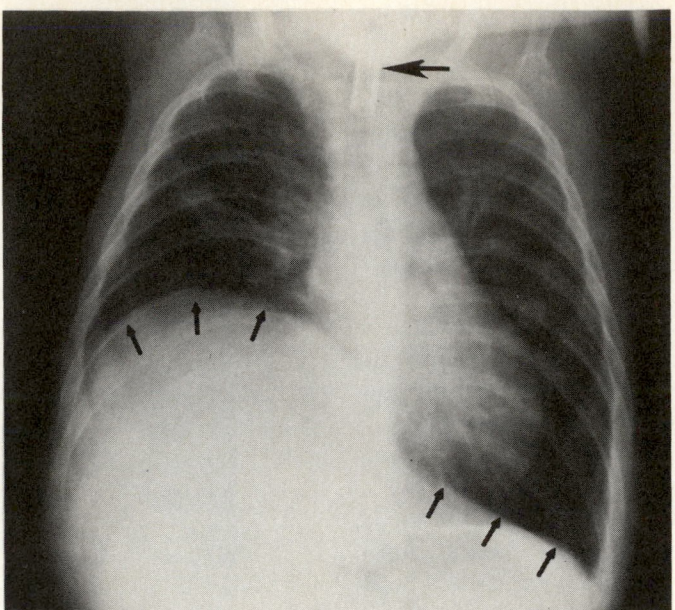

Fig. 5-3 Paralysis of the right hemidiaphragm. This infant has congenital paralysis of the right hemidiaphragm. During the first days of life the infant demonstrated respiratory distress and asymmetric movement of the chest wall. The chest radiograph revealed significant elevation of the right hemidiaphragm (*small arrows* on patient's right). The infant ultimately required a tracheostomy (*wide arrow*). Note that the pulmonary vascularity appears more prominent in the right (compressed) lung; this is because the right lung is not expanded fully. The left lung is hyperexpanded, and the left hemidiaphragm is depressed and flattened as a result (*small arrows* on patient's left). The number of ribs visible in this infant's right and left lung fields may be counted to compare the relative lung expansion bilaterally. You may wish to compare the appearance of the child's hemidiaphragm to Fig. 5-1.

Chest radiograph courtesy Dr. H. Rex Gardner, Rush Presbyterian-St. Luke's Medical Center, Chicago, Ill.

may be seen in the child with hypoventilation, abdominal distention, ascites, or obesity.

If the image of the diaphragm is not apparent, it is because the silhouette between the air density of the lungs and the tissue density of the diaphragm is obscured. This usually occurs because of atelectasis or accumulation of free pleural fluid along the diaphragm (Fig. 5-4). Note that accumulation of subpleural fluid may closely resemble diaphragmatic elevation when an AP film is taken with the patient upright.

The diaphragm can appear to be unusually flat and depressed in any condition that increases the volume of the lung or the contents of the hemithorax. The patient's diaphragm will be unilaterally flattened and displaced downward if the child has a significant unilateral pneumothorax or if the child has unilateral lung disease and hyperexpansion of one lung (see Fig. 5-3 and look at the infant's left hemidiaphragm).[15]

The structures below the diaphragm should also be examined. There is usually some air in the child's stomach (in fact, the absence of gastric air in the neonate is one of the pathognomonic signs of esophageal atresia).[12] The gastric bubble should appear under the patient's left hemidiaphragm. If the gastric bubble is present under the patient's right hemidiaphragm, situs inversus (abdominal organs located on opposite sides from their usual locations) is present. It is extremely important to be aware that the child has situs inversus since the nurse may be checking placement of the child's nasogastric tube or palpating the liver for evidence of hepatomegaly. In addition, situs inversus may be associated with cardiac malpositions, congenital heart disease, or asplenia.[10,13] There should normally be no free air in the peritoneal cavity, although air is usually present in the child's stomach, intestines, and colon.[11]

The newborn with diaphragmatic hernia has severe respiratory distress. The chest radiograph reveals circumscribed air density within the chest (usually the left hemithorax). This air is caused by the presence of loops of air-filled bowel in the chest (Fig.

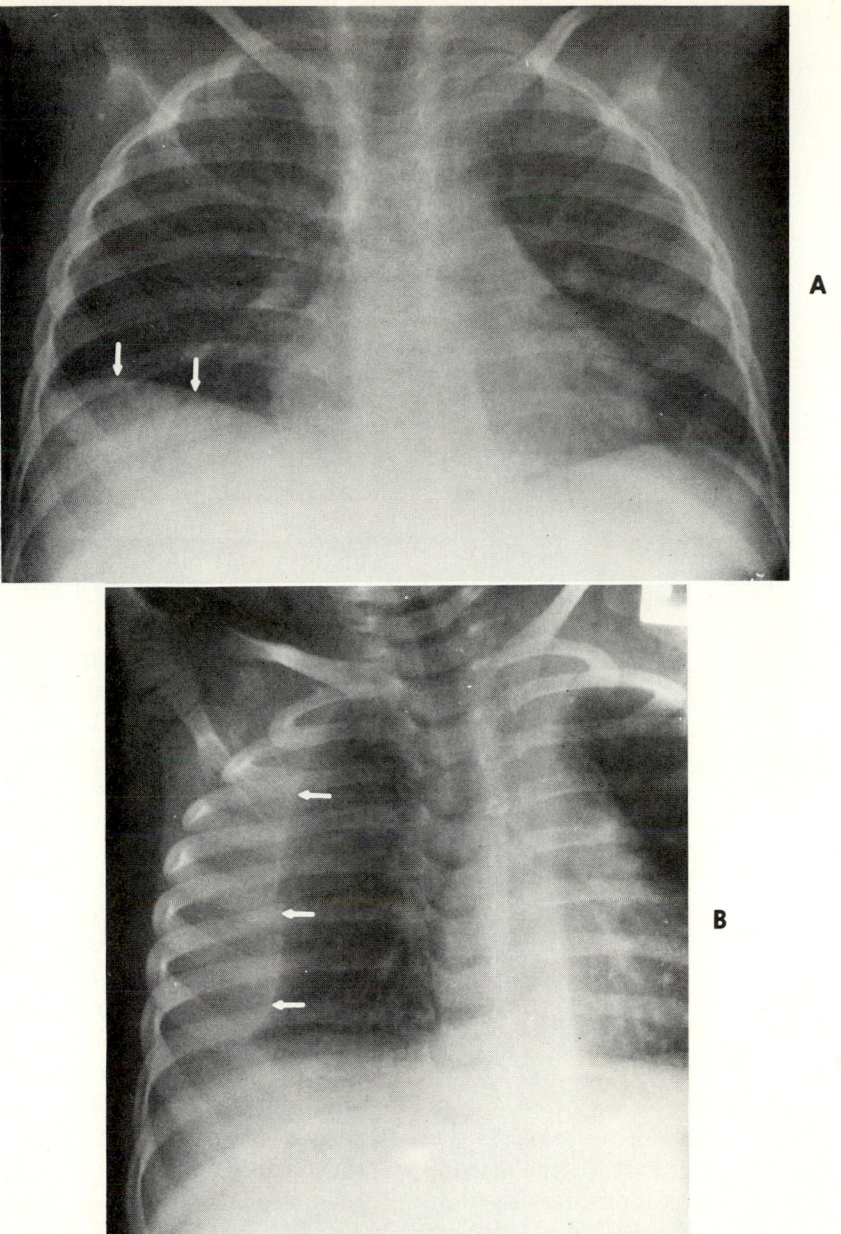

Fig. 5-4   Pleural effusion. These films were obtained when this 3-year-old child developed tachypnea and increased respiratory effort several days following repair of a double outlet right ventricle. The nurse noted a significant decrease in breath sounds over the right lung fields, particularly the right middle and lower lobes. The right lung fields were dull to percussion. The radiograph was ordered to differentiate between atelectasis and pleural effusion. **A,** The upright AP film. Despite an apparently good inspiratory film, the right lung field is smaller than the left. This could represent diaphragmatic elevation as a result of atelectasis. It could also represent free pleural fluid accumulation along the diaphragm. The hilar pulmonary vascular markings are somewhat hazy; this is consistent with either atelectasis or compression of the right lung by subpulmonic fluid. The right costophrenic angle is blunted, so the diagnosis of pleural effusion was favored and a decubitus film was ordered to confirm the diagnosis. **B,** The decubitus film. The film was taken with the child lying on his right side so that any free right pleural fluid should have accumulated along that side. Now the fluid level is easily appreciated *(arrows).*

Chest radiographs courtesy Dr. Andrew K. Poznanski, Children's Memorial Hospital, Chicago, Ill.

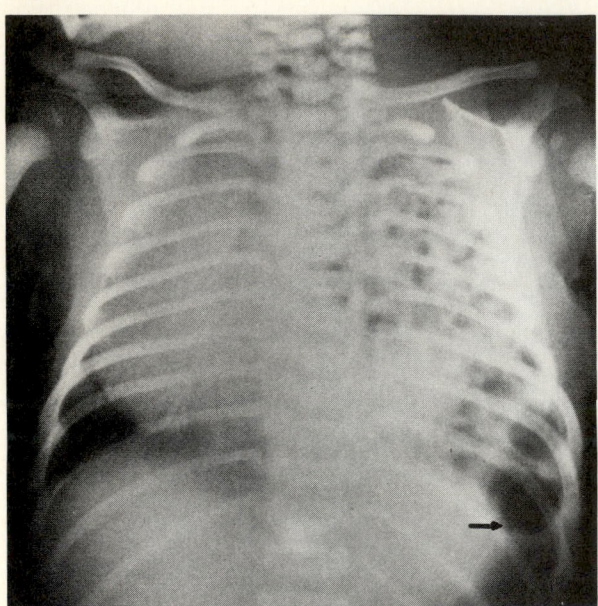

Fig. 5-5 Diaphragmatic hernia. This newborn was transported to the critical-care unit with extreme respiratory distress for evaluation of a mass in the right side of the chest. This radiograph accompanied the infant. The fluid-density "mass" in the infant's right side of the chest is the heart, which has been displaced from the left chest. The loculated shadows in the left chest are cast by the air-filled bowel that has moved up from the abdomen into the chest as the result of a left diaphragmatic hernia. You can see that the bowel is continuous from the abdomen into the chest (arrow).

Chest radiograph courtesy Dr. Andrew K. Poznanski, Children's Memorial Hospital, Chicago, Ill.

5-5). The bowel not only compresses the lung on the involved side, but it shifts the heart to the noninvolved (usually right) hemithorax, compressing that lung also. Until the bowel fills with air, the infant with a diaphragmatic hernia may be thought to have a mass in the left chest. Therefore it is important to look for abnormal structures below the diaphragm and to attempt to recognize abdominal contents abnormally located above the diaphragm.

The *pleura* is a double-layered serous membrane; one layer lines the inside of the thoracic cavity, and the other layer adheres to the outside of the lung.[2] The space between these two layers (the pleural cavity) is normally collapsed so that the two layers cast only a small (thin) shadow on the radiograph.[15] However, if free fluid or air accumulates in the chest, an air-fluid interface or a fluid density may be observed—between the bony thorax and the lung—in the pleural cavity. In addition, if the pleura thickens

as the result of pleural reaction (following surgery or other irritation) or the collection of loculated (encapsulated) fluid, the pleura will cast a thicker light shadow on the radiograph.

When the pleura is examined, it is important to follow it (and any visible pleural space) around the entire margin of each lung. Since free pleural fluid tends to accumulate in dependent portions of the chest, it will be noted along the diaphragm in an upright film and behind the lungs in a supine film. As a result small collections of fluid on an upright film can obscure the costophrenic angle (the angle produced by the lateral downward curve of each hemidiaphragm), whereas more significant collections of fluid tend to obscure the diaphragm and make it appear elevated.[4]

Free pleural fluid on a supine film may seem to opacify the lung fields; thus it is often difficult to distinguish from pulmonary congestion.[4] In this case an upright or lateral decubitus film is usually obtained (see Fig. 5-4 and the discussion of pleural effusions later in this chapter). Fluid may also accumulate in the minor fissure (between the right middle and upper lobes); this fluid accumulation can often be observed on both AP and lateral films.[4] Fluid accumulation in the major fissure (which separates the right upper and middle lobes from the right lower lobe) is best seen on a lateral film.

A pneumothorax will produce an air-tissue interface in the pleural cavity since the pneumothorax contains only air (and, as a result, no pulmonary vascular markings), whereas the lung contains air, tissues, and vessels. The presence of a significant pneumothorax will cause partial or complete collapse of the adjacent lung (see Fig. 5-2 and the discussion of pneumothorax later in this chapter). Note that free pleural air will accumulate in the highest portions of the chest so that the location of the air will depend on the patient's position. In an upright film free pleural air is often observed above the apexes of the child's lungs, whereas in a supine film the air may accumulate along the front and sides of the lung and along the diaphragm (Fig. 5-6).

Pleural thickening or a loculated (encapsulated) pleural effusion will create a fluid shadow in the chest that does not change when the patient's position changes.

The *costophrenic angle* is a sharp angle formed bilaterally from the downward curve of the lateral diaphragm seen on an AP (or a PA) film. The base of the lower lobes of the lung dip into this recess bilaterally.[15] Obliteration or blunting of this angle can occur with accumulation of relatively small amounts of free pleural fluid. The angle can also be blunted if pleural reaction or thickening is present.[15]

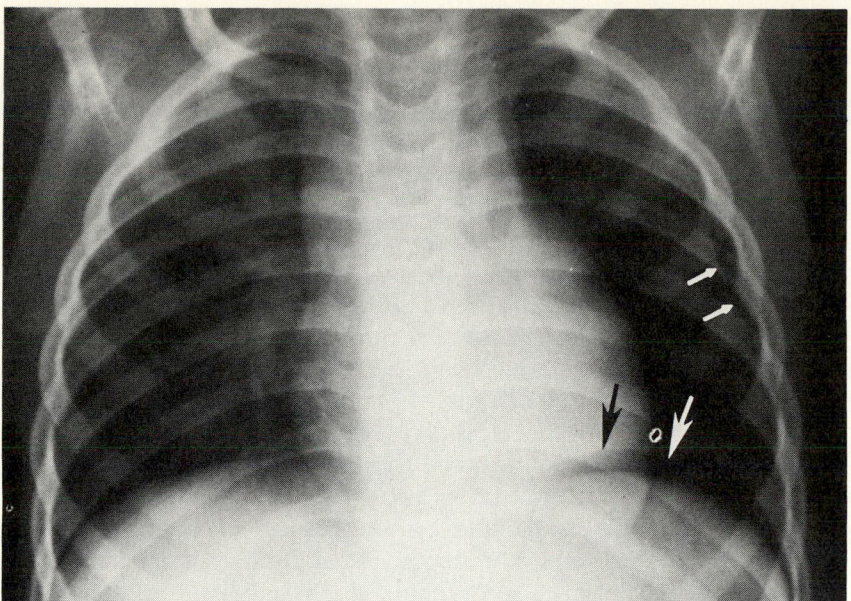

Fig. 5-6 Pneumothorax. This film was obtained following removal of a left pleural (chest) tube to rule out pneumothorax (caused by entry of air into the chest as the tube is pulled out of the chest). The presence of a pneumothorax was strongly suspected because the child's respiratory rate increased, and the nurse noted decreased breath sounds over the left lung fields, particularly over the left lower lobe. The film was taken with the child *supine*. This is important to know because air would tend to accumulate along the diaphragm and in the anterior chest. The pneumothorax is, in fact, visible along the diaphragm *(wide arrows)*, although the air/lung interface can be seen along the periphery of the left chest *(small arrows)*.

Chest radiograph courtesy Dr. H. Rex Gardner, Rush Presbyterian-St. Luke's Medical Center, Chicago, Ill.

The *mediastinum* consists of the trachea, the two bronchi, the esophagus, the ascending aorta, the aortic arch (and major branches), the main pulmonary artery (and the proximal right and left pulmonary arteries), the major veins of the heart, the heart, and the thymus. Since most of these structures contain fluid, the radiographic appearance of the mediastinum is that of a single fluid density between the lungs. Since the trachea contains air, a dark vertical radiolucent column identifies its position within the mediastinum.

The trachea should be straight, and often it is located slightly to the right of the patient's midline. The posterior portion of the aortic arch creates a knob or curve that is usually seen just to the left of the patient's spine. If the aorta archs to the right instead of to the left, the aortic knob may be superimposed on the shadow of the patient's spine on the AP projection, and the trachea is displaced to the patient's left. The incidence of congenital heart disease is higher in patients with a right aortic arch,[17] although this arch can be seen on otherwise normal individuals.

The aortic knob and the trachea will be displaced if a mediastinal shift occurs. When significant atelectasis is present, the trachea and aortic knob are usually displaced *toward* the area of collapse (see the discussion of atelectasis later in this chapter).[15] However, if a large pleural effusion or pneumothorax is present, the trachea and aortic knob will be displaced *away from* the involved lung and toward the unaffected side (see the discussions of pleural effusion and pneumothorax later in this chapter).

The *trachea* is identified by a straight vertical air density just to the right of the patient's midline.

As noted previously, it may appear to buckle to the right on an expiratory film, or it may be displaced toward an area of atelectasis or away from a pneumothorax or pneumomediastinum. The trachea bifurcates into the right and left mainstem bronchus at approximately the level of the patient's fourth rib. The carina, a portion of the lowest tracheal ridge, is located at the bifurcation of the trachea and is used as a landmark in radiographic assessment of endotracheal tube placement (see the discussion on evaluation of line and tube placement later in this chapter). The angle of branching of the left main bronchus is normally more acute than the right main bronchus. For this reason, aspirated substances most frequently enter the right bronchial tree.[14]

The *heart* is normally located in the left chest. If the child has dextrocardia or dextroversion, the heart will be located in the center of the chest or in the right chest, and the presence of other congenital heart lesions is more likely.[16] The cardiac shadow on the AP film is created largely by the shadow of the superior vena cava, the right atrium, the aortic knob, the main pulmonary artery, the left pulmonary artery, and the left ventricle.[6] The right ventricle and left atrium do not normally contribute to the margin of the heart shadow in this view. The size of the heart is quantified by calculation of a ratio of the heart to chest width, called the cardiothoracic ratio. To obtain the cardiothoracic ratio, the heart is measured between vertical lines drawn at its widest margins and the chest is measured at the costophrenic angles on the inside of the rib cage. The cardiothoracic ratio in newborns is normally up to 0.55. In older infants and children up to 6 years of age, a ratio of 0.45 is normal. Between 6 and 12 years of age, a cardiothoracic ratio of up to 0.44 is normal.[6] As a convenient rule, the cardiothoracic ratio in children is normally 0.5, plus or minus 5% to 6%, and it is normally larger in neonates and smaller in older children.[11]

Cardiac enlargement will increase the cardiothoracic ratio. It is important to note that cardiac chamber *hypertrophy* may not appreciably alter heart size since the cardiac shadow is determined by the outer border of the heart chambers and is not influenced by the thickness of chamber walls. Cardiomegaly that is apparent on the radiograph is caused by an increase in cardiac chamber volume; thus it is most often a result of cardiac *dilation*.[9]

Right atrial enlargement may appear as a displacement of the lateral border of the heart toward the patient's right. The right atrial portion of the right heart margin may also appear to be more convex.

Right ventricular enlargement may be difficult to appreciate from the AP film alone. When this ventricle enlarges, the rest of the heart is displaced posteriorly and cephalad (upward). Frequently, this increases the transverse diameter of the heart and pushes the cardiac apex outward and upward (like the upturned toe of a shoe or boot), although this is not an invariable radiologic finding.[6,9] Right ventricular enlargement may also be appreciated from a lateral chest film because the enlarged (anterior) right ventricle will fill the retrosternal space and rest against the sternum; it may, however, be difficult to differentiate between the retrosternal thymus and the retrosternal right ventricle in small infants.[6,9]

Left atrial enlargement may be difficult to appreciate since the left atrium normally does not form a distinct portion of the cardiac margin. With left atrial enlargement, the left heart border below the aortic knob may straighten or even become convex instead of concave. In addition, the posterior enlargement of this chamber can elevate the left mainstem bronchus so that the angle of the tracheobronchial bifurcation is widened.[6] A double density may also be observed in the center of the cardiac shadow[9] (Fig. 5-7).

Left ventricular enlargement generally increases the transverse diameter of the heart and extends the left heart border toward the left chest wall. Commonly, left ventricular enlargement will displace the cardiac apex downward as well as outward so that it rests on the diaphragm.[6,9]

After cardiovascular surgery the mediastinum and cardiac silhouette may be enlarged as the result of bleeding or fluid accumulation around the site of surgery. If the cardiac silhouette widens dramatically in the presence of tachycardia, signs of pulmonary and systemic venous engorgement, and decreased systemic perfusion, the development of cardiac tamponade should be suspected.[8,15] However, it is important to note that the cardiac silhouette may remain small despite the presence of tamponade if the pericardial sac does not distend.[8]

Cardiac enlargement is often seen when the child has congestive heart failure. Heart failure, often biventricular in children, may produce a global enlargement of all heart chambers. Pulmonary vascular markings will also be increased (see Fig. 5-7 and Chapter 3 for further discussion).

The most reliable way to evaluate changes in heart size by radiograph is by comparison of the most recent film with several previous films made under the same conditions. Also, clinical assessment should always be correlated with radiographic findings.

The *great vessels* may be enlarged or reduced in size as the result of congenital heart defects. If the

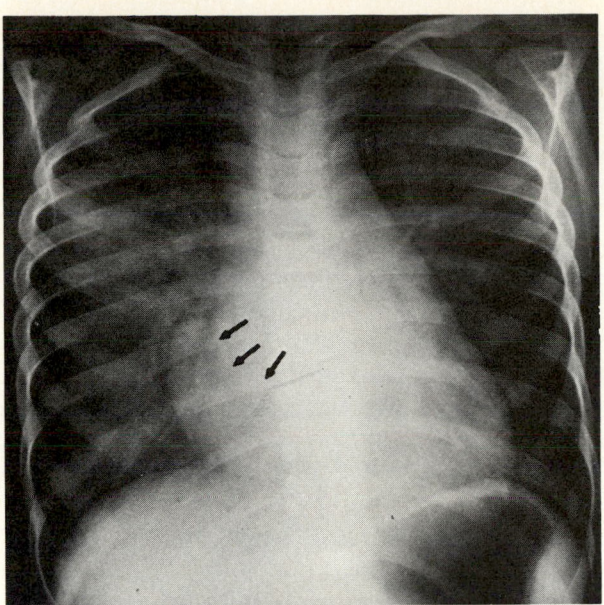

Fig. 5-7 Severe congestive heart failure with pulmonary edema. This 5½-year-old boy with known mitral insufficiency was admitted to the critical-care unit with tachypnea and increased respiratory effort. On physical examination, a heart rate of 137 with a gallop rhythm was noted. The respiratory rate was 54 with moderate retractions. Breath sounds were adequate and equal bilaterally, and rales were noted, particularly over the left lung fields. The liver was palpable 6 cm below the right costal margin. The child has cardiomegaly (cardiothoracic ratio of 0.6). The double density seen behind the heart *(wide arrows)* is caused by the *large* left atrium. Pulmonary interstitial markings are very prominent and hazy through both lung fields. Kerley B lines are noted in the base of the right lung *(small arrows).*

Chest radiograph courtesy Dr. Andrew K. Poznanski, Children's Memorial Hospital, Chicago, Ill.

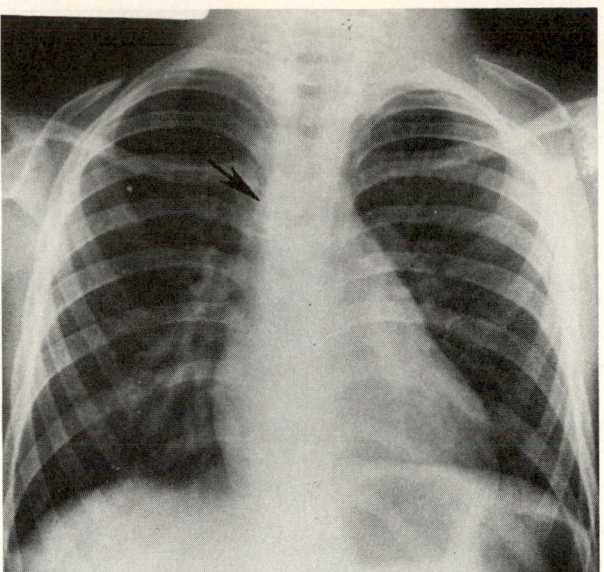

Fig. 5-8 Intracardiac left-to-right shunt. This is a radiograph of a 5-year-old boy who has been diagnosed as having a ventricular septal defect. Because the child demonstrated no symptoms, the defect was thought to be moderate in size. Cardiomegaly is not evident on the chest radiograph (cardiothoracic ratio of 0.5). Pulmonary vascular markings are prominent, particularly in the hilar area; this is consistent with increased pulmonary blood flow caused by a left-to-right intracardiac shunt. This child also has a *right* aortic arch *(arrow).* On catheterization, the child was found to have a moderate ventricular septal defect and significant pulmonary hypertension.

Chest radiograph courtesy Dr. Andrew K. Poznanski, Children's Memorial Hospital, Chicago, Ill.

child has a thoracic coarctation of the aorta, a characteristic E configuration of the aortic silhouette may be seen (because of the coarctation). The aortic knob may also be prominent in the presence of coarctation of the aorta, patent ductus arteriosus, or aortic valvular stenosis.[5]

The child with an intracardiac left-to-right shunt or a patent ductus arteriosus may demonstrate a very large and convex main pulmonary artery shadow on radiograph, because of large pulmonary blood flow (Fig. 5-8). Pulmonary valve stenosis can result in poststenotic dilation of the main pulmonary artery.

Some congenital heart defects, such as severe tetralogy of Fallot or pulmonary atresia, are associated with a small main pulmonary artery. In this case

a concavity of the upper portion of the left heart border may be observed since an extremely small main pulmonary artery will not produce the normal convexity below the aortic knob. This concavity can make the mediastinum appear to be very narrow since the upper heart shadow is created only by the aorta instead of by the pulmonary artery and aorta. Many of these children also have a right aortic arch so that the aortic knob is located to the right of the patient's trachea. This will further decrease the fullness of the left heart border.

The borders of the heart and great vessels should be sharp. Since the cardiac silhouette is created by the contrast between the fluid density of the heart and the air density of the lung, obliteration of the heart border is most often caused by opacification of portions of the lung that are in anatomic contact with the heart or great vessels. This loss of a normal silhouette on radiograph is referred to as the *silhouette sign*.[4] Loss of the cardiac silhouette most often results from congestion or atelectasis of areas of the lung in anatomic contact with the heart; it can also occur as the result of pleural fluid accumulation, lung inflammation, or a lung mass.

To determine the reason for appearance of the silhouette sign, the nurse must know which areas of the lung are in direct contact with the heart or great vessels; these are summarized in Table 5-1.

Obliteration of the margins of the upper portion of the right side of the heart border and ascending aorta can occur as the result of opacification of the right upper lobe. Opacification of the right middle lobe can result in loss of most of the right side of the heart border. Since the right lower lobe is posterior and not in direct contact with the heart, opacification of the right lower lobe will overlap the heart border but will not obliterate it.

If the margin of the aortic knob is indistinct, the left upper lobe is generally opacified. Atelectasis or pneumonia of the left lingula will obliterate most of the left side of the heart border. Since most of the left lower lobe is posterior and not in direct contact with the heart, left lower lobe opacification will overlap the heart but will not obliterate its silhouette.[4]

The *lung fields* on the chest radiograph are largely radiolucent since air does not absorb or block much of the x-ray beam. The fibrous tissues of the lung do not normally produce radiographic shadows, although some of the blood-filled arteries and veins will produce fluid density shadows.

The right lung is larger and is normally divided into the upper, middle, and lower lobes. Although the thin fissures between the lobes are usually not visible, the minor fissure (between the right upper and

right middle lobes) is occasionally seen as a thin white line on the chest film. The left lung is smaller because the left chest also contains the heart. The left lung contains two lobes, the left upper and left lower lobes. The left lung homologue of the right middle lobe is called the lingula.

The radiolucent lung fields should contain no significant opacifications (other than those created by pulmonary vasculature) or fluid levels. If an opacification is present, it must be further described and localized (see the discussions of pneumonia, atelectasis, and pleural effusion later in the chapter). If a pulmonary opacification obliterates a heart border, it can be localized if the nurse knows which lung segments are in direct contact with specific portions of the heart (see Table 5-1).

As already noted, the air-filled bronchi normally are not visible on the chest radiograph. Visualization of a bronchus is called an *air bronchogram*; the bronchus is visible only if it is in direct contact with an intrapulmonary structure of water or fluid density. It can be seen as the result of pneumonia, atelectasis, pulmonary edema, consolidation, infarction, or certain chronic pulmonary lesions.[4] In addition, an air bronchogram can be seen within the mediastinum in the radiographs of normal infants and young children because portions of their lobar bronchi lie within the tissues of the mediastinum. Thus while an air bronchogram is almost invariably associated with intrapulmonary disease in adults, it may be a normal finding in the mediastinum of infants and young children.[4]

The *hili* of the lungs contain the pulmonary artery and vein for each lung, as well as the right and left main bronchi. Since the bronchi do not normally produce a radiographic shadow, the shadow of the

Table 5-1 Significance of the silhouette sign: areas of the heart and great vessels in direct contact with the lungs[4]

Obliterated heart border or structure	Opacified lung segment
Upper portion of the right heart border and the ascending aorta	Right upper lobe (RUL)
Most of the right heart border	Right middle lobe (RML)
Aortic knob	Left upper lobe (LUL)
Most of the left heart border	Left lingula

right and left hili are produced by the right and left pulmonary arteries and veins and their major branches. In the vast majority of patients, the left hilum is slightly higher than the right hilum.[4,15] The hili may be enlarged because of increased pulmonary blood flow and pulmonary *arterial* engorgement; this may be the result of a congenital heart defect such as a ventricular septal defect or a patent ductus arteriosus (Fig. 5-8). The hili may also be enlarged because of pulmonary *venous* engorgement (as the result of congestive heart failure or pulmonary venous obstruction). Often there may be enlargement of both pulmonary arteries and veins (e.g., when the child with a large ventricular septal defect develops congestive heart failure). Enlargement of the hili may also be caused by lymph node enlargement.

The hilum of a lung can be displaced toward an area of lung collapse or away from a significant pneumothorax or pleural effusion.[4]

Pulmonary edema, pulmonary hemorrhage, overwhelming infection, aspiration pneumonitis, and pulmonary venous obstruction can cause *perihilar infiltrations*[14]; as a result the lung hili become more radiopaque and hazy (Fig. 5-9). The surrounding lung tissue may be more radiopaque with a reticular appearance (caused by interstitial edema). Occasionally, the lung fields are radiolucent, creating a dark halo around the hazy opacity of the hili.

Pulmonary edema, infectious pneumonitis, and pulmonary venous obstruction often produce diffuse changes that are symmetric bilaterally. Aspiration pneumonitis and partial pulmonary venous obstruction can produce unilateral or localized opacifications. Pulmonary edema can also be segmental.[14] Further evaluation of the pulmonary vascularity is made by examination of the peripheral pulmonary vascular markings.

The *peripheral pulmonary vascular markings* are normally not very prominent and can generally be seen only in the proximal two thirds of the lung fields. Prominent pulmonary vascularity can result from the presence of an intracardiac shunt (causing increased pulmonary blood flow), pulmonary venous obstruction, pulmonary hypertension, and increased collateral blood flow to the lungs. Although each of these problems theoretically can produce distinct radiographic changes, it is often difficult to differentiate among them by interpretation of an AP film alone. The radiologist may be able to differentiate between the radiographic appearance of pulmonary arterial engorgement and that of pulmonary venous engorgement, but this is often not possible in the critical-care unit. These points of differentiation will be reviewed later, but they may not always be apparent.

Intracardiac shunt lesions such as a large ventricular septal defect or patent ductus arteriosus will initially produce a dilation of apical vessels on an upright film (these vessels are normally not very prominent when the child is upright). With greater increase in pulmonary blood flow, the lung hili and the pulmonary arteries and veins become uniformly prominent as the result of increased pulmonary blood flow and possible increased pulmonary pressure (see Fig. 5-8).[1,3] Occasionally, the child with anemia or an arteriovenous fistula will develop pulmonary hypervascularity that mimics the appearance of a shunt lesion.

When the newborn has pulmonary venous obstruction because of left heart disease or total anomalous pulmonary venous return below the diaphragm, he often does not develop redistribution of pulmonary blood flow. Instead, lung fields become more radiopaque as a result of venous congestion, and the lung fields have a uniform reticulated or "ground-glass" appearance caused by interstitial edema and pulmonary venous dilation (see Fig. 5-9, *B*).

When the older infant or child has pulmonary venous obstruction (e.g., because of left heart failure or left heart obstruction), blood flow in the lungs is redistributed. Normally, when the patient is upright, blood flow in the bases of the lungs is greater than flow to the apexes. With an increase in pulmonary venous pressure, blood flow is shifted to the upper portions of the lungs, causing a prominence of apical pulmonary venous markings.[9] With progressive pulmonary venous engorgement, the lung hili and all vascular markings begin to become hazy and indistinct as a result of the development of interstitial edema. The hili may be particularly opaque.[3] *Kerley-B lines* may be seen when pulmonary venous engorgement is severe. These lines appear as thin, radiopaque, horizontal streaks in the lung bases that are thought to represent lymphatic channels in the interlobular septa of the lungs (see Fig. 5-7).[3,9,15] If pulmonary venous pressure increases further, transudation of fluid into the alveoli can occur. This produces fluffy, diffuse opacification of both lung fields. Air bronchograms may be visible (Fig. 5-10, *A* and *B*).

When the child develops pulmonary hypertension with increased pulmonary vascular resistance, the hilar and *proximal* pulmonary vessels often appear to be prominent, but *peripheral* pulmonary vascular markings can be absent. This radiographic appearance of the pulmonary vessels is often referred to as the "pruned tree" configuration.[3] Since chest radiographs are not the chief method used to confirm or rule out the diagnosis of pulmonary hypertension, the observation of findings consistent with pulmonary

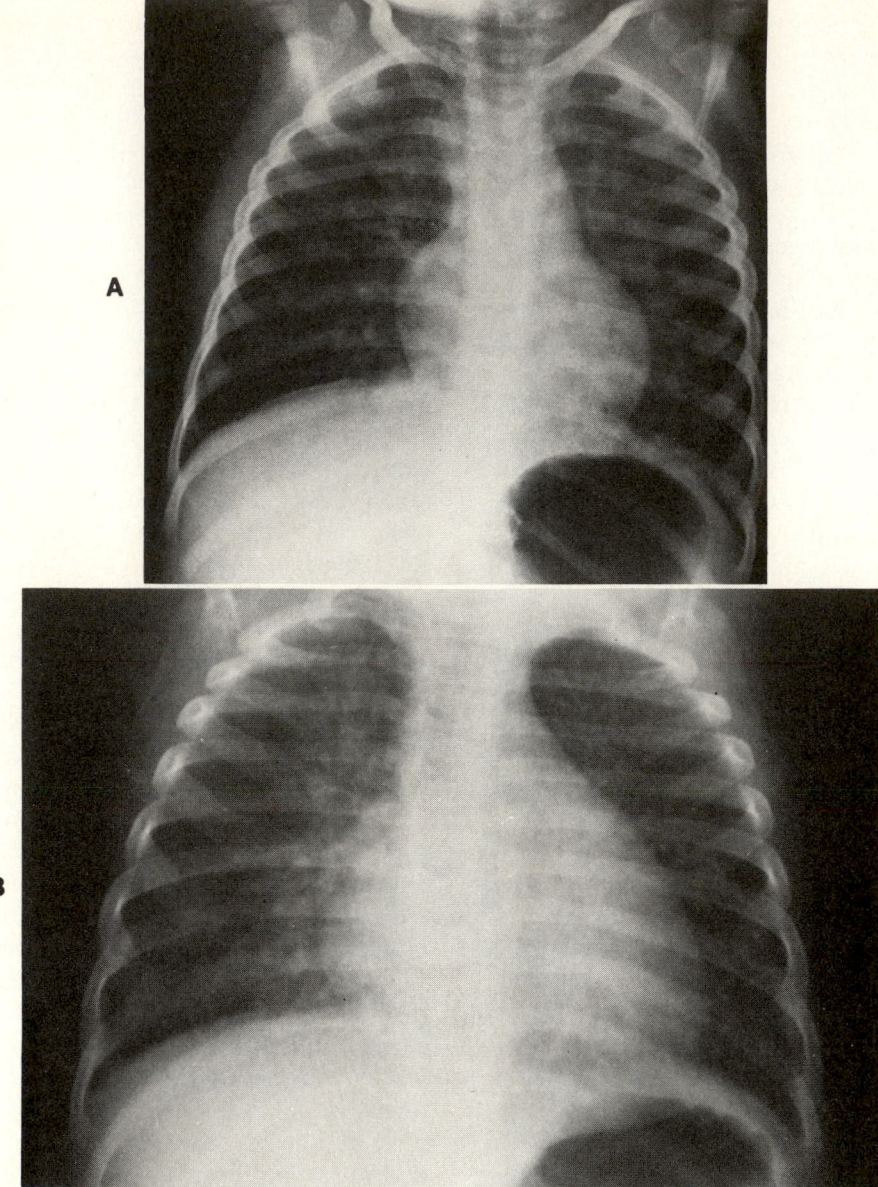

Fig. 5-9 Pulmonary edema in the child. **A,** This child was admitted to the critical-care unit after near-drowning. The child resumed spontaneous breathing a few minutes after being withdrawn from the swimming pool. The child continued to breath spontaneously, although tachypnea and increased respiratory effort were noted. The chest radiograph reveals a normal heart size. The pulmonary interstitial markings are all increased and hazy and are particularly prominent surrounding the hilum of the lungs (the halo effect is seen). The edema resolved within 24 hours. **B,** This infant was admitted with a history of "breathing difficulty." The child was tachypneic with increased respiratory effort. Lung aeration was equal and adequate bilaterally, although rales were noted bilaterally. Signs of congestive heart failure were noted. The chest x-ray reveals generalized cardiomegaly (cardiothoracic ratio of 0.58) and pulmonary venous congestion. Pulmonary vascular markings are increased and hazy throughout the lung fields, giving the lungs a reticulated appearance. This infant had a diffuse cardiomyopathy of unknown etiology.

Chest radiograph *A,* courtesy Dr. Andrew K. Poznanski, Children's Memorial Hospital, *B,* courtesy Dr. H. Rex Gardner, Rush Presbyterian-St. Luke's Medical Center, Chicago, Ill.

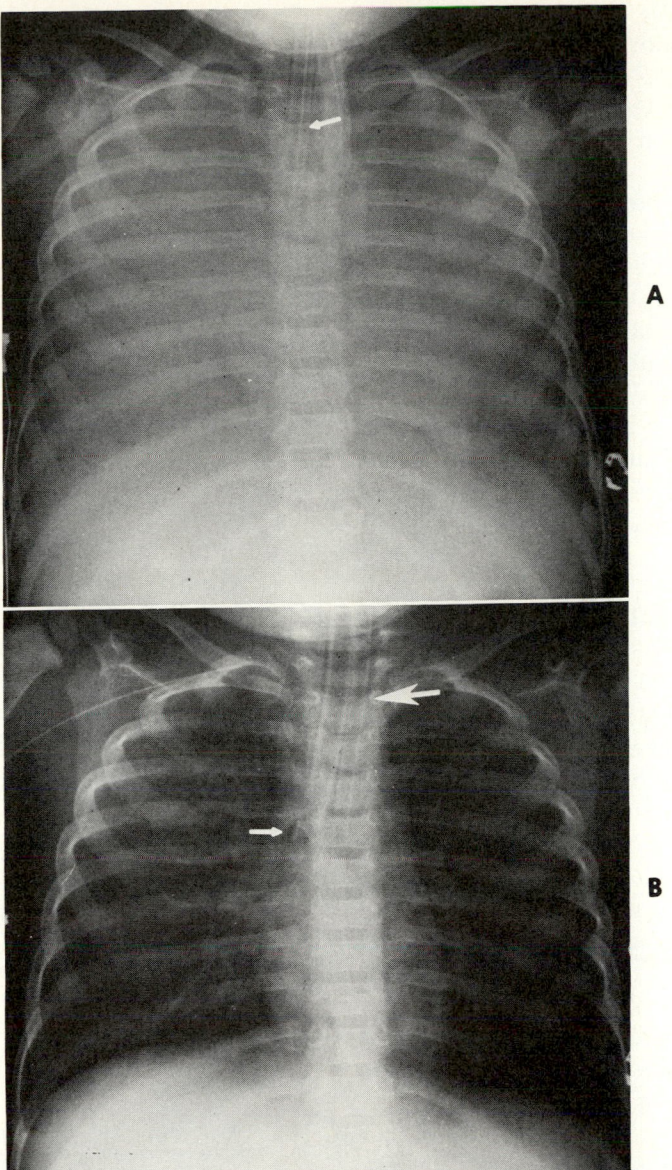

Fig. 5-10 Pulmonary edema. This toddler developed acute cardiorespiratory failure during neurosurgery. Although the child was intubated *(arrow)*, it was difficult to hand ventilate the child, and large amounts of frothy exudate were suctioned from the endotracheal tube. Blood gases revealed hypoxemia and acidosis. **A,** This chest film was obtained in the operating room immediately following resuscitation. Diffuse opacification of both lung fields is seen. The cardiac silhouette is barely discernable. This film is consistent with diffuse pulmonary edema with alveolar exudate. **B,** This chest film was obtained in the intensive care unit, after the child was mechanically ventilated and after a positive end-expiratory pressure (PEEP) of 10 cm H_2O was provided. Although pulmonary interstitial markings are still prominent, there is obvious improvement in lung aeration. Since the PEEP has been instituted, the lungs appear hyperinflated, and both diaphragms are flattened. A nasogastric tube is present *(small arrow)*. The ET tube is just beyond the carina and in the right mainstem bronchus *(wide arrow)*. The child's neck is flexed (because the chin is visible at the top of the film), displacing the tip of the ET tube downward; the tube should probably be withdrawn approximately 1 to 1½ cm.

Chest radiographs courtesy Dr. Andrew K. Poznanski, Children's Memorial Hospital, Chicago, Ill.

hypertension should be used only to provide an index of suspicion. Many children with significant pulmonary hypertension have normal chest radiographs (see Fig. 5-8).[3]

Occasionally, children with severe long-standing obstruction of pulmonary arterial blood flow (caused, e.g., by uncorrected or palliated pulmonary atresia) develop prominent bronchial collateral vessels that proliferate, thus increasing the absolute amount of pulmonary blood flow. These vessels can be very dense, but they often do not follow any pattern. These children would also be expected to have a normal or diminutive main pulmonary artery shadow and small right and left hili.[3]

When pulmonary artery blood flow is reduced, the lung fields appear to be abnormally radiolucent (or "empty"), since they do not contain the normal opacities produced by pulmonary vessels. The main pulmonary artery and the hili may also be small.[3]

■ RADIOGRAPHIC EVALUATION OF LINE PLACEMENT

If the child is intubated, the position of the ET tube should probably be checked first. The radiopaque tip of the tube should be located approximately 1 to 2 cm above the child's carina or approximately at the level of the child's third rib. Since the position of the ET tube relative to the carina will change with a change in the head position, it is important to note the position of the child's head when the radiograph is taken. The tip of the ET tube will be displaced *downward*, or further into the trachea, when the child's neck is *flexed* (see Fig. 5-10, *B*) and it will move *upward* if the child's neck is *extended* or if the head is turned to one side (Fig. 5-11).[7]

If the tip of the ET tube is positioned too near the carina (especially if it is near the carina despite extension of the child's neck), it can easily slip into the child's right mainstem bronchus. Unintentional intubation of the right mainstem bronchus soon results in hyperinflation of the right lung and hypoventilation and possible atelectasis of the left lung (Fig. 5-12, *A* and *B*). If the tip of the ET tube is too far above the carina, the tube may inadvertently slip out of the trachea with very little patient movement.

The location of any central venous, pulmonary artery, or intracardiac lines should be assessed. These lines should be traced along their entire length since they may migrate distally or advance to undesirable areas (Fig. 5-13). For example, during percutaneous insertion of a subclavian venous line, the catheter may advance through the jugular vein into the head instead of into the superior vena cava. The right atrial

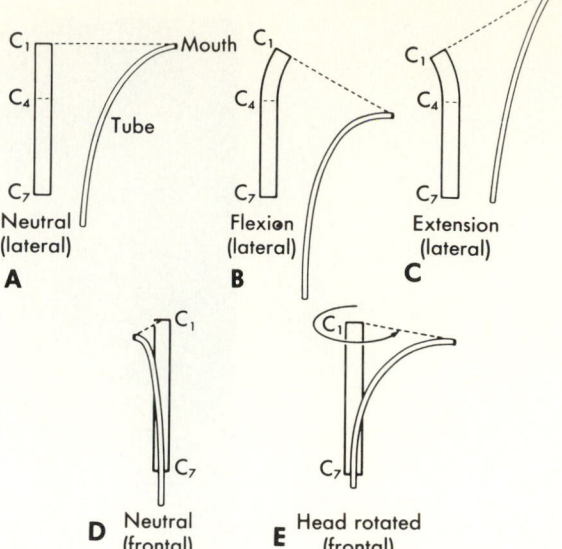

Fig. 5-11 Proposed mechanism of endotracheal tube movement with changes in head position. This schematic diagram depicts the proposed movement of the ET tube as head position changes. The first four cervical vertebrae (C_1 to C_4) primarily provide neck flexion and extension and head rotation. The lower cervical spine (C_4 to C_7) is fairly fixed. A functional lever arm is present within the skull, between the anterior maxilla and the front cervical spine; this lever serves to move the ET tube. **A**, Neutral position, lateral view. **B**, Flexion of neck, lateral view. Neck flexion has pushed the ET tube downward (caudad). **C**, Extension of neck, lateral view. The ET tube has been pulled upward by the lever arm effect. **D**, Neutral position, frontal view. **E**, Lateral rotation, frontal view. Rotation of the head laterally also displaces the ET tube upward and away from the carina.

From Donn, S.M., and Kuhns, L.R.: Mechanisms of endotracheal tube movement with change of head position in the neonate, Pediatr. Radiol. 9:39, Springer-Verlag New York, Inc., 1980.

catheter may drop into the right ventricle (this will be obvious from pressure measurements and waveform tracings), or it may rest against the tricuspid valve. The pulmonary artery line (Swan-Ganz catheter) can migrate distally and become "wedged" in a small pulmonary arteriole. Therefore it is important that the nurse check the location of all catheters and discuss apparent abnormal location of these catheters with a physician.

The location of the nasogastric tube should also be assessed. Although its location should be known from clinical assessment, occasionally the nasogastric tube will migrate, especially if it is taped inadequately or if there is excessive patient movement.

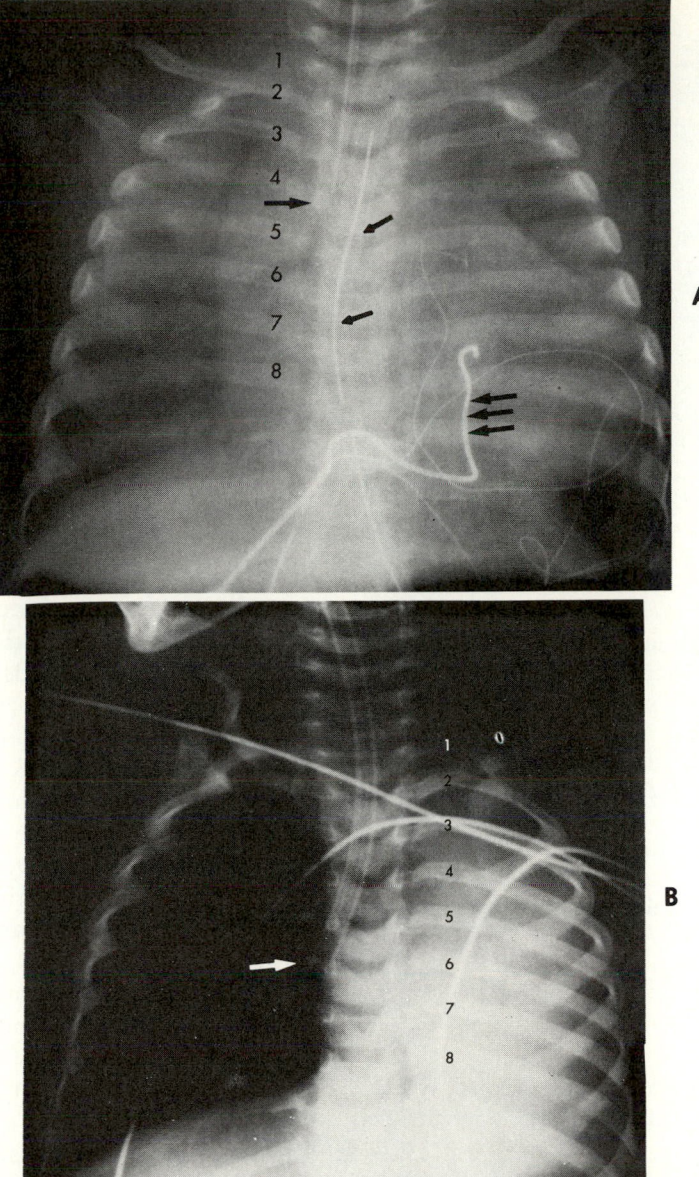

Fig. 5-12 Evaluation of ET tube placement. **A,** This radiograph of a 2-year-old child was taken immediately after she returned from cardiovascular surgery. The heart is enlarged (cardiothoracic ratio of 0.67), and pulmonary vascular markings are diffusely increased and hazy. An ET tube is in place, and the tip lies just above the carina, at the level of the third and fourth ribs *(wide arrow).* Since the child's head is not visible on the film, the neck is not flexed, so the tip of the tube has not been displaced downward by head position. The tube should be withdrawn approximately 0.5 cm to prevent migration of the ET tube to the right mainstem bronchus with neck flexion. A mediastinal chest tube is in place *(thin arrows),* and an epicardial pacer wire is also visible *(three small arrows).* **B,** This radiograph was ordered when the nurse noted that breath sounds were decreased over the child's left lung fields. It was suspected that the child's ET tube may be at the carina or in the right main-stem bronchus. Before the film could be taken, the child developed marked cyanosis and hypotension. No breath sounds could be heard over the left chest, and the child's left chest did not move during hand ventilation. The chest film was quickly taken and revealed that the ET tube was in the right mainstem bronchus *(arrow).* This has produced hyperinflation of the right lung (note increased radiolucency) and total collapse of the left lung (note complete opacification of the left chest). This left lung collapse produced profound hypoxemia and cardiovascular collapse. The child's neck is slightly flexed (the chin is visible at the top of the film), so this has displaced the ET tube downward even further. The tube was immediately withdrawn 2.5 cm, and the left lung reexpanded.

Chest radiographs courtesy Dr. H. Rex Gardner, Rush Presbyterian-St. Luke's Medical Center, Chicago, Ill.

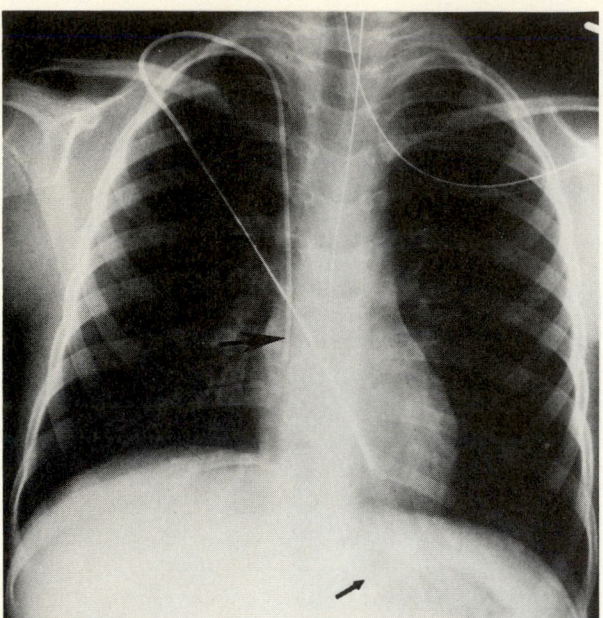

Fig. 5-13 Evaluation of line placement. This 10-year-old child has just returned from major abdominal surgery. Chest expansion is good and equal bilaterally, and lungs are clear to auscultation. Vital signs are stable. The chest radiograph is unremarkable. The heart size is normal (cardiothoracic ratio is 0.4). Pulmonary vascular markings are normal. A central venous pressure line is in place. It has been inserted by percutaneous stick into the subclavian vein, and threaded into the right atrium *(wide arrow).* A nasogastric tube is also in place *(thin arrow).*

The presence and location of any pacing wires should also be verified. Occasionally, a pacer wire is dislodged or fractured (see Fig. 5-12, *A*).

Lateral chest radiographs should also be used to evaluate tube placement. As noted earlier in the chapter, AP or PA films are most useful for evaluation of the lateral relationships of structures (Fig. 5-14, *A*). However, this view can occasionally be misleading because it does not enable evaluation of the AP relationships of structures. The lateral view provides extremely valuable information when evaluating tube placement, since it does allow evaluation of the AP relationships of structures (Fig. 5-14, *B*).

■ **COMMON RADIOGRAPHIC ABNORMALITIES OBSERVED IN PEDIATRIC CRITICAL CARE**

The preceding discussion has focused on the systematic review of a chest radiograph, including a brief discussion of abnormalities. Since the critically ill child may develop pneumonia, atelectasis, or accumulation of free pleural fluid or air and since these problems require specific changes in nursing care, they will be discussed further here.

The term, "air space disease" applies to the presence of abnormal (nonair) densities in the lung. These densities can be localized or diffuse and generally indicate the development of lung disease, atelectasis, or tumor or the accumulation of exudate, transudate, or blood in the lung.[14] Often it may be difficult to differentiate between opacification produced by intrapulmonary (air space) disease and that produced by pleural space fluid accumulation. The following discussion includes identifying characteristics of each problem and clues to differentiating among them.

Pneumonia can initially produce a patchy infiltration with fluffy margins. The presence of an air bronchogram within the infiltrate can confirm the impression that the opacification is caused by intrapulmonary disease.[14] If the pneumonia causes obliteration of the cardiac border, the pneumonia must be in contact with the heart (Fig. 5-15, *A*). The portion of the heart that is obliterated will help localize the pneumonia (see Table 5-1).[4]

Frequently, pneumonia will later cause more segmental or lobar disease, with more homogenous opacification of the involved area of the lung.[14] The child may develop air trapping with resultant depression of the diaphragm and increased radiolucency of the lung fields.

Some pneumonias can be recognized by their characteristic radiographic appearance and clinical history. Most infectious pneumonia in children, regardless of origin, begins with local or alveolar involvement (difficult to differentiate from interstitial disease) before progressing to lobar disease. Lobar consolidation frequently occurs as the result of pneumococcal pneumonia. *Haemophilus pneumoniae* is nearly always associated with a pleural effusion. Epiglottitis can also accompany this disease. *Staphylococcus pneumoniae* occurs more commonly in infants less than 1 year of age; it more commonly involves the right lung and may cause development of pneumatoceles (localized collections of intrapulmonary air) or abscesses. *Streptococcus, Klebsiella,* and *Haemophilus pneumoniae* may also be associated with empyema (a purulent pleural space infection) or pneumatocele formation.[14]

Aspiration pneumonia usually develops in the portion of the lung that is dependent at the time of aspiration. The radiographic changes following the aspiration are related to irritation and inflammation caused by the aspirated material and to the develop-

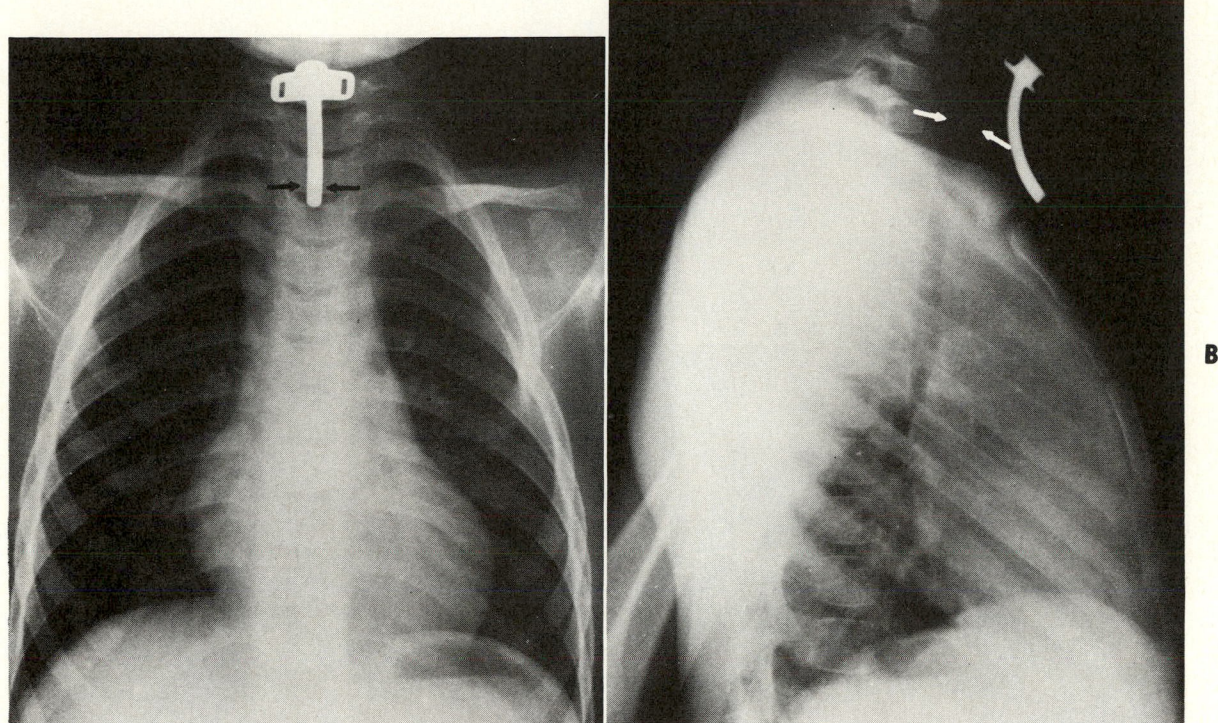

Fig. 5-14   These chest films of a 6-year-old boy
were obtained after the nurse changed the boy's
tracheostomy tube and was unable to insert a
suction catheter more than 2 to 3 cm through the
new tube. The child complained of difficulty
"getting air," although air movement was adequate
bilaterally by auscultation. **A,** AP view. Lung
expansion appears adequate, and the tracheostomy
tube seems to be located in the midline, in the
center of the air density of the trachea *(arrows).*
Fortunately, a lateral film was also taken. **B,** Lateral
view. The air density of the trachea is seen
(arrows), and it is clear that the tracheostomy tube
has been placed subcutaneously and that it is not in
the trachea at all.

Chest radiographs courtesy Dr. Andrew K. Poznanski, Children's
Memorial Hospital, Chicago, Ill.

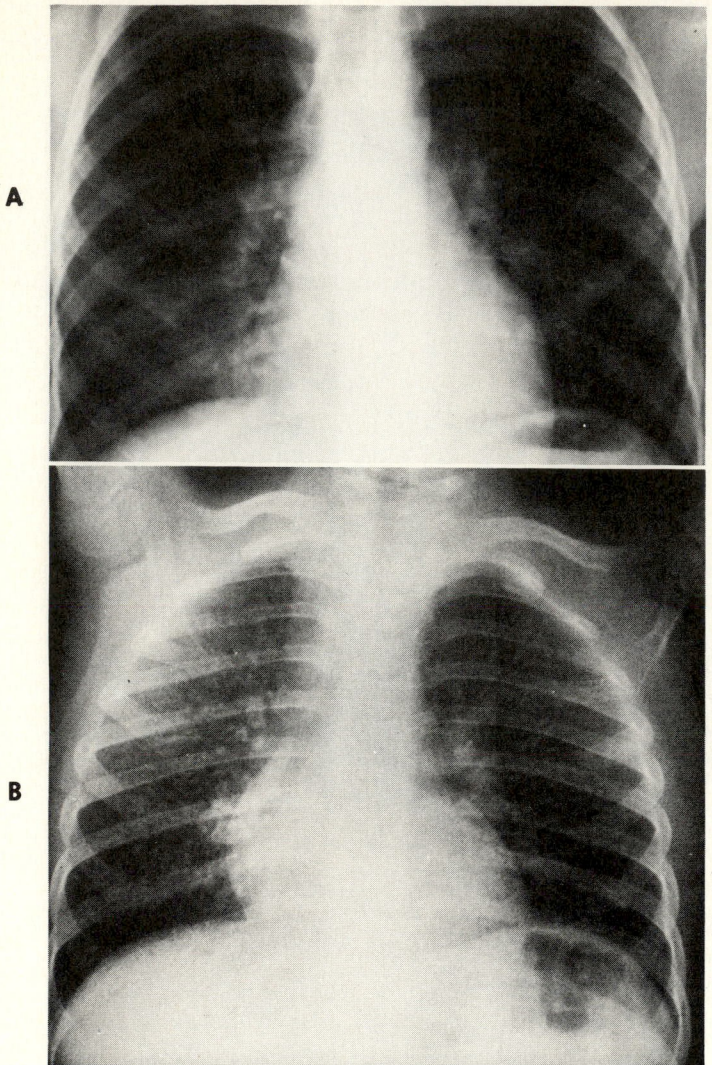

Fig. 5-15 Pneumonia. **A,** This radiograph of a 15-year-old young man was taken when he was admitted with fever, tachypnea, and rhonchi heard over the right middle lobe. The right heart border is obliterated by the fluffy opacification produced by right-middle lobe pneumonia. **B,** This chest film of a 3-year-old girl was obtained when she developed fever, progressive tachypnea, increased respiratory effort, and cyanosis in room air. Because the girl was known to have acute lymphoblastic leukemia, the diagnosis of pneumocystis carinii was suspected. The diffuse distribution of the disease creates both perihilar and alveolar changes, and it creates the reticular appearance in the lung fields. The child required a lung biopsy to confirm the diagnosis.

Chest radiograph *A,* courtesy Dr. H. Rex Gardner, Rush Presbyterian-St. Luke's Medical Center, and *B,* courtesy Dr. Andrew K. Poznanski, Children's Memorial Hospital, Chicago, Ill.

ment of the pneumonia. Aspiration pneumonia characteristically produces patchy opacification in the lung bases, and perihilar infiltrations.[14]

Bronchopneumonia produces perihilar congestion. Pneumonia produced by *Pneumoncystis carinii* (most frequently seen in immunologically compromised patients) initially produces perihilar congestion and then peripheral intrapulmonary involvement. The disease soon assumes an alveolar and interstitial distribution (see Fig. 5-15, *B*).

Atelectasis also produces intrapulmonary opacification as the result of collapse of a portion of the lung (Fig. 5-16). Atelectasis is usually produced by obstruction of an airway (caused by a mucous plug, exudate, or foreign body), compression of the airway by another thoracic structure (such as enlarged lymph nodes, large heart, or tumor), or significant hypoventilation. Since atelectasis represents loss of lung volume (collapse), other intrathoracic structures usually shift toward an area of atelectasis. The trachea, mediastinum, hilum, and any visible intrapulmonary septa all shift toward the atelectatic area. In addition, the hemidiaphragm on the involved side is elevated, and the intercostal spaces on that side narrow. The uninvolved lung may become hyperinflated, and as a result the intercostal spaces on the uninvolved side widen and the hemidiaphragm may be flattened.[4] An air bronchogram may be noted within the opacified area, although the visualized bronchi are often crowded together because of lung collapse.

Pleural fluid accumulation can be a result of pleural effusion, a chylothorax, hemothorax or hydrothorax, or a pleural reaction. Free pleural fluid characteristically assumes a dependent position so that in the upright chest film it generally accumulates in the subpulmonic area, along the diaphragm. With small amounts of fluid accumulation, the costophrenic angles are blunted, and the diaphragm appears to be elevated (see Fig. 5-4). If fluid accumulation continues, an air-fluid interface will be seen in the up-

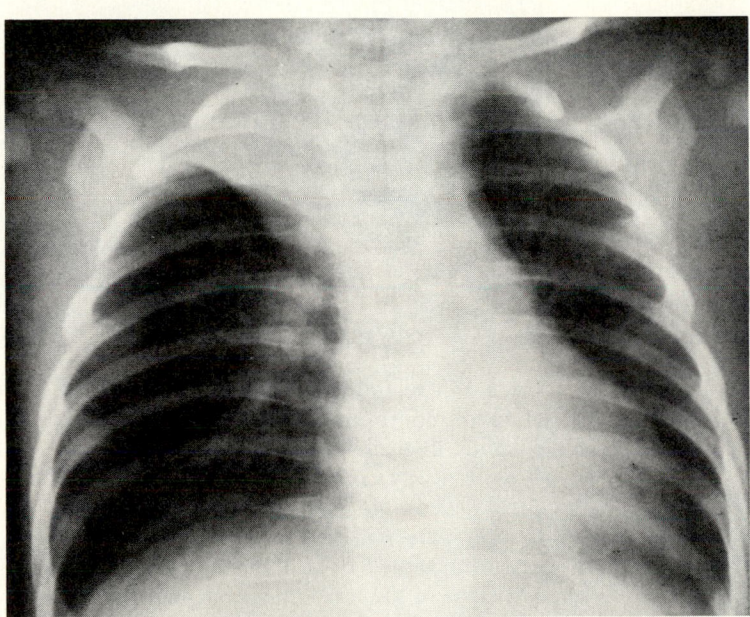

Fig. 5-16 Atelectasis. This chest film was taken when the nurse noted tachypnea and decreased breath sounds over this 3-year-old child's right upper lobe 2 days following gastrointestinal surgery. The opacification of the right upper lobe is readily apparent. Since atelectasis represents collapse of a portion of the lung, other structures have shifted toward the involved area. The right hemidiaphragm is higher, and the hilum of the right lung is shifted upward. The minor fissure, which separates the right upper and middle lobes, serves to demarcate the lobar atelectasis.

Chest radiograph courtesy Dr. H. Rex Gardner, Rush Presbyterian-St. Luke's Medical Center, Chicago, Ill.

right film wherever the fluid level occurs. Fluid may also accumulate between lobes of the lung on the involved side and along the side of the lung.

If the free pleural fluid continues to accumulate, the entire hemithorax can be filled. This produces complete opacification of that hemithorax, with compression of the underlying lung and flattening of the involved hemidiaphragm.[14] The trachea, mediastinum, and hilum are usually shifted away from significant fluid accumulation since this represents an increase in intrathoracic lung volume (unless concurrent atelectasis is present on the involved side).

If the child is supine when the chest film is taken, free pleural fluid will accumulate along the dorsal surface of the chest. This will produce a diffuse opacification within the involved thorax that may be difficult to differentiate from interstitial lung disease. An upright film or a lateral decubitus film will help differentiate free pleural fluid from intrapulmonary disease. Since the lateral decubitus view enables visualization of smaller amounts of fluid, that view is often specifically requested to confirm the presence of free pleural fluid (see Fig. 5-4).

Abnormal areas of radiolucency may also be observed on the chest film as collections of air within soft tissues or surrounded by tissues. They are most frequently caused by a pneumothorax, pneumomediastinum, lung abscess, pneumatocele, or emphysema.

Unilateral hyperlucency is most often a result of a *pneumothorax*. A small pneumothorax is not readily observed on an inspiratory chest film. Since in an expiratory film the child's lung volumes are smaller, the normal pulmonary vascular markings are crowded together (see Fig. 5-1, *A* and *B*). Thus the difference between the vascularized lung fields and the avascular, radiolucent pneumothorax is intensified. A pneumothorax may also be more readily discerned if the patient is upright while the film is taken since free pleural air will rise toward the apexes of the lungs. If the child is supine when the film is taken, free pleural air will tend to collect along the diaphragm and the anterior aspects of the thorax so that it may not be seen as easily (compare Figs. 5-2 and 5-6). In addition, the interface between the pneumothorax and the lung will be in the same plane as the chest film; therefore a distinct border (or density contrast) between the two will not be apparent. However, the pneumothorax should be suspected if an extremely radiolucent area (lacking in vascular markings) is noted along the diaphragm.

If the pneumothorax is significant, the underlying lung will collapse, and the trachea and medias-

tinum will be compressed and shifted away from the side of the pneumothorax. Since the pneumothorax occupies volume, the hemidiaphragm on the involved side of the chest will often be flattened or displaced downward.

Lung abscesses and pneumotoceles can develop as a result of pneumonia. They both produce more localized collections of air within the lungs. The increased radiolucency from an absess occurs as the re-

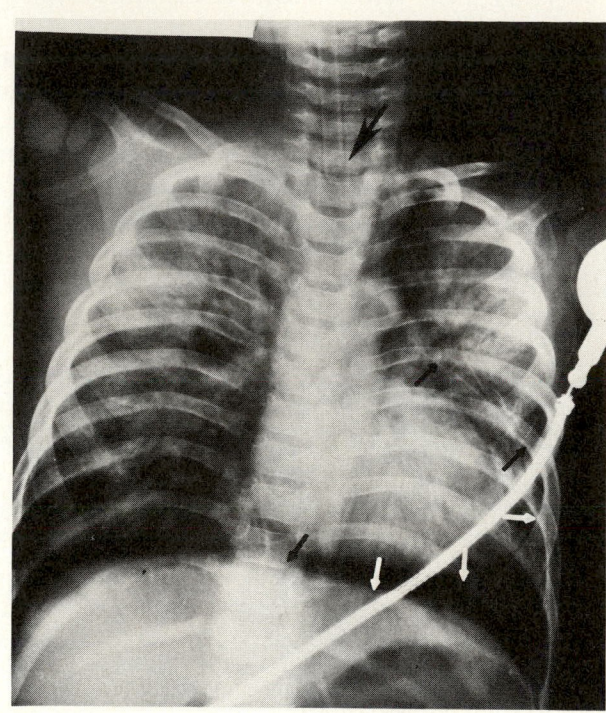

Fig. 5-17 Pneumopericardium. This is a chest film of an 18-month-old infant with known complex cyanotic heart disease. An aortopulmonary shunt was surgically created; after surgery the child developed progressive signs of congestive heart failure, including respiratory distress and hepatomegaly. The child's symptoms progressed, and signs of low cardiac output and pulmonary edema were noted. Rales were present on auscultation. The child was returned to surgery for reduction of the shunt size, but this produced no improvement in clinical condition. The chest radiograph reveals diffuse severe pulmonary edema; pulmonary vascular markings are prominent and hazy throughout the lung fields, resulting from both pulmonary arterial and venous congestion. A pneumopericardium is present; it is seen as a dark air density surrounding the heart (*arrows*). The child has an endotracheal tube in place that is too high (*thick arrow*).

Chest radiograph courtesy Dr. Andrew K. Poznanski, Children's Memorial Hospital, Chicago, Ill.

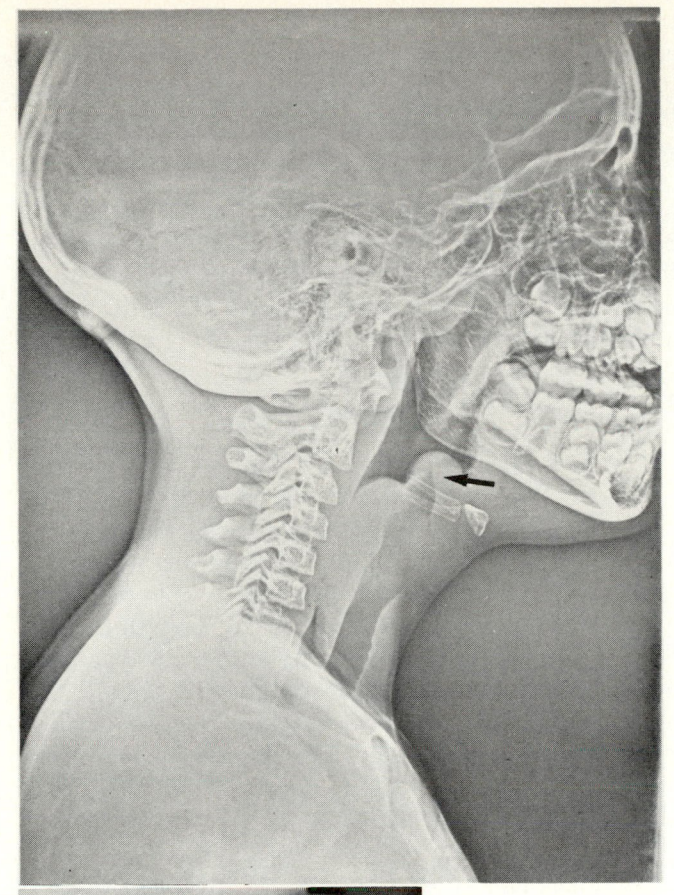

A

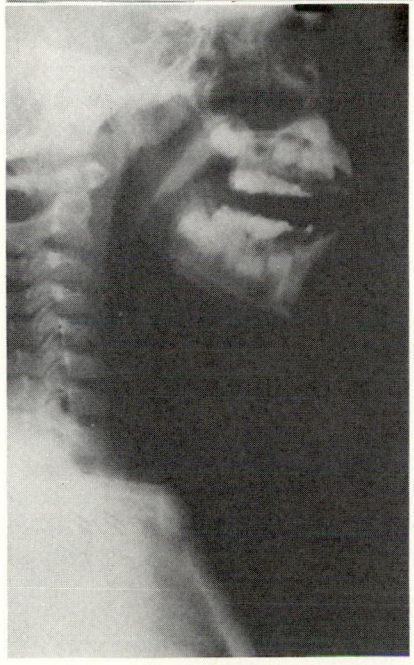

B

Fig. 5-18 Diagnosis of epiglottitis. **A,** Xeroradiogram. This radiographic exposure and film combination depicts the structures of the upper airway in sharp contrast. Obstruction of the upper airway by the enlarged epiglottis is apparent. The child also demonstrates laryngeal and subglottic edema. Because this technique requires greater radiation exposure than routine radiographs, it is rarely used. **B,** Lateral radiograph. Upper airway obstruction by the enlarged epiglottis is again visible. Although less detail is apparent when compared to the xeroradiogram, this film is also diagnostic with approximately one-seventh of the radiation exposure required for a xeroradiogram. **C,** This schematic drawing of the upper airway depicts the site of airway compromise in epiglottitis. Note the normal caliber of the airway at the cricoid cartilage; this confirms the diagnosis of epiglottitis and rules out the diagnosis of croup.

Xeroradiogram courtesy Dr. H. Rex Gardner, Rush Presbyterian–Saint Luke's Hospital, Chicago, Ill. *B* and *C* from Morriss, F.C.: Epiglottitis. In Levin, D.L., Morriss, F.C., and Moore, G.C.: A practical guide to pediatric intensive care, ed. 2, St. Louis, 1984, The C.V. Mosby Co.

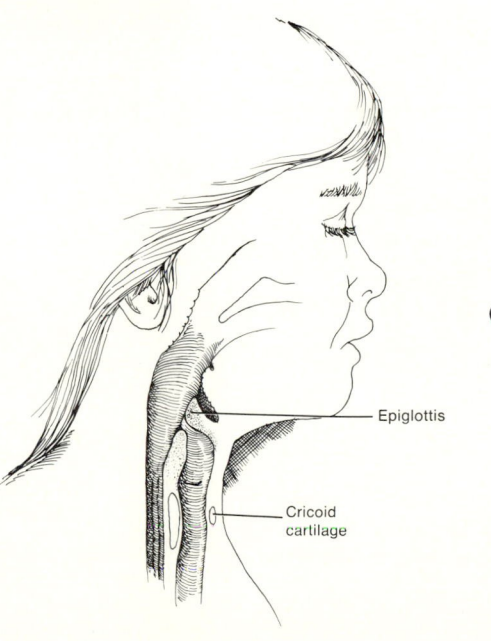

C

Epiglottis

Cricoid cartilage

sult of necrosis. The pneumotocele can also occur as the result of necrosis or air trapping.[14]

Emphysematous changes in the lungs can also cause localized, circumscribed areas of increased radiolucency within the lungs. The emphysematous lung is distended, and air trapping occurs. The diaphragm on the involved side is flattened, and the trachea and mediastinum are shifted away from the involved side.

A *pneumopericardium* is a collection of air within the pericardial sac surrounding the heart. It is usually easily recognized because it appears as a radiolucent border between the radiopaque pericardial sac and the radiopaque heart (Fig. 5-17).

The child with a diaphragmatic hernia may also demonstrate abnormal densities within the thorax. This child generally has hypoplasia of both lungs. The lung on the side of the diaphragmatic defect is compressed by abdominal contents during fetal life. The heart and other abdominal contents shift to the uninvolved side, thus compressing the other lung during fetal life. Even after repair of the diaphragmatic hernia, the small lungs may not completely fill the thorax, so radiolucent areas will surround the lung.

■ SPECIAL TECHNIQUES
■ Xeroradiography

Xeroradiography is a special radiographic technique, that involves use of specially coated x-ray films to obtain radiographic films with far greater resolution of images than standard films. Although xeroradiography is currently still used for mammography in adults, it is not commonly used in the pediatric setting since it requires greatly increased radiation exposure. Whereas xeroradiograms were previously obtained in pediatric patients to confirm the diagnosis of epiglottitis, they are now almost exclusively used to detect the presence and location of nonmetallic foreign bodies. The diagnosis of epiglottitis and other information previously obtained by xeroradiography is now obtained by good standard radiographic exposure (Fig. 5-18).[11]

■ Fluoroscopy

Fluoroscopy is a form of examination that records the radiographic images rapidly (at approximately 50 frames per minute) to provide a dynamic image of the structures examined; it is similar to an "x-ray movie." Fluoroscopy is used whenever structure or organ movement (such as the diaphragm) needs to be evaluated. It may also be used for localization of pathology before spot filming.[11] Since the examination records movement with rapid filming techniques, it does not provide the sharp resolution for evaluation of anatomic features that is possible with spot films.

Fluoroscopy is generally performed in the radiology department, although it may be performed at the bedside of the critically ill patient. Videotapes of the fluoroscopic examination are usually made to allow later viewing and analysis. Gonadal shielding is required for the child and for the attendant nurse.

■ CONCLUSION

Chest radiographs are a valuable adjunct to assessment of the critically ill patient when they are used in conjunction with a thorough clinical examination. If the nurse develops a systematic method of reviewing the radiograph and if she is able to recognize abnormal densities in the chest, she will be able to confirm clinical impressions and better evaluate progress and complications of therapy. Since the nurse is often the first person to see the chest radiograph, it is important that she be able to recognize significant changes or indications of serious problems.

ACKNOWLEDGMENT

Dr. Andrew K. Poznanski from Children's Memorial Hospital and Dr. H. Rex Gardner from Rush Presbyterian-St. Luke's Medical Center (both of Chicago, Illinois) have provided invaluable assistance in the preparation of this chapter. They both have freely shared their radiographic teaching files and expertise.

REFERENCES

1. Beguery, P., and Remy, J.: Simple radiologic investigation of congenital heart diseases during childhood. In Kaufmann, H.J., editor: Clinical practice in pediatric radiology, vol. 1: Heart and great vessels, New York, 1979, Masson Publishing USA, Inc.
2. Crouch, J.E.: Functional human anatomy, ed. 3, Philadelphia, 1978, Lea & Febiger.
3. Elliott, L.P.: Radiologic evaluation of the patient with congenital heart disease, Cardiovasc. Clin. **4:**194, 1972.
4. Felson, B., Weinstein, A.S., and Spitz, H.B.: Principles of chest roentgenology: a programmed test, Philadelphia, 1965, W.B. Saunders Co.
5. Fink, B.W.: Congenital heart disease: a deductive approach to its diagnosis, Chicago, 1975, Year Book Medical Publishers, Inc.
6. Hoeffel, J.C., and Pernot, C.: Radiologic anatomy of the heart and great vessels. In Kaufmann, H.J., editor: Clinical practice in pediatric radiology, vol. 1: Heart and great vessels, New York, 1979, Masson Publishing USA, Inc.

7. Kuhns, L.R., and Poznanski, A.K.: Endotracheal tube position in the infant, J. Pediatr. **78:**991, 1971.

8. Logue, R.B.: Etiology, recognition and management of pericardial disease. In Hurst, J.W., editor: The heart, arteries, and veins, ed. 5, New York, 1982, McGraw-Hill, Inc.

9. Milledge, R.D., and Edwards, F.K.: X-ray examinations of the heart. In Wenger, N.K., Hurst, J.W., and McIntyre, M.C., editors: Cardiology for nurses, New York, 1980, McGraw-Hill, Inc.

10. Moller, J.H., and others: Congenital cardiac disease associated with polysplenia, Circulation **36:**789, 1967.

11. Poznanski, A.K.: The chest. In Practical approaches to pediatric radiology, ed. 2, Chicago, 1984, Year Book Medical Publishers, Inc.

12. Raffensperger, J.G.: Esophageal atresia and tracheoesophageal fistula. In Swenson's pediatric surgery, ed. 4, New York, 1980, Appleton-Century-Crofts.

13. Ruttenberg, H.D., and others: Syndrome of congenital cardiac disease with asplenia, Am. J. Cardiol. **16:**387, 1964.

14. Siegle, R.L., and Rabinowitz, J.G.: Radiographic patterns of thoracic disease in the infant and child. In Rabinowitz, J.G., editor: Pediatric radiology, Philadelphia, 1978, J.B. Lippincott Co.

15. Squire, L.F.: Fundamentals of roentgenology, Cambridge, Mass., 1964, Harvard University Press.

16. Stanger, P., Rudolph, A.M., and Edwards, J.E.: Cardiac malpositions: an overview based on a study of sixty-five necropsy specimens, Circulation **56:**159, 1977.

17. Swischuck, L.E.: Plain film interpretation in congenital heart disease, Baltimore, 1979, The Williams & Wilkins Co.

18. Tinker, J.H.: Understanding chest x-rays, Am. J. Nurs. **76:**54, 1976.

CHAPTER SIX

Neurologic Disorders

JUDY HARR

MARY FRAN HAZINSKI

Care of the critically ill child with neurologic problems is both challenging and rewarding. It requires knowledge of neuroanatomy, neurophysiology, and normal growth and development. In addition, the nurse must have the ability to accurately assess the patient's condition by comparing patient behavior with designated norms. Since the critically ill child with neurologic disease is often admitted *in extremis*, the medical team usually does not have the benefit of adequate historical data. As a result the accuracy of the nurse's observations and the rapidity of her responses are crucial to the successful treatment of the child.

This chapter provides an overview of relevant neurologic anatomy, physiology, and pathophysiology. In addition, it provides the information required to perform precise assessment and appropriate interventions for the critically ill child with neurologic disease.

■ Essential Anatomy and Physiology

■ THE AXIAL SKELETON

The *axial skeleton* consists of the bones of the skull and vertebral column and protects the underlying structures of the central nervous system. The bones of the skull are divided into regions that form the wall of the cranial cavity and that cover the uppermost aspects of the brain and face. The frontal, occipital, temporal, and paired parietal bones form the *cranial vault.* The floor of this vault is composed of three bony compartments—the anterior, middle, and posterior *fossae.* The anterior fossa contains the frontal lobes of the brain; the middle fossa contains the upper brainstem and the pituitary gland; and the posterior fossa contains the lower brainstem. These fossae and the parts of the brain they contain are often used to designate areas of injury or disease; such a designation allows location of the problem as well as delineation of the brain functions that may be affected. Since, for example, injury to the area of the posterior fossa potentially disrupts the critical brainstem functions, damage in this area is usually more life-threatening than damage to the anterior fossa.

Blood vessels and cranial nerves enter and leave the skull through small openings or *foramina.* It is useful to know the course of the cranial nerves so that clinical signs and symptoms can be readily correlated with areas of cranial injury (Table 6-1). The posterior fossa contains a large foramen, the *foramen magnum,* through which the brainstem and spinal cord join. Lesions in this area, such as those produced by cervical neck trauma, can interrupt vital brain functions and nerve pathways to and from the brain. Cerebrospinal fluid (CSF) also flows through the foramen magnum as it passes from the brain to the spinal cord and back again.

At birth the skull plates are not fused, and they are separated by nonossified spaces, called *fontanelles.* The anterior fontanelle is the junction of the coronal, sagittal, and frontal bones. The posterior fontanelle represents the junction of the parietal and occipital bones (Fig. 6-1). Normally, the posterior fontanelle closes at approximately 2 months of age; the anterior fontanelle closes at approximately 16 to 18 months of age. If the brain does not grow, as in patients with microcephaly, the cranial bones may fuse early. Conversely, premature fusion of cranial bones, known as *craniosynostosis,* can result in microcephaly because brain growth is inhibited. If the infant develops a space-occupying lesion or an increase in intracranial pressure, the fontanelles will bulge. If intracranial volume or pressure is chronically increased

Table 6-1 Course of the cranial nerves

Foramina	Bones involved	Structures passing through
1. Olfactory	Cribriform plate of ethmoid	Olfactory nerves (I)
2. Optic	Sphenoid	Optic nerves (II)
3. Superior orbital fissure	Sphenoid	Oculomotor (III), trochlear (IV), ophthalmic of trigeminal (V), abducens (VI) nerves
4. Inferior orbital fissure	Sphenoid, maxilla, palatine, zygomatic	Maxillary nerve (V), infraorbital vessels
5. Rotundum	Sphenoid	Maxillary nerve (V)
6. Ovale	Sphenoid	Mandibular nerve (V)
7. Spinosum	Sphenoid	Middle meningeal vessels
8. Lacerum	Sphenoid, temporal, occipital	Meningeal branch of the ascending pharyngeal artery, internal carotid artery
9. (Internal acoustic meatus)	Petrous portion of temporal	Facial (VII) and vestibulocochlear (VIII) nerves, internal auditory artery
10. Jugular	Petrous temporal and occipital	Glossopharyngeal (IX), vagus (X), and accessory (XI) nerves, internal jugular vein
11. (Hypoglossal canal)	Occipital bone	Hypoglossal nerve (XII)
12. (Carotid canal)	Petrous temporal	Internal carotid artery
13. Stylomastoid	Temporal—between mastoid and styloid processes	Facial nerve (VII)
14. (Condyloid canal)	Occipital	Vein to transverse sinus
15. Foramen magnum	Occipital	Medulla oblongata and its membranes, accessory nerves, vertebral arteries
16. Mastoid	Mastoid portion of temporal	An emissary vein

From Crouch, J.E.: Functional human anatomy, ed. 3, Philadelphia, 1978, Lea & Febiger.

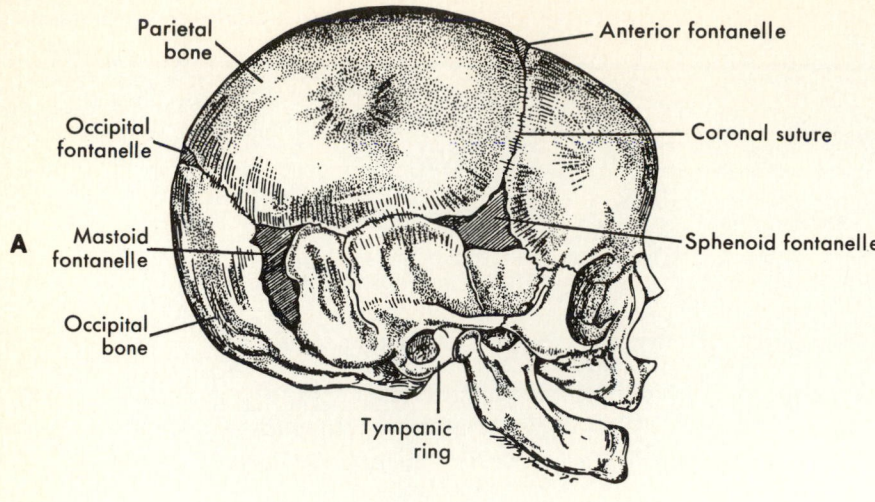

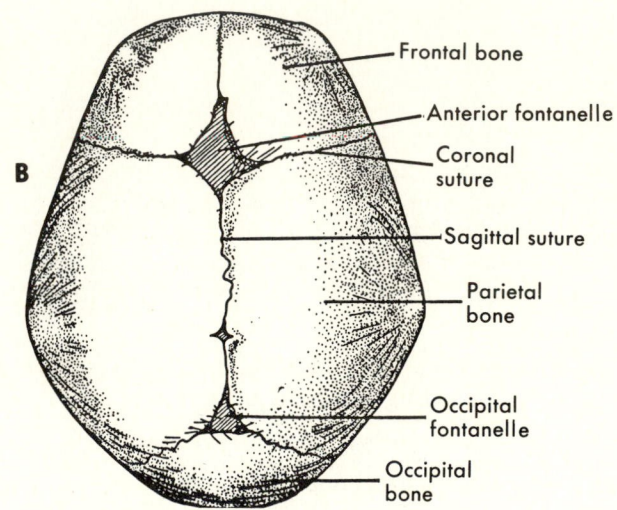

Fig. 6-1 Infant skull. **A,** Lateral view. **B,** Superior view.

From Conway, B.L.: Pediatric neurologic nursing, St. Louis, 1977, The C.V. Mosby Co.

or if it increases gradually over a period of time, the bones of the skull may separate even after fusion; such separation can occur in a child up to 12 years of age.

At birth the brain is approximately 25% of the adult volume; by 2 years of age, approximately 75% of adult brain volume has been achieved. The cranium itself continues to expand until about the age of 7, when most brain differentiation has been completed. This growth of the brain can be indirectly assessed through measurements of the head circumference. These measurements should always be plotted on a growth chart since they can aid in the detection of excessive or inadequate head and brain growth, which may reflect neurologic disease.

■ THE MENINGES

Three highly vascular membranes, the meninges, surround the brain and spinal column. The outermost membrane, the *dura mater* consists of tough connective tissue that lines the endocranial vault. The dura mater is folded into tents of tissue immediately underneath the skull cap. The most familiar of its many folds, is the fold that roofs the posterior fossa; this is called the *tentorium cerebelli.* This fold serves as an anatomic landmark, and intracranial lesions are usually divided into those that occur above the tentorium cerebelli (supratentorial lesions) and those that occur below the tentorium cerebelli (infratentorial lesions). The dura not only lines the endocranium, but it also lines the vertebral column. It descends through the foramen magnum to the level of the second sacral vertebra and ends as a blind sac.

The next membrane, the *arachnoid*, consists of spiderlike tissue from which it gains its descriptive name. The arachnoid membrane is separated from the dural membrane by the *subdural space*, which contains cerebral vessels. Since these vessels traverse the subdural space with relatively little support, serious head trauma can cause rupture of these vessels and development of a subdural hematoma. This space does allow for some cerebral expansion or collection of hematoma without cerebral compression, but the critical capacity is rather small. Beneath the subdural space the arachnoid membrane follows the contour of the brain and spinal cord to the end of the spinal cord root.

The *pia mater* is the third and the innermost membrane. It consists of highly vascular tissue that is separated from the arachnoid membrane by a space called the *subarachnoid space*. This space contains cerebrospinal fluid and provides for two major CSF collecting chambers. The largest chamber, the *cisterna magna* (also called the cisterna cerebello-medullaris), is located between the cerebellum and the medulla. The smallest, the *lumbar cistern*, is located at the level of the sacrum. Since this space contains cerebrospinal fluid, obstruction of the subarachnoid space will cause obstruction to the flow of cerebrospinal fluid.

■ **THE BRAIN**

The brain is contained within the cranial vault and extends through the foramen magnum. It is composed of distinct structures, each having a specific function. The brain is divided into three major areas, the *cerebrum*, the *brainstem*, and the *cerebellum*. The cerebrum consists of the cerebral hemispheres, the thalamus, hypothalamus, basal ganglia, and the olfactory and optic nerves. The brainstem consists of the pons, the medulla, the thalamus, and the third ventricle.[42] The cerebellum is the final major division of the brain (Table 6-2 lists the divisions of the brain and their major functions). Each of these brain divisions will be presented separately in the following pages.

■ **The cerebrum**

The cerebral cortex. The cerebral cortex consists of the convoluted gray matter that forms the outermost layer of the brain. It is made up largely of specialized neurons that process and respond to specific sensory stimuli. The cortex receives electrical discharges from other neurons and converts them into ideas or actions. The cortex is divided into five anatomic divisions: the frontal, parietal, temporal, occipital, and limbic divisions. The cortical neurons are specialized so that within each major division of the brain specific areas are devoted to specific functions. Fifty-two specialized areas have been identified and numbered according to histologic appearances and functions. If brain injury is identified in one of these areas, the sensory or functional impairment that will result may be predicted. Conversely, a lesion can often be localized according to the motor functions or sensations that the patient has lost.

The cerebral cortex performs the highest functions of the human brain; as a result it continues to develop beyond infancy and childhood. The newborn responds to the environment with simple awareness and reflex behavior. During infancy, individual sensations, sights, and sounds can be stored in memory in the cerebral cortex, and the infant learns to associate these sights and sounds with events or feelings. As the infant develops into a toddler, higher cortical functions, such as imagination and language, become apparent. Thus there is tremendous growth of cortical function during the early years of life. Most developmental and neurologic assessment tools evaluate only basic reflexes and motor skills of the young infant and toddler, and it is not until the preschool and the early childhood years that cognitive functions and learning can be documented.

The *cerebral hemispheres* are two mirror-image portions of the brain that consist largely of the cerebral cortex and fiber tracts. In general the cerebral hemispheres govern functions of and receive sensations from the contralateral side of the body. Thus the right cerebral hemisphere governs movement of and receives sensory input from the left side of the body. The left cerebral hemisphere governs movement of and receives sensory input from the right side of the body. Most humans have one side of the brain that is considered dominant; right-handed people are thought to have a dominant left side of the brain, and left-handed people are thought to have a dominant right side of the brain. The dominant hemisphere is primarily involved in verbal, analytical, and cognitive functions, and the nondominant side is involved with nonverbal, geometric, spatial, visual, musical, and synthetic functions.[15] To a certain extent, if one side of the brain is injured, the other side of the brain can be taught to assume the dominant functions. This is thought to be especially true when the injury occurs during infancy or early childhood because cerebral dominance is not fully established until approximately 3 years of age.

Table 6-2 Basic brain divisions and functions

Division	Contents	Function
Cerebrum	Cerebral hemispheres	Integration of sophisticated sensory and motor activities and thoughts
	Cerebral cortex	
	Frontal lobes	Reception of smell, memory banks, and higher intellectual processes
	Parietal lobes	Sensory discrimination, localization of body awareness (spatial relationships), and speech
	Temporal lobes	Auditory functions and emotional equilibrium
	Occipital lobes	Vision and memory of events
	Limbic lobes	Primitive behavior, moods, and instincts
	Basal ganglia	Transmission of motor tracts, linking pyramidal pathways
	Corpus collosum	Provision of intricate connection between cerebral hemispheres
Brainstem	Midbrain	Hypothalamic response to neuroendocrine stimuli
	Pons	Origin of cranial nerves V, VI, VII, VIII
	Medulla	Vital center activity (cardiac, vasomotor, respiratory centers); origin for cranial nerves IX, X, XI
Cerebellum	White and gray matter	Muscle and proprioceptive activity, balance, and dexterity

The cerebral hemispheres are connected by nerve fibers called the *corpus callosum.* These nerve fibers allow the brain to function as a single unit despite the fact that it is divided into two hemispheres.

The basal ganglia. The *basal ganglia* are paired masses of gray matter deep within the cerebral hemispheres. They contain nuclei of neurons and networks of tracts that control motor function. These basal ganglia send information to the motor cortex through the thalamus to inhibit unintentional movement. Thus the basal ganglia serve as a regulatory center for the *extrapyramidal motor system.* This system selects motor messages from lower pathways for interpretation upward to the cerebral cortex. This provides for influence over motor activities, skeletomuscular control, rhythmic movement, and maintenance of an erect posture. Interference with neurotransmission to this area is evidenced by disturbances of intentional movement. The uptake by the brain of bilirubin during infancy, known as kernicterus, af-

fects this area specifically and can result in the development of cerebral palsy.

The thalamus and hypothalamus. The *thalamus* is located at the uppermost aspect of the brain and is comprised of tracts of gray matter. This gray matter modifies messages that come from the basal ganglia and cerebellum and transmits the corrected information upward to the cerebral cortex. All sensory impulses, with the exception of those from the olfactory nerve, are received by the thalamus. These impulses are then associated, synthesized, and relayed through thalamocortical tracts to specific cortical areas. The thalamas is the center for primitive appreciation of pain, temperature, and tactile sensations.

Lying beneath the thalamus and near the optic chiasm is the *hypothalamus.* This is the chief region for subcortical integration of sympathetic and parasympathetic activities. The hypothalamus secretes hormones that are important in the control of visceral activities, maintenance of water balance and sugar and fat metabolism, regulation of body temperature, and secretion from the endocrine glands. The hypothalamus is the source of two hormones: *vasopressin* (antidiuretic hormone, or ADH) and *oxytocin.* These hormones are synthesized by the hypothalamus and transmitted in nerve tracts to a small mass of tissue suspended below the hypothalamus called the posterior *pituitary gland* (or neurohypophysis). Vasopressin and oxytocin are then released by the posterior pituitary gland as needed. The anterior pituitary gland, called the *adenohypophysis,* secretes hormones that control glands throughout the body; these hormones include growth hormone (somatotrophin), adrenocorticotropic hormone (ACTH), thyroid-stimulating hormone (TSH), melanocyte-stimulating hormone, follicle-stimulating hormone (FSH), luteinizing hormone releasing factor (LHRF), and prolactin.

Injury to or disease of the hypothalamus or the pituitary can produce a wide variety of neuroendocrine problems and can result in fluid and electrolyte imbalance and growth disturbances.

■ The brainstem

The *brainstem* is located at the base of the skull and consists of the *midbrain,* the *pons,* and the *medulla.* The *midbrain* is a short segment between the hypothalamus and the pons. It contains the cerebral peduncles and the corpus quadrigemina. The midbrain is made up of fibers that connect the upper and lower brainstem. It is the origin of the oculomotor and trochlear cranial nerves. The midbrain is the center for reticular activity, which serves to assimilate all sensory input from the lower neurons before it is relayed to the cortex. It is because of this relay that the cortex can maintain consciousness, arousal, and sleep.

The *pons* is a round structure located in the posterior portion of the brainstem. It contains fiber tracts that connect the medulla oblongata and cerebellum with upper portions of the brain. It is the origin for the abducens, facial, trigeminal, and acoustic cranial nerves. Disturbances within this area often produce signs of abducens malfunction as evidenced by the development of strabismus and visual hemiplegias.

The *medulla oblongata* lies between the pons and the spinal cord at the level of the foramen magnum. It is a virtual pyramid of tracts crossing and transmitting messages to and from the spinal pathways for interpretation and reaction by the cortex. The medulla is the origin for the glossopharyngeal, vagus, spinal accessory, and hypoglossal cranial nerves. Critical regulatory centers for cardiovascular and respiratory functions are found within this portion of the brain. The most serious form of cranial injury results in the loss of medullary control of respirations and cardiac output. A blow to the back of the head can result in respiratory arrest, labile blood pressure, and decreased cardiac output. Because specific posture is controlled by the medulla, medullary injury can produce decorticate and decerebrate posturing. Loss of medullary function can also be evidenced by a decreased gag reflex or swallowing difficulties since the glossopharyngeal and the vagus nerves originate in the medulla. Any disease or injury to the medulla can be life-threatening.

■ The cerebellum

The *cerebellum* is located in the posterior fossa, directly below the occipital lobe. It consists of two hemispheres that contain gray matter, and it joins with the basal ganglia and the reticular system. Spatial orientation, fine motor movements, balance, and dexterity are controlled by visual, auditory, and proprioceptive stimuli that are fed into the cerebellum. The cerebral cortex can exert voluntary control over the cerebellum by virtue of cognitive nerve pathways that adjust movement.

■ The ventricles

The four *ventricles* of the brain are cavities that begin in the cerebral hemispheres and channel downward into the brainstem. They are designed specifically for the production and distribution of cerebrospinal fluid. The first two ventricles are called the *lateral* ventricles, and each is located in a cerebral hemisphere. These ventricles communicate with the third ventricle through *foramen of Monro* at the level of the thalamus. The third ventricle joins the fourth ventricle through a channel known as the *sylvian aqueduct.* This fourth ventricle is located at the level of the pons and medulla. From this last chamber rise three foramina that open into the subarachnoid space to allow distribution of the cerebrospinal fluid around the brain and spinal cord. Insult or injury to areas surrounding the CSF pathway can cause acute or chronic CSF flow obstruction and can result in the development of hydrocephalus.

■ THE CRANIAL NERVES

The *cranial nerves* are twelve pairs of nerves that rise from the brain; each has a specific function. Cranial nerve functions can be lost as a result of lesions near the origin of the cranial nerves or as a result of direct injury to the cranial nerves themselves. When the functions of the nerves are tested, the location and degree of specific CNS disease or injury can be determined. For example, pupil inequality and a unilateral sluggish pupil response to light can occur with uncal herniation of the brain (lateral herniation of the temporal lobe through the tentorial notch) and with compression and stretching of the oculomotor nerve. The ability to evaluate cranial nerve function and to assess signs of dysfunction becomes extremely important when the patient is comatose or unresponsive (see Table 6-3 for a listing of cranial nerve origins and functions) (see Fig. 6-2 for an illustration of the origins of these nerves).

Table 6-3   Cranial nerve functions

Cranial nerve	Frequency of involvement	Functional involvement	Test	Abnormal findings
I. Olfactory	Uncommon	Fracture of cribriform plate or in ethmoid area	Application of simple odors such as peppermint to one nostril at a time	Anosmia
II. Optic	Common	Direct trauma to orbit or globe; fracture involving optic foramen	Light flashed in affected eye	Loss of both direct and consensual pupillary constriction
			Light flashed in normal eye	Direct and consensual pupillary constriction
		Pressure on geniculocalcarine tract; laceration or intracerebral clot in temporal, parietal or occipital lobes (rarely from subdural clot)	Hand brought suddenly toward eye from the side	Absence of the blink reflex indicates a visual field defect (always homonymous)
III. Oculomotor	Very common	Pressure of herniating uncus on nerve just before it enters cavernous sinus or fracture involving cavernous sinus	Light flashed in affected eye	Unreactive pupil, ptosis, eye turned down and out
			Light flashed in normal eye	Direct pupil reflex absent; consensual reflex present
				Direct pupil reflex present; consensual reflex absent
IV. Trochlear	Uncommon	Injury near course of nerve around brainstem or fracture of orbit	Isolated involvement requires special equipment	Eye fails to move down and out
V. Trigeminal	Uncommon	Direct injury to terminal branches, particularly second division in roof of maxillary sinus	Sensation First division—above eye and cornea	Loss of sensation of pain and touch; paresthesias

Table 6-3 Cranial nerve functions—cont'd

Cranial nerve	Frequency of involvement	Functional involvement	Test	Abnormal findings
V. Trigeminal—cont'd			Second division—upper lip Third division—lower lip and chin	Palpated masseter and temporalis fail to contract
			Motor function Ability to bite down or chew	
VI. Abducens	Uncommon	Injury near course of nerve around brainstem	Lateral eye movement	Eye fails to move laterally
VII. Facial	Common	Peripheral Laceration or contusion in parotid region	—	Paralysis of facial muscles; eye remains open; angle of mouth drops; forehead fails to wrinkle
		Peripheral Fracture of temporal bone	—	As above plus associated involvement of acoustic nerve and chorda tympani (dry cornea and loss of taste on ipsilateral two-thirds of tongue)
		Supranuclear intracerebral clot	Ability to wrinkle forehead	Forehead wrinkles because of bilateral innervation of frontalis; otherwise paralysis of facial muscles as above
VIII. Acoustic	Common	Fractures of petrous portion of temporal bone; cranial nerve VII also often involved	For children and uncooperative patients, hands are clapped close to ear	Startle reflex
			Weber test: tuning fork held at middle of forehead	Sound not heard by involved ear
IX. Glossopharyngeal	Rare	Brainstem injury or deep laceration of neck	Motor power of stylopharyngeus—impractical to test	Loss of taste posterior one third of tongue
			Cotton applicator touched to soft palate	Loss of sensation on affected side of soft palate

Continued.

Table 6-3 Cranial nerve functions—cont'd

Cranial nerve	Frequency of involvement	Functional involvement	Test	Abnormal findings
X. Vagus	Rare	Brainstem injury or deep laceration of neck	Inspection of soft palate, laryngoscopy	Sagging of soft palate; deviation of uvula to normal side; hoarseness from paralysis of vocal cord
XI. Spinal accessory	Rare	Laceration of neck	Hand placed on side of chin—ability to push against hand	Palpated sternocleidomastoid fails to contract
			Ability to shrug shoulders	Palpated upper fibers of trapezius fail to contract
			Ability to stretch hands out toward examiner	Affected arm seems longer (scapula not "anchored")
XII. Hypoglossal	Rare	Neck laceration usually associated with major vessel damage	Ability to stick out tongue	Tongue protrudes toward affected side; dysarthria

■ THE SPINAL CORD

The *spinal cord* is a cylindrical structure composed of neurons and nerve fibers that joins the brainstem at the foramen magnum and extends to the level of the second lumbar vertebra. There are 31 pairs of spinal nerves, which are distributed along the entire spinal cord (Fig. 6-3). All of these nerves are multifibered and transmit impulses between the central nervous system (CNS) and the rest of the body. When a portion of the spinal cord is viewed in cross section, it is clear that the cord does not completely fill the vertebral column; it is surrounded by the pia mater, the cerebrospinal fluid, the arachnoid, and the dura mater. The spinal cord contains gray and white material. The gray matter consists of cell bodies and cell nuclei, and the white matter consists of nerve fibers. The gray matter in the spinal cord is shaped like a butterfly with anterior and posterior projections called the anterior and posterior horns, or, respectively, the ventral or dorsal root. Lower motor neurons from the periphery carry impulses to the posterior horn (the dorsal root) of the spinal column where they synapse or communicate with other neurons that will carry information up the spinal column or to other neurons at the same level of the spinal column. Lower motor neurons are located in the anterior horn (the ventral root) of the spinal column. The lower motor neurons receive input from the brain as well as from other neurons within the spinal cord; they affect motor activity.

Some spinal cord reflexes do not require any input from the brain. For example, when the patellar tendon is tapped with a reflex hammer, the rapid stretch of the muscle will ultimately produce a reflexive contraction of the rectus femorus without the participation of higher CNS structures. Occasionally, stimulus of a sensory neuron on one side of the body will result in movement on the opposite side of the body. For example, if the right hand is placed on something hot, that hand will automatically be withdrawn, and the left hand and left leg will often also be extended to allow the body to withdraw from the painful stimulus. These behaviors can all occur at the spinal cord level, and they may continue despite injury to the cerebral cortex. If damage to the brain or higher levels of the spinal cord does occur, however, it can also result in loss of inhibition to the lower motor neurons and cause flaccid or spastic paralysis.

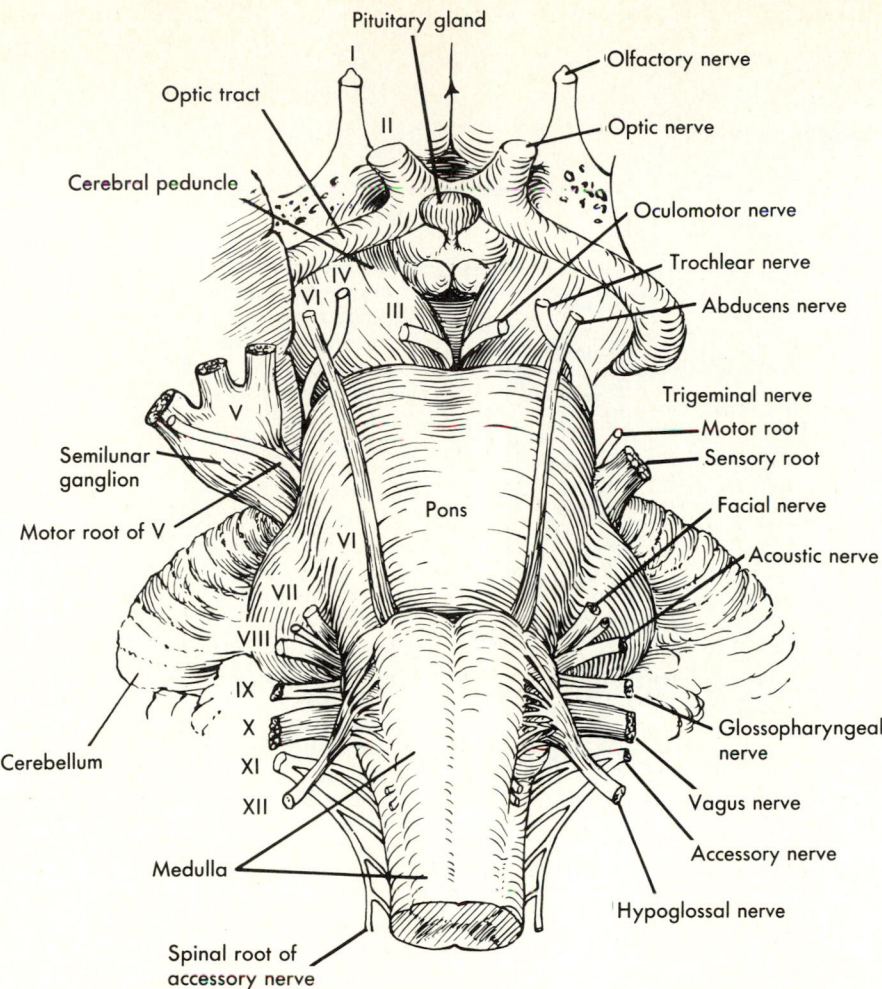

Fig. 6-2 Origins of the cranial nerves from the brain.

From Chusid, J.G.: The cranial nerves. In Correlative neuroanatomy and functional neurology, ed. 18, Los Altos, Calif., 1982, Lange Medical Publications.

■ **CENTRAL NERVOUS SYSTEM CIRCULATION**
■ **The cerebral circulation**

The brain requires a constant supply of oxygen so that carbohydrates may be metabolized as an energy source. In addition, adequate circulation is necessary to remove carbon dioxide and other metabolites from the brain. The brain requires approximately 18% of the total body oxygen content, and it receives approximately 25% of the child's cardiac output.[15] The healthy brain of the child consumes 5.1 cc of oxygen per 100 gm of brain per minute; as a result, if the brain is deprived of oxygen for even a few minutes, brain ischemia occurs. Since cells of the central nervous system do not regenerate, cerebral ischemic injury may not be reparable, and if the injury is severe, brain death will result.[15,42]

Cerebral arterial circulation rises from the two vertebral arteries and from the right and left internal carotid arteries. The internal carotid arteries enter the skull anteriorly and end in the anterior cerebral and the middle cerebral arteries; they supply approximately 85% of cerebral blood flow. The vertebral arteries enter the skull posteriorly and join to form the basilar artery, which ultimately bifurcates to form two posterior communicating arteries (Fig. 6-4). The junction of the two internal carotid arteries, the two anterior and two posterior cerebral arteries, and the posterior and anterior communicating arteries form *Circle of Willis* at the base of the brain. This arterial configuration is present in approximately half

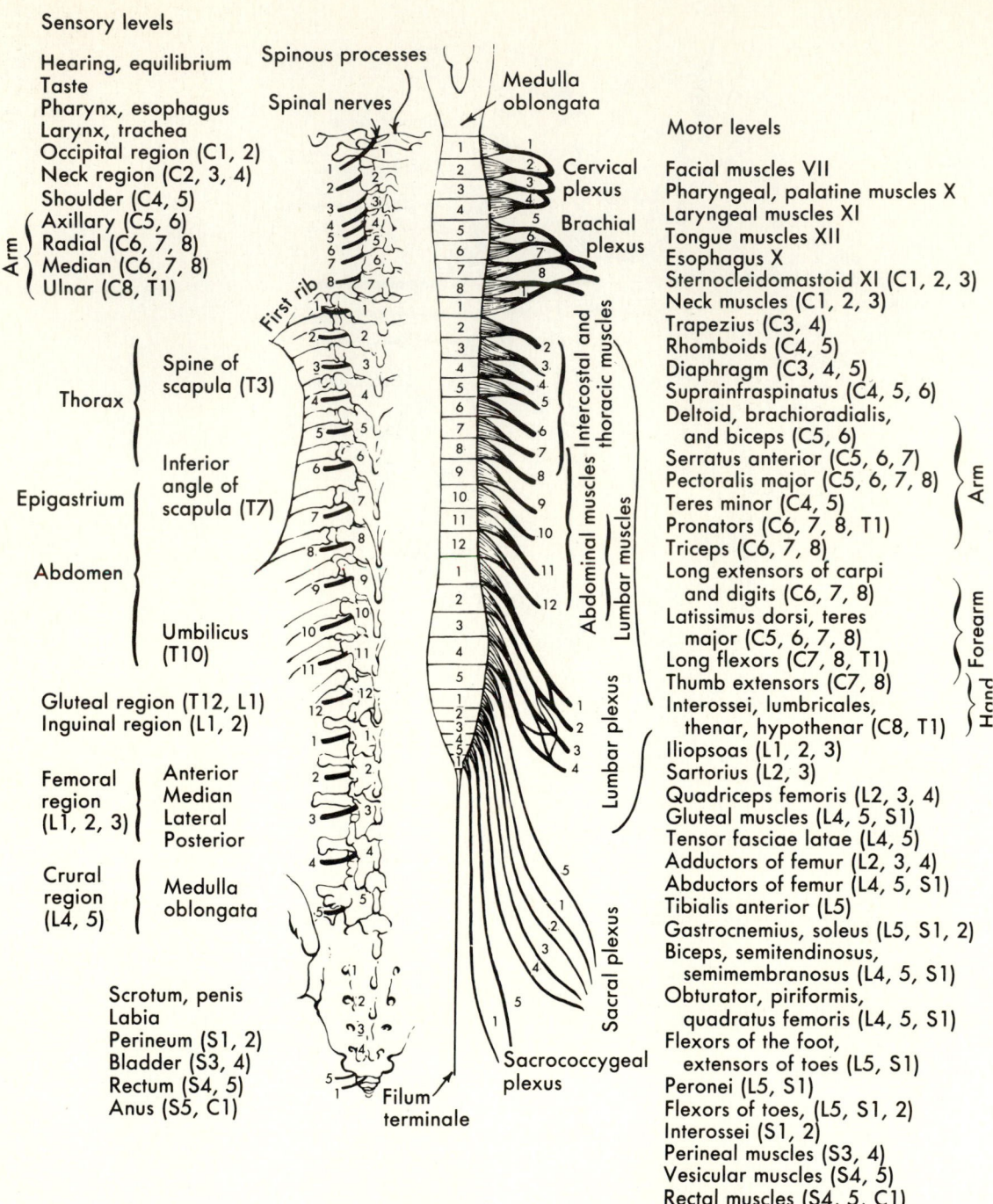

Sensory levels

Hearing, equilibrium
Taste
Pharynx, esophagus
Larynx, trachea
Occipital region (C1, 2)
Neck region (C2, 3, 4)
Shoulder (C4, 5)

Arm {
Axillary (C5, 6)
Radial (C6, 7, 8)
Median (C6, 7, 8)
Ulnar (C8, T1)
}

Thorax {
Spine of scapula (T3)

Inferior angle of scapula (T7)
}

Epigastrium

Abdomen

Umbilicus (T10)

Gluteal region (T12, L1)
Inguinal region (L1, 2)

Femoral region (L1, 2, 3) {
Anterior
Median
Lateral
Posterior
}

Crural region (L4, 5) {
Medulla oblongata
}

Scrotum, penis
Labia
Perineum (S1, 2)
Bladder (S3, 4)
Rectum (S4, 5)
Anus (S5, C1)

Spinous processes
Spinal nerves
Medulla oblongata
First rib
Filum terminale

Cervical plexus
Brachial plexus
Intercostal and thoracic muscles
Abdominal muscles
Lumbar muscles
Lumbar plexus
Sacral plexus
Sacrococcygeal plexus

Motor levels

Facial muscles VII
Pharyngeal, palatine muscles X
Laryngeal muscles XI
Tongue muscles XII
Esophagus X
Sternocleidomastoid XI (C1, 2, 3)
Neck muscles (C1, 2, 3)
Trapezius (C3, 4)
Rhomboids (C4, 5)
Diaphragm (C3, 4, 5)
Suprainfraspinatus (C4, 5, 6)
Deltoid, brachioradialis, and biceps (C5, 6)
Serratus anterior (C5, 6, 7)
Pectoralis major (C5, 6, 7, 8)   } Arm
Teres minor (C4, 5)
Pronators (C6, 7, 8, T1)
Triceps (C6, 7, 8)
Long extensors of carpi and digits (C6, 7, 8)
Latissimus dorsi, teres major (C5, 6, 7, 8)   } Forearm
Long flexors (C7, 8, T1)
Thumb extensors (C7, 8)
Interossei, lumbricales, thenar, hypothenar (C8, T1)   } Hand
Iliopsoas (L1, 2, 3)
Sartorius (L2, 3)
Quadriceps femoris (L2, 3, 4)
Gluteal muscles (L4, 5, S1)
Tensor fasciae latae (L4, 5)
Adductors of femur (L2, 3, 4)
Abductors of femur (L4, 5, S1)
Tibialis anterior (L5)
Gastrocnemius, soleus (L5, S1, 2)
Biceps, semitendinosus, semimembranosus (L4, 5, S1)
Obturator, piriformis, quadratus femoris (L4, 5, S1)
Flexors of the foot, extensors of toes (L5, S1)
Peronei (L5, S1)
Flexors of toes, (L5, S1, 2)
Interossei (S1, 2)
Perineal muscles (S3, 4)
Vesicular muscles (S4, 5)
Rectal muscles (S4, 5, C1)

Fig. 6-3 Motor and sensory innervation from the spinal cord.

From Chusid, J.G.: The spinal nerves. In Correlative neuroanatomy and functional neurology, ed. 18, Los Altos, Calif., 1982, Lange Medical Publications.

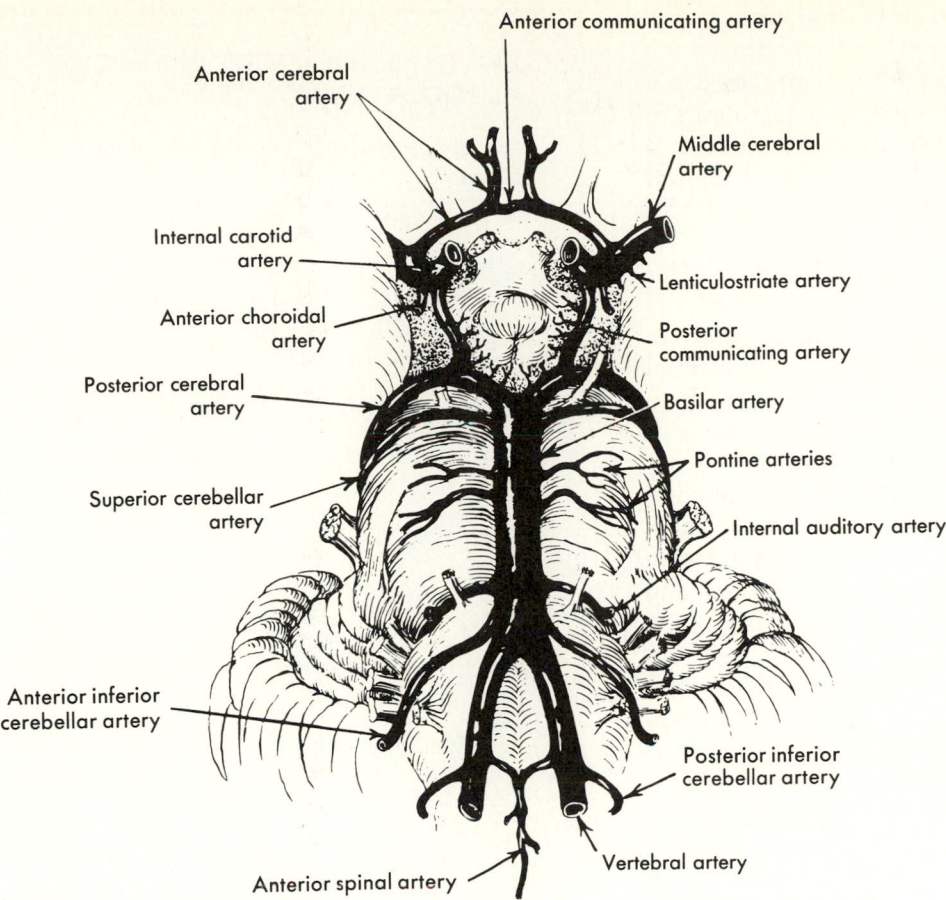

Anterior communicating artery

Anterior cerebral artery

Middle cerebral artery

Internal carotid artery

Lenticulostriate artery

Anterior choroidal artery

Posterior communicating artery

Posterior cerebral artery

Basilar artery

Pontine arteries

Superior cerebellar artery

Internal auditory artery

Anterior inferior cerebellar artery

Posterior inferior cerebellar artery

Anterior spinal artery

Vertebral artery

Fig. 6-4 The cerebral circulation, including the circle of Willis.

From Chusid, J.G.: The brain. In Correlative neuroanatomy and functional neurology, ed. 18, Los Altos, Calif., 1982, Lange Medical Publications.

of all adults.[55] Those patients with an alternative form of arterial circulation are classified as having anomalous cerebral circulation, although these differences in the arterial circulation are usually not significant. Congenital anomalies of one or both carotid arteries or of the internal carotid system have been demonstrated. In many of these patients, the development of collateral circulation early in life prevents any compromise in cerebral circulation.[14]

The cerebral venous circulation is unique in that the cerebral veins have no valves, and they do not follow the course of the cerebral arteries.[42] Venous drainage from the brain flows primarily into large vascular channels within the dura, known as *dural sinuses*, that ultimately drain into the internal jugular vein.

A cerebrovascular accident (CVA or stroke) can occur in children as the result of congenital malfor-

mations of the cerebral arterial or venous circulation. The most common of these cerebrovascular anomalies are telangiectasis and arteriovenous malformation. *Telangiectases* are small groups of dilated capillaries that can develop anywhere in the brain. These capillaries usually do not produce symptoms unless or until they rupture. *Arteriovenous malformations* are abnormal connections between cerebral arteries and veins. They most commonly include branches of the middle cerebral artery. Since arterial blood flows directly into the vein without passage through a capillary bed, the veins receive high-volume, high-pressure blood flow. This results in dilation and sclerosis of the veins. It also produces an increase in cerebral venous return and can produce cardiac enlargement and congestive heart failure. If the thin-walled veins rupture, a large intracranial hemorrhage and death can result.

■ Factors affecting the cerebral circulation

Cerebral blood flow is normally maintained at a constant level as the result of constant adjustments of the tone (and resistance) in the cerebral arteries. If systemic arterial pressure increases, cerebral arterial vasoconstriction will minimize the pressure rise in the cerebral arterial circulation. Conversely, if systemic arterial pressure falls, cerebral vasodilation will maximize the amount of cerebral blood flow and minimize the pressure fall in the cerebral circulation. However, if the rise or fall in the systemic arterial pressure exceeds the limits of autoregulatory compensation, further changes in arterial pressure will affect the cerebral perfusion.

Cerebral blood flow is also affected by cerebral venous pressure. If cerebral arterial pressure falls, venous pressure will also fall, so the "blood pressure head" (the difference between cerebral arterial and venous pressures) remains the same and cerebral blood flow is not reduced.

Another important factor affecting cerebral blood flow is local or systemic hypercapnia. If carbon dioxide accumulates in the brain or if the arterial carbon dioxide tension rises, cerebral arterial vasodilation occurs and cerebral blood flow increases. Hydrogen ion accumulation or acidosis is another potent cerebral vasodilator. Cerebral hypoxia or a fall in systemic oxygen tension will also produce cerebral vasodilation, although not to the same extent as hypercapnia. Other factors that produce a net increase in cerebral blood flow include anemia, a significant rise in systemic arterial pressure and/or a fall in cerebral venous pressure, administration of vasodilator drugs, and hyperthyroidism. Cerebral blood flow will also increase if a hemangioma or arteriovenous malformation is present or if CSF pressure is abnormally low. Seizures can produce an increase in cerebral blood flow as the result of local tissue hypoxia, carbon dioxide production, or patient Valsalva's maneuver (see the box that follows and Table 6-4).

Cerebral blood flow can be reduced if CSF pressure (and intracranial pressure) is increased or if cerebral venous pressure rises and/or systemic arterial pressure falls dramatically. Severe *hypocapnia* (Pa_{CO_2} less than 21 to 23 torr) or hyperoxia can also produce cerebral vasoconstriction. Polycythemia and hypothyroidism are also known to reduce cerebral blood flow.[15]

If cerebral blood flow is severely reduced, local cerebral metabolism is compromised as the result of hypoxia. Severe ischemia and anoxia results in a loss of cerebral cellular metabolic functions. If the hy-

---

FACTORS AFFECTING CEREBRAL BLOOD FLOW[15,42]

Factors resulting in increased cerebral blood flow

Increased carbon dioxide tension

Hypoxia

Increased systemic arterial pressure (severe)

Anemia

Hyperthyrodism

Reduced cerebral venous pressure

Seizures

Administration of vasodilator drugs

Factors resulting in decreased cerebral blood flow

Increased intracranial pressure

Profound hypocapnia

Severe hypotension

Increased cerebral venous pressure

Polycythemia

Hypothyroidism

Administration of vasoconstrictor drugs

---

poxia continues, cerebral edema results in a further compromise in cerebral blood flow and perpetuation of the cerebral ischemia—cerebral edema cycle. Unless this process is interrupted, brain death will rapidly result.

Cerebral perfusion pressure (CPP) is the difference between the cerebral arterial pressure and the intracranial pressure, as noted below:

$$\text{Cerebral perfusion pressure (CPP)} = \text{Mean systemic arterial pressure} - \text{Mean intracranial pressure}$$

The normal range of cerebral perfusion pressure is approximately 80 to 100 mm Hg, and a minimum cerebral perfusion pressure of 50 mm Hg is required for any cerebral blood flow to occur. The cerebral perfusion pressure may fall if the mean systemic arterial pressure is reduced or if the mean intracranial pressure rises (or if both occur simultaneously). The cerebral perfusion pressure can rise if the mean systemic arterial pressure rises or if the mean intracranial pressure falls (or if both occur simultaneously). In some

Table 6-4 Autoregulation of cerebral blood flow

Factors affecting cerebral blood flow	Autoregulation intact		Damaged autoregulation	
	Cerebral blood volume	Cerebral perfusion	Cerebral blood volume	Cerebral perfusion
↑Local tissue pH	↓	Adequate		
↓Local tissue pH	↑	Adequate		
↑Pa_{CO_2}	↑	Adequate	↑	Inadequate
↓Pa_{CO_2}	↓	Adequate	↓	Inadequate
↓Pa_{O_2}	↑	Adequate		Inadequate
↑Systemic arterial blood pressure	Normal	Adequate	↑	Inadequate
↓Systemic arterial blood pressure	Normal	Adequate	↓	Inadequate
↑Intracranial pressure	↓	Adequate initially, inadequate late	Variable	Compromised

From Morriss, F.C.: Increased intracranial pressure. In Levin, D.L., Morriss, F.C., and Moore, G.C., editors: A practical guide to pediatric intensive care, ed. 2, St. Louis, 1984, The C.V. Mosby Co.

tertiary care centers, a documented cerebral perfusion pressure of less than 40 mm Hg for 20 or more minutes in a normothermic patient is thought to be compatible with brain death.

■ **The blood-brain barrier**

The *blood-brain barrier* is the name given to the unique relationship between the cerebral capillary walls and the glial astrocyte cells. The astrocytes occupy the space between the relatively impermeable cerebral capillaries and the tissues of the central nervous system. The decreased permeability of the capillaries and the glial investment around the capillaries can protect the cerebral tissue from exposure to wide fluctuations in acid-base balance or ionic composition, and it can prevent the entry of antigenic or toxic material into the brain.[15] However, because the blood-brain barrier *is* freely permeable to water, rapid changes in the patient's level of hydration or intravascular volume can affect cerebral hydration and

function. Many drugs, including some water-soluble contrast agents and some antibiotics, do not cross the blood-brain barrier.

The immature brain does not have adequate development of glial cells; therefore the blood-brain barrier is incomplete in the young infant. As a result the neonate can develop kernicterus as the result of hyperbilirubinemia, and the neonatal brain may be more affected by circulating toxins.[31]

■ **The spinal cord circulation**

The arterial supply of the spinal cord begins from paired spinal arteries that rise from the vertebral arteries at the level of the foramen magnum. In addition, the spinal cord is perfused from branches of the intercostal arteries that rise from the thoracic aorta. This spinal cord circulation can be injured during thoracic surgery (especially repair of coarctation of the aorta), resulting in spinal cord damage and paralysis.

■ THE CEREBROSPINAL FLUID CIRCULATION

The cerebrospinal fluid is a clear, colorless liquid that is produced in the ventricles and in specialized capillaries within the central nervous system. Cerebrospinal fluid circulates in the ventricles, the subarachnoid space, and the central canal of the spinal cord; it provides buoyancy to reduce the effective weight of the brain, and it cushions the central nervous system from injury.

Cerebrospinal fluid is not merely a filtrate of plasma. It contains water, oxygen, carbon dioxide, sodium, potassium, chloride, glucose, a small amount of protein, and an occasional lymphocyte. The CSF chloride concentration is normally 115 to 125 $\mu g/L$. The CSF glucose concentration is approximately half that of the serum glucose concentration; it is usually 40 to 80 mg/100 ml. The normal protein concentration is 14 to 45 mg/100 ml (higher normal values are present in neonates), and there are usually less than 10 white blood cells per mm³ present.[84] Red blood cells are only present in a CSF sample if a traumatic spinal tap was performed or if the patient has suffered a cerebral hemorrhage. Generally, cerebrospinal fluid is hypertonic to blood, but its changes in osmolality will parallel those of blood (i.e., an increase in serum osmotic pressure will soon be followed by an increase in CSF osmotic pressure). Abnormalities of CSF composition can aid in the diagnosis of some CNS diseases (see Tables 6-5 and 6-6).

Cerebrospinal fluid is formed primarily by the choroid plexuses, which are collections of capillaries located on the floor of each lateral ventricle, as well as in the third and fourth ventricles. Additional cerebrospinal fluid is formed by ependymal cells lining the ventricles and meninges and by blood vessels of the brain and spinal cord. CSF formation requires both active transport and simple diffusion between the existing cerebrospinal fluid and the secreting surfaces.

In the child, approximately 504 ml of cerebro-

Table 6-5 Normal results of cerebrospinal fluid analysis

	Neonates		Patients >6 mo of age
	Preterm	Term	
WBC/mm³			
Mean	9	8	0
± 2 SD	0-25	0-22	0-4
PMNs* (%)	57	61	0
Protein (mg/100 ml)			
Mean	115	90	<40
Range	65-150	20-170	
Glucose (mg/100 ml)			
Mean	50	52	>40
Range	24-63	34-119	
CSF/blood glucose (%)			
Mean	74	81	50
Range	55-150	44-248	40-60

From Hieber, J.P.: Encephalitis/meningitis. In Levin, D.L., Morriss, F.C., and Moore, G.C.: A practical guide to pediatric intensive care, ed. 2, St. Louis, 1984, The C.V. Mosby Co.
*Polymorphonuclear leukocytes.

Table 6-6   Cerebrospinal fluid findings with central nervous system disease

Entity	Appearance	Pressure (in mm water)	Cells (per μl)	Protein	Miscellaneous cerebrospinal fluid findings
Normal lumbar	Clear and colorless	70-200	0-5	15-45 mg/dl	Glucose 50-75 mg/dl
Normal ventricular	Clear and colorless	70-190	0-5 (lymphocytes)	5-15 mg/dl	BUN 10-35 mg/dl
Traumatic tap	Bloody; supernatant fluid clear	Normal	Red blood cells	4 mg/dl rise per 5000 red cells	Bloody; supernatant fluid clear
Cerebral hemorrhage					
Ventricular Subarachnoid	Bloody; supernatant fluid yellow	Slightly increased	Red blood cells	As above	Blood equal in all 3 specimens
Meningitis					
Acute purulent (bacterial)	Clear, cloudy, milky, or xanthochromic; occasional clot formation	Greatly increased (250-700)	Polymorphonuclear cells, usually over 1000	Increased	Glucose decreased early; chloride decreased late; organisms on smears and culture
Viral	Clear	Normal or increased	0-few hundred (mostly lymphocytes)	Increased	Glucose usually normal
Acute tuberculous	Opalescent to turbid; faint fibrin web or pellicle formation	Moderately increased (200-450)	10-500 (lymphocytes)	Increased	Chlorides decreased early, often before decrease of glucose; smear, culture, and guinea pig inoculation for organisms
Brain tumor	Usually clear and colorless	Increased	Normal or increased	Increased	Findings depend on location and type of tumor
Brain abscess	Clear and colorless	Greatly increased	Polymorphonuclear cells normal or increased	Increased	Pressure may go as high as 600-700 mm water

Modified from Chusid, J.G.: The cerebrospinal fluid. In Correlative neuroanatomy and functional neurology, ed. 18, Los Altos, Calif., 1982, Lange Medical Publications.

Continued.

Table 6-6   Cerebrospinal fluid findings with central nervous system disease—cont'd

Entity	Appearance	Pressure (in mm water)	Cells (per μl)	Protein	Miscellaneous cerebrospinal fluid findings
Subdural hematoma	Classically yellow, but often clear and colorless	Usually increased	Normal	Normal or slightly increased	—
Encephalitis	Clear and colorless	Normal	Normal or increased (mostly lymphocytes)	Normal or slightly increased	Serologic tests of value in viral infections
Uremia	Clear and colorless	Slightly increased	Normal	Normal or slightly increased	Spinal fluid BUN increased
Lead encephalopathy	Clear or slightly cloudy	Increased	Lymphocytes	Normal or slightly increased	Lead in spinal fluid
Arterial hypertension (hypertensive encephalopathy)	Clear	Normal or increased	Normal	Normal or slightly increased	Choked disk may suggest brain tumor
Epilepsy (idiopathic)	Normal fluid	Normal	Normal	Normal	—
Multiple sclerosis	Normal fluid	Normal or low	Normal or increased	Normal or increased (increased gamma globulin)	Negative serology
Poliomyelitis, acute	Opalescent, may be faintly yellow; delicate fibrin web	Slightly increased	Slightly increased	Slightly increased (for a few weeks)	Preparalytic stage, 80% polymorphonuclear cells; paralytic state, mononuclears
Spinal cord tumor					
Partial block	Clear and colorless	Normal	Normal	Slightly increased	—
Complete block (Froin's syndrome)	Yellow	Normal or low	Slightly increased	Marked rise (200-600 mg/dl)	Coagulation may occur
Diabetic coma	Clear and colorless	Decreased	Normal	Normal or slightly increased	Glucose elevated; may reach 200-300 mg/dl

spinal fluid are secreted daily.[84] The amount of cerebrospinal fluid formed is affected by cerebral metabolism, cerebral perfusion pressure, blood pressure, and changes in the serum osmotic pressure. An increase in the cerebral perfusion pressure or systemic arterial blood pressure usually results in an increase in CSF formation. An increase in the serum osmotic pressure can ultimately result in an increase in the CSF osmotic pressure. Once formed, the cerebrospinal fluid flows from both lateral ventricles through the *foramina of Monro* into the third ventricle. From there, the fluid passes through the *cerebral aqueduct*, also known as the *sylvian aqueduct*, into the fourth ventricle. Some of the cerebrospinal fluid then passes through the two lateral *Luschka's foramina* into the subarachnoid space to bathe the brain; the remaining fluid passes through *Magendie's foramen* and enters the subarachnoid space to circulate around the spinal cord. Most of the cerebrospinal fluid is ultimately reabsorbed by venous sinuses that project into the sub-

arachnoid space, known as the *arachnoid villi* (Fig. 6-5). An obstruction in the flow of cerebrospinal fluid, an increase in its production, or a decrease in its reabsorption will result in a condition known as *hydrocephalus*. This condition will result in an increase in head circumference in the infant, and can produce increased intracranial pressure in the older child or adult.

The normal CSF pressure is 40 to 180 mm H_2O in the quiet, resting child. This pressure is not static, however, and it normally varies during the cardiac and respiratory cycles, and normally increases transiently during crying, sneezing, or Valsalva's maneuver. This pressure can be measured from the central canal of the spinal cord (during a lumbar puncture), through catheterization of a lateral ventricle, or by insertion of a bolt into the subarachnoid space. All of these procedures measure CSF pressure, and they are thought to represent the intracranial pressure. If the CSF pressure remains above 200 mm H_2O (or 18

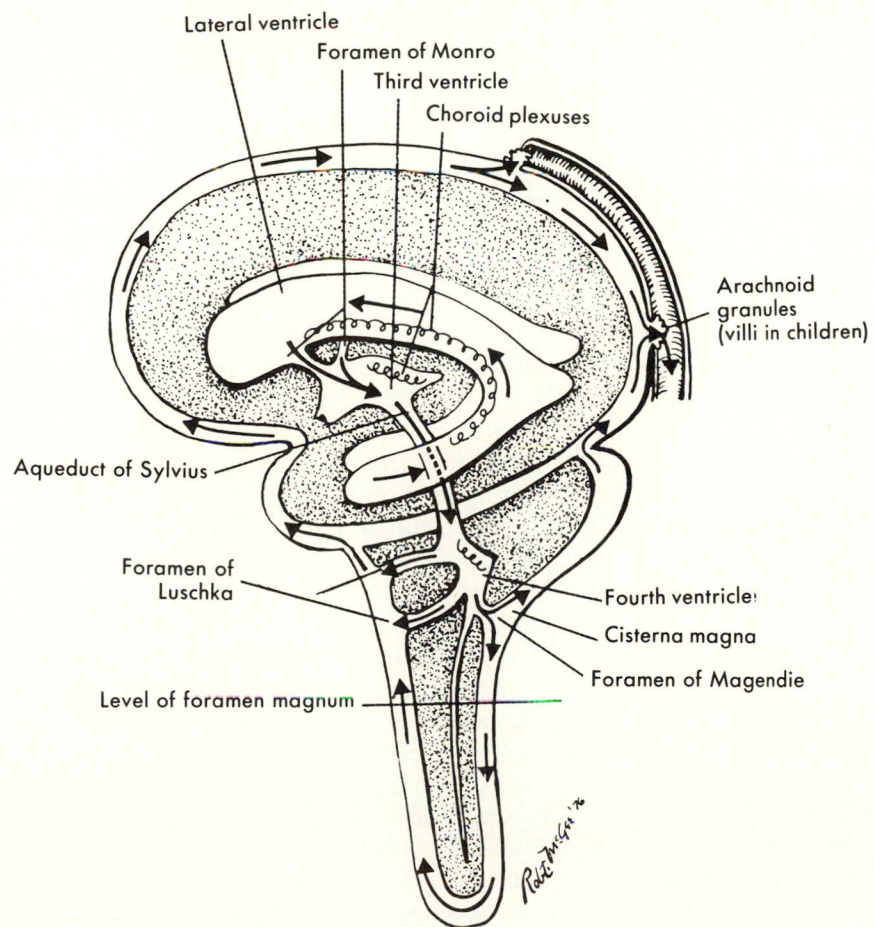

Fig. 6-5 Cerebrospinal fluid circulation.

From Whaley, L.F., and Wong, D.L.: Nursing care of infants and children, ed. 2, St. Louis, 1983, The C.V. Mosby Co.

mm Hg), it is considered elevated.[42] It is important to note that intracranial pressure is *not necessarily uniform* throughout the child's brain, spinal cord, subarachnoid space, and ventricular system; therefore the CSF pressure does not always reflect the pressure in all areas of the cranium. Measurements of the cerebrospinal fluid pressure in the subarachnoid space or ventricles are most helpful in that they document *trends* in the child's intracranial pressure in response to treatment.

■ INTRACRANIAL PRESSURE (ICP)

Once the cranial sutures fuse, the skull is a rigid structure. The cranium normally contains the *brain*, the cerebral arterial and venous *blood*, and the *cerebrospinal fluid*. These three materials are relatively noncompressible, and they occupy a relatively fixed space. The brain occupies the largest portion (80%) of the intracranial space; it is essentially noncompressible, but it is somewhat movable within the cranium. Cerebral blood normally comprises approximately 7% to 10% of the total intracranial volume. An increase in cerebral blood volume can occur as the result of increased cerebral arterial flow or cerebral venous obstruction. A decrease in cerebral blood volume occurs as the result of a decrease in cerebral arterial flow. If cerebral blood flow is severely reduced, brain ischemia, damage, or death will result. Cerebrospinal fluid normally comprises 7% to 10% of the total intracranial volume; this volume will increase if CSF flow is obstructed, if CSF production is increased, or if CSF reabsorption is reduced. The cerebrospinal fluid is thought to be material most easily displaced from the cranium as compensation for an increase in brain or cerebral blood volume.

The intracranial volume is equal to the sum of the volumes of the brain, the cerebral blood, and the cerebrospinal fluid within the cranium.

Intracranial volume (constant after suture fusion) =
    Brain volume + Blood volume + CSF volume

The intracranial pressure is the pressure exerted by these substances. The normal intracranial pressure is approximately 80 to 180 mm H_2O (0 to 15 mm Hg).[28] However, it is not normally static; it can be transiently increased by anything that acutely increases superior vena caval pressure, such as a cough, Valsalva's maneuver, or movement from an upright to a reclining position. Cerebral blood flow is normally constant over a wide range of systemic arterial blood pressure, but it can be affected by changes in the arterial carbon dioxide tension, oxygen tension, pH, or severe increases in intracranial pressure.

Mild or gradual increases in intracranial volume can produce a compensatory decrease in the volume of other intracranial contents: the brain can be slightly compressed or displaced, cerebrospinal fluid can be displaced from the subarachnoid space, cerebrospinal fluid reabsorption can be increased, or blood volume can decrease. If these adjustments occur, even significant increases in intracranial volume can be tolerated without a rise in intracranial pressure. Once the limits of intracranial compensation have been reached, however, even a small increase in intracranial volume will produce a significant rise in the intracranial pressure.[35] When intracranial pressure is high, cerebral blood flow can be severely reduced.[9,42] Even though the infant's skull is expandable, sudden increases in intracranial volume can produce an increase in intracranial pressure. This results in brain ischemia and cerebral edema, perpetuating the rise in intracranial pressure and resulting in brain death.

The etiology and pathophysiology of increased intracranial pressure and the assessment and treatment of the child with an increase in intracranial pressure will be discussed further in the following section.

■ Common Clinical Conditions

■ INCREASED INTRACRANIAL PRESSURE
■ Etiology

Increased intracranial pressure is present when the child's measured intracranial pressure is persistently greater than normal or when the child demonstrates clinical signs and symptoms compatible with the diagnosis of increased intracranial pressure. Since intracranial contents include the brain, cerebral blood, and cerebrospinal fluid, an increase in the volume of any of these substances can produce an increase in intracranial pressure. In addition, the development of a mass lesion (such as a tumor) can also increase intracranial pressure. Since normal intracranial pressure is equal to 80 to 180 mm H_2O (0 to 15 mm Hg), an intracranial pressure greater than 200 to 275 mm H_2O (18 to 20 mm Hg) is considered increased. It is important to note, however, that most clinical methods of measuring intracranial pressure are only able to measure the CSF pressure at one area of the central nervous system; as a result the measurement can be misleading since intracranial pressure is not uniform or static.

When brain volume, blood, or CSF volume increases, the effect on the intracranial pressure will depend on the magnitude as well as the rate of the volume increase. If intracranial volume increases slowly (such as occurs with a slow-growing tumor), there is more time for compensatory changes in other intracranial content, and the change in intracranial pressure may be minimal. If, however, intracranial volume increases suddenly, such as occurs following rupture of a cerebral aneurysm or development of an epidural hematoma, compensatory mechanisms may be ineffective, and intracranial pressure can rise sharply.

Since intracranial volume and pressure can increase as the result of an increase in volume of the brain, blood, or cerebrospinal fluid or as the result of a mass lesion, these causes of intracranial pressure will be considered separately.

Cerebral edema. Cerebral edema is swelling of the brain that occurs as the result of injury. Two forms of cerebral edema are most commonly recognized: cytotoxic cerebral edema and vasogenic cerebral edema. *Cytotoxic cerebral edema* is the more common form of cerebral edema seen in pediatric critical-care patients. It is the result of swelling of the cellular elements of the central nervous system caused by hypoxia, poisons, or hypoglycemia. *Vasogenic cerebral edema* occurs as the result of increased cerebral capillary permeability and is most often the result of focal trauma or irritation. *Hyperemic cerebral edema* has been recently recognized in children following head trauma and is thought to result from increased cerebral blood flow.[12,65]

Increased cerebral blood volume. Cerebral blood volume can increase as the result of cerebral arterial vasodilation, arteriovenous malformations, or intracranial bleeding. A rise in the child's arterial carbon dioxide tension is the most potent cerebral vasodilator; hypoxemia also produces cerebral vasodilation but not to the same extent as hypercapnia. The combination of hypercapnia and hypoxemia is also an extremely potent cerebral arterial vasodilator.

Arteriovenous malformations are the most common noncongenital, nontraumatic cause of intracranial hemorrhage in children.[9] Head trauma can result in the development of epidural, subdural, or intracerebral hematomas (see the section on head trauma for further information). Premature neonates with respiratory distress syndrome are particularly at risk for the development of intraventricular hemorrhage related to anoxic or ischemic injury, hypercapnia, or positive-pressure ventilation.[38]

Increased CSF volume. An increase in CSF volume (hydrocephalus) can occur as the result of blockage of the CSF flow (often referred to as "obstructive" hydrocephalus), increased CSF production (which can

occur as the result of some CSF tumors), or decreased CSF reabsorption.

Obstructive hydrocephalus can be congenital in origin, or it can develop as the result of birth trauma, meningitis and subsequent scarring, or compression of the sylvian aqueduct as a result of cerebral tumors. Nonobstructive hydrocephalus can occur when a rare choroid plexus tumor develops that secretes large amounts of cerebrospinal fluid.

Mass lesions. Intracranial tumors are one of the most common forms of childhood malignancy. Most commonly, the tumors are infratentorial, located near or in the brainstem, and most contain glial cells.[16,68] The most common types of tumors occurring during childhood include astrocytomas, medulloblastomas, and ependymomas; these tumors are located in the posterior fossa.

Fast-growing tumors may produce early signs of increased intracranial pressure, and other tumors may produce negligible symptoms until cerebellar, brainstem, or cranial nerve involvement is apparent (see the section on intracranial tumors later in this chapter).

■ Pathophysiology

Initially, as intracranial volume increases, cerebrospinal fluid is reabsorbed more quickly or it is displaced to the subarachnoid space of the spinal column. If the infant's sutures have not fused, the skull can expand to accomodate a gradual increase in intracranial volume. This skull expansion can occur even after the bones of the cranium are fused, and it has been reported as late as 12 years of age.[9]

If intracranial volume continues to increase despite maximal displacement of cerebrospinal fluid or if it occurs too rapidly for compensatory mechanisms to occur, the brain may be shifted so that local pressure is relieved. This shifting of the brain is called *herniation*; the consequences of the herniation depend on its severity and location.

Transtentorial herniation occurs when part of the brain herniates downward around the tentorium cerebelli. This herniation can occur in the anterior or posterior portion of the brain, and it may be unilateral or bilateral. Transtentorial herniation will initially produce unilateral or bilateral pupil dilation with decreased response to light and impeded upward gaze. It may also produce obstruction of the sylvian aqueduct; this results in CSF accumulation and a further increase in intracranial pressure. If large portions of the brain herniate across the tentorial notch, death can result from compression of vital brain structures.

Temporal lobe herniation (or uncal herniation)

occurs when the temporal lobe herniates laterally across the tentorial notch. This produces compression of the third cranial nerve and unilateral pupil dilation. If the brain continues to herniate through the tentorial notch, flaccid paralysis, pupil dilation, and death result.

The *cerebellar tonsils* can herniate through the foramen magnum, without the development of any symptoms. However, some patients will develop a stiff neck, upper arm and shoulder paresthesias, a change in the respiratory pattern, or a wide fluctuation in heart rate.[42]

Brainstem herniation through the foramen magnum results in compression of the vital cardiorespiratory centers and death.

As noted in the previous section (see the discussion on intracranial pressure in the section on essential anatomy and physiology), an increase in intracranial volume can be tolerated to a point because of the displacement of cerebrospinal fluid or shifting of the brain. Beyond that point, further small increases in intracranial volume can result in significant increases in intracranial pressure (see Fig. 6-6). When this occurs, cerebral veins are compressed and cerebral venous pressure rises. This results in an increase in

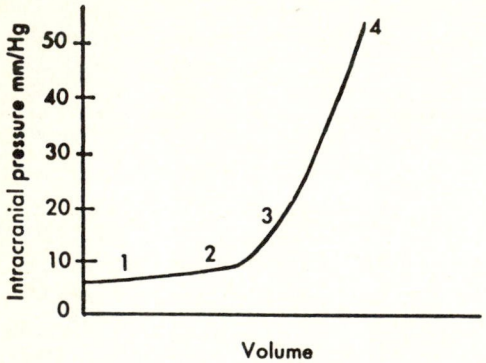

Fig. 6-6 Intracranial compliance curve demonstrates the changes in intracranial pressure *(vertical axis)* that occur with increases in intracranial volume *(horizontal axis)*. *1,* The patient's intracranial volume is increasing, but the pressure does not rise because of a compensatory decrease in the volume of other intracranial compartments. *2,* A further increase in intracranial volume produces only a mild elevation in intracranial pressure; however, any additional increase in intracranial volume will produce a significant rise in intracranial pressure. *3,* Intracranial volume has increased only a small amount, yet intracranial pressure has risen sharply. *4,* Further small increases in intracranial volume (such as that produced by hypercapnia and cerebral vasodilation) produce large increases in intracranial pressure.

cerebral blood volume and a further increase in intracranial pressure. As intracranial pressure rises, cerebral blood flow is reduced, and cerebral ischemia occurs. In addition, brain herniation can develop. Finally, inadequate cerebral perfusion or massive cerebral herniation will result in death.

Specific pathophysiology of cerebral edema, increased cerebral blood volume, increased CSF volume, and mass lesions is discussed separately in the following pages.

Cerebral edema. *Cytotoxic cerebral edema* develops most commonly after the patient has sustained cerebral hypoxia, ischemia, or trauma. These injuries result in increased intracellular sodium and water content and in cellular swelling. This swelling may be exacerbated by the water retention occurring as the result of development of the syndrome of inappropriate ADH secretion. When cytotoxic cerebral edema is present, the cerebral edema is diffuse.

Vasogenic cerebral edema is characterized by increased capillary permeability and increased extracellular fluid volume. Although vasogenic cerebral edema can surround localized areas of ischemia, it most commonly develops around lesions such as abscess, hemorrhage, tumor, or infarct. It can also be seen when the child develops meningitis, lead poisoning, or other metabolic derangements.[38]

Increased cerebral blood volume. Cerebral blood flow is normally maintained at a relatively constant pressure despite wide ranges in the arterial blood pressure (this is known as autoregulation). Small variations in cerebral blood flow do occur, however, with changes in the arterial oxygen and carbon dioxide levels and with changes in intrathoracic or systemic venous pressures. Hypercapnia and acidosis are potent cerebral vasodilators, and hypoxia is a mild vasodilator. Anything that increases intrathoracic pressures (such as the use of high inspiratory pressures or high positive end-expiratory pressures during mechanical ventilation) tends to impede cerebral venous return and to increase cerebral blood volume. Valsalva's maneuver also reduces cerebral venous return in the same manner.

Intracranial hemorrhage and epidural, subdural or intracerebral hematomas will produce a rapid increase in cerebral blood volume and a sudden rise in intracranial pressure as the result of the accumulation of blood.[42]

Increased CSF volume. Increased CSF volume, hydrocephalus, may occur as the result of congenital or acquired obstruction of the CSF pathway. Congenital hydrocephalus occurs most commonly as the result of an obstruction of the foramina of Monro or Magendie called an Arnold-Chiari malformation; this is often seen in association with meningomyelocele. Acquired hydrocephalus can result from intravascular hemorrhage, cerebral trauma, or an infection that results in clot formation or scarring around the foramina of Monro or Magendie or around the sylvian aqueduct. Acquired hydrocephalus can also occur as the result of tumors that compress the sylvian aqueduct, or that include the choroid plexus and cause excessive CSF production.[21]

When hydrocephalus develops during infancy, the gradual accumulation of fluid causes separation of the cranial bones and enlargement of the head. This skull expansion usually prevents the development of increased intracranial pressure. When hydrocephalus develops in the older child, the cranial bones are fused and they do not readily separate. As a result ventricular expansion produces a rise in intracranial pressure. With gradual, progressive accumulation of cerebrospinal fluid, separation of the cranial sutures may develop in children up to 12 years of age.[9]

Mass lesions. Malignant or benign tumors can produce a rise in intracranial pressure as the result of an increase in intracranial volume. Children with slow-growing tumors usually demonstrate localized signs of brain or cranial nerve compression before overt signs of increased intracranial pressure develop because the mass grows slowly and compensatory mechanisms (such as a decrease in CSF volume and a shifting of the brain) can occur.

■ Clinical signs and symptoms

The child with increased intracranial pressure characteristically demonstrates an alteration in the level of consciousness, pupil dilation with decreased reactivity to light, alterations in heart rate, blood pressure, and respiratory rate or pattern, and abnormal motor activity and reflexes. The child may complain of headache or nausea, and he may vomit, particularly in the morning or after moving from a reclining to an upright position. Since the infant or child will usually not be able to articulate his symptoms, the recognition of the development of increased intracranial pressure will usually depend largely on the quality of the nurse's assessments. If, of course, an intracranial pressure monitoring device is in place, this measurement is used in conjunction with the clinical assessment to determine the severity of the intracranial hypertension.

Alterations in level of consciousness. Evaluation of the child's *level of consciousness* is probably the single most important aspect of assessment of the critically ill child with neurologic problems. This assessment will be made more readily if adequate information about the child's normal activities is obtained from the primary caretaker and recorded in the nursing care plan. The nurse should be familiar with the names of the child's family members, pets, or favorite stuffed animals. This will become critical when the nurse attempts to determine the verbal child's orientation to time and place and short- and long-term memory. For example, if a child reports that, "Oscar was flying around my room at home," the nurse would be concerned if Oscar is the child's brother, but she would probably be reassured if Oscar is the child's pet parakeet that frequently escapes from the cage. The nurse should also determine the names of any imaginary friends that the child has since it may be absolutely normal for the child to talk to an invisible friend.

The nurse must carefully evaluate the infant's or child's behavior. Excessive irritability is a very common and nonspecific sign in the critically ill child. Lethargy is almost always abnormal, and is a more specific and crucial indicator of deterioration of neurologic function. However, interpretation of behavior should be made only with an appreciation of the patient's normal behavior and routines. Because an infant is expected to be irritable when hungry, tired, or overstimulated, it is important to be aware of normal feeding times and nap times and to attempt to

---

Table 6-7   Glasgow coma scale

Response	Score*
Eye opening	4 Spontaneous
	3 To speech
	2 To pain
	1 None
Best verbal	5 Oriented
	4 Confused
	3 Inappropriate
	2 Incomprehensible
	1 None
Best motor	6 Obeys commands
	5 Localizes pain
	4 Withdraws
	3 Flexion to pain
	2 Extension to pain
	1 None

*Total possible score = 15.

prevent constant stimulation of the infant. It is normal, also, for the infant to be comforted when held and to be quiet and sleepy after feeding. It would be abnormal for an infant to cry or sleep constantly. A high-pitched cry is also usually abnormal. The child is expected to be sleepy if he has been awake all night in the emergency room. However, it would be extremely abnormal for the same child to sleep while a venipuncture is performed. Thus the nurse should be able to evaluate the activity of the infant or child in the context of surrounding events and environmental stimulation.[41]

The nurse should use consistent terminology and a consistent rating scale when evaluating the child's level of consciousness so that changes in the child's activities will be easily recognized. The Glasgow Coma Scale evaluates motor activity, verbal responses to questions, and motor responses to simple commands to enable objective appraisal of the child's level of consciousness (Table 6-7). Similar scales may be incorporated into a nursing flow sheet or observation chart (Fig. 6-7).

Signs of decreased level of consciousness in infants with increased intracranial pressure include lethargy, decreased eye contact with caretaker, poor visual tracking, and a change in feeding behavior (including anorexia). The child with a decreased level of consciousness resulting from increased intracranial pressure may be very irritable or lethargic, may be confused about where he is, may forget his name or the name of family members or pets, or may appear drowsy.[41] *Decreased response to painful stimuli is abnormal in the child of any age and should be reported to a physician immediately.*

Pupillary changes. The pupils are normally the same size bilaterally, and they normally constrict briskly in response to light as the result of innervation by the third cranial (oculomotor) nerve. When increased intracranial pressure develops, the oculomotor nerve is compressed by either general expansion of the brain, an intracranial lesion, or herniation of the brain; this results in pupil dilation and decreased or absent pupil constriction in response to light. When the intracranial herniation or lesion is unilateral, the pupil dilation will occur on the same side as the lesion. The child may also complain of blurred vision or diplopia.[42]

Unilateral *ptosis* may be present. This may occur in conjunction with ipsilateral pupillary dilation as the result of compression of the oculomotor nerve. If unilateral ptosis is noted with ipsilateral pupil constriction, *Horner's syndrome* may be present. This syndrome consists of unilateral ptosis, miosis (small pupil), and anhydrosis (lack of sweat on that side of

the face). Horner's syndrome is the result of unilateral interruption of sympathetic nervous system fibers, and it can occur following cardiovascular surgery near the aortic arch. It is important to differentiate between ptosis caused by third nerve compression and that caused by Horner's syndrome since the former indicates the presence of increased intracranial pressure (requiring immediate treatment) and the latter requires no treatment. When the third cranial nerve is compressed, the pupil *will not constrict* normally in response to light. When Horner's syndrome is present, the involved pupil is constricted, but both pupils should still react (constrict) in response to light.

Some clinical conditions or medications can modify pupil size or response to light. When the patient has unilateral blindness, the involved pupil will not constrict in response to light. Pupil constriction (or *miosis*) can occur as the result of hemorrhage in the pons, poisoning, or administration of morphine. Pupil dilation will occur as the result of hypothermia, as the result of administration of atropine or of very large doses of sympathomimetic drugs such as dopamine or epinephrine, or as the result of pain. Changes in pupillary response to light with altered levels of consciousness are summarized in Fig. 6-8.

Papilledema. *Papilledema* is edema of the optic nerve or disc that results from increased intracranial pressure and compression of these structures. When an ophthalmoscope is used to examine the retina, the optic disc appears indistinct, and the retinal veins are engorged and pulseless. Papilledema develops when intracranial pressure has been elevated for 48 hours or more; therefore, when papilledema is present, it is a reliable indicator of the presence of increased intracranial pressure. When it is absent, however, the diagnosis of an acute increase in intracranial pressure cannot be ruled out.[9,59]

When mild papilledema is present, the child's vision should be normal. With progressive compression of the optic disc, however, hemorrhages can develop in the optic disc, and the child may complain of headaches, blurred vision, or diplopia.

Alterations in blood pressure and heart rate. The best cardiovascular sign of increased intracranial pressure is the *Cushing reflex*. This reflex is initiated as the result of increased intracranial pressure and the resultant increase in CSF pressure and possible ischemia of the vasomotor center.[42] This reflex consists of an increase in systolic arterial blood pressure (as an attempt to maintain cerebral perfusion pressure) and bradycardia. The increase in systolic arterial blood pressure produces a widening of the pulse pressure. The Cushing reflex is usually associated with a de-

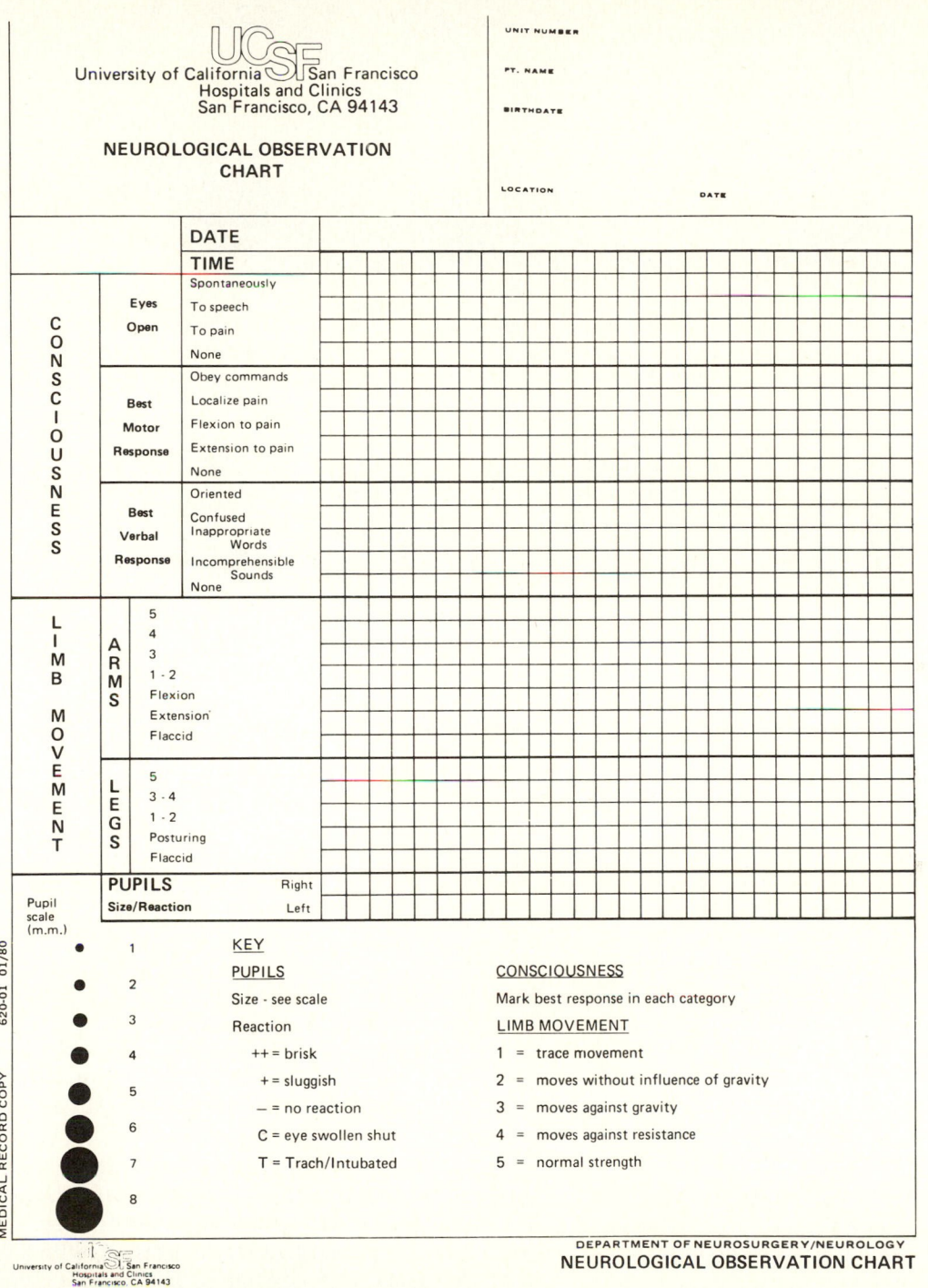

Fig. 6-7 Neurologic observation chart, University of California at San Francisco.

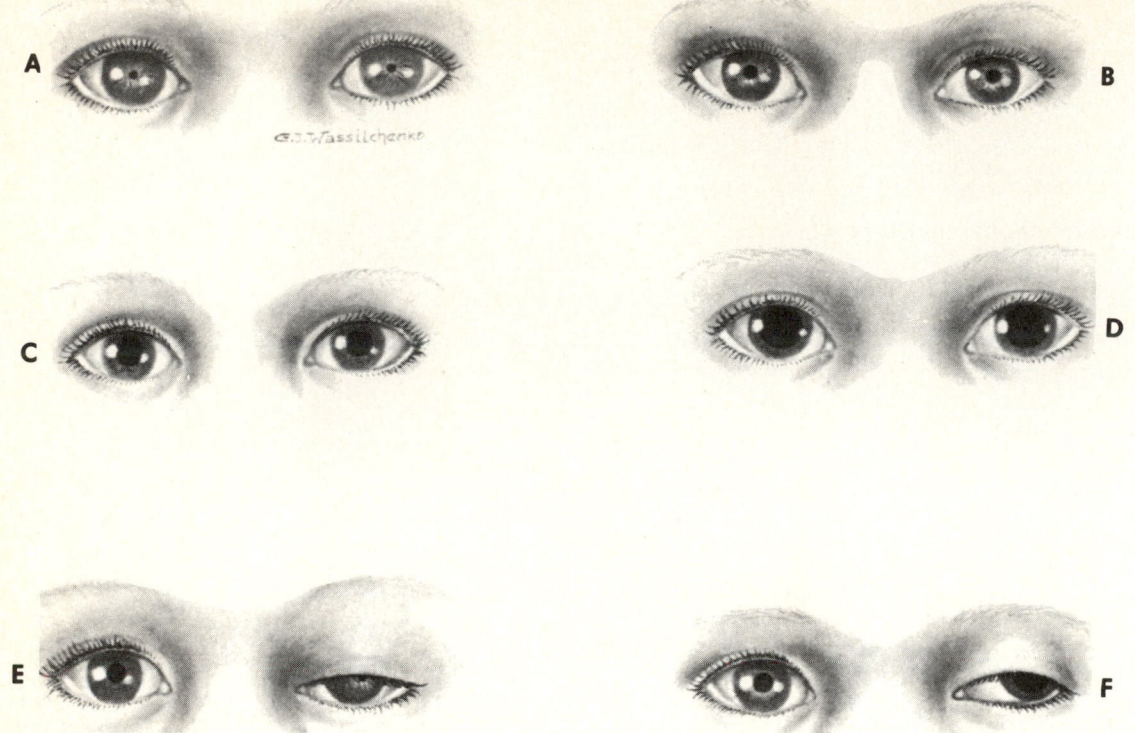

Fig. 6-8 Variations in pupil size with neurologic disorders. **A,** Bilateral small pupils or miosis. This can develop as the result of hemorrhage in the pons or as the result of administration of morphine sulfate or other barbiturates. **B,** Pinpoint pupils can also be observed as the result of barbiturate administration, poisoning, or brainstem dysfunction. **C,** Bilateral fixed pupils are usually observed as the result of third cranial nerve dysfunction following transtentorial cerebral herniation. **D,** Fixed and dilated pupils are commonly thought to indicate brainstem damage, although they may be observed in the hypothermic patient or in the patient who has received large doses of atropine or extremely large doses of sympathomimetic drugs. **E,** Ptosis with ipsilateral pupillary constriction usually occurs as the result of unilateral interruption of sympathetic nervous system fibers (Horner's syndrome). Both pupils should still react to light. **F,** Ptosis with ipsilateral eye abduction and pupil dilation often indicates significant cranial nerve (third and sixth) dysfunction as the result of ipsilateral brain lesion or transtentorial herniation.

From Whaley, L.F., and Wong, D.L.: Nursing care of infants and children, ed. 2, St. Louis, 1983, The C.V. Mosby Co.

crease in respiratory rate and depth or apnea.[56] It is important to note that this reflex does not develop completely until intracranial pressure is significantly elevated. Earlier signs of increased intracranial pressure may include tachycardia and fluctuations in arterial blood pressure. A late sign of increased intracranial pressure is hypotension (see Tables 6-8 and 6-9 for normal ranges of blood pressure and heart rates in children).

Alterations in respiratory rate and pattern. The patient with increased intracranial pressure may demonstrate a wide variety of respiratory patterns. When intracranial pressure rises and the Cushing reflex is initiated, the patient will classically develop apnea. However, other breathing patterns may also be noted Cheyne-Stokes respirations are defined as alternating hyperpnea and bradypnea. This means that the patient initially breathes faster and deeper, then more shallowly, than demonstrates a long respiratory pause before beginning the cycle again. Cheyne-Stokes respirations may be observed in patients with encephalopathies or cerebrovascular disease. *Central neurogenic hyperventilation* is present when the patient breathes at a constant, rapid rate despite the presence of adequate arterial oxygenation and hypocapnea. This hyperventilation usually indicates the presence of cerebral hypoxia or ischemia or of a midbrain or pontine lesion. Other abnormal breathing patterns include apneustic breathing (prolonged inspiration and expiration), cluster breathing (irregular

Table 6-8 Normal pediatric blood pressure ranges

Age	Systolic (mm Hg)	Diastolic (mm Hg)
Newborn—12 hr (less than 1000 gm)	39-59	16-36
Newborn—12 hr (3 kg)	50-70	25-45
Newborn—96 hr	60-90	20-60
Infant	74-100	50-70
Toddler	80-112	50-80
Preschooler	82-110	50-78
School-age child	84-120	54-80
Adolescent	94-140	62-88

The above ranges were taken from the tenth to ninetieth percentile ranges determined by the following studies: de Swiet, M., Fayers, P., and Shinebourne, E.A.: Systolic blood pressure in a population of infants in the first year of life: the Brompton study, Pediatrics 65:1028, May 1980; National Heart, Lung, and Blood Institute's Task Force on Blood Pressure Control in Children, Pediatrics 59(suppl. 5):797, 1977; and Versmold, H., and others: Aortic blood pressure during the first 12 hours of life in infants with birth weight 610 to 4220 gms, Pediatrics 67:107, May 1981.

breathing associated with apnea), and ataxic breathing (very irregular breathing).

Regardless of the respiratory rate or pattern demonstrated by the patient, it is essential that the nurse ensure that the patient's arterial oxygen saturation and carbon dioxide removal are adequate since hypercapnia and hypoxia can both contribute to cerebral vasodilation and increased cerebral blood flow. Although such an increase in blood flow may be well tolerated by a normal patient, it may contribute to an increase in intracranial pressure in the patient with cerebral edema or cerebral trauma. Thus the nurse should report development of respiratory insufficiency to a physician immediately.

Children with increased intracranial pressure may develop *neurogenic* pulmonary edema. This pulmonary edema develops suddenly and without warning (see Chapter 5 and Fig. 5-10 for representative radiographs of a child who developed acute neurogenic pulmonary edema). The mechanism for the development of this pulmonary edema is unclear, but it seems to be related to increased systemic and pulmonary artery pressure, which develops in response to the intracranial hypertension. Pulmonary edema usually produces respiratory failure (hypoxemia and

Table 6-9 Normal heart rates in children*

Age	Beats per minute
Infant	120 to 160
Toddler	90 to 140
Preschooler	80 to 110
School-aged child	75 to 100
Adolescent	60 to 90

*Your patient's normal range should always be considered. Also, the heart rate will normally increase in the presence of fever or stress, and it will decrease during sleep or vagal stimulation.

hypercapnia) with decreased lung compliance and increased respiratory effort (see the section on respiratory failure in Chapter 4).

Changes in motor function and reflexes. The infant or child with increased intracranial pressure can demonstrate decreased motor function, as well as abnormal posturing or reflexes. With progressive neurologic deterioration, flaccid paralysis will result.

When a neurologic injury or lesion is unilateral, the child may demonstrate hemiparesis or hemiplegia on the side contralateral to that of the injury. The development of *decorticate rigidity* (Fig. 6-9) indicates ischemia of or damage to the cerebral hemispheres. It is characterized by flexion of the elbows, wrists, and fingers, and by extension of the legs and ankles with plantar flexion of the feet. All four extremities are tightly abducted. The development of *decerebrate posturing* indicates the presence of a diffuse metabolic cerebral injury or the development of ischemia of or damage to more primitive areas of the brain, including the diencephalon, midbrain, or pons. In general, a progression from decorticate rigidity to decerebrate posturing usually indicates progression of the extent of the neurologic injury. However, a patient may occasionally alternate between decorticate rigidity and decerebrate posturing. This seems to result from variations in cerebral blood flow to the brainstem and the cerebral hemispheres. The physician should be notified immediately of the presence of either decorticate or decerebrate posturing. The physician should also be notified if the patient with decorticate rigidity develops decerebrate posturing.

Babinski's reflex is present or positive if the toes fan out and if the great toe flexes when the sole of the foot is stroked from the heel to the toes and around to the ball of the foot. Although positive Babinski's reflex is *normal* in the infant before he has begun walking, a positive Babinski's reflex is *abnormal* in any child who has begun walking, and it may indicate the presence of increased intracranial pressure.

All children should withdraw from painful stimuli. Lack of such withdrawal usually indicates a depressed level of consciousness, paresthesia, or paralysis and should be reported to a physician immediately.

The infant or child who develops increased intracranial pressure may demonstrate very few spontaneous movements and may be unable to perform motor skills previously demonstrated. For example, the 9-month-old infant may be unwilling or unable to sit without assistance, although he sat alone days earlier. The child may demonstrate an abnormal gait, or he may be unwilling to walk without assistance. Deterioration may also be demonstrated in the child's

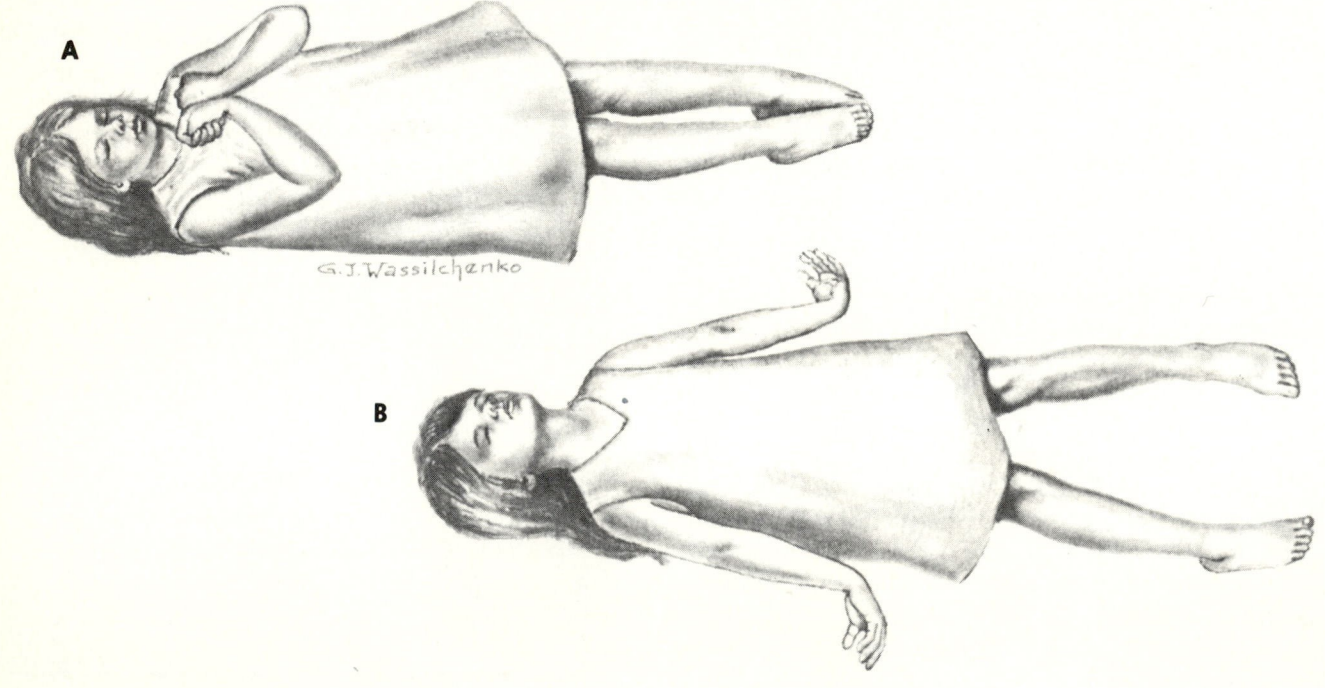

Fig. 6-9 Abnormal posturing. **A,** Decorticate rigidity, and **B,** decerebrate posturing.

From Whaley, L.F., and Wong, D.L.: Nursing care of infants and children, ed. 2, St. Louis, 1983, The C.V. Mosby Co.

Table 6-10   Normal age for attainment of major developmental milestones

Age	Motor skill	Language	Adaptive behavior
4-6 wk	Head lifted from prone position and turned from side to side	Cries	Smiles
4 mo	No head lag when pulled to sitting from supine position Tries to grasp large objects	Sounds of pleasure	Smiles, laughs aloud, and shows pleasure to familiar objects or persons
5 mo	Voluntary grasp with both hands Plays with toes	Primitive sounds: "ah goo"	Smiles at self in mirror
6 mo	Grasps with one hand Rolls prone to supine Sits with support	Range of sounds greater	Expresses displeasure and food preferences
8 mo	Sits without support Transfers objects from hand to hand Rolls supine to prone	Combines syllables: "baba, dada, mama"	Responds to "No"
10 mo	Sits well Creeping Stands holding Finger-thumb opposition in picking up small objects	—	Waves "bye-bye," plays "patty-cake" and "peek-a-boo"
12 mo	Stands holding Walks with support	Says 2 or 3 words with meaning	Understands names of objects Shows interest in pictures
15 mo	Walks alone	Several intelligible words	Requests by pointing Imitates
18 mo	Walks up and down stairs holding Removes clothes	Many intelligible words	Carries out simple commands
2 yr	Walks up and down stairs by self Runs	2- to 3-word phrases	Organized play Points to some parts of body

From Rudolph, A.M.: Pediatrics, ed. 17, New York, 1982, Appleton-Century-Crofts.

ability to coordinate movements or to carry out simple commands. To best evaluate such changes in the child's motor skills, it is essential that the nurse be familiar with the normal sequence of achievements of developmental milestones (see Table 6-10) and that she familiarize herself with the child's previous motor skills.

Although seizures are not a primary sign of increased intracranial pressure, they can develop in the child with neurologic disease or injury. Since status epilepticus will compromise cerebral perfusion and worsen ischemia, it is important that the nurse recognize the development of seizures and that a physician be notified. Because nystagmus, pupil changes, or wide fluctuations in blood pressure may be the only clinical signs of seizures in the child receiving paralyzing agents, an electroencephalogram (EEG) may be necessary to confirm or rule out the presence of seizures (see the section on status epilepticus later in this chapter).

Other signs of increased intracranial pressure. The infant with increased intracranial pressure is often extremely lethargic with a high-pitched cry. The infant's anterior fontanelle is usually full and tense. The scalp veins may appear distended, and the infant's eyes may be deviated downward ("sunset eyes"). The infant may become extremely irritable when his head is moved or his neck is flexed, and he may be uninterested in feeding or may vomit frequently. As intracranial pressure increases further, the nurse may be able to palpate spaces between the cranial bones as the cranial sutures widen.

The child with intracranial hypertension may complain of headache, nausea, vomiting, blurred vision, or *diplopia*. The child may demonstrate mood swings, and he may also be more lethargic with periods of confusion. Slurred speech is not uncommon. Clinical signs of increased intracranial pressure are summarized in the box on signs and symptoms of increased intracranial pressure in infants and children.

Intracranial pressure monitoring. The most reliable method for determining the presence and degree of intracranial hypertension is through measurement of the intracranial pressure. This is most frequently accomplished through insertion of a subarachnoid screw or bolt or through insertion of an intraventricular catheter. Other less frequently used methods of monitoring the intracranial pressure include use of a subarachnoid sensor or a fontogram.[45]

The subarachnoid screw or bolt can be inserted at the bedside or in the operating room. The bolt is then connected to a standard transducer system, and the pulsations in the cerebrospinal fluid are converted to a pressure by the transducer. Use of the bolt is contraindicated in infants because it is likely to crack

---

SIGNS AND SYMPTOMS OF INCREASED INTRACRANIAL PRESSURE IN INFANTS AND CHILDREN[41,42]

Infants
  Lethargy
  Poor feeding, anorexia, or vomiting
  Tense, bulging fontanelle
  High-pitched cry
  Increased head circumference (may be absent if increased ICP is acute)
  Separation of cranial sutures (if increased ICP is persistent)

Children
  Irritability or lethargy
  Anorexia, nausea, or vomiting
  Headache
  Diplopia or blurred vision
  Papilledema (after 48 hr)
  Separation of cranial sutures (if increased ICP is chronic)

Late signs
  Altered level of consciousness
  Unilateral or bilateral pupil dilation and sluggish response to light
  Tachycardia, then bradycardia
  Systolic hypertension and widened pulse pressure
  Alterations in respiratory rate and pattern leading to apnea

the thin skull of the infant. If an *intraventricular* monitoring system is desired, a polyethylene catheter is inserted through a burr hole and threaded into the anterior horn of the lateral ventricle in the patient's nondominant hemisphere.[42] The catheter is then connected to a sterile transducer system *and* to a sterile collection chamber (Fig. 6-10). If the intraventricular pressure rises, fluid may be drained from the ventricle with a physician's order. If the intraventricular catheter remains in place, the child should be placed in reverse isolation, and sterile technique should be used whenever the drainage system is handled (per physician order or hospital policy). This system is also referred to as an *extraventricular drainage system.* For further information about intracranial pressure monitoring equipment see the section on intracranial pressure monitoring in Chapter 9.

Helpful diagnostic tests. Intracranial pressure monitoring and careful clinical assessment provide the most useful information about the child's neurologic status. In addition, the EEG may be used during barbiturate therapy to assess cerebral activity. Computerized axial tomography (CAT or CT scan) is extremely helpful in localizing mass lesions or intracranial bleeding or in determining the presence of diffuse cerebral edema or infarction (see the section diagnostic tests later in this chapter for further discussion of EEG and CT or CAT scan). When the

child's intracranial pressure has risen sharply and when cerebral ischemia is suspected, a cerebral perfusion scan may be performed to evaluate adequacy of cerebral blood flow. When brainstem herniation or severe cerebral ischemia have developed, this can be documented by the perfusion scan.

■ **Medical treatment and nursing interventions**

Care of the child with increased intracranial pressure requires constant assessment of the child's clinical status, acute reduction of intracranial pressure by reduction of intracranial volume, prevention of further increases in intracranial pressure, and preservation of cerebral metabolic functions.

Assessment. If an intracranial pressure monitoring device is in place, the intracranial pressure should be monitored continuously (see the section on intracranial pressure monitoring in Chapter 9). In addition, it is helpful if an arterial catheter is inserted so that the arterial pressure can also be displayed continuously on an oscilloscope. When both of these measurements are available, the child's cerebral perfusion pressure should be calculated hourly and whenever a change in the child's condition develops. The following formula is used.

Cerebral perfusion pressure = mean arterial pressure − ICP

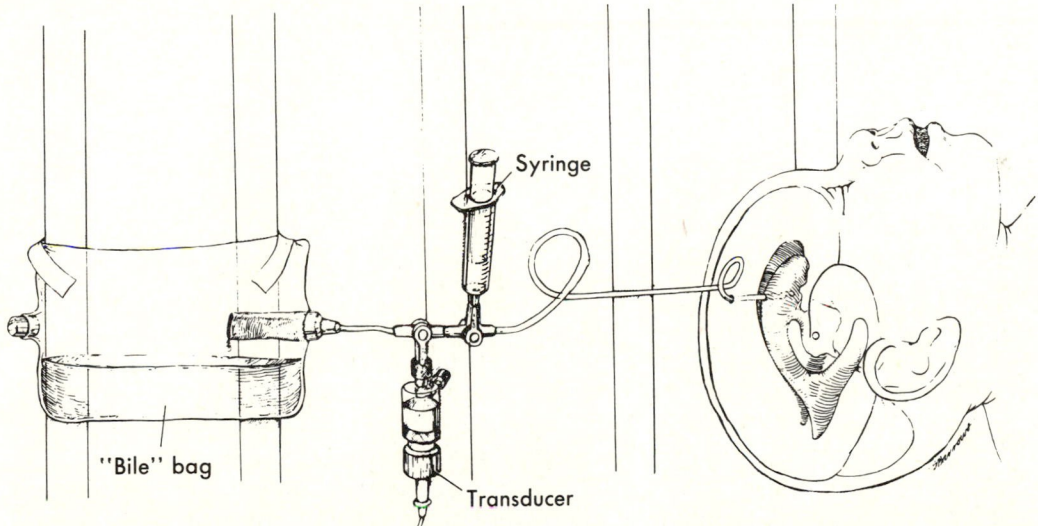

Fig. 6-10 Intraventricular pressure monitoring system. This system uses a catheter in the frontal horn of the right lateral ventricle, which is connected to a transducer, drainage bag, and syringe. The system is "closed," so that contamination is minimized. Appropriate stopcock adjustments allow for measuring of intraventricular pressure, drainage of cerebrospinal fluid, or flushing of the ventricular catheter (with physician order). The bag is positioned at a prescribed height in relation to the lateral ventricle since lowering of the bag will enhance cerebrospinal fluid drainage and raising the bag will reduce this drainage.

From Sklar, F.H., Patz, J., and Stein, P.: Intracranial pressure measurements and ventricular taps. In Levin, D.L., Morriss, F.C., and Moore, G.C., editors: A practical guide to pediatric intensive care, ed. 2, St. Louis, 1984, The C.V. Mosby Co.

Although the child with increased intracranial pressure may initially be capable of breathing spontaneously, the child is usually intubated, paralyzed, and sedated so that the arterial carbon dioxide and oxygen tensions can be controlled. The arterial carbon dioxide tension should be maintained between 25 to 29 mm Hg, and the arterial oxygen tension should be maintained at 80 to 100 mm Hg (60 to 80 mm Hg in the infant) since hypercapnia and, to a lesser extent, hypoxia are potent cerebral vasodilators. Hand ventilation should be performed before endotracheal suctioning and whenever the child's intracranial pressure rises; this will reduce the child's arterial carbon dioxide tension and prevent cerebral vasodilation and increased intracranial pressure. A nasogastric tube should also be placed to decompress the stomach since gastric distention can compromise diaphragmatic movement and produce hypoventilation.

If the child's measured intracranial pressure rises sharply, if the cerebral perfusion pressure falls to near 60 mm Hg, or if clinical signs of neurologic deterioration develop, a physician should be notified, and the nurse should hand ventilate the child at a relatively rapid respiratory rate to reduce the carbon dioxide tension (per unit policy or physician order).

Throughout the child's care, the nurse should thoroughly assess the child's neurologic status for clinical signs of deterioration (see the previous section on clinical signs and symptoms). The level of consciousness (if the child is not paralyzed or sedated), pupillary size and response to light, blood pressure, heart rate, respiratory rate and pattern (if the child is not receiving controlled mechanical ventilation), motor function, muscle tone, and reflexes should be checked hourly and whenever the child's clinical appearance changes. A physician should be notified immediately of any deterioration in the patient's clinical status.

In addition to careful assessment of the child's neurologic status, the nurse should closely monitor evidence of the child's systemic perfusion and respiratory function. If the child's cardiac output and systemic perfusion are good, peripheral pulses will be strong, the child's extremities will be warm with pink nailbeds and brisk capillary refill, and the child's urine output will total 1.0 ml/kg body weight/hour. Insertion of a central venous pressure line is desirable since measurement of the central venous pressure will enable evaluation of the child's circulating blood volume. Although it is necessary to maintain adequate hydration to maximize systemic and cerebral perfusion, a high central venous pressure (above 5 to 8 mm Hg) is to be avoided since it will impede cerebral venous return.

The child's respiratory function must be adequate to prevent the development of hypercapnia or hypoxia. Atelectasis, endotracheal (ET) tube obstruction or dislodgement, or hypoventilation must be avoided in these patients. Vigorous chest physical therapy, prolonged suctioning, stimulation of vigorous cough, and use of the head-down position for bronchial drainage are contraindicated in these patients, however, since they may contribute to a rise in intracranial pressure. The goal of pulmonary toilet should be maintenance of a clear airway.

When an intracranial pressure monitoring device is used, the nurse should be able to verify functioning of the system (see the section on intracranial pressure monitoring in Chapter 9). There are three distinct pressure waveforms, designated A, B, and C, that can be appreciated when the intracranial pressure waveform is displayed on an oscilloscope (Fig. 6-11 demonstrates these waveforms). *A waves* are commonly called *plateau waves*, and they usually range in amplitude from 50 to 100 mm Hg. These plateau waves usually appear when the patient already has elevated intracranial pressure; they represent a further critical rise in the intracranial pressure as the result of hypercapnia, hypoxia, or cerebral edema. Because the appearance of A waves is extremely worrisome and is usually associated with other signs of neurologic deterioration, a physician should be notified immediately if they are observed. *B waves* are rhythmic, low-amplitude waves that fluctuate during the respiratory cycle. These waves usually range in amplitude between 20 to 50 mm Hg, and they are usually associated with sleep or developing coma. *C waves* are also rhythmic, low-amplitude waves. They do not vary during the respiratory cycle, although they will reflect systemic arterial pulsations. The clinical significance of *C waves* is not clear.[42,45,82]

Transducers used for intracranial pressure monitoring *must not* be connected to standard infusion devices since solution should never be routinely infused into the subarachnoid space or ventricles. Occasionally, a physician may specifically order instillation of a small amount of solution into the intracranial pressure catheter, but such instillation should only be performed with a specific order and in the presence of a physician (see Fig. 6-10). When the child has increased intracranial pressure, the addition of even a small amount of fluid in this manner can produce a sharp critical rise in intracranial pressure.[35] Occasionally, the intracranial pressure monitoring tubing is filled with an antibacterial solution (such as one containing gentamicin) as a prophylactic measure against infection. It is important to note that this

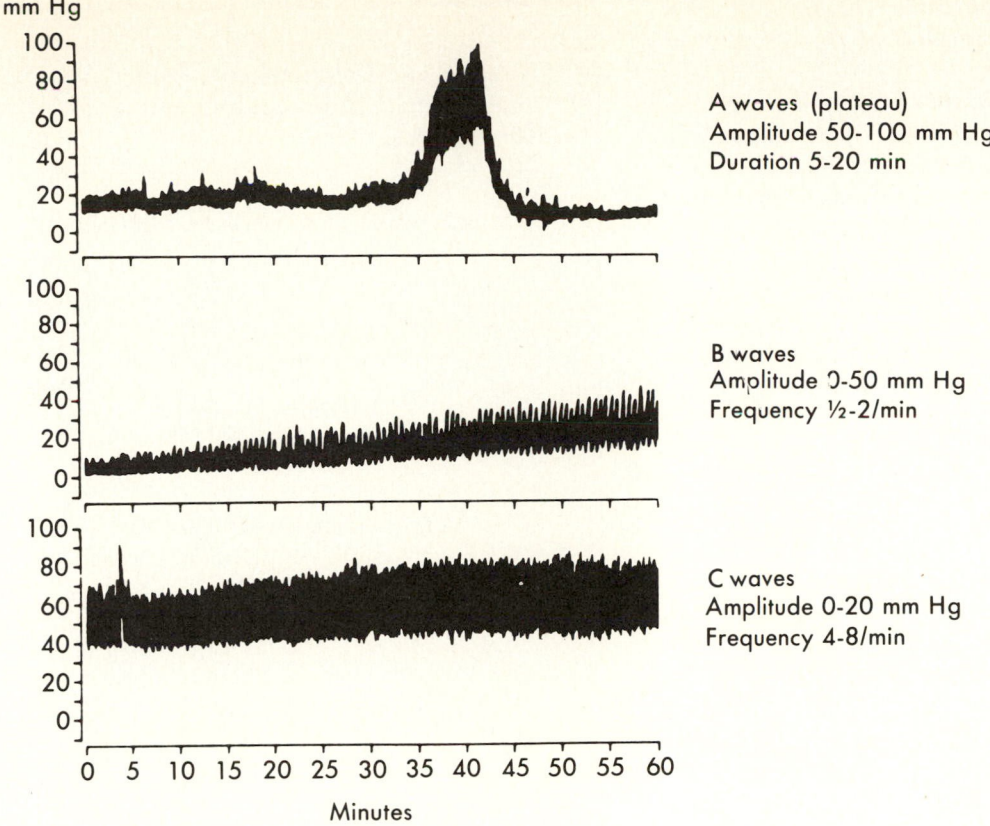

Fig. 6-11 Intracranial pressure waves.

From Taylor, F.A., and others: Symptoms caused by intracranial pressure waves, J. Neurosurg. Nurs. **9**:145, Dec. 1977.

solution is intended to remain in the tubing, rather than be used for irrigation.

The intracranial pressure monitoring system is intended for use as a guide to therapy. Since intracranial pressure is not uniform or static, the intracranial pressure recorded by the monitoring device should be used in conjunction with a careful clinical assessment to determine trends in the child's neurologic condition. Rarely are single absolute values as important as such trends. Whenever intracranial pressure monitoring is performed, the physician should write specific orders regarding response to changes in the intracranial pressure. For example, the physician may request that the child be hyperventilated, using a hand ventilator, if the intracranial pressure rises above 20 to 25 mm Hg for 3 or more minutes or if the cerebral perfusion pressure falls below 55 to 60 mm Hg. These orders eliminate ambiguity about the patient's care and protect the patient, nurse, and physician. The physician should be notified immediately of any deterioration in the child's clinical status, an increase in the child's intracranial pressure, dampen-ing of the intracranial pressure waveforms, or malfunctions of the intracranial pressure system.

Acute reduction of intracranial pressure. *Reduction in cerebral blood volume* is acutely accomplished through *hyperventilation.* Since hyperventilation is the most effective short-term method of reducing intracranial pressure, it should be performed immediately if the intubated child's intracranial pressure rises or if cerebral perfusion pressure falls to critical levels. As noted earlier, full ventilatory control should be assured so that the arterial P_{CO_2} can be maintained at 25 to 29 mm Hg and so that the arterial P_{O_2} can be maintained between 80 to 100 mm Hg (60 to 80 mm Hg in neonates). Use of paralyzing agents such as intravenous pancuronium (0.1 mg/kg) or d-tubocurarine (0.2 to 0.4 mg/kg loading dose and 0.125 to 0.35 mg/kg as needed every hour) with morphine sulfate (0.1 mg/kg every 3 to 4 hours) will prevent patient agitation or resistance to mechanical ventilation.[59] Pancuronium bromide is the most popular paralyzing agent used in children; it has minimal cardiovascular effects, and it can easily be reversed with neostigmine (Prostigmin).[50] Tachyarrhythmias have been reported following use of this drug, however.[5]

Reduction in CSF volume is necessary if hydrocephalus is present. This is achieved by surgical insertion of a ventriculoperitoneal shunt (or other form of ventricular drainage). If the child has such a shunt in place, it is important to know if the shunt must be regularly "pumped" to maintain function. The shunt may become obstructed or malfunction, or it may become disconnected during the immediate postoperative period or several months or years after insertion, resulting in a gradual or sudden increase in intracranial pressure.

Even if excess CSF volume is *not* present, reduction in CSF volume may be attempted to reduce intracranial volume and pressure. This can be accomplished if an intraventricular catheter is in place. Cerebrospinal fluid may be intermittently withdrawn by a physician to reduce intracranial pressure. A drainage system can also be assembled to allow continuous drainage of cerebral spinal fluid. With this type of extraventricular drainage, the collection chamber is maintained at a constant prescribed level below the head; the lower the collection chamber, the more rapid the CSF drainage. Excess drainage is to be avoided since upward herniation of the brain can occur. If an extraventricular drain is in place, the child is placed in reverse isolation, and strict sterile technique is used whenever the drainage system is manipulated (per physician order or unit policy).

Reduction in cerebral edema is accomplished through fluid restriction, diuretic therapy, administration of colloids and blood products, and occasional use of hypertonic agents or steroids. IV fluid therapy is calculated to provide approximately one half to two thirds of calculated maintenance fluid requirements (Table 6-11) in the form of 5% or 10% glucose in 0.2 or 0.45 normal saline. Administration of hypotonic solutions is to be avoided since water tends to diffuse into injured brain cells and since ADH secretion during the immediate postoperative period will produce maximal renal water retention.

Five percent albumin or fresh frozen plasma may be administered to provide colloid or treat hypovolemia, and packed red blood cells should be used to maintain a normal hemoglobin concentration.

Diuretics are administered to promote renal excretion of free water. Furosemide is the intravenous diuretic of choice since it not only reduces body water but decreases venous tone and reduces production of cerebrospinal fluid.[65] Intravenous furosemide (0.5 to 2.0 mg/kg/dose) usually produces a prompt diuresis. Before administration of any diuretic, a urinary cath-

---

Table 6-11   Calculation of daily maintenance fluid requirements for children

Child's weight	Kilogram body weight formula
Newborn (0-72 hr old)	60-100 ml/kg
0-10 kg	100 ml/kg (may increase up to 150 ml/kg if renal and cardiac function adequate)
11-20 kg	1000 ml for the first 10 kg + 50 ml/kg for each kg over 10 kg
21-30 kg	.500 ml for the first 20 kg + 25 ml/kg for each kg over 20 kg

Body surface area formula: 1500 cc/m² body surface area/day provides normal maintenance fluid requirements.

---

eter should be inserted or a dry, weighed diaper should be placed under the child so that the timing and volume of diuretic response can be accurately recorded.

Throughout the child's care, the child's serum osmolality is monitored closely. A serum osmolality of approximately 300 mOsm is desirable because it promotes fluid shifts from the intracellular to the intravascular space. A serum osmolality of greater than 320 mOsm is to be avoided, however, since it is associated with excessive cellular fluid loss and renal damage.[54,65]

Previously, large doses of hypertonic agents were repeatedly administered to patients with increased intracranial pressure in an effort to increase serum osmolality. Recently, it has been thought that children with head trauma develop excessive cerebral blood flow. Administration of hypertonic agents in these patients can actually be harmful since an increase in cerebral intravascular volume (as a result of fluid shift from the cellular to the vascular space) temporarily results in a further increase in intracranial pressure. Thus administration of hypertonic agents in these patients is now usually avoided. Administration of hypertonic agents is also contraindicated in patients with active cerebral bleeding since movement of the hypertonic agent into the brain tissue would tend to draw more fluid into that tissue. Therefore use of hypertonic agents in the treatment of intracranial hypertension is primarily reserved for patients with an intracranial mass lesion or those patients with increased intracranial pressure unresponsive to other medical therapy.

When a hypertonic agent is administered, *mannitol* (0.15 to 0.3 gm/kg every 1 to 2 hours) is often the agent of choice. Continuous infusion therapy of 0.05 to 0.15 gm/kg/hour may be ordered during the initial 48 hours of therapy.[12] Frequent administration of low doses of mannitol is thought to increase the serum osmolality without significantly increasing cerebral blood volume. Higher doses of mannitol (up to 1.5 to 2.0 gm/kg every 4 to 6 hours) are reserved for emergency control of intracranial pressure that is producing rapid clinical deterioration.

Urea (30%) is occasionally administered (1.0 gm/kg every 4 to 6 hours). Contraindications to urea therapy include the presence of kidney or liver disease, as well as those contraindications common to any hypertonic agent. This drug should only be infused into a large vein or central venous line since tissue sloughing can occur if the drug enters the subcutaneous tissue. Side effects of urea administration include nausea, vomiting, headaches, syncope, dizziness, and hypotension.

Concentrated intravenous glucose solutions (D_{25} or D_{50}) are relatively benign solutions that may also be infused to increase intravascular osmolality. These solutions should be infused into a central venous line to prevent vascular irritation.

Steroids may be administered in an attempt to minimize later development of cerebral edema. Dexamethasone (0.5 to 1.0 mg/kg intravenously or intramuscularly as an initial dose, then 0.25 to 0.5 mg/kg/day in four doses) or prednisone (1.5 to 2.0 mg/kg/day orally) are the steroids of choice. Peak effect of the steroid will be approximately 12 to 18 hours after administration; this renders the drug ineffective for acute management of increased intracranial pressure. Whenever steroids are administered, the nurse should monitor for side effects, including gastrointestinal bleeding, glycosuria, and susceptibility to infection. When steroids are discontinued, they should be tapered slowly.[12,65]

Dimethyl sulfoxide (DMSO) is an anti-inflammatory agent that has been used in approved clinical research centers for the treatment of extremely high intracranial pressure unresponsive to conventional forms of medical management. Use of this drug, even on a limited research basis, is highly controversial. Hazardous fumes may be expired by the patient receiving DMSO, causing nausea and vomiting in persons caring for the patient. Since DMSO is a solvent, use of nonplastic IV tubing and stopcocks is necessary. Further investigation of this drug is currently underway.[75]

Prevention of further increases in intracranial pressure. Further increases in intracranial pressure can be prevented by maintenance of adequate ventilatory support, administration of analgesics, proper patient positioning, and provision of general supportive care.

Ventilatory support should be adequate, and hypoventilation, hypercapnia, and hypoxia are to be prevented. This requires excellent hand ventilation and suctioning technique and good pulmonary toilet.

The head of the child's bed should be elevated to promote cerebral venous return. The child's head should be supported in the midline, and flexion or rotation of the neck is to be avoided since this can obstruct venous return. The child's central venous pressure should be adequate to maintain systemic perfusion but not excessive; a central venous pressure over 5 to 8 mm Hg can reduce cerebral venous return. Provision of positive pressure ventilation with high-peak inspiratory pressures or administration of high levels of positive end-expiratory pressures will also slow cerebral venous return. Stool softeners should be administered to prevent bowel impaction or straining (and Valsalva's maneuver) during defecation.

The child should receive adequate analgesia in addition to paralyzing agents. Pain can cause hypoventilation and Valsalva's maneuver, which can produce a rise in intracranial pressure. Fever should be treated with antipyretics to reduce metabolic rate and oxygen consumption. If infection is suspected, appropriate blood, wound, and catheter cultures should be obtained.

The child should receive adequate caloric intake in the form of parenteral alimentation (see Chapter 7). This will promote wound healing and speed recovery.

Preservation of cerebral metabolic functions. If the intracranial pressure remains high and cerebral perfusion pressure is compromised despite maximal medical therapy, a neurosurgeon may create burr holes in the skull to allow decompression of the cranium. If massive cerebral trauma has been sustained, a skull flap may be removed to allow brain swelling without compression. Most commonly in a tertiary care center, however, the patient with a severe or sustained increase in intracranial pressure is placed in a barbiturate coma with hypothermia to reduce cerebral metabolic requirements, cerebral blood flow, and intracranial pressure. In addition, it is thought that barbiturate administration in the child with increased intracranial pressure will maintain cerebral cellular membrane stability and allow the brain to tolerate short periods of ischemia.[65]

Thiopental, pentobarbital, or phenobarbital may be used to induce the coma; pentobarbital is used most frequently in children. Initially, a loading dose of 2.0 to 5.0 mg/kg is administered, and the dosage is increased as needed until the EEG is isoelectric (or nearly so). Serum pentobarbital levels are then obtained, and the drug dosage is adjusted to maintain a serum pentobarbital level of 20 to 40 µg/ml (or 2.0 to 4.0 mg/dl). This usually requires hourly doses of 0.5 to 3.0 mg/kg/hour or an equivalent bolus dose.[12]

As the pentobarbital is administered, the nurse must carefully monitor the child's blood pressure. Volume expanders and vasopressors should be readily available since many patients will develop significant hypotension during induction with pentobarbital. Because the hypotension results from decreased systemic vascular resistance it will be exacerbated in those patients who are hypovolemic (please see the section on low cardiac output in Chapter 3), and it will usually respond to the administration of colloids or low-dose dopamine infusion.[65] Hypotension is also more likely to occur if high doses of pentobarbital are administered.

A pentobarbital coma is usually maintained for 48 to 72 hours following cerebral injury or ischemia; this seems to be the interval during which cerebral edema is maximal.[65] If necessary, however, the coma may be maintained for 2 to 3 weeks.[12] During this time, meticulous attention must be given to pulmonary toilet, positioning, skin care, and nutrition since the child is totally dependent upon the health care team for complete physical care. Because all of the child's cranial nerve reflexes are abolished, it is difficult to assess the child's neurologic function in a conventional manner. Brainstem evoked responses (BERs) may still be monitored, however (see the section on electroencephalogram later in this chapter).

Barbiturate therapy is tapered gradually when the child's intracranial pressure no longer rises as the barbiturate dosage is reduced.[59] Throughout the weaning process, the nurse should monitor the child's neurologic status carefully; seizures may occur during pentobarbital weaning, and the child's intracranial pressure may rise sharply if significant cerebral injury remains. Either of these clinical signs should be reported to a physician immediately.

Hypothermia is used in conjunction with the barbiturate coma to reduce cerebral metabolic requirements and to minimize cerebral injury.[77] The child is placed on a cooling mattress and the rectal temperature is maintained between 30° to 32° C. Dur-

ing the cooling, the child must be intubated and mechanically ventilated to prevent respiratory depression, and he should be paralyzed to prevent shivering. Continuous (30 to 100 µg/kg/hour) or intermittent (0.1 mg/kg/dose) doses of morphine sulfate should be administered to prevent pain and anxiety.

Hypothermia decreases the rate of hepatic and renal excretion of drugs; therefore drug requirements are reduced when hypothermia is used. A serum potassium concentration of 2.5 to 3.0 mEq/L is usually adequate to prevent hypokalemic cardiac arrhythmias, and a serum potassium concentration above this level may reflect a relative hyperkalemia.[66]

Rewarming should be accomplished *slowly*, without the use of warming blankets. If the child is rewarmed rapidly, barbiturates can be rapidly mobilized from fatty tissue, and cardiorespiratory depression can occur.

Weaning from ventilatory support. As the child's condition improves, he may be gradually allowed to waken, move, and begin weaning from ventilatory support. Only one change in treatment should be made at a time to allow thorough evaluation of the child's response before a second change is made. If the child's intracranial pressure again begins to rise, a physician should be notified immediately and resumption of paralysis and mechanical support may again be required. Development of hypercapnia, hypoxia, and hypoventilation must still be avoided in these patients since these can still result in a rise in intracranial pressure.

Psychosocial support. Throughout the child's care, the child and family will require sensitive support. While the child is unstable, it is often necessary to focus complete attention on the technical aspects of the child's care; however, the psychosocial aspects can obviously not be neglected. If the nurse feels unable to allow time or attention for supportive interaction with the family, an additional nurse, chaplain, or social worker should be called to provide the parents with the support they will need. Throughout the child's care, the child should receive explanations of all procedures performed and of all things he will see, feel, or hear. *Paralyzed or comatose children are still able to hear;* therefore the staff should minimize technical discussions near the bedside and avoid discussion of a poor prognosis in the child's presence. Too often, the child is treated as if he is unconscious when he is merely immobile. As the child becomes able to move, simple signals should be devised to allow the child to communicate, and all signals should be carefully recorded in the nursing care plan.

As the child recovers, he should receive repeated explanations of where he is and how he is progressing since he will often be disoriented when waking from a sound sleep. It is natural for the child to be frightened during this time.

If the child will require extended rehabilitative therapy, such therapy should be initiated as soon as possible so that the child's progress or discharge from the unit are not unnecessarily delayed. If the child is not expected to recover, each member of the health care team should be aware of the prognosis, the information provided to the family, and the family's response to this information, so that consistent and constructive intervention can be planned (see the section on cerebral death later in this chapter).

■ **COMA**
■ **Etiology**

Normal responsiveness to environmental stimulation requires normal function of the cerebral hemispheres and the reticular system. A normal state of consciousness is existence of awareness of the environment, the ability to be aroused from sleep, and orientation (as appropriate) to time, place, and person. A decreased level of consciousness is present if the child is abnormally lethargic or confused or if the child is not appropriately oriented to time and place. *Stupor* is a state of decreased consciousness from which the child can be aroused only through application of strong external stimuli. *Coma* is a state of decreased consciousness from which the child cannot be aroused despite provision of strong external stimuli. Coma can be described more specifically as the lack of eye opening and verbal response for 6 or more hours following a cerebral insult.[12,63]

Coma in children can occur as the result of any of the following disorders: CNS inflammation, cerebral edema, head injury, intracranial bleeding, intracranial tumors or other mass lesions, hypoxia, hypercapnia, acid-base imbalance, electrolyte imbalance (such as hyponatremia or hyperglycemia), disturbances of water balance, or Reye's syndrome. Coma in children can also result from ingestion of excessive amounts of therapeutic drugs (such as aspirin, barbiturates, antihistamines, and ferrous sulfate) and from ingestion of "street" drugs (including phencyclidine [PCP], methaqualone [Quaaludes], diazepam [Valium], and heroin).

It is probably helpful to divide the causes of coma into structural and toxic or metabolic problems. *Structural coma* results from actual physical injury to the brain, and treatment is aimed at preventing or limiting cerebral edema and the development of increased intracranial pressure. *Toxic* or *metabolic coma* results from electrolyte or acid-base imbal-

ances, liver or renal failure, or the ingestion of toxic substances. Treatment of this type of coma is aimed at removing or neutralizing the toxin.[23,63]

■ **Pathophysiology**

Although coma can result from a variety of causes, the pathophysiology and treatment of any comatose patient is similar. When the child is comatose, brain function is depressed and loss of consciousness occurs. When coma persists, critical cardiorespiratory functions often require support.[63]

One of the most popular methods for staging of coma, the Huttenlocher staging, is commonly used in the clinical setting. This method describes the progression from "light" coma to brain death.[63] Such staging methods are useful because they allow objective determination of the severity of the child's condition as well as objective criteria for assessment of the child's improvement. If the child has Reye's syndrome, the Lovejoy staging criteria can be used (see the section on Reye's syndrome later in this chapter). Because most scales for staging neurologic function in coma are very similar, the choice of staging criteria will depend on the physician and on the preference of the health care team (see the box below).

■ **Clinical signs and symptoms**

The comatose child demonstrates no observable response to external stimuli. In addition, abnormal posturing can be observed. The child may demonstrate impaired cranial nerve function, loss of oculocephalic and oculovestibular reflexes, and progressive brainstem dysfunction. Ultimately, cardiorespiratory compromise may develop.

Assessment of the comatose child should include all aspects presented in the section on clinical

---

HUTTENLOCHER STAGING OF COMA

Stage 1	Lethargy, confusion, or listlessness; vomiting may be present
Stage 2	Agitation, delirium, disorientation; decorticate rigidity may be present
Stage 3	Coma—total unresponsiveness; decerebrate posturing is often present
Stage 4	Cessation of brainstem function; flaccid muscle tone is noted

signs and symptoms of increased intracranial pressure. The child's level of consciousness should be constantly evaluated. The child's pupil size and reaction to light should be assessed hourly and whenever the child's clinical condition changes. Although there are no characteristic changes in pupil response associated with coma, characteristic changes may occur as the result of the underlying cerebral insult or as the result of the development of increased intracranial pressure (see Fig. 6-8 and Table 6-12 for examples of variations in pupil size with altered levels of consciousness).

Assessment of cranial nerve function is necessary since evaluation of higher brain function is impossible in the unresponsive child. Thorough cranial nerve evaluation is often specifically performed by the physician, although the nurse frequently assesses function of the oculomotor nerve (third cranial nerve) when evaluating pupil constriction to light, of the acoustic nerve (eighth cranial nerve) when speaking to the child, and of the glossopharyngeal and vagus nerves (ninth and tenth cranial nerves—producing a gag reflex) when suctioning the child. (See Table 6-13 for a summary of clinical methods used to evaluate cranial nerve function and Table 6-3 for a review of cranial nerve functions.)

Two reflexes that may be absent in the comatose child are the *oculocephalic reflex* and the *oculovestibular reflex*. The oculocephalic reflex is commonly referred to as testing of "doll's eyes." This test must not be performed on any patient suspected of having a cervical fracture. The reflex is evaluated when the child's head is sharply turned from the midline to one side and then turned to the other side with the eyes open. If the child's brainstem is intact, the normal doll's eyes reflex is present, and the eyes will seem to move in the direction opposite that of the head movement; thus, if the patient's head is turned sharply to his left, the patient's eyes will deviate toward the right. When the doll's eyes reflex is absent, the eyes are fixed in the middle of their sockets and they appear to move with the head in the direction of

Table 6-12 Reflex responses in altered states of consciousness

Level of CNS lesion	Level of consciousness	Pupillary size and reactivity	Oculocephalic and oculovestibular reflexes	Respiratory pattern	Motor responses
Thalamus	Lethargy, stupor	Small, reactive	Increased or decreased	Cheyne-Stokes*	Normal posture, tone slightly increased
Midbrain	Coma	Midposition, fixed	Absent	Central neurogenic hyperventilation†	Decorticate,‡ tone markedly increased
Pons	Coma	Pinpoint	Absent	Eupnea§ or apneustic breathing‖	Decerebrate,¶ flaccid
Medulla	Coma	Small, reactive	Present	Ataxic breathing	No posturing, flaccid

From Morriss, F.C.: Altered states of consciousness. In Levin, D.L., Morriss, F.C., and Moore, G.C.: A practical guide to pediatric intensive care, ed. 2, St. Louis, 1984, The C.V. Mosby Co.
*Cheyne-Stokes respiration: type of regular periodic breathing characterized by crescendo-decrescendo breaths interspersed with periods of apnea.
†Central neurogenic hyperventilation: hyperventilation with forced inspiration and expiration.
‡Decorticate posturing: upper extremities flexed against chest, lower extremities extended.
§Eupnea: normal breathing.
‖Apneustic breathing: pattern of breathing in which there is cessation of respiration in inspiratory position, usually rhythmical.
¶Decerebrate posturing: arms and legs extended with arms internally rotated, neck extended.

Table 6-13 Clinical evaluation of cranial nerve function*

Cranial nerve	Clinical evaluation	Etiology of abnormal findings
I. Olfactory	In a young infant or child, function can be tested by placing a substance with a strong scent near the nose; a positive reaction is movement of the head away from the substance or a facial grimace; the older child can be asked to identify familiar odors	Loss of smell (anosmia) is frequently associated with frontal lobe tumors or basilar skull fractures
II. Optic	The infant or child should be able to track the course of a beam of light or of a brightly colored object with both eyes; the older child may be asked to read a few sentences from a book and from a sign across the room; central and peripheral vision in both eyes must be evaluated	Loss of optic function is frequently associated with tumors along the optic nerve tract
III. Oculomotor IV. Trochler VI. Abducens	These nerves are evaluated simultaneously because together they control eye movement; when tested separately, both pupils should constrict in response to light; both eyes should move simultaneously in the same direction to track an object horizontally and vertically	Loss of these cranial nerve functions commonly occurs with insult to the brainstem or transentorial herniation and results in absence of the doll's eyes reflex
V. Trigeminal	Sensory function is tested by gentle application of warm, cold, and sharp objects against the face; the corneal reflex is present if light application of a cotton swab against the cornea produces a blink response; the motor function of this nerve is intact if the patient can chew	Loss of function of this nerve is common in patients with coma or brainstem insult
VII. Facial	The facial nerve is probably intact if the child's facial expressions at rest and during cry are symmetrical	Loss of facial nerve function can result from a pontine or temporal lobe lesion or tumor, or it may be noted following a temporal or basilar skull fracture
VIII. Acoustic	Patient blink, grimace, or startle response to an unseen sound stimulus verifies the function of the acoustic component of this nerve; an intact acoustic nerve is required for the oculovestibular reflex ("calorics")	Acoustic nerve dysfunction occurs as the result of brainstem injury

*Refer to Table 6-3 for additional information.

Continued.

Table 6-13 **Clinical evaluation of cranial nerve function—cont'd**

Cranial nerve	Clinical evaluation	Etiology of abnormal findings
IX Glossopharyngeal X. Vagus	When these nerves are intact, the child should gag following stimulation of the posterior pharynx with a tongue blade or suction catheter; the ability to swallow and speak without hoarseness also indicates normal vagus nerve function	Loss of function of these nerves is common following head or neck injury or as the result of ascending peripheral neuropathies; loss of the gag reflex increases the patient's risk of aspiration
XI. Accessory	This nerve is evaluated by noting the strength and symmetry of head and neck movement, especially the ability to lift the head	Loss of function may be related to injury to the neck
XII. Hypoglossal	If this nerve is intact, the older child should be able to move his tongue on request	Fasciculations and tremors of the tongue are suggestive of hypoglossal nerve atrophy or injury that tends to occur as the result of lower motor neuron disease or neck injuries

head movement. Loss of the doll's eyes reflex indicates the presence of a severe lesion in the area of the brainstem.[7,42]

The elicitation of the *oculovestibular reflex* is commonly referred to as "calorics." Testing of this reflex is usually performed by a physician, and it is contraindicated in the patient with a ruptured tympanic membrane. The test is performed by instilling 10 to 20 ml of ice water into the external auditory ear canal while the head is elevated at a 45 to 60 degree angle. If the brainstem is intact, both eyes should deviate toward the side of the irrigation. This deviation often occurs with nystagmus. If the child's eyes do not deviate toward the side of the irrigation, brainstem injury is present.

The *corneal reflex* should also be tested in the comatose child. Normally, gentle stroking of the eyelashes or of the peripheral portion of the cornea with a wisp of cotton will produce a brisk blink response. If no blink is seen, brainstem injury is probably present.[23]

The *tonic neck reflex* is normally present in infants between 2 and 6 months of age. This reflex can be elicited by rapidly turning the infant's head to the side while the infant is supine. When the tonic neck reflex is present, the ipsilateral arm and leg will ex-

tend, while the contralateral arm and leg will flex (Fig. 6-12). Persistence of this reflex beyond 9 months of age usually indicates neurologic disease or injury.

Deep tendon reflexes (such as the patellar reflex) may be checked by the physician. The nurse or physician should attempt to elicit *clonus* by flexing the wrists and ankles; clonus is present if the extremities then rhythmically flex and contract. Exaggerated deep tendon reflexes or sustained clonus or spasticity may be present if the child is fatigued, but they may also indicate the presence of upper motor neuron lesions (cerebral cortex injury) or diffuse metabolic disorders.[7]

The child's posture and limb movements should also be carefully evaluated. The development of decorticate rigidity or decerebrate posturing should be reported to a physician. Decerebrate posturing usually indicates damage to lower (more basic) brain centers; however, some comatose patients demonstrate alternating decorticate rigidity and decerebrate posturing (see Fig. 6-9).

Limb movements should be described as purposeful, nonpurposeful, or consistent with seizure activity. Purposeful movements can be documented if the child specifically withdraws an extremity from painful stimulation. To elicit this withdrawal, it is

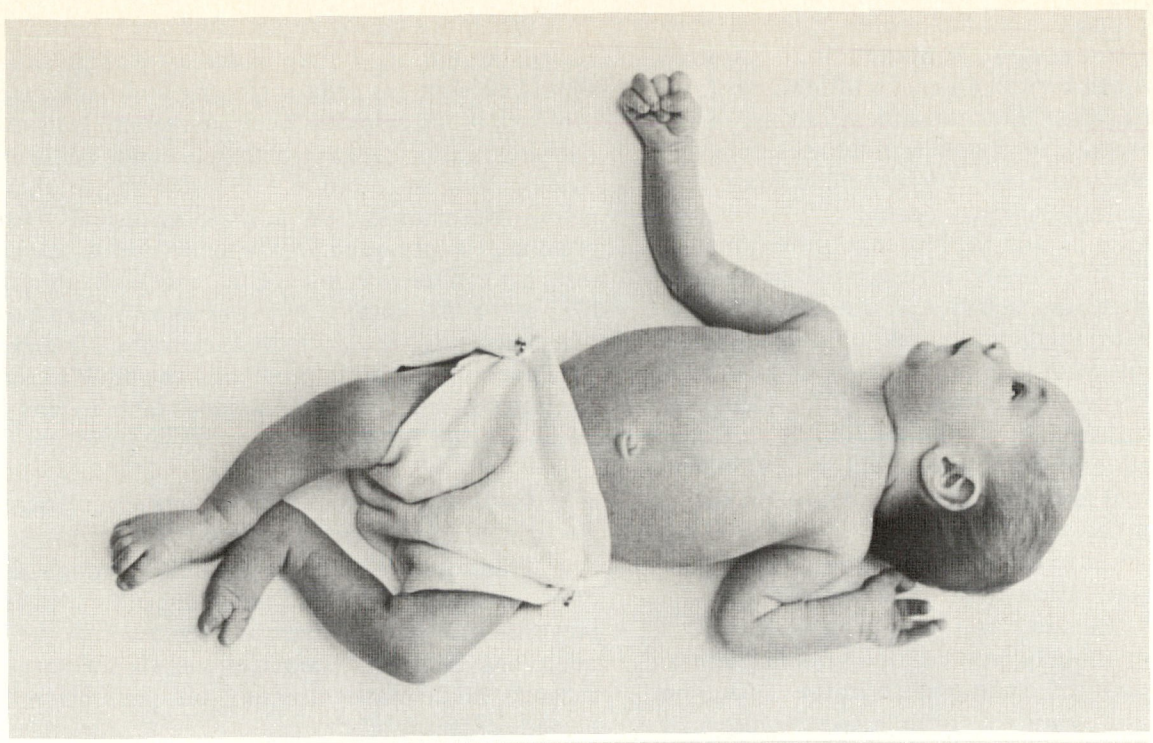

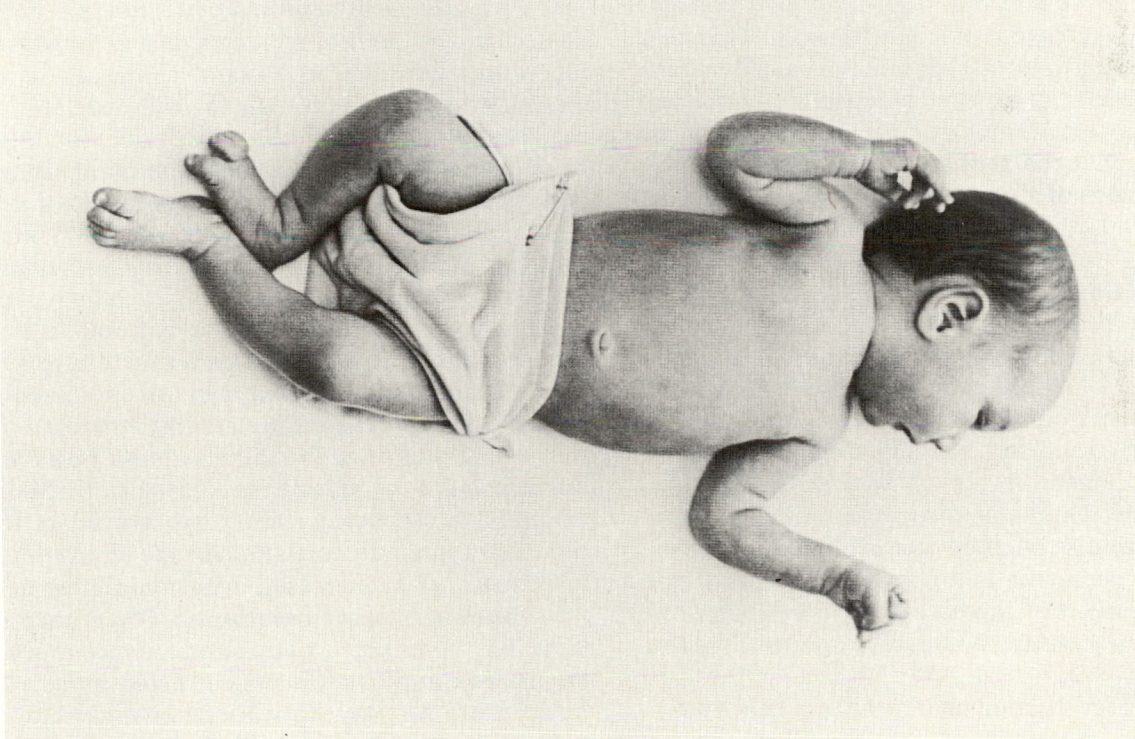

Fig. 6-12. Tonic neck reflex. Turning of the head to one side while the infant is supine produces ipsilateral extension and contralateral flexion of the extremities.

Mead Johnson & Company, Evansville, Indiana 47721.

important to pinch the *medial* aspect of the extremity; purposeful movement is present if the limb is abducted or withdrawn from the midline (and from the painful stimulus). Flexion and adduction of extremities in response to painful stimuli are not necessarily purposeful and may represent decorticate posturing.[23]

Rhythmic or bizarre movements of the limbs or eyes should be thoroughly investigated since they may represent seizure activity. If the child has received paralyzing medication, seizures may be impossible to confirm or rule out without an EEG. It is important to recognize seizures and to document their frequency, duration, and severity since status epilepticus can compromise cerebral perfusion and result in cerebral ischemia (see the section on status epilepticus later in this chapter).

The child's respiratory rate and pattern and the adequacy of ventilation must be carefully assessed. Major abnormalities in respiratory pattern have been summarized previously (see the material on alterations in respiratory rate and pattern in the section on clinical signs and symptoms of increased intracranial pressure). The most common respiratory patterns observed in the comatose patient include Cheyne-Stokes respirations (alternating bradypnea and hyperpnea), central neurogenic hyperventilation (constant rapid respiratory rate in the absence of hypercapnia or hypoxemia), apneustic breathing (prolonged inspiration and expiration), cluster breathing (very irregular breathing associated with apnea), and ataxic breathing (extremely irregular breathing). (See Table 6-12 for correlation of abnormal breathing patterns with levels of cerebral injury.)

Regardless of the respiratory pattern observed, the nurse must ensure that the child's ventilation is adequate. Arterial blood gases should be monitored, and the child's color and systemic perfusion should be assessed. Clinical signs of hypoxemia include tachycardia and peripheral vasoconstriction, and late signs of hypoxemia include cyanosis and hypotension. Since hypercapnia and hypoxia can contribute to the development of increased cerebral blood flow and intracranial pressure, respiratory distress must be avoided.

Thorough evaluation of the child's respiratory status includes assessment of cough and gag reflexes. The presence of these reflexes implies that the glossopharyngeal (ninth cranial) and vagus (tenth cranial) nerves are intact. The patient requires these reflexes to maintain a patent airway and to prevent aspiration of secretions. The child who does not possess adequate cough and gag reflexes will probably require insertion of an ET or tracheostomy tube and frequent pharyngeal suctioning.

When any child is admitted with coma of unknown origin, the first urine specimen obtained should be sent for drug screening and toxicology. In addition, blood samples are drawn for analysis of arterial blood gases, serum electrolyte concentrations (including glucose), and blood cultures. A thorough neurologic examination is performed, and a lumbar puncture is obtained. Additional useful diagnostic tests for evaluation of the comatose child include an EEG and a CT scan. These studies may help confirm the presence of local or diffuse cerebral injury, and they may be helpful in predicting the child's recovery (see the section on diagnostic tests later in this chapter for further information).

■ **Medical treatment and nursing interventions**

The comatose child requires thorough assessment of neurologic and cardiorespiratory function, prevention or early detection of any deterioration in neurologic function, support of vital functions, maintenance of adequate nutrition, and prevention of the hazards of immobility.

Assessment of neurologic function has been discussed in the preceding section. It is important to report any deterioration in clinical status to a physician. If the child is at risk for the development of increased intracranial pressure, the nurse should continuously monitor evidence of the child's systemic perfusion, including urine output, warmth of extremities, strength of peripheral pulses, and briskness of capillary refill, as well as the child's level of consciousness, pupil response to light, blood pressure, heart rate, respiratory rate and pattern, and motor function or posturing. If the patient develops signs of poor systemic perfusion or signs of increased intracranial pressure (including lethargy, increase in systolic blood pressure, widening of pulse pressure, and bradycardia), a physician should be notified immediately, and the nurse should hyperventilate the patient using a hand ventilator (see the section on medical treatment of increased intracranial pressure).

Support of vital functions. The comatose patient may be unable to cough effectively to keep the oropharynx and trachea unobstructed by secretions. In addition, he may have ineffective gag and uncoordinated swallow reflexes, which increases the risk of aspiration of vomitus or mucus. As a result it is the nurse's responsibility to keep the patient's airway patent and free of secretions. The pharynx should be suctioned as needed, and the patient should be positioned so that secretions pool in the side of the patient's mouth, instead of in the pharynx. The tongue of the unconscous patient can obstruct the pharynx when the patient is supine; therefore the head of the patient's bed should be elevated, and the patient's head should be turned to the side (unless increased intracranial pressure is present). If secretion control or maintenance of a patent airway becomes difficult, intubation may be required.

If the child is breathing spontaneously, the nurse must constantly assess the adequacy of the child's ventilation. Air movement should be adequate and equal bilaterally, and signs of increased respiratory effort (retractions, nasal flaring, or grunting) should be absent. The head of the child's bed should be elevated and a small linen roll should be placed under the child's shoulders to extend the airway and promote maximal inspiratory effort. If the comatose child is apneic, use of an apnea alarm or constant attendance by a nurse is necessary. Mechanical ventilatory assistance should probably be initiated if apnea continues. This assistance is also provided if hypercapnia, hypoxia, or inadequate inspiratory effort develops.

Even after institution of mechanical ventilatory support, the child will require excellent pulmonary toilet with use of strict aseptic technique. The child should receive supplemental ventilation before and immediately after suctioning to prevent carbon dioxide retention and hypoxia during the suctioning; this is especially important if the child is at risk for the development of increased intracranial pressure.

If the child has severe pulmonary dysfunction and hypoxia, attempts should be made to determine the position of the child associated with the best arterial oxygen saturation and most efficient carbon dioxide removal. Dependent portions of the lung will receive the greatest blood flow, while the best aerated portions of the lung are often the nondependent lung segments. As a result the nurse should document the child's position when blood gases are drawn in an attempt to determine what effect, if any, the child's position has on oxygenation and carbon dioxide elimination.

Since the comatose patient will usually not become agitated or restless when hypoxic and since he is unable to articulate complaints, the nurse must quickly recognize signs of poor systemic perfusion or inadequate respiratory function. She must ensure that adequate cardiorespiratory function is maintained during the patient's recovery.

When the child is comatose or when he receives a paralyzing agent, venous pooling of blood occurs.[5] This can cause a relative hypovolemia. The child may require administration of additional IV fluids to maintain an adequate central venous pressure and systemic perfusion.

If the comatose child is always kept in the recumbent position, orthostatic hypotension can result

when the child initially resumes the upright position.[61] In addition, the recovering child may be extremely frightened when immobilized in the supine position, with caretakers looming overhead. Therefore, if possible, the child should be placed in the semi-Fowler's position several times each day. This position allows the child a different view of the unit as he begins to waken, helps prevent the development of orthostatic hypotension, and allows maximal diaphragmatic excursion and chest expansion. This positioning can be provided for the small infant through elevation of the head of the crib mattress or use of an upright "infant seat."

The child's hourly fluid intake and daily weight should be assessed carefully. Urine output should average 1.0 ml/kg/hour if fluid intake is adequate. If the child's fluid intake or output is inadequate, this should be discussed with a physician.

Maintenance of adequate nutrition. As soon as the comatose child is admitted to the intensive care unit, consideration should be given to the provision of needed calories and fluid. Usually fluid requirements can easily be provided in the form of IV solutions. If inadequate caloric intake is provided, the child will develop a negative nitrogen balance and protein deficiency, wound healing will be delayed, the infant will not be able to make brown fat needed to generate heat, and general recovery will be delayed. Therefore some form of enteral or parenteral alimentation must be planned.

If nasogastric feedings are attempted, they should begin with small amounts of elemental formula, and the amount and concentration should be advanced slowly as tolerated. Continuous nasogastric feeding may be attempted initially, then the child can be advanced to *small* bolus feedings. During this time, the nurse should measure and record the residual formula remaining in the stomach after feeding, and should assess the abdominal girth and firmness throughout the feeding. It may not be possible for the comatose child to tolerate enteral feedings because immobilization may produce a paralytic ileus. If gastric distention, diarrhea, vomiting, or gastric reflux develops, enteral feedings should be discontinued, and parenteral alimentation should be instituted (see the section on parenteral alimentation in Chapter 8).

Care should be taken to monitor the child's acid-base and electrolyte status without constant drawing of blood for sampling. The child's daily electrolyte requirements should be provided, and electrolyte concentrations should be checked at regular intervals or with changes in the patient's condition.

Stool softeners should be provided as needed to prevent constipation or bowel impaction. Stool output should be charted consistently so that the health team does not suddenly realize that the child has not had a bowel movement for several days. Use of glycerine suppositories or enemas may be required occasionally to promote evacuation of stools.

Prevention of the hazards of immobility. When the neurologic status of the comatose child is stable, a referral should be made to an occupational or physical therapist. Passive range-of-motion exercises should be initiated on a regular basis, and splints or ankle pads constructed as needed to prevent ankle and wrist contractures, footdrop, and pressure sores.

The comatose child requires excellent skin care. Eggshell or water mattresses or new microsphere air flow suspension mattresses (Clinitron*) aid in the prevention of pressure sores over bony prominences. The child's skin should be completely inspected at least once every shift. Any reddened areas should be gently massaged to promote circulation and reduce ischemia. The skin should be kept as dry as possible, and the sheets should be free of wrinkles. The development of skin breakdown signals inadequate attention to skin care.

Since the comatose patient often requires insertion of multiple monitoring lines and drainage or other tubes, he is at risk for the development of infection. Although good handwashing technique is one of the best ways to avoid transmission of infection, hospital personnel often do not wash their hands before and after each patient contact.[3] It is important that strict handwashing technique be employed when handling the patient or patient lines and tubes, and that aseptic technique be used when suctioning the ET tube or changing a central venous pressure dressing. All skin puncture sites should be inspected at least once each shift, and wound drainage, wound fluctuance, erythema, or odor should be reported to a physician. Other signs of infection include an elevation in white blood cell count and fever. In small children, a decrease in platelet count may indicate the presence of sepsis and the development of disseminated intravascular coagulation (see Chapter 8). If infection is suspected, appropriate wound, serum, or catheter cultures should be obtained, and antibiotics should be administered as indicated.

The comatose child usually has bowel and bladder incontinence. However, a urinary catheter should not be inserted merely to simplify urine collection. Diapers, condom catheters, or padded rubberized sheets may be used to allow urine measurement and minimize linen changing. If use of a urinary catheter

*Clinitron: Support Systems International, Charleston Heights, SC 29405.

is required to enable ongoing evaluation of renal function and urine output, the child should receive meticulous catheter and meatus care. If the nurse notices cloudy or foul-smelling urine, a physician should be notified, and urinalysis and urine culture (and Gram's stain, if indicated) should be ordered.

If the child does not have an intact blink reflex, a prescribed ophthalmic ointment should be applied to lubricate the cornea and prevent corneal abrasions. It may be necessary to patch the eyes to protect the corneas. If this is done, both the child and the family should be told about the purpose of the patches before they are placed.

The child's mouth should be lubricated and cleaned several times each shift to prevent the development of gingivitis or dental caries. The child's mouth and lips should be kept clean, even if they are covered with the tape holding the ET or nasogastric tube in place.

Psychosocial support. The comatose child may hear any or all of the conversations held near the bedside. Therefore all hospital staff should be careful to avoid terminology that could be misinterpreted by the child, and discussions of a pessimistic prognosis should be avoided near the patient's bed. At all times the nurse should assume that the comatose child is able to hear and that he may be frightened. The nurse should begin and end her shift by speaking gently to the child and orienting him to time and place. Throughout the day the nurse should talk to the child about the time of day and should prepare the child any time treatments or procedures are performed and any time the child will be moved. As the child is recovering, he may be alert, yet unresponsive to his surroundings, and unable to ask questions; therefore the nurse should plan to review the child's progress (as appropriate) daily and provide the child with encouragement. The child should be told of recent pleasant news about family members.

The family will require consistent information and support from the health care team, and a realistic prognosis should be provided. If the child's recovery is doubtful, it will be necessary to prepare the family for the news, yet convey continued concern about the child's care. The family should never be made to believe that the medical team has "given up" on their child unless or until the child meets the legal definition of brain death. If withdrawal of support is considered, the family should be allowed to discuss the decision, but they should not be made to feel that they are responsible for discontinuation of medical care (see the section on cerebral death later in this chapter).

Recent studies have documented the presence of

predictors of cerebral recovery following prolonged coma during childhood. The clinical findings most consistently associated with neurologic sequelae and poor prognosis following coma include: absence of spontaneous respirations, flaccidity, fixed pupils, presence of decorticate or decerebrate posturing, the presence of deep coma (stage 3 or 4) for longer than 2 weeks, and the presence of prolonged elevations in intracranial pressure.[12,57,63] Children, as a rule, demonstrate faster and more complete recovery from coma than do adults. However, it is important to note that the child's brain is growing rapidly (particularly through the age of seven), making it extremely difficult to predict the degree of permanent neurologic damage that will result from a neurologic injury. Neurologic sequelae are often not manifest for months or years after the insult has occurred.[51]

Care of the comatose child can be extremely depressing and frustrating. Yet, if there is to be hope of recovery, the child will require excellent nursing care throughout the period of coma and during recovery.

■ **HEAD TRAUMA**
■ **Etiology**

Approximately 200,000 children are hospitalized yearly as the result of head trauma, and approximately 4000 children die yearly, many within the first few hours following injury. Because most head injuries in children are sustained during automobile accidents, most are traumatic impact injuries. Other causes of head trauma during childhood include those produced by child abuse and those resulting from falls or sports injuries.[13,37,65,72]

■ **Pathophysiology**

The rigid cranium and the CSF cushion can protect the child's brain from injury during minor trauma. However, if distortion of the skull, shear injury, actual tissue damage, intracranial hemorrhage, or cerebral edema develop, the child is at risk for the development of increased intracranial pressure. Thus the child with head trauma often requires assessment and treatment of the primary (or direct) injury, as well as careful assessment and treatment of other secondary injuries.

The types of cerebral injuries occurring with head trauma include concussions, contusions, skull fractures, vascular injuries, and cerebral edema. The pathophysiology of each lesion will be discussed separately below.

Concussion. A *concussion* is a moderate cerebral injury. It results from a blow to the head or a shearing rotational injury of the brain within the skull that produces no structural brain damage. The concussion is more likely to occur if the head moves freely after impact, so an *acceleration/deceleration* injury is produced that places shearing stresses on the brainstem and results in injury to the reticular activating system. This produces loss of consciousness for a few seconds or several hours. Following the impact, the CSF pressure rises transiently and electroencephalographic evidence of slow brain wave activity can be noted.[42] The diagnosis of concussion is only made if the patient regains consciousness and demonstrates no other deterioration in clinical status.[6,42,65,72]

Contusion. A *cerebral contusion* is a localized brain injury that consists of bruising, hemorrhage, and edema of brain tissue.[6] The hemorrhage may be epidural, subdural, or subarachnoid (see the section on vascular injuries that follows), and it may produce an increase in intracranial pressure or loss of consciousness. The injury can occur directly beneath the site of impact (the coup injury) or on the side of the brain opposite the impact (the contrecoup injury). The *contrecoup* injury is thought to occur as the brain strikes the skull on the side of the head opposite the initial impact. The severity of the cerebral contusion depends upon the amount of direct tissue injury, bleeding, and edema that results. Approximately 10% of children with cerebral contusions will develop *posttraumatic seizures.*[71]

Skull fractures. A skull fracture is a break in the continuity of the cranial bones that may or may not be associated with displacement of the bone fragments.[6] Skull fractures are present in approximately one fourth of all patients hospitalized with head injury. Even if the fracture itself is benign, it may be associated with damage to the underlying brain tissue, meninges, or blood vessels.

A *simple* or *linear skull fracture* constitutes approximately three fourths of all skull fractures in children.[71] In this form of skull fracture, the bone fragments remain approximated and the dura mater is not pierced.

A *depressed skull fracture* is present when one or more bone fragments are indented below the normal contour or table of the cranium. As a result the skull is "indented," and the brain tissue below the fracture is injured. A hematoma may cover the area of injury, and a cerebral contusion may be present below the fracture. The dura is usually not pierced when a depressed skull fracture is present.

A *compound skull fracture* exists when a scalp laceration and depressed skull fracture are present, allowing direct communication from the scalp through the skull and into the cranium. The dura is often pierced when a compound fracture is present, and the skull fragment can actually be displaced into brain tissue.

Basilar skull fractures are those that involve a break in the posteroinferior portion of the skull. This type of fracture usually does not produce cerebral tissue damage, but it does frequently produce dural tears. As a result basilar skull fractures are most commonly associated with leakage of cerebrospinal fluid. When a dural tear and CSF leak are present, contamination of the cerebrospinal fluid by ascending upper respiratory tract infection is also possible and can result in the development of meningitis. Basilar skull fractures can occur over the paranasal sinuses of the frontal bone, over the temporal bone, or over the entrance of the internal carotid artery into the skull. A fracture over the internal carotid artery can result in hemorrhage or in the development of an aneurysm or fistula.[42]

Vascular injuries. Vascular injuries that occur as the result of head trauma can produce epidural hematoma, subdural hematoma, or a subarachnoid hemorrhage. Each of these vascular injuries are discussed separately in this section.

An *epidural hematoma* refers to accumulation of blood between the skull and the dura. It usually results from a low-velocity direct blow to the skull and is most often associated with a skull fracture. The bleeding produced is most often the result of a tear of the middle meningeal artery caused by a temporal lobe skull fracture. Since the hematoma often develops from arterial bleeding, the accumulation of blood between the skull and the dura can be rapid. Children with epidural hematomas characteristically demonstrate a lucid period that lasts several hours after the head injury; then suddenly they demonstrate decreased responsiveness and unilateral pupil dilation (usually ipsilateral to the hematoma) as the result of supratentorial herniation. If the hematoma continues to expand, the child will lose consciousness and develop a sharp and severe increase in intracranial pressure. Mortality may be as high as 10% among children with epidural hematoma because the possibility of a progressive injury is not appreciated or because the severity of the child's symptoms are not immediately recognized.[71]

A *subdural hematoma* is defined as the accumulation of blood between the dura and the arachnoid membranes. A subdural hematoma is often classified as acute, subacute, or chronic. An *acute subdural hematoma* usually develops following a severe head injury or cerebral laceration, and results in accumulation of blood within hours of the injury. A *subacute subdural hematoma* occurs early after a less severe

cerebral contusion, and usually produces a rise in intracranial pressure that prevents the patient from regaining consciousness following the head injury.[6,42,76] A *chronic subdural hematoma* develops weeks or months after a relatively minor head injury. These injuries usually produce a venous tear, and blood accumulates in the subdural space very slowly. Subdural hematomas are often present bilaterally, and they are frequently present in victims of child abuse under the age of 2 years. Subdural hematomas produce CNS symptoms as the result of blood accumulation and an increase in intracranial pressure. Symptoms can also appear as the result of lacerations and contusions of underlying brain tissue and resultant vasogenic cerebral edema.[12] Many patients who sustain subdural hematomas demonstrate seizure activity acutely or as a late result of the injury. In addition, the patients often develop cerebral edema and increased intracranial pressure. Subdural hematomas are responsible for almost 10% of all CNS bleeding.[71]

A *subarachnoid hemorrhage* occurs as the result of severe head injury. The hemorrhage occurs when subarachnoid vessels are torn as a result of shear forces produced during a massive head injury. The child with a subarachnoid hemorrhage can rapidly demonstrate seizures or develop increased intracranial pressure. Since subarachnoid hemorrhages are frequently seen in abused children, the observer should assess the child carefully for evidence of other injuries, including healed fractures or retinal hemorrhages.

Cerebral edema. An increase in brain volume occurs most commonly as the result of hyperemia or as the result of an increase in cerebral blood flow that occurs during the first 24 hours following injury.[12,65] The child may develop a form of cytotoxic or vasogenic cerebral edema following direct cerebral or vascular injury or as the result of hypoxia or other complications of trauma or hemorrhage. The pathophysiology of cerebral edema is reviewed in detail in the section on increased intracranial pressure earlier in this chapter.

■ **Clinical signs and symptoms**

Clinical signs and symptoms of the major forms of head injury are discussed separately in this section. A review of the initial assessment of the child with head trauma is included at the beginning of the following section on medical and surgical treatment and nursing interventions.

Concussion. The patient who sustains a concussion loses consciousness for a variable period of time. This loss of consciousness is usually associated with a brief slowing of respirations (possibly accompanied by apnea), bradycardia, and hypotension. The patient may demonstrate depressed reflexes (such as the corneal and gag reflexes) and reduced response to painful stimuli.[42] All reflexes should be present, however.

When the patient wakes up, he slowly becomes oriented to his surroundings (over a period of hours or days), and he is gradually able to respond to questions and commands. Patients often suffer temporary memory loss, called *traumatic amnesia.* Following a concussion, there is no evidence of further neurologic injury. Patients occasionally complain of headache, malaise, vertigo, anxiety, or fatigue for several days or weeks following a concussion; these symptoms are known as *postconcussion syndrome.*[6,42,65]

The *pediatric concussion syndrome* has recently been described. This clinical pattern follows an apparently minor head injury. The child loses consciousness and awakens with no apparent neurologic damage. However, during a period of several minutes or hours, the child's level of consciousness again deteriorates and vomiting may develop. Ultimately the child loses consciousness and demonstrates unilateral or bilateral pupil dilation, decerebrate posturing, and a positive Babinski's reflex. The syndrome may progress to coma or death, or the child may spontaneously recover after several days.[65] Obviously, this syndrome is caused by more extensive neurologic injury than a mere concussion. However, since the initial presentation and recovery are identical to those seen with a concussion, it is important that the child with a concussion be observed closely for later signs of neurologic deterioration.

Contusion. The clinical signs and symptoms that occur as the result of a cerebral contusion are dependent upon the extent of the cranial injury, the volume of bleeding present, and the amount of cerebral edema that occurs. The associated hemorrhage may be epidural, subdural, or subarachnoid (see the section on vascular injuries that follows). The resultant cerebral edema may produce increased intracranial pressure.

The patient who suffers a cerebral contusion may or may not lose consciousness. Mild motor and sensory weakness or coma may result. Since at least 10% of children with cerebral contusion do develop posttraumatic seizures, most are hospitalized following the injury for observation.[71]

Skull fractures. The clinical signs and symptoms associated with any skull fracture will depend on the location of the fracture and on the extent of the underlying cranial injury. Most skull fractures are diagnosed by radiographic examination, rather than by clinical examination, since the vast majority of skull fractures are linear (the bone fragments remain approximated). Depressed or compound skull fractures should be suspected whenever the contour of the patient's head is altered or whenever an obvious indentation in the skull is observed or palpated. If a depressed skull fracture is located over the saggital or lateral sinus, profuse bleeding may develop from injury to these venous channels, and hypovolemic shock may result.

If a basilar skull fracture is present, the patient may develop a CSF leak from the floor of the brain into the nose or ears. Although the CSF leak itself is not harmful, it indicates that communication is present between the upper respiratory tract and the subarachnoid space. Thus the patient is at risk for the development of ascending infection of the central nervous system (meningitis). Detection of such a CSF leak is extremely difficult; various bedside techniques have been described, but none is reliable and all can provide false-positive results. For example, if a yellow halo forms around seroussanguineous drainage that has been collected from the nose or ear and placed on filter paper, this drainage is thought to be produced by cerebrospinal fluid; however, plasma frequently can produce a similar halo. Nasal or ear drainage can be tested for glucose with chemical reagent strips (Labstix*); theoretically, the presence of glucose in the drainage indicates that cerebrospinal fluid is present; however, nasal drainage can also contain glucose. If confirmation of the CSF drainage is desired, radioactive albumin may be injected into the subarachnoid space during a lumbar puncture; if this albumin appears in the nose or ear, the presence of a CSF leak will be confirmed. In general, the possibility of a CSF leak is present in any child with a basilar skull fracture, so the child is usually admitted to the hospital for observation. Signs of deterioration of clinical status or signs of CNS infection (including fever, irritability, nuchal rigidity, and leukocytosis) should be reported to a physician immediately. Other signs associated with basilar skull fracture include the presence of ecchymotic lesions over the mastoid (Battle's sign) or around the eyes (racoon sign) and palsies of the first, seventh, and eighth cranial nerves.[6,42,71,81]

Vascular injuries. The patient with the classic presentation of an *epidural hematoma* sustains a head injury, briefly loses consciousness, awakens and appears alert, then suddenly develops a headache, a decreasing level of consciousness, and signs of increased intracranial pressure.[71] Actually, approxi-

*Labstix: Ames Company, Elkhart, Ind. 46514

mately one third of children sustaining an epidural hematoma lose consciousness and do not awaken spontaneously, and another one third of affected children never lose consciousness.[12] Thus the actual clinical presentation of the child with an epidural hematoma can be misleading. An epidural hematoma should be suspected in any child who develops headache, decreased level of consciousness, and dilation of one pupil. The pupil usually dilates on the side of the injury—however, since an epidural hematoma can result from a contrecoup injury, the pupil contralateral to the side of injury may dilate. As the child's symptoms progress, he will demonstrate decerebrate posturing, and approximately half of the involved children may develop hemiparesis (usually on the side contralateral to that of pupil dilation). If immediate surgical decompression of the hematoma is not provided, the child will develop bilateral pupil dilation, respiratory depression, bradycardia, apnea, and death from increased intracranial pressure.[12] The child may also develop a fever.[42] The best diagnostic test to confirm the presence of an epidural hematoma is a CAT or CT scan. Since the hematoma is often located directly under the skull fracture, plain skull radiographs may be adequate to localize the hematoma in a severely ill child. In some hospitals, angiography is also performed.[12] (See the section in this chapter on diagnostic tests for further information.)

The patient with an *acute subdural hematoma* may have a severe diffuse neurologic injury, and bilateral hematomas. Approximately two thirds of all children with subdural hematomas lose consciousness immediately following the cranial trauma. Frequently, the child demonstrates focal signs of injury, such as unilateral pupil dilation, focal seizures, or hemiparesis. Since most of these patients sustain additional cerebral injuries, including cerebral lacerations, contusions, and intracerebral hematomas, intracranial hypertension can develop rapidly and progress to serious levels. Diagnosis of a subdural hematoma can be confirmed with a CT scan or angiography. These studies are extremely important since they can help determine the indication for surgery.[12]

The patient with a *chronic subdural hematoma* may develop a headache and progressive decrease in level of consciousness weeks or months after a relatively minor head injury. Since the hematoma is present for a long period of time, papilledema can be observed. The ipsilateral pupil will be large with sluggish response to light. Hemiparesis can ultimately develop.[42]

The patient with a *subarachnoid hemorrhage* may develop increased intracranial pressure rapidly. The child with this form of hemorrhage may demon-

strate nuchal rigidity, headache, and gradual deterioration in level of consciousness. If temporal lobe herniation occurs, ipsilateral pupil dilation and hemiparesis will be noted.[42]

Cerebral edema. Signs of development of cerebral edema are those associated with increased intracranial pressure. Since these have been summarized several times in this chapter, the reader is referred to the section on clinical signs and symptoms of increased intracranial pressure earlier in the chapter.

■ Medical and surgical treatment and nursing interventions

When the child with head trauma is admitted to the critical-care unit, ventilatory function, systemic perfusion, neurologic impairment, and the presence of other injuries must be assessed rapidly and thoroughly. During the initial assessment, intervention is provided to maintain vital functions until the extent of the child's injuries is ascertained. Once the child is somewhat stable, he may be prepared for neurosurgery or monitored and treated for increased intracranial pressure, coma, status epilepticus, or other complications of the neurologic injury. During this time, the child will require careful fluid therapy, provision of adequate nutrition, and prevention of infection. In addition, the nurse must provide calm reassurance for the child and support for the family.

Initial assessment and treatment of the child with head trauma. When the child with head trauma is admitted to the critical-care unit, first priority must be given to establishing and maintaining adequate ventilation and systemic perfusion. Since increased intracranial pressure can cause apnea and since hypoventilation and hypercapnia can contribute to increased intracranial pressure, there is adequate reason why insufficient ventilation may develop and why effective ventilation must be maintained.

The child's neck should be extended to reduce upper airway obstruction only if a cervical vertebral fracture has been ruled out. If the child is severely injured, an ET tube will be placed to ensure the presence of a patent airway, and, if necessary, ventilatory support will be provided. A nasogastric tube should also be placed to decompress the stomach and prevent vomiting during the initial assessment. The head of the child's bed should be elevated to maximize diaphragmatic excursion (if the child is breathing spontaneously) and enhance cerebral venous return.

Careful assessment should be made of the child's systemic perfusion. Extremities should be warm with pink nailbeds and brisk capillary refill.

Peripheral pulses should be strong, and the child's blood pressure should be appropriate for his age (see Table 6-8). Hypotension is rarely caused by head injury; if it is present, hypovolemic shock should be suspected.[13] Tachycardia may indicate the presence of hemorrhage or the development of increased intracranial pressure; it may also indicate that the child is frightened or in pain. If hypovolemic low cardiac output is present, it should be treated immediately (see the section on low cardiac output in Chapter 3). As soon as possible, a large bore central venous line should be inserted to allow measurement of the central venous pressure and administration of blood products, colloids, medications, or IV fluids.

Since head trauma is frequently associated with injury of other major organs, care should be taken to assess for signs of abdominal trauma (see the section on gastrointestinal bleeding in Chapter 8), hemothorax, flail chest, and pneumothorax (see the discussion of these problems in Chapter 4). Since a serum hematocrit will be among the first blood studies ordered and reported, the suspicion of hemorrhage can be quickly reinforced if significant anemia or a rapidly falling hematocrit is documented. Cerebrovascular injury alone can usually not account for a significant blood loss, unless a massive intracranial hemorrhage (and increased intracranial pressure) develops. The child's circulating blood volume should be calculated; the blood volume totals approximately 80 ml/kg in infants and 75 ml/kg in children (see Table 3-9 for precise formula). All blood lost or drawn from the infant or young child for laboratory analysis should be recorded, and this blood should be replaced when it totals 5% to 7% of the child's total circulating blood volume.

Once adequate cardiopulmonary function has been established, the nurse should perform a careful neurologic assessment. This includes an evaluation of the child's level of consciousness and pupil size and response to light, measurement of heart rate, arterial blood pressure, and respiratory rate, evaluation of the respiratory pattern (if any), and careful assessment of motor activity and reflexes.

The normal child will be awake, alert, and frightened in the hospital. The comatose child is unresponsive to external stimulation. Clarification of degrees of responsiveness is possible if a standard rating scale, such as the Glasgow Coma Scale, is used by everyone in the critical-care unit. (See Tables 6-7 and the box [p. 395] on the Huttenlocher staging of coma for criteria and staging of coma.)

The child's pupil size and responsiveness to light should be evaluated frequently. The pupils are normally of equal size, and they should react briskly to light. Morphine sulfate will cause pupil constriction, and atropine and large doses of dopamine will produce pupil dilation. The presence of fixed and dilated pupils during initial evaluation of the child with a head injury is often regarded as a poor prognostic sign; however, children that have fixed pupils after a head injury have a far better rate of recovery than do adults.[12]

Although the classic "Cushing's reflex" (bradycardia, elevation in systolic blood pressure with widening of pulse pressure, and apnea) is thought to herald the development of increased intracranial pressure, children rarely demonstrate such "classic" findings. Often, the child is tachycardic and hypertensive. The widening of the pulse pressure and the respiratory depression are usually only late signs of deterioration in neurologic status.

The presence of any seizures should be reported immediately to a physician, and the child should be protected from injury during any seizure activity. Status epilepticus should be treated since it compromises cerebral blood flow. Any abnormal posturing (such as decerebrate rigidity or decorticate posturing—see Fig. 6-9) should also be reported to a physician.

As soon as the patient is stable, the nurse should attempt to evaluate the child's cranial nerve functions. In addition, some assessment of the child's oculocephalic ("doll's eyes") and oculovestibular reflexes should be made. If brainstem injury is present, the patient's *oculocephalic reflex* is often abnormal, and the eyes will behave as though fixed in their sockets, despite turning of the head. As mentioned earlier, the *oculovestibular reflex* ("calorics") is tested by infusion of iced water into the external ear of the comatose patient by a physician. If brainstem injury is present, the eyes will not deviate toward the side of the infusion.

Another major reflex to be tested is the *corneal reflex.* If the eyelashes or the outer edge of the child's eye is stroked with a sterile cotton applicator, the child should blink. If this blink is absent, brainstem injury is probably present, and the child will require regular application of ophthalmic ointment and eye patching to prevent corneal drying and lacerations.

When the child is stable, CAT (or CT) scans and skull films may be performed to aid in evaluation of the extent of the head injury (see the section on diagnostic tests in this chapter). A nurse should always accompany the child to the CT scan to monitor the child's level of consciousness and cardiorespiratory function, and she should always bring a hand ventilator and mask or ET tube adapter and other appropriate supportive equipment.

The association of neurologic assessment findings most consistently linked to a poor prognosis in children who have sustained head trauma includes the following: absence of spontaneous ventilation, decerebrate rigidity or flaccid paralysis, bilateral fixed and dilated pupils, and absence of oculocephalic and oculovestibular reflexes.[12,13,65]

A urinary catheter should be inserted if multisystem trauma or shock is present. The nurse should report any difficulty inserting the catheter or the presence of bloody urine to a physician immediately since these may indicate the presence of genitourinary trauma. The child's urine output should average 1.0 ml/kg/hour if fluid intake is adequate. Inadequate urine output can be the result of prerenal failure (such as occurs with inadequate systemic perfusion), renal failure (as the result of tubular injury), or postrenal failure (such as occurs with urethral obstruction). Oliguria should be promptly investigated and treated (see the section on renal failure in Chapter 7). Administration of diuretics or hyperosmotic agents may be necessary if increased intracranial pressure develops.

In addition to assessment of major organ function, the nurse should assess the child carefully for the presence of fractures or major lacerations that may require sutures. The child's skin should be thoroughly inspected for any signs of edema, contusions, petechiae, or hematomas, and the scalp should be palpated for evidence of depressed or compound skull fractures.

Throughout the assessment and treatment of the infant and young child it is imperative that the patient be kept warm since cold stress can increase oxygen consumption and produce peripheral vasoconstriction and poor skin color. The child's skin and rectal temperature should be closely monitored; a high rectal temperature and low skin temperature can indicate the presence of poor systemic perfusion, and fever may indicate the presence of an epidural hematoma or infection.[44]

During the initial assessment and treatment of the child with head trauma, it may be impractical to allow the parents to remain at the bedside, and it may be difficult to arrange the time to speak with them. Most parents understand the need for the nurse to give undivided attention to the physical care of the child, but the parents will also appreciate any brief report the nurse can provide about the child's condition or the progress of treatment. The parents are often reassured to hear the types of treatment the child is receiving since this indicates that the situation is not hopeless. If the nurse is unable to spend time with the family, a social worker, chaplain, or patient ombudsman should be called.

Later management. Once the child is stable, treatment of the child's specific injury can be undertaken. The following discussion reviews those most common forms of pediatric head injury (those discussed earlier in this section) and reviews the most common medical and surgical treatment required. (See also Appendix A.)

Concussion. Concussions usually require no treatment. However, since the history of loss of consciousness followed by recovery and responsiveness can also be consistent with that of development of an epidural hematoma, the child is usually admitted to the hospital for observation. As noted earlier, children occasionally complain of headache, dizziness, malaise and fatigue for days or weeks following a concussion. It is important that the parents be aware of this *postconcussion syndrome* so that the child will not be suspected of malingering. However, the child should not be specifically made aware of the likelihood of such symptoms since this may suggest that the symptoms will be an expected part of the child's behavior.

Since some physicians have noted the progressive development of severe neurologic deterioration soon after a relatively minor head injury and apparent concussion (pediatric concussion syndrome), the nurse should assess the child's level of consciousness frequently. Signs of increased intracranial pressure should be reported to a physician immediately (see the section on clinical signs and symptoms of increased intracranial pressure earlier in this chapter), and treatment of increased intracranial pressure must be prompt.

Contusion. The appropriate treatment of a cerebral contusion is determined by the extent of the primary cerebral injury and the severity of secondary injuries, such as hemorrhage or cerebral edema. Treatment of skull fractures, epidural and subdural hematomas, and subarachnoid hemorrhage is discussed later. (Treatment of cerebral edema is elaborated in the section on treatment of increased intracranial pressure.) Approximately 10% of children with cerebral contusion will develop posttraumatic seizures beginning hours, months, or years after the head injury.[71]

Skull fractures. The vast majority of children with simple or linear skull fractures require no treatment. The child should, however, be observed carefully for signs of development of an epidural or subdural hematoma.[6]

Depressed skull fractures are surgically elevated if the skull fragment is 5 mm or more below the contour of the skull or if serious underlying cerebral injury or hemorrhage is present. Before any surgery is performed, the child's cardiorespiratory status should be thoroughly assessed and the appropriate support should be provided. If the depressed skull fracture is located near the saggital or lateral sinus, this venous channel might tear, causing profuse external or intracranial bleeding. In this case, the child will require immediate treatment of hypovolemic shock (see the section on low cardiac output in Chapter 3), and immediate surgical control of the bleeding site. The surgeon will also elevate the depressed bone fragment and debride the wound.

When a *compound* skull fracture is present, surgical elevation and repair is also necessary. Since portions of the scalp or other foreign material can enter the wound (and the intracranial space), careful debridement of the wound will be necessary. In addition, the surgeon will repair any tears in the dura that are observed.[6,42]

The child with a basilar skull fracture should be hospitalized for observation. Since CSF drainage from the nose or ear indicates communication between the subarachnoid space and the nasal passages or external ear, the child is at risk for the development of meningitis. Antibiotic therapy is initiated if CSF drainage occurs. Occasionally, children develop chronic CSF leakage as the result of entrapment of the dura between skull fragments during healing. This may produce chronic meningitis and may eventually require surgical repair.

When any child is admitted with a skull fracture, the nurse should watch for the development of seizures, hemorrhage, or increased intracranial pressure.

Vascular injuries. When the child with an *epidural hematoma* develops a decreased level of consciousness, immediate surgical decompression of the hematoma is required or death will result. A CT scan, skull radiograph, or angiogram should aid in the diagnosis of a subdural hematoma before deterioration in the child's clinical status.[12] (See the section on diagnostic tests at the end of this chapter for further information.) Surgical repair is accomplished by the creation of burr holes in the scalp that allow evacuation of the hematoma, immediate reduction in intracranial pressure, and repair of any vascular tear. A craniectomy may also be performed, although this necessitates later repair.[12] Before surgery, the child requires prevention or minimization of the increased intracranial pressure resulting from the hematoma. After surgery, approximately one fifth of patients will demonstrate elevation in intracranial pressure requiring aggressive medical management.[12] The perioperative mortality is proportional to the degree of neurologic deterioration that develops preoperatively; if

surgical decompression is performed before significant herniation or pupil dilation occurs, the perioperative mortality will be less than 10%. If, however, significant elevation in intracranial pressure, brain herniation, and ischemia develop before surgical relief is provided, perioperative morbidity and mortality will be high.[12]

Care of the patient with *acute subdural hematoma* requires careful assessment for and prevention of increased intracranial pressure and cerebral herniation. The indication for surgery in these patients is controversial. Removal of a localized clot will acutely reduce the intracranial pressure. However, many children with subdural hematoma also have diffuse hyperemic and vasogenic cerebral edema that may be aggravated by surgery and that may continue to progress even after removal of the hematoma. In any event, the child with a subdural hematoma will require aggressive management of increased intracranial pressure. Because extremely high intracranial pressure measurements have been recorded in both operated and nonoperated patients, initiation of hypothermia and a barbiturate coma may be ordered.[12] Mortality following a subdural hematoma is significant, and both morbidity and mortality seem to be closely related to the patient's level of consciousness at the time of surgery (if operated) and the degree and duration of intracranial hypertension.[12]

The child with a *subarachnoid hemorrhage* can rapidly develop an increase in intracranial pressure. Immediate surgical control of the bleeding site is required, and close observation for signs of postoperative elevation of intracranial pressure is necessary. These patients usually have a poorer prognosis than those with diffuse posttraumatic cerebral edema.[12]

Intracerebral hemorrhage can be the most damaging form of cerebral vascular injury because it results in a rapid increase in intracranial pressure as well as in direct damage to surrounding brain tissue. When the diagnosis of an intracerebral hemorrhage is confirmed by CT scan or arteriography, immediate surgery is performed. The bleeding site is controlled, the clot is evacuated, and the area is debrided. Often, however, access to the area of bleeding is achieved only by incision or resection of underlying brain tissue. Thus perioperative morbidity is high, and postoperative management is often complicated by increased intracranial pressure, seizures, and motor or sensory deficits.[12,42]

Cerebral edema. The child with head injury usually develops hyperemic cerebral edema for 24 to 48 hours after the injury. In addition, direct cerebral injury may produce vasogenic cerebral edema, and cytotoxic cerebral edema can result from hypoxia secondary to hypovolemic shock.[65] Thus children with head injury have a high risk of development of increased intracranial pressure, and the child should be transferred to or cared for at a trauma center familiar with intracranial pressure monitoring and management of intracranial hypertension. Medical and nursing management of this complication has been discussed previously (see the section on medical treatment and nursing interventions of increased intracranial pressure).

Psychosocial support. The child with head injury can be extremely agitated as the result of fear, pain, or increased intracranial pressure. It is important that the nurse be able to provide calm, efficient care, and that she be able to continue her assessment of the child while providing both physical and emotional support to the child. She is also the best person to recognize changes in the child's level of consciousness and separate these signs from those produced by fear, pain, or exhaustion.

The parents may feel extremely guilty if the child's injury occurred during an automobile accident while one of them was driving the car or if the child was injured as the result of a fall or sports activity; parents are often inclined to think that they could or should have prevented the injury. If the child's injury is the result of child abuse, the parents may feel distraught and guilty. If child abuse is suspected, it is important that the hospital child abuse team be notified so that the parents are supported adequately, the child is protected during recovery, and appropriate family counseling or legal action is taken.

If the child's neurologic status deteriorates and if cerebral death develops, the parents require gradual and consistent preparation and support (see the section on cerebral death later in this chapter).

■ **STATUS EPILEPTICUS**
■ **Etiology**

Status epilepticus is characterized by a prolonged or frequently repeated seizure activity that effectively creates a fixed and lasting epileptic condition.[69] In clinical practice, status epilepticus is defined as "a single generalized tonic-clonic seizure or a series of generalized tonic-clonic seizures lasting 30 minutes or longer without intervening return of consciousness."[74]

The most common causes of status epilepticus in children include high fever secondary to a non-central nervous system infection and sudden discontinuation of an anticonvulsant drug. Approximately one fifth of children with status epilepticus have a chronic encephalopathy or seizure disorder. In ap-

proximately half of the children who develop status epilepticus, no specific cause can be identified.[2] The remaining causes of status epilepticus in children include (in decreasing order of frequency): acute encephalopathy (such as occurs as the result of meningitis or encephalitis), metabolic disorders (including hypoxia, acidosis, sepsis, dehydration, hypocalcemia, hypoglycemia, hyponatremia, and hypernatremia), ingestion of toxic substances, and head injury.[74] Causes of status epilepticus at various ages may also be categorized. Metabolic disorders or intraventricular hemorrhage are more likely to be the cause of repetitive or prolonged seizures during the neonatal period. High fever, toxic ingestion, and pre-existant seizure disorders are more common causes of status epilepticus during later infancy and early childhood. Status epilepticus during adolescence is often caused by metabolic disorders, toxic ingestions, and head injury.[60] Three fourths of all documented episodes of status epilepticus occur in children under 3 years of age.[29]

■ **Pathophysiology**

The presence of status epilepticus constitutes a medical emergency since sustained convulsions can produce cerebral anoxic or ischemic damage and can result in permanent brain damage or death.[60]

Seizures are characterized by spontaneous, repetitive, electrical discharge from abnormal neurons. If this activity is spread throughout the subcortical area, a *generalized* seizure and bilateral tonic-clonic activity will occur; this can be associated with loss of consciousness or coma. If the abnormal electrical activity remains localized within a small area of the cerebral cortex, a *focal* seizure will occur, producing unilateral tonic-clonic activity. Localized seizure activity can affect adjacent neurologic tissue so that the focal seizure becomes a generalized seizure; this progressive seizure activity is known as a *jacksonian seizure.*

Sustained seizure activity increases the adenosine triphosphate (ATP) requirements of neurons since the constant electrical activity requires an extremely active sodium-potassium pump. In addition, the constant muscle contraction and relaxation produced by tonic-clonic seizures will increase tissue oxygen requirements. Thus cerebral and tissue metabolic requirements are maximal at this time. In addition, seizures may cause Valsalva's maneuver and result in increased resistance to cerebral venous return; this may increase the intracranial pressure in the patient with cerebral edema or increased intracranial volume.[80] If cerebral blood flow cannot increase sufficiently to meet cerebral cell substrate requirements, cerebral ischemia and death can result. If tissue oxygenation is not maintained adequately, hypoxemia, lactic acidosis, and hypoglycemia can develop.[60]

Some clinical conditions may predispose the child to the development of seizures. These include fatigue, pain, specific photic stimuli (usually rapidly and regularly flickering lights or images), or hypervolemia, with rapid infusion of hypotonic fluids.[29]

■ Clinical signs and symptoms

Whenever seizure activity is suspected, the nurse should note the time of the onset of the seizure activity, any precipitating factors, any progression of the seizure, and its duration. Although it is best for the nurse to describe (rather than label) the seizure activity, a few descriptive terms are widely used.

Generalized myoclonic (or tonic-clonic) status epilepticus is characterized by bilateral muscular contractions that occur continuously or in a series lasting for hours or days. This form of status epilepticus is generally related to degenerative brain disease, toxic encephalopathy, and anoxic brain damage. The EEG usually reveals the presence of many spikes with slow background activity.[29,74]

Generalized absence status epilepticus is associated with periods of confusion and with a decreased level of consciousness or stupor that is *not* associated with any abnormal muscle activity. This form of status epilepticus most commonly develops in children with persistent *petit mal* seizures. It is rarely associated with acute CNS pathology. The EEG shows bilateral, regular, generalized, symmetrical spikes.[29,74]

Focal motor status epilepticus is produced by a localized area of cortical injury or by metabolic disease. It produces rapid, focal, clonic movements of one part or one side of the body without loss of consciousness. The EEG reveals focal spikes.[29,74]

Without an EEG the presence of seizure activity or of status epilepticus is impossible to ascertain in the paralyzed patient. The critically ill child who receives paralyzing agents usually has severe neurologic, cardiac, respiratory, or multisystem disease; therefore this is the patient most at risk for the development of cerebral injury, anoxia, or metabolic imbalances that may produce seizures. However, when a child receives paralyzing agents, myoclonic or tonic-clonic muscle activity will be suppressed and seizure activity will not be apparent. In these patients, the only evidence of seizure activity may be tachycardia or alternating tachycardia and bradycardia, wide fluctuations in blood pressure, poor sys-

temic perfusion, nystagmus, or rapid alterations in pupil size. Therefore it is extremely important that an EEG be obtained whenever seizures are suspected in the paralyzed child so that status epilepticus does not develop or progress undetected.

■ Medical treatment and nursing interventions

Treatment of the child with status epilepticus requires maintenance of vital functions, abolition of the seizures, and elimination of any precipitating factors.

Maintenance of vital functions. Systemic perfusion and cerebral oxygenation must be maintained. If the child is breathing spontaneously, he should be positioned to prevent upper airway obstruction and to maximize diaphragmatic excursion; a roll should be placed under the child's shoulders to extend the neck, and the head of the bed should be elevated approximately 30 degrees. If the child's aeration is adequate and if there is no obvious oral bleeding from lacerations of the mouth or tongue, there is no need to stick anything in the patient's mouth. Forced insertion of a tongue blade or airway may produce broken teeth or oral lacerations. Placement of an oral airway is recommended, however, if the child is biting his tongue or cheek, causing oral bleeding.

If the child becomes apneic or if he demonstrates inadequate aeration or respiratory distress, bag and mask ventilation should be provided until intubation is accomplished. Before intubation is attempted, a nasogastric tube should be placed to allow emptying and decompression of the stomach so that vomiting does not occur during the intubation. It is extremely important that all members of the health care team be notified if paralyzing agents or sedatives are administered during the intubation since these will affect (or eliminate) motor activity and neurologic responses after the intubation.

During the seizure activity, the child should be placed on a flat soft surface with no hard or sharp objects nearby. The patient's bed is an appropriate surface, although the side rails should be padded.

Careful assessment and maintenance of systemic perfusion must be provided throughout the episode of status epilepticus. Hypotension or bradycardia must be treated promptly since they can result in inadequate systemic and cerebral perfusion. (See the section on treatment of low cardiac output in Chapter 3.) A large bore venous catheter should be inserted as quickly as possible to allow infusion of IV fluids and medications, and blood samples should be obtained for analysis of arterial blood gases and electrolytes (including glucose, calcium, and blood urea nitrogen). If the child has just been admitted to the critical-care unit, a urine specimen should be obtained for toxicology screening.

A rapid neurologic examination must be performed to determine if there is a possible reversible or accelerating neurologic problem that is causing the status epilepticus. Increased intracranial pressure, brain herniation, and intracranial hemorrhage can all produce seizures. If signs of intracranial hypertension are present, treatment of this problem should be provided at the same time the status epilepticus is treated.

Correction of any existing metabolic derangements is performed as quickly as possible. This may result in abolishment of the seizure activity. Occasionally, hypertonic glucose (D_{25}—1.0 to 2.0 ml/kg or D_{50}—0.5 to 1.0 ml/kg), 10% calcium gluconate (100 to 200 ml/kg to a maximum of 2.0 gm), or calcium chloride (20 to 50 mg/kg to a maximum of 1.0 gm) may be ordered empirically before serum electrolyte analysis is available since hypoglycemia and hypocalcemia are relatively common and rapidly treatable causes of seizures in critically ill children.

The infant's rectal temperature should be measured since febrile convulsions are also relatively common during infancy. If a high fever (above 40° C) is present, administration of an antipyretic suppository (such as acetaminophen) and use of a cooling blanket are required to slowly reduce the child's temperature.

Anticonvulsant therapy. The most popular drugs for treatment of status epilepticus include diazepam, phenobarbital, phenytoin, and paraldehyde. The choice of drug will depend on physician preference and on the previous effectiveness of the drug on the patient. Each of the drugs will be reviewed separately in this section. The drugs should be administered intravenously (rather than intramuscularly) to ensure maximal absorption and rapid CNS penetration.

Diazepam (Valium) is used widely in the initial treatment of seizures. The initial dose of 0.1 to 0.5 mg/kg (maximum 10 mg) is usually administered by slow IV push over several minutes. The drug should be effective within minutes; peak diazepam concentrations are reached in the brain within 1 to 5 minutes. Since the *serum* half-life of the drug is only approximately 7 minutes, the dosage may be repeated at 15 minute intervals. Side effects of diazepam include hypotension, cardiac arrest, laryngospasm, respiratory depression, respiratory arrest, sedation, and localized vascular irritation (at the site of infusion). Disadvantages of this drug are its relatively short effective period and the possible cardiorespiratory depressant effects.[6,60,74]

Phenobarbital enjoys wide use in treatment of seizures in children because it has a relatively long serum half-life and a wide therapeutic range. Phenobarbital is often administered with diazepam during treatment of status epilepticus because they seem to act synergistically. If phenobarbital is administered with diazepam, a lower dose (5.0 mg/kg; maximum dose 390 mg) of phenobarbital may be given initially by slow IV push. This dose is usually repeated twice (at 20-minute intervals) even if the seizures are controlled to provide a total initial dose of 15.0 mg/kg and establish a therapeutic serum level (15 to 40 μg/ml). Peak concentrations of phenobarbital can develop in the brain within minutes, although the drug is usually not maximally effective for 30 to 60 minutes. Side effects of phenobarbital include respiratory depression, bronchospasm, apnea, bradycardia, hypotension, and sedation. Occasionally, phenobarbital produces CNS irritability in children. The major disadvantage of this drug is the long-term sedation it produces because it makes further neurologic evaluation difficult.[6,60,74]

Phenytoin (Dilantin) is the primary nonsedative anticonvulsant used in children. If status epilepticus is not controlled after the initial infusion of diazepam and phenobarbital, phenytoin (10 to 15 mg/kg; maximum 1250 mg) may be slowly administered alternatively with the phenobarbital at 20-minute intervals.[60] The onset of the phenytoin action is approximately 10 minutes, and the therapeutic serum range (10 to 25 μg/ml) will usually be maintained for 24 hours. Phenytoin is incompatible with many IV drugs, so the IV tubing should be carefully flushed before and after the drug is administered. Side effects of phenytoin include depression of myocardial function, heart block, bradycardia or other arrhythmias, and cardiac arrest. The major disadvantage of this drug is the potential for cardiovascular compromise.[6,60,74]

Paraldehyde is used to treat status epilepticus that is refractory to other drugs. It can be administered intravenously or rectally. If the drug is administered intravenously, the initial dose (0.15 ml/kg of 4% solution) may be administered as a bolus or as a slow infusion (over 1 hour). The advantage of the infusion is that the dosage can be tapered if seizures are controlled before the entire dose is administered. Paraldehyde should only be prepared from freshly opened vials since it deteriorates rapidly when exposed to air. In addition, it must be drawn up in and administered from a glass syringe with a metal-hubbed needle. If paraldehyde is administered rectally, 0.3 ml/kg are provided in the form of a suspension enema. Side effects of the drug include potential cardiac, respiratory, renal, and hepatic toxicity, although these rarely occur. Paraldehyde is excreted through the lungs, making the drug extremely useful in patients with renal failure. A disadvantage of the drug is its strong odor.[6,60,74]

Lidocaine is used occasionally to treat intractable status epilepticus in adults; it has only recently been used in children on an experimental basis. Caution should be used if lidocaine administration is provided since it can produce seizures at higher dosages.[74]

If the above medications are unsuccessful in controlling the status epilepticus, a barbiturate anesthetic, such as thiopental sodium (Pentothal: 2.0-4.0 mg/kg) may be administered.[60] (See the discussion of barbiturate coma in the section on treatment of increased intracranial pressure earlier in the chapter.) Barbiturates should only be administered if the child is intubated and if adequate ventilatory support is provided. Volume expanders and vasopressors should be at the bedside since hypotension may develop during barbiturate administration.

Please refer to Table 6-14 for a summary of anticonvulsant therapy for status epilepticus. Once the child's continuous seizures are controlled, maintenance anticonvulsant therapy should be planned. Generally, phenobarbital (4.0-6.0 mg/kg/24 hours orally or intramuscularly) is prescribed for infants and young children, and phenytoin (5.0 to 8.0 mg/kg/24 hours intravenously, then orally after therapeutic blood levels are established) is prescribed for older children and adolescents.[6,60,74]

■ SYNDROME OF INAPPROPRIATE ANTIDIURETIC HORMONE SECRETION
■ Etiology

The syndrome of inappropriate antidiuretic hormone (SIADH) secretion can develop in any patient who sustains injury to or compression of the pituitary or hypothalamus. This occurs most commonly as the result of head injury, intracranial hemorrhage, encephalopathies (including Guillain-Barré syndrome, meningitis, and encephalitis), hydrocephalus, increased intracranial pressure, or neurosurgery with intracranial manipulation. Syndrome of inappropriate ADH secretion can also occur in patients who develop ADH-secreting tumors, following ingestion of some drugs, and in patients who experience a sudden and significant temporary fluid loss.[34] Finally, the syndrome has also been reported following redistribution of intravascular volume, perceived intravascular fluid loss, or regional hypovolemia. This may follow the development of cirrhosis and splanchnic sequestration of fluid, pulmonary hypertension (and other diseases resulting in decreased pulmonary venous return to the left atrium), or repair of mitral valve insufficiency or stenosis (and decompression of the left atrium).[26,57]

Table 6-14 Anticonvulsant therapy for status epilepticus in children[29,30,60,74]

Drug	Trade name	Dosage	Peak effect	Therapeutic serum drug level
Diazepam	Valium	0.1-0.5 mg/kg IV (maximum 10 mg)	1-5 minutes (half-life 7 minutes)	—
Phenobarbitol	—	5 mg/kg/dose IV for 3 doses (maximum 390 mg)	½-1 hour (range 24 hours)	15-40 μg/ml
Phenytoin	Dilantin	10-15 mg/kg IV (maximum 1250 mg)	10 minutes (range 24 hours)	10-25 μg/ml
Paraldehyde	—	.15 ml/kg IV (may be repeated) or 0.3 ml/kg rectally	Immediate	—

■ **Pathophysiology**

ADH is formed by the supraoptic and paraventricular nuclei in the hypothalamus. It is transported to the posterior lobe of the pituitary where it is released in response to an increase in intravascular osmotic pressure (to above 280 to 285 mOsm/kg), hypovolemia (and decreased left atrial stretch), a decrease in pulse pressure, pain, fear, or anxiety.[26,57] Because ADH increases the permeability of the renal distal tubule and collecting ducts to water, less free water is excreted in the urine, urine volume is reduced, and urine concentration is increased. This should result in a decrease in serum osmolality and an increase in blood volume. If ADH levels remain elevated and if the patient continues to receive normal amounts of water, serum hypoosmolality and hyponatremia will develop. The urine volume will often be reduced, but the urine osmolality and sodium concentration will be high. If the syndrome of inappropriate ADH secretion continues, water intoxication and hyponatremic seizures can develop from movement of water from the intravascular space into cerebral tissue. (See the sections on hyponatremia, syndrome of inappropriate ADH secretion and water intoxication in Chapter 7.)

■ **Clinical signs and symptoms**

The diagnosis of the syndrome of inappropriate ADH secretion can only be made in the absence of adrenal or renal disease and in the presence of otherwise normal pituitary function. The patient with SIADH has a true *hyponatremia*, not merely a dilutional reduction in serum sodium concentration, and persistent high urinary excretion of sodium despite the presence of serum hyponatremia. The urine volume is often less than 1 ml/kg/hour, and urine osmolality is high (although it may be less than or greater than the serum osmolality).[34,57] Signs of water intoxication, including lethargy, stupor, seizures, and coma may also develop if the syndrome of inappropriate ADH secretion progresses undetected.

■ **Medical treatment and nursing interventions**

The diagnosis of the syndrome of inappropriate ADH secretion is confirmed when the patient responds to fluid restriction with correction of the hyponatremia. When this syndrome is suspected, the child's total fluid intake is restricted to 30% to 75% of maintenance fluid requirements (see Table 6-11); more severe fluid restriction is occasionally necessary if significant hyponatremia is present.

A 24-hour urine collection may be ordered to allow quantification of urine sodium losses so that precise sodium replacement can be ordered. This replacement is calculated at 80% of urinary sodium losses with a solution containing 75 mEq/L of sodium chloride and 30 mEq/L of potassium chloride.[34] However, since fluid restriction should produce an immediate reduction in urine sodium losses, the 24-hour urine analysis may provide clinical results that are no longer applicable to the child's clinical condition. If the child demonstrates profound hyponatremia or signs of significant water intoxication (including deterioration in level of consciousness or seizures), administration of hypertonic saline (3.0 to 5.0 ml/kg of 3% sodium chloride) and a loop diuretic (such as furosemide, 1.0 to 2.0 mg/kg) may be ordered to increase the serum sodium concentration and to eliminate excess intravascular water.[34,52,57] Throughout this therapy the child's level of consciousness, level of hydration, total fluid intake and output, daily weight, and serum and urine chemistries should be carefully monitored. The child's weight should fall as the result of urinary excretion of excess intravascular water, his serum sodium concentration should rise, and his level of consciousness should improve.

Occasionally, a child demonstrates chronic syndrome of inappropriate ADH secretion. In this case, administration of lithium carbonate or demeclocycline (Demethyl chlorotetracycline) may be prescribed since these drugs inhibit the ADH effect on the renal collecting ducts. (See the sections on treatment of hyponatremia, syndrome of inappropriate ADH secretion, and water intoxication in Chapter 7.)

■ **DIABETES INSIPIDUS (DI)**
■ **Etiology**

Diabetes insipidus occurs most often as the result of decreased production of ADH (vasopressin), but it can also occur as the result of decreased renal response to vasopressin. Diabetes insipidus resulting from decreased production of ADH is also known as central or neurogenic diabetes insipidus. A defect in the kidneys' ability to respond to ADH is known as nephrogenic diabetes insipidus. The following discussion will pertain only to central or neurogenic diabetes insipidus (for a presentation of nephrogenic diabetes insipidus, see the section on diabetes insipidus in Chapter 7).

Central diabetes insipidus is often seen in pediatric patients who sustain head injuries, CNS infections, or intraventricular hemorrhage, or in those who undergo neurosurgical procedures.[53]

■ Pathophysiology

When ADH is not synthesized by the hypothalamus, circulating ADH levels are negligible. As a result the renal collecting tubules remain relatively impermeable to water so that no free water is reabsorbed from the collecting tubules. Large amounts of water are lost in the urine, even in the presence of increased serum osmolality or hypovolemia. The intravascular volume is quickly depleted, and hemoconcentration produces significant hypernatremia. As fluid shifts from the cellular to the vascular space as the result of an osmotic gradient, that fluid is also lost in the urine. Intravascular hypovolemia stimulates aldosterone secretion so that sodium and water is reabsorbed by the renal proximal tubule. The sodium reabsorption further increases the serum sodium concentration, and the water reabsorption by the proximal tubule has negligible effect on the serum osmolality or on the patient's intravascular volume.

If the child is ambulatory and old enough to obtain fluid independently, he can compensate for the diabetes insipidus with ingestion of large quantities of fluid. However, if the child's fluid intake is limited to IV therapy, diabetes insipidus can quickly produce hypovolemia, hypernatremia, and serum hyperosmolality.

■ Clinical signs and symptoms

The major sign of diabetes insipidus is polyuria—excretion of large amounts of very dilute urine, with low osmolality, low sodium concentration, and very low specific gravity. It is extremely important that the onset of diabetes insipidus be detected immediately since the critically ill child can quickly become hypovolemic and hypernatremic. If the child is awake, alert, and communicative, he will frequently complain of thirst.

If the child's enormous urinary fluid losses are not quickly replaced, hypovolemic shock can develop. As the child's intravascular volume is depleted, the central venous pressure will fall, mucous membranes will appear to be parched, the patient may act irritable, and tachycardia will be noted. The infant's anterior fontanelle will be depressed. Initially, the extremities will feel cool, and as hypovolemia worsens, the peripheral pulses become weak, capillary refill time is prolonged, and hypotension and metabolic acidosis develop. (See the section on clinical signs and symptoms of low cardiac output in Chapter 3.)

■ Medical treatment and nursing interventions

Acute management of the child with central or neurogenic diabetes insipidus requires rapid replacement of urinary fluid and electrolyte losses and provision of exogenous ADH in the form of vasopressin (Pitressin).

When the critically ill child develops diabetes insipidus, it is important that good venous access be achieved; two large bore venous catheters should be inserted to allow measurement of the central venous pressure and administration of fluids and medications. If hypovolemic shock is present, the child should receive a bolus of 10 ml/kg of glucose ($D_{2\frac{1}{2}}$) and 0.45 normal saline over 15 to 30 minutes.[53] This fluid bolus should be repeated until the child's central venous pressure reaches 3.0 to 5.0 mm Hg and until systemic perfusion improves (extremities will be warmer, peripheral pulses stronger, and capillary refill more rapid).

When diabetes insipidus is present, it is imperative that accurate records of fluid intake and output be maintained to enable appropriate fluid replacement. The child's urine output should be totaled every 30 minutes to 1 hour. The volume of the urine loss is then replaced over the next 30 minutes or 1 hour (the interval before the next urine volume measurement) in the form of glucose ($D_{2\frac{1}{2}}$) and $\frac{1}{16}$ or $\frac{1}{8}$ normal saline.[53] Throughout the replacement therapy, the nurse should carefully assess the child for evidence of hypovolemia and report any such findings to a physician immediately. To monitor the effectiveness of the volume replacement, simultaneous urine and serum sodium, potassium, chloride, and osmolalities should be measured. The urine specific gravity should be measured and recorded at least hourly.[53]

If the child has vasopressin-sensitive (central) diabetes insipidus, administration of vasopressin is indicated. This vasopressin can be given as an intramuscular injection or as an intravenous or subcutaneous infusion. However, if the vasopressin is administered intramuscularly (0.2 ml/dose IM every 1 to 3 days as needed) or subcutaneously in the aqueous form (1.0 to 3.0 ml/day divided in 3 doses), the absorption may be slow and inconsistent, and the injection site may remain painful for several days. Therefore IV administration of aqueous vasopressin is often preferred. The vasopressin may be administered slowly in a single dose (0.5 to 1.0 ml/day of the 20 U/ml aqueous solution, divided into 3 doses and increased as needed according to patient response) or in a continuous drip infusion totaling 15 mU/hour. To prepare this infusion, a dilution of 2.0 mU/ml is *care-*

fully prepared from the original ampule containing 20 units/ml.[34,53] Once the infusion is started, the child's urine volume and specific gravity should be measured every 15 minutes, and urine and serum sodium, potassium, chloride, and osmolality should be measured every hour.

A positive response to any vasopressin administration will include a decrease in urine volume (to less than or equal to 1.0 ml/kg/hour) and a rise in urine specific gravity (to greater than 1.010) and osmolality (to 280 to 300 mOsm/ml). If there is no response to an intramuscular, subcutaneous, or intravenous vasopressin dose, the dose may be repeated on the order of a physician. If there is no response to a continuous infusion of 15.0 mU/hour, the dose can be doubled to total 30.0 mU/hour or up to 60 mU/hour as needed.[53] Throughout vasopressin administration, the nurse should observe the patient closely for evidence of tachycardia, bradycardia, hypertension, hypotension, or other signs of hypersensitivity. Abdominal cramping may also follow vasopressin administration.

A synthetic analogue of vasopressin, 1-deamino-8-D-arginine-vasopressin (DDAVP) has been developed that can be administered via a nasal spray; this form of vasopressin, which has fewer systemic effects than other forms of vasopressin, has reduced the need for subcutaneous, intravenous, or intramuscular vasopressin administration. The initial dose of DDAVP in a child with diabetes insipidus is usually between 1.0 to 5.0 mg. The dose must be administered into the posterior nasal area rather than to the nasal pharynx. The most effective dose of DDAVP is only roughly dependent on the weight or age of the patient; each patient will set his own pattern for duration of response, varying from 8 to 20 hours.[8] A positive response to DDAVP administration is a decrease in urine volume and an increase in urine osmolality (as noted earlier). If the patient is vasopressin-responsive after any form of vasopressin therapy, replacement IV fluids will require tapering to prevent water intoxication as urine volume falls.

It is difficult to supply enough calories for growth when the child has polydipsia. A diet low in sodium and potassium and low in protein is important to reduce renal solute load. Starch, butter, oil, and vitamins are important food sources, but fruits and vegetables rich in mineral salts should be avoided. Growth for the child with nephrogenic diabetes insipidus is often less than normal, and if the diagnosis has not been made until multiple episodes of dehydration and hypernatremia have been sustained, developmental and growth retardation may be permanent.

■ CEREBRAL DEATH

Occasionally, despite vigorous medical or surgical therapy, the child with serious CNS disease or trauma develops severe intracranial hypertension and brain herniation with irreversible cerebral ischemia and cessation of cerebral and cranial nerve function. With the sophisticated cardiorespiratory support equipment available, it is possible to maintain the body's vital functions despite the presence of cerebral death. As a result it is sometimes necessary to consider discontinuation of aggressive medical support to allow the child to die.[64]

There is no universal legal definition of death. In some states, statutes exist that define death in the narrowest of terms, as the cessation of cardiorespiratory function. In other states, however, statutes allow the patient with cessation of brain function to be declared legally dead. Individual hospitals have also established protocols for the declaration of cerebral death and for the discontinuation of life support systems.[1,17,63] It is extremely important that all members of the health care team be familiar with the legal definition of death in the state and hospital in which they practice. The most widely used clinical criteria for declaration of brain death are included in the box that follows.

When the child is assessed for the presence or absence of brain function, a few conditions must be met. The diagnosis of brain death must be made by a physician not directly involved in the child's care; this is usually a consulting neurologist. The diagnosis cannot be considered until the child's cardiorespiratory status is stable (e.g., hypovolemic shock or tension pneumothorax should be corrected) and until potential metabolic causes of cerebral depression (such as hypoglycemia, hyperkalemia, or high serum levels of sedative drugs) have been eliminated. In addition, hypothermia cannot be present. Two independent assessments are usually performed 6-24 hours apart. The documentation of the assessments must be complete, and all criteria must be met simultaneously.

The decision to withdraw life support systems should not be made only on the basis of established criteria. Consideration should be given to legal precedents, hospital protocol, ethical standards of the community, and the wishes of the child's parents or primary caretakers. The opinions of family members must be solicited, but the family must never be made to feel that *they* are deciding to hasten the child's death. When the health care team has developed good rapport with the family and kept family members realistically informed about the child's condition, the possibility of cerebral death should not come as a to-

CRITERIA FOR THE DIAGNOSIS OF CEREBRAL DEATH*

I. The Harvard Criteria†
   A. Unresponsive coma
      Absence of receptivity and responsivity to even the most painful externally applied stimuli
   B. Apnea and lack of spontaneous movement
      Absence of spontaneous respiratory effort during a minimum of 1 hour of continuous observation; absence of spontaneous respiratory effort when mechanical respiratory support is withdrawn for a 3-minute interval (the patient's arterial P_{CO_2} must be normal and the patient must be ventilated with room air for 10 minutes before the trial)
   C. Absence of cephalic reflexes
      Pupils are fixed and dilated; corneal, gag and swallow, oculocephalic, and oculovestibular reflexes are absent; no posturing is observed; as a rule, tendon reflexes cannot be elicited
   D. Isoelectric EEG
      Two EEGs run at standard gains, each with 10 to 20 minutes of continuous recording time must be isoelectric; the EEGs should be repeated at least 24 hours apart
   E. Absence of hypothermia or drug-induced cerebral depression
      The body or rectal temperature must be above 32° C; the patient may not be under the influence of CNS depressant drugs
II. Collaborative Study[17]
   A. Prerequisite conditions
      Absence of sedative drug intoxication, normothermia, absence of cardiovascular shock, and absence of a remedial condition should be documented for a minimum of 6 hours before consideration of cerebral death; these conditions should be absent during 30 minutes of continuous observation and at least 6 hours after the onset of coma or apnea
   B. Cerebral unresponsivity
      Purposeful responses are not present (e.g., withdrawal from pain); movements of spinal reflex origin may be present
   C. Apnea
      Absence of spontaneous respiratory effort is confirmed during 15 continuous minutes of mechanical ventilatory support; if uncertainty exists, the patient may be temporarily removed from support and apnea confimed
   D. Electrocerebral silence
      The EEG should be made at gains of $2 \mu v = 1$ mm and it should be read by a competent electroencephalographer; if causes of reversible coma can be eliminated with assurance, a single recording is acceptable
   E. Additional criteria
      Absence of cephalic or spinal reflexes; fixed pupils may also be present
   F. Confirmation of cerebral death *may* be made with documentation of the absence of cerebral blood flow

*References 1, 17, 63, 64.
†These conditions must persist for a minimum of 24 hours.

tal surprise to the family, and the wishes of family members about aggressive life support are often well known. Once the child meets all of the established criteria of brain death, the family should be informed that, by medical definitions, the child is dead. If state statutes also support the definition of brain death, the parents can be told that the child meets both medical and legal definitions of death. These statements of fact can help clarify the child's condition and prevent later family guilt about the decision to terminate life support.

Once the health care team has made the diagnosis of brain death and the decision to terminate life support, one of the child's attending physicians should *write* a specific "no code," "do not resuscitate," or "disconnect ventilator" order to allow enactment of the decision. Often, once life support equipment is terminated, the child's heart continues to beat for several minutes or hours before cardiorespiratory arrest occurs. The waiting period can be extremely stressful to the critical-care staff and to the family. The nursing staff should make every effort to support the family during this time, and chaplains or nurse counselors may be able to provide assistance.

Please refer to Chapter 2 for a review of the child's concept of death, the effect of death of the child on the family, and staff stressors in pediatric critical care.

■ Postoperative Care of the Pediatric Neurosurgical Patient

Care of the child following neurosurgery requires maintenance of vital functions, assessment of neurologic function, recognition and treatment of potential complications of neurosurgery, regulation of fluid and electrolyte balance, and provision of support necessary to meet the child's and family's emotional needs.

A firm basis for postoperative assessment is provided by a thorough preoperative assessment of the child. This enables the nurse to quickly recognize changes in the child's condition or level of response to stimuli. Thus the following discussion begins with an elaboration of the preoperative assessment.

■ PREOPERATIVE ASSESSMENT

The nurse must obtain as much information as possible about the child's behavior from the parents or primary caretaker. If the child is transported to the hospital by medical personnel, information should be obtained from the medical team previously involved in the care of the child. Information should also be obtained from medical records, from a copy of the nursing care plan from the transferring hospital, and from the parents or primary caretaker (in person or by telephone).

It is important to be familiar with the child's normal motor activity, self-comforting measures, communication and motor skills, sleep patterns, feeding preferences, and behavior when frightened or angry; all of this information will be helpful during the postoperative period. The names of family members, special friends, and pets and favorite activities should be noted on the nursing care plan to enable evaluation of level of consciousness through questions about familiar people or things.

The nurse should also note the presence and severity of any preexistent neurologic symptoms such as seizures, coma, blindness, cranial nerve palsies, delayed developmental milestones, abnormal posturing or motor activity, or abnormal or absent reflexes since these may be present or exacerbated after surgery. This information allows establishment

of a baseline for evaluation of postoperative progress or deterioration. The preoperative head circumference should be recorded in the care plan of any infant whose cranial sutures are not yet fused.

The child's *level of consciousness* should be evaluated carefully. Whenever possible, the nurse should use terms that describe rather than classify the patient's behavior to avoid confusion. When the child is older and responsive, the nurse should ask the child specific questions about his name, age, birthday, and normal activities. Alert, accurate answers are normal; confused answers and lack of response to painful stimuli are clearly abnormal. During infancy, evaluation of level of consciousness will be made through observation of the infant's cry, response to auditory and tactile stimuli, and feeding and sleeping behavior. A high-pitched, breathless cry is considered abnormal in an infant; extreme lethargy or poor feeding is also considered abnormal.

The child's *motor ability* should also be assessed. This includes head control, grasp, strength of movement of extremities, and symmetrical withdrawal of the arms and legs following painful stimulus. The older child should be able to move his head and squeeze the observer's fingers upon request, and hand use and strength should be relatively symmetrical and equal bilaterally. The nurse should observe the child's gait and note any limp or unsteadiness.

The child's *reflexes* should be evaluated preoperatively. The nurse should inspect the child's pupil size and pupillary response to light. The presence of papilledema (usually confirmed by a physician) should also be noted. (See the section on clinical signs and symptoms of increased intracranial pressure in this chapter.) If time permits, the nurse should observe or perform an assessment of the child's cranial nerve function (see Table 6-13). The evaluation of some reflexes (such as the oculomotor or oculovestibular) will not be necessary in an alert, mobile, responsive child, but it becomes extremely important in the comatose child with increased intracranial pressure. Thus the complexity and depth of the assessment will be determined by the child's general condition.

The child's *cardiovascular function* must be evaluated carefully preoperatively. The skin should be well perfused with age-appropriate blood pressure, strong peripheral pulses, warm extremities, pink nailbeds and mucous membranes, brisk capillary refill, and adequate heart rate and circulating blood volume. Poor systemic perfusion can quickly result in a decrease in level of consciousness, and it can complicate intracranial hypertension. The child's normal heart rate and blood pressure should be noted carefully preoperatively for comparison with postoperative values (see Tables 6-8 and 6-9 for normal pediatric blood pressure and heart rate ranges). If the child has increased intracranial pressure preoperatively, see the section on clinical signs and symptoms of increased intracranial pressure in this chapter.

The child's *respiratory status* is assessed carefully preoperatively because neurologic disease can produce characteristic respiratory patterns (such as Cheyne-Stokes respirations), apnea, or respiratory arrest. It is important to note the presence and strength of the child's gag and cough reflexes since this will indicate the child's potential ability to handle respiratory secretions and oral or enteral feedings postoperatively. If the child has increased intracranial pressure, central hypoventilation, or apnea preoperatively, it is wise to obtain a preoperative arterial sample for blood gas analysis. This will allow correction of any serious hypercapnia or hypoxemia and will also provide a basis for comparison of ventilatory function during the postoperative period.

The child's *fluid balance* and *general nutrition* should also be assessed preoperatively. The child admitted with the syndrome of inappropriate ADH secretion will demonstrate hyponatremia and water intoxication (with potential cerebral edema). The child with diabetes insipidus may demonstrate massive intravascular volume depletion and hypernatremia. Careful evaluation of the child's preoperative fluid balance will aid in both perioperative and postoperative fluid administration. It is extremely helpful if the child's normal feeding behavior, food preferences, and sleep patterns are documented on the nursing care plan so that attempts can be made to provide these postoperatively.

If neurosurgery is planned on an elective basis, the child (as age-appropriate) should receive preoperative teaching so that he will be prepared for the sights, sounds, and sensations he will encounter during postoperative care. The parents should be included in these sessions so that they can clarify some of the child's concerns and reassure the child that they will be present throughout the child's postoperative care (see the section on preparation of children and adolescents for procedures and surgery in Chapter 2).

If the child is admitted to the critical-care unit as the result of trauma, intracranial hemorrhage, or sudden disease, it is extremely helpful if the nurse can spend a few moments with the parents and family before they enter the intensive care unit. This can help the parents to be somewhat prepared for the sights and sounds of the critical-care unit. If the child

has had major multisystem trauma, the family will require preparation regarding the child's altered appearance. Too often the medical team welcomes the parents to the bedside of a recently stabilized child with the comment, "He looks good," when the parents are confronted with the sight of a bruised or bloodied, puffy, unconscious child covered with tubes and bandages. The parents should be reassured that the child is not aware of his appearance, and that the phrase "looks good" refers to his neurologic status and vital functions. If at all possible, the child should be bathed (however quickly) and partially covered with a colorful blanket so that the parents' first sight of the child will not be overwhelming.

■ **PREPARATION FOR THE CHILD'S POSTOPERATIVE CARE (SET-UP)**

It is imperative that all equipment necessary for postoperative care be assembled at the bedside and ready for use before the child returns from neurosurgery. All IV fluids should be prepared and "flushed" through appropriate infusion pumps. Arterial and central venous pressure line transducers, manifolds, flush systems, and an intracranial pressure monitoring system should be prepared per unit policy or physician order. A pediatric ventilator should be readied for use; if the surgeons are planning to have the child breathing spontaneously and extubated at the end of the surgery, a high-humidity hood, tent, face mask or face tent can be prepared with the ventilator on "stand-by" status. A hand ventilator, mask, airway, and oxygen source should be ready at the bedside, and the appropriate size of ET tube should be taped to the child's bed. Pediatric intubation equipment should be readily available and resuscitation drugs should be nearby. Drugs used in the prevention or treatment of increased intracranial pressure (such as vasopressors, furosemide, or mannitol), those used to control status epilepticus (such as diazepam, phenobarbital, and phenytoin), and those used to ensure complete ventilatory control (d-tubocurarine or pancuronium) should be available in the unit. It is helpful if an emergency drug sheet is prepared with calculation of the patient's specific emergency drug dosages based on body weight (see Fig. 6-13 for an example of this drug sheet).

■ **POSTOPERATIVE CARE**
■ **Initial assessment**

As the child returns from neurosurgery and as the nurse receives a report from the surgical team, she

Pediatric emergency drug sheet

Patient name:———————— Age:———— Weight:————

Drug	Comes as	Average dose*	Patient's dose
Atropine sulfate	0.1 mg/ml 10 ml syringe	0.1 mg/kg (0.1 ml/kg) maximum single dose: 0.4 mg	mg ml
Atropine sulfate and Neostigmine methylsulfate	1 mg/ml—1 ml 1 mg/ml—10 ml	Dose: 0.05 ml/kg mixture Mix: atropine 1 mg, neostigmine 2.5 mg, normal saline 1.5 ml	ml
Sodium bicarbonate	1 mEq/ml 10 or 50 ml syringe	2 mEq/kg per single dose (2 ml/kg)	mEq ml
Calcium chloride (1.4 mEq/ml) 27% calcium	100 mg/ml 100 ml amp or syringe	10 mg/kg 0.1 ml/kg	mg ml
Calcium gluconate (0.48 mEq/ml) 9% calcium	100 mg/ml 10 ml amp or syringe	30 mg/kg 0.3 ml/kg	mg ml
50% glucose	500 mg/ml 50 ml vial	Dilute to 25% (250 mg/ml) Dose: 2 ml/kg	ml
Dopamine (Intropin)	40 mg/ml 5 ml amp	Dilute 200 mg in 250 ml D_5W = (800 μg/ml) Infuse 6 μg/kg/min	μg/min gtt/min
Epinephrine (Adrenalin)	0.1 mg/ml (1:10,000) 10 ml syringe	0.01 mg/kg 0.1 ml/kg	mg ml
Isoproterenol (Isuprel)	0.2 mg/ml (1:5000) 5 ml amp	Dilute 1 mg in 250 ml D_5W = (4 μg/ml) Infuse 0.1 μg/kg/min	μg/min gtt/min
Lidocaine (Xylocaine) (Bolus)	20 mg/ml 10 ml syringe	1 mg/kg 0.05 ml/kg	mg ml
Lidocaine (Xylocaine) (Infusion)	40 mg/ml 25 ml vial	Dilute 100 mg in 250 ml D_5W = (400 μg/ml) Infuse 20 μg/kg/min	μg/min gtt/min
Naloxone (Narcan)	0.4 mg/ml 1 ml amp	0.01 mg/kg 0.025 ml/kg	mg ml
Edrophonium Cl (Tensilon)	10 mg/ml 10 ml amp	0.2 mg/kg 0.02 ml/kg	mg ml

Developed by Linda R. Bernstein, Pharm. D. with the cooperation of the U.C.S.F. Intensive Care Unit medical and nursing staffs, January, 1979.
*Use intravenous route unless otherwise directed.

Fig. 6-13 Pediatric emergency drug sheet.

should be rapidly assessing the child's respiratory function or the adequacy of ventilatory support, systemic perfusion, and evidence of neurologic compromise. First priority must be given to establishment of vital functions.

If the child is breathing spontaneously, he should be positioned so that the neck is *extended* (not flexed or hyperextended). The head of the child's bed should be elevated approximately 30 degrees to maximize chest expansion and diaphragmatic excursion and to enhance cerebral venous return.[80] The child's aeration should be equal and adequate bilaterally, and the respiratory rate should be appropriate for the child's age and clinical condition (see Chapter 4 for further information). Obviously, a respiratory rate of 50 can be appropriate in a crying, vigorous infant, but this rate is fairly rapid for an adolescent. Conversely, a respiratory rate of 12 in a sleeping but arousable adolescent may be perfectly normal, but it is too slow for an infant. Evidence of respiratory distress such as retractions, nasal flaring, grunting, stridor, apnea, gasping, or cyanosis should be reported immediately to a physician because inadequate ventilation can produce hypercapnia and hypoxia and result in increased intracranial pressure. In addition, apnea may be a sign of increased intracranial pressure. Therefore, if inadequate ventilation develops, the child should be hand ventilated with a bag and mask until intubation can be accomplished and mechanical ventilation provided. As soon as possible, an arterial sample should be drawn for blood gas analysis to confirm or rule out the presence of hypercapnia, hypoxemia, or acidosis. Based on the blood gas results, ventilatory support should be initiated or adjusted.

The nurse should quickly assess the child's *systemic perfusion*. The extremities should be warm, peripheral pulses strong, nailbeds pink, and capillary refill brisk. The blood pressure should be appropriate for age; hypotension or hypertension should be reported immediately to a physician. Hypotension may be the result of bleeding or hypovolemia and can result in a fall in the child's cerebral perfusion pressure (cerebral perfusion pressure equals mean arterial pressure minus intracranial pressure). Hypertension may be an early sign of increased intracranial pressure; if this develops, it should not be corrected (unless an *extremely* high blood pressure raises concern about the development of hypertensive encephalopathy) because it may be helping to maintain the cerebral perfusion pressure. The nurse should monitor for a rising intracranial pressure (if an intracranial pressure monitoring device is in place) or clinical signs of increased intracranial pressure whenever arterial hypertension develops. If an arterial line was not inserted during surgery and if the child is critically ill, the nurse should request the insertion of an arterial catheter to enable continuous monitoring of the arterial blood pressure and sampling of blood for laboratory analysis. If the child requires frequent venipunctures for sampling, vigorous crying can result in a rise in intracranial pressure every time blood samples are drawn.

The child's heart rate should be monitored closely. Although bradycardia is often noted as one of Cushing's triad of signs of increased intracranial pressure, tachycardia may be an early sign of the development of intracranial hypertension. The heart rate should be appropriate for age *and* clinical condition; if the child is apprehensive, crying, or febrile, tachycardia is expected.

The child's *neurologic status* should be quickly but thoroughly assessed. Pupils should be equal and reactive to light; pupil inequality or sluggish response to light should be reported immediately to a physician since these signs can indicate the development of increased intracranial pressure and cerebral herniation. When pupil size and responsiveness is checked, the nurse should assess the *corneal reflex* and notify a physician if it is absent.

Decorticate rigidity or decerebrate posturing should be reported to a physician immediately. Absence of gag and cough reflex during suctioning and absence of swallow should also be reported since this indicates cranial nerve (ninth and tenth) dysfunction. The child should withdraw an extremity when a painful stimulus is applied; lack of this withdrawal should also be reported to a physician.

The child should be monitored at all times for seizure activity since seizures can frequently develop following intracranial surgery.[80] If paralyzing agents are administered postoperatively, seizures may progress unrecognized. Therefore whenever seizures are suspected in the paralyzed child or whenever unexplained fluctuations in heart rate or blood pressure, poor systemic perfusion, nystagmus, or alternating dilation and constriction of pupils develop, a physician should be notified and an EEG should be obtained (per physician order).

If an intracranial pressure monitoring system is in place, it should be attached to the bedside monitoring equipment immediately, and both the intracranial pressure and the calculated cerebral perfusion pressure should be recorded on the vital sign sheet. The nurse should obtain specific orders to perform hyperventilation if the intracranial pressure increases above 25 to 30 mm Hg or if the cerebral perfusion pressure falls near or below 55 to 60 mm Hg. The physician may also provide more specific orders about furosemide or mannitol administration.

■ Maintenance of vital functions

As noted earlier, adequate ventilatory function must be maintained. If the child has increased intracranial pressure postoperatively, the surgeon will request that the child remain intubated and receive paralyzing agents (d-tubocurarine, 0.5 to 0.7 mg/kg IV bolus and 0.125 to 0.35 mg/kg IV every hour as a bolus or by constant infusion; or pancuronium, 0.1 mg/kg IV) and total mechanical ventilatory support.[59] The child's arterial P_{CO_2} should be maintained between 25 to 29 mm Hg, and the P_{O_2} beween 80 to 100 mm Hg (60 to 80 mm Hg in neonates); this requires provision of adequate sedation and paralysis and careful pulmonary toilet. Hyperventilation should be performed before and after endotracheal suctioning, and suctioning should be brief with careful assessment of the child's color, arterial blood pressure, and intracranial pressure (if monitored). Suctioning should be discontinued and hyperventilation performed if the child develops bradycardia, hypotension, hypertension, or increased intracranial pressure (see the section on treatment of increased intracranial pressure in this chapter).

If the child is relatively stable and if he is breathing spontaneously upon arrival in the intensive care unit, the nurse's goals are then maintenance of adequate respiratory function and detection of early signs of respiratory insufficiency.

A nasogastric tube should be inserted to decompress the stomach and prevent vomiting and aspiration. This is especially important when the patient demonstrates absence of cough and gag reflex.

Assessment of systemic perfusion, heart rate, and blood pressure should continue throughout the postoperative care. Extreme tachycardia, bradycardia, and systolic hypertension with a widened pulse pressure should be reported to a physician immediately since these signs may indicate the development of increased intracranial pressure. Following neurosurgery, most children receive approximately 50% to 75% of maintenance fluid requirements (see Table 6-11). in the form of 5% or 10% glucose and 0.2 to 0.45 normal saline. If this fluid volume is inadequate to replace insensible losses, bleeding, and urine output, hypovolemia may develop. Since poor systemic perfusion can compromise cerebral perfusion, hypovolemia and hypotension should be promptly treated. Occasionally, systemic *vasopressors* may be required

to increase the mean arterial pressure (even to levels above normal) to raise the cerebral perfusion pressure in the face of a high intracranial pressure (see the section on treatment of increased intracranial pressure in this chapter). However, since these children tend to retain fluids as the result of ADH secretion or the syndrome of inappropriate ADH secretion, aggressive fluid administration is also unwise. If a central venous catheter is in place, the child's central venous pressure should be monitored, and a central venous pressure of approximately 3 to 8 mm Hg should be maintained with specific physician order.

■ Neurologic assessment

The nurse who cares for the pediatric neurosurgical patient must be able to perform a rapid but thorough neurologic assessment and to detect or prevent potential complications of neurosurgery. These potential complications include: increased intracranial pressure, status epilepticus, the syndrome of inappropriate ADH secretion, diabetes insipidus, drainage of cerebrospinal fluid from the nose or ears, and CNS infection. In most cases, a thorough neurologic examination and accurate measurement of vital signs and fluid intake and output should alert the nurse to the development of any of these complications.

Since assessment, pathophysiology, and treatment of each of the major postoperative complications has been discussed previously, the following discussion is designed to highlight important parts of the neurologic examination of the critically ill child and to provide a brief discussion of major complications of neurosurgery. For more detailed information about these complications, please refer to the section on common clinical conditions in this chapter.

Highlights of the neurologic examination. The *level of consciousness* is one of the most important aspects of the neurologic examination of a nonsedated, nonparalyzed infant or child.[62] Since the infant is unable to communicate verbally, the nurse must evaluate the baby's alertness and response to his environment. The alert infant will awaken to auditory or tactile stimuli, will visually track bright objects or lights, will cry in response to painful stimuli, will be comforted when held or fed, will suck vigorously, and will sleep peacefully. The critically ill infant may be extremely irritable, reacting strongly to even mild stimulation. He will have a high-pitched cry, will not be comforted when held or fed, will only sleep or feed for short periods, and will seem to hold extremities rigidly. Lethargy is, however, a more specific sign of neurologic disease. When lethargy is present, the infant is difficult to arouse at all times, seems uninterested in his surroundings, has poor muscle tone and weak suck, and does not demand feedings.

Evaluation of the level of consciousness in the nonsedated, nonparalyzed child can rely heavily on the child's response to questions. Sluggish or confused responses are usually signs of a decreased level of consciousness. However, if the child is suffering from sleep deprivation, drowsiness and confusion can be appropriate. Whenever possible, the questions used to evaluate the child's alertness should include questions about familiar family members or activities (using information obtained from the parents or primary caretaker) since the child is more likely to respond to questions if he feels he is not being "tested." Rating of the child's level of consciousness should be performed using a standard rating scale (see Table 6-7 and Fig. 6-7).

The child's *pupil size and response* to light are extremely sensitive indicators of intracranial events. With the development of increased intracranial pressure and brain herniation, one or both pupils dilate and begin to constrict sluggishly to light. When the child receives any drugs that may cause pupil dilation (such as atropine or large doses of dopamine), this should be noted in bold letters in the flow sheet. The pupils will dilate (but remain reactive) in response to pain (see Fig. 6-8 for variations in pupil size that can result from neurologic disorders).

As noted earlier, *assessment of the child's vital signs* is another important part of the neurologic examination. Signs of increased intracranial pressure in children can include tachycardia, bradycardia, systolic hypertension and widening of the pulse pressure, respiratory depression, or apnea.

The child's *motor function and reflexes* should be assessed carefully. Decorticate rigidity and decerebrate posturing are abnormal (see Fig. 6-9). A positive Babinski's reflex is abnormal once the infant has begun walking. The child should withdraw extremities in response to pain, and he should have corneal, gag, and cough reflexes. If the child has been awake and alert and if he is old enough to follow commands, the nurse can assess muscle strength by asking the child to move all extremities and to squeeze her fingers with both hands. When asking the child to move extremities, it is important that strength of *antigravity* muscles be tested, to avoid overestimation of the child's motor strength. The nurse should ensure that the child does move all four extremities equally and appropriately, and is able to sense light touch and pain. Evaluation of coordination can be made by asking the child to touch the nurse's index finger and his

nose—even toddlers will perform this activity if the nurse presents it as a game. Seizure activity should be reported to a physician, and status epilepticus must be treated promptly.

Many of the cranial nerves can be evaluated while other nursing care is performed (see Table 6-13). For example, the glossopharyngeal (ninth cranial) nerve and vagus (tenth cranial) nerve are probably intact if he coughs and gags during suctioning and if the child swallows. The child may complain of headaches, nausea, malaise, vomiting, blurred vision, diplopia, and poor feeding; these may be "soft" symptoms of increased intracranial pressure in the child and should be reported to a physician. The infant's *head circumference* should be measured (unless a large head dressing is in place) on return from surgery and once each shift thereafter since increasing head circumference can develop in the infant with a gradual increase in intracranial volume (e.g., hydrocephalus or subdural empyema).

Postoperative complications. *Increased intracranial pressure* results from an increase in the volume of blood, brain, or cerebrospinal fluid within the relatively fixed skull. The child's cerebral blood volume can increase as the result of hemorrhage, cerebral venous obstruction, or cerebral arterial dilation, the brain size can increase as the result of cerebral edema, and the CSF volume can increase as the result of hydrocephalus. Although an increase in intracranial volume can develop initially without a rise in intracranial pressure, once a critical volume is reached, further small increases in intracranial volume will produce significant increases in intracranial pressure (see the section on pathophysiology of increased intracranial pressure).

Signs and symptoms of increased intracranial pressure are reviewed in the box on signs and symptoms of increased intracranial pressure in infants and children on p. 388 of this chapter. They include a decrease in the level of consciousness, pupil dilation and sluggish response to light, decreased reflexes, hypertension, bradycardia or tachycardia, altered respiratory pattern, and, ultimately respiratory depression and death. If intracranial pressure monitoring is used, this will confirm and quantify the level of intracranial hypertension.

Treatment of increased intracranial pressure includes acute reduction in cerebral blood volume through hyperventilation, administration of diuretics, and occasional use of hypertonic agents. Reduction of CSF volume can be accomplished through insertion of a ventriculoperitoneal shunt (if hydrocephalus is present) or through gradual withdrawal of small amounts of cerebrospinal fluid through an extraventricular drain (with specific order from and supervision by a physician). If all other methods of treatment fail, the child may be placed in a hypothermic barbiturate coma to reduce cerebral metabolic requirements and preserve cerebral function until the acute cerebral injury is reduced. (See the section on treatment of increased intracranial pressure earlier in this chapter.)

Status epilepticus is repetitive or continuous seizure activity for 20 to 30 minutes or more without return to consciousness. Since status epilepticus can result in a reduction in cerebral perfusion and in an increase in intracranial pressure, it must be treated immediately.

When the child receives paralyzing agents during the postoperative period, it becomes impossible to clinically assess seizure activity. Therefore the presence of seizures or status epilepticus should be considered if any paralyzed child demonstrates wide fluctuations in blood pressure or otherwise unexplained deterioration in clinical status. An EEG will be necessary to rule out the presence of seizures in these children.

An individual seizure does not require treatment. Status epilepticus, however, must be treated immediately. In children, diazepam (0.1 to 0.5 mg/kg/intravenously), phenobarbital (5.0 mg/kg intravenously), phenytoin (10 to 15 mg/kg intravenously) and paraldehyde (0.15 ml/kg intravenously or 0.3 ml/kg rectally) are used most commonly (see Table 6-14 and the section on treatment of status epilepticus for further information). Serum drug levels of any anticonvulsant administered (except diazepam) and paraldehyde should be monitored.

The syndrome of inappropriate ADH secretion occurs when there is injury to or compression of the pituitary or when there is redistribution of intravascular water with perceived volume loss. The syndrome of inappropriate ADH secretion frequently develops following neurosurgery. Clinical signs and symptoms of this syndrome include hyponatremia, persistently high urine sodium concentration, high urine osmolality, and (often) low urine volume.

Treatment of the syndrome of inappropriate ADH secretion includes water restriction to 30% to 70% of maintenance fluid requirement. If the serum sodium concentration is dangerously low or if neurologic signs of water intoxication (lethargy, irritability, etc.) are present, hypertonic saline administration (3.0 to 5.0 ml/kg of 3% sodium chloride) may be ordered.

Diabetes insipidus most commonly occurs as the result of decreased production of ADH, and it results in loss of enormous amounts of free water in the urine. If diabetes insipidus is not immediately recognized in the pediatric postoperative patient, fluid depletion, dehydration, and neurologic deterioration can occur. Clinical signs of diabetes insipidus include excretion of large (often 200 to 300 ml every 15 to 30 minutes) quantities of dilute urine. If the child becomes fluid depleted, he can quickly become hypotensive and hypernatremic.

Treatment of diabetes insipidus is accomplished through assessment for and treatment of any hypovolemia, replacement of ongoing urinary losses, and administration of vasopressin (see the discussion of treatment of diabetes insipidus in the section on common clinical conditions in this chapter).

■ General supportive care and prevention of infection

Fluids and nutrition. During the child's care, the serum electrolytes and osmolality and urine output, specific gravity, and osmolality should be monitored to determine fluid and electrolyte replacement requirements. Clinical signs of the child's level of hydration should also be monitored closely. A well-hydrated child has moist mucous membranes, adequate urine output (1.0 ml/kg/hour), tearing with cry, and evidence of good systemic perfusion. The infant's fontanelle will not be depressed if hydration is appropriate. The dehydrated infant will demonstrate dry mucous membranes, decreased urine output with increased specific gravity, poor skin turgor, and an elevation in blood urea nitrogen. With more severe levels of dehydration, hemoconcentration produces a rise in serum electrolyte concentrations and signs of circulatory compromise. The dehydrated infant will have a sunken fontanelle (see Chapter 7 and Chapter 8 for further information).

Intravenous fluids containing 5% to 10% glucose will not provide for the child's maintenance caloric requirements. Therefore it is necessary for plans to be made to provide parenteral alimentation if the child does not tolerate oral or enteral feedings within a few days.

The physician may request that the child's serum osmolality be maintained between 280 to 320 mOsm/kg by administration of blood products, colloids, or small doses of mannitol.[65] In this case, regular measurement of the serum osmolality will be required.

Analgesia. Adequate relief of pain during the postoperative period is extremely important. If the child is breathing spontaneously, codeine (0.5 to 1.0 mg/kg/dose po, subcutaneously, or rectally) is usually the preferred analgesic since it does not produce the respiratory depression associated with morphine sulfate or meperidine. If the child is intubated and mechanically ventilated, morphine sulfate (0.1 mg/kg/dose intravenously) or meperidine (0.5 to 1.0 mg/kg/dose intravenously or intramuscularly) may be administered. If the child becomes agitated, increased intracranial pressure should be ruled out before it is assumed that analgesia or sedation is needed.

Prevention of infection. The child is usually placed on prophylactic antibiotics surrounding the time of surgery to reduce the risk of operative infection. This risk is also minimized with good hand-washing technique and wound care during the postoperative period. The incidence of postoperative infection is increased, on the other hand, if the surgery was performed to repair cerebral contusion or skull penetration by a foreign object or if the child develops leakage of cerebrospinal fluid from the nose or ears (see the discussion on treatment of head trauma in the section on common clinical conditions in this chapter). The child's temperature and white blood cell count should be monitored for evidence of infection and appropriate blood, wound, and catheter cultures should be drawn (as ordered) if infection is suspected.

Treatment of fever. Fever should be treated with antipyretics such as aspirin (10 mg/kg orally or rectally every 4 hours) or acetaminophen (10 mg/kg/dose orally or rectally every 4 hours). Sources of infection should be ruled out if high or persistent fever develops. Use of a hypothermia mattress is often necessary to reduce fever if antipyretics are not effective.

Prevention of the hazards of immobility. The comatose or paralyzed child can quickly develop atelectasis, stasis of pulmonary secretions, contractures, and other hazards of immobility unless the nurse provides good pulmonary toilet, passive range-of-motion exercises, and other preventive care (for further information see the discussion of treatment of coma in the section on common clinical conditions in this chapter).

■ **Psychosocial support**

Neurosurgery is usually extremely frightening for the child and parents. In recent years, the general public has become much more aware that a patient can be maintained by equipment in a vegetative state. Many parents have expressed the willingness to cope with their child's physical handicap as long as a chronic vegetative state does not develop. Thus the prospect of neurosurgery and its possible complications can be extremely threatening. If the child requires surgery as the result of head trauma, the parents may be overwhelmed by the suddenness and severity of the injury and by guilt for not having prevented it.

If possible before the surgery, the nurse should obtain as much information as possible about the parents' and child's understanding of and response to the child's condition. If the parents have major misconceptions, the nurse can attempt to clarify them; it is wise, however, to request that a physician clarify the child's clinical condition, postoperative complications, and alternatives to surgery since it is legally necessary for these explanations to be provided by a physician in order for the parents to give an informed consent to surgery.

During the surgery, it is helpful for the nurse to keep the parents informed about the surgical progress. It is not necessary for the parents to be made aware of each aspect of the surgical technique or specifics of dissection, suturing, or debridement, but it is helpful for the parents to know of the general progress of the surgery. The nurse can also provide the parents with interim reports of the child's condition during surgery—this must, however, be done very carefully, with the consent and participation of the surgeon. Such interim reports can reduce the parents' anxiety during the waiting period, and it can also allow the nurse time to prepare the family for bad news if the child's condition deteriorates during surgery. If the family's first hint of trouble comes when the surgeon arrives to inform them of the child's death, they can be overwhelmed by grief or anger and be too shocked to respond or ask questions.

Following surgery, the parents will require support when visiting the child for the first time. They will also need consistent reports of the child's condition and prognosis throughout postoperative care. The child will require gentle care and encouragement (see Chapter 2 for further information).

Table 6-15 provides a summary of important aspects of nursing care of the postoperative pediatric neurosurgical patient.

Text continued on p. 436.

Table 6-15   Nursing care of the postoperative pediatric neurosurgical patient

Nursing diagnosis	Expected outcomes	Nursing activities

A. Possible compromise of cardiorespiratory function related to anesthesia, surgical complications, or increased intracranial pressure	1. Patient will demonstrate appropriate heart rate, respiratory rate, and blood pressure for age and clinical condition (see Tables 6-8 and 6-9); abnormal vital signs will be reported to physician immediately
	2. Patient will demonstrate evidence of adequate systemic perfusion as assessed by:
	  a. Appropriate blood pressure
	  b. Warm extremities
	  c. Strong peripheral pulses
	  d. Pink nailbeds and mucous membranes
	  e. Brisk capillary refill
	  f. Urine output of 1 ml/kg/hr
	3. Patient will demonstrate adequate and equal lung expansion bilaterally (whether breathing spontaneously or with mechanical ventilatory assistance), and adequate arterial blood gases (ABGs) as determined by health care team, with no evidence of nasal flaring, retractions, stridor, or grunting; any symptoms of respiratory distress will be reported to physician immediately
		1. Obtain a summary of the patient's condition and the surgery performed, if possible, before the child returns from surgery; if sedatives, atropine, or large doses of sympathomimetic drugs were administered during surgery, note this on the care plan since these may alter neurologic assessment findings
		2. Upon child's return from the operating room, position child so the neck is extended, the head is in the midline, and the head of the bed is elevated
		3. Obtain vital signs and report excessive tachycardia, bradycardia, hypertension, hypotension, or respiratory distress to physician immediately (use patient's preoperative vital signs as a guide)
		4. Assess indirect evidence of systemic perfusion as follows:
		  a. Peripheral pulses should be strong
		  b. Extremities should be warm
		  c. Nailbeds and mucous membranes should be pink
		  d. Capillary refill should be brisk
		  e. Urine output should average 1 ml/kg/hr if fluid intake is adequate
		Notify physician if signs of inadequate systemic perfusion are present; if low cardiac output is present, refer to Chapter 3
		5. Assess child's respiratory function
		  a. Auscultate lung fields bilaterally; aeration should be equal and adequate
		  b. Check color of mucous membranes and nailbeds; cyanosis indicates the presence of hypoxemia
		  c. If child is breathing spontaneously, note respiratory rate and effort; assess for presence of nasal flaring, retractions, stridor, or grunting, which may indicate increased respiratory effort

Table 6-15   Nursing care of the postoperative pediatric neurosurgical patient—cont'd

Nursing diagnosis	Expected outcomes	Nursing activities

A. Possible compromise of cardiorespiratory function related to anesthesia, surgical complications, or increased intracranial pressure—cont'd		d. Assess signs of spontaneous respiratory effort; if child is breathing spontaneously, observe for abnormal respiratory patterns (see Table 6-12) or apnea
		
		If child is receiving mechanical ventilatory support, observe for abdominal or chest movements or negative or lowered airway pressures indicative of patient initiation of respirations.
		
		If respiratory function is inadequate, notify physician and begin hand ventilation with bag and mask if patient is extubated; if mechanically ventilated patient demonstrates signs of respiratory distress, ensure patency of ET tube, provide hand ventilation, and notify physician
		6. Obtain ABG sample (as ordered); Request physician order elaborating preferred ABG ranges, and notify physician of blood gas results not consistent with the desired results (see nursing diagnosis B for further information), and adjust ventilatory support accordingly (as ordered or per unit policy)
		7. Administer paralyzing agents as ordered to maintain effective mechanical ventilatory support
		8. Ensure that patient's airway remains patent through provision of appropriate pulmonary toilet
		9. Insert a nasogastric tube if needed (and per unit policy or physician order) to decompress stomach and allow maximal diaphragmatic excursion
		10. Perform a brief neurologic assessment; note the following:
		  a. If child is not sedated and is recovering from anesthesia, he should become progressively more alert and oriented
		  b. Pupils should be equal and should react briskly to light
		  c. Corneal reflex (blink) and gag reflex should be present

Continued.

Table 6-15 Nursing care of the postoperative pediatric neurosurgical patient—cont'd

Nursing diagnosis	Expected outcomes	Nursing activities
A. Possible compromise of cardiorespiratory function related to anesthesia, surgical complications, or increased intracranial pressure—cont'd		d. Decorticate or decerebrate posturing are abnormal e. Seizure activity should not be present If abnormal neurologic signs are noted, notify physician immediately; if increased intracranial pressure is suspected, begin hyperventilation with hand ventilator in attempt to reduce intracranial pressure (see nursing diagnosis B) 11. Provide IV fluids as ordered (usually, 50%-75% of child's maintenance fluid requirements are provided in the form of 5%-10% glucose in 0.2 normal saline); total all fluid intake and output and discuss imbalance with physician (see Table 6-11 for daily maintenance fluid requirements)

B. Possible decrease in cerebral perfusion, cerebral herniation, or death as a result of increased intracranial pressure (ICP)	1. ICP (if monitored) will be maintained at 5-15 mm Hg
	2. Child will demonstrate no evidence of deterioration in neurologic status, as indicated by the following:
	  a. Decreased level of consciousness
	  b. Unilateral or bilateral pupil dilation or sluggish response to light
	  c. Tachycardia, severe bradycardia, or hypertension with widened pulse pressure
	  d. Apnea, decreased respiratory rate, or abnormal breathing patterns
	  e. Decorticate or decerebrate posturing
	  f. Abnormal or absent reflexes
	3. Cerebral perfusion pressure will be maintained ≥60 mm Hg
		1. If ICP monitoring device is in place, connect transducer to monitoring system and ensure that system is calibrated and functioning properly
		  a. Obtain physician order for desired ICP range
		  b. Obtain physician order for performance of hyperventilation if ICP increases above 20-25 mm Hg (or as per physician order)
		Notify physician of a high or rising ICP and begin hyperventilation (as ordered)
		2. If ICP monitoring device is in place, monitor ICP and calculate *cerebral perfusion pressure* (CPP)
		CPP = Mean arterial pressure − ICP
		Notify physician of falling CPP or CPP of ≤55-60 mm Hg
		3. Monitor for signs of increased ICP including:
		  a. Decreased level of consciousness (and lack of responsiveness to stimuli)
		  b. Unilateral or bilateral pupil dilation with sluggish response to light
		  c. Decreased corneal or gag reflexes or sluggish withdrawal from painful stimuli

Table 6-15 Nursing care of the postoperative pediatric neurosurgical patient—cont'd

Nursing diagnosis	Expected outcomes	Nursing activities
B. Possible decrease in cerebral perfusion, cerebral herniation, or death as a result of increased intracranial pressure (ICP)—cont'd		d. Tachycardia or bradycardia e. Hypertension with widened pulse pressure f. Decreased respiratory rate or apnea Notify physician immediately if these develop and begin hyperventilation (with hand ventilation) as ordered or as per unit policy 4. Maintain mechanical ventilatory support (as ordered) so hypercapnia, acidosis, and hypoxemia are prevented; physician will often request that mechanical ventilatory support be provided to maintain the following ABG results: a. $Paco_2$: 25-29 mm Hg b. Pao_2: 80-100 mm Hg (60-80 mm Hg in child) c. pH: 7.40-7.50 Notify physician of a deterioration in ABGs and provide hand ventilation as needed to maintain them 5. Maintain fluid restriction as ordered; calculate child's maintenance fluid requirements (see Table 6-11) and discuss with physician if child is receiving >75% of maintenance fluid requirements, or if fluid intake exceeds total fluid output 6. Measure serum and urine osmolality q 4-6 hr or as ordered by physician; notify physician of a serum osmolality <280 mOsm/L, >320 mOsm/L, or osmolality outside of the range ordered by physician 7. Administer IV furosemide (0.5-2.0 mg/kg/dose) as ordered, and monitor patient diuretic response; notify physician if diuresis does not follow furosemide administration or if urine output is less than following previous doses 8. Administer colloid, plasma, or other blood components as ordered to maintain serum osmolality; maintain serum hematocrit at approximately 40%-45%

Continued.

Table 6-15   Nursing care of the postoperative pediatric neurosurgical patient—cont'd

Nursing diagnosis	Expected outcomes	Nursing activities
B. Possible decrease in cerebral perfusion, cerebral herniation, or death as a result of increased intracranial pressure (ICP)—cont'd		9. Administer small doses of mannitol (or other hypertonic agent) as ordered: 　a. 0.15-0.3 gm/kg q 1-2 hr 　b. 0.05-0.15 gm/kg/hr by continuous infusion 　c. 1.5-2.0 gm/kg q 4-6 hr (this dose is no longer used routinely) 10. Administer steroids as ordered: 　a. Usually, dexamethasone (initial dose of 0.5-1.0 mg/kg IV, then maintenance dose of 0.25-0.5 mg/kg/day in 4 doses) or prednisone (1.5-2.0 mg/kg/day orally) are ordered 　b. If steroids are given, monitor for side effects including gastrointestinal bleeding, glycosuria, and susceptibility to infection 　c. Steroids should be tapered slowly, not discontinued abruptly 11. If hypothermic barbiturate coma is ordered: 　a. Ensure that adequate mechanical ventilatory support is provided 　b. Ensure that volume expanders and vasopressors are readily available and monitor for hypotension, tachycardia, and bradycardia that may complicate pentobarbitol coma 　c. Administer barbiturate as ordered: pentobarbitol 2.0-5.0 mg/kg (loading dose) then doses of 0.5-3.0 mg/kg/hr as needed to maintain appropriate serum pentobarbitol level 　d. Monitor serum pentobarbital levels; notify physician of levels <2.0-4.0 mg/dl (or 20-40 μg/ml) 　e. Maintain hypothermia as ordered through use of cooling blanket; administer paralyzing agents as needed to prevent shivering; note that serum potassium concentration should be maintained at a lower level (2.5-3.0 mEq/L) when hypothermia is present

Table 6-15 Nursing care of the postoperative pediatric neurosurgical patient—cont'd

Nursing diagnosis	Expected outcomes	Nursing activities

B. Possible decrease in cerebral perfusion, cerebral herniation, or death as a result of increased intracranial pressure (ICP)—cont'd		f. Inform child and family (as needed) about purpose of coma—attempt to prepare parents for sight of child in coma and for fact that child feels cold
		g. When child is weaned from barbiturate therapy, monitor child carefully for signs of increased ICP and report these to physician immediately
		12. When child's condition stabilizes, wean from ventilatory support (per physician order); during weaning monitor for signs of increased ICP or respiratory distress and notify physician immediately if they develop
		13. Administer analgesics as needed (per physician order)
		  a. Morphine sulfate: 0.1 mg/kg/IV dose q 3-4 hr (or meperidine 0.5-1.0 mg/kg/IV dose q 3-4 hr)
		    NOTE: Since morphine sulfate can cause respiratory depression, it should be administered cautiously in the child breathing spontaneously
		  b. If child is breathing spontaneously, codeine (0.5-1.0 mg/kg/dose po, subcutaneously, or rectally) is the preferred analgesic since it does not cause respiratory depression
		  c. If child is in barbiturate coma, morphine sulfate may be given by continuous infusion (30-100 μg/kg/hour)

C. Possible status epilepticus related to irritable cerebral focus, withdrawal of previous anticonvulsant therapy, or fluid or electrolyte imbalance	1. Patient will demonstrate no clinical evidence of status epilepticus; if continuous seizures do develop, they will be promptly recognized and treated
	2. If EEG is performed, no evidence of status epilepticus will be present
		1. Monitor child's muscle tone and movements; notify physician of any suspected seizure activity
		  a. If seizure activity continues uninterrupted for 20 min, status epilepticus is present, and anticonvulsant therapy must be provided immediately
		  b. When any seizures are observed, nurse should record their duration, progression, and any precipitating or alleviating factors

Continued.

Table 6-15 Nursing care of the postoperative pediatric neurosurgical patient—cont'd

Nursing diagnosis	Expected outcomes	Nursing activities
C. Possible status epilepticus related to irritable cerebral focus, withdrawal of previous anticonvulsant therapy, or fluid or electrolyte imbalance—cont'd		c. It is necessary to protect patient from harm during seizure; head should be positioned so that neck is extended to maintain a patent airway; nothing should be forced into patient's mouth unless teeth are producing lacerations of and bleeding from tongue and cheek; if this is the case, attempts should be made to insert an airway or tongue blade between the teeth 2. If child is receiving paralyzing agents, tonic-clonic activity will be suppressed; therefore status epilepticus can be masked; signs of seizures in the paralyzed patient can include: a. Tachycardia or bradycardia b. Wide fluctuations in blood pressure c. Sudden unexplained clinical deterioration d. Nystagmus or rapid changes in pupil size If these signs develop in the child receiving paralyzing agents, notify physician immediately so that status epilepticus may be ruled out 3. If status epilepticus develops, check serum electrolyte concentrations and ABGs (as ordered) to exclude a possible metabolic cause of the seizures; any imbalances should be corrected immediately 4. Administer appropriate IV anticonvulsant therapy as ordered to treat the status epilepticus: a. diazepam: 0.1-0.5 mg/kg/dose (maximum 10 mg) b. phenobarbitol: 5.0 mg/kg/dose (maximum 390 mg) may be repeated at 20 minute intervals twice c. phenytoin: 10-15 mg/kg/dose (maximum 1250 mg) d. paraldehyde: 0.15 ml/kg IV (may be repeated) If any of these drugs are administered, monitor for side and toxic effects and check serum levels of the drugs as ordered or per unit policy (see the material on status epilepticus in the section on common clinical conditions in this chapter)

Table 6-15 Nursing care of the postoperative pediatric neurosurgical patient—cont'd

Nursing diagnosis	Expected outcomes	Nursing activities

D. Possible fluid or electrolyte imbalance related to surgery and to potential syndrome of inappropriate ADH secretion or diabetes insipidus	1. Patient will demonstrate moist mucous membranes, good skin turgor, good systemic perfusion, and urine output of 1.0 ml/kg/hr
	2. Patient will not demonstrate evidence of serum electrolyte imbalance (including hyponatremia or hypernatremia)
	3. Patient will not demonstrate decreased urine output, decreased level of consciousness, or hyponatremia (consistent with syndrome of inappropriate ADH secretion and water intoxication)
		1. Measure child's fluid intake and output hourly
		  a. Provide approximately 50%-75% of maintenance fluids (per physician order) in the form of 5%-10% glucose and 0.2 normal saline (see Table 6-11)
		  b. Measure urine specific gravity and osmolality (and serum osmolality, if ordered)
		  c. Notify physician of urine volume exceeding fluid intake, or urine output <1 ml/kg/hr
		2. Monitor for signs of the syndrome of inappropriate ADH secretion, including:
		  a. Decreased serum sodium concentration
		  b. High urine sodium concentration
		  c. High urine osmolality
		  d. Low urine volume
		  e. Irritability or lethargy (signs of water intoxication)
		  Notify physician if these signs develop
		3. If the syndrome of inappropriate ADH secretion is present:
		  a. Restrict fluid intake to 30%-70% of maintenance fluid requirements (as ordered)
		  b. Correct hyponatremia slowly with 3.0-5.0 ml/kg of 3% sodium chloride (as ordered)
		  c. Monitor the child's serum sodium concentration and neurologic status closely
		4. Monitor for signs of diabetes insipidus, including:
		  a. Increased urine volume that greatly exceeds fluid intake
		  b. Urine specific gravity <1.005-1.010
		  c. Clinical signs of intravascular volume depletion, such as tachycardia and peripheral vasoconstriction
		  d. Dry mucous membranes, depressed anterior fontanelle (in the infant), poor skin turgor, and irritability

Continued.

Table 6-15 Nursing care of the postoperative pediatric neurosurgical patient—cont'd

Nursing diagnosis	Expected outcomes	Nursing activities
D. Possible fluid or electrolyte imbalance related to surgery and to potential syndrome of inappropriate ADH secretion or diabetes insipidus—cont'd		5. If central diabetes insipidus is present: a. Correct any existing hypovolemia with infusion of 10 ml/kg of glucose solutions containing small amounts of sodium chloride (per physician order) b. Develop plan to provide hourly or half-hourly replacement of urine fluid losses c. Administer vasopressin as ordered and assess patient response (should include a decrease in urine volume and an increase in urine concentration)
E. Possible infection related to: 1. Contamination of operative site (such as occurs with a compound skull fracture) 2. Contamination of ventricular drainage system or other ICP monitoring device 3. Poor wound healing (related to steroid therapy) 4. Continued CSF leak through dural tear 5. Poor nutritional status	1. Patient will not demonstrate any of the following signs of infection: a. Fever greater than 38.5° C b. Elevated white blood cell count c. Wound erythema, fluctuance, or drainage If the above signs are noted, a physician will be notified immediately and appropriate cultures will be drawn and treatment will be initiated 2. If the patient demonstrates signs of continuous CSF drainage from the ear or nose, physician will be notified immediately	1. Monitor child's temperature and white blood cell count and notify physician of fever or leukocytosis 2. Maintain good handwashing technique before and after each patient contact 3. Use aseptic technique when handling any of the equipment related to the ICP monitoring device (if in place) 4. If ventricular drainage system has been placed, place patient in reverse isolation (per physician order or unit policy) 5. Check the appearance of all skin puncture and catheter sites; notify physician of any erythema, fluctuance, or drainage, and obtain appropriate skin or catheter cultures as ordered 6. Check appearance of craniotomy incision; report any erythema, fluctuance, or drainage to physician 7. If CSF drainage from the ears or nose is suspected, record this fact clearly in the nursing care plan since this places the child at risk for the development of CNS infection; report any signs of CNS infection (including fever, leukocytosis, nuchal rigidity, or irritability) to physician 8. Administer antibiotics as ordered and monitor for side effects

Table 6-15 Nursing care of the postoperative pediatric neurosurgical patient—cont'd

Nursing diagnosis	Expected outcomes	Nursing activities
F. Possible nutritional compromise related to: 1. Prolonged coma and inability to take oral feedings 2. Prolonged immobility 3. Inadequate caloric intake 4. Anorexia, nausea, or vomiting resulting from CNS disease or increased intracranial pressure	1. Patient will demonstrate small but steady weight gain, with good wound healing and good skin turgor	1. Calculate child's maintenance fluid and caloric requirements and speak with physician if child is not receiving them (see Chapter 8) 2. If child is unconscious or critically ill, discuss plans for IV alimentation with physician 3. Assess child's gag and swallow reflex and bowel sounds, and notify physician if all are present and adequate; in this case, continuous nasogastric feedings may be ordered 4. If patient begins to receive nasogastric feedings, assess for signs of intolerance, including: a. Vomiting b. Abdominal distention c. "Residual" formula remaining in stomach for longer than 1 hr d. Diarrhea Notify physician if these signs develop, and reduce volume or concentration of feeding as ordered
G. Possible skin breakdown or contractures related to: 1. Immobility 2. Poor nutritional status 3. Inadequate attention to skin care	1. Patient will demonstrate no signs of skin breakdown over bony prominences 2. Patient will maintain full range-of-motion in all joints	1. Begin physical therapy (PT) program (with physician order, and appropriate consultation) within 2 days of surgery if child remains immobile or comatose: a. Note PT plan on nursing care plan b. Provide active (if feasible) as well as passive range-of-motion exercises 2. Keep sheets dry and wrinkle free 3. Obtain sheepskin, eggshell or water mattress (per hospital policy) to reduce pressure on skin over bony prominences 4. Keep skin dry and turn patient frequently; massage skin to stimulate skin blood flow
H. Possible patient and family anxiety related to child's surgery or prognosis	1. Patient will not demonstrate harmful behavior	1. Provide child (as appropriate) and family with realistic and consistent information; record specific descriptive terms in the nursing care plan so they can be reinforced by all members of the health care team

Continued.

Table 6-15 Nursing care of the postoperative pediatric neurosurgical patient

Nursing diagnosis	Expected outcomes	Nursing activities
H. Possible patient and family anxiety related to child's surgery or prognosis—cont'd	2. Patient (as appropriate) and family will indicate comprehension of the need for the child's surgery, the surgery performed, and the child's prognosis by repeating this information accurately to other members of the health care team 3. Family members will not demonstrate behavior that interferes with the child's physical care or coping mechanisms	2. Attempt to be present when physicians speak to the patient or family regarding the surgery or the child's prognosis so that this information can be reinforced by the nursing staff 3. Provide time to prepare the child (as age-appropriate) before moving him, or before any painful or noisy treatments are performed 4. Assume that the child is able to hear at all times; provide appropriate explanations, and avoid discussing a child's poor prognosis around the child's bedside 5. Provide the child with long, uninterrupted sleep periods to prevent sleep deprivation 6. Talk to the child frequently about the day, date, and time of day to help the child orient himself to time and place 7. As the child's condition improves, provide new physical therapy routines or small rewards (such as stars or stickers on a calendar) to give the child tangible evidence of improvement 8. If the child's prognosis is poor, begin to prepare the family gradually, allowing them time to cope with new information; prepare the child, as age appropriate (see Chapter 2)

■ Specific Diseases

■ INTRACRANIAL TUMORS
■ Etiology

The incidence of CNS tumors in children is approximately 2.5 per 100,000 children annually. Tumors of the brain are second only to leukemia as a cause of neoplasms in children, and they account for nearly 20% of all pediatric neoplasms.[4,16,68,87]

Tumors are abnormal swellings or masses that can arise from any tissue in the body. Their cause is unknown, although the role of hereditary factors and environmental carcinogens continues to be explored. Although few tumors are present from birth, many tumors of childhood arise from inappropriate development of primitive neuroepithelial cells.[16] Tumors are most frequently diagnosed in children 5 to 10 years of age.[68]

■ Pathophysiology

Intracranial tumors in children produce an increase in intracranial volume and, in the absence of an expanding skull, will produce a rise in intracranial pressure. In addition, the tumor causes compression of surrounding brain tissue, compromising important cerebral functions.

Tumors are classified according to their location, degree of malignancy, and histologic features. Classification by location enables more straightforward prediction of the clinical consequences of tumor expansion and the possibility and risks of surgical excision of the tumor; thus this classification will be used (see the box above). *Supratentorial* tumors involve the cerebral hemispheres and all structures located above the tentorium cerebelli. *Infratentorial* tumors are those that involve the brainstem and cerebral structures located below the tentorium cerebelli.

Classification of tumors by cell type allows some predictions to be made about speed of the tumor growth and spread and about recurrence risks. It is important to note that intracranial tumors in children may be malignant by *position* as well as by cell type. This means that the tissue itself is not malignant but that the effect of tumor growth on surrounding tissues can produce serious neurologic compromise or death as a result of compression or erosion of vital brain tissue.

In the following section, the most common intracranial tumors in children are discussed. This discussion includes clinical consequences of tumor growth.

Supratentorial tumors. The two most common supratentorial tumors in children are the astrocytoma and the craniopharyngioma. The *astrocytoma* is the most common of all supratentorial tumors; it is responsible for approximately 28% of all intracranial tumors in children.[22] It arises from abnormal proliferation of the cerebral astrocytes. Astrocytomas can develop in the frontal, temporal, and central parietal areas of the cerebral hemispheres, and tumor growth can extend across the corpus callosum from one parietal lobe to the other. These tumors can also invade the brainstem or third ventricle.

Astrocytomas can be slow-growing or rapid-growing tumors, and tumor specimens can be graded on a scale of one to four according to the degree of cell differentiation present in the tumor.[16] When an astrocytoma is located above the tentorium, it is usually diffuse, and it expands into surrounding tissue or along long nerve fiber tracts. Expansion through metastases (transfer to other organs) is rare.

The *craniopharyngioma* is responsible for approximately 10% of all intracranial tumors in children.[68] It occurs as the result of growth of displaced neuroepithelial cells. The tumor consists of a solid mass or cyst that contains fluid, cellular debris, and calcified material. It develops within or just above the sella turcica (the skull pouch containing the pituitary) or within the third ventricle. Thus as the craniopharyngioma grows, obstruction of the foramen of Monro, the optic chiasm, the pituitary, or the hypothalamus occurs, producing hydrocephalus, visual disturbances, fever, hypoglycemia, diabetes insipidus, or occasional hypotension.[68]

Infratentorial tumors. Infratentorial tumors account for nearly two thirds of all pediatric brain tumors and for nearly half of all tumors in children. These tumors usually are detected more rapidly because they can quickly produce changes in vital body functions. The two most common forms of infratentorial tumors in children are brainstem gliomas and medulloblastomas; astrocytomas and ependymomas are responsible for a smaller proportion of the tumors.

Brainstem gliomas are cysts that compress the cranial nerves, the pons, and medulla. If the glioma expands into the cerebellum, relatively large growth can be accommodated without symptoms of cerebellar compression. The first symptoms of the brainstem glioma are usually those of cranial nerve dysfunction. Initially, compression of the abducens nerve (sixth cranial nerve) will cause nystagmus, then facial nerve (seventh cranial nerve) compression will cause a facial palsy, and oculovestibular nerve (eighth cranial nerve) compression will result in hearing loss. As the glossopharyngeal and vagus nerves (ninth and tenth cranial nerves) become involved, the child will develop hoarseness and difficulty swallowing. Increased intracranial pressure develops during the terminal stages of tumor expansion, producing headache, vomiting, and other signs of intracranial hypertension. The prognosis of this tumor is extremely poor, and many children do not survive a year beyond diagnosis because surgical excision of the tumor is impossible.

The *medulloblastoma* is the most malignant of the posterior fossa tumors because it grows rapidly and tends to recur after surgical excision; it is responsible for approximately one fourth of all primary intracranial tumors in children.[22] The tumor rises from neuroepithelial cells. It is usually a soft, gray mass that extends from the medulla into the fourth ventricle, subarachnoid space, third ventricle, or spinal column, along CSF pathways. Symptoms that are often present include stiff neck or neck pain, increased intracranial pressure, obstructive hydrocephalus, ataxia, and fatigue. Hypotension or hypertension may develop as the result of compression of the medulla, and backache, limb weakness, or loss of bladder control will indicate spinal cord involvement. Medulloblastomas occur most commonly in children 1 to 5 years of age.[68]

Astrocytomas can also grow in the brainstem, although they are usually confined to the pons. They produce sequential and multiple cranial nerve palsies, ataxia, and pyramidal (voluntary movement) dysfunction; headache and diplopia also occur frequently. The mean age at diagnosis of brainstem astrocytoma is 7 years, and survival is usually less than 2 years despite aggressive therapy.[68]

Ependymomas account for approximately 7% of all intracranial tumors in children.[22] This tumor rises from neuroepithelial cells, and it forms a fleshy gray mass that most frequently obstructs the fourth ventricle, producing hydrocephalus and cranial nerve palsies.

■ **Clinical signs and symptoms**

Intracranial tumors in children may grow to a large size without producing significant symptoms until they invade vital brain tissue or cause increased intracranial pressure. This is because the child's skull can expand to accomodate a gradual increase in intracranial volume and because testing of cognitive functions, fine motor skills, and sensation is very difficult in the infant and young child.

Signs and symptoms of any *neoplasm* in the child include a change in size, appearance, or growth patterns; swellings, lumps, or masses; vague pains or persistent irritability; a change in feeding patterns or bowel or bladder function; unexplained clumsiness or stumbling; or unexplained or persistent bleeding.[4] General signs of an intracranial tumor during childhood include signs of increased intracranial pressure, headache, emesis, anorexia, ataxia, cranial nerve palsies, nystagmus, paresis, seizure activity, or hydrocephalus.

The signs of increased intracranial pressure in the child with an intracranial tumor include papilledema, an altered level of consciousness, visual disturbances (diplopia and blurring of vision), headache, and emesis. The headache is characteristically intermittent but progressive. It tends to be present after awakening, and it often is associated with vomiting. The child usually does not feel nauseated before vomiting. If vomiting or headache are persistent, anorexia may develop.

As the tumor grows, an infant will develop a bulging fontanelle, and he may demonstrate torticollis as the result of asymmetric compression of neck muscles by the tumor. Nuchal rigidity may also be noted.[16]

If the tumor compresses the sixth cranial nerve or if brain herniation develops as the result of increased intracranial pressure, the child may develop strabismus, diplopia, or blurring of vision. Ataxia or nystagmus will develop if the tumor compresses or erodes the cerebellum.[16] Paresis will develop if the tumor compresses the brainstem or pyramidal tract. Seizures are rarely an early sign of an intracranial tumor, although they can develop late in the clinical course. If hydrocephalus is present, the tumor is obstructing the CSF pathway.

The best means of diagnosing an intracranial tumor is through a thorough neurologic examination and a CAT scan (see the section on common diagnostic tests). A plain skull radiograph may demonstrate characteristic changes associated with some tumors (e.g., calcification near the sella turcica that occurs with a craniopharyngioma), but often the films are not helpful. Arteriography may be performed to better locate and define the tumor.

■ **Medical and surgical treatment and nursing interventions**

Care of the child with an intracranial tumor requires decompression of intracranial hypertension (see the discussion of treatment of increased intracranial pressure in the section on common clinical conditions), surgical resection if possible, and initiation of antineoplastic therapy. Radiation therapy is prescribed most often for intracranial tumors, although chemotherapy has recently been found to be helpful in the treatment of some intracranial tumors in children.[16] The child is usually hospitalized in the critical-care unit following neurosurgery or for management of sepsis or infections secondary to chemotherapy-induced immunosuppression (see the section on pneumonia in Chapter 4 for further information).

The child and family will require long-term physical and emotional support. If the tumor initially produced vague clinical signs and symptoms, the parents may have ignored the child's initial complaints—this can later cause a great deal of parental guilt and frustration. Unless deterioration is rapid, the child will require surgery, or radiation or chemotherapy with frequent hospitalizations. The child may, in fact, have a chronic neurologic disease and the family will require prolonged treatment and support.[47] An excellent resource regarding nursing care of the child with cancer has been edited by Fochtman and Foley.[25] The reader is referred to this text for specific information about the tumors, their treatment, administration and complications of chemotherapy and radiation therapy, and prognosis of specific tumors.

■ **MENINGITIS**
■ **Etiology**

Meningitis is an acute inflammation of the meninges and cerebrospinal fluid. It occurs far more commonly in children than in adults; it occurs most frequently in children between 1 month and 5 years of age.[32] Meningitis is most commonly produced by bacteria (called purulent meningitis) or viruses (usually called aseptic meningitis), although it can also result from fungi, parasites, or yeasts.

The bacterial organisms most likely to produce meningitis in children include *Haemophilus influenzae*, *Neisseria meningitidis*, and *Streptococcus pneumoniae*. These forms of meningitis are usually associated with extension of a localized infection, resulting in transient bacteremia and CNS spread of the organism. Staphylococcal meningitis occurs most commonly after neurosurgery or after a skull fracture with a dural tear.[10,33]

■ **Pathophysiology**

Once the pathogen invades the central nervous system, it can act as a toxin, stimulating an inflammatory response. Cerebral vascular endothelial dam-

age can produce cerebral vasculitis, thrombosis, or infarction. Invasion of cerebral cortical tissue can produce cerebral edema and inflammation that can result in increased intracranial pressure and the development of subdural empyema. Edema or scarring of the outlet of the third ventricle produces stenosis of the sylvian aqueduct and results in obstruction to CSF flow and hydrocephalus.

■ **Clinical signs and symptoms**

In the infant less than 3 to 6 months of age, the diagnosis of meningitis is difficult because the signs of meningeal irritation are vague. The infant may be extremely irritable or lethargic with a history of poor feeding, vomiting, and fever. Seizures may also occur. If intracranial pressure is high, the anterior fontanelle will be full, and it may be tense. Although the presence of nuchal rigidity (stiff neck) provides an index of suspicion, it is often not present in the young infant.[33] The diagnosis is only confirmed by the results of the spinal tap.

The child with meningitis usually complains of headaches and photophobia (extreme sensitivity to light). Nuchal rigidity, neck pain, and sensitivity to touch are also present.

When meningitis is suspected, a complete blood cell count with white blood cell differential, glucose, electrolytes, and blood cultures should be obtained. This will help detect evidence of localized infection or sepsis. However, a lumbar puncture is usually required to confirm the diagnosis of meningitis. During the lumbar puncture, CSF samples are drawn. From these samples a culture, Gram's stain, and cell count will be performed, and protein and sugar levels will be measured. The general appearance of the fluid and the opening and closing CSF pressures should be noted in the nursing record. When bacterial meningitis is present, the glucose concentration of the cerebrospinal fluid is low, but the protein content is high; in addition, there will be a large number of cells present in the fluid, predominantly polymorphonuclear neutrophils. The culture and Gram's stain will be positive. When aseptic (viral or fungal) meningitis is present, the CSF glucose concentration is usually normal, and the protein content is only slightly elevated. In aseptic meningitis, there may be a moderate or large number of cells, predominantly polymorphonuclear leukocytes, early in the course and lymphocytes later in the course. The Gram's stain is usually negative, and the serologic culture is usually positive for virus.[10,33,43] (See Table 6-6 for further information about CSF findings.)

Since meningitis may be present in conjunction

with a local infection or sepsis, appropriate additional urine, serum, or wound cultures should be obtained as indicated.

In any child with untreated meningitis, symptoms may rapidly progress from mild irritability and fever to high fever, seizures, decreased level of consciousness, and coma.[33] Thus the effectiveness of treatment can be directly related to the speed of diagnosis and the early initiation of appropriate treatment.[58]

■ Medical treatment and nursing interventions

The treatment of meningitis includes the prompt initiation and uninterrupted administration of appropriate IV antimicrobial agents. This requires insertion of an IV catheter that is carefully taped and maintained. Usually, initial doses of broad-spectrum antibiotics are administered even before the results of the CSF cultures and sensitivities have been obtained. The infant or child is usually given nothing by mouth until his condition has stabilized. Accurate measurement of fluid intake and output and serum electrolyte concentrations is important since many children will develop the syndrome of inappropriate ADH secretion during or after the meningitis (see the discussion of this syndrome in the section on common clinical conditions in this chapter).

The infant's head circumference should be measured on admission and at least every 8 hours since subdural effusions and obstructive hydrocephalus can develop after meningitis and can be detected by an increase in head circumference. The infant or child with meningitis should be isolated until 24 hours of antibiotic therapy have been administered.[18]

The antibiotics of choice for treatment of meningitis of undetermined cause in the infant less than 2 months of age include intravenous gentamicin (2.5 mg/kg, then 1.85 mg/kg every 6 hours to total 7.5 mg/kg/day) and intravenous ampicillin sodium (100 mg/kg, then 50 mg/kg every 4 hours). If the infant is older than 2 months, the same dose of intravenous ampicillin is administered in conjunction with intravenous chloramphenicol succinate (25 mg/kg, then 25 mg/kg every 6 hours). Once the causative agent is identified, it is treated with specific antibiotics based on its sensitivities (Table 6-16). Recently, some *H. influenzae*, type B organisms have been found to be resistent to penicillin and ampicillin. This resistance can be determined by culture and by lactamase production tests; if the tests are positive, the ampicillin or the chloramphenicol may be discontinued and the remaining antibiotic continued as long as antibiotic

therapy is necessary. The recommended duration of continuous IV antibiotic treatment is 10 to 14 days or longer (chloramphenicol may be given orally during the last 5 days of therapy). Additional days of therapy are indicated if the patient fails to demonstrate clinical improvement or if additional CSF findings indicate partially-treated meningitis. Throughout therapy the nurse must monitor for side effects of the antibiotics.[18,33]

Some physicians will repeat the lumbar puncture after the child has received 24 to 36 hours of antibiotic therapy to evaluate the effectiveness of therapy. Other physicians recommend a repeat lumbar puncture just before the child completes the course of antibiotics. In any event, a repeat lumbar puncture should be performed whenever the child deteriorates clinically or whenever there is any question of the effectiveness of the antibiotics. CSF findings should return to normal (other than a mild elevation in lymphocyte count) before treatment is discontinued.[33,43]

If the infant or child has viral meningitis, supportive care is provided. Antibiotic administration is usually not indicated unless a concurrent bacterial infection is present.

Any child with meningitis should receive approximately 70% of maintenance fluids, and the nurse should assess the child carefully for signs of the syndrome of inappropriate ADH secretion (see the section on common clinical conditions in this chapter for more information). Antipyretics should be administered to reduce fever and to decrease the risk of febrile seizures. If seizures develop and progress to status epilepticus, prompt anticonvulsant therapy is essential (see the discussion of status epilepticus in the section of common clinical conditions in this chapter). If the child is septic, disseminated intravascular coagulation (DIC) may develop (see the section on disseminated intravascular coagulation in Chapter 8).

Throughout the first days of therapy, the infant or child should be watched closely for signs of increased intracranial pressure, continued fever, or neurologic deterioration (see the section on common clinical conditions in this chapter). These findings should be reported to a physician immediately. If the child does develop signs of increased intracranial pressure, intracranial pressure monitoring and diuresis may be required (see the section on increased intracranial pressure in the section on common clinical conditions in this chapter).

Long-term sequelae of meningitis in infants and children include hydrocephalus, seizures, sensory

Table 6-16 Recommended treatment for pyogenic meningitis

Organism	Drug	Comment
Etiology undetermined >2 months of age	Chloramphenicol succinate (25 mg/kg, then 25 mg/kg q6hr) and ampicillin sodium (100 mg/kg, then 50 mg/kg q4hr)	Both drugs should be started (they must not be mixed in the IV line; they must be administered consecutively) until causative organism is known
<2 months of age	Gentamicin or tobramycin (2.5 mg/kg, then 1.9 mg/kg q6hr) and ampicillin sodium (100 mg/kg, then 50 mg/kg q4hr)	
Haemophilus influenzae	Chloramphenicol succinate (25 mg/kg, then 25 mg/kg q6hr) and ampicillin sodium (100 mg/kg, then 50 mg/kg q4hr)	Both drugs should be started (see preceding comment about administration); one of them should be discontinued as soon as sensitivity of *H. influenzae* to ampicillin is established (using beta-lactamase test)
Neisseria meningitidis, Streptococcus pneumoniae, beta-hemolytic streptococci (group A or B)	Penicillin G sodium (100,000 IU/kg, then 50,000 IU/kg q4hr) or ampicillin sodium (100 mg/kg, then 50 mg/kg q4hr)	Some strains of *S. pneumoniae* show relative resistance to penicillin; sensitivity should be determined in the laboratory
Staphylococcus aureus	Methicillin (100 mg/kg, then 50 mg/kg q4hr)	Staphylococci should be checked for sensitivity and tolerance to methicillin
*Escherichia coli**	Gentamicin or tobramycin (2.5 mg/kg, then 1.9 mg/kg q6hr) and ampicillin sodium (100 mg/kg, then 50 mg/kg q4hr)	—
*Salmonella**	Chloramphenicol succinate (25 mg/kg, then 25 mg/kg q6hr) or ampicillin sodium (100 mg/kg, then 50 mg/kg q4hr) or both	Both drugs should be started; one should be discontinued as soon as sensitivities are determined
*Pseudomonas aeruginosa**	Tobramycin (2.5 mg/kg, then 1.9 mg/kg q6hr) and carbenicillin or ticarcillin (100 mg/kg, then 60 mg/kg q4hr)	—

Adapted from Rudolph, A.M., Pediatrics, ed. 17, New York, 1982, Appleton-Century-Crofts.
*Meningitis resulting from these gram-negative organisms is generally resistant to treatment; ventriculitis occurs commonly, and the prognosis is poor.

impairment, learning disability, cranial nerve palsies, hearing and sight impairment, and cerebral atrophy.[32,33]

■ **ENCEPHALITIS**
■ **Etiology**

Encephalitis is an inflammation of the brain. It can be associated with other CNS infections, such as meningitis, or it can be related to viral illness, such as rabies or herpes simplex. Encephalitis may appear during the course of an acute viral illness, or it may follow an infection such as measles, chicken pox, or rubella,[73] or vaccination (such as pertussis). The term "encephalitis" is used to indicate an infective or inflammatory cerebral disorder. The term "encephalopathy" is used to refer to any neurologic disorder of unknown or noninfectious cause associated with a change in level of consciousness, irritability, seizures, and motor or sensory deficit.[73] The following section refers to care of the child with encephalitis; for a summary of the management of the child with encephalopathy see the section on Reye's syndrome later in the chapter.

■ **Pathophysiology**

Encephalitis seems to be produced by entrance of a toxic or infectious agent into the brain. This produces an inflammatory response that is associated with cerebral edema, cellular damage, and transient neurologic dysfunction.

■ **Clinical signs and symptoms**

The child with encephalitis demonstrates symptoms during or immediately after an acute viral illness or following exposure to a toxic or inflammatory agent. The child usually complains of a headache, and he may demonstrate irritability, lethargy, a change in level of consciousness, nuchal rigidity, visual, auditory, and speech disturbances, seizures, or loss of consciousness. Most children with encephalitis are 5 to 14 years of age and most do not have high fevers.[20,42]

A lumbar puncture is usually performed to rule out a bacterial cause of the neurologic symptoms; it reveals normal CSF pressure, normal or increased cell count (lymphocytes may be present in increased quantity), normal or slightly increased protein concentration, and normal glucose concentration. The CSF culture and Gram's stain will yield no bacterial growth, but serologic tests may aid in the diagnosis of a viral agent (see Table 6-6). An EEG will reveal diffuse cortical inflammation, and a CT scan will fail to demonstrate a localized area of infection.[42]

■ **Medical treatment and nursing interventions**

Treatment of encephalitis is largely supportive. Antibiotic administration is not indicated since the disease is viral or toxic in origin. If the toxic agent can be identified (e.g., a drug) and if an antidote is available, this should be administered.

The child with encephalitis is monitored closely for signs of neurologic deterioration that may indicate greater inflammation or the development of increased intracranial pressure. Analgesics that do not produce respiratory depression (e.g., codeine) may be prescribed to relieve a persistent or severe headache. If the child complains of sensitivity to light or noise, provision of a private room or isolated bedspace is usually necessary so that the room light can be reduced and the noise kept to a minimum.

The child with encephalitis may demonstrate mild symptoms and a rapid recovery, or he may develop progressive neurologic deterioration and die. The prognosis depends on the causative agent and on the general health of the patient.[42,73]

■ **BRAIN ABSCESS**
■ **Etiology**

A brain abscess is an isolated intracranial collection of purulent fluid that is most commonly located in the cerebral hemispheres or the cerebellum. It usually develops after a bacteremia, but it can also occur as a result of chronic sinusitis or following a skull fracture. Children with cyanotic congenital heart disease (especially those older than 2 years) or those with bacterial endocarditis are at increased risk for the development of brain abscesses.

■ **Pathophysiology**

The pathogen enters the cerebral circulation at the site of intracranial surgery or compound skull fracture or as the result of a systemic or blood-borne infection. Abscesses can also spread into adjacent cerebral tissue from middle ear or mastoid infections.

The infected tissue is initially localized and is quickly invaded by white blood cells. Over a period of several weeks, necrotic tissue within the abscess liquifies, and the abscess becomes encapsulated by fibroblasts.[42] As the abscess grows, it can produce signs of increased intracranial pressure. If it ruptures, it can produce diffuse meningoencephalitis.

■ Clinical signs and symptoms

The child with a brain abscess may be asymptomatic during the initial period, or he may demonstrate nonspecific signs and symptoms including headache, fever, malaise, vomiting, confusion, seizures, motor, sensory or speech deficits, and leukocytosis. As the brain abscess enlarges, it produces signs of increased intracranial pressure, including a progressive headache, decreased level of consciousness, pupil dilation with sluggish or absent response to light (especially if uncal herniation develops), papilledema, cranial nerve deficits, and seizures. With enlargement of the abscess, progressive signs of increased intracranial pressure will develop (the signs are summarized in the section on clinical signs and symptoms of increased intracranial pressure earlier in this chapter).

A brain abscess may also produce some localized symptoms. If the child has a frontal lobe abscess, contralateral hemiparesis, frontal headache, aphasia, or seizures may be present. Temporal lobe abscesses can produce a temporal lobe headache and contralateral facial weakness. A cerebellar abscess often produces a postoccipital headache, nystagmus, ipsilateral ataxia, and limb weakness.[42]

A lumbar puncture will reveal an extremely high CSF pressure, a normal or increased cell count (with polymorphonuclear lymphocytes), an increased protein concentration, and a normal glucose concentration (see Table 6-6). The brain abscess can be localized with a CT scan, an EEG, and an arteriogram (see the section on diagnostic tests later in this chapter for further information).

■ Medical and surgical treatment and nursing interventions

Prompt initiation and continued administration of IV antibiotics is the treatment of choice for a brain abscess. The most common pathogens include anaerobic streptococci, *S. aureus*, and *E. coli*. As a result adminstration of penicillin G (200,000 to 400,000 IU/kg/day) or intravenous ampicillin (100 mg/kg, then 50 mg/kg every 4 hours) plus intravenous chloramphenicol (25 mg/kg, then 25 mg/kg every 6 hours) is usually ordered until the specific abscess pathogen is identified. Treatment of increased intracranial pressure may also be required (see the section on medical treatment of increased intracranial pressure earlier in this chapter).

If the abscess appears to be well encapsulated, surgical excision may be attempted. If complete excision is not possible, aspiration of the abscess and irrigation with antimicrobials may be performed one or more times.

Throughout the child's care it is important that the nurse monitor for signs of neurologic deterioration since increased intracranial pressure may develop and progress rapidly. Even with aggressive medical and surgical treatment of brain abscess, mortality is significant, and survivors may have neurologic deficits and seizures.[42]

■ REYE'S SYNDROME
■ Etiology

Reye's syndrome is a multisystem disease that is characterized by a severe encephalopathy with fatty degeneration and infiltration of the viscera (especially the liver) following recovery from a viral illness. Positive confirmation of Reye's syndrome is made by a liver biopsy, which reflects hepatic fatty degeneration. The cause of Reye's syndrome is unknown. Research has attempted to determine predictors of the disease or links between events occurring during the child's antecedent illness and the development and severity of the syndrome. Several retrospective studies have recently revealed an epidemiologic association between salicylate ingestion during the antecedent viral illness and later development of Reye's syndrome; children who were given aspirin during the viral illness seem to be more likely to develop Reye's syndrome than similar children who received acetaminophen or nothing.[67] Although these findings are not conclusive, they were compelling enough for the American Academy of Pediatrics to recommend that aspirin not be administered to children with influenza or varicella.[27]

■ Pathophysiology

Liver cellular mitochondrial damage interrupts the normal pathways for detoxification of waste products; these disrupted pathways include the urea cycle. The urea cycle is responsible for the breakdown of serum ammonia to urea, which is then excreted (see Fig. 8-20 in Chapter 8). As the disease progresses and as this cycle remains incomplete, serum ammonia rises (the normal range is 0 to 80 μg/dl or 0 to 48 μmol/L). These ammonia levels and other unknown factors become toxic to the body and may contribute to the development of cerebral dysfunction. Decreased mitochondrial function triggers alternate pathways to supply the cells with needed oxygen and glucose; pyruvic acid is converted to lactic acid, and metabolic acidosis develops. The child often becomes hypoglycemic and dehydrated, particularly if vomiting develops, and hyperventilation may produce a respiratory alkalosis.

Fluid and electrolyte imbalance (including dehydration, hypoglycemia, and acidosis) and coagulopathies result from liver dysfunction. Neurologic complications are the result of the development of toxic encephalopathy, cerebral edema (cytotoxic edema), and increased intracranial pressure; these problems seem to be related to hyperammoniemia, hypoglycemia, possible direct effects of the antecedent viral illness, and other unknown factors.

■ Clinical signs and symptoms

Reye's syndrome occurs most commonly in children 6 to 12 years of age, and signs and symptoms usually occur 4 to 7 days after a systemic viral illness. The child may develop mild symptoms such as malaise, nausea, and vomiting followed by complete recovery, or he may demonstrate progressive deterioration and coma over the course of a few hours. As a result it is helpful to consider the child's neurologic symptomatology in terms of staging of the disease described by Huttenlocher or Lovejoy.[50] Since staging of the coma is so closely linked with treatment and prognosis, the Lovejoy and Huttenlocher staging criteria will be elaborated in the following discussion.

The Huttenlocher staging, which involves four stages, is used for staging of coma in any patient, including the patient with Reye's syndrome.

In the *first stage* the child may be mildly confused or listless and apathetic, and vomiting is present. Occasionally, the child may become sleepy and unresponsive. The child in *stage two* is restless, ir-

ritable, disoriented, and combative. These children can quickly become unresponsive, and decorticate rigidity may be noted. Hyperpnea, tachycardia, fever, and pupil dilation are often observed at this time. In the *third stage* the child is totally unresponsive, and decerebrate posturing may be present. In *stage four* brainstem function (including cranial nerve function and oculocephalic and oculovestibular reflexes) is absent. The child is apneic with fixed and dilated pupils and flaccid paralysis.[20]

The Lovejoy staging is a five-stage rating system that is based on the Huttenlocher staging with the addition of liver function studies and EEG findings.[48,50] (These findings are summarized in the box below.)

In the *first stage* the child begins to vomit, and is lethargic. Laboratory evidence of liver dysfunction can be obtained. If an EEG is performed, it will reveal rhythmic slowing (Type 1 EEG).

In the *second stage* the child becomes agitated, delirious, and combative. Reflexes are hyperactive and hyperventilation is present. The child will still withdraw an extremity from a painful stimulus. Serologic evidence of abnormal liver function continues to be present, and the EEG demonstrates dysrhythmic slowing (Type 2 EEG).

In the *third stage* the child is unresponsive and comatose with decorticate rigidity and hyperventilation. Brainstem reflexes (including brisk pupillary constriction in response to light and oculovestibular and oculocephalic reflexes) remain intact (see the section on clinical signs and symptoms of coma earlier in this chapter for further information). Liver function studies are abnormal, and dysrhythmic EEG slowing is present (Type 2 EEG).

In the *fourth stage* the child is comatose, and

LOVEJOY STAGING OF COMA IN REYE'S SYNDROME[48,50]

Stage 1   Vomiting, lethargic; serologic evidence of liver dysfunction; EEG—rhythmic slowing, dominant theta waves, rare delta waves

Stage 2   Agitated, delirious, combative; hyperactive reflexes and hyperventilation; withdraws extremity from painful stimuli; serologic evidence of liver dysfunction; EEG—dysrhythmic slowing, dominent delta waves, some theta waves

Stage 3   Unresponsive, comatose; decorticate rigidity and hyperventilation; intact brainstem reflexes; serologic evidence of liver dysfunction; EEG—dysrhythmic slowing, dominent delta waves, some theta waves

Stage 4   Unresponsive, comatose; oculocephalic and oculovestibular reflexes absent; pupils dilated and fixed; decerebrate posturing; minimal serologic evidence of liver dysfunction; EEG—disorganized, monorhythmic, polyrhythmic delta waves, or isoelectric

Stage 5   Comatose; flaccid extremities, absence of spontaneous respirations; no withdrawal from painful stimuli; absent deep tendon reflexes; liver function normal; EEG—isoelectric oculocephalic ("doll's eye's") and oculovestibular ("calorics") reflexes are no longer present. The pupils are dilated and fixed, and decerebrate posturing is present. Serologic evidence of liver dysfunction is present, although it may show improvement. The EEG demonstrates severe cerebral dysfunction, including disorganized monorhythmic or polyrhythmic delta waves (Type 3 EEG) or an isoelectric EEG (Type 4 EEG).

In the *fifth* stage the child is comatose with flaccid extremities and absence of spontaneous respirations. There is no withdrawal from painful stimuli, and deep tendon reflexes are absent. Liver function may return to normal, and an isoelectric EEG is present (Type 4 EEG).

Cerebral dysfunction is the most severe but not the only clinical consequence of Reye's syndrome. The child also demonstrates evidence of liver dysfunction, including an elevation in serum glutamic-oxaloacetic transaminase (SGOT), serum glutamic-pyruvic transaminase (SGPT), and blood ammonia levels. The prothrombin (PT) and partial thromboplastin (PTT) times will be prolonged. The serum concentrations of uric acid, lactate, pyruvate, amino acids, free fatty acids, and serum enzymes, including lactic dehydrogenase (LDH), amylase and lipase are usually elevated.[20] The child's serum glucose concentration may be normal initially, but it can decrease rapidly as a result of poor intake, vomiting, and stress. In infants and young children significant hypoglycemia may be noted on admission.

While initial blood samples will be drawn on admission to support the diagnosis of Reye's syndrome, the child's neurologic status should be rapidly assessed, and treatment should be taken immediately to reduce any existing intracranial hypertension. The child may demonstrate signs and symptoms of early stages of Reye's syndrome without progression, or he may progress through the latter stages of coma; the progression may be gradual or fulminant. Thus the value of rapid recognition and prompt and effective treatment of Reye's syndrome cannot be underestimated.

Reye's syndrome must be differentiated from other disorders that can produce coma and liver failure. These include severe hypoglycemia, drug ingestion (including salicylate toxicity or phenobarbital or phenothiazine ingestion), and toxic exposure (such as lead encephalopathy).

■ **Medical treatment and nursing interventions**

The following information pertains largely to management of the neurologic problems associated with Reye's syndrome. For a discussion of treatment of the complications of liver dysfunction the reader is referred to the section on Reye's syndrome in Chapter 8.

When the child is admitted with a presumptive diagnosis of Reye's syndrome, the nurse should perform a thorough but rapid neurologic assessment. A large bore IV line is inserted, and hypovolemia or poor systemic perfusion should be treated as needed (see the section on low cardiac output in Chapter 3). Aggressive fluid administration is, however, contraindicated in these patients, especially if signs of increased intracranial pressure are present. If the child is apneic or demonstrates signs of deep coma or intracranial hypertension, an ET tube will be inserted and hyperventilation performed in an attempt to reduce cerebral blood volume and intracranial pressure. If the child is demonstrating deep coma, lack of response to painful stimuli, and decerebrate posturing, many physicians will institute intracranial pressure monitoring (see the discussion of intracranial pressure monitoring with increased intracranial pressure earlier in this chapter). Blood should be drawn for appropriate serologic tests, and the child's first urine specimen should be sent for toxicology screening if the diagnosis of Reye's syndrome is uncertain. The child's vital signs and neurologic function should be assessed continuously, and the physician should be notified of any deterioration in clinical status. If an intracranial pressure monitoring device is placed, the child's intracranial pressure and cerebral perfusion pressure should be recorded hourly and whenever a change in intracranial pressure or mean arterial pressure develops (cerebral perfusion pressure = mean arterial pressure − intracranial pressure).[39]

The thrust of medical and nursing care is to prevent or reduce intracranial hypertension. The child with Reye's syndrome has a combined vasogenic, cytotoxic, and hyperemic cerebral edema; this must be effectively treated to prevent fatal increases in intracranial pressure.[20] If intracranial pressure monitoring is initiated, the nurse should obtain specific orders to maintain the intracranial pressure below 20 to 25 mm Hg with hyperventilation as necessary. This hyperventilation provides the most effective acute treatment of intracranial hypertension.[78] The child's arterial carbon dioxide tension should be maintained between 25 to 29 mm Hg, and his arterial oxygen tension should be maintained between 80 to 100 mm Hg (60 to 80 mm Hg in neonates) through mechanical ventilation. Diuretics may be ordered to reduce cerebral edema by eliminating excess free water through the urine, and hypertonic solutions (such as 25% to 50% glucose), blood products, or colloids may be administered to maintain the serum osmolality between 280 to 320 mOsm/L. Small doses of mannitol may also be ordered if other hypertonic agents are ineffective. Corticosteroids may be prescribed to reduce vasogenic cerebral edema. If all other methods of controlling intracranial hypertension fail, the child may be placed in a pentobarbital coma with hypothermia to reduce cerebral metabolic requirements until the cerebral edema subsides.[70] This treatment is reviewed in detail in the discussion of medical treatment and nursing interventions of increased intracranial pressure earlier in this chapter.

The child with Reye's syndrome may require additional glucose or calcium supplements, and blood component therapy may be required to correct coagulopathies produced by liver dysfunction. These therapies are discussed in detail in the section on medical treatment and nursing interventions of Reye's syndrome in Chapter 8 (see also Table 3-10 for a review of treatment of coagulopathies).

If the child with Reye's syndrome is admitted before coma or signs of increased intracranial pressure develop, the child should be placed in a quiet area with parents present and a nurse in constant attendance. This nurse must be able to reduce the child's and the family's anxiety and to detect signs of neurologic deterioration as soon as they begin to develop. This disease is frightening to the child, the family, and the medical team because it can produce mild neurologic symptoms or rapid, progressive, and fatal neurologic dysfunction. With the development of more sophsticated intracranial pressure monitoring and better supportive therapy, survival rates following Reye's syndrome are improved. However, the incidence of significant neurologic sequelae is high.[78,79] Thus the parents and child will require a great deal of consistent information and support throughout the child's hospitalization and continued medical follow-up after discharge.

■ **GUILLAIN-BARRÉ SYNDROME**
■ **Etiology**

Guillain-Barré syndrome is the association of a precedent infection, progressive motor weakness, and elevated CSF protein content. The precedent illness may be an upper respiratory infection or a viral illness such as varicella, rubella, or enterovirus. This syndrome can also occur as a toxic response to viral vaccinations. The disease occurs most commonly in children 4 to 10 years of age.[11,88]

The cause of Guillain-Barré syndrome is unknown, but it seems to be related to an autoimmune or inflammatory process that produces inflammation of nerves and nerve roots.

■ **Pathophysiology**

The inflammation of the nerves and nerve roots involves the endodural and epidural blood vessels. Initially, the myelin becomes edematous; demyelinization then develops, producing decreased speed and intensity of peripheral nerve conduction. Nerve degeneration can also occur.[11]

■ **Clinical signs and symptoms**

Clinical signs and symptoms produced by this syndrome are determined by the severity and extent of nerve involvement. The patient with Guillain-Barré syndrome usually contracts an upper respiratory illness, a virus such as varicella, or receives a viral immunization approximately 3 weeks before the onset of symptoms.[11] The child may complain of limb paresthesia or pain but soon demonstrates weakness of the lower extremities and possible loss of deep tendon reflexes. Over a period of several days or weeks, the motor weakness ascends to include the arms and possibly the cranial nerves. If the intercostal muscles are paralyzed, the child will require ventilatory assistance. Glossopharyngeal and vagus nerve dysfunction develop in approximately half of all involved patients and produce impairment of gag and swallow reflexes.

During the initial stages of the illness, the child may demonstrate autonomic instability, including wide fluctuations in blood pressure, diaphoresis, vasoconstriction, pupil dilation and constriction, and cardiac arrhythmias.[11,88] The cerebrospinal fluid is usually normal except for an elevation in CSF protein content.

Recovery from Guillain-Barré syndrome usually begins approximately 4 weeks after the onset of symptoms. Although complete recovery occurs in approximately three fourths of all involved children, approximately 5% to 7% of affected patients die, and 10% to 15% are left with significant neurologic sequelae.[11,88]

■ **Medical treatment and nursing interventions**

Treatment of the child with Guillain-Barré syndrome is largely supportive. Thorough and frequent neurologic evaluation should be performed, including assessment of limb movement and strength and assessment of cranial nerve function (see Table 6-13). Respiratory support should be initiated if clinical evidence of respiratory failure develops, including hypercapnia ($Paco_2$ more than 50 mm Hg), hypoxemia (Pao_2 less than 50 mm Hg during room air breathing) or decreased aeration. In addition, intubation and ventilatory support should be initiated if the child develops difficulty in coughing or swallowing or slurring of speech since these signs usually indicate cranial nerve involvement and usually precede the development of respiratory arrest. Mechanical ventilatory support is also required if the maximal inspiratory force is less than −20 cm H_2O, if the vital capacity is less than 15 ml/kg, or if the forced expiratory volume is less than 10 ml/kg.[86] (Other clinical signs and symptoms of respiratory failure are discussed in Chapter 4.) Weaning from ventilatory support will be undertaken as respiratory function improves.

The child with Guillain-Barré syndrome requires careful monitoring of cardiovascular function and systemic perfusion. Arrhythmias and hypotension should be treated whenever they result in a compromise of systemic perfusion (see Chapter 3 for further information).

Supportive care includes provision of adequate caloric intake (nasogastric or parenteral alimentation may be required), passive and active range-of-motion exercises, and good skin care. Some physicians recommend administration of adrenocorticotrophic hormone (ACTH) or prednisone (2 mg/kg/day), although their efficacy has not been proven.[11,88]

Although recovery from Guillain-Barré syndrome is likely, the uncertainty of the disease progression and the loss of function can be extremely frightening to the child and family. In addition, the child may be hospitalized for a prolonged period of time. Therefore the child should be assigned consistent caretakers who will best be able to recognize changes in clinical status and provide the patient and family with consistent information and support.

■ Common Diagnostic Tests

One of the best methods of evaluating the neurologic function in the child is a thorough neurologic examination. However, in the critically ill or unresponsive child, it is often difficult to determine the severity of a neurologic injury or deficit, and it may be difficult to separate signs of neurologic disease from neurologic depression associated with failure of other body systems. As a result a few diagnostic studies can provide additional important information about the child's diagnosis, clinical status, or prognosis.

■ LUMBAR PUNCTURE
■ Definition and purpose

A lumbar puncture or spinal tap is performed by introducing a needle into the subarachnoid space of the lumbar spinal canal. The needle is inserted through a stylet into the interspace between the third and fourth lumbar vertebrae; when the lumbar puncture is performed at this level, damage to the spinal cord is avoided.[42,85]

The lumbar puncture may be performed to measure CSF pressure, to examine the cerebrospinal fluid, or to introduce medication, air, or radiopaque contrast material into the subarachnoid space. The lumbar puncture will aid in the diagnosis of intracranial or intraventricular hemorrhage if blood is present in the cerebrospinal fluid. The fluid can be sent for culture, Gram's stain, cell count, and glucose and protein content to aid in the diagnosis of CNS infection or inflammation. In addition, anesthesia or antibiotics may be introduced into the subarachnoid space to reduce pain or treat infection, respectively. Finally, injected air or radiopaque contrast material can be used to outline subarachnoid structures or identify CSF obstructions or leaks. In the pediatric critical-care unit, the lumbar puncture is used most often to confirm the diagnosis of CNS infection.[42,85]

■ Procedure

The lumbar puncture is quite safe when it is performed correctly by an experienced physician. Before the procedure, the child should be examined carefully for signs of increased intracranial pressure. If these are present in the *infant*, the lumbar puncture may proceed with caution if a CSF sample is absolutely necessary to treat the child's CNS disease. If, however, signs or suspicion of increased intracranial pressure are present in the *older child* with fused cranial sutures, the lumbar puncture may be postponed since the sudden release of cerebrospinal fluid and pressure by the lumbar puncture can result in herniation of the medulla through the foramen magnum.

The procedure should be explained carefully to the child (as age-appropriate). The child is placed in the knee-chest position, either sitting up or lying on his side with his neck flexed toward the knees; this position provides maximal separation of the vertebral bodies. Occasionally, however, some modification of position may have to be made if the child is intubated or has major trauma and fractures. The child should be held firmly to prevent excessive movement during the lumbar puncture.[42,85]

Once the child is positioned, the back is draped and the puncture area is identified and scrubbed with a surgical preparation (such as an iodine solution), and the remainder of the procedure is performed using strict aseptic technique. Xylocaine is infiltrated intradermally around the area of puncture to provide local anesthesia. The needle and stylet are then firmly inserted into the subarachnoid space; frequently, a sharp sound is heard when the dura is pierced.[85]

As soon as the subarachnoid space is entered, the opening CSF pressure is obtained with a manometer. A few drops of cerebrospinal fluid are then allowed to drain from the stylet. Additional cerebrospinal fluid is collected in three or more sterile sampling tubes as follows:

Tube 1—Culture and Gram's stain analysis

Tube 2—Protein and sugar analysis

Tube 3—cell count

Additional tubes as needed for viral cultures or other special studies

The appearance of the cerebrospinal fluid in the test tube should be noted. If red blood cells were present in the initial drops of cerebrospinal fluid as the result of a traumatic tap, the fluid should be clear by the time the final tube is filled. If, on the other hand, intracranial hemorrhage is present, the final CSF collection tube will still contain red blood cells. CSF *cloudiness* is usually abnormal and often indicates the presence of infection. *Xanthochromia* (yellow discoloration of the cerebrospinal fluid) may be noted as the result of hyperbilirubinemia or the presence of hemolyzed red blood cells. Changes in the CSF content with common CNS diseases have been included in Table 6-6.[42,85]

Before the lumbar puncture is completed, a measurement of the CSF closing pressure is made, the stylet is withdrawn, and a small dressing is placed over the area of the puncture site. The opening and closing pressures may be used to calculate an *Ayala's index* as follows:

$$\text{Ayala's index} = \frac{\text{Quantity of fluid removed} \times \text{Spinal closing pressure}}{\text{Initial pressure}}$$

The normal range of Ayala's index is 5.5 to 6.5. An Ayala's index of greater than 7.0 is often indicative of the presence of a large CSF reservoir, such as occurs in hydrocephalus. An Ayala's index of 5.0 or less usually indicates a subarachnoid obstruction.

■ **Nursing responsibilities and complications**

It is the nurse's responsibility to prepare the child (as age-appropriate) for the procedure, and to position, monitor, and comfort him throughout the procedure. In addition, the nurse must ensure that all CSF samples are correctly labeled and sent for analysis.

The most serious (although unusual) complication of a lumbar puncture is brainstem herniation.

Therefore, during and after the lumbar puncture, the nurse should monitor for signs of deterioration of neurologic status that may indicate brainstem herniation. These signs include decreased responsiveness, tachycardia or bradycardia, unilateral or bilateral pupil dilation with sluggish constriction to light, hypertension with widening pulse pressure, apnea, and abnormal posturing. These signs should be reported to a physician immediately, and efforts should be made to acutely reduce intracranial pressure (see the discussion of increased intracranial pressure earlier in this chapter).

Additional complications of the lumbar puncture include severe headache and bleeding from the puncture site.[42] Many physicians request that the child be kept in a reclining position for 4 to 6 hours after the procedure to reduce the possibility and severity of headaches. Analgesics should be given as needed and per physician order.[49]

■ **ELECTROENCEPHALOGRAPHY (EEG)**
■ **Definition and purpose**

The electroencephalogram (EEG) is a recording of the electrical potentials that arise from the brain. These potentials can be quantified, localized, and compared with established, normal EEGs for the patient's age to aid in the diagnosis of seizure activity or CNS injury or dysfunction.[42,83] Specific changes in the EEG of the child with Reye's syndrome can be used to stage the child's symptoms and to monitor the child's progress or deterioration. An isoelectric (flat) EEG in the nonhypothermic, nonsedated patient is one of the criteria for diagnosis of cerebral death.

■ **Procedure**

The EEG is recorded by placement of approximately 17 to 21 electrodes on the surface of the frontal, parietal, occipital, and temporal areas of the scalp and over the ear. These electrodes are fixed with an acetone-soluble paste to prevent electrode movement during the study. The EEG is performed when the patient is reclining and still. When this study is required in critically ill patients, it is generally performed in the critical-care unit.

The EEG is usually recorded continuously for 20 minutes; longer recordings will be necessary if additional studies (such as measurement of brainstem evoked auditory potentials) are requested. Since the cerebral electrical activity must be magnified to provide a visible recorded signal, patient movement and electrical (equipment) artifact must be reduced to a minimum. Since extraneous or sudden noise or lights can stimulate cranial nerve electrical activity, they should be minimized during the recording. In the event that the child is alert and mobile, sedation may be required.

The EEG is usually recorded during sleep (or coma), and the recording is often continued during hyperventilation and with photic (rhythmic light flash) stimulation. The sleep EEG allows analysis of baseline activity; hyperventilation is used to accentuate abnormal EEG findings. A 2-minute, rhythmic, light flash (photic stimulation) may be performed in an attempt to induce seizure activity during the recording.

Brainstem evoked responses have been tested recently to evaluate cranial nerve responses and early evidence of cranial nerve damage. This is particularly useful in the newborn or comatose patient when specific response to a specific stimulus is difficult or impossible to detect. The brainstem evoked auditory response is obtained by recording electrical activity over the auditory pathway after provision of a standard auditory stimulus. If the acoustic *nerve* itself is damaged, early conduction of the impulse *through* the nerve will be prolonged or diminished; this can occur, for example, as a complication of drug therapy and resultant ototoxicity. If *brainstem* disease or dysfunction is present, conduction of the auditory impulse through the nerve will be normal, but the time required for the impulse to travel *between* the auditory nerve and the brainstem will be prolonged.

■ **Nursing responsibilities and complications**

Before the EEG is obtained, the procedure should be described to the child (as age-appropriate) and parents. Important points to emphasize include the fact that the procedure is painless, and (if applicable) that the child will be given medication to make him drowsy. In addition, the child should be told that some special soap (acetone) is used to clean the hair after the procedure since the acetone has a distinctive and noxious odor. If the child is awake and alert, the nurse should administer a sedative or chloral hydrate as ordered by a physician.

During the EEG, it is important that the nurse avoid touching or stimulating the patient more than is absolutely necessary for safe care. Lights should be dimmed, and noises should be reduced to a minimum. The nurse should remain near the child's bedside throughout the EEG to answer questions, provide hyperventilation as requested, and monitor the child throughout the procedure.

There are no complications of the standard EEG.

■ **SKULL ROENTGENOGRAPHY (SKULL FILMS)**
■ **Definition and purpose**

Skull roentgenography (or skull radiographs or films) evaluates cranial bone relationships and densities and the size and shape of the skull. Skull films are helpful in the diagnosis of skull deformities or fractures, head injuries, and bone erosion or calcification secondary to space-occupying lesions. Skull films, however, are often not helpful in the diagnosis of a brain tumor.[24] A complete roentgenographic study of the skull includes anteroposterior and lateral views of the skull and an oblique anteroposterior view or other special angles as indicated by the child's presumed diagnosis.

■ **Procedure**

Preferably skull films are obtained in the radiology department so that the patient's head can be immobilized and so that good quality radiographs can be obtained. If this is impossible, portable radiographs are obtained in the critical-care unit. The x-ray technician will assist in positioning the child appropriately for each film.

■ **Nursing responsibilities and complications**

Explanations should be provided to the child (as age-appropriate) and family about the need for radiographs and about any special positioning that is required. The nurse should monitor the child closely throughout the procedure. If an intracranial pressure monitoring system is in place, the nurse should monitor the effect of changes in head position on the child's intracranial pressure and suggest modifications in these positions as needed to maintain the intracranial pressure at appropriate levels. The procedure is painless. The only complication of skull roentgenograms is the small amount of radiation emitted.[24,36]

■ **CEREBRAL ANGIOGRAPHY**
■ **Definition and purpose**

In cerebral angiography, the injection of a radiopaque contrast agent into the cerebral arterial system enables radiographic visualization of cerebral circulation.[36,45] The progress of the contrast material through the cerebral circulation is recorded with radiographs for further study. Angiography is helpful in the diagnosis of intracranial tumor, hematoma, arterial aneurysm, and arteriovenous fistula.

■ Procedure

Contrast material (usually an iodine-containing material) is injected into a selected cerebral vessel—usually into the internal carotid artery. Sequential roentgenograms of the head are then taken. This procedure is usually performed in the radiology department.

■ Nursing responsibilities and complications

The procedure should be carefully explained to the child and parents. It is usually best to limit the child's explanation to only those things that he will see, hear, or feel; most often, the child is either frightened or intrigued by the x-ray equipment.

Since the child will be transported to the radiology department for the angiography, the nurse is responsible for monitoring the child's condition during transport to and from the radiology department and throughout the procedure itself.

A reaction to the contrast agent can occur following angiography; this can include fever, a rash, and hypotension similar to that occurring with anaphylaxis. If an active cerebral hemorrhage is present or develops during the procedure, the contrast agent can enter cerebral tissue, producing a cerebral vascular accident, seizures, increased intracranial pressure, cerebral arterial thrombosis, dysphagia, or visual difficulty.[42] In addition, injection of the contrast material directly into the internal carotid artery may stimulate the carotid baroreceptors, causing compensatory bradycardia and hypotension.[42]

■ COMPUTERIZED TOMOGRAPHY (CT SCAN)
■ Definition and purpose

Computerized axial tomography (CAT or CT scan) consists of a series of skull radiographs analyzed and reconstructed by a computer to form a pictorial image of the intracranial contents.[40] The scan is obtained using an x-ray beam in motion that obtains a series of radiographic films in predetermined planes. These films are converted to images similar to those that would be produced if radiographs could be obtained of separate layers of the brain. The images produced by the scan allow differentiation of intracranial spaces and normal gray and white matter (Fig. 6-14).

The CAT or CT scan is a reliable, painless, safe, and noninvasive method of visualizing a variety of neurologic disorders, including space-occupying lesions, hematomas, hemorrhage, hydrocephalus, brain abscess, and cortical atrophy. This scan has eliminated or reduced the need for many other more invasive diagnostic neurologic tests[36]; it is especially useful in the treatment of children with head trauma.

■ Procedure

This procedure must be performed in the neuroradiology department. The child is positioned supine on a mobile platform that is then moved toward the scanner so that the child's head is ultimately positioned within the scanner. A portion of the scanner will move around the child's head so that the x-ray beam is directed at many different angles; hundreds of radiographs are obtained and reconstructed during the scan.

The entire CT scan takes approximately 20 to 30 minutes. Occasionally, contrast agents are administered intravenously immediately before the scan to enable better visualization of intracranial structures.[40]

■ Nursing responsibilities and complications

The nurse will prepare the child for the procedure (including a discussion of the noises that the child will hear during the scan) and monitor the child during the procedure itself. Since the child must be kept absolutely still throughout the procedure, sedation or chloral hydrate are usually administered (per physician order) before the procedure is begun.

During the procedure, health care personnel and x-ray technicians may be positioned behind a lead screen to minimize stray radiation exposure. Therefore it will be necessary for the nurse to periodically check the child and ensure proper functioning of the child's IV equipment and mechanical ventilatory support; in addition, the child should be viewed continuously during the procedure.

There are no complications associated with the CAT scan. The radiation exposure is approximately equivalent to that produced during a series of skull films.[42] If a contrast agent is injected before the scan, the nurse must monitor for signs of a reaction to the contrast material or for evidence of complications similar to those occurring after cerebral angiography.

REFERENCES

1. Ad Hoc Committee of Harvard Medical School to examine the definition of brain death: A definition of irreversible coma, JAMA 205:85, 1968.
2. Aicardi, J., and Chevrie, J.J.: Convulsive status epilepticus in infants and children, Epilepsia 11:187, 1970.
3. Albert, R.K., and Candie, F.: Handwashing patterns in medical intensive care units, N. Engl. J. Med. 304:1465, 1981.

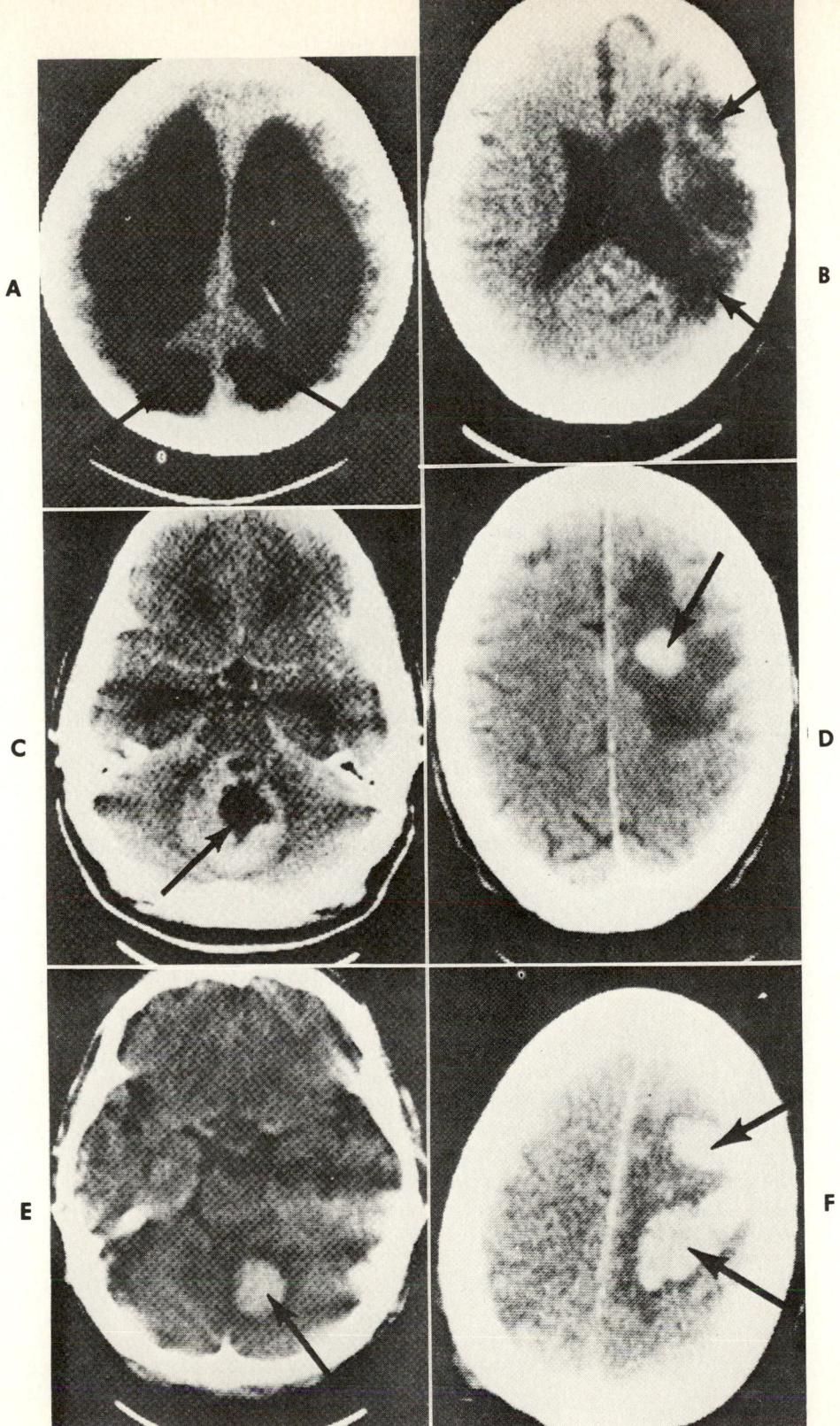

Fig. 6-14 Representative examples of abnormal computerized axial tomograms (CT scans). **A,** Ventricles *(arrows)* are grossly dilated as the result of hydrocephalus. **B,** Cerebral hemiatrophy is present in a patient with a history of previous subarachnoid hemorrhage *(arrow)*. **C,** Arrow indicates the location of a brain tumor, which was proved to be a cerebellar medulloblastoma. **D,** Frontal lobe brain tumor *(arrow)*. **E,** Cerebellar hemorrhage *(arrow)*. **F,** Intracerebral hemorrhage *(arrows)* developed as the result of severe head injury.

Courtesy G.P. Ballweg and reproduced with permission from Chusid, J.G.: Radiologic examination. In Correlative neuroanatomy and functional neurology, ed. 18, Los Altos, Calif., 1982, Lange Medical Publications.

4. American Cancer Society: Cancer in children, New York, 1964, The Society.

5. Anderson, E.F., and Rosenthal, M.H.: Pancuronium bromide and tachyarrhythmias, Crit. Care Med. **3**:13, 1975.

6. Barber, J.M., and Budassi, S.A.: Neurologic emergencies. In: Mosby's manual of emergency care, St. Louis, 1979, The C.V. Mosby Co.

7. Barness, L.A.: The neurological examination. In: Manual of pediatric physical examination, ed. 5, Chicago, 1981, Year Book Medical Publishers Inc.

8. Becker, D., and Foley, T.: 1-deamino-8-D-arginine vasopressin in the treatment of central diabetes insipidus in childhood, J. Pediatr. **92**(6):1011, 1978.

9. Bell, W.E.: Increased intracranial pressure: diagnosis and management, (monograph), Curr. Prob. Pediatr. **7**:1, February 1978.

10. Bell, W.E.: Bacterial meningitis. In Rudolph, A.M., editor: Pediatrics, ed. 17, Norwalk, Conn., 1982, Appleton-Century-Crofts.

11. Blaw, M., and Levin, D.L.: Guillain-Barré syndrome. In Levin, D.L., Morriss, F.C., and Moore, G.C., editors: A practical guide to pediatric intensive care, ed. 2, St. Louis, 1984, The C.V. Mosby Co.

12. Bruce, D.A., Gennarelli, T.A., and Langfitt, T.W.: Resuscitation from coma due to head injury, Crit. Care. Med. **6**:254, 1978.

13. Bruce, D.A., and Schut, L.: Management of acute craniocerebral trauma in children, Contemp. Neurosurg. **10**:1, 1979.

14. Capildeo, R.: Cerebrovascular disease. In Rose, F.C., editor: Paediatric neurology, Oxford, 1979, Blackwell Scientific Publications Inc.

15. Chusid, J.G.: The brain. In: Correlative neuroanatomy and functional neurology, ed. 18, Los Altos, Calif., 1982, Lange Medical Publications.

16. Cleaveland, M.J.: Tumors of the central nervous system. In Fochtman, D., and Foley, G.V., editors: Nursing care of the child with cancer, Boston, 1982, Little, Brown & Co.

17. Collaborative study: An appraisal of the criteria of cerebral brain death, JAMA **237**:982, 1977.

18. Conway, B.L.: Pediatric neurologic nursing, St. Louis, 1977, The C.V. Mosby Co.

19. Conway, B.L.: Expanding intracranial and spinal cord lesions and related disorders. In: Pediatric neurologic nursing, St. Louis, 1977, The C.V. Mosby Co.

20. DeVivo, D.C.: Acute encephalopathies of childhood. In Rudolph, A.M., editor: Pediatrics, ed. 17, Norwalk, Conn., 1982, Appleton-Century-Crofts.

21. Eckstein, H.B.: Hydrocephalus. In Rose, F.C., editor: Paediatric neurology, Oxford, 1979, Blackwell Scientific Publications Inc.

22. Falwell, J.R., and others: Central nervous system tumor in children, Cancer **40**:3123, 1977.

23. Finklestein, S., and Ropper, A.: The diagnosis of coma: its pitfalls and limitations, Heart Lung **8**:1059, 1979.

24. Fish, I.: Diagnostic tools in neurology, Pediatr. Ann. **7**:438, 1975.

25. Fochtman, D., and others: The treatment of cancer in children. In Fochtman, D., and Foley, G.V., editors: Nursing care of the child with cancer, Boston, 1982, Little, Brown & Co.

26. Friedman, A., and Segar, W.: Antidiuretic hormone excess, J. Pediatr. **94**:521, 1979.

27. Fulginitti, V.A., and others: Special report from the Committee on Infectious Diseases: aspirin and Reye syndrome, Pediatrics **69**:810, 1982.

28. Ganong, W.: Review of medical physiology, ed. 11, Los Altos, Calif., 1983, Lange Medical Publications.

29. Gardner-Thorpe, C.: The epilepsies. In Rose, F.C., editor: Paediatric neurology, Oxford, 1979, Blackwell Scientific Publications Inc.

30. Goodman, L., and Gillman, A.: The pharmacologic basis of therapeutics, ed. 7, New York, 1982, Macmillan Publishing Co., Inc.

31. Green, S.H.: Neurophysiology. In Godfrey, S., and Baum, J.D., editors: Clinical paediatric physiology, Oxford, 1979, Blackwell Scientific Publications Inc.

32. Green, S.H., and George, R.H.: Bacterial meningitis. In Rose, F.C., editor: Paediatric neurology, Oxford, 1979, Blackwell Scientific Publications Inc.

33. Grossman, M.: Meningitis. In Rudolph, A.M., editor: Pediatrics, ed. 17, Norwalk, Conn., 1982, Appleton-Century-Crofts.

34. Gruskin, A.B.: Serum sodium abnormalities in children, Pediatr. Clin. North Am. **29**:907, 1982.

35. Guertin, S.R., and others: Intracranial volume-pressure response in infants and children, Crit. Care Med. **10**:1, 1982.

36. Guinto, F.C., and Stevens, E.A.: Neuroradiologic examination. In Farmer, T.W.: Pediatric neurology, ed. 3, Philadelphia, 1983, Harper and Row, Publishers Inc.

37. Hahn, J.F.: Cerebral edema and neurointensive care, Pediatr. Clin. North Am. **27**:587, 1980.

38. Hall, D.: Neonatal neurology. In Rose, F.C., editor: Paediatric neurology, Oxford, 1979, Blackwell Scientific Publications Inc.

39. Haller, J.: Intracranial pressure monitoring in Reye's syndrome, Hosp. Pract. **15**:101, 1980.

40. Hammock, M.K., and Milhorat, T.H.: Cranial computed tomography in infancy and childhood, Baltimore, 1981, Williams & Wilkins.

41. Hausman, K.A.: Critical care of the child with increased intracranial pressure, Nurs. Clin. North Am. **16**:647, 1981.

42. Hickey, J.V.: The clinical practice of neurological and neurosurgical nursing, Philadelphia, 1981, J.B. Lippincott Co.

43. Hieber, J.P.: Encephalitis/meningitis. In Levin, D.L., Morriss, F.C., and Moore, G.C., editors: A practical guide to pediatric intensive care, ed. 2, St. Louis, 1984, The C.V. Mosby Co.

44. Jones, C.: Glasgow coma scale, Am. J. Nurs. **79**:1551, 1979.

45. Katkis, J.: An introduction to monitoring intracranial pressure in critically ill children, Crit. Care Quarter. **3**:1, June 1980.

46. Katz, R.L., and Katz, G.H.: Clinical considerations in the use of muscle relaxants. In Katz, R.L., editor: Muscle relaxants, New York, 1975, American Elsevier.

47. Krulik, T.: Helping parents of children with cancer during the midstage of illness, Cancer Nurs. **5:**441, 1982.

48. Levin, D.L.: Reye's syndrome. In Levin, D.L., Morriss, F.C., and Moore, G.C., editors: A practical guide to pediatric intensive care, ed. 2, St. Louis, 1984, The C.V. Mosby Co.

49. Levin, D.L., Morriss, F.C., and Moore, G.C., editors: A practical guide to pediatric intensive care, ed. 2, St. Louis, 1984, The C.V. Mosby Co.

50. Lovejoy, F.H., and others: Clinical staging in Reye's syndrome, Am. J. Dis. Child. **128:**36, 1974.

51. Margolis, L.H., and Shaywitz, B.A.: The prolonged coma in childhood, Pediatrics **65:**477, 1980.

52. Marks, J.F.: Inappropriate secretion of antidiuretic hormone. In Levin, D.L., Morriss, F.C., and Moore, G.C., editors: A practical guide to pediatric intensive care, ed. 2, St. Louis, 1984, The C.V. Mosby Co.

53. Marks, J.F.: Central diabetes insipidus. In Levin, D.L., Morriss, F.C., and Moore, G.C., editors: A practical guide to pediatric intensive care, ed. 2, St. Louis, 1984, The C.V. Mosby Co.

54. Mattar, J.A., and others: A study of the hyperosmolar state in critically ill patients, Crit. Care Med. **1:**293, 1973.

55. McCormick, W.F., and Schochet, S.S.: Atlas of cerebrovascular disease, Philadelphia, 1976, W.B. Saunders Co.

56. McGillicuddy, J.E., and others: The relation of cerebral ischemia, hypoxia, and hypercarbia to the Cushing response, J. Neurosurg. **48:**730, 1978.

57. Mendoza, S.: Syndrome of inappropriate anti-diuretic hormone secretion, Pediatr. Clin. North Am. **23:**681, 1976.

58. Menkes, J.: Textbook of child neurology, Philadelphia, 1980, Lea & Febiger.

59. Morriss, F.C., and Cook, J.D.: Increased intracranial pressure. In Levin, D.L., Morriss, F.C., and Moore, G.C., editors: A practical guide to pediatric intensive care, ed. 2, St. Louis, 1984, The C.V. Mosby Co.

60. Morriss, F.C., and Cook, J.D.: Status epilepticus. In Levin, D.L., Morriss, F.C., and Moore, G.C., editors: A practical guide to pediatric intensive care, ed. 2, St. Louis, 1984, The C.V. Mosby Co.

61. Olson, E.: The hazards of immobility, Am. J. Nurs. **67:**780, 1967.

62. Paine, R., and Oppe, T.: Neurological examination of children. In: Clinics in developmental medicine, vols. 20 and 21, London, 1966, William Heinemann Medical Books Ltd.

63. Plum, F., and Posner, J.B.: The diagnosis of stupor and coma, ed. 3, Philadelphia, 1980, F.A. Davis Co.

64. Powner, D.J., and Grevnik, A.: Triage in patient care: from expected recovery to brain death, Heart Lung **8:**1103, 1979.

65. Raphaely, R.C., and others: Severe pediatric head trauma, Pediatr. Clin. North Am. **27:**715, 1975.

66. Reitz, B.A., and Ream, A.K.: Uses of hypothermia in cardiovascular surgery: pharmacology. In Ream, A.K., and Fogdall, R.P., editors: Acute cardiovascular management: anesthesia and intensive care, Philadelphia, 1982, J.B. Lippincott Co.

67. Reye's Syndrome Working Group, National Surveillance of Reye Syndrome 1981: Update: Reye's syndrome and salicylate usage, Morbid. Mortal. Week. Rep. **31:**53, 1982.

68. Richardson, A.: Intracranial tumors. In Rose, F.C., editor: Paediatric neurology, Oxford, 1979, Blackwell Scientific Publications Inc.

69. Roger, J., Lob, H., and Tassinari, C.A.: Status epilepticus. In Vinkin, P.J., and Bruyn, G.W., editors: Handbook of clinical neurology, Amsterdam, 1974, North-Holland Publishing Co.

70. Rogers, E.L., and Rogers, M.C.: Fulminant hepatic failure and hepatic encephalopathy, Pediatr. Clin. North Am. **27:**701, 1980.

71. Rosman, N.: Pediatric head injuries, Pediatr. Ann. **7:**55, 1978.

72. Rosman, N., and others: Acute head trauma in infancy and childhood, Pediatr. Clin. North Am. **26:**707, 1979.

73. Ross, E.M., and Bellman, M.H.: Encephalitis and encephalopathy. In Rose, F.C., editor: Paediatric neurology, Oxford, 1979, Blackwell Scientific Publications Inc.

74. Rothner, A.D., and Erenberg, G.: Status epilepticus, Pediatr. Clin. North Am. **27:**593, 1980.

75. San Francisco General Hospital, Protocol for use of intravenous DMSO in the management of intracranial pressure, San Francisco, 1980.

76. Seelig, J.M., and others: Traumatic acute subdural hematoma, N. Engl. J. Med. **304:**1511, 1980.

77. Severinghaus, J.W.: The physiology of induced hypothermia, National Research Council, Washington, pub. no. 451, 1956.

78. Shaywitz, B., Rothstein, P., and Venes, J.: Monitoring and management of increased intracranial pressure in Reye's syndrome: results in 29 children, Pediatrics **66:**198, 1980.

79. Shaywitz, B.A., and others: Long-term consequences of Reye's syndrome: a sibling-matched, controlled study of neurologic, cognitive, academic, and psychiatric function, J. Pediatr. **100:**41, 1981.

80. Sklar, F.H.: Neurosurgery: perioperative principles. In Levin, D.L., Morris, F.C., and Moore, G.C., editors: A practical guide to pediatric intensive care, ed. 2, St. Louis, 1984, The C.V. Mosby Co.

81. Swischuk, L.: Childhood head injuries and the skull roentgenogram, Pediatr. Ann. **4:**10, 1975.

82. Taylor, F., and Schutz, H.: Symptoms caused by intracranial pressure waves, J. Neurosurg. Nurs. **9:**36, Dec. 1977.

83. Van Allen, M.: Pictorial manual of neurological tests, Chicago, 1969, Year Book Medical Publishers, Inc.

84. Waring, W.W., and Jeansonne, L.O.: Normal cerebrospinal fluid. In: Practical manual of pediatrics, ed. 2, St. Louis, 1982, The C.V. Mosby Co.

85. Weiner, H.L., Bresnan, M.J., and Levitt, L.P.: Lumbar puncture. In: Pediatric neurology for the house officer, ed. 2, Baltimore, 1982, Williams & Wilkins.

86. Yeh, T.S., and Holbrook, P.R.: Monitoring during assisted ventilation in children. In Gregory, G.A., editor: Respiratory failure in the child, Clinics in Critical Care Medicine, New York, 1981, Churchill Livingstone Inc.

87. Young, J.L., Jr., and Miller, R.W.: Incidence of malignant tumors in U.S. children, J. Pediatr. **84:**254, 1975.

88. Ziter, F.A.: Childhood neuropathies. In Rudolph, A.M., editor: Pediatrics, ed. 17, Norwalk, Conn., 1982, Appleton-Century-Crofts.

Renal Disorders

JEANETTE KENNEDY

The kidney is the organ most responsible for maintenance of stable extracellular fluid volume and composition. During a variety of conditions, the kidney adjusts the amount and type of acids and ions that are secreted and absorbed from blood plasma.

■ Essential Anatomy and Physiology

■ KIDNEY STRUCTURE
■ Gross anatomy

The kidneys lie anterior and lateral to the twelfth thoracic and first, second, and third lumbar vetebrae and behind the abdominal peritoneum (thus they are retroperitoneal structures). The kidneys are surrounded by double layers of fascia, called the peri-renal fat or the adipose capsule; this fat holds the kidneys in place (Fig. 7-1). The left kidney is usually slightly higher than the right. The average length of the adult kidney is 11.5 cm (4½ inches), the average width is 5 to 7.5 cm (2 to 3 inches), and the thickness averages 2.5 cm (1 inch). The medial aspect of each kidney is curved away from the midline; at the center of this concavity is the hilus, and this is where the renal artery and nerves enter the kidney and where the renal vein and ureter exit the kidney. Surrounding each kidney is a strong, fibrous capsule, which becomes the outer lining of the renal calyces, the renal pelvis, and the ureter.

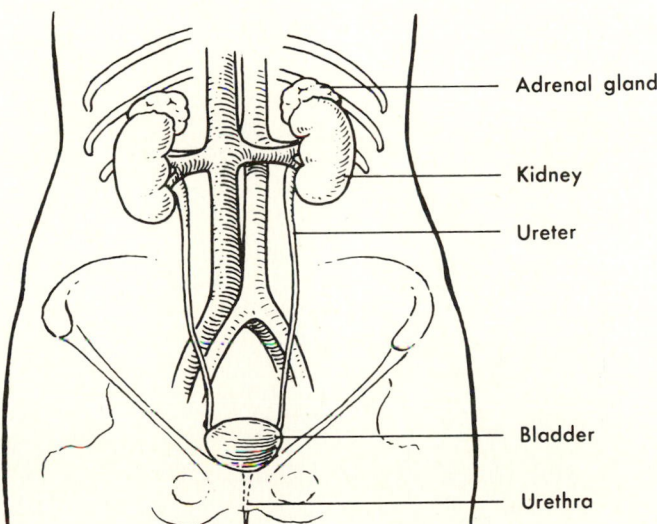

Fig. 7-1 Components of the urinary system.

From Brundage, D.J.: Nursing management of renal problems, ed. 2, St. Louis, 1980, The C.V. Mosby Co.

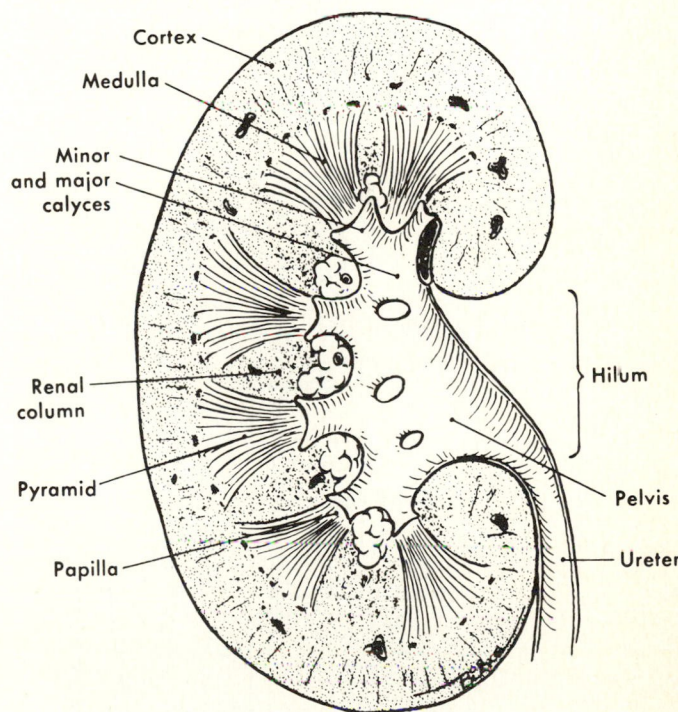

Fig. 7-2 Cross section of the kidney.

From Brundage, D.J.: Nursing management of renal problems, ed. 2, St. Louis, 1980, The C.V. Mosby Co.

A longitudinal section of the kidney shows the three general areas of renal structure: the cortex, the medulla, and the pelvis (Fig. 7-2).

The renal cortex is the outer portion of the kidney. It has a granular appearance and extends in fingerlike projections into the medullary areas. The cortex contains all the glomeruli, the proximal and distal convoluted tubules, and the first portions of the loop of Henle and the collecting ducts.

The renal medulla is composed predominately of collecting ducts that progress from smaller ducts to larger ducts as they approach the renal pelvis. These collecting ducts give the medulla a striated, pyramid-like appearance, with the apex of the pyramid pointing toward the renal pelvis and the base pointing toward the renal cortex.

The renal pelvis is the expanded upper end of the ureter, and it subdivides to form the major and minor calyces. These calyces receive urine that will flow from the kidney to the bladder.

The functioning unit of the kidney is the nephron, which consists of a vascular component, a tubular component, and the collecting ducts (Fig. 7-3). Each kidney contains approximately 1 to 1¼ million distinct nephrons. Eighty-five percent of all nephrons originate in the outermost area of the cortex and have relatively short loops of Henle, which extend only into the outer medulla. The remaining nephrons originate in the inner cortical area immediately adjacent to the medulla. These "juxtamedullary" nephrons have long loops of Henle that extend deep into the medulla and lay parallel to the medullary collecting ducts (Fig. 7-4).

■ **Renal vasculature**

Each kidney is supplied with systemic arterial blood from a single artery. The two renal arteries receive about 20% of the total cardiac output. Each renal artery branches from the aorta at the level of the second or third lumbar vertebra. Each artery divides into an anterior and posterior arterial vessel, then continues to branch into small arterial vessels; some of these arterioles will supply nutrients to the renal medulla, cortical tissue, and capsule. Other arterioles will enter the glomerular capsule. The *afferent arteriole* enters the glomerular capsule and perfuses the glomerulus. This glomerulus consists of a tuft of capillaries that allow filtration through the capillary membranes. The glomerular capillaries do not recombine into venous channels, but instead they reform into a second arteriole, called the *efferent arteriole*. Since arterioles are present at either end of the glomerulus, constriction or dilation of these arterioles will alter the resistance of flow through the glomerular capillaries and thus will regulate glomerular filtration.

The efferent arterioles form a network of capillaries that surround the convoluted tubules and loop of Henle. These peritubular capillaries then converge into venules that will return renal venous blood to the systemic circulation via the inferior vena cava.

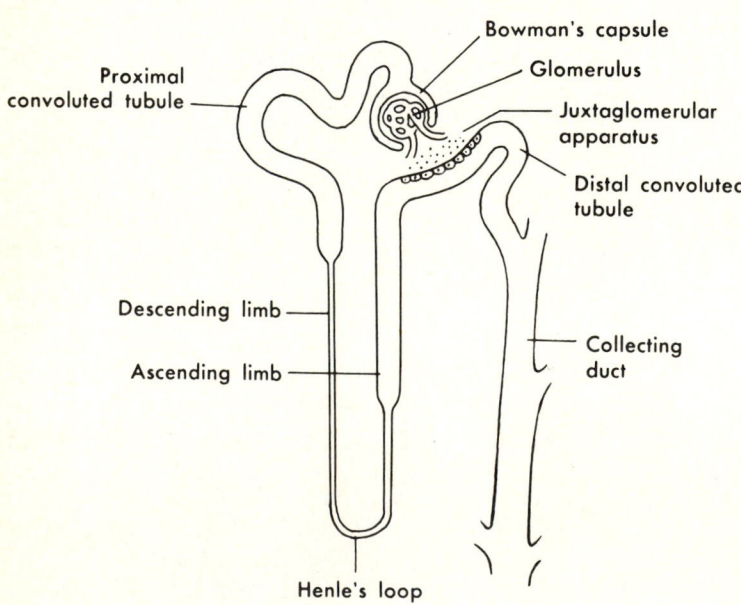

Fig. 7-3 Components of the nephron.

From Brundage, D.J.: Nursing management of renal problems, ed. 2, St. Louis, 1980, The C.V. Mosby Co.

The juxtamedullary nephrons have the same vascular network as cortical nephrons; in addition, however, the vasa recta hairpin-loop capillary vessels are present. They run parallel to the medullary loop of Henle and collecting ducts. The vasa recta ultimately reforms with juxtamedullary peritubular capillaries into the venous channels, returning blood to the systemic circulation.

■ Renal tubules and collecting ducts

The tubular component of the nephron begins in the renal cortex as a single layer of flat epithelial cells, which surrounds the glomerulus and is known as *Bowman's capsule.* Filtered fluid from the glomerulus will enter this portion of the tubule. Leading from Bowman's capsule is a coiled tubule called the *proximal convoluted tubule* (PCT). The luminal cells of the PCT are cuboidal in shape and have a brush border on the inner luminal surface; these PCT cells

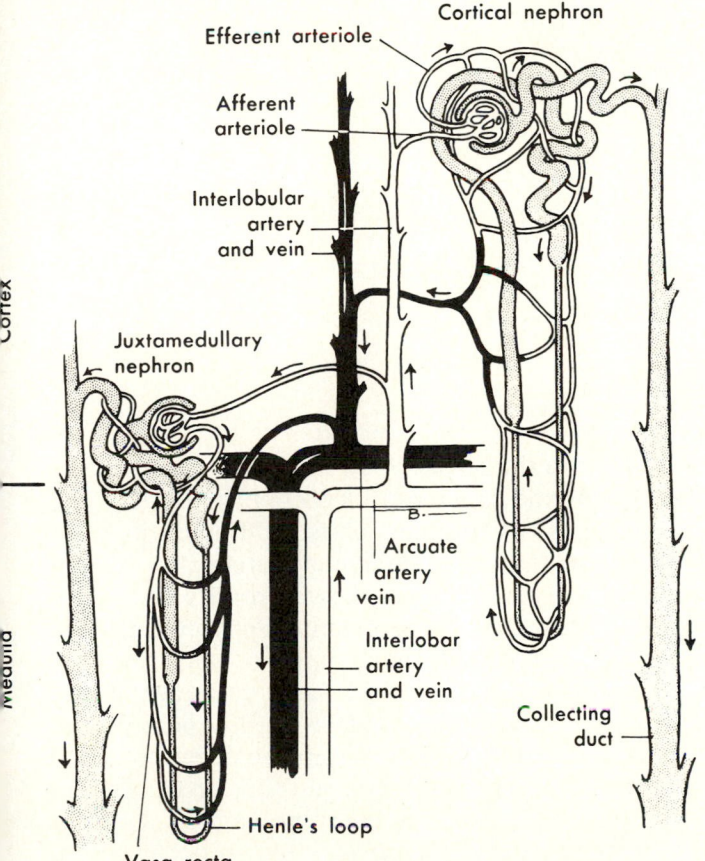

Fig. 7-4 Location of cortical and juxtamedullary nephrons and their blood supply.

From Brundage, D.J.: Nursing management of renal problems, ed. 2, St. Louis, 1980, The C.V. Mosby Co.

are continuous with the epithelial cells of Bowman's capsule. The appearance of the proximal convoluted tubule changes as it descends toward the renal medullary area. The tubular lumen narrows and the cells become flattened as the tubule makes a hairpin turn, called the *loop of Henle.* As the loop of Henle ascends from the medulla into the renal cortical areas, the tubular cells enlarge and again become cuboidal. Once the tubule enters the renal cortex, it again becomes convoluted, forming the *distal convoluted tubule* (DCT). The cells of the inner layer of the DCT have no brush border. Just beyond the distal convoluted tubule, the tubule straightens and joins a collecting duct (Fig. 7-5). Collecting ducts are the terminus of many distal tubules; they are formed in the inner and outer renal cortex. These small collecting ducts then enter the renal medulla, where they join to form larger ducts, which in turn drain into a minor calyx in the renal pelvis. Ultimately, fluid from the renal pelvis will flow into the ureter and will enter the bladder.

■ Ureters

The two ureters conduct urine from the renal pelvis to the urinary bladder. They are located behind the peritoneum and they descend through the pelvic cavity, crossing over the common iliac arteries. Both ureters enter the posterior-lateral aspect of the bladder, where they traverse the bladder wall at an oblique angle. This oblique entry serves as a valve to prevent the back flow of urine into the ureters during bladder contraction. In addition, the ureteral entrance into the bladder (the uretero-vesicular junction) is closed by a fold of mucous membrane.[84]

Each ureteral wall has three layers: an inner epithelial lining, a middle muscular layer, and the outer fibrous layer that is continuous with the renal capsule. The middle muscular portion of the ureter consists of both a circular and a longitudinal muscle layer. The circular muscles propel the urine toward the bladder by peristaltic contractions, and they generate enough pressure to overcome the resistance caused by the oblique ureteral insertions into the bladder. Contraction of the longitudinal fibers serves to open the lumen of the ureters. These ureteral muscle fibers are innervated by fibers from the aortic, spermatic or ovarian, and hypogastric plexuses.[65]

■ The bladder and urethra

The urinary bladder is a hollow, muscular organ that stores the urine. There are three openings in the bladder wall, caused by the entrance of the two

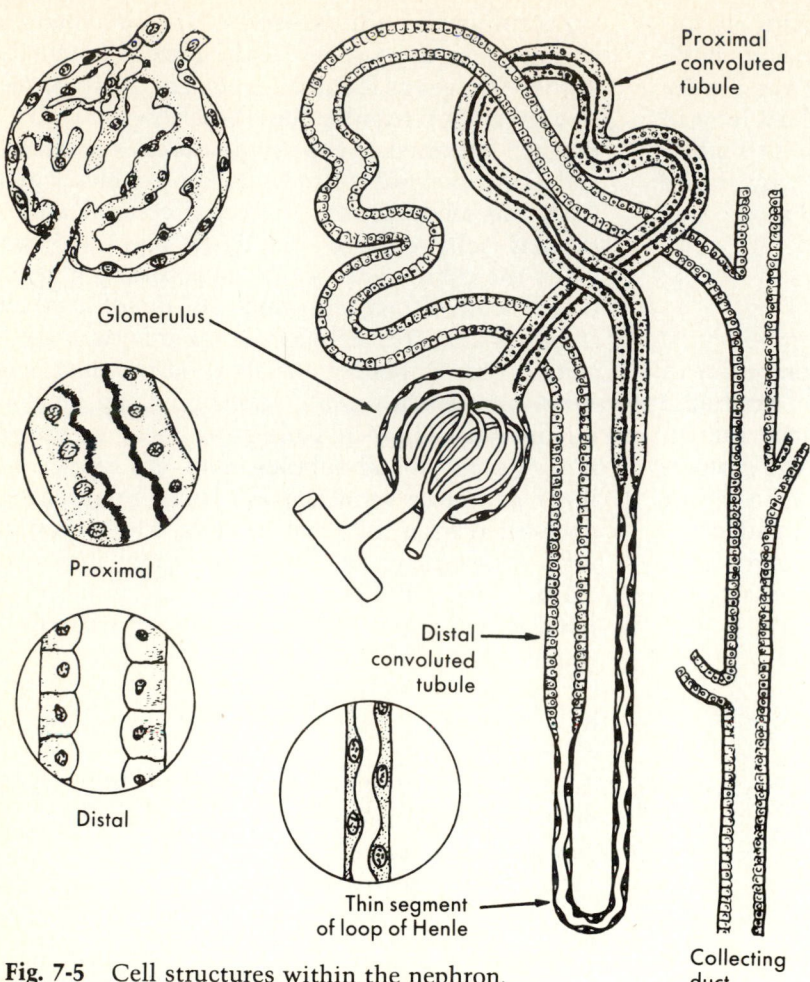

Proximal
convoluted
tubule

Glomerulus

Proximal

Distal

Distal
convoluted
tubule

Thin segment
of loop of Henle

Collecting
duct

Fig. 7-5 Cell structures within the nephron.

From Pitts, R.F.: Physiology of the kidney and body fluids, 3rd edition. Copyright © 1974 by Year Book Medical Publishers, Inc., Chicago. Adapted from Smith, H.W., The kidney (New York: Oxford University Press, 1935).

ureters and the exit of the urethra. These openings form the corners of a triangle, called the trigone. There is a dense area of smooth (involuntary) muscle around the neck of the bladder at the orifice of the urethra; this muscle constitutes the internal sphincter. The urethra extends from the urinary bladder to the body surface. When the urethra passes through the muscles of the pelvic floor, striated (voluntary) circular muscles form an external sphincter.

Micturation is the emptying of the stored urine from the bladder. The process involves both voluntary and involuntary nervous system activities in children (beyond 2 to 3 years of age) and adults. Once an adequate volume of urine has accumulated in the bladder, the bladder wall stretches, stimulating afferent nerves that carry impulses to the central nervous system. Efferent nerves from the central nervous system return impulses through the pelvic and hypogas-

tric nerves to the bladder wall muscle and the neck of the bladder and cause contraction of the bladder and relaxation of the internal sphincter. In addition, impulses from the central nervous system through the pudendal nerves innervate the voluntarily controlled external sphincter. If the external sphincter also relaxes, the bladder will then empty.

Appropriate contraction and voluntary intermittent emptying of the bladder requires both inhibitory and facilitory impulses from the upper pons, the hypothalamus, the midbrain, and the cortex. The inhibitory centers prevent constant voiding, and the facilitory centers allow micturation to occur voluntarily. If the inhibitory centers are injured, the patient can demonstrate an *uninhibited neurogenic bladder* and nearly constant urination.

Reflex bladder contraction and sphincter relaxation also require the presence of intact afferent nerves from the bladder to the second and third sacral spinal cord level and intact efferent nerves (including the hypogastric nerves, the pelvic nerve, and the pudendal nerve) from the first through third sacral spinal level. If afferent nerves from the bladder to the spinal cord are injured or malformed, the patient can develop an atonic bladder, with loss of voluntary sphincter control. When an atonic bladder is present, the bladder fills to capacity; then overflow voiding begins. If the spinal cord is damaged *above* the sacral spinal level, the patient initially loses all micturition reflexes as a result of loss of inhibitory and facilitory reflexes from the brain. Later, however, simple spinal reflexes can return, and the patient can void when bladder distention is sufficient. In this case, the bladder reflex will be initiated at that volume of urine that is usually present in the bladder during the patient's convalescent period.[36]

■ GLOMERULAR FUNCTION
■ Filtration kinetics

The kidney receives its sympathetic nerve supply from the tenth through twelfth thoracic nerves and its parasympathetic nerve supply from branches of the vagus nerve. Innervation involves the renal blood vessels only, rather than the renal tubules. Adjustment in the diameter of either or both the afferent and efferent arterioles will affect the amount of fluid filtered in the glomerulus. As with any capillary, filtration of fluid in the glomerulus is affected by pressure gradients across the capillary bed and the intrinsic properties of the glomerular capillary membrane.

Hydrostatic pressure is the pressure generated by the pumping action of the heart; this is maintained or altered by the resistance within the arterial system. Capillary hydrostatic pressure in most capillaries is higher at the arterial end of the capillary than at the venous end of the capillary. This difference favors *filtration* of fluid outward from the vascular space at the arterial end and probably favors *reabsorption* of fluid at the venous end. However, since the glomerulus has an afferent arteriole at the proximal end and an efferent arteriole at the distal end, the glomerular capillary pressure is higher than in other capillary beds and is approximately equal to systemic arterial pressure. This favors fluid filtration out of the vascular space. The amount of glomerular capillary pressure can be altered by constriction or relaxation of the afferent or efferent arteriole.

Intravascular colloid osmotic pressure (or oncotic pressure) is the pressure generated by dissolved proteins, ions, and other particles that are normally present in the blood. Larger particles, such as proteins,

cannot readily move across a capillary membrane, so they exert an osmotic pressure of approximately 30 mm Hg, which opposes hydrostatic filtration from the vascular space.[67]

The hydrostatic pressure present in Bowman's capsule is equal to the hydrostatic pressure surrounding the glomerulus, and it is approximately 15 mm Hg; this pressure opposes fluid filtration from the glomerulus. Since tubular fluid is normally a protein free plasma filtrate, colloid osmotic pressure in Bowman's capsule is normally lower than plasma oncotic pressure (Fig. 7-6).

Net filtration pressure (NFP) within the nephron, then, is the *difference* between forces favoring filtration (largely resulting from capillary hydrostatic pressure) and forces opposing filtration (largely caused by intravascular colloid osmotic pressure and the hydrostatic pressure within Bowman's capsule):

NFP = (forces favoring filtration) − (forces opposing filtration)

NFP = (capillary hydrostatic pressure) − (intravascular colloid osmotic pressure and Bowman's capsule hydrostatic pressure)

Any change in the hydrostatic pressure in either Bowman's capsule or in the capillaries, or changes in serum colloid osmotic pressure can change the net filtration pressure and may result in a change in the glomerular filtration rate (GFR). For example, obstruction of a ureter increases resistance to urine drainage from the renal pelvis; this increases pressure in the tubules and in Bowman's capsule and opposes filtration. The loss of a large volume of hypotonic fluid caused by diarrhea or increased insensible losses during fever will produce dehydration and hemoconcentration; this increases the colloid osmotic pressure. If the child develops severe hypotension, capillary hydrostatic pressure will fall. These changes oppose filtration and reduce the amount of glomerular filtrate.

Capillary hydrostatic pressure, as noted above, is determined not only by the strength of cardiac contraction but by the resistance in the arterioles.[82] The relationship of flow, pressure, and resistance is described by the following equation:

$$\text{Organ blood flow (Q)} = \frac{P}{R}$$

P = mean arterial pressure − venous pressure for that organ

R = resistance to flow

The equation predicts that an increase in mean arterial pressure will increase organ blood flow, if the resistance to flow remains constant. In the kidney,

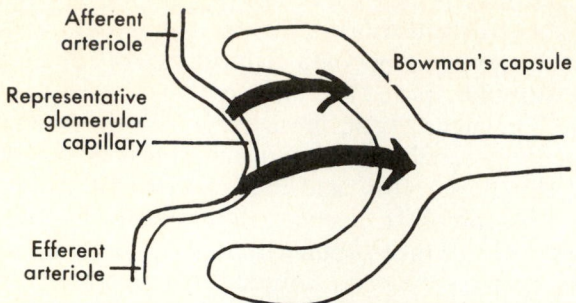

FACTORS FAVORING FILTRATION

Capillary hydrostatic pressure

Tubular (Bowman's capsule) oncotic
pressure

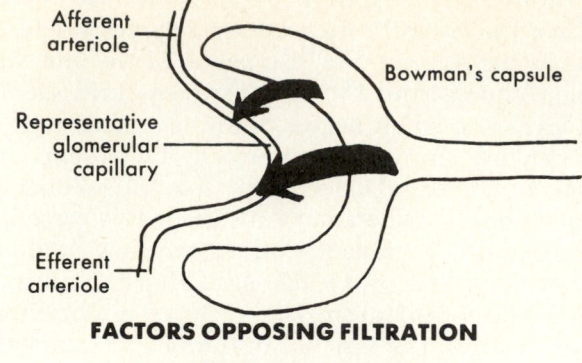

FACTORS OPPOSING FILTRATION

Capillary oncotic pressure

Tubular (Bowman's capsule)
hydrostatic pressure

Fig. 7-6 Starling capillary forces operating within the glomerular capillary. Factors that *favor* filtration from capillary into Bowman's capsule include capillary hydrostatic pressure (regulated by afferent and efferent renal arterioles) and tubular oncotic pressure. Factors that *oppose* filtration from capillary into Bowman's capsule include capillary oncotic pressure (which is normally essentially zero, since proteins should not be filtered) and pressure in Bowman's capsule (which is normally negligible).

resistance to flow *does not* remain constant during changes in systemic arterial blood pressure. Instead, when mean arterial pressure increases, the afferent arterioles constrict; this constriction restricts renal blood flow (RBF) and prevents transmission of the entire increase in arterial pressure to the glomerulus. When arterial pressure falls, the sympathetic innervation to the afferent and efferent arterioles increases arterial tone and increases resistance to flow into and out of the glomerulus. This can maintain the glomerular filtration rate at near normal levels despite a fall in renal blood flow. This ability to respond to changes in flow into and out of the glomerulus allows the kidney to maintain solute and volume regulation at relatively constant levels despite changes in systemic arterial blood pressure and renal blood flow; this ability is termed "autoregulation." When arterial blood pressure is extremely high or low, autoregulation fails, and renal blood flow becomes simply proportional to arterial pressure.

■ **Glomerular filtration rate**

Renal function can be evaluated by measuring the volume of glomerular filtrate formed during a specific period of time. The quantity of ultrafiltrate formed per unit of time is the glomerular filtration rate (GFR). The measurement of GFR is accomplished by simultaneous measurements of the concentration of a specific substance in both the plasma and in the urine. The substance used must have certain physical properties; it must be freely filtered at the glomerulus, must not be reabsorbed once it is filtered, and must not be broken down, synthesized, or secreted by the renal tubules. This means that all of the substance that is filtered from the vascular space at the glomerulus remains in the urine and can be measured. *Inulin* is one such substance. It is not normally present in the blood, so it must be intravenously infused if assessment of inulin clearance is required. The inulin is administered at a constant rate, and the plasma level of inulin is measured. Urine is collected for a precise period of time, usually 1 or 2 hours, and the volume of the urine and the urinary inulin concentration are measured. The ratio between the plasma and urine concentrations of inulin and the urine volume formed per unit of time defines the GFR.

$$GFR = \frac{\text{Urine concentration of inulin} \times \text{Volume of urine per minute}}{\text{Plasma inulin concentrations}}$$

$$GFR = \frac{U_{IN}V}{P_{IN}}$$

Since inulin is not normally present in the body, use of a naturally occurring substance to calculate the GFR is often preferable; such a substance is *creati-*

nine. Creatinine is formed by the muscles and is released at a near-constant rate into the bloodstream so that its plasma concentration changes negligibly during a 24-hour period in the normal patient. A sample drawn at any time during the 24-hour urine collection period will accurately reflect plasma levels. The use of creatinine to estimate GFR will result in a slightly higher estimation of the filtration rate than when inulin is used, because minute amounts of creatinine are secreted by the renal tubules into the filtrate. The discrepancy is very small, however, so creatinine clearance is the most common method of assessing GFR.

Glomerular filtration rates are expressed as ml/minute/m² body surface area. This allows a comparison between the renal function of children and that of adults. The child's GFR is approximately 55 to 65 ml/minute/m² and will approach adult values (120 ml/minute/1.73 m²) by 3 years of age. When the amount of fluid filtered by the glomerulus is expressed as a fraction of the total renal plasma flow (600 ml/minute/1.73 m² in the adult), the percentage of the circulating plasma that has filtered into Bowman's capsule can be estimated. This ratio is termed the *filtration fraction* and equals approximately 20% of total renal plasma flow. Plasma that is not filtered continues through the glomerulus into the capillary system surrounding the tubules.

The glomerular filtrate in Bowman's capsule is an ultrafiltrate of the blood. Its composition, like interstitial fluid from other capillaries, is usually free of proteins and cells. Animal micropuncture studies have established that all of the solutes (such as ions and amino acids) measured in the glomerular filtrate are present in virtually the same concentrations as their free, unbound concentrations in the plasma. If a substance is bound, even partially, to protein, its glomerular filtration will be restricted, since proteins cannot normally pass through the glomerular capillary membrane.

The urine that is ultimately formed by the kidneys is not merely an ultrafiltrate of plasma, since this would soon deplete the body of solutes and water. To modify the volume and content of the urine, the tubules selectively reabsorb and secrete substances.

■ **TUBULAR FUNCTION**
■ **Reabsorption**

Passive and active reabsorption. Reabsorption of substances from the renal tubular fluid is described as passive if no energy is required. Passive reabsorption occurs if a substance is reabsorbed as the result of an electrical gradient or concentration gradient. Active reabsorption, or active transport, moves sub-

stances against a concentration or electrochemical gradient; active reabsorption requires energy expenditure by the transporting cells. Both active and passive reabsorption from the renal tubules require diffusion of substances through the tubular luminal cell membrane. Once the substances enter the cell, they traverse the cytoplasm of the tubular cell, and exit through the cell membrane on the opposite side into the interstitial fluid. These substances can then pass into the adjacent peritubular capillaries for return to the systemic venous circulation. If energy is required at any of these steps, the process is considered active transport. Sodium, chloride, glucose, and bicarbonate are important substances that are actively reabsorbed, while water is passively reabsorbed.

Thresholds and transport maximums (Tm). Many of the active transport mechanisms of the tubules are limited in the amount of reabsorption of a particular substance that is possible in a given amount of time. This transport maximum (Tm) is relatively fixed for each substance, although it can be affected by hormones or drugs. The *renal threshold* of a substance is that plasma and filtrate concentration at which some of the active transport tubular carriers become saturated. Once the renal plasma threshold is reached, *some* of the substance will begin to appear in the urine, because it cannot all be reabsorbed from the filtrate. The *tubular transport maximum* (Tm) is reached when *all* of the tubular carriers for that substance are saturated. Any further increase in the serum and filtered concentration of the substance beyond the Tm will produce a proportional increase in the urine concentration of the substance.

Glucose is a familiar substance that can be used to illustrate this concept of renal plasma threshold and tubular transport maximum. Under normal conditions, glucose is not excreted in the urine: all of the glucose filtered by the glomerulus is reabsorbed by the tubules and returned to the blood. When serum glucose levels exceed approximately 180 mg/dl, some glucose tubular carriers are saturated and glucose begins to appear in the urine. The appearance of the glucose in the urine indicates that the *renal threshold* for glucose reabsorption has been reached. If the serum glucose exceeds approximately 300 mg/dl, all of the tubular carriers are saturated, and the Tm for glucose has been reached. The difference between the renal plasma threshold and the transport maximum for glucose is caused by the different transport maximums of the individual nephrons and tubules.

For many substances, there is a large difference between the normal serum concentration of a substance and the renal threshold and transport maximum of that substance. This indicates that the kidney conserves the substance but does not specifically regulate its serum concentrations. Once the serum concentration of the substance far exceeds the homeostatic requirements, then that substance will be lost into the urine. Glucose is one substance that is conserved by the kidneys, though the specific serum glucose concentration is not determined by the kidneys.

If the renal threshold and transport maximum are approximately equal to the daily filtered load of a substance, then the kidneys participate in regulation of the serum level of the substance. In such a case, a slight increase or decrease in plasma and filtered concentration of the substance will result in a change in its rate of renal reabsorption and excretion, and serum levels will return to normal. The renal threshold and transport maximum for phosphate are very close to the normal daily filtered load of phosphate, so serum phosphate levels are closely regulated by kidney tubular function. Phosphate transport and reabsorption will, in turn, also be affected by serum calcium levels and by levels of parathyroid and adrenal cortical hormones.[69]

Since many of the active transport mechanisms will transport two or more substances, saturation of carrier sites can occur either in the presence of excessive amounts of one substance or by the presence of a second substance that competes for the same transport mechanism. For example, many of the diuretics exert their effects by blocking solute reabsorption in the kidney tubules.

■ Secretion

Though most substances enter the tubules through filtration, other substances can actually be *secreted* into the urine by the tubules. Like tubular reabsorption, tubular secretion can be either an active or a passive transport process. Substances dissolved in the serum of the peritubular capillaries cross into the tubular cell and can then be transported into tubular lumen and excreted into the urine. Substances most commonly secreted by the tubules include organic acids and bases, food additives, and many drugs and chemicals. There is a transport maximum for secretion of only a few substances, so secretory functions of the tubules may be less limited than reabsorptive functions.

■ Reabsorption and secretion in the proximal tubule

The selective reabsorption of solute begins in the proximal tubules. Approximately two thirds to seven eighths of the glomerular filtrate is reabsorbed

in the proximal tubule.[66] The most important function of the proximal tubule is the reabsorption of approximately 65% of the filtered sodium and water. In addition, this portion of the tubule is responsible for reabsorption of almost 100% of the filtered glucose and amino acids, 65% of the filtered potassium, and 90% of the bicarbonate and phosphate. The proximal tubule is largely responsible for reabsorption of water and electrolytes; it neither concentrates nor dilutes the urine.

Sodium. Sodium is freely filtered at the glomerulus, so its concentration in the proximal glomerular filtrate is identical to its plasma concentration. Sodium is reabsorbed by an active transport mechanism; the mechanism is carrier mediated and requires energy, so that sodium can move against a gradient. Sodium is not secreted into the tubules. Once sodium is filtered, it moves passively through the extremely sodium-permeable brush border of the proximal tubular cell. It diffuses across this cuboidal cell to the opposite cell membrane, which is impermeable to sodium. This cell membrane actively pumps sodium out of the tubular cell into the surrounding interstitial space. The diffusion of sodium from the tubular lumen to the tubular cell and the active transport of sodium out of the tubular cell creates an osmotic gradient between the tubule and the interstitial space. Since the epithelium of the proximal tubule is highly permeable to water, water will follow the movement of the sodium ion. As water moves out of the tubule, the relative concentration of other solutes within the tubular lumen will increase. This establishes a concentration gradient for those substances between the tubular lumen and the interstitial area. As a result, solutes such as chloride, calcium, and urea will passively diffuse out of tubules into the tubular cells and interstitial area.

Diffusion and transport of the sodium ion from the tubule also creates an electrical gradient between the tubular lumen and the inside of the tubular cell; the tubular cell becomes more positively charged and the tubular lumen becomes more negatively charged. As a result, negatively charged substances such as chloride are reabsorbed passively in the proximal tubule as a result of the electrochemical gradient created by active sodium transport.

As the ultrafiltered fluid reaches the end of the proximal tubule, 65% of the filtered sodium and water has been reabsorbed into the renal interstitial areas, predominantly through the active transport of sodium. Since water is being reabsorbed at almost the same rate as the sodium is being pumped out of the proximal tubule, the osmolality of the proximal tubular fluid will be virtually the same as the plasma osmolality (normally around 300 mOsm/L).

Renal sodium and water reabsorption in the proximal tubule as well as in the loop of Henle varies proportionately with the glomerular filtration rate. Increases in GFR are automatically accompanied by an increase in sodium reabsorption. This coupling between the quantity of filtrate and the amount of reabsorption is termed *glomerulotubular* balance. This balance means that if renal blood flow remains constant, and if the glomerular filtration rate increases, sodium (and water) reabsorption will increase. Conversely, if renal blood flow remains constant and the glomerular filtration rate falls, sodium (and water) reabsorption will be decreased. This mechanism maintains sodium balance despite changes in the GFR. If there is a *severe* reduction in renal arterial pressure *and* glomerular filtration rate, sodium will be almost completely reabsorbed from the proximal tubule.

Bicarbonate and hydrogen ion. Sodium and bicarbonate ions in the glomerular filtrate enter the proximal tubule, where sodium passively diffuses into the proximal tubular cells as a result of a concentration gradient, and then is actively transported out of the tubular cell. Positively charged hydrogen ions will be actively pumped from the tubular cells *into* the tubular lumen in exchange for the positively charged sodium ions that are moving *out* of the tubule. Thus electrical balance is maintained.

Once the hydrogen ion enters the tubular lumen, it combines with the bicarbonate in the filtrate to form carbonic acid. The carbonic acid in the tubule quickly disassociates to form carbon dioxide and water; the carbon dioxide easily diffuses back through the tubular lumen cell membrane where its recombination with water is catalyzed by carbonic anhydrase, and carbonic acid is again formed. Subsequent disassociation of the carbonic acid within the tubular cell again forms the hydrogen ions (which the cell will again actively secrete in exchange for sodium ions) and bicarbonate ions (which will passively diffuse out of the tubule cell into the peritubular interstitial fluids as the result of a concentration and electrical gradient).

As a result of this process, for every bicarbonate ion that combines with a hydrogen ion in the lumen of the tubule, a bicarbonate ion will ultimately diffuse into the peritubular plasma (Fig. 7-7). This secretion of hydrogen ions and reabsorption of bicarbonate ions occurs along the length of the renal tubules, but 90% of the bicarbonate reabsorption occurs in the proximal tubule. Since the kidney is responsible for bicarbonate reabsorption and is also responsible for generating new bicarbonate ions, the kidney plays an important role in regulation of acid-base balance. (See the section on renal regulation of acid-base balance later in this chapter.)

Potassium. Potassium is freely filtered by the glomerulus into the tubular ultrafiltrate, so that the tubular concentration of potassium is equal to the serum potassium concentration in the postglomerular vessels. The tubular reabsorption of potassium is an active transport process that occurs in all segments of the tubule, except for the descending limb of the loop of Henle. The active transport of the potassium ion from the tubule into the tubular cell occurs against a concentration gradient (potassium concentration is relatively low within the tubule and relatively high within the tubular cell). Nearly all of the filtered potassium is reabsorbed by the proximal tubule, and the remaining potassium is reabsorbed in the ascending limb. The proximal reabsorption of the filtered potassium occurs at a constant rate, and does not alter despite the presence of serum hyperkalemia or hypokalemia. The net result is that there is a continuous loss of potassium from the urine even when no potassium is being administered to the patient.

Calcium. Very little calcium is excreted in the urine. Forty percent of the total serum calcium is bound to serum proteins, such as albumin, and is not able to pass through the glomerular capillary membrane, so it is not filtered in the glomerulus. The remaining 60% of total serum calcium is filtered and is present in the filtrate as either ionized calcium (the biologically active form) or as complex calcium (calcium bound in reactions with other ions). Calcium reabsorption parallels sodium reabsorption in the proximal tubule: 80% to 90% of filtered calcium is reabsorbed in the proximal tubule and loop of Henle. Like sodium, only 10% of filtered calcium enters the distal tubule for concentration adjustments. Calcium reabsorption is controlled by parathyroid hormone.

Urea. Urea is a small molecule that is formed by the liver during detoxification of ammonia (NH_3). Ammonia is a very reactive and toxic end-product of protein metabolism. Since urea is a small molecule, it is easily filtered from the glomerulus; its concentration in the filtrate is equal to its plasma concentration. Urea is not actively reabsorbed but passively follows the proximal tubule osmotic reabsorption of water, so that approximately half of the filtered urea is reabsorbed. The amount of urea reabsorbed directly parallels the amounts of sodium and water reabsorbed; when water reabsorption is high, a larger percentage of the filtered urea is reabsorbed.

Drugs. The glomerulus is nonselective in its filtration of solutes, because the glomerular membrane does not restrict the passage of small mole-

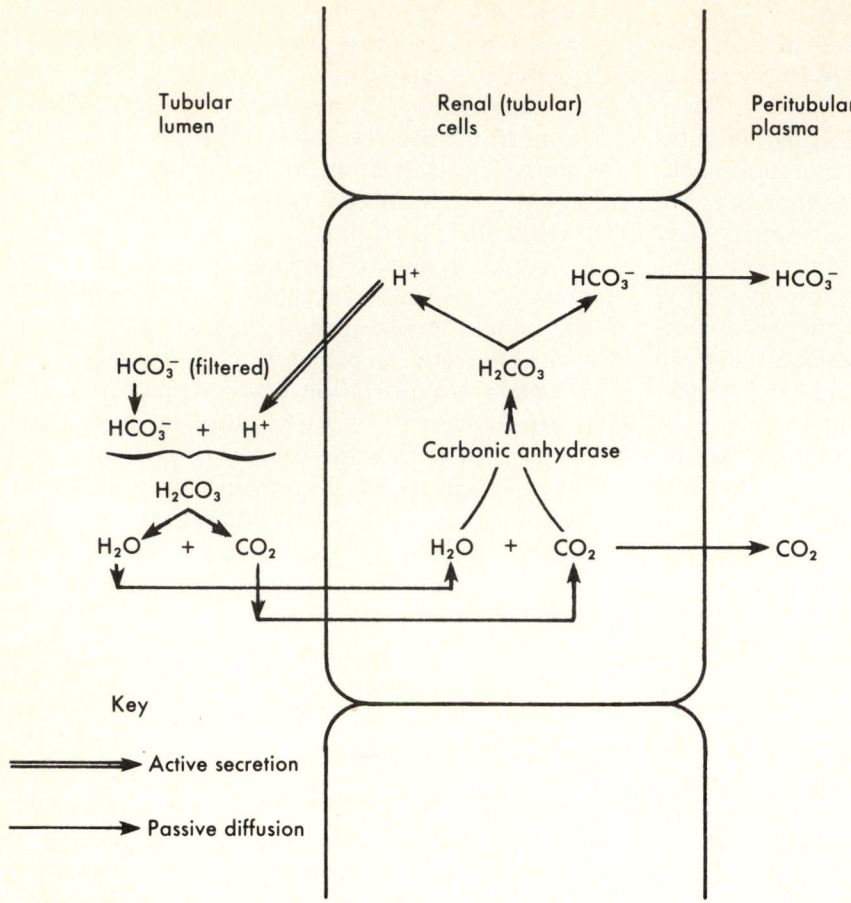

Fig. 7-7 Mechanism of bicarbonate reabsorption. Filtered bicarbonate combines with hydrogen ion that is secreted by renal tubules and carbonic acid is formed. The carbonic acid quickly dissociates into water and carbon dioxide, which can diffuse into renal tubular cells. Inside renal tubular cells, water and carbon dioxide can again join to form carbonic acid, because reaction is catalyzed by carbonic anhydrase. Carbonic acid then dissociates to yield hydrogen ion (which can again be secreted by tubular cells) and bicarbonate ion, which diffuses into peritubular plasma and ultimately returns to vascular space.

cules. Most drugs are of a small molecular size, and only a fraction of the drugs are bound to serum albumin, so most will filter into the tubular fluid. Changes in the GFR or in the degree of protein binding will alter the amount of drug present in the glomerular filtrate. Protein binding of a drug in turn can be influenced by competition between drugs for the same binding sites. If there is competition between drugs, a larger proportion of both drugs will be present in the unbound state, so the glomerular filtration of the drugs will be increased.[89]

Many drugs are also actively secreted from the peritubular blood into the tubular lumen. The drugs most commonly secreted include those that form either a weak acid or a weak base, so that they are partially ionized when the serum pH is normal. Other organic cations can be secreted into the proximal tubule through carrier mediation; these substances have a tubular secretion maximum.

Reabsorption of a drug from the proximal tubule is dependent upon the function of the renal tubular epithelium. This epithelium functions like a lipid barrier: it permits nonionized lipid-soluble molecules to diffuse across it, but it is relatively impermeable to

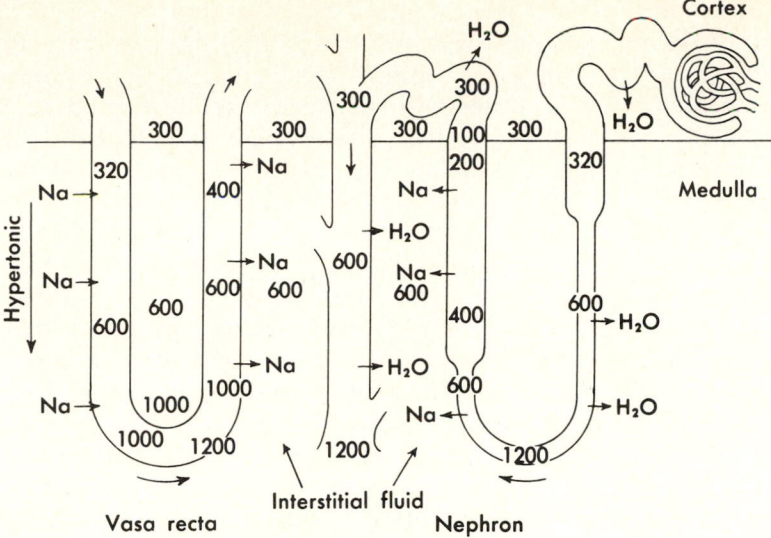

Fig. 7-8 Countercurrent mechanism for concentrating urine within loop of Henle. Numbers represent osmotic concentrations (in mOsm/L) of tubular fluid, blood, and interstitial fluid.

From Brundage, D.J.: *Nursing management of renal problems,* ed. 2, St. Louis, 1980, The C.V. Mosby Co.

ionized compounds. Weak acids in an aqueous solution exist in balance as both a nonionized acid and as an anion. The ratio of nonionized molecules to anion will depend upon the pH of the solution (in this case, the glomerular filtrate) and upon the tendency of that acid to dissociate. As the filtrate passes down the proximal tubule and water is reabsorbed, the concentration of the weak acid is increased, causing an increase in its diffusion back into the plasma (as the result of the concentration gradient). This reabsorption is enhanced because the tubular epithelium is permeable to the nonionized component. As a result, renal excretion of a drug often requires that it first be converted in the liver to an ionic metabolite; this transformation increases the water solubility of the drug, which diminishes tubular reabsorption and enhances urinary excretion.

■ **The loop of Henle**

When sodium and water are reabsorbed from the proximal tubule, the volume of the glomerular filtrate is significantly reduced. However, since the sodium and water are reabsorbed at approximately the same rate, the osmolality of the filtrate remains unchanged as it passes through the proximal tubule; it is neither concentrated nor diluted. The function of the loop of Henle is to remove more solute and water from the filtrate.

The loop of Henle, located within the renal cor-

tex and the medulla, provides a *countercurrent mechanism* for urine concentration. The *descending* limb of the loop of Henle does not actively transport sodium or chloride, but it is very *permeable* to sodium and water. The *ascending* limb of Henle's loop, on the other hand, has an active pump, is permeable to sodium, and is relatively *impermeable* to water. As sodium and chloride are pumped from the ascending limb into the interstitial space, the interstitial fluid surrounding the loop of Henle and the collecting ducts will become very hypertonic. As the urine filtrate passes down the descending limb of the loop of Henle, water freely passes from the tubule into the interstitial fluid, as the result of the osmotic gradient between the tubule and the hypertonic interstitial fluid. Thus, as the filtrate passes through the descending limb, it becomes progressively more concentrated. The osmolality may increase from 300 mOsm/L to 1200 mOsm/L between the beginning of the descending limb and the tip of the loop of Henle (Fig. 7-8).

As the filtrate begins to pass through the *ascending* limb of the loop of Henle, chloride is actively pumped out of the tubule, sodium follows passively, and water remains in the tubule. As a result of this solute loss from the tubule, the osmolality of the filtrate again falls. Consequently the fluid arriving in the distal tubule has a lower osmolality than the fluid entering the loop of Henle and a lower osmolality than the interstitial fluid.

The loop of Henle will remove approximately

25% of the filtered sodium and 15% of filtered water from the tubule, leaving approximately 10% of the filtered sodium and 20% of the filtered water to enter the distal tubule.

The blood vessels surrounding the loop of Henle also form a hairpin loop structure, called the *vasa recta.* The vasa recta consists of capillaries that run parallel to the loops of Henle and collecting ducts. As these capillaries follow the loop of Henle into the area of the medulla made highly concentrated by the tubular countercurrent mechanism, water moves out of capillaries into the interstitum, and sodium and chloride from the interstitium move into the capillaries, as the result of the osmotic gradient.

The vasa recta is not actively involved in generating a concentration gradient; it merely reflects the gradient created by the loop of Henle. This capillary loop mechanism is termed a *countercurrent exchanger;* the term exchanger is descriptive of its passive nature. By this mechanism the solute and water in the interstitial fluid from the loops of Henle and the collecting ducts are carried away, and the medullary osmotic gradient is maintained.

■ The distal tubule and collecting ducts

The distal tubule arises from the ascending limb of the loop of Henle; its thick cellular structure is distinct from the thin segment of the ascending loop. Thick cuboidal cells continue up through the renal cortical area to a point where the distal tubule is in direct contact with the afferent arteriole of its own glomerulus. At this junction the distal tubule cells become more densely packed and more columnar, and the muscle cells of the arteriole enlarge and have a granular appearance. This point of contact between the distal tubule and the glomerular afferent arteriole is called the *juxtaglomerular apparatus.*

Beyond the juxtaglomerular apparatus, the distal tubule joins the collecting duct. The collecting duct will in turn descend from the renal cortex, through the medulla, to the renal calyces.

The filtrate present in the early distal tubule has a lower osmolality and lower sodium concentration than the plasma and the surrounding interstitial fluid. As the urine filtrate passes through the distal tubule and the collecting ducts, more water will be removed, so that the urine finally excreted will be far more concentrated. The final urine concentration accomplished in the distal tubule and the collecting ducts depends on the active transport of sodium out of the distal tubule and on the relative impermeability of the collecting ducts to water.

The distal tubule is the site of final adjustments in the urine sodium and potassium content. The distal tubule actively reabsorbs approximately 10% of the filtered sodium. This active transport process occurs against a high electrochemical gradient, is influenced by the volume and character of the fluid arriving from the loop of Henle, and is influenced by certain hormones, especially aldosterone.

A major clue to the control of sodium reabsorption was found when the observation was made that patients with diseased or absent adrenal glands and resultant aldosterone insufficiency often had profound hypovolemic shock and large amounts of sodium present in the urine. The quantity of sodium excreted in the urine when aldosterone is absent totals approximately 2% of the total filtered sodium. Thus aldosterone is responsible for the reabsorption of a very small but significant portion of the sodium filtrate.

Aldosterone is secreted by the adrenal cortex in response to pituitary adrenal corticotropic hormone (ACTH) secretion and a variety of other stimuli. A fall in the pulse pressure, decreased distension of the right atrium, and an increased serum potassium concentration all stimulate aldosterone secretion.[67] An important stimulus for aldosterone is also angiotensin formation; this occurs as the result of renin release by the juxtaglomerular apparatus (see discussion of the juxtaglomerular apparatus). Aldosterone stimulates epithelial cellular transport of sodium, not only in the renal tubular epithelium but also along the intestinal lumen and in sweat and saliva. Increased aldosterone levels increase the active reabsorption of sodium and decrease potassium reabsorption. The increased sodium reabsorption produces water reabsorption; this increases intravascular volume and reduces the juxtamedullary secretion of renin. The reduction in potassium tubular reabsorption produces increased potassium excretion in the urine and should result in a fall in serum potassium concentration. These responses to aldosterone should in turn reduce the stimulus for aldosterone secretion (Fig. 7-9).

Antidiuretic hormone (ADH, or *vasopressin*) secretion also affects the final concentration of urine. ADH is formed by the supraoptic and paraventricular nuclei in the hypothalamus and is transported to the posterior lobe of the pituitary, where it is released in response to an increase in intravascular osmotic pressure. Once the serum osmolality exceeds approximately 280 mOsm/L, ADH is secreted. It is also secreted in response to significant (10% to 15%) volume depletion, a fall in blood pressure, painful stimuli, fear, and exercise. If sodium concentrations rise or mannitol is administered, ADH is secreted. Ad-

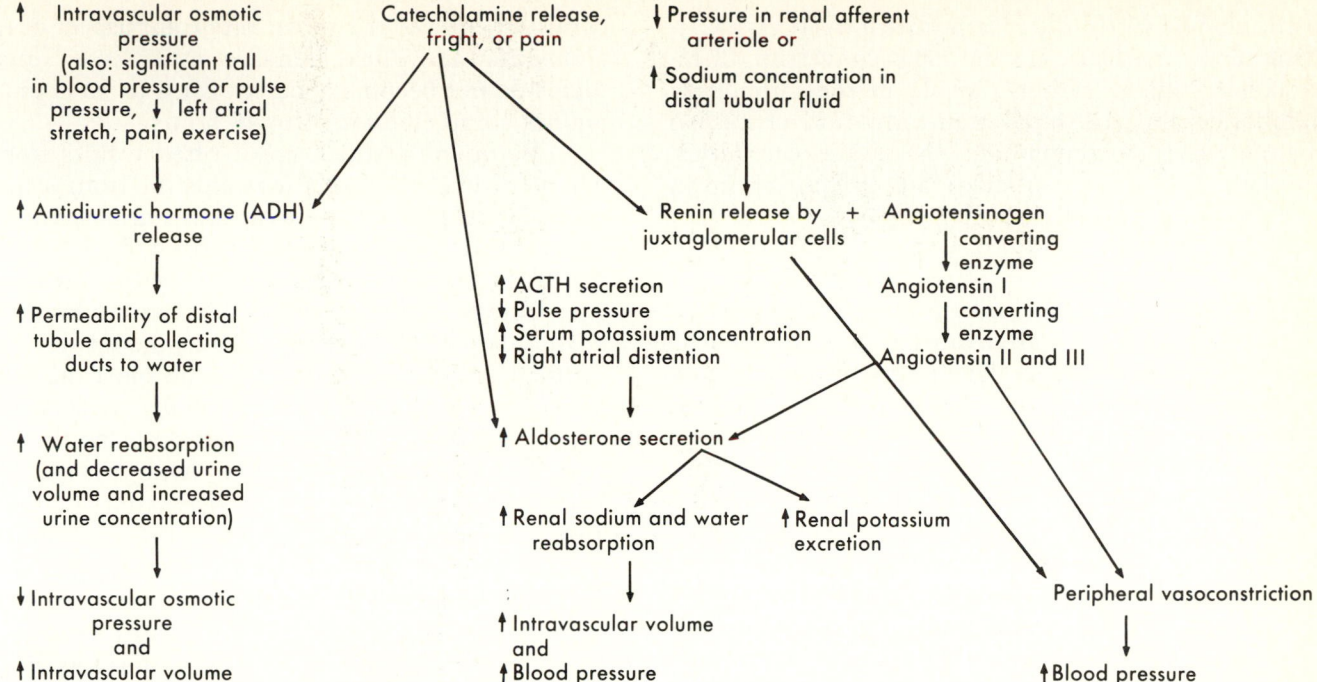

Fig. 7-9 Renal response to changes in extracellular fluid volume and concentration.[68,71]

ministration of hypertonic glucose, on the other hand, often inhibits ADH secretion.[71] The predominant stimulus for ADH secretion is, however, a rise in serum osmolality in the blood vessels in the hypothalamus.

If ADH is present, the distal tubule and collecting ducts become highly permeable to water. As the collecting ducts descend through the hypertonic interstitium in the renal medulla, water will pass from the collecting ducts into the medullary interstitium. As a result of ADH secretion then, urine volume is reduced and urine concentration is increased.

If ADH levels are low, the distal tubule and collecting ducts are relatively impermeable to water, so the urine filtrate in the collecting duct will have the same low osmolality as it passes through the renal medulla into the renal calyces. Thus low ADH levels result in the secretion of larger quantities of dilute urine.

■ **The juxtaglomerular apparatus**

The juxtaglomerular cells are located in the renal afferent arteriole just adjacent to the distal convoluted tubule. These cells form and secrete the protein enzyme, renin, in response to a fall in the pressure in the afferent arteriole, an increase in sodium concentration in the distal tubular filtrate, sympathetic nerve impulses, an increase in circulating cate-

cholamines, and a variety of other impulses. When renin is secreted into the bloodstream, it reacts with angiotensinogen, a protein synthesized by the liver, and angiotensin I is formed. Angiotensin I is converted by a plasma enzyme to angiotensin II. Angiotensin II produces peripheral vasoconstriction and an increase in aldosterone secretion (and ultimately, increased sodium and water reabsorption). These effects should produce an increase in pressure in the afferent arteriole and an increase in intravascular volume (Fig. 7-9). Angiotensin I and II are destroyed by angiotensinase, an enzyme secreted by many organs (including the kidney, intestine, and liver) and present in the plasma.[67]

■ **Renal regulation of acid-base balance**

The regulation and correction of acid-base balance involves the intracellular and extracellular buffer systems, the respiratory exchange of gases, and the ability of the kidney to excrete or to reabsorb acids and bases.

The carbonic acid buffering system. All of the body fluids contain buffers. These are compounds that combine with any acid or base in such a manner that they keep the acid or base from significantly altering the serum or tissue pH. One buffer that is present in all body fluids is the bicarbonate buffering system. This system consists of a very weak acid, carbonic acid (H_2CO_3), and bicarbonate ion (HCO_3^-). Carbonic acid will facilitate the rapid conversion of bicarbonate ion to carbon dioxide in the pulmonary capillaries and the rapid transformation of carbon dioxide into bicarbonate in the tissue capillaries. Carbonic acid and bicarbonate are in equilibrium in the following relationship:

$$CO_2 + H_2O \rightleftharpoons H_2CO_3 \rightleftharpoons H^+ + HCO_3^-$$

The carbon dioxide tension is primarily regulated by the lungs, and the bicarbonate ion concentration is regulated by the kidneys. The pulmonary regulatory mechanisms are initiated almost immediately, but the renal compensatory mechanisms are activated over a period of several hours or days.

These compensatory mechanisms protect the body from the effect of exposure to either a strong acid or a strong base. When excess hydrogen ion is present, the hydrogen ion combines with a bicarbonate ion to form carbonic acid, which is excreted in the lungs as carbon dioxide.

Carbon dioxide is constantly formed as an end product of metabolism. Normally, the lungs eliminate carbon dioxide at approximately the same rate as it is formed. A number of other acids are formed during normal metabolism. Large amounts of phosphoric acid and smaller quantities of sulfuric acid and ketoacids will enter the extracellular fluid; most of this acid will eventually be buffered and excreted by the kidneys.

Renal compensatory mechanisms for acidosis. *Respiratory acidosis* results from inadequate excretion of carbon dioxide by the lungs. This increase in carbon dioxide drives the carbon dioxide-bicarbonate reaction to the right as indicated below:

$$H_2O + CO_2 \rightleftharpoons H_2CO_3 \rightleftharpoons H^+ + HCO_3^-$$

This produces an increase in hydrogen ion concentration and acidosis. Initially, this increase in the hydrogen ions will be buffered by plasma buffer systems and plasma proteins (2% to 3%), by extracellular chloride exchanges for intracellular bicarbonate (29%), and by intracellular sodium (37%) and potassium (14%) exchanges for extracellular hydrogen ions (these hydrogen ions become bound by protein and organic phosphates).

The renal compensatory mechanisms for respiratory acidosis include increased reabsorption of filtered bicarbonate from the renal tubules, excretion of additional hydrogen ion through the formation of "titratable acids," the formation of new bicarbonate, and the excretion of ammonia. Since plasma bicarbonate concentration will need to be increased in the presence of respiratory acidosis, generation of new bi-

carbonate will be the most important aspect of renal compensation. These renal compensatory mechanisms do not become apparent for 6 to 12 hours and are not completed for 24 to 48 hours.

Metabolic acidosis most often results from an excess of hydrogen ions (or acids) or from a loss of bicarbonate. The excess hydrogen ion concentration can result from incomplete oxidation of fatty acids (as occurs in diabetic ketoacidosis or salicylate poisoning), lactic acid production as the result of hypoxia, or accumulation of inorganic acids as the result of renal failure (see the box, opposite). The most rapid compensatory mechanism for metabolic acidosis is an increase in carbon dioxide elimination by the lungs. If metabolic acidosis persists, renal compensatory mechanisms will be initiated. When metabolic acidosis is present, plasma bicarbonate concentration is reduced; therefore the amount of bicarbonate filtered and reabsorbed in the kidneys is also reduced. As a result, other urinary buffers such as the formation of "titratable acid," secretion of ammonia, and the creation of "new" bicarbonate will play a greater role in renal compensation for metabolic acidosis.

The mechanism for tubular reabsorption of bicarbonate has been reviewed previously (see the section on bicarbonate and hydrogen ion under reabsorption and secreton in the proximal tubule earlier in this chapter). In summary, hydrogen ion can be secreted into the tubular lumen; this hydrogen ion combines with bicarbonate ion present in the filtrate in the tubule, and carbonic acid is formed. This acid quickly dissociates to form carbon dioxide and water; these substances can freely diffuse out of the tubular lumen into the tubular cell, where they reform into carbonic acid. This carbonic acid in the tubular cell then dissociates into hydrogen ion and bicarbonate ion. Bicarbonate ion is ultimately reabsorbed into the vascular space, and hydrogen ion can again be utilized to reabsorb another bicarbonate ion (see Fig. 7-7). It is important to note that this reabsorption of bicarbonate ions does not result in the excretion of hydrogen ions; instead the hydrogen ions are merely utilized to aid in the bicarbonate reabsorption. Ordinarily, the amount of hydrogen ion secreted by the tubular cell is equal to the amount of bicarbonate ion reabsorbed.

The major stimulus for increased bicarbonate reabsorption from the tubules is an increase in hydrogen ion concentration in the tubular cells (such as occurs when respiratory acidosis develops). However, bicarbonate reabsorption is also affected by changes in potassium and chloride concentrations. Bicarbonate reabsorption by the renal tubules is enhanced in the presence of intracellular *hypokalemia*. When

CAUSES OF METABOLIC ACIDOSIS

Gastrointestinal loss of HCO_3^-
    Diarrhea
    Small-bowel or pancreatic drainage or fistula
    Ureterosigmoidostomy, obstructed ileal loop
      conduit
    Anion-exchange resins

Renal loss of HCO_3^-
    Carbonic anhydrase inhibitors
    Renal tubular acidosis (RTA)

Increased acid production
    Diabetic ketoacidosis
    Lactic acidosis
    Starvation
    Alcoholic ketoacidosis
    Inborn errors of metabolism
    Nonketotic hyperosmolar coma

Miscellaneous
    Dilutional acidosis
    Addition of HCl or its congeners
    Hyperalimentation acidosis

Ingestion of toxic substances
    Salicylate overdose
    Paraldehyde poisoning
    Methyl alcohol ingestion
    Ethylene glycol ingestion

Asphyxia

Failure of acid excretion
    Acute renal failure
    Chronic renal failure

Hypovolemia

---

intracellular hypokalemia is present, hydrogen ions move into the cells. This increases the amount of hydrogen ion in the tubular cells and enhances hydrogen ion secretion into the tubule. It also enhances bicarbonate reabsorption, even in the presence of alkalosis. Thus a *hypokalemic alkalosis* occurs and urine pH is low. If the hypokalemia is aggressively treated and/or a *hyperkalemia* results, potassium will replace hydrogen ion in the renal tubular cells and will be secreted by the tubular cells in place of hydrogen ion. This will reduce the hydrogen ion secretion so that bicarbonate formation is reduced. In this case, an alkaline urine is excreted that contains a large amount of potassium. This inverse relationship between potassium and hydrogen ion secretion by the renal tubules is thought to result from the fact that they compete for the same secretory mechanism in the renal tubules.[68]

Bicarbonate reabsorption is also affected by chloride concentration. When hypochloremia develops, bicarbonate reabsorption increases; if hyperchloremia develops, bicarbonate reabsorption is decreased. Thus there is also a reciprocal relationship between bicarbonate and chloride concentrations and reabsorption.

When body buffering mechanisms are activated to buffer hydrogen ions during acidosis, the bicarbonate ion stores may be depleted, so that the quantity of bicarbonate ions present in the glomerular filtrate is reduced. This limits the amount of bicarbonate available to combine with hydrogen ions (which are being secreted by the tubular cell in exchange for sodium ions). In this case, the hydrogen ions secreted by the tubules combine with phosphate or other organic buffers present in the urine, and a nondissociating acid is formed. Thus the excess hydrogen ions are excreted in the urine (see Fig. 7-10). When hydrogen ions are excreted in this way, a quantity of nondissociating acid can be measured in the urine, so this buffering mechanism is known as the formation of "titratable acid." To measure the quantity of hydrogen ion present in the urine combined with phosphate or other organic buffers, sodium hydroxide (NaOH) is titrated into the urine sample. The number of milliequivalents of sodium hydroxide required to restore the urine pH to 7.4 is equal to the number of milliequivalents of hydrogen ions that are present in combination with the buffers. This quantity of hydrogen ion is referred to as the *titratable acid* present in the urine.

When titratable acid is formed and excreted in the urine, hydrogen ions are actually eliminated, and bicarbonate ions are formed as a byproduct of the reaction (see Fig. 7-10). These bicarbonate ions can then be added to the plasma as the "new" bicarbonate to increase the plasma buffering capability. The capacity of the kidneys to form titratable acid and to generate new bicarbonate is limited, since the kidney cannot excrete a urine with a pH lower than approximately 4.4. In addition, the rate of excretion of titratable acid will be limited by the amount of phosphate and other inorganic buffers present in the glomerular filtrate. As a result, additional hydrogen ions will be excreted through another renal buffering mechanism, the formation of ammonia.

Amino acids are reabsorbed from glomerular fil-

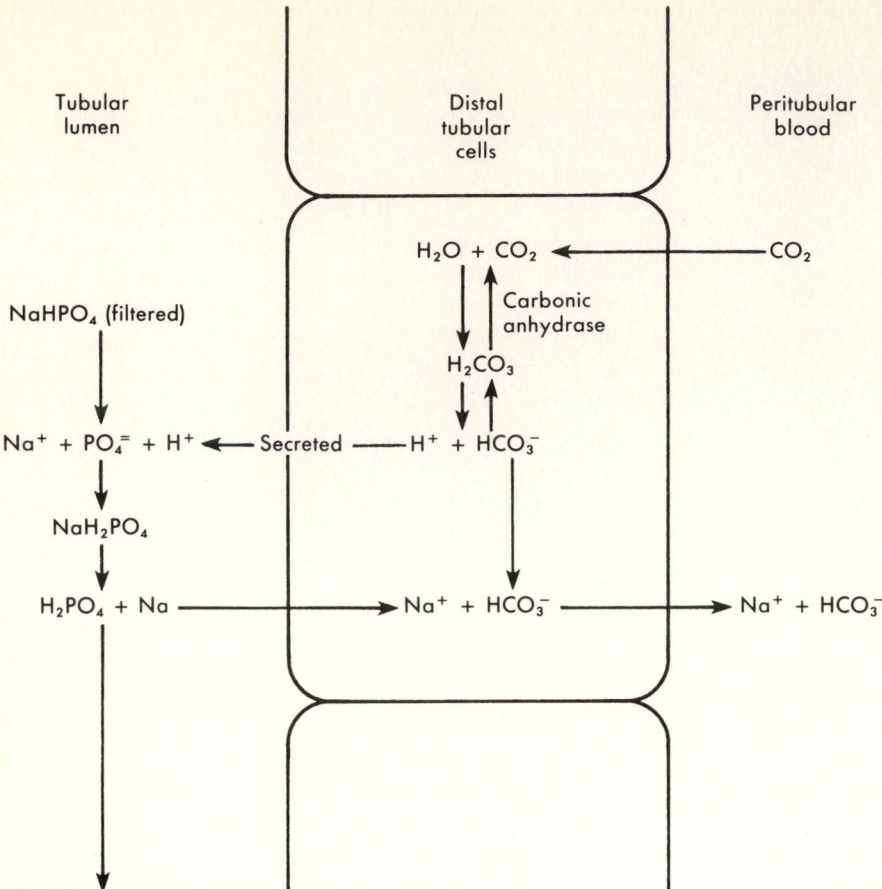

Fig. 7-10 Mechanism for formation of titratable acid in renal tubular cells. Carbon dioxide diffuses from peritubular blood into distal tubular cells, where it combines with water (with carbonic anhydrase as catalyst) to form carbonic acid. Carbonic acid dissociates into bicarbonate ion (which diffuses out of tubular cell and ultimately diffuses back into peritubular blood) and hydrogen ion, which is secreted into renal tubule. In renal tubule, the hydrogen ion is exchanged for sodium ion; hydrogen ion combines with phosphate to form hydrogen phosphate, which is excreted. Sodium ion diffuses into renal tubular cells and ultimately diffuses into peritubular blood.

trate by the tubular cells. They are then deaminated in the cells, so the free base, ammonia, is created. Ammonia (NH_3) is a nonionized, lipid-soluble substance; hence it easily diffuses across cell membranes into both the tubular lumen and the blood. The intratubular NH_3 reacts with hydrogen ion to form ammonium ion (NH_4^+). Since ammonium ion (NH_4^+) is an ionized, lipid-insoluble substance, it is trapped within the tubular lumen and excreted in the urine.

There are other urinary buffers that occasionally appear in the tubular fluid in sufficient quantities to act as significant buffers. In uncontrolled diabetes mellitus, incomplete carbohydrate metabolism produces large amounts of ketoacids. At plasma pH levels, these ketoacids almost completely dissociate to yield their anions and hydrogen ions. The hydrogen ion is buffered by serum buffers. The dissociated anions are filtered into the glomerular filtrate, but because their concentration is so great, they are only partially reabsorbed. As a result, these organic anions are available to buffer some of the hydrogen ion being secreted by the tubules, although this buffering capability is very limited.

Renal compensatory mechanisms for alkalosis. *Respiratory alkalosis,* a very uncommon primary event, results from excessive removal of carbon dioxide. This decrease in carbon dioxide drives the carbon dioxide-bicarbonate reaction to the left, as indicated below:

$$H_2O + CO_2 \leftrightarrows H_2CO_3 \leftrightarrows H^+ + HCO_3^-$$

This produces alkalosis because the carbonic acid and hydrogen ion concentrations will be reduced. Buffer systems in the body will result in the release of lactic acid, the exchange of extracellular bicarbonate for chloride, and the movement of hydrogen ion from the intracellular to the intravascular space, in exchange for sodium and potassium ion shifts. Intracellular hydrogen ion stores are reduced, so less hydrogen ion is available for tubular secretion; this results in increased secretion of bicarbonate ion into the urine.

Metabolic alkalosis can be caused by either increased bicarbonate concentration or loss of hydrogen ions. As noted above renal reabsorption of bicarbonate is enhanced in the presence of hypokalemia or hypochloremia. These conditions reduce the kidneys' ability to excrete bicarbonate in the urine. Thus hypokalemia or hypochloremia can produce a metabolic alkalosis or can reduce renal compensation for the alkalosis. The presence of a metabolic alkalosis can also increase potassium excretion in the urine; this can further enhance the metabolic alkalosis. This form of hypokalemic and/or hypochloremic alkalosis may be seen after vigorous diuresis with a drug such as furosemide, since this drug produces both potassium and chloride loss in the urine.

Another relatively common cause of metabolic alkalosis in pediatric patients is the loss of hydrochloric acid associated with vomiting. This acid loss is often complicated by increased urinary loss of potassium, so the alkalosis may develop and progress more rapidly. In these patients, the alkalosis will not improve until potassium is administered.

When metabolic alkalosis develops, respiratory compensation is initiated almost immediately. This produces a decrease in alveolar ventilation and carbon dioxide retention. When the plasma carbon dioxide tension rises, more carbonic acid, hydrogen ion, and bicarbonate will be present. If renal compensatory mechanisms are intact, excess bicarbonate is excreted in the form of sodium bicarbonate. Sodium is excreted in exchange for the hydrogen ion, which is reabsorbed. This produces increased bicarbonate excretion and enhanced hydrogen ion reabsorption.

■ Calcium regulation

The regulation of extracellular ionized calcium concentration is normally maintained within very narrow limits by renal compensatory mechanisms and by adjustments in bone deposition or demineralization and vitamin D reabsorption in the gastrointestinal tract. Serum ionized calcium concentrations are also affected by serum albumin concentrations and acid-base balance.

The precise regulation of extracellular calcium levels is necessary, because calcium imbalance may exert a profound effect on neuromuscular excitability and cardiovascular function. In addition, calcium plays an important role in the chemical reactions necessary for thrombin formation and coagulation. Finally, calcium ions react with phosphate ions to form bone salts; these bone salts give the bones rigidity.

Approximately 99% of the total body calcium stores are deposited in the bones and the remaining 1% of calcium stores reside in the blood plasma and the interstitial fluid. If a serum pH is normal, approximately 40% of the total plasma calcium is bound to the serum albumin. This protein-bound calcium does not enter into chemical reactions and does not filter into the glomerular filtrate. The remaining 60% of the total plasma calcium is present in the ionized form; this constitutes the biologically active form of calcium. Whenever serum calcium levels are evaluated, it is important to correlate the total serum calcium level with the concentration of the serum proteins. An increase in the serum levels of albumin and globulin will increase that portion of the total serum calcium bound to proteins and will reduce the amount of ionized calcium in the plasma. For each 1 gm/dl increase in serum *albumin* levels, 0.8 mg/dl of calcium is removed from its ionized state and is bound to the albumin. Increases in serum *globulin* levels, however, will lower the ionized calcium concentration by only 0.16 mg/dl. If serum albumin and globulin concentrations are reduced, a relatively greater portion of the patient's total serum calcium will be present in the ionized form. As a result, the patient with a low total serum calcium concentration *and* a reduction in serum albumin may have a normal ionized calcium concentration.

Changes in the serum pH will also affect the amount of calcium bound by proteins. An increase of 0.1 in serum pH will increase protein-bound calcium by 0.12 mg/dl. Conversely, when the serum pH is lowered, more calcium is removed from its protein binding sites and is available for participation in chemical reactions. Thus, when a decreased serum calcium concentration is present in the patient with alkalosis, the ionized calcium concentration is probably very low. On the other hand, if the serum calcium concentration is low in the patient with acidosis, ionized calcium levels may not be significantly reduced.

The maintenance of a normal serum calcium level requires regulation of the amounts of calcium absorbed from the gastrointestinal tract, the amounts filtered and reabsorbed by the kidneys, and the mobilization or deposition of calcium phosphate and other minerals in the bone matrix. All three of these methods of regulating calcium are controlled by parathyroid hormone, which is secreted by the four parathyroid glands. When serum ionized calcium levels fall, parathyroid hormone will be released. This parathyroid hormone will increase the renal reabsorption of calcium and the gastrointestinal absorption of calcium. It will also increase the movement of calcium (and phosphate) from the bone into the extracellular fluid (ECF). In addition, parathyroid hormone release will decrease renal tubular reabsorption of phosphate, resulting in a lowered phosphate concentration in the extracellular fluid.

Renal regulation of calcium. Renal calcium reabsorption is active and occurs throughout the nephron. Normally, only 1% of filtered calcium is excreted in the urine, although this amount can be altered by changing either the filtered load of calcium or its rate of reabsorption. If calcium intake is increased, the plasma calcium concentration increases. This increase in plasma calcium will be reflected in an increased amount of calcium filtered into the tubule and increased calcium excretion in the urine. The renal capacity to excrete calcium is compromised by a reduction in GFR, volume depletion, and chronic expansion of the ECF associated with mineralocorticoid administration.

The rate of calcium reabsorption from the tubules can also be altered. When parathyroid hormone is secreted, renal calcium excretion is reduced and urinary excretion of sodium is enhanced. Calcium retention is also increased by the chronic administration of thiazide diuretics; these drugs produce a distal tubular natriuresis, so sodium is excreted and calcium is retained.

Gastrointestinal absorption of calcium. The gastrointestinal absorption of calcium occurs as the result of an active transport system, which is controlled by parathyroid hormone. Under normal conditions, the intestinal handling of calcium involves the formation of the insoluble precipitate calcium phosphate, resecretion of large masses of calcium by the cells of the intestinal epithelium, and finally a net absorption of approximately 10% of the ingested calcium. When serum calcium concentrations fall and parathyroid hormone is released, intestinal absorption of calcium will increase somewhat as the result of the parathyroid hormone release. More importantly, parathyroid hormone will stimulate renal activation of vitamin D_3. The presence of activated vitamin D_3 will greatly accelerate gastrointestinal absorption of ingested calcium.

Mobilization of calcium from bone. Approximately 99% of the body's calcium stores are deposited in the bone matrix as hydroxyapatite. Every time calcium is deposited, phosphate is deposited also, and when bone is reabsorbed, both calcium and phosphate are released into the body fluid. Bone is continually being broken down (reabsorbed) under the influences of cells called osteoclasts and simultaneously reformed under the influences of a different cell group called osteoblasts. When parathyroid hormone levels are increased, the osteoclasts are stimulated to increase the breakdown of the bone structure; this liberates calcium and phosphate and raises the serum concentrations of both. Since parathyroid hormone also enhances renal calcium reabsorption but reduces phosphate absorption, the ultimate effect of parathyroid hormone release is an increase in serum ionized calcium concentration. The full effect of parathyroid hormone in bone reabsorption does depend upon the simultaneous presence of vitamin D_3, which must be activated in the kidneys.

■ Prenatal and postnatal development of renal function

During fetal life, the placenta performs many of the functions of the kidney, so renal malformations may not cause fetal distress. Urine secretion into the amniotic fluid begins during the ninth through twelfth weeks of gestation. Most kidney growth occurs during the last 20 weeks of gestation, and the glomerular filtration rate increases rapidly between the twenty-eighth and thirty-fifth weeks of gestation.[35] All of the nephrons of the mature kidney are formed by the twenty-eighth week of gestation.[70]

After birth, kidney size increases in proportion to body length. Kidney weight doubles in the first 10 months of life, more as the result of proximal tubular growth than because of increase in glomerular size. The glomerular filtration rate also increases significantly after birth; the GFR of the full-term neonate (per square meter of body surface area) is approximately equal to one third the GFR of an adult. The GFR doubles during the first 2 weeks of life and is approximately equal to adult values by the first year of life.[8] Renal perfusion also doubles during the first weeks of life.[70]

Immediately after birth the neonate normally demonstrates a high urine volume with low osmolality. This is thought to be the result of diuresis of excess body water. Since increased systemic arterial pressure and systemic vascular resistance also result in an increase in renal blood flow (RBF) and glomerular filtration rate during this time, these factors may also be responsible for the high urine volume. Beyond the first several hours of life, urine volume normally falls, and urine concentration gradually rises.[80]

The newborn kidney is able to excrete amino acids and conserve sodium and glucose as well as the adult kidney. The ability of the newborn kidney to excrete free water and to concentrate urine is less than that of the adult kidney, however.[35,81] As a result, the infant kidney may be less able to excrete a hypotonic urine in response to water loading and may be unable to excrete a very concentrated urine in response to dehydration.

Regulation of acid-base balance by the newborn kidney is relatively efficient,[35] although there is less ability to secrete hydrogen ions or fixed acid than the adult kidney. As a result, renal compensation for metabolic acidosis may be limited during the neonatal period. Dehydration, hypotension, and hypoxemia all produce a marked fall in the infant's glomerular filtration rate,[6,33] so renal function may quickly become compromised during critical illness.

■ COMPOSITION AND DISTRIBUTION OF BODY WATER
■ Body water distribution

Water is the largest constituent of body weight. In the premature infant, up to 80% to 85% of body weight is body water; in the full-term infant, approximately 70% of body weight is water. In young adults body water constitutes approximately 65% of body weight in males, and 52% of body weight in females. The percentage of body weight that is water does vary according to amount of body fat that is present. Since fat is essentially water free, the more fat the individual has, the smaller the proportion of total body weight is water. This relationship between water content and weight is important to consider during assessment of levels of hydration, consideration of fluid and solute losses and replacement requirements, and calculation of medication dosages.

Body water is divided between the intracellular and extracellular compartments. Intracellular water usually constitutes approximately 55% of total body water, and extracellular water constitutes approximately 45% of total body water. During infancy, however, a larger proportion of the body water is extracellular, and approximately one half of the infant's extracellular fluid is exchanged daily.[61] Extracellular water consists of plasma (7.5%), interstitial fluid and lymph (20%), bone water (7.5%), and connective tissue water (25%). A small fraction (2.5%) of extracellular fluid is present as *transcellular* fluid; this fluid includes cerebrospinal fluid, intraocular, pleural, peritoneal, and synovial fluid, and the digestive secretions. These fluids are separated from the extracellular fluid by specialized epithelial cells, and the fluid content in each of these compartments is modified from plasma.[85,89] Each of the body's water compartments contains different concentrations of electrolytes that are characteristic for that compartment (Table 7-1).

■ Serum osmolality

Osmotic pressure in each fluid is measured in milliosmoles (mOsm). It is the force exerted by particles in solution that will draw water across a semipermeable membrane. Osmotic activity depends upon the number of particles present and is not affected by the particle size or electrical charge. The *normal serum osmolality* is approximately 272 to 294 mOsm/L. Sodium and its chief anions, chloride and bicarbonate, account for 90% of the total osmolality of the plasma. The serum osmolality can be calculated by adding the concentrations of the solutes per unit of solvent; these solutes include sodium, potassium, calcium, magnesium, sulfate, creatinine, glucose, protein, and urea. For simplicity, the total serum osmolality can be estimated utilizing the serum concentrations of sodium, glucose, and blood urea nitrogen (BUN) in the following formula[15]:

$$2 \times \text{Sodium concentration (mEq/L)} \quad \underline{\qquad}$$
$$\frac{\text{Glucose concentration (mg/dl)}}{18} \quad \underline{\qquad}$$
$$\frac{\text{Blood urea nitrogen (mg/dl)}}{2.8} \quad \underline{\qquad}$$
$$\text{TOTAL serum osmolality (mOsm/L)} = \underline{\qquad}$$

■ Changes in body fluid composition and distribution during critical illness

The critically ill infant or child has a tendency to retain fluids because antidiuretic hormone and aldosterone secretion are usually increased. Catecholamine release, hypotension, fright, or pain can all stimulate antidiuretic hormone (ADH, or vasopres-

Table 7-1 Composition of intracellular and extracellular body fluids

Extracellular		Intracellular
137 mEq/L	Na	10 mEq/L
5 mEq/L	K	141 mEq/L
5 mEq/L	Ca	0 mEq/L
3 mEq/L	Mg	62 mEq/L
103 mEq/L	Cl	4 mEq/L
28 mEq/L	HCO_3	10 mEq/L
4 mEq/L	Phosphates	75 mEq/L
1 mEq/L	SO_4	2 mEq/L
90 mg %	Glucose	0-20 mg %
30 mg %	Amino acids	200 mg %
0.5 gm %	Cholesterol	2-95 gm %
	Phospholipids	
	Neutral fat	
35 mm Hg	P_{O_2}	20 mm Hg
46 mm Hg	P_{CO_2}	50 mm Hg
7.4	pH	7.1

sin), renin, and aldosterone release. ADH release is also known to be stimulated by any condition that reduces left atrial pressure (including hemorrhage, positive-pressure ventilation, and severe pulmonary hypertension), and it is also stimulated by administration of general anesthetics, morphine, or barbiturates.[29,48]

ADH secretion promotes water reabsorption by the renal tubules and collecting ducts, so intravascular volume will increase and intravascular osmotic pressure will fall. Aldosterone secretion enhances renal sodium and water reabsorption; this also results in an increase in intravascular volume. As a result of the actions of these hormones, the postoperative patient often demonstrates decreased urine volume and increased urine concentration. Since the newborn kidney has limited ability to concentrate urine, the neonate may demonstrate decreased urine volume and only moderate urine concentration.

Postoperative fluid administration must be tailored to prevent fluid overload or sodium imbalance.[37] Most commonly, hypotonic sodium chloride solutions (0.2 NaCl or 0.45 NaCl) are administered with 5% or 10% glucose. Urine volume should be monitored closely and should average ≥1 ml/kg/hour, if fluid administration totals half of maintenance fluid requirements or more. If severe fluid restriction is imposed, urine volume may average 0.5 to 1.0 ml/kg/hour. Urine concentration should be evaluated through measurement of urine specific gravity and

osmolality. The specific gravity of the urine reflects the combined weight of all of the particles in the urine. The specific gravity of water is 1.000, and the specific gravity of normal urine ranges from 1.003 to 1.030. The higher the solute content of urine, the higher will be the specific gravity. The urine *specific gravity* usually correlates with the *urine osmolality*. However, if an excessive number of *large* particles is present in the urine as the result of glycosuria or proteinuria or as the result of the use of radiographic contrast agents or mannitol, the urine specific gravity will increase disproportionately to its true osmolality. Since the urine osmolality best indicates the renal ability to concentrate urine above the serum osmolality, it is a more reliable indicator of renal function than the measurement of the urine specific gravity.

Some drugs or solutions used in the evaluation or treatment of critically ill patients may be nephrotoxic. Antibiotics such as the cephalosporins, the aminoglycosides, and the sulfonamides may be nephrotoxic in infants and children.[35,45] Alpha-adrenergic medications that produce renal vasoconstriction can result in decreased renal perfusion and oliguric renal failure. Indomethacin administration to promote constriction of the neonatal ductus arteriosus can produce a fall in glomerular filtration rate or a decrease in urine output.[14] The use of hypertonic angiographic contrast agents can result in renal vein thrombosis, medullary hypoperfusion, renal ischemia, and renal insufficiency.[35] Since these agents have an osmolality of 1300 to 1940 mOsm/kg water, they should be administered carefully, in low doses, to only well-hydrated infants. Their use in children should also be restricted if circulatory compromise or renal insufficiency is present.

■ DIURETICS

Diuretics are agents that increase urine volume. The primary effect of such drugs is to decrease tubular reabsorption of sodium and chloride; this in turn will decrease water reabsorption indirectly. Diuretics usually do not exert a primary effect on water reabsorption itself. The diuretics may be classified according to their renal site of action. The osmotic agents, mercurial diuretics, and carbonic anhydrase inhibitors are proximal tubule diuretics, which are seldom used. The more popular thiazides, sulfonamide derivatives, and potassium-sparing diuretics act in the distal tubule. Furosemide (Lasix) and ethacrynic acid exert their effect on the loop of Henle (see the box on the right).

■ Proximal tubule diuretics

The osmotic agents such as mannitol, urea, and glucose exert their effects as a result of their high osmolality. Once these agents are filtered through the glomerulus, they pull additional free water into the filtrate. This retards sodium and water reabsorption in the proximal tubule and results in increased volume of glomerular filtrate and urine. Hypertonic glucose and mannitol are not the drugs of choice for routine diuresis. However, they can be extremely useful in promoting diuresis in the child with marginal renal function, since their effect is produced as soon as they are filtered through the glomerulus, and they do not depend on renal tubular excretory or reabsorptive functions. Mannitol administration does increase renal medullary blood flow and it may reduce the incidence of acute tubular necrosis.[45]

Immediately after any osmotic agent is administered intravenously, it can produce a temporary but significant increase in intravascular volume. This increase occurs because the intravenous osmotic agent pulls water from the extravascular to the intravascular space. Use of these agents is usually contraindicated in patients with congestive heart failure or hypervolemia, since this may further increase intravascular volume. However, these drugs can be extremely useful in the treatment of patients with cerebral edema (see Chapter 6).

Mercurial diuretics are very powerful diuretics

CLASSIFICATION OF DIURETICS BY NEPHRON SITE OF ACTION

Filtration diuretics
Aminophylline
Glucocorticoids

Proximal tubular diuretics
Mannitol
Acetazolamide

Loop of Henle diuretics
Ethacrynic acid
Furosemide

Distal tubular diuretics
Potassium-losing
Thiazides
Chlorthalidone
Metolazone (?)
Potassium-retaining
Triamterene
Spironolactone

---

that decrease reabsorption of sodium in the proximal tubule. Since mercurial diuretics are ineffective when they are administered orally, they must be given parenterally. Therefore these drugs are rarely used, since there are several more effective oral and parenteral diuretics available.[79]

Carbonic anhydrase inhibitors limit the rate at which the proximal cells hydrate carbon dioxide to carbonic acid. Therefore less hydrogen ion is available beyond the proximal tubule cell to exchange for sodium, so sodium reabsorption is reduced and a diuresis results. This reduced hydrogen ion-sodium exchange also limits the amount of urinary bicarbonate returned to the blood (as sodium bicarbonate) and a mild metabolic acidosis may result.[19]

■ Distal tubule diuretics

The thiazide diuretics block the reabsorption of sodium and chloride in the cortical segment of the distal tubule. Thus they do not interfere with the nephron's ability to concentrate the urine, but they do limit the excretion of a maximally dilute urine. All of the thiazide diuretics produce significant potassium and calcium loss in the urine. Since thiazide diuretics can depress the glomerular filtration rate, thiazide administration can result in a reversible rise in blood urea nitrogen. Thiazide diuretics are promptly absorbed from the gastrointestinal tract and usually produce diuresis within 1 hour. The effects of the drugs usually last 12 to 24 hours, then they are excreted in the urine. Patients who receive thiazide diuretics may require simultaneous administration of a potassium supplement to prevent hypokalemia.

Potassium-sparing diuretics constitute a separate class of diuretics, and include spironolactone, triamterene, and amiloride. These drugs block distal tubule sodium reabsorption and interfere with sodium-potassium exchange and with the sodium-hydrogen ion exchange. Consequently sodium (and water) is excreted, and potassium and hydrogen ion are reabsorbed. Spironolactone is an aldosterone antagonist and does not depress the GFR, while triamterene and amiloride may depress the GFR significantly.[19] These drugs are not as potent as other diuretics, so they are best used in conjunction with other diuretics such as the thiazides or furosemide.

■ **Loop of Henle diuretics**

The loop diuretics, furosemide (Lasix) and ethacrynic acid (Edecrin), are the most potent and popular of the diuretics used in the care of critically ill children. Both drugs will exert a diuretic effect, even in patients responding maximally to other diuretics, and they will be effective despite a decrease in glomerular filtration rate.[89] Both drugs can be administered intravenously, and they have a rapid onset. They block chloride and sodium reabsorption in the ascending limb of the loop of Henle; this results in large quantities of sodium in the filtrate of the distal tubule that overwhelm the various sodium exchange mechanisms and result in a loss of water and salt. This diuresis also results in increased potassium, hydrogen, and calcium ion loss. The large diuresis often produces a decrease in plasma volume, which may result in a contraction alkalosis. The increased hydrogen ion excretion that results from administration of loop diuretics can further contribute to the alkalotic state (see the box). In large doses, both furosemide and ethacrynic acid may cause an increase in renal blood flow with accompanied increase in perfusion to the outer renal cortical areas. These drugs are very useful in patients with marginal renal perfusion or in patients with cardiovascular and renal disease.[19] Both drugs have been associated with ototoxicity, although the reported incidence of this complication seems to be higher with ethacrynic acid. The ototoxicity may not be reversible, even after the drug is discontinued. Patients receiving only furosemide or ethacrynic acid may require potassium supplementation to prevent hypokalemia. The peak effects, actions, and dosages of the most powerful pediatric diuretics are included in Table 7-2.

■ **Common Clinical Conditions**

■ **DEHYDRATION: HYPERNATREMIC**

The osmolality of the intravascular fluid compartment is determined by the concentration of solute (chiefly sodium) dissolved in the plasma solvent (water). The loss of free water or the gain of solute will produce an increase in the amount of solute per unit of solvent. This will result in an increase in the osmolality in the intravascular space. As the serum osmolality increases, an osmotic gradient is created between the intracellular and the intravascular space. Water is drawn from the intracellular spaces into the intravascular space; this reduces the intracellular fluid volume. If the serum osmolality is increased by glucose in the nondiabetic patient, there will be little change in body water distribution because the glucose freely enters cells. Sodium, on the other hand, is actively pumped out of cells and sodium movement often affects water movement, so an increase in intravascular sodium content can produce a significant fall in intracellular water.

■ **Etiology**

Hypernatremic (or hypertonic) dehydration results from loss of both fluid and electrolytes; in this type of dehydration, however, loss of free water exceeds the loss of sodium and other solutes. Hypertonic dehydration in children can occur as the result of diarrhea, vomiting, burns, high fever, diabetes insipidus, inappropriate parenteral alimentation (with insufficient administration of free water), aggressive dialysis, administration of large amounts of sodium

---

FACTORS CONTRIBUTING TO METABOLIC ALKALOSIS WITH ADMINISTRATION OF LOOP DIURETICS

Losses of:
potassium
chloride
hydrogen

Increased:
titratable acid
ammonium
"new" bicarbonate added to plasma
contraction of plasma volume

Table 7-2 Diuretic dosages in children

Drug (Trade name)	Action	Dosage	Peak effect	Effect on serum K+
Furosemide (Lasix)	Inhibits NaCl transport in ascending limb of Loop of Henle and proximal and distal tubules	1-2 mg/kg/IV dose or 1-4 mg/kg/oral dose	Immediate (IV) ½-4 hours (oral)	$\downarrow\downarrow\downarrow$
Ethacrynic acid (Edecrin)	Same as furosemide (above)	1 mg/kg/IV dose or 2-3 mg/kg/oral dose	Few minutes (IV) ½-8 hours (oral)	$\downarrow\downarrow\downarrow$
Chlorothiazide (Diuril)	Inhibits tubular reabsorption of Na+ primarily in the distal tubule but also in the Loop of Henle; also inhibits H₂O reabsorption in cortical diluting segment of ascending limb of Loop	20-40 mg/kg/day (oral)	2-4 hours	$\downarrow\downarrow$
Spironolactone (Aldactone)	Aldosterone antagonist (inhibits exchange of Na+ for K+ in distal tubule)	1.5-3.3 mg/kg/day (oral)	1-4 days, and persists for days beyond discontinuation	K+ is "saved"
Hydrochlorothiazide + Spironolactone (Aldactazide)	(See above discussion for aldosterone antagonist.) Hydrochlorothiazide inhibits Na+ reabsorption in distal tubule and in Loop of Henle and inhibits H₂O reabsorption in cortical diluting segment of ascending limb of Loop	1.65-3.3 mg/kg/day (oral)	2-4 hours (as a result of thiazide component), but persists for days beyond discontinuation (as a result of spironolactone component)	— (remains approximately unchanged)

Adapted from Hazinski, M.F.: Critical care of the pediatric cardiovascular patient, Nurs. Clin. North Am. 16:677, 1981.

bicarbonate or mannitol, or increased respiratory insensible water loss. Diabetic ketoacidosis can also produce hypertonic dehydration as the result of the osmotic diuresis produced by the glycosuria. In addition, hypernatremic dehydration during infancy can result from administration of infant formula prepared with too much salt or from formula inappropriately mixed from concentrate.

■ Pathophysiology

Since hypernatremic dehydration is caused by proportionately greater free water loss than sodium loss, the serum sodium concentration and serum osmolality will increase, even though total body sodium concentration is decreased. The increase in intravascular osmolality stimulates antidiuretic hormone (ADH) and aldosterone secretion. ADH secretion increases free water reabsorption, but aldosterone secretion increases both water and sodium reabsorption.[22]

If the fluid loss is significant and reduces intravascular volume and compromises systemic perfusion, aldosterone secretion increases significantly. This produces further sodium and water reabsorption and results in the perpetuation of the hypernatremia.

Once the osmolality of the fluid in the intravascular space increases, fluid shifts from the cells into the vascular space, as the result of osmosis. As a result, the fluid lost in hypertonic dehydration is largely intracellular. The most important tissues to be damaged by such a fluid loss are the cells of the brain. If hypertonic dehydration develops gradually, the brain can generate intracellular solutes, called "idiogenic osmoles." These solutes exert osmotic force within brain cells and can prevent massive water loss from the brain into the hypertonic intravascular space. If, however, hypertonic dehydration develops quickly, water shift from the brain into the vascular space can be significant, and it can result in cerebral damage, including subdural effusions, cerebral thrombosis, or cerebral hemorrhage.[72] In many of these patients, seizures develop during the period of rehydration (see the section on pathophysiology of dehydration in Chapter 8).

Dehydration can produce a fall in glomerular filtration rate. Renal tubular injury can also occur as the result of dehydration and can produce a loss of renal concentrating ability.[72]

■ Clinical signs and symptoms

Hypertonic dehydration produces fluid shifts from the intracellular to the intravascular space. As a result, the intracellular fluid loss is greater than the intravascular fluid loss, so signs of circulatory compromise do not appear until late in the clinical course. The clinical signs and symptoms most commonly seen as the result of hypertonic dehydration include those of weight loss, altered skin turgor or appearance, and signs of central nervous system irritability.

The child's eyes will appear sunken and dark. Dehydrated infants less than 16 to 18 months of age can have marked depression of the anterior fontanelle. The child with hypertonic dehydration may have adequate skin turgor, though the skin may feel "doughy" over the abdomen, and the skin color is grey. Mucous membranes will be dry. The infant or child with hypertonic dehydration is often extremely irritable and may demonstrate hyperactive reflexes.

Initially, the diagnosis of this form of dehydration may be difficult to separate from that of meningitis, since both may include a history of fever and irritability. However, a more detailed history may reveal a cause for the dehydration, and an elevation in serum sodium concentration will confirm the diagnosis. In many children, the serum sodium concentration may exceed 150 mEq/L. If a spinal tap is performed as part of a septic workup, cerebrospinal fluid protein level is often elevated.[72]

Urinalysis can reveal proteinuria, hyaline or granular casts, white blood cells, and red blood cells. These findings should disappear after the patient is successfully rehydrated, unless intrinsic renal disease or renal damage has occurred (see also the section on clinical signs and symptoms of dehydration in Chapter 8).

Infants and children with hypertonic dehydration often develop metabolic acidosis. Because of this, potassium can shift into the vascular space, producing a normal or high serum potassium concentration, despite a total body deficit of potassium. Once the acidosis is corrected, the child's serum potassium concentration usually falls significantly.

Since the intravascular volume will be maintained at cellular expense, a 10% weight loss is usually not associated with clinical signs of shock, so extremities will be warm and pulses strong. When fluid losses total more than 10% of body weight, signs of poor systemic perfusion (tachycardia, poor peripheral pulses, oliguria or anuria, cool extremities, poor capillary refill, and metabolic acidosis) are likely to be present. The child with severe hypertonic dehydration is severely ill and requires prompt and skillful treatment.

■ Medical treatment and nursing interventions

Acute medical management of hypertonic dehydration is aimed at *gradual* correction of the fluid and electrolyte deficit and prevention of central nervous system complications.

Before therapy is begun, an accurate weight should be obtained, and a large bore venous catheter should be inserted. It is imperative that the intravenous catheter be secured adequately, so that it will remain in place as long as possible. It is often extremely difficult to gain venous access in these critically ill patients, so the catheters should be maintained carefully. Before large dressings or armboards are taped in place, they should be weighed on a clean scale, so their weight can be used in evaluation of the child's daily weight gain or loss. The child should be weighed daily on the same scale at the time of day by, preferably, the same nurse. Initially, the child is weighed every 8 hours, then daily. The scale used and the weighing times should be recorded on the nursing care plan. A weight change of 50 gm/24 hours in an infant, 200 gm/24 hours in a child, or 500 gm/24 hours in an adolescent should be discussed with a physician, and the patient's fluid balance should be carefully assessed.

The placement of a urinary catheter with aseptic technique is mandatory when the child has moderate or severe dehydration, since this will enable evaluation of urine output, renal function, and response to therapy. For small infants, a sterile #5 French feeding tube securely taped and connected to a closed sterile connector can be used for urinary drainage. Urine output should total 10 ml/m²/hour or 1 ml/kg/hour once rehydration is achieved.

The first urine specimen obtained should be sent for urinalysis, culture, sensitivity, colony count, sodium, potassium, chloride, and osmolality. Only when urine output has been established, and laboratory reports have confirmed that potassium levels are not elevated, can potassium be added to IV solutions. With restoration of adequate circulation, as evidenced by adequate urine flow, improved renal function will allow renal correction of acidosis.

The infant or child is *gradually* rehydrated with fluids containing both free water and small amounts of sodium. It is important to note that too rapid a reduction of the serum sodium concentration may produce seizures. It is thought that such seizures may occur as the result of a rapid fluid shift from the vascular space back into the brain, causing cerebral edema. As a result, it is recommended that children with hypernatremic dehydration be rehydrated during approximately 48 hours, so that their serum sodium concentration does not fall by more than 10 mEq/24 hours.[72] Throughout therapy, the child should be assessed carefully for seizure activity or other signs of a change in neurologic status. Such findings should be reported to a physician immediately, and tapering of fluid administration may be necessary.

If the child is demonstrating signs of poor systemic perfusion (tachycardia, peripheral vasoconstriction, poor capillary refill, oliguria, or hypotension), a single rapid fluid infusion (10 to 20 ml/kg) may be ordered, utilizing any of the following solutions:

1. 5% glucose and 0.9% saline
2. 20 ml 25% albumin added to each 80 ml of 5% glucose and 0.9% saline
3. 0.45% saline plus 24 mEq/L sodium bicarbonate and 53 mEq/L of sodium chloride

This initial infusion should result in improvement of systemic and renal perfusion, so that fluid and electrolyte replacement can then be accomplished more gradually.

When any type of dehydration is present, the fluid deficit can be easily and accurately estimated by the difference between the child's weight before illness and the admission weight. Any acute weight loss represents the amount of water lost; 1 gm weight loss is produced by 1 ml of fluid loss. If the weight before illness is not available, the estimation of the dehydration status must be made from clinical appearance and laboratory data.

Estimation of the degree of dehydration from clinical appearance provides the health care team with a reasonable guide for volume therapy. Dehydration is classified as mild, moderate, or severe, for infants and young children. The following definitions of these categories are used:

> *Mild dehydration:* a loss of less than 5% of body weight or approximately 50 ml/kg
>
> *Moderate dehydration:* a loss of 5% to 10% of body weight, or approximately 100 ml/kg
>
> *Severe dehydration:* a loss of 10% to 15% of body weight, or approximately 150 ml/kg

Since total body water and extracellular fluid volume represent a smaller percentage of body weight in older children and adolescents, mild dehydration is present with a 3% loss of body weight, moderate dehydration is present with a 6% loss of body weight, and severe dehydration is present if fluid losses total 9% of body weight in these patients.

The following clinical signs and symptoms have been utilized to differentiate mild, moderate, and severe dehydration. It is important to note that these percentages and clinical signs correlate best when *isotonic dehydration* is present. If hypertonic dehydration is present, the child's intravascular volume is maintained at the expense of the intracellular volume. As a result, the fluid deficit associated with each of these groups of signs and symptoms is probably higher than that listed.

When the child has mild (less than 5%) isotonic dehydration, the mucous membranes and the skin are dry. The child's temperature may be low, unless a concurrent bacterial infection is present. Tachycardia is present, but peripheral perfusion and blood pressure are normal, and the respiratory rate is appropriate for age. When moderate (approximately 5% to 10%) isotonic dehydration is present, the child will appear to be ill. The fontanelle and the eyes will be depressed and mucous membranes will be dry. Severe (10% to 15%) isotonic dehydration will be associated with signs of poor systemic perfusion. The child will be tachycardic, peripheral pulses will be diminished in intensity, extremities will be cool, the skin color will be pale or mottled, urine output is less than 0.5 to 1.0 ml/kg/hour or anuria is present, and hypotension may be noted (see Chapter 8 for further discussion of dehydration).

Once the fluid deficit is calculated, the replacement is planned over a 48-hour period. As a result, the child's hourly IV rate will total $\frac{1}{48}$ of the deficit, plus maintenance fluids, plus any unusually large ongoing fluid losses. The following case study illustrates the calculation of maintenance and replacement fluid therapy in the child with hypernatremic (hypertonic) dehydration. For an illustration of calculation of fluid therapy for the child with isotonic or hypotonic dehydration, please see Chapter 8. (Please note that these case studies involve similar patients with different forms of dehydration and are meant to illustrate the differences in approach to fluid therapy.)

CASE STUDY

A 9-kg, 10-month-old infant is admitted with a history of vomiting and diarrhea, which began soon after the mother started mixing the child's formula from powdered concentrate. The infant has a sunken fontanelle, dry and pale mucous membranes, and cool extremities. The skin turgor is good, although the skin over the abdomen is "doughy". Peripheral pulses are strong and equal bilaterally, capillary filling time is brisk, and blood pressure is normal for age. The infant's urine output is less than 0.5 ml/kg/hour. The infant acts extremely irritable, and all extremities are rigidly extended at rest. The infant's serum sodium concentration is 154 mEq/L. The infant's weight before the illness was 10 kg.

Degree of deficit:	1 kg of 10 kg (10%)
Fluid deficit:	1 kg or 1000 ml
Type of dehydration:	Hypernatremic or hypertonic
Replacement plan:	1000 ml to be replaced during next 48 hours at 20.8 ml/hour for 48 hours

Normal maintenance fluid requirement:	100 ml/kg/24 hours or 1000 ml/24 hours or 41.7 ml/hour for 24 hours

Therefore, if the infant's intravenous fluid rate totals 20.8 ml + 41.7 ml/hour during the first 48 hours of therapy, the infant's fluid deficit will be replaced within 48 hours (unless additional losses occur), and the infant will also receive maintenance fluid therapy.

NOTE: The intravenous fluids used to replace fluid losses should contain *some* sodium. The infant's serum sodium concentration should not fall by more than 10 mEq/24 hours, so it should return to a normal range after 48 hours of therapy.

It is *necessary that water replacement be accomplished slowly when the child has hypertonic dehydration* to avoid rapid water uptake by the brain and other cells. Throughout therapy, the nurse should assess the child closely for evidence of seizures or other signs of neurologic injury. If seizures are present before treatment is begun, or if the child's spinal fluid contains blood or elevated protein levels, a cerebral injury (resulting from cerebral hemorrhage, cerebral thrombosis, or subdural effusion) is strongly suspected. If seizure activity is initially noted after therapy is begun, cerebral edema or intracranial hemorrhage must be suspected. Cerebral edema caused by water intoxication most commonly produces seizures within 4 to 24 hours after initiation of fluid replacement and is more likely to occur if the child's serum sodium concentration is reduced too rapidly.[34] If seizures develop, the physician should be notified immediately. Intravenous administration of hypertonic (3%) saline (3 to 5 ml/kg) or mannitol (0.5 to 1 gm/kg) will usually be ordered. These solutions increase intravascular osmolality and will halt the fluid shift from the vascular to the cellular space, and will draw fluid back into the vascular space. As a result, they should reduce cerebral edema, and usually they are effective in controlling seizures related to fluid shifts.[51] If the seizures are uncontrolled by the administration of the hypertonic saline or the mannitol, cerebral hemorrhage should be suspected, and efforts should be made to reduce intracranial pressure (see the section on increased intracranial pressure in Chapter 6).

Throughout fluid therapy, the child's tolerance of the fluid replacement and the child's urine output should be carefully assessed. Once rehydration is achieved, the child's urine output should total 1 ml/kg/hour, and blood urea nitrogen concentration and serum creatinine should be normal.

Treatment of hypertonic dehydration resulting from diabetes insipidus is reviewed in the section on specific diseases, diabetes insipidus, later in this chapter.

■ DEHYDRATION: HYPOTONIC
■ Etiology

Hypotonic dehydration occurs when the child's sodium losses exceed free water losses or when salt-poor solutions are administered. The most common causes of hypotonic dehydration in children include gastroenteritis and inappropriate intravenous therapy. Less common causes include gastric suction with inadequate replacement of removed electrolytes, inappropriate ADH secretion, and water enemas. Gastroenteritis produces fluid, sodium, potassium, chloride, hydrogen, and/or bicarbonate losses through vomiting and diarrhea. Inappropriate intravenous therapy can produce hypotonic dehydration when the severely dehydrated child is partially rehydrated with inadequate amounts of intravenous sodium chloride, or when small amounts of water are given to replace gastrointestinal fluid losses.

■ Pathophysiology

Since sodium and chloride are largely distributed in the intravascular space, loss of salt can reduce intravascular osmolality. As a result, water moves from the intravascular to the intracellular space and circulating blood volume is reduced. As with any type of dehydration, the amount of dehydration can be classified as mild, moderate, or severe, according to the quantity of fluid lost or the child's clinical appearance. As noted previously, mild dehydration represents up to 5% weight loss and a loss of up to 50 ml/kg body weight. Moderate dehydration represents 5% to 10% weight loss, or a loss of up to 100 ml/kg body weight. Severe dehydration represents a 10% to 15% weight loss, or as much as 150 ml/kg.

■ Clinical signs and symptoms

When the child has hypotonic dehydration, the degree of deficit can be accurately estimated from the child's clinical appearance. When the child has mild dehydration, the eyes appear sunken, the mucous membranes are dry, and the infant's fontanelle is usually depressed. The child may be tachycardic, but the blood pressure and respiratory rate will be normal. The child looks ill and skin turgor is poor (the skin remains "tented" after it is pinched). The child is often irritable.

Moderate (up to 10%) dehydration is associated with signs of peripheral circulatory failure. The child is tachycardic and tachypneic, and the skin is cool and often clammy. Peripheral pulses may be decreased in intensity and urine output is reduced. The child's mucous membranes are dry and his eyes are sunken. The infant's fontanelle will be depressed. As the child's clinical status deteriorates, the blood pressure will fall, and the child may become unresponsive.

Severe (10% to 15%) dehydration is a life-threatening condition. The infant or child has hypovolemic shock, and signs of low cardiac output, including metabolic acidosis, are present (see the section on low cardiac output in Chapter 3).

When hypotonic dehydration is present, the child's serum sodium concentration is reduced and serum osmolality is low (see Table 7-3 for a summary of these signs and symptoms).

■ Medical treatment and nursing interventions

If the child with hypotonic dehydration has signs of circulatory failure, the immediate goal of therapy is restoration of adequate circulating blood volume. As soon as the diagnosis is made, one or more large bore central venous catheters are inserted, and a rapid infusion of normal saline or lactated Ringer's solution (10 to 20 ml/kg body weight) is given. This bolus of fluid may be repeated two or three times if necessary to ensure acceptable blood pressure and systemic perfusion. As the child's circulating blood volume is expanded, the heart rate should decrease to a more normal range and urine output should improve.

Once the child's blood pressure and systemic perfusion are adequate, treatment is aimed at replacing the solute losses and administering needed fluid. When the child has hyponatremic dehydration, the replacement fluids utilized are usually normal saline or half-normal saline. The replacement of the fluid losses are calculated so that the fluid deficit is replaced within the first 24 hours of therapy. The first half of the deficit is corrected during the first 8 hours of therapy, and the remaining half of the deficit is replaced in the subsequent 16 hours of therapy. This replacement fluid is always administered *in addition to* the child's normal fluid requirements. Throughout therapy, the child's clinical appearance, urine output, and fluid losses should frequently be evaluated so that fluid administration can be adjusted as necessary.[51]

Additional information regarding treatment of hypotonic dehydration is provided in the section on dehydration in Chapter 8.

Table 7-3 Assessment of degree of dehydration in isotonic fluid losses

Clinical parameters	Mild	Moderate	Severe
Body weight loss			
Infant	5% (50 ml/kg)	10% (100 ml/kg)	· 15% (150 ml/kg)
Adult	3% (30 ml/kg)	6% (60 ml/kg)	9% (90 ml/kg)
Skin turgor	slightly ↓	↓↓	↓↓↓
Fontanelle	may be flat or depressed	depressed	significantly depressed
Mucous membranes	dry	very dry	parched
Skin color	normal	pale gray	mottled
Urine output	slightly ↓	mild oliguria	marked oliguria
Azotemia	absent	present	present and severe
Pulse	± ↑	↑	↑↑
Blood pressure	normal	± normal	reduced
Sensorium	normal	lethargic	semicoma, convulsions

The above must be modified for age and for hypertonic or hypotonic dehydration.

■ **HYPONATREMIA, SYNDROME OF INAPPROPRIATE ANTIDIURETIC HORMONE SECRETION (SIADH), AND WATER INTOXICATION**
■ **Etiology**

The infant or child may develop a low serum sodium concentration as a result of increased losses of sodium, increased intake of free water, or decreased intake of sodium. The most common causes of hyponatremia in children include inappropriate antidiuretic hormone secretion, adrenal insufficiency, aggressive administration of diuretics or insufficient sodium intake or administration.

The SIADH occurs with some frequency following neurosurgery or in pediatric patients with infections of the central nervous system or malignant neoplasms. Normal secretion of antidiuretic hormone (ADH, or vasopressin) occurs in response to increased intravascular osmotic pressure, a significant fall in blood pressure, a fall in intravascular volume, decreased left atrial stretch, catecholamine secretion,

fright, or pain (see the section on the distal tubule and collecting ducts at the beginning of this chapter). Antidiuretic hormone increases the permeability of the collecting ducts to water, so more water is reabsorbed, a more concentrated urine is excreted, and more free water ultimately returns to the vascular space. If ADH levels are elevated, and the patient continues to take or receive normal amounts of water, hyponatremia will develop. When ADH secretion continues despite the presence of hyponatremia, the patient has "the syndrome of inappropriate ADH secretion." This syndrome is defined as the association of serum hypoosmolality and hyponatremia, urine hyperosmolality, high urine sodium concentration, and clinical improvement following water restriction.[29,60] The clinical manifestations of inappropriate ADH secretion are consistent with those produced by water intoxication.[49]

Inappropriate ADH secretion (or ADH excess) can be seen in postoperative patients, especially if hemorrhage, trauma, or significant fluid loss has occurred. Children who develop meningitis, encephalitis, hydrocephalus, increased intracranial pressure, head trauma, subarachnoid hemorrhage, brain tumor, or coma may also develop SIADH. This syndrome may be seen in patients with cirrhosis and splanchnic sequestration (see Chapter 8), congestive heart failure, pulmonary hypertension, pneumonia, and ADH-secreting tumors, and in those patients recovering from repair of mitral stenosis.[29,55,60] Patients who demonstrate ADH excess will continue to secrete ADH despite a fall in serum osmolality, and they will continue to excrete sodium in the urine despite the presence of serum hyponatremia.

There are occasions when a laboratory report of low serum sodium concentration can be misleading. These "pseudohyponatremic" states are associated with serum that is hyperlipidemic, hyperproteinemic, or hyperglycemic. When hyperlipidemia or hyperproteinemia are present, the lipid or protein displaces fluid from the serum specimen and decreases the relative volume of water and electrolytes in any liter of plasma. As a result, the measured serum sodium concentration will appear to be low. The *amount* of sodium may actually be normal, although its concentration in milliequivalents per liter of plasma is reduced. Hyperlipidemia of this degree is usually easily recognized because the plasma appears milky white.

When the child is hyperglycemic, the high glucose concentration increases the serum osmolality, drawing fluid into the vascular space; this can artificially reduce the serum sodium concentration. These patients may have a normal serum sodium content, even though the serum sodium concentration is low. They are protected from the effects of serum hypoosmolality by the increase in osmotic effect resulting from the elevated serum glucose.

■ Pathophysiology

When hyponatremia is present from any cause, serum hypoosmolality may develop. This can cause a fluid shift from the intravascular to the intracellular space, and cerebral edema can result.

Whenever the child's serum sodium concentration is abnormal, or when the child is dehydrated, the child's serum osmolality should be calculated. This osmolality calculation will help differentiate between hyponatremia associated with intravascular hypoosmolality and that associated with normal or elevated intravascular osmolality and will help dictate the appropriate therapy. The following case study illustrates the usefulness of this calculation.

CASE STUDY

A child is admitted to the Intensive Care Unit with diabetic ketoacidosis and a serum glucose con-

centration of 900 mg/dl. The child's serum sodium concentration is 125 mEq/L and blood urea nitrogen (BUN) is 28. Calculate the child's serum osmolality.

$2 \times$ Sodium concentration (mEq/L)	$2(125)$
$\dfrac{\text{Glucose concentration (mg/dl)}}{18}$	$\dfrac{900}{18}$
$\dfrac{\text{Blood urea nitrogen (mg/dl)}}{2.8}$	$\dfrac{28}{2.8}$

TOTAL serum osmolality (mg/dl) = 310 mOsm/L

This child does *not* have serum hypoosmolality, despite the fact that the serum sodium is low. In fact, this child's serum osmolality is high. As a result, instead of fluid restriction, this child will require administration of some free water and sodium.

■ Clinical signs and symptoms

When hyponatremia alone is present, the patient may become irritable and may demonstrate seizures, abdominal cramps, or diarrhea. Since water diffuses from the hypoosmotic intravascular space to the intracellular space, "fingerprinting" may be noted over the sternum. In this case, when the fingers are pressed firmly on the patient's sternum, the fingerprint marks will remain indented even after pressure is removed. This indicates the presence of increased plasticity of the tissues resulting from increased intracellular water.[61] Patients who develop hyponatremia and hypoosmolality are at risk for the development of seizures and cerebral edema. As a result, their neurologic status should be monitored closely, and signs of irritability, lethargy, seizures, or increased intracranial pressure should be reported to a physician immediately.

When the syndrome of inappropriate ADH secretion (SIADH) is present, the following signs and symptoms will be noted[29,55,60]: serum hyponatremia *and* serum hypoosmolality, continued urine sodium excretion, high urine osmolality, absence of appropriate cause of ADH secretion (such as hemorrhage or hypovolemia), normal adrenal function, and normal renal function. The child's urine volume is usually low, though this is not an invariable finding.

■ Medical treatment and nursing intervention

Whenever a patient develops sodium imbalance, changes in serum osmolality, or disorders of aldosterone or antidiuretic hormone release or effect, a simultaneous serum and urine osmolality should be measured, and the child's serum sodium concentration should be followed closely. The child will also require very accurate documentation of total fluid intake and output and daily weights. The type and volume of fluids provided should be reevaluated frequently in light of changes in the child's clinical status.

Since serum hypoosmolality can produce cerebral edema, the patient requires frequent, thorough assessments of neurologic function. If irritability, seizures, or signs of increased intracranial pressure develop, a physician should be notified immediately. Serum electrolytes and serum and urine osmolality should be checked, so hyponatremia or other electrolyte imbalances can be treated immediately. If hyponatremia is producing symptoms, it may be treated with hypertonic (3%) saline (3 to 5 ml/kg provides 1.5 to 2.5 mEq/kg).[55]

If the child has the syndrome of inappropriate ADH secretion (SIADH) and demonstrates seizures or other severe symptoms, hyponatremia and water intoxication can be treated acutely by administration of hypertonic saline (3 to 5 ml/kg of 3% NaCl) and furosemide (1 to 2 mg/kg). These drugs increase the serum sodium concentration and eliminate excess free water. However, they only provide a transient increase in serum sodium concentration if excess ADH secretion continues.

The treatment of choice for the syndrome of inappropriate ADH secretion (SIADH) is *fluid restriction*. Fluid intake may be restricted to 30% to 75% of maintenance requirements, according to the degree of hyponatremia and hypoosmolality present.

If the SIADH is chronic, lithium chloride or demethylchlortetracycline may be administered, since these drugs inhibit the action of ADH on the permeability of the collecting ducts. However, since these drugs have significant side effects, their use is not indicated for the child with acute transient SIADH.[29,34,55]

■ POTASSIUM DEFICIT

Potassium is the chief intracellular cation; its intracellular concentration averages about 145 mEq/L, although the extracellular (intravascular) concentration is only approximately 5 mEq/L. The magnitude of the gradient between intracellular and extracellular potassium concentration is largely responsible for the size of the membrane potential in excitable muscles (such as the heart) and nerves. As a result, precise regulation of serum potassium concentration is necessary.

■ Etiology

Potassium deficit is present when the serum potassium concentration totals less than 3.5 to 4.5 mEq/

L. This can occur as a result of true potassium losses or because potassium has shifted from the intravascular space. Since the intravascular potassium concentration represents only a small proportion of the total body potassium, the serum potassium concentration should only be interpreted after consideration of the child's clinical status and acid-base balance. A true potassium deficit in the critically ill patient is most commonly encountered following use of diuretics, especially thiazide diuretics. Since gastrointestinal fluids all contain significant amounts of potassium in the form of potassium chloride salt, vomiting, diarrhea, intestinal fistulas of the small intestine or colon, ileostomy drainage, or gastric suctioning can all result in potassium losses as well as loss of hydrogen ion and chloride.[30] Hypokalemia is also associated with severe hypochloremia and the potassium-wasting Bartter's syndrome.

Potassium may also be lost as the result of increased renal excretion. This occurs as the result of metabolic alkalosis, renal tubular acidosis, and diabetic ketoacidosis. Metabolic alkalosis especially enhances potassium excretion since the potassium is substituted for the hydrogen ion that is reabsorbed from the urine filtrate.

■ Pathophysiology

Since the intracellular potassium ion concentration is high, this potassium provides a large reservoir for maintaining normal intravascular potassium concentration, despite the loss of intravascular potassium. When the serum potassium level begins to decline, a portion of the intracellular potassium, known as the "exchangeable potassium," is available to move from the cells to maintain the intravascular potassium concentration. Only when this amount of "exchangeable" potassium is depleted will further intravascular potassium losses result in a fall in the serum potassium concentration. At this point, serum hypokalemia reflects not only a low serum potassium concentration but also a low total body potassium concentration.

The serum potassium concentration is also affected by changes in the patient's acid-base status. When metabolic acidosis develops and the intravascular hydrogen ion concentration rises, hydrogen ion will move from the intravascular to the intracellular space as the result of a concentration gradient. In exchange for the hydrogen ion, potassium ions will move from the intracellular to the extracellular (including intravascular) space to maintain cellular electrical neutrality. As a result, *metabolic acidosis will cause an elevation in the child's serum potassium concentration,* even though the child's total body potassium concentration has not changed. *When acidosis is corrected, the child's intravascular potassium concentration falls,* because hydrogen ions move out of the cells and back into the vascular space, and they are replaced by potassium ions, which move out of the vascular space and into the cells. If the acidosis persists until renal compensatory mechanisms are activated, the hydrogen ions will be excreted by the kidneys and bicarbonate reabsorption will be enhanced.

Since potassium ions shift into the vascular space when acidosis develops, a mild elevation in serum potassium concentration is normal when the child is acidotic. However, the serum potassium concentration normally will fall with correction of the acidosis. Consequently, a child with hypokalemia in the presence of acidosis will require a potassium supplement, since the potassium concentration will fall even farther as the child's acidosis is corrected.

When the child develops *alkalosis, the serum potassium concentration will fall,* because hydrogen ions move out of the cells into the vascular space and are replaced by potassium ions, which move out of the vascular space and into the cells. *When metabolic alkalosis is corrected, the serum potassium concentration will rise* as the potassium ions return to the vascular space. As a result, if the child has a mild serum hypokalemia with alkalosis, administration of a potassium supplement may not be necessary, since the potassium concentration will rise as the alkalosis is corrected.

Hypokalemia may perpetuate metabolic alkalosis, particularly if either condition is chronic. When the serum potassium concentration is low, potassium ions will be reabsorbed by the proximal tubules in exchange for the excretion of hydrogen ions. As a result, it may be necessary to treat the child's hypokalemia in order for the alkalosis to be corrected.

■ **Clinical signs and symptoms**

A decrease in serum potassium concentration increases the magnitude of the gradient between intracellular and extracellular potassium concentrations; this hyperpolarizes excitable tissues. Symptoms of a true potassium deficit include the development of muscle weakness and diminished reflexes. Cardiac arrhythmias infrequently occur as the result of mild hypokalemia during childhood. With severe hypokalemia, however, ventricular irritability may produce premature ventricular contractions. In addition, the electrocardiogram may reveal flattened "T" waves and S-T segment depression. The child may

also demonstrate vomiting and a paralytic ileus.[61]

Chronic hypokalemia also produces changes in renal concentrating ability, and polyuria is often present. The kidney has little ability to conserve potassium when body potassium stores become low; as a result, urinary potassium excretion will remain greater than 20 mEq/L once hypokalemia has persisted for 10 to 20 days.

■ **Medical treatment and nursing interventions**

If the child with hypokalemia is nauseated and vomiting, intravenous potassium replacement should be provided. If vomiting continues, in fact, oral feedings should be discontinued, since vomiting will aggravate potassium, hydrogen ion, and chloride losses. Before any potassium supplement is administered, the child's renal function should be carefully assessed, and urine output should be adequate. Potassium supplements are calculated at approximately 2 to 4 mEq/kg/24 hours. If the child is moderately or severely hypokalemic, 0.5-1.0 mEq/kg of potassium chloride may be slowly administered as an intravenous infusion over 1 to 2 hours; this solution should be diluted adequately and administered slowly enough so that a bolus infusion of the potassium is prevented (since this can produce arrhythmias). If the potassium is infused through a peripheral intravenous catheter, its concentration should not exceed 30 to 40 mEq/L[90]; stronger concentrations may produce vascular irritation or burns.

■ **POTASSIUM EXCESS**
■ **Etiology**

Potassium excess may occur as the result of excess administration of potassium or as the result of intravascular accumulation of potassium ions caused by changes in acid-base balance, significant cell destruction (and release of intracellular potassium), or reduced renal excretion of potassium ions. Any rise in serum potassium concentration in the normal patient is usually transient, since the kidney is able to excrete potassium ion and return the serum potassium level to normal. If, however, the rate of potassium ion accumulation exceeds the rate of renal potassium ion excretion, the serum potassium concentration will increase.

■ **Pathophysiology**

As noted above, acidosis will increase the intravascular potassium ion concentration. As the hydrogen ions move from the vascular space into the cells, potassium ions will move from the cells into the vascular space. Each time the arterial pH falls by 0.1, the serum potassium concentration can be expected to increase by 0.6 to 0.8 mEq/L. As the acidosis is corrected, the serum potassium concentration should fall again.

Alkalosis can artificially lower the serum potassium concentration (see preceding discussion). Therefore, if the serum potassium concentration is high despite the presence of alkalosis, hyperkalemia is probably present.

One of the most common causes of hyperkalemia in the critically ill patient is decreased renal excretion of potassium ion. When the child has chronic renal failure, the serum potassium concentration can remain normal as long as the child does not have an excess load of potassium (which can occur as the result of increased potassium intake, acidosis, or potassium release from injured cells).

If the child has acute renal failure and decreased urine volume, the child's serum potassium concentration may rise quickly, particularly if acidosis or cell injury is present.

■ **Clinical signs and symptoms**

The manifestations of hyperkalemia are primarily neuromuscular, since the membrane potential in excitable tissue is determined by the ratio of the extracellular to the intracellular potassium concentration. Increased serum potassium levels may cause muscle cells to remain polarized (in tetany) or depolarized (flaccid). The patient usually demonstrates generalized muscle weakness; this weakness usually produces flaccidity rather than muscle fatigue upon exertion.

Hyperkalemia can produce some characteristic changes in the electrocardiogram. Initially, a tall peaked T wave develops; this is followed by a widening of the QRS complex and decreasing amplitude of the R wave. As the serum potassium concentration continues to rise, the P-R interval is prolonged, then the amplitude of the P wave decreases, and finally, the P wave disappears. Ultimately, the patient's rhythm deteriorates into a classic sine wave. Ventricular arrhythmias or fibrillation may occur at any point during this progression.

■ **Medical treatment and nursing interventions**

The best way to prevent complications of hyperkalemia is to identify those patients at risk for the development of hyperkalemia, so that potassium administration can be curtailed. Since hyperkalemia

can result from increased potassium administration, cell release during catabolism, or impaired renal excretion of potassium, patients with severe dehydration, extensive trauma, burns, prolonged surgery, shock, sepsis, hemorrhage, or transfusion reaction are all at risk for the development of hyperkalemia. Whenever the child demonstrates oliguria or anuria, potassium excretion is reduced or eliminated, so the child may rapidly develop hyperkalemia unless potassium administration is quickly reduced. These children require frequent assessment of serum potassium concentrations and assessment for signs of potassium excess. In addition, the child's fluid intake and output and acid-base status should be monitored, since these also affect serum potassium concentrations.

Once the child's serum potassium concentration approaches 7 mEq/L, there is a high risk of serious or fatal cardiac arrhythmias. As a result, vigorous attempts should be made to reduce the intravascular potassium concentration. This may be accomplished through expansion of the extracellular fluid space, administration of calcium, increase in the movement of potassium into the cells, and removal of potassium from the body. Each of these methods will be discussed separately below.

Children may develop serum hyperkalemia as the result of contraction of intravascular volume or hemoconcentration (such as occurs as the result of hypovolemic shock or severe dehydration). In this case, reexpansion of the intravascular volume should produce a dilutional reduction in the child's serum potassium concentration. Usually, 0.9% sodium chloride is administered (10 ml/kg body weight) to expand the intravascular volume, though any potassium-free solution may be utilized.

Calcium gluconate or calcium chloride may also be administered, since it transiently counteracts the adverse effects of hyperkalemia on neuromuscular membranes.[86] Most commonly, 0.5 ml/kg of 10% calcium gluconate will be administered intravenously over 2 to 4 minutes. During the calcium infusion, the nurse should monitor for side effects of the calcium, including bradycardia. Since the calcium infusion does not affect the serum potassium concentration its protection of neuromuscular membranes lasts only approximately 30 minutes. However, during that time, additional attempts may be made to reduce the potassium concentration.

Since the presence of alkalosis produces a shift of potassium ions from the intravascular space into the cells, sodium bicarbonate may be administered (2.5 mEq/kg) over a 30 to 60 minute period to alkalinize the serum and enhance the potassium shift.[87] The sodium bicarbonate is usually diluted to half strength before administration to infants and young children to prevent vascular trauma and to avoid the development of increased intravascular osmolality. This administration of the sodium bicarbonate does not reduce the total body potassium, but it can temporarily reduce the serum potassium concentration; the effects begin within one half hour and last for several hours.

Cellular uptake of potassium from the extracellular (intravascular) fluid is enhanced with the infusion of glucose and insulin. This is one of the most effective methods of reducing hyperkalemia in critically ill children. Fifty percent glucose (1 ml/kg) plus insulin (0.1 unit/kg) may be given, or a 20% to 50% glucose infusion (0.5 to 1.0 ml/kg of 50% glucose or 2.5 to 5.0 ml/kg of 20% glucose) plus regular insulin (0.1 unit/kg) may be administered. Often the glucose infusion itself will be effective in reducing the intravascular potassium concentration, since potassium will enter the cells with the glucose. The administration of the insulin will enhance the movement of both glucose and potassium into the cells (see the upcoming section on acute renal failure).

The glucose and insulin administration should begin to reduce the serum potassium concentration within one half hour, and should be effective for several hours. Since this infusion also does not eliminate any of the potassium ions from the body, its effects are temporary.

Removal of potassium from the body can be accomplished via the gastrointestinal tract, since potassium present in the intestinal fluids is in equilibrium with the interstitial and intravascular potassium concentration. Therefore, if hyperkalemia is present, there is a high potassium concentration in the intestinal fluids. The ion exchange resin, sodium polystyrene sulfonate (Kayexalate), will exchange potassium for sodium ions on an ion-for-ion basis when it is administered orally or as a retention enema. Oral Kayexalate is administered as a 20% suspension in a 5% glucose solution. The dosage is 0.5 gm/kg and it may be repeated as often as two or three times in 24 hours.[85] Since the greatest exchange of sodium for potassium occurs in the large intestine, an oral dosage of 1.0 gm/kg (given in divided doses) can reduce the serum potassium 1 mEq/L over a 24-hour period. The enema dosage is somewhat higher and usually totals 2 gm/kg, given once or twice a day. For oral use, Kayexalate is suspended in water or glucose water as 3 to 4 ml of fluid per gm of resin (one teaspoonful of resin is slightly more than 3 gm). For rectal administration, 1 gm of resin per 6 to 8 ml of a 20% sorbitol solution is prepared. Since the serum sodium will rise following Kayexalate administration, fluid retention

may develop. If all other measures to reduce serum potassium concentration fail, the child may be dialyzed (see the section on care of the child during dialysis later in this chapter).

■ ACUTE RENAL FAILURE

Acute renal failure (ARF) is a sudden loss of kidney function. Since the kidney has a wide variety of excretory and regulatory functions, ARF can result in the accumulation of by-products of metabolism, the loss of regulation of electrolyte concentration, and/or acid-base imbalance. When nitrogenous by-products of metabolism accumuate in the blood, *azotemia*, or *uremia*, is present. The magnitude of the azotemia and more often the serum level of creatinine are the two indicators most often used to estimate the degree of renal impairment. ARF is defined as a BUN greater than 80 mg/100 ml and a serum creatinine concentration greater than 1.5 mg/dl. Other characteristics of ARF include disturbances in fluid balance and acid-base status, hyperkalemia, and decreased urine volume (less than 300 ml/m²/day).[39]

Renal failure may occur as the result of primary kidney disease, or it may occur as a complication of diseases of other body systems or of other structures within the genitourinary system. As a result, the causes of acute renal failure are most commonly classified according to the location of the primary disorder. The most common categories utilized to describe these causes are prerenal, postrenal, and renal. Theoretically, prerenal and postrenal causes of ARF do not involve damage to the renal parenchyma. If this is true, then, reversal of these causes should allow renal function to return to normal. However, severe prerenal or postrenal failure can produce damage to the nephron unit, so relief of the prerenal and postrenal causes of ARF may not always reestablish normal renal function. For the sake of consistency, the following discussion is organized according to the classifications of prerenal, postrenal, and renal causes of ARF, although the reader is cautioned against utilizing these divisions too strictly.

■ Etiology

Critically ill neonates develop acute renal failure as the result of hypoxia, shock, and sepsis.[6,56] It may also occur as a complication of umbilical artery or vein catheterization and subsequent thrombosis of the aorta, the renal artery, or the renal vein.[39] Critically ill children most commonly develop acute renal failure as a complication of major surgical procedures, drug toxicity, or toxic ingestions.[2,25,91] For convenience, the most common causes of ARF are divided into prerenal, postrenal, and renal causes and are discussed separately below.

Prerenal azotemia is associated with conditions that reduce renal perfusion. This can occur directly, as the result of an embolism or thrombosis of the renal artery, or it may be caused by intravascular fluid loss, sepsis, cardiovascular disease, hypoxemia, or shock. In each case, renal blood flow and renal perfusion are compromised, the glomerular filtration rate falls, and ARF develops. A fall in renal blood flow and the glomerular filtration rate is frequently encountered among patients with moderate to severe dehydration, but the reduced perfusion rarely causes intrinsic damage to the renal parenchyma. Usually, correction of the underlying cause of prerenal ARF rapidly restores renal function.

Postrenal causes of acute renal failure include any disorders that obstruct urine flow and prevent the elimination of urine. The obstruction to flow must involve both of the ureters (since a single normal kidney can adequately maintain fluid and electrolyte balance), or it must produce a decrease in function. Obstruction to urine flow may occur as the result of compression by an extrarenal mass, such as a Wilms' tumor or a neuroblastoma. Blood clots, calculi, inflammation or edema, or posterior insertions of the urethras into the bladder are a few of the conditions that may prevent urine flow into the bladder or prevent adequate bladder evacuation.

Renal ARF may be secondary to a chronic prerenal or postrenal problem, it may involve chemicals that have a toxic effect upon the kidney, or it may be associated with glomerulonephritis. Acute renal failure of this nature is frequently termed *acute tubular necrosis* (ATN) and it may develop after profound circulatory disturbances, hypoxemia, septicemia, or accidental ingestion of drugs or poisons. Approximately 60% of ARF in children is associated with acute tubular necrosis.[25]

Acute renal failure in the neonate can be associated with renal structural anomalies. Since the placenta performs the excretory functions of the kidneys, neonates with significant renal malformations can have normal plasma electrolyte concentrations at birth. Ninety percent of all healthy newborns excrete urine within the first 24 hours of life, and 99% excrete urine within the first 48 hours of life.[21] Therefore failure of micturation in the first 2 days of life is strongly suggestive of severe congenital renal anomalies. A history of oligohydramnios, limb deformities, and characteristic facial features suggest the presence of Potter's syndrome, which includes renal dysplasia or bilateral renal agenesis. Many neonates with oligo-

hydramnios also have associated pulmonary hypoplasia.

■ Pathophysiology

The most common prerenal cause of ARF is an acute reduction in renal perfusion. This can occur as the result of hypovolemia, hypotension, or other forms of shock or from renal artery or aortic thrombosis.

Postrenal failure can develop as the result of obstruction of the ureters or urethra that, in turn, obstruct urine flow. This increases the pressure in the ureters and can ultimately increase the hydrostatic pressure in the collecting ducts and renal tubules. Once the hydrostatic pressure in Bowman's capsule is increased, the glomerular filtration rate will fall, tubular reabsorption will be enhanced, and oliguria or anuria will develop. Once the obstruction to urine flow is relieved, a natriuresis can persist for 2 days to 2 weeks and renal function may ultimately be restored.

If both pre- and postrenal causes of ARF have been ruled out, the cause of the ARF is assumed to be injury to the nephron itself. This nephron damage can occur through direct damage to the glomeruli, the tubules, or the renal vasculature. Glomerular damage is more commonly associated with the glomerulonephropathies or hemolytic uremic syndrome, while tubular damage is more commonly a result of ischemia or nephrotoxins. Damage to the renal vasculature may occur as the result of umbilical artery or vein catheterization in the neonate, but it is an uncommon cause of acute renal failure in children.[39,62]

Tubular lesions caused by nephrotoxins temporarily disrupt the tubular structure, because they produce necrosis of the tubular epithelium down to, but not including, the supporting basement membrane. Ischemic lesions may affect any segment of the nephron, and injured areas may be interspersed with normal segments of tubular epithelium. Healing of both ischemic and nephrotoxic injury occurs through reepithelialization. If the basement membrane is intact, tubular morphology can be reestablished after healing. If the basement membrane has been fragmented, however, the lack of supportive structure prevents regrowth of organized tubules. Connective tissue may extend through the ruptured basement membrane and fibrosis can replace the tubules. Because of the unpredictability of tubular healing, it is impossible to predict the rate of recovery of nephron function following ischemic or nephrotoxic injury.[87]

Although the precise pathophysiology of acute

renal failure is not understood, almost all theories include a severe reduction in renal blood flow by 50% to 75%.[25] As a result, glomerular filtration rate and renal cortical blood flow are reduced. This stimulates renin and aldosterone secretion, and produces sodium and water retention and decreased urine volume. The development of ARF, however, usually indicates the presence of renal tubular damage as well as reduced renal blood flow. In addition, there may be destruction of the glomerular capillary membrane, increased tubular permeability, or obstruction of the tubules.[52]

■ Clinical signs and symptoms

Acute renal failure is characterized by oliguria (urine output less than 300 ml/m²/day), a blood urea nitrogen greater than 80 mg/dl, and a serum creatinine of greater than 1.5 mg/dl. Since the newborn infant has a comparatively low rate of urea production and a relatively large amount of body water, the newborn's rise in BUN may be limited to approximately 5 mg/dl/day.[87] Anuria is uncommon among children with acute renal failure, and it often indicates unrelieved prerenal or postrenal problems or obstruction to urine flow. Occasionally, children who develop ARF may develop nonoliguric renal failure.[53] This disorder would be characterized by a rise in serum BUN and creatinine without a fall in urine volume; in fact, polyuria may be present.

Once ARF develops, the kidney's ability to regulate fluid volume and potassium, calcium, and glucose concentrations is seriously impaired. In addition, the kidney's regulation of acid-base balance is reduced. Finally, many patients with ARF may develop anemia and coagulopathies, and they are at risk for the development of gastrointestinal hemorrhage and infection.[25] As a result, assessment of the child with ARF must include assessment of reversible causes of renal failure, as well as assessment of possible signs and symptoms of complications of the ARF.

If oliguria develops among patients with ARF and fluid administration is not tapered appropriately, hypervolemia will develop. This can particularly complicate the management of children with cardiovascular problems and may also produce hypertension. To evaluate the child's fluid status, the nurse should assess for signs of congestive heart failure, including hepatomegaly, high central venous pressure, periorbital edema, tachycardia, and increased respiratory effort or oxygen requirements. The child's mucous membranes will be moist, and ascites or edema of dependent areas or extremities may also be noted. When the infant is younger than 16 to 18 months of age, the fontanelle should be palpated; it will be full or tense. The child will also have evidence of a positive fluid balance when fluid intake, output, and insensible water loss are calculated. In addition, the child's weight will increase. If these signs are noted, the child probably is hypervolemic.

Signs of inadequate intravascular volume include dry mucous membranes, poor skin turgor, low (less than 5 mm Hg) central venous pressure, and (late findings) hypotension and decreased systemic perfusion. The child may also have a negative fluid balance when total fluid intake less output and insensible losses are calculated. When these clinical signs are present, the child may have a low intravascular volume and may require fluid administration. It is important to note that the child's intravascular volume may be inadequate despite the administration of adequate fluids and the presence of edema, if the child is losing fluid from the vascular space or peritoneal cavity (this is known as "third spacing" of fluid and may be seen in the child with sepsis, burns, or ascites).

Hyperkalemia is one of the most serious complications of acute renal failure, since it can result in fatal cardiac arrhythmias. Hyperkalemia develops because the child's renal excretion and regulation of potassium are impaired, and potassium release from cells is increased because of cellular catabolism. Normally, the serum potassium level rises within 2 to 3 days after an acute reduction in the glomerular filtration rate.[31] However, the rate of potassium rise will be accelerated in the presence of acidosis (because of the shift of potassium into the vascular space), hemolysis, infection, gastrointestinal bleeding, or trauma. Adverse effects of hyperkalemia are enhanced as the result of hypocalcemia, hypomagnesemia, and use of digitalis.[25] Signs of hyperkalemia have been reviewed previously (see the section on clinical signs and symptoms of hyperkalemia earlier in this chapter) and include generalized muscle weakness, peaking of the T wave on ECG, ventricular arrhythmias, heart block, and ventricular fibrillation.

Hypocalcemia develops frequently among patients with ARF, because renal activation of vitamin D is reduced, and renal clearance of phosphate is impaired. Hypocalcemia is more likely to develop following administration of stored whole blood or packed cells preserved with citrate, phosphate, and dextran (CPD), because ionized calcium can precipitate with the phosphate.[25] Signs of hypocalcemia include a low serum calcium concentration, decreased cardiovascular function (including arrhythmias and evidence of decreased cardiac contractility), muscle cramps, tetany, and seizures.[61]

Hypoglycemia is more likely to develop in critically ill infants, because they have high glucose needs and low glucose stores. Signs of hypoglycemia include a low serum glucose concentration, irritability, and (late findings) seizures or poor systemic perfusion.

Metabolic acidosis often develops in children with ARF, since the kidney is less able to secrete hydrogen ions, form titratable acids or ammonia, or reabsorb bicarbonate ions. Metabolic acidosis can be caused by poor systemic perfusion, and it can quickly compromise cardiac contractility and worsen systemic perfusion.

Anemia and bleeding can be serious problems in the critically ill pediatric patient with ARF. These children often have thrombocytopenia and thrombocytopathia (decreased platelet function). These coagulopathies may become apparent as the result of abnormalities found in a coagulation screening panel or because of the development of petechiae or ecchymoses. Gastrointestinal hemorrhage occurs in a significant number of patients with ARF, and stress ulcers may also be noted.[25]

Since *infection* can produce such serious complications in the child with ARF, the child should be watched closely for evidence of fever (or hypothermia in infants), lethargy, irritability, localized signs of infection (such as erythema or drainage from venous access sites or wounds), an elevation in white blood count, or presence of white blood cells or glucose in the urine.

During initial assessment of the child with ARF, it is important to attempt to differentiate between pre- or postrenal causes of the ARF that are reversible and ARF caused by renal parenchymal damage. If prerenal azotemia is present, the urine sodium concentration will be low (less than 10 to 20 mEq/L), and the urine osmolality will be greater than the serum osmolality (the urine osmolality should be above 500 mOsm and the serum osmolality should be below 300 mOsm). The serum blood urea nitrogen will be increased out of proportion to the serum creatinine, because the urea is a small molecule that is reabsorbed as the kidneys reabsorb sodium and water. As a result, in prerenal azotemia, the ratio of serum BUN to creatinine will be greater than $10:1$. The most accurate test to separate prerenal azotemia from ARF resulting from renal factors is the *fractional excretion of filtered sodium* (FE_{Na}). This is calculated as follows:

$$\text{Fractional excretion Na (\%)} = \frac{\dfrac{\text{Urine sodium concentration}}{\text{Plasma sodium concentration}}}{\dfrac{\text{Urine creatinine concentration}}{\text{Plasma creatinine concentration}}} \times 100$$

When prerenal azotemia is present, the FE_{Na} is less than 1% (2.5% in neonates), while it is greater than 1% to 3% when ARF is caused by renal damage.[16,39]

When acute renal failure results from renal damage, the child's urine is usually not concentrated, and it often contains casts of renal tubular cells. If the urine is positive when tested for blood using lab sticks, but contains no red blood cells on microscopic examination, hemoglobinuria or myoglobinuria should be suspected.[25,39] See Table 7-4 for summary of the differences between prerenal and renal failure.

If the newborn has developed renal failure, it is important to determine whether or not the neonate has voided, since lack of micturation within the first 48 hours of life is associated with renal anomalies. Other clinical signs frequently indicative of renal anomalies in the neonate include persistent bladder distention, ascites, ambigious genitalia, epispadias, single umbilical artery, hypospadias, abnormalities of the abdominal muscles (prune belly) or off-set or low-set ears.

■ Medical treatment and nursing interventions

Assessment of fluid balance and prerenal factors. An important part of the treatment of ARF in children is early detection, so that fluid overload can be prevented and drug and potassium accumulation can be minimized. Whenever any critically ill child becomes oliguric, acute renal failure should be suspected; once it is suspected, immediate efforts should be made to determine and eliminate any reversible causes of the renal failure.

The child's fluid balance should be assessed. This requires insertion of a large-bore venous catheter. If possible, a central venous line should also be inserted, because it will allow measurement of central venous pressure and it will provide venous access for blood sampling. An indwelling urinary drainage catheter should be inserted to allow continuous determination of urine volume and to allow urine collection for analysis.

Indirect evidence of the child's systemic perfusion should be assessed carefully, since hypovolemia or shock can be a frequent prerenal cause of ARF among critically ill children. The child's mucous membranes and nailbeds should be pink and extremities should be warm. The child's heart rate, respiratory rate, and blood pressure should be appropriate for age and clinical condition. Peripheral pulses should be strong. The child's central venous pressure should be 3 to 5 mm Hg. If the child has pale mucous membranes or nailbeds and cool extremities, peripheral vasoconstriction secondary to low cardiac output may be present. Low cardiac output is also character-

Table 7-4 Laboratory tests in differential diagnosis of prerenal and renal failure[26,39]

	Prerenal	Renal
Urine specific gravity	>1.018	≤1.010
Urine osmolality	>500	<400
Urine creatinine (mg/dl)	>100	<70
Creatinine urine: plasma ratio	>30	<20
Urea urine: plasma ratio	>14	<10
Urine urea	>2000	<400
Urine sodium (mEq/L)	<20	>30
Urine potassium (mEq/L)	30-70	<20-40
Urine Na:K ratio	<1.0 usually 0.2	0.8-1.0

ized by tachycardia, tachypnea (unless the child is mechanically ventilated) and, ultimately, hypotension. Peripheral pulses are usually diminished in intensity, a metabolic acidosis is often present, and oliguria is noted (see the section on clinical signs and symptoms, low cardiac output, in Chapter 3). If the low cardiac output results from hypovolemia, the child's central venous pressure will be less than 5 mm Hg. If hypovolemia is suspected, a fluid challenge of 10 to 20 ml/kg of isotonic fluid (normal saline or albumin) may be prescribed. If the hypovolemia results from hemorrhage, isotonic fluid may be administered initially, although blood products will later be required.

If the child's blood pressure and systemic perfusion improve following fluid administration, but urine output does not increase, furosemide (1 to 4 mg/kg/dose) or mannitol (0.2 to 0.5 gm/kg) may be prescribed. These drugs should stimulate a urine output of 6 to 10 ml/kg over a 1- to 3-hour period, unless renal failure is caused by intrinsic renal damage or postrenal causes. If urine output does not improve, administration of other potentially nephrotoxic diuretic agents should be avoided, since this may increase renal damage.[31] In this case, fluid and potassium administration should be limited, and dosages of any drugs excreted by the kidneys should be reevaluated and adjusted as needed.

If oliguria is associated with poor systemic perfusion and a high central venous pressure (above 5 mm Hg), the renal failure may be the result of low cardiac output resulting from heart (pump) failure. In this case, the child's electrolyte and acid-base status should be carefully assessed, since hypoglycemia, hypocalcemia, and acidosis can all depress cardiovascular function. In the absence of such disorders, the child may require administration of a sympathomimetic inotropic agent. The drug of choice for the oliguric patient with low cardiac output resulting from pump failure is dopamine, since this drug produces selective dilation of the renal artery and increased renal blood flow and glomerular filtration rate when it is administered in low (1 to 4 μg/kg/minute) doses. Higher doses of dopamine (>8 to 10 μg/kg/minute), however, can produce alpha-adrenergic effects, resulting in renal vasoconstriction and decreased renal blood flow and urine output. Additional sympathomimetic drugs such as dobutamine (1 to 10 μg/kg/minute) or isoproterenol (0.05 to 0.5 μg/kg/minute) may also be administered. If systemic perfusion remains poor, systemic vasodilators such as sodium nitroprusside (0.5 to 8 μg/kg/minute) or nitroglycerin (0.1 to 10 mg/kg/minute) may be required (see the section on medical treatment and nursing interventions, low cardiac output, in Chapter 3). If administration of sympathomimetic agents or vasodilators results in an increase in systemic perfusion and blood pressure without a concurrent rise in urine output, furosemide (1 to 4 mg/kg/dose, though up to 5 to 10 mg/kg may be given in a single dose) or mannitol (0.2 to 0.5 gm/kg) may be administered. Some authors advise against use of mannitol for treatment of ARF, since it may precipitate intravascular volume overload.[39] If urine output does not improve within 1 to 3 hours after administration of either diuretic, the child is presumed to have renal failure and renal parenchymal damage.

Occasionally, the child's urine output may increase following a period of oliguric prerenal failure, only to begin a phase of nonoliguric renal failure. As a result, the urine specific gravity and osmolality should be monitored in an attempt to assess renal concentrating abilities in addition to assessment of urine volume. If the child does develop nonoliguric renal failure, water and salt depletion may occur, since these are lost in the urine. Additional electrolytes, including calcium, potassium, and hydrogen ions may be lost with high urine flow, so the child's serum electrolyte and acid-base status should also be monitored closely.

Serum electrolytes, BUN, creatinine, albumin, total protein, calcium, magnesium, phosphorus, uric acid, plasma osmolality, colloid osmotic pressure, and arterial blood gases should all be monitored when ARF is present.

Fluid therapy. If the child with ARF demonstrates signs of fluid overload, the child's fluid intake should be restricted to insensible water losses plus urine and nasogastric output. Too often these children receive repeated boluses of fluid in an unsuccessful attempt to increase urine output, and instead, hypervolemia develops. Repeated administration of osmotic diuretics should also be avoided once the patient has failed to respond to them, because these agents will increase intravascular volume and serum osmolality. Infants require approximately 35 ml/kg/day (or 300 ml/m²/24 hours) for insensible losses, and children who weigh more than 10 kg require 15 to 20 ml/kg/day.[25] The child's insensible water losses are increased in the presence of fever or during periods of catabolism, because more metabolic water is produced. If the child is mechanically ventilated with adequate inspired humidity, water losses through the respiratory tract should be negligible. For further information about insensible fluid losses in children, see Table 8-2 in Chapter 8.

During strict fluid regulation, *all* sources of fluid intake should be calculated, including fluids required to flush monitoring lines and administer medications. Types of fluids administered should be deter-mined by the child's electrolyte and acid-base balance.

If hypervolemia produces cardiovascular compromise, and oliguria persists, the child may require dialysis for removal of excess fluid.

Potassium balance. The child's serum potassium concentration should be assessed frequently, especially if the child develops concurrent acidosis, bleeding, or infection. Potassium administration should be curtailed unless significant hypokalemia is present. Hyperkalemia should be promptly treated. If the serum potassium concentration is greater than 5.5 mEq/L and less than 7.0 mEq/L and the electrocardiogram is normal, sodium polystyrene sulfonate (Kayexalate) can be administered orally (1 gm/kg in divided doses) or rectally (as an enema—0.5 gm/kg/dose), and oral and IV sources of potassium are withdrawn. If the serum potassium concentration exceeds 7 mEq/L, or if there are ECG abnormalities (such as peaked T waves, bradycardia, or heart block), the hyperkalemia must be treated on an urgent basis, utilizing any of the following mechanisms (see the section on medical treatment and nursing interventions for potassium excess earlier in this chapter).

1. *Intravenous infusion of 10% calcium gluconate:* 0.5 ml/kg over 2 to 4 minutes. This attempts to counteract the adverse effects of hyperkalemia on the neuromuscular membranes. The nurse should monitor for bradycardia during this infusion.

2. *Intravenous infusion of a sodium bicarbonate drip:* 1 to 3 mEq/kg (average of 2.5 mEq/kg) over 30 minutes. This attempts to alkalinize the serum and results in a shift of potassium from the vascular space into the cells. The bicarbonate solution is generally diluted 1:1 with sterile water to reduce its osmolality. NOTE: The bicarbonate solution should *not* be mixed with the calcium gluconate, since a precipitate will form.

3. *Intravenous infusion of concentrated glucose or glucose and insulin:* 0.5 to 1 ml/kg of 50% glucose plus 0.1 unit/kg of regular insulin. This increases cellular uptake of potassium ions. NOTE: Please also see the opposite box for additional methods of calculating and preparing the glucose and insulin infusion.

As previously noted (see the section on hyperkalemia earlier in this chapter), these solutions do not remove potassium from the body, they merely transiently lower the serum level by increasing cellular uptake of potassium. Potassium must be removed either through the use of sodium polystyrene sulfo-

---

ADMINISTRATION OF GLUCOSE AND INSULIN TO REDUCE CRITICAL HYPERKALEMIA

Standard 0.5-1 ml 50% glucose/kg body weight + 0.1 unit regular insulin/kg body weight

Ratio method Premature infant: 0.5-1 ml 50% glucose/kg + 1 unit regular insulin/12 gm glucose infused

or

0.5-1 ml 50% glucose/kg + 0.02-0.04 units regular insulin/kg

Child: 0.5-1 ml 50% glucose/kg + 1 unit regular insulin/8 gm glucose infused

or

0.5-1 ml 50% glucose/kg + 0.03-0.04 units regular insulin/kg

Adult: 0.5-1 ml 50% glucose/kg + 1 unit regular insulin/4 gm glucose infused

or

0.5-1 ml 50% glucose/kg + 0.06-0.125 units regular insulin/kg

---

nate or through dialysis (see the section on dialysis later in this chapter).

Calcium and phosphorus therapy. Hypocalcemia should be prevented, since it can depress cardiovascular function and can exacerbate cardiac arrhythmias resulting from hyperkalemia. Significant hypocalcemia is usually treated with infusions of 10% calcium gluconate (in doses of 100 to 200 mg/kg, with a maximum dose of 2 gm) or calcium chloride (in doses of 20 to 50 mg/kg, with a maximum dose of 1 gm). The calcium should always be administered slowly to prevent bradycardia. Since patients with rhabdomyolysis and myoglobinuria tend to deposit calcium in damaged muscle, calcium infusion in children with ARF should be restricted to those children with signs of significant or symptomatic hypocalcemia or to those with severe hyperkalemia.

Most patients with ARF develop hyperphosphatemia. When hyperphosphatemia is present in conjunction with a normal serum calcium concentration, the calcium and phosphorus may precipitate. As a result, it is often wise to prevent hyperphosphatemia initially, before the patient develops hypocalcemia, or before mild hypocalcemia becomes severe. Hyperphosphatemia can be prevented with administration of a phosphate-bending gel or solution such as aluminum hydroxide (Amphojel, 15 to 30 ml every 4 hours by mouth or through nasogastric tube).

Glucose therapy and nutrition. The infant's heelstick serum glucose concentrations should be checked frequently, so that hypoglycemia can be promptly treated. When severe hypoglycemia develops, hypertonic glucose solutions are administered (50% glucose: 0.5 to 1 ml/kg/dose; 25% glucose: 1 to 2 ml/kg/dose; these hypertonic solutions may be diluted to half-strength before administration).

If the child can tolerate oral or nasogastric feedings, these should be instituted as soon as possible to prevent excess protein catabolism. If oral or nasogastric feedings are impossible, parenteral alimentation should be instituted within the limits of the child's daily fluid restriction. Any form of nutrition should provide calories in the form of glucose or essential amino acids to minimize accumulation of metabolic waste products.[25] The child's daily caloric requirements will still total approximately 50% to 75% of normal daily maintenance requirements when ARF is present, since a larger portion of the child's calories are utilized for basal requirements and growth (see Table 7-5 for daily caloric requirements). Administration of adequate nutrition has been shown to reduce mortality and promote recovery of patients with ARF,[1] so this aspect of care cannot be overemphasized.

Metabolic acidosis. The child's arterial blood gases should be monitored as needed to assess adequacy of arterial oxygen saturation as well as arterial pH. Acidosis should be corrected as needed through administration of sodium bicarbonate. The bicarbonate is administered in doses of 1 to 4 mEq/kg, or the dosage is calculated from the child's base deficit (provided with blood gas results from some laboratories):

$$\text{Base deficit} \times \text{kg body weight} \times 0.3 = \underline{\hspace{2cm}} \text{ mEq } NaHCO_3 \text{ administered}$$

Sodium bicarbonate is diluted to half-strength before administration to neonates and young infants, because of its high osmolality.[10] Since the buffering action of sodium bicarbonate results in the formation of carbon dioxide, it is essential that the child who receives bicarbonate have adequate ventilatory function, or a respiratory acidosis may develop.[64] If possible, an attempt is made to limit the total daily dosage of sodium bicarbonate to a maximum of 8 mEq/kg/24 hours, since greater dosages are thought to be associated with an increased risk of intracranial hemorrhage. Since sodium bicarbonate does contain sodium, its administration may enhance water retention and edema.

Acidosis causes a shift of the potassium ion into the vascular space, so it often causes an elevation in serum potassium concentration. As a result, acidosis should be prevented in the patient with ARF because it will worsen existing hyperkalemia.

Prevention of hematologic complications. Since ARF can produce anemia and coagulopathies, the child should be assessed frequently for the presence of petechiae, ecchymoses, gastrointestinal bleeding, or other sources of bleeding. Blood samples should be drawn frequently to measure the child's platelet count, prothrombin time (PT), and partial thromboplastin time (PTT), and appropriate blood components should be administered as needed (see the section on cardiovascular disorders and Table 3-10 in Chapter 3 for summary of blood component therapy for children with bleeding). Prophylactic administration of cimetidine may be prescribed (5 mg/kg intravenously every 8 hours) to prevent gastrointestinal

bleeding. Antacids may also be administered through a nasogastric tube to reduce the risk of stress ulcer formation.

If the child does develop a coagulopathy, all bodily secretions should be tested for the presence of blood. The number of venipunctures and injections prescribed should be minimized, and pressure should be applied for 5 to 15 minutes (or longer, if necessary) to any puncture sites to reduce the risk of hematoma.

The child's hematocrit should be measured daily, and a sudden fall in the hematocrit should be verified and reported to a physician immediately, since it may be the result of bleeding. The child should receive transfusions of packed red blood cells to maintain a satisfactory hematocrit (infants: above 40% to 45%; children: above 30% to 35%) according to physician order and unit policy and within the child's fluid restrictions.

Hypertension. When the child with ARF develops hypervolemia, hypertension can result. This hypertension can be exacerbated by the high plasma renin activity that accompanies some renal disorders. If the hypertension becomes severe, neurologic complications (such as hypertensive encephalopathy) and cardiovascular compromise can occur.

Antihypertensives will be prescribed if the infant or child demonstrates severe hypertension or moderate hypertension with symptoms. A continuous infusion of sodium nitroprusside (0.5 to 8 μg/kg/minute) or nitroglycerin (0.1 to 10 μg/kg/minute), parenteral diazoxide (5 mg/kg/IV dose), or hydralazine (0.2-3.6 mg/kg/dose IV or IM as often as every 4 hours) may control the systemic arterial blood pressure. Reserpine (0.04 to 0.07 mg/kg/dose to a maximum dose of 1 mg IM every 4 to 6 hours) may also be administered. Oral drugs that may be prescribed include hydralazine (1 to 3 mg/kg/day, not to exceed 20 mg/dose), prazosin (10 to 25 μg/kg/dose every 6 hours), propranolol (0.5 to 2 mg/kg/day given in three divided doses), or methyldopa (10 to 50 mg/kg/day).[41]

Infection control. The child with ARF is often nutritionally compromised and usually requires insertion of multiple catheters and tubes for hemodynamic monitoring, urine drainage, or dialysis. In addition, the child is examined frequently every day by many physicians and nurses. It is therefore imperative that each member of the health care team adopt flawless handwashing technique, before and after examination of the child, to reduce the child's risk of nosocomial infection.

The physician should be notified if the child develops a fever or any localizing signs of infection (such as wound drainage). Blood cultures should be obtained if bacteremia is suspected.

Table 7-5 Nutritional requirements for infants and children

Age	cal/kg/24 hours
0-6 months	120
6-12 months	100
12-36 months	90-95
4 years-10 years	80
>10 years, male	45
>10 years, female	38

Nutrient	Percent of total daily calories	
Carbohydrates	40%-45%	combined 85%-88%
Fat	40%	
Protein	20%	

Adjustment of medication dosages. When the child develops renal failure, the dosages of all drugs the child is receiving, especially drugs excreted by the kidney, should be reevaluated. The actual dosage of the drug can be reduced, or the interval between drug administration can be increased in light of the child's reduced glomerular filtration rate. An excellent review of guidelines for drug therapy in renal failure has been written[13] and should be consulted to determine relative portion of renal and nonrenal modes of excretion of specific drugs. (See Appendix B.)

If the rate of nonrenal excretion of a specific drug is known and the child's creatinine clearance is known, the daily excretion of a specific drug (and hence the daily replacement dosage needed) can be estimated. If drug levels are available, these should also be utilized to evaluate drug metabolism and drug replacement requirements. To determine the maintenance dose of digoxin required by the child with heart disease and renal failure, a formula is available from the American Society of Hospital Pharmacists.[59] This formula should be utilized cautiously since creatinine clearance does not always accurately reflect renal function. (For further information about digitalization, see Chapter 3, Table 3-4.)

Dosage adjustments should be made very carefully in those drugs with potentially toxic metabolites (e.g., partial metabolism of sodium nitroprusside results in thiocyanate and cyanide formation). Drug levels should be assessed frequently in these patients. Even after the dosage of a drug has been reduced, the nurse must be alert for evidence of drug toxicity; this requires a knowledge of side and toxic effects of each drug that the child is receiving. Of course, if dialysis is instituted, the medication dosages will again require readjustment.

Psychosocial aspects. When the child develops ARF, the child and the family are usually very frightened. At the very time that the nurse must provide her most thorough observations and skilled care, the child and family are most in need of reassurance and support. If the child's physical care requires the nurse's undivided attention, the nurse should request assistance from a colleague or from additional supportive staff (such as a chaplain, social worker, or patient ombudsman). The child requires explanations and preparation for uncomfortable treatments or procedures (as age appropriate), gentle handling, and soothing verbal and nonverbal interaction. (See Chapter 2 for further information).

See Table 7-6 for a summary of nursing care of the patient with ARF.

Indications for dialysis. If the infant or child with ARF continues to deteriorate despite aggressive medical management, peritoneal dialysis or hemodialysis may be required. The indications for dialysis are listed in the following section on care of the child during dialysis. The differences between peritoneal dialysis and hemodialysis in children and the techniques of dialysis are also reviewed in the following section.

Text continued on p. 503.

Table 7-6 Nursing care of the child with acute renal failure

Nursing diagnosis	Expected outcomes	Nursing activities
A. Potential acute renal failure (ARF) related to poor systemic perfusion (prerenal failure)	1. Urine output will total 1-2 ml/kg/hr (or 10 ml/m² body surface area/hr) 2. Urine osmolality and specific gravity will reflect appropriate urine concentration when urine volume is low (<1 ml/kg/hr) 3. Child's blood urea nitrogen (BUN) and creatinine will remain within normal limits	1. Assess indirect evidence of child's systemic perfusion: blood pressure should be appropriate for age; peripheral pulses should be strong; extremities should be warm; mucous membranes and nailbeds should be pink; capillary refill should be brisk If above conditions are not noted, child may be developing low cardiac output, and physician should be notified immediately

Care plan contributed by Mary Fran Hazinski, R.N., M.S.N.

Continued.

Table 7-6 Nursing care of the child with acute renal failure—cont'd

Nursing diagnosis	Expected outcomes	Nursing activities
A. Potential acute renal failure (ARF) related to poor systemic perfusion (prerenal failure)—cont'd	4. Child will demonstrate adequate blood pressure for age (see Chapter 3), strong peripheral pulses, brisk capillary refill, and warm extremities	2. Measure urine output q hr, and compare amount with child's hourly fluid intake; notify physician immediately if urine output is <1-2 ml/kg/hr, or if fluid intake greatly exceeds fluid output
		3. Record urine osmolality and specific gravity q 4-8 hr or as ordered by physician; notify physician if urine osmolality and specific gravity do not rise when urine volume falls
		4. Monitor color of urine; notify physician of cloudy or rusty urine (hemolyzed red blood cells may be present in urine and may be contributing to a decrease in urine output)
		5. If low cardiac output is present, administer fluid challenge, correct any electrolyte or acid-base imbalance, administer inotropic or chronotropic agents, or administer vasodilators as ordered by physician (see section on low cardiac output in Chapter 3); notify physician immediately if urine output does not improve as systemic perfusion improves
		6. Administer fluid bolus (10-20 ml/kg) as ordered by physician if decreased urine output is thought to be related to hypovolemia; notify physician of urine response
		7. Administer furosemide (1-4 mg/kg/dose) and/or mannitol (0.25-0.5 gm/kg/dose) intravenously if urine output does not improve after fluid bolus; notify physician of urine response to these medications
		8. Send urine specimen to laboratory for culture, osmolality, sodium, BUN, and creatinine measurements, as ordered by physician; if measurement of urinary electrolytes, BUN, or creatinine is ordered, blood sample must be drawn at same time urine is collected, to allow analysis of serum creatinine and calculation of urine creatinine clearance
		a. If prerenal failure is present, serum BUN will usually begin to rise before the serum creatinine

Table 7-6 Nursing care of the child with acute renal failure—cont'd

Nursing diagnosis	Expected outcomes	Nursing activities
A. Potential acute renal failure (ARF) related to poor systemic perfusion (prerenal failure)—cont'd		b. When hypovolemia is present and responsible for prerenal failure, urine sodium content will fall to <20 mEq/L, because sodium will be actively reabsorbed by the kidneys; urine osmolality will exceed 500 mOsm/L since the kidneys will reabsorb water from urine 9. If urine flow does not increase as rehydration is accomplished and systemic perfusion improves, check urine osmolality again; if urine osmolality remains near 300 mOsm/L with a urine specific gravity of approximately 1.010, calculate *renal failure index* (RFI) as follows: $$RFI = \frac{\text{Urine sodium}}{\dfrac{\text{Urine creatinine}}{\text{Plasma creatinine}}} \times 100$$ An RFI of <1 is associated with *prerenal* failure; an RFI of >2 is associated with *nephrotic* (renal tubular) damage NOTE: Calculation of the RFI can provide misleading results if diuretics or mannitol have been administered since such drugs will increase urine sodium content regardless of renal tubular function 10. Ensure proper urinary catheter function; if catheter obstruction is suspected, irrigate catheter with 5-25 ml of bacteriostatic normal saline (per unit policy or physician order); the irrigant should then be withdrawn or amount injected into catheter should be subtracted from child's urine output for that hr 11. Tape urinary catheter and position tubing so that tension on catheter is avoided and gravity drainage is facilitated; position tubing so that dependent loops are eliminated

Continued.

Table 7-6 Nursing care of the child with acute renal failure—cont'd

Nursing diagnosis	Expected outcomes	Nursing activities
B. Potential hypervolemia and cardiovascular compromise related to oliguria and excessive fluid administration	1. Patient will not demonstrate any signs of hypervolemia: a. High central venous pressure b. Hepatomegaly c. Periorbital or other systemic edema d. Tachycardia e. Hypertension f. Tachypnea or increased ventilatory support requirements g. Full fontanelle (in infants <16-18 mo) h. Increased oropharyngeal or endotracheal secretions i. Reduced serum electrolyte concentrations and reduced hematocrit caused by hemodilution 2. Patient will not demonstrate excessive weight gain: >50 gm/24 hr in infants; >200 gm/24 hr in children; >500 gm/24 hr in adolescents If such weight gain is noted, physician will be notified and child's fluid intake will be adjusted	1. Measure and record patient's total fluid intake and output q hr; notify physician immediately if urine output is <1-2 ml/kg/hour or <10 ml/m²/hr 2. Maintain fluid and sodium restriction as ordered once acute renal failure is suspected 3. Administer diuretics as ordered and notify physician of urine output following diuretic administration; if furosemide is administered, monitor child's serum potassium and chloride concentration since hypochloremia may be caused by furosemide therapy (hypochloremia can then contribute to development of metabolic alkalosis and decreased renal response to furosemide) 4. Monitor for signs of hypervolemia (see expected outcomes); notify physician if these signs appear; if hypervolemia is compromising cardiovascular function, peritoneal or hemodialysis may be required to remove excess fluid 5. Measure child's daily or twice-daily weight and notify physician of excessive weight gain (see expected outcomes); to ensure that accurate weights are obtained: a. Weigh child on same scale each time (scale used should be specified in the nursing care plan) b. Weigh child at the same time of day—consider timing of diuretic administration and meals (e.g., child should not be weighed one morning before breakfast or before his diuretic response to furosemide, and weighed the next day after breakfast or after a diuresis in response to furosemide) c. If bulky dressings or armboards are to be placed on the child, weigh these items before they are placed, or weigh comparable items and note their weight next to child's recorded weight on the nursing flow sheet

Table 7-6   Nursing care of the child with acute renal failure—cont'd

Nursing diagnosis	Expected outcomes	Nursing activities
C. Potential hyperkalemia related to decreased renal potassium excretion and continued potassium accumulation as result of cell catabolism	1. Patient will demonstrate serum potassium concentration of 3.5-4.5 mEq/L; if hyperkalemia develops, physician will be notified	1. Monitor child's serum potassium concentration, and notify physician of high or rapidly rising potassium concentration
		2. Monitor for clinical signs of hyperkalemia, including arrhythmias (especially peaking of T wave or premature ventricular contractions, ventricular tachycardia, or fibrillation), diarrhea, and muscle weakness
		If hyperkalemia is suspected, draw blood sample for analysis of serum potassium concentration (per unit policy or physician order), notify physician, and be prepared to institute emergency cardiopulmonary resuscitation if ventricular fibrillation develops
		3. Administer *calcium gluconate* 10% solution (50-200 mg/kg over 2-5 min) as ordered to counteract the adverse effects of hyperkalemia on neuromuscular membranes—monitor for bradycardia during calcium infusion
		4. Administer *sodium bicarbonate* drip (1-3 mEq/kg) over 30 min as ordered, to encourage a shift of potassium from the vascular space into the cells; *do not* mix sodium bicarbonate with calcium gluconate since these substances are incompatible and precipitate will form in IV tubing
		5. Administer *concentrated glucose or glucose plus regular insulin* as ordered to increase cellular uptake of potassium; usually 0.5-1.0 ml/kg of 50% glucose is ordered; this may be followed by approximately 1 U of regular insulin/4 gms of glucose administered (this usually amounts to approximately 0.1 unit of regular insulin/kg); see the box on administration of glucose and insulin to reduce critical hyperkalemia in the section on acute renal failure earlier in this chapter, for further details

Continued.

Table 7-6   Nursing care of the child with acute renal failure—cont'd

Nursing diagnosis	Expected outcomes	Nursing activities
C. Potential hyperkalemia related to decreased renal potassium excretion and continued potassium accumulation as result of cell catabolism—cont'd		6. If hyperkalemia persists, a sodium polystyrene sulfonate (Kayexalate) enema is often ordered; this sodium polystyrene sulfonate is administered as a 20% suspension in a 5% glucose solution, in a dosage of 0.5 g/kg (this may be repeated 2-3 times in 24 hr); an oral dose (1.0 g/kg in divided doses) may be ordered to reduce the serum potassium 1 mEq/L/24 hr 7. If hyperkalemia persists at dangerous levels (>6.5 mEq/L or a level that causes arrhythmias), dialysis is required to reduce child's potassium concentration 8. If ventricular fibrillation develops, begin cardiopulmonary resuscitation, and defibrillate per unit policy and physician order (1-4 watt-seconds/kg)
D. Potential hypocalcemia related to decreased renal excretion of phosphate, calcium-phosphate precipitation, and decreased renal activation of vitamin D	1. Patient will maintain normal serum calcium concentration NOTE: Since amount of ionized calcium depends on serum albumin concentration and pH, serum calcium concentration should only be interpreted after consideration of these variables 2. Patient will not demonstrate clinical signs of hypocalcemia, including: a. Evidence of poor cardiac contractility (see low cardiac output in Chapter 3) b. Seizures c. Complaint of muscle cramps or tingling of extremities d. Tetany	1. Monitor patient's serum calcium concentration—interpret concentration in light of child's serum albumin concentration and pH since these factors influence amount of ionized calcium present in serum as follows: a. Amount of *ionized calcium* is *increased* in presence of *acidosis* (and *decreased* in presence of *alkalosis*) b. Amount of *ionized calcium* is *increased* in presence *low serum albumin concentration* (and *decreased if serum albumin concentration is high*) Notify physician of hypocalcemia or normal serum calcium concentration in the presence of alkalosis or high serum albumin concentration 2. Administer calcium supplements as ordered: Calcium gluconate—100-200 mg/kg (maximum dose 2 gm) Calcium chloride—20-50 mg/kg (maximum dose 1 gm) Do not administer calcium at a rate exceeding 100 mg/min or bradycardia may result; monitor infusion site carefully since calcium infusion may produce vascular irritation 3. Monitor for clinical signs of hypocalcemia, including seizures, tetany, patient complaints of tingling of extremities or muscle cramps

Table 7-6 Nursing care of the child with acute renal failure—cont'd

Nursing diagnosis	Expected outcomes	Nursing activities
E. Patient may develop hypoglycemia related to high glucose needs and low glucose stores (this problem most commonly occurs in infants with acute illness)	1. Patient will demonstrate normal serum glucose concentration	1. Monitor patient serum glucose concentration or heelstick glucose concentration; notify physician of hypoglycemia 2. If hypoglycemia develops, administer concentrated glucose solution as ordered (usually 0.5-1.0 ml/kg of 50% glucose or 1-2 ml/kg of 25% glucose) administer this solution through large bore venous catheter and monitor for signs of vasculitis (solution may be diluted to half-strength before administration) 3. Monitor for clinical signs of hypoglycemia, including decreased systemic perfusion (as a result of poor cardiac contractility) or seizures; these signs are more likely to occur in infant, rather than in older child 4. Calculate child's maintenance caloric requirements (see Table 7-5) and discuss inadequate caloric intake with physician

F. Potential metabolic acidosis related to poor systemic perfusion associated with prerenal failure and/or decreased renal ability to excrete hydrogen ions	1. Patient will have normal serum pH without evidence of respiratory compensation for metabolic acidosis	1. Monitor child's arterial blood gases, and notify physician of development of acidosis
		2. If metabolic acidosis develops, administer sodium bicarbonate as ordered:
		  a. If base excess is available with blood gas results, appropriate bicarbonate dose can be calculated according to following formula:
		
		  $$\text{Base excess} \times \text{weight in kg} \times 0.3 = \underline{\hspace{2cm}} \text{ mEq NaHCO}_3$$
		
		  b. If a base deficit can not be used to calculate bicarbonate dose, 1-4 mEq of sodium bicarbonate may be ordered
		  c. Total bicarbonate dose should preferably not exceed 8 mEq/24 hr since higher doses can increase risk of intracranial hemorrhage
		  d. Since buffering action of sodium bicarbonate results in the formation of carbon dioxide, it is imperative that respiratory function be adequate or be supported adequately to prevent development of hypercapnia and possible respiratory acidosis

Continued. ■

Table 7-6 Nursing care of the child with acute renal failure—cont'd

Nursing diagnosis	Expected outcomes	Nursing activities
F. Potential metabolic acidosis related to poor systemic perfusion associated with prerenal failure and/or decreased renal ability to excrete hydrogen ions—cont'd		3. If metabolic acidosis develops, monitor child's serum potassium concentration since acidosis enhances a potassium ion shift into vascular space, and can contribute to development of hyperkalemia
G. Possible drug toxicity related to decreased renal excretion of drugs or drug metabolites	1. Patient will not demonstrate clinical or laboratory evidence of drug toxicity	1. Once renal failure develops, review patient's drug dosages and administration schedule, and discuss these with physician 2. Assess child carefully for clinical signs of drug toxicity, and notify physician if these appear
H. Increased risk of infection related to multiple invasive monitoring lines, poor caloric intake, and poor nutritional status	1. Patient will demonstrate no leukocytosis, fever, or localizing signs of infection (including wound erythema, exudate, or culture-positive drainage)	1. Monitor patient's temperature and white blood cell count, and notify physician of elevation in either 2. Check all skin puncture sites twice daily and notify physician of presence of any erythema, drainage, or fluctuance of wound edges; obtain cultures of urine, skin puncture sites, and/or blood if infection or sepsis is suspected (per physician order or unit policy) 3. Administer antibiotics as ordered; check dosage in light of renal function (see nursing diagnosis G) and monitor for side effects
I. Potential child and family anxiety related to child's condition	1. Child will be able to cooperate with treatment plan, and will not demonstrate any self-destructive behavior 2. Family members will demonstrate understanding of child's illness, prognosis, and treatment, and will be able to participate in a constructive way	1. Provide child (as age-appropriate) and family with consistent explanations and support (see Chapter 2) 2. Provide child with positive reinforcement and encouragement throughout care 3. Provide explanations (as age-appropriate) before any treatments are performed 4. Plan some activities that will allow child (as age-appropriate) to demonstrate anger, frustration, or sadness; encourage expression of these feelings if child seems willing to discuss them

■ Care of the Child During Dialysis

■ DIALYSIS IN CHILDREN

As noted in the previous section, dialysis is indicated for the child with ARF when aggressive medical management has failed to control hypervolemia, hypertension, bleeding, electrolyte imbalance, or acid-base imbalance. Dialysis is also indicated when the child's cardiovascular or neurologic function deteriorates as the result of electrolyte imbalance and uremia.

The indications for dialysis include the following[41]:

1. Hypervolemia with congestive heart failure, uncontrolled hypertension, or hypertensive encephalopathy
2. Deterioration in neurologic status
3. Bleeding unresponsive to blood component therapy
4. Biochemical alterations (these criteria are not absolute):
   a. Serum potassium concentration above 6.5 to 7 mEq/L, despite maximal medical therapy and administration of sodium polystyrene sulfonate exchange resin
   b. Persistent metabolic acidosis, particularly in the presence of hypervolemia or hyperkalemia
   c. Metabolic alkalosis
   d. BUN greater than 125 to 150 mg/dl
   e. Serum sodium concentration above 160 mEq/L
   f. Serum calcium concentration above 12 mg/dl
5. Acute poisonings or drug toxicity, including ingestion of the following substances:
   a. Salicylates
   b. Phenytoin
   c. Barbiturates
   d. Heavy metals
   e. Other poisons

Both hemodialysis and peritoneal dialysis utilize osmotic and concentration gradients between the child's blood and the dialysate to reduce the child's intravascular volume and to alter intravascular electrolyte concentrations. The content of the *dialysate,* or dialysis solution, will determine the specific changes made in the child's volume and electrolyte status. When peritoneal dialysis is utilized, the peritoneal membrane itself acts as the semipermeable membrane, which allows diffusion of electrolytes and water between the peritoneal capillaries and the dialysate. Peritoneal dialysis is especially effective in children because the surface area of the child's peritoneal membrane per kilogram of body weight is approximately twice as large as the surface area of the adult's peritoneal membrane.[27,41]

Peritoneal dialysis can be accomplished slowly, so that rapid shifts in intravascular volume and electrolyte concentrations can be avoided. The dialysis is accomplished through insertion of a peritoneal catheter, so it is not necessary to insert an arterial or large venous catheter solely for the dialysis.

Hemodialysis utilizes an artificial semipermeable membrane and dialysate located outside of the patient's body. An arterial catheter or catheter in an arteriovenous fistula or graft is utilized, and the child's blood is passed through the dialysis machine through layers or hollow strands of a semipermeable membrane. The osmolality and electrolyte content of the dialysate, located on the other side of the semipermeable membrane, will affect the volume of fluid removed and the alterations in the child's electrolyte concentration during the dialysis. Hemodialysis is much more efficient than peritoneal dialysis in the child or the adolescent, if good circulatory access is possible. However, such circulatory access can be very difficult to obtain in the infant or young child. In addition, the hemodialysis circuit volume cannot exceed 10% of the child's circulating blood volume.[63] As a result, most hemodialysis equipment is inappropriate for use in infants. Hemodialysis is, however, especially effective for removal of lipid-soluble drugs after accidental ingestion in the older child.

■ ACUTE PERITONEAL DIALYSIS

When the decision to begin peritoneal dialysis (PD) is made, informed consent is obtained from the parents by the physician. The results of serum chemistries obtained within the previous 8 hours should be available at the bedside, and the child's weight is obtained before dialysis. If the child is very small, the predialysis weight should be obtained after the peritoneal catheter is in place and dressings applied.

There are no absolute contraindications to peritoneal dialysis. If the child has had recent abdominal surgery, smaller dialysate volumes may be used; if the child has preexisting peritonitis, treatment can be accomplished through use of intraperitoneal antibiotics. It is important to note, however, that peritoneal losses of protein will be increased as the result of peritoneal infection.

■ Bedside placement of peritoneal catheter

If the peritoneal dialysis is expected to be required for only a short time, the catheter placement may be performed at the bedside rather than in the operating room. The following supplies will be required:

1. Two pediatric peritoneal dialysis catheters with trocars, Y tubing, a peritoneal dialysis tray, and a water bath warmer or warming pad with thermometer. Acetic acid is usually added to the warming bath to reduce the growth of bacteria.

2. Acute PD is accomplished with 4 or 6 2-liter bottles of dialysate containing either 1.5% glucose or 4.25% glucose. *These are warmed to body temperature before infusion* (to prevent hypothermia).

3. A patent urinary catheter must be in place. If the child's catheter has been in place for several days, it may be wise to replace it to ensure patency. This ensures the emptying of the bladder and reduces the risk of bladder perforation when the PD catheter is placed.

4. Laboratory results obtained within the previous 8 hours should include hemoglobin (Hgb), hematocrit (Hct), BUN, electrolytes, glucose, phosphorus, uric acid (if appropriate, as in uric acid nephropathy associated with chemotherapy), a PT, PTT, and platelet count, as well as a type and cross match for a unit of blood (or packed cells).

5. One thousand units of sodium heparin are added to each 2-liter bottle of dialysate, unless frank abdominal bleeding is present. Heparin crosses the peritoneal membrane poorly, and its presence in the dialysate will reduce fibrin formation and assist in maintaining peritoneal catheter patency.

6. Two 16-gauge catheters and two short sets of extension tubing. These are used to infuse a volume of solution into the peritoneum to increase the peritoneal space and reduce the risk of bowel perforation.

7. Two small (1 ml) syringes and lidocaine (Xylocaine) without epinephrine

8. Sterile gloves, masks, and gowns

9. Sterile dressings and tape

10. Tubes for culture of the peritoneal fluid. The first outflow is cultured, then cultures are obtained of fluid from every sixth pass.

When the decision for dialysis is first considered, the preparation of the child must begin. The

discussion should be appropriate for the child's age and comprehension, and it should involve the physician, family, and nurse. The nurse must attempt to understand what significance the procedure might have for the child and address those points directly. It is very important that the parents understand and support the child throughout the dialysis. The parents and the nurse must be comfortable with the facts before attempting to discuss them with the child. Often a sedative will be prescribed for the child to

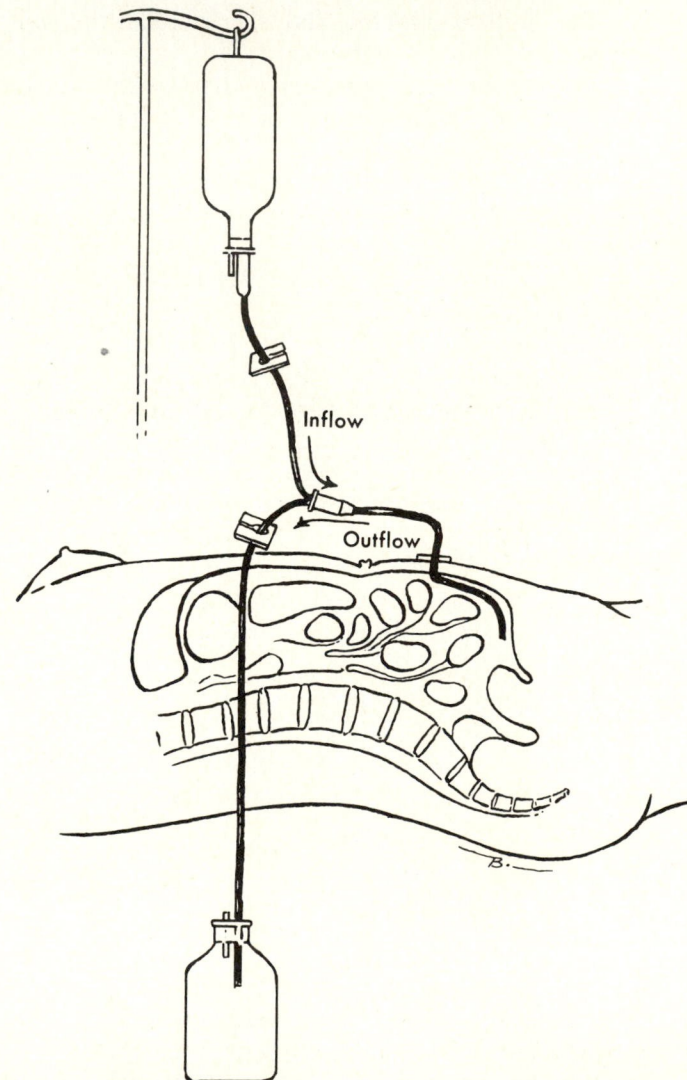

Fig. 7-11 Diagram of peritoneal dialysis, showing placement of peritoneal catheter. During dialysate *inflow*, clamp on upper tubing is open, and clamp on lower tubing is closed. During dialysate *outflow*, clamp on upper tubing is closed, and clamp on lower tubing is open.

From Brundage, D.J.: Nursing management of renal problems, ed. 2, St. Louis, 1980, The C.V. Mosby Co.

reduce the child's pain and anxiety during the procedure.

A surgical preparation of the abdomen is performed, usually involving a 5- to 10-minute scrub with povidone-iodine (Betadine). Local anesthetic is infiltrated along the lower quadrant of the abdominal wall. The 16-gauge catheter (Medicut) is inserted into the peritoneal cavity, and a volume of solution is infused to expand the peritoneal space. The PD catheter is then placed, the outflow tubing is closed, and dialysate (warmed to approximately 37° C) is infused to total 30 to 50 ml/kg (Fig. 7-11).

The child's blood pressure, temperature, respiratory rate, and pulse rate are obtained every 15 minutes for 1 hour, then every hour once the child is stable. Changes in the child's level of consciousness and activity level should be noted and reported to a physician, since these may indicate serious fluid or electrolyte disturbances (see the box below for the protocol for acute peritoneal dialysis in children).

The dialysate remains in the peritoneal space for 30 to 60 minutes, then the outflow connection is opened and the fluid is slowly drained. All subsequent weights obtained are obtained at the end of the outflow cycle, when the peritoneal cavity is empty.

The dialysate solutions contain a chemical concentration similar to that of the plasma except for the absence of potassium and the increased glucose concentrations (Table 7-7). Because hyperkalemia is usually present when dialysis is initiated, the absence of potassium in the dialysate creates a concentration gradient, which promotes potassium movement from the serum into the peritoneal fluid. After four to six

PROTOCOL FOR ACUTE PERITONEAL DIALYSIS IN CHILDREN

Part I: Beginning Acute Peritoneal Dialysis

PURPOSE: To standardize the procedure for Acute Peritoneal Dialysis, thereby decreasing the opportunities for contamination.

GENERAL INFORMATION

1. Definition—Peritoneal Dialysis is the use of the peritoneum as a dialyzing membrane to remove fluid and diffusible toxins from the body through the process of osmosis and diffusion.
2. The peritoneal cavity, implanted catheter, attached administration set tubing, and the dialysate solution are the major components of a closed, sterile system.
3. Peritoneal dialysis may be set up and performed by an RN or LPN II.
4. Patients on peritoneal dialysis are susceptible to peritonitis.
5. Aseptic technique must be maintained whenever the closed system of peritoneal dialysis is opened.
6. Check the following in the patient Kardex prior to initiating a bath:
   a. Dialysate solution
   b. Dialysis exchange frequency
   c. Dialysis exchange volume
   d. Special needs for individual patient
7. The peritoneal dialysis administration set, in-line burette, and catheter site dressing should be changed every 24 hours.
8. Daily cultures should be obtained from the first outflow of a new peritoneal dialysis administration set.
9. When spiking a new peritoneal dialysate bottle, the nurse must wear mask and glove.
10. The peritoneal dialysis flowsheet must be used to record intake and output, following the instructions provided on the form.

EQUIPMENT
1. Peritoneal dialysis solution.
2. IV pole.
3. Peritoneal dialysis catheter (for pediatric use).
4. Peritoneal dialysis administration set (Y-type with drainage bag).
5. In-line burette (in ICUs only).
6. Catheterization tray.
7. Straight urinary catheter (appropriate size).
8. One cutdown tray.
9. Sterile suture (as ordered).
10. Two 16-gauge Medicuts.
11. Four gauze 4 × 4's—two gauze 2 × 2's.
12. Sterile gloves (appropriate sizes and number for those involved).
13. Masks (enough for everyone within 6' of procedure).
14. Sterile specimen container.
15. Graduated cylinder.
16. Betadine swab.
17. Betadine solution.
18. Xylocaine 1%.
19. Infant size hyperthermia pad.
20. Tape.
21. Peritoneal dialysis flowsheet.

Modified from Nursing Procedures, Critical Care, The Children's Memorial Hospital, Chicago, Illinois, 1983.

Continued.

PROTOCOL FOR ACUTE PERITONEAL DIALYSIS IN CHILDREN—cont'd

PERITONEAL DIALYSIS SET-UP AND CATHETER INSERTION

Steps in procedure	*Points of emphasis*
1. Obtain patient weight and record.	Have patient in hospital gown.
2. Gather all equipment.	Allow time to obtain supplies from Pharmacy Central Supply and Respiratory Therapy.
3. Set up infant hyperthermia mattress with temperature set at 32° C or 90° F.	Dry heat is the preferred technique for warming dialysate.
4. Wash hands thoroughly.	

5. Open the following packages:
  a. Peritoneal dialysis Administration set, (Y-Type with drainage bag).
  b. In-line burette (ICU only).	

6. Open sterile glove pack.	
7. Put on mask.	Maintain sterile technique during assembly.
8. Remove protective cap on the dialysate bottle, but not the rubber diaphragm.	
9. Put on gloves, remove the rubber diaphragm.	
10. Spike bottle with in-line burette and then assemble peritoneal dialysis administration set according to manufacturer's directions.	An in-line burette is used to provide accuracy of exchange volume.
11. Prime tubing and close all the clamps.	
12. Wrap all connections with Betadine swabs and 2 × 2 gauze, tape securely.	On most set-ups, there is only one connection.
13. Wrap dialysate bottle in infant hyperthermia mattress and begin warming the solution.	Warmed dialysate is less irritating during installation, and it increases solute clearance and controls heat loss.
14. Assist or perform straight urinary catheterization and obtain urine specimen if applicable.	This is done to remove residual urine in the bladder, thereby decreasing the chance of bladder injury during catheter insertion.
15. Assist physician with gowning and gloving.	
16. Assist physician with insertion of catheter according to his instructions.	Each person within 6 ft. of the procedure should wear a mask.
17. Apply dry sterile dressing to insertion site.	In the ICUs—weigh sterile gauze 4 × 4. The gauze is weighed prior to use to determine fluid loss, should the catheter insertion site leak. Record gauze weight on a sign near the bedside for future reference.
18. Wrap catheter and administration set connection with Betadine swab and gauze 2 × 2, tape securely.	

DOCUMENTATION

1. Record the urinary catheterization results appropriately.
2. Document the following information regarding the Peritoneal Catheter Insertion procedure.
   a. Patient/parent teaching done.
   b. Medications administered for the procedure.
   c. Physician performing the procedure.
   d. Patient tolerance of the procedure.
   e. Insertion site appearance, i.e., dry sterile dressing applied.

FOLLOW-UP

1. Observe catheter insertion site for leakage.

Part II: Continuation of Acute Peritoneal Dialysis

PROCEDURE

Steps in procedure	*Points of emphasis*
1. Obtain temperature, pulse, respirations, blood pressure.	Obtain base line vital signs prior to initiating the procedure and thereafter, when the abdomen is empty.
2. Check that the drainage clamp is closed.	Check that all air has been removed from the instillation tubing.

PROTOCOL FOR ACUTE PERITONEAL DIALYSIS IN CHILDREN—cont'd

Part II: Continuation of Acute Peritoneal Dialysis—cont'd

PROCEDURE

Steps in procedure	*Points of emphasis*
3. Open instillation clamp and allow the prescribed amount of dialysate solution to flow into the abdomen.	Adjust rate so that instillation is accomplished in 5-15 minutes, and as rapidly as the patient can tolerate.
4. Close instillation clamp.	Do not allow air to flow into the abdomen; this can cause distention and discomfort and it can impede dialysate drainage.
5. Allow solution to remain in abdomen for prescribed period of time.	
6. Open drainage clamp leading to drainage bag at the scheduled time.	Drainage should be complete in 5-10 minutes. Repositioning the patient facilitates drainage.
7. When drainage is complete, clamp and obtain vital signs.	Vital signs should be obtained when the abdomen is empty.
8. Open drainage bag outflow port, and drain into graduated cylinder.	
9. Clamp drainage bag outflow port.	
10. Repeat steps 2-9 at prescribed intervals.	

DOCUMENTATION

1. Accurately record intake and output on the Peritoneal Dialysis flowsheet
2. Document any untoward patient reactions in the Nurse's Notes and the action taken

FOLLOW-UP OBSERVATION OF NURSING CARE

1. Observe catheter insertion site for leakage.
2. Observe the following signs and symptoms of peritonitis and notify physician if they are observed.

a. Cloudy dialysate outflow
b. Fever
c. Abdominal pain and tenderness
d. Alteration in level of consciousness, including irritability or lethargy (may indicate dysequilibrium syndrome or cerebral edema)
e. Change in the child's volume status (e.g., evidence of hyper- or hypovolemia)

Table 7-7 Peritoneal dialysis solutions (2-liter volumes)*

	1.5% Dextrose	2.5% Dextrose	4.25% Dextrose
Dextrose in water	15 gm/L	25 gm/L	42.5 gm/L
Sodium	132 mEq/L	132 mEq/L	132 mEq/L
Calcium	3.5 mEq/L	3.5 mEq/L	3.5 mEq/L
Magnesium	1.5 mEq/L	1.5 mEq/L	1.5 mEq/L
Chloride	102 mEq/L	102 mEq/L	102 mEq/L
Lactate	35 mEq/L	35 mEq/L	35 mEq/L
Total osmolality	347 mOsm/L	398 mOsm/L	486 mOsm/L
Approximate pH	5.5	5.5	5.5

*Diamed, Travenol Laboratories, Inc.

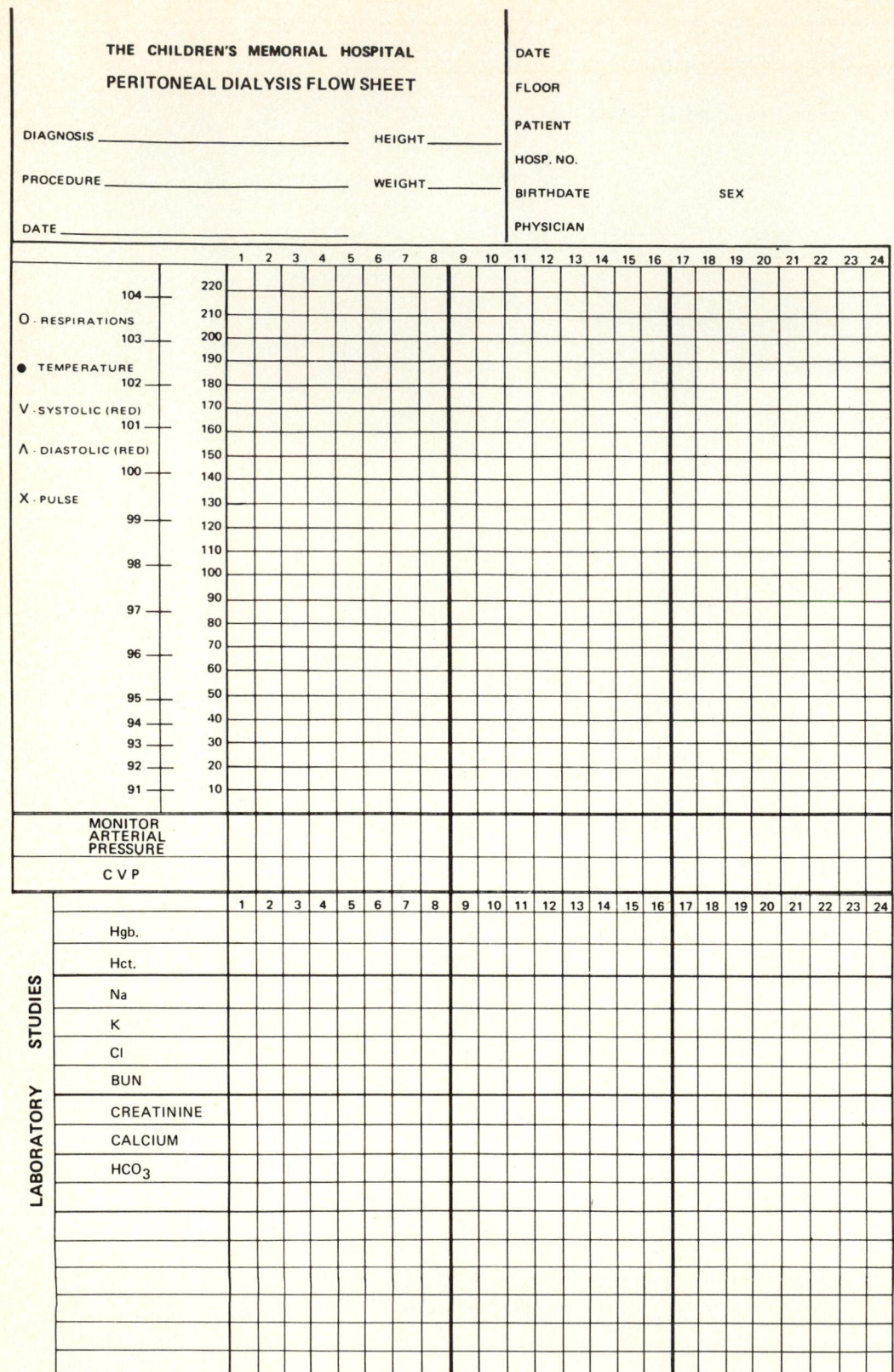

Fig. 7-12 Sample flow sheet for use during peritoneal dialysis.

From The Children's Memorial Hospital, Chicago, 1983.

																																		DATE AND TIME
																																			SOLUTION AND ADDITIVES
																																			BOTTLE NUMBER
																																			BATH NUMBER
																																			TIME SOLUTION STARTED
																																			TIME CLAMPED
																																			DRAINAGE STARTED
																																			DRAINAGE COMPLETED
																																			AMOUNT IN
																																			AMOUNT RETURNED
																																			HOURLY * PERITONEAL BALANCE
																																			RUNNING PERITONEAL BALANCE
																																			INTRAVENOUS FLUIDS
																																			REPLACEMENT & IRRIGATION FLUIDS
																																			GASTRIC INTAKE
																																			HOURLY TOTAL FLUID INTAKE
																																			URINE
																																			GASTRIC LOSS
																																			OTHER FLUID LOSSES
																																			HOURLY TOTAL FLUID LOSSES
																																			HOURLY * FLUID BALANCE
																																			HOURLY ** BODY BALANCE
																																			TOTAL BODY BALANCE

Fig. 7-12, cont'd   For legend see opposite page.

Continued.

INTRUCTIONS

Record BOTTLE NUMBER and BATH NUMBER
Record TIME SOLUTION STARTED
Follow Step 4 in Procedure
Record TIME CLAMPED, when DRAINAGE STARTED and COMPLETED

AMOUNT IN MINUS AMOUNT RETURNED = HOURLY PERITONEAL BALANCE
+(Positive) = Amount of Solution Retained in Peritoneum
−(Negative) = Amount of Drainage in Excess of Dialysis Solution
Example: (+75 plus −75 = 0)

HOURLY PERITONEAL BALANCE + previous RUNNING PERITONEAL BALANCE = RUNNING
PERITONEAL BALANCE

Record and total all fluids IN for one hour.
Record and total all fluids OUT for one hour.
HOURLY TOTAL FLUID INTAKE + HOURLY TOTAL FLUID LOSSES = HOURLY FLUID BALANCE
* HOURLY PERITONEAL BALANCE + *HOURLY FLUID BALANCE = **HOURLY BODY BALANCE
** HOURLY BODY BALANCE + PREVIOUS TOTAL BODY BALANCE = TOTAL BODY BALANCE

Form #75053
(N-76)

TREATMENTS			

PATIENT OBSERVATION RECORD

Date & Time		Date & Time	

Fig. 7-12, cont'd   Sample flow sheet for use during peritoneal dialysis.

dialysis cycles, if the serum potassium has begun to decrease, small amounts of potassium may be added to the dialysate to a maximal concentration of 8 mEq/2 L. This should prevent the development of hypokalemia. The glucose concentration in the dialysate is either 1.5%, 2.5%, or 4.25%. It is the osmotic pressure caused by the glucose in the dialysate that will draw fluid from the vascular space into the peritoneal cavity; the 4.25% glucose concentration solution will remove more fluid than the 1.5% solution because it has a higher osmolality. The peritoneum will also allow glucose to leave the peritoneal space and enter the vascular space as the result of a concentration gradient; this will increase the child's serum glucose levels. In the nondiabetic patient, endogenous production of insulin will usually be sufficient to prevent hyperglycemia.

Since fluid is being removed from the vascular space, the nurse should frequently assess the child's volume status. Signs of hypovolemia include tachycardia, a low central venous pressure, and signs of poor systemic perfusion (such as decreased intensity of pulses, pale mucous membranes, and cool extremities). The development of hypotension will indicate critical hypovolemia.

If edema is present, peritoneal dialysis will not immediately abolish all fluid excess, but as fluid is removed from the vascular compartment, the intravascular proteins and sodium ions will draw water out of the edematous tissues.

■ Calculation of fluid balance during peritoneal dialysis

While the child receives peritoneal dialysis, two records of total fluid intake and output must be strictly maintained. One set of figures records the dialysate infused and the dialysate recovered at the end of each cycle (Fig. 7-12). The amount infused should equal the amount recovered; if less dialysate is recovered than was infused, the nurse should check for signs of catheter or tubing obstruction (see the upcoming section on catheter dysfunction/obstruction). If additional dialysate cannot be recovered, the difference between the amount infused and the amount recovered is recorded as a *positive* fluid balance, and a physician should be notified if this continues.

During the initial cycles of peritoneal dialysis, *more* dialysate solution may be recovered than was infused. This indicates removal of some excess intravascular fluid that is present as the result of the child's underlying renal disease. When this occurs, the amount of fluid recovered in excess of the amount infused should be recorded as a *negative* number,

since this represents excess fluid loss for the child. If this fluid loss continues, a physician should be notified; it may be necessary to reduce the osmolality of the dialysate to prevent excessive fluid loss and dehydration.

The time and the duration of each infusion and drainage cycle, as well as the duration of the dwell time, should be recorded. Since maximum solute transfer occurs during the first 30 to 60 minutes that the dialysate is in the peritoneal cavity, the dwell time is rarely longer than this.[18] The temperature of the dialysate should also be measured and recorded; this temperature should be as close as possible to 37° C to improve the efficiency of the dialysis and to minimize the child's heat loss and discomfort.[18,41]

The second portion of the child's fluid balance record includes a total of all of the child's fluid intake and output. The net dialysis balance should also be considered as part of this total. It is extremely important that this record be strictly maintained, since it will aid in the evaluation of the child's progress and in determination of changes required in the dialysis technique.

When dialysis is begun, adjustment in drug dosages and administration schedules are again required, since many drugs are removed by dialysis.

■ Potential complications

Peritonitis. As many as one third of children who receive peritoneal dailysis develop peritonitis; the risk may be even higher among infants less than 2 years of age.[41] The clinical signs and symptoms of peritonitis during peritoneal dialysis include fever, leukocytosis, diffuse abdominal pain, and a cloudy dialysate return. Paralytic ileus and constipation may also develop. Because of the high risk of this infection, a sample of outflow dialysate solution should be obtained every 24 hours and whenever peritonitis is suspected. The dialysate sample should be centrifuged, and a gram stain, cell count, and culture and sensitivity are also obtained. Fungal as well as bacterial infections are best avoided by scrupulous attention to sterile technique during the catheter insertion process and aseptic technique during exchanges. When the outflow collection bottle is examined, care must be exercised that the bottle is not raised above the level of the bed, since this allows reflux of dialysate back into the peritoneum.

Catheter dysfunction/obstruction. When dialysate solution will not flow either into or out of the peritoneal cavity, it is most likely because of an external kink or an internal plug in the tubing. If external causes are eliminated and flow does not resume, the physician may attempt to remove the catheter plug. Before the catheter is disconnected from the tubing, a 5-minute povidone-iodine (Betadine) scrub is done on the connection of the peritoneal catheter to the dialysate tubing. Clamps are placed on both the PD catheter and the dialysis tubing, they are then disconnected, and the PD catheter is gently flushed. Aspiration of the catheter is generally contraindicated, since it is thought that aspiration is very likely to occlude the catheter ports with omentum. The old dialysate tubing may be reconnected if it has been kept sterile (e.g., wrapped in dry sterile 4 × 4 gauze) during the manipulation. If this tubing is to be reused, make sure that no fluid leaks out of the system. If a solid column of fluid is maintained in the tubing, air does not enter the tubing and fluid does not drain out of the tubing.

In most forms of catheter obstruction, dialysate will flow freely into the peritoneal cavity but will not drain freely from the peritoneal cavity. Very commonly, the catheter floats upward above the level of dialysate, or the catheter becomes wrapped in the omentum. Catheter obstruction may also be caused by constipation, which locks the catheter into a position that restricts drainage. Once the bowel is evacuated, dialysis can proceed. If the child is repositioned or turned from side to side, drainage can often be restored.

Sluggish outflow may also be caused by loops in the dialysis tubing that hangs off the edge of the bed. The collection bottle and tubing should be repositioned so that the tubing falls straight down from the bed to the collection bottle; any extra tubing should be coiled on the bed.

Pain. Almost all patients with new peritoneal catheters will have pain during the initial dialysis infusions and outflows. The pain experienced upon inflow may be relieved by slowing the rate of infusion or by infusing smaller dialysate volumes. Pain may also be caused by encasement of the catheter in a false passage; this causes the dialysate to fill only a small area of the peritoneal cavity instead of spreading throughout the peritoneal space. That small area can distend and become painful. If the catheter has been immobilized so that the dialysate flow is directed at the same point in the peritoneal cavity, it usually causes pain in the lateral or posterior peritoneal wall. It may be possible to float the catheter to another position when the abdomen is filled; occasionally, insertion of a new catheter may be necessary. Painful inflow may also be related to extremes of dialysate temperature.

The patient rarely complains of pain only during the outflow of dialysate; instead, the pain is usually during dialysate *inflow*. Therefore, its causes are those previously mentioned. Pain at the *end* of out-

flow will occur when the abdomen is completely emptied, and it can be abolished by stopping the outflow when a small volume of solution remains in the peritoneal cavity. The presence of this residual solution also diminishes the likelihood of omentum entering the catheter.

Miscellaneous complications. *Bloody dialysate return* is a common observation during the initial 24 to 48 hours following catheter implantation; it is usually self-limiting, and heparin should still be added to the dialysate solution. If the amount of blood present seems excessive, serial dialysate hematocrits may be obtained to quantify the amount of blood present. Transfusion may be required if excessive blood loss through the dialysate occurs.

Leakage around the catheter is encountered more commonly when catheters are placed under urgent conditions at the bedside; it seldom occurs in surgically placed or chronic catheters. Whenever leakage occurs, the nurse should check for overfilling of the abdomen by feeling the tenseness of the abdomen at the end of inflow. The abdomen should not feel rigid. The catheter insertion wound should also be reassessed to determine if the catheter is slipping out of its correct placement. If leakage occurs, weighed sterile dressings are aseptically packed around the catheter, changed when soaked, and weighed again to measure the leakage volume. The physician is notified and a smaller volume of dialysate inflow may be ordered.

Leakage into the abdominal subcutaneous tissues is occasionally encountered. The most likely places for accumulation of this fluid is in the most dependent perineal areas of the penis or scrotum. Subcutaneous leaks are usually of small volumes and they usually reabsorb. If, however, a large volume subcutaneous leak occurs into closed tissue areas like the penis or scrotum, it may be necessary to replace the catheter.

Pulmonary complications. Since peritoneal dialysis results in abdominal fullness, it may compromise diaphragmatic excursion, resulting in hypoventilation and atelectasis. This tendency to hypoventilate, especially in the lower lobes, is accentuated when the child is in the supine position. The nurse should frequently listen to the child's breath sounds and should perform chest physical therapy if areas of atelectasis are noted. If the child is awake, old enough, and cooperative, he should be encouraged to cough and take deep breaths or perform inspiratory exercises (with instruments such as blow bottles or spirometers) to prevent atelectasis. The infant may require frequent "rib-springing" exercises to encourage deep breathing (see Chapter 4 for a discussion of this form of therapy). The head of the child's bed should also be elevated to maximize diaphragmatic excursion and chest expansion.

Fluid or electrolyte imbalance. *Hypertonic dehydration* and hemoconcentration may develop if too much water is taken off too rapidly with peritoneal dialysis. This can result in hypernatremia and can exacerbate hyperkalemia. If dehydration is suspected, the nurse should assess the child's level of hydration and systemic perfusion. If the serum sodium concentration is elevated and the child is dehydrated or hypovolemic, free water may be administered in the form of glucose and water or hypotonic sodium chloride solutions. The osmolality of the dialysate solu-

tion should be reduced before the peritoneal dialysis is resumed.

Hypokalemia may develop if a hypokalemic dialysate is utilized after the serum potassium concentration has fallen. If this occurs, small dosages of potassium can be added to the dialysate, or small amounts of potassium chloride may be administered intravenously (0.5 to 1.0 mEq/kg over several hours).

Hypoproteinemia may develop if peritoneal dialysis is required for several days, since 0.2 to 8.0 gm of protein is lost per liter of dialysate recovered.[18] As a result, the child's total protein and albumin

---

CONTINUOUS AMBULATORY PERITONEAL DIALYSIS PROCEDURE

A. Dialysate Exchange Procedure

(For use with the Travenol Model 3 (5C4157) Prep Kit)

PURPOSE: To maintain a sterile pathway for fluid flowing in and out of the peritoneal cavity while performing an indwelling dialysate exchange.

GENERAL INFORMATION

1. The peritoneal cavity, implanted and attached tubing, and the dialysate bag are the major components of a closed sterile system.
2. All connections of the CAPD system should remain closed and as clean as possible.
3. Each connection should be adequately disinfected prior to opening and/or closing.
4. Exposure time during an opening of the system should be kept to an absolute minimum.
5. Maximum precautions to avoid contamination should be observed during any opening of the system.

6. The dialysate exchange procedure is the most frequent opening of the closed sterile system. The goal of this procedure as written is to incorporate the above general guidelines in order to prevent bacterial contamination and includes a safety margin for human carelessness.

EQUIPMENT

1 Bag dialysate as ordered by physician
1 Travenol Model 3 Prep Kit
2 White outlet port clamps
1 Pair sterile gloves
1 Mask for everybody in the room (within 10 feet of the patient)
Scale if the patient is to be weighed when the dialysate is drained
Blood pressure equipment if a B/P is to be taken
Means for warming the dialysate bag

PROCEDURE

Steps in procedure	Points of emphasis
1. Select an area free of drafts where you will not be disturbed during the procedure.	To decrease the chance of airborn bacterial contamination.
2. Warm fresh dialysate bag using an approved method.	Warmed dialysate is more comfortable during inflow and more effective when dwell time is short. Dry heat is an approved method. Water baths are a source of potential contamination. Microwaves are not recommended.
3. Place supplies you will need on a clean work surface.	
4. Wash your hands thoroughly.	Hands should be washed before starting any procedure. This decreases chances of contamination.
5. Unfold empty dialysate bag attached to catheter and place bag below patient's waist but not directly on the floor.	Bag may be placed on the floor if placed on a clean cloth or pad. Bag should be 2-3 feet below abdomen for purpose of gravity drainage.
6. Open roller clamp on the tubing going to the bag and drain fluid from patient completely. Record time on flow sheet.	Time is recorded on dialysis flow sheet to determine usual amount of time needed to drain.

This procedure has been compiled by Misiewicz, L., CAPD Nurse, Children's Memorial Hospital, Chicago, Illinois, May, 1983. Modified from L. Misiewicz and Children's Memorial Hospital.

Continued.

CONTINUOUS AMBULATORY PERITONEAL DIALYSIS PROCEDURE—cont'd

PROCEDURE—cont'd

Steps in procedure

7. When fresh dialysate is warmed, remove protective outer wrapping. (Wrap removed by pharmacy in hospital.) Dry bag if it is wet.
8. Examine the dialysate bag. Check for:
   a. Clarity of fluid
   b. Leaks—straighten ports and squeeze the bag firmly.
   c. Blue protector shield on spike port.
   d. Proper dextrose concentration.
   e. Expiration date.
   f. Note whether medications were added or need to be added.
9. If you are adding medications, do so at this time.
10. Place white outlet port clamp on fresh bag and position bag on work surface with ports extending just over the edge of the surface.
11. When the dialysate is completely drained from the patient, close the roller clamp and note time on dialysis flow sheet.
12. Place white outlet port clamp on used dialysate bag and position used bag on work surface next to fresh dialysate bag.
13. Open package of sterile gloves. Inner wrapper is to be used as a sterile field.
14. Open Travenol Model 3 Prep Kit and remove contents.
15. Tape medication port back on fresh dialysate bag if you desire.
16. Put mask on yourself, the patient, and all others in the room or within 10 feet of the patient.
17. Open prep kit inner packet and deposit connection shield on sterile field. (Inner glove wrapper.)
18. Remove connection shield from used dialysate bag.
19. Remove blue spike port shield from fresh bag. Be careful not to contaminate the exposed port tip.
20. Put on sterile gloves.

21. Remove the spike from the used bag grasping the outlet port clamp behind the rim. Carefully turn and gently pull the spike from the port.
22. Carefully insert the spike into the port of the new dialysate bag. Push and twist the spike all the way into the port right up to the shoulder of the container.

23. Place the new connection shield around the outlet port connection and snap shut. Note: The rectangular opening of the shield fits over the flange of the spike tubing.

24. You may remove your mask at this time if desired.
25. Remove the outlet port clamp from the fresh dialysate bag.
26. Elevate the dialysate bag and open the roller clamp to allow the dialysate to fill the peritoneal cavity.
27. Watch the bag closely. When a small amount of fluid (about 10 cc) remains, close the roller clamp. Record time infusion completed on flow sheet and type of solution infused.

28. Fold the infused dialysate bag around the tubing-bag union and coil the tubing over the bag.

Points of emphasis

A wet bag can lead to contamination of the tip when the blue protector is removed.

DO NOT USE DIALYSATE BAG
—if dialysate is not clear.
—if leaks in container are present.
—if expiration date has passed.
—if blue protector shield is not securely on spike port.
If the dialysate is cloudy, outdated, or if the container is not intact, the dialysate may be contaminated.

In hospital all medications must be added by pharmacy.
Outlet port clamp is used to grip bag during spike insertion. Extending ports over the edge prevents contamination with the work surface.

Avoid contamination by positioning the wrapper so you will not have to reach over it.

Port will stay out of the way during spike insertion.

Prevent airborn bacterial contamination.

Carefully drop shield onto sterile field without touching it.

Shield should not be reused.
Tip must remain sterile. If it is contaminated, a new bag must be prepared.
Perform the next three steps without touching any nonsterile objects (other than those specified) with your gloves. This is the most crucial time. Hold the spike securely—do not let it touch anything. Avoid contamination.

Minimize the time the spike is exposed to air but be careful not to contaminate. Pushing the spike into the new port takes effort as the fittings must be snug to prevent accidental disconnections.
If the rectangular end opening of shield is not placed over the flange, the shield will not be securely in place and can move, leaving the connection site exposed and open to possible contamination.
The system is now closed and the connection protected.

Keeping a small amount of solution in the bag eliminates the chance of air getting into the abdomen or the system getting airlocked, making outflow difficult. Also a small amount of fluid in the bag makes it easier to flatten the bag before folding it up.
Avoid sharp bends that may weaken and lead to cracks in the tubing.

CONTINUOUS AMBULATORY PERITONEAL DIALYSIS PROCEDURE—cont'd

PROCEDURE—cont'd

Steps in procedure	*Points of emphasis*
29. Secure the folded bag to the patient using a pouch-like device. Avoid tugging on the catheter.	Tension on the catheter may cause exit site irritation or trauma which may lead to infection.
30. Examine the drained dialysate. Report: Cloudy or hazy fluid Fibrin strands in the fluid Bloody or pink fluid	Cloudy fluid is an early sign of peritonitis. When fibrin or bleeding is present, clotting may occur in the catheter.
31. If the dialysate is cloudy or hazy, obtain a specimen for: Culture Sensitivity Gram's stain Cell count	A white blood cell count of greater than 100 neutrophils per mm^3 is usually indicative of bacterial peritonitis. Gram's Stain can often detect bacteria in the peritoneum and assist in the selection of antibiotics.
32. Clean the work area.	
33. Measure and record the amount of dialysate drained. Dispose of drained dialysate in a toilet.	Should the patient have peritonitis, the dialysate should be disposed of so that it will not contaminate others.

DOCUMENTATION: All significant data regarding the CAPD Exchange should be recorded on the CAPD Flow Sheet. In addition to the time, solution used, and volume drained, it is helpful to record the patient's weight and any abnormal vital signs or pertinent data.

FOLLOW-UP EVALUATION: The effectiveness of the dialysis is determined by evaluating the exchange volume balances and the patient's weight together with the patient's overall physical condition. Peritonitis will occur occasionally despite the strictest precautions to prevent it. An acceptable rate of peritonitis, at centers in North America where CAPD is done, is one to two cases of peritonitis for every patient year.

REFERENCES

Going Home With Confidence. Procedures for Continuous Ambulatory Peritoneal Dialysis—Staff Program. Travenol Labs., Deerfield, IL., 1979.

CAPD Update. Continuous Ambulatory Peritoneal Dialysis. Edited by Moncrief and Popovich, New York, 1981, Masson Publishing, USA, Inc.

B. Instructions for daily exit site and catheter care

The Tenckhoff Catheter and the site where it exits from the patient's skin must be cared for daily to prevent bacterial infection. A bacterial infection of the exit site may spread to the catheter and possibly to the peritoneum, where a more serious infection may develop.

Care of the exit site and the catheter should be performed during a daily bath or shower. The Tenckhoff Catheter, titanium adapter connection and the transfer tubing should be washed up to the point where the connection shield covers the tubing-bag connection. The entire tubing may be submerged in water but care should be taken not to wet either the connection shield or the dialysate bag, as water may become a pathway for contamination. It is recommended that the dialysate bag be secured outside the tub or shower to prevent it from getting wet.

The following steps outline the required daily care.

1. During the bath or shower wash the exit site and catheter with regular bath soap.
2. Rinse the abdominal area, exit site, and tubing with tap water.
3. Inspect the exit site. If dried or crusty drainage remains, use hydrogen peroxide on a 4 × 4 gauze or a cotton tipped applicator to cleanse thoroughly.
4. Pour a small amount of Betadine scrub on a 4 × 4 gauze, wet it with tap water, and wash the exit site and tubing.
5. Rinse off the Betadine scrub with fresh tap water.
6. Dry around the exit site with a sterile 4 × 4.
7. Towel dry the remainder of the body with a clean towel.
8. Cover the exit site with a band-aid or 2 × 2 gauze to prevent trauma to the exit site from rubbing against clothing.
9. Tape the Tenckhoff Catheter to the skin, in alignment with the mid-line incision and exit site, to prevent trauma to the internal cuff from accidental pulling on the catheter.

Redness, swelling and purulent drainage at the exit site are signs of an infection. If an infection is suspected, notify the CAPD staff as soon as possible.

should be monitored, and the nurse should assess for signs of peripheral edema. If hypoproteinemia develops, the child may require administration of amino acids.

Hyperglycemia may develop if concentrated glucose dialysate solutions are required to eliminate large amounts of free water. The child's serum glucose concentration (and the infant's heelstick glucose) should be monitored closely, and hyperglycemia (or hypoglycemia) should be reported to a physician. It may be necessary to reduce the glucose concentration of the dialysis. If the patient is diabetic, it may be necessary to provide additional insulin.

Throughout the dialysis period, the child's electrolyte and acid-base balance should be monitored closely. If the child develops electrolyte or acid-base imbalances, these should be discussed immediately with a physician.

■ Removal of the catheter

When the PD catheter is removed, it is done so using sterile technique. While one individual withdraws the catheter, a second individual should maintain tension on the purse string stitch that was placed during the catheter insertion. The suture is drawn tight as the catheter is withdrawn. The catheter tip should be sent to the laboratory for culture. Antibiotic ointment is applied, then sterile dressings are placed over the catheterization site.

■ EXTENDED PERITONEAL DIALYSIS OR CONTINUOUS AMBULATORY PERITONEAL DIALYSIS (CAPD)

Some patients with ARF will require peritoneal dialysis for a long period of time (longer than 5 to 10 days). In these patients, a permanent cuffed peritoneal catheter can be surgically placed, so that ambulatory peritoneal dialysis can be performed.

■ Method

Continuous Ambulatory Peritoneal Dialysis (CAPD) is a form of continuous dialysis that does not require bed rest or hospitalization. CAPD utilizes a cuffed peritoneal dialysis tube and disposable plastic bags of dialysate. Approximately 4 to 5 exchanges are performed daily, and each exchange volume totals approximately 30 to 50 ml/kg (or 0.5 to 2 L total). The exchange time is approximately 4 to 6 hours, which is much longer than the exchange time during acute peritoneal dialysis.[4] However, during the exchanges, the empty dialysate bag is clamped and strapped to the patient's abdomen, and the patient is free to be

relatively active. At the end of each exchange period, the empty dialysate bag is placed at a level lower than the patient's abdomen, the drainage tubing is unclamped, and the bag is filled from the dailysate in the patient's abdomen. The bag of used dialysate is then discarded, and a new disposable bag is obtained for use in the next exchange (see the box on pp. 513-515 for the procedure for continuous ambulatory peritoneal dialysis).

CAPD is not the dialysis method of choice in the acutely ill child, when excess intravascular volume or high serum potassium concentration is life threatening. However, CAPD has a definite place in the management of the child with chronic renal failure. It allows excellent regulation of fluid and serum electrolyte concentrations when it is utilized on a daily basis. Children who receive CAPD require less frequent blood transfusions than children who receive chronic hemodialysis, and their serum urea nitrogen and phosphorus levels may be better controlled than children receiving hemodialysis; however, renal osteodystrophy and hyperphosphatemia do persist.[3,76] Recent evidence indicates that children with chronic renal failure who are managed with CAPD achieve 75% to 100% of normal growth for age. This is significantly higher than the growth of children who receive hemodialysis,[3,80] although catch-up growth has not been achieved.

Children receiving CAPD have very few dietary restrictions, since their relatively continuous dialysis can remove excess fluid and allow constant regulation of electrolyte and acid-base balance. As a result, children receiving CAPD may be better nourished than those who require intermittent forms of dialysis. Control of hypertension is also excellent when children with renal failure receive CAPD.

■ Complications

The most frequent complications associated with CAPD are mechanical problems and infection. The mechanical problems are related to cuff erosion and fluid leaks, and the infectious problems are related to peritonitis.

The cuffed peritoneal catheter can erode the abdominal wall. This can cause a fluid leak and require catheter replacement.[76] Hernias can develop from subcutaneous fluid leaks around the dialysis incision, and these hernias often require surgical repair.

The incidence of peritonitis among children receiving CAPD varies widely in clinical reports, but it ranges from 0.8 to 1.81 episodes per patient-year.[3,5,11,27,76] Many patients also develop local infections around the catheter site.[76]

When selecting patients for CAPD, it is ob-

Text continued on p. 522.

Table 7-8 Complications of continuous ambulatory peritoneal dialysis
A. Complications of dialysis

Complication	Probable causes	Signs and symptoms	Corrective action

1. Fluid overload	Inaccurate assessment of the patient's dry weight
	Imbalance of intake and output
	Excessive oral fluid intake
	Inadequate ultrafiltration (removal of fluid) through dialysis
		Hypertension (↑ B/P)
		Edema (swelling)
		Shortness of breath*
		Increase in weight
		Congestive heart failure and/or pulmonary edema*
			Notify CAPD Staff.
			Most probable course of action:
			  Decrease fluid intake.
			  Increase the use of 4.25% glucose dialysate.
			Extra exchanges with 4.25% glucose dialysate.‡
			Accurate I & O.

2. Dehydration	Inaccurate assessment of the patient's dry weight
	Removal of too much fluid from patient
	Inadequate fluid intake
	Abnormal fluid loss
		Hypotension*
		Cramping in patient fingers, feet, or toes
		Orthostatic drop in blood pressure
		Dizziness
		Decrease in body weight
			Notify CAPD Staff.
			Most probable course of action:
			  Hold exchanges until B/P is higher.
			  Use 1.5% glucose dialysate.
			Accurate I & O.
			Increase oral fluid administration to patient.
			Restrict activity until B/P is higher.
			Bed rest.

3. Constipation	Side effect of inadequate oral intake, bedrest Side effect of taking antacids	No bowel movement Poor drainage of peritoneal fluid from patient†	Regulate bowels with stool softener, cathartic, or diet if patient is taking oral nourishment. Chart bowel movements and size accurately. Enemas only if necessary. Soap suds only. NOT FLEETS‡
4. Diarrhea	Many, including "flu," medications, liquid or tube feedings, diet Peritonitis	May lead to dehydration	Assess if cloudy fluid or other symptoms of peritonitis are present.† Treat the cause with doctor's order. Monitor serum electrolytes.‡

This table has been modified from Pamela Balzar, RN, Clinical Educator, Mount Sinai Hospital, Milwaukee, and revised by Larry Misiewicz, RN, CAPD Nurse, Children's Memorial Hospital, Chicago. Reproduced with permission.
*This condition constitutes an emergency, and a physician should be notified immediately.
†This condition is urgent, but not emergent; please contact the CAPD staff as soon as possible.
‡This corrective action should only be performed after instructions from the CAPD staff.

Continued.

Table 7-8 Complications of continuous ambulatory peritoneal dialysis—cont'd

A. Complications of dialysis

Complication	Probable causes	Signs and symptoms	Corrective action
5. Nausea and vomiting	Many causes including peritonitis Inadequate dialysis	May lead to dehydration	Assess if cloudy fluid or other symptoms of peritonitis are present.† Treat the cause with doctor's order. Physical exam in clinic.

6. Muscle cramps	Patient has had too much fluid removed
	Too rapid removal of fluid, usually when using all 4.25% glucose dialysate
	Electrolyte imbalance
		Cramping in legs, feet, hands	Report to CAPD Staff.
			Assess weight, blood pressure.
			Relief measures:
			  Apply heat to cramping area.
			  Rub cramp vigorously.
			  Apply pressure to foot or hand.
			Check serum electrolytes and calcium.‡

7. Abdominal cramping	Dialysate temperature too cold Dialysate draining too fast Many others, including peritonitis	Abdominal cramps associated with an exchange usually subside soon after the exchange is completed Persistent pain (lasting over 1 hour) may indicate a more serious condition*	Assess if cloudy fluid or other symptoms of peritonitis are present.† Warm dialysate with heating pad prior to administration. Adjust in/out flow to a more comfortable rate with roller clamp. Notify CAPD Staff if pain persists.

8. Air in the peritoneal cavity	Infusion of air with the dialysate	Shoulder pain
		Seeing the air infuse into the peritoneal cavity
		Note: Air in the peritoneal cavity is usually not dangerous (in contrast to air in an IV or in hemodialysis lines).
			Try to remove air from peritoneal cavity:
			  Lay patient on back.
			  Elevate hips on several pillows.
			  Open roller clamp as usual to drain peritoneal fluid.
			  Air should flow out.
			Notify CAPD Staff if pain persists.

9. Blood in the peritoneal fluid Pink tinged fluid	Rupture of tiny peritoneal capillaries Possible serious abdominal injury	Pink fluid (you can still see through the bag)	Pink fluid usually clears up in two or three exchanges without treatment.

Table 7-8 Complications of continuous ambulatory peritoneal dialysis—cont'd
A. Complications of dialysis

Complication	Probable causes	Signs and symptoms	Corrective action
Bloody fluid with blood clots	Many causes including peritonitis		Check blood pressure and pulse. Observe patient. Hematocrit on peritoneal fluid.‡ May add heparin as ordered to prevent clotting of peritoneal catheter.‡
		Bloody fluid (you cannot see through the bag), clots may be present*	Call CAPD Staff Immediately.*
10. Protein loss	Large amount of protein is lost through the peritoneal membrane	Check serum total protein and albumin Cloudy peritoneal fluid	Diet as advised by renal dietician. Protein supplements as ordered by physician.
11. Peritonitis†	Break in sterile technique Exit site infection Endogenous source	Cloudy fluid Abdominal pain Nausea and vomiting Fever Combination of any of the above	Notify CAPD Staff.† Save last bag of dialysate drained in refrigerator. Obtain culture, sensitivity, Gram's stain and cell count from last bag *before* adding antibiotics. Take vital signs and weigh patient between exchanges. Add antibiotics as ordered to dialysate.‡
12. Fibrin in the peritoneal fluid	Physiological response to a foreign body in the peritoneal cavity Peritonitis	White strands floating freely in the peritoneal fluid Protein clumps	Notify CAPD Staff. Heparin 500-1000 units per liter should be added to dialysate to prevent clotting of the catheter.
13. Weakness	Anemia Hypotension Lack of exercise Protein deficiency Fluid weight gain	Lethargy Increased sleep Muscle weakness Increased weight over dry weight	Complete blood count. Check fluid balance. Increase exercise. Increase protein intake.‡ Weigh between exchanges.
14. Dizziness	Low blood pressure Pulling off too much fluid or too quickly	Weight is less than dry weight Low blood pressure	Take blood pressure. Weigh patient.

Continued.

Table 7-8 Complications of continuous ambulatory peritoneal dialysis—cont'd

A. Complications of dialysis

Complication	Probable causes	Signs and symptoms	Corrective action
	Postural (orthostatic) hypotension	Loss of balance	Check fluid balance, evaluate medications. Replace fluid and salt. Instruct patient to stand up more slowly. Call CAPD Staff.

B. Technical complications of the peritoneal dialysis system

Complication	Probable causes	Corrective action
1. Fluid will not outflow	Kink in the tubing Airlock in the tubing Fibrin clot in the catheter Omentum caught in catheter Constipation No fluid in the peritoneal cavity Roller clamp left closed or outlet port clamp left closed	Check spike bag connection, tubing, and catheter for kinks, clamps or any obstruction. Open clamp on drain line, and ask patient to bear down, as if he were having a bowel movement. This will increase the pressure in the abdomen. Change the patient's position, (side to side, knees up, etc.). Assess for constipation. If unable to establish an outflow, attach a new bag of dialysate with heparin added. Inflow approximately 100-200 cc. If outflow begins, stop inflow and allow outflow to continue. If inflow/outflow cannot be established, notify the CAPD Staff.†
2. Fluid will not flow into patient	Kink in tubing Air in tubing Fibrin clot Constipation	Check spike/bag connection, tubing, and catheter for kinks or clamps on the line. Raise the bag as high as possible and gently squeeze to get an inflow started. Assess if patient is constipated. Change the patient's position. Respike a new bag of dialysate and repeat above. Call CAPD Staff.

Table 7-8 Complications of continuous ambulatory peritoneal dialysis—cont'd

B. Technical complications of the peritoneal dialysis system

Complication	Probable causes	Corrective action
3. Inadequate outflow (less than volume instilled)	Reabsorption of the fluid into the vasculature Clotted catheter Malposition of the catheter Fluid will reabsorb on long exchanges, particularly when using 1.5% glucose	Outflow should never exceed 25 minutes. Slow outflow should be treated before catheter is nonfunctioning.† Keep accurate intake and output. Monitor weight between exchanges. Assess abdomen for tenseness or fullness. Notify CAPD Staff if output is consistently short of amount infused and the patient's weight is increasing.
4. Spike contamination Broken spike Hole in transfer tube Accidental disconnection of transfer tube from catheter	Break in technique Excessive wear on transfer tube or spike	Do not proceed with the exchange. Clamp off transfer tubing. Proceed with a tubing change or decontamination procedure. Prophylactic antibiotics may be given if it is thought the patient may have received fluid that was contaminated.‡ Notify CAPD Staff.†
5. Leaking bag of dialysate	Rough handling of bags Manufacturing or packaging defect	Check bag carefully before using. Discard any questionable bags. If a patient receives any fluid from a defective bag, prophylactic antibiotics may be given—notify CAPD Staff for advice.‡

C. Complications of the peritoneal dialysis catheter

Complication	Signs and symptoms	Corrective action
1. Exit site infection†	Exit site is red, swollen and tender to the touch Purulent drainage noted on the old dressing	Notify CAPD Staff. Obtain a culture and sensitivity of the exit site.‡ Begin appropriate antibiotics.‡ Assess if catheter care is being done correctly.

Continued.

Table 7-8 Complications of continuous ambulatory peritoneal dialysis—cont'd
C. Complications of the peritoneal dialysis catheter

Complication	Signs and symptoms	Corrective action
		Soak exit site twice daily.
		Watch for signs of peritonitis.
		Catheter may need to be removed if infection becomes serious.
2. Leaking from exit site†	Wet dressings	Notify CAPD Staff.
	You can see fluid dripping out of exit site	Bed rest.
		Smaller exchange volumes—only infuse part of each bag of dialysate.‡
		Catheter may need to be replaced.
3. Crack or tear in catheter*	Visually inspect the catheter; a tear may be seen	Stop dialysis and clamp the catheter with a plastic clamp as near the exit site as possible.
	Fluid leaking	Notify CAPD Staff immediately.
4. Catheter comes out of the patient*	Catheter will not inflow or outflow	Stop dialysis.
	Catheter is no longer in the patient	Notify CAPD Staff immediately.
	Leaking at the exit site	DO NOT attempt to reinsert the catheter.

viously very important that the child and the parents be reliable and able to follow the established protocol. Children or families must be taught the dialysis technique, and they should be instructed to contact the CAPD nurse whenever they experience abdominal pain, inflow or outflow occlusion, inflammation of the catheter site, a feeling of weakness or dizziness when standing, hypotension, cloudy dialysate outflow, catheter disconnection or contamination, fever, excessive weight gain, edema, or other illness (please refer to Table 7-8 for a summary of complications of CAPD).

Because the dialysate dwells in the peritoneum for a long time, and the risk of peritonitis is relatively high in children receiving CAPD, it is often recommended that only the CAPD nurse perform any in-hospital CAPD that the child requires. This minimizes the child's exposure to multiple people and contaminants and may reduce the risk of peritonitis.

■ HEMODIALYSIS
■ Method

Hemodialysis is one of the most efficient artificial methods of removing nitrogenous wastes from the body and of restoring fluid, electrolyte, and acid-base balance. Hemodialysis does require removal of blood from the body. The blood is drawn from an artery, an arteriovenous fistula, or a cannula or graft and is pumped into a dialyzer (Figs. 7-13 and 7-14). The blood and dialysate solution are separated by a semipermeable membrane. Nitrogenous wastes pass from the blood into the dialysate as the result of a concentration gradient. Free water or other solvent can be drawn from the blood, and electrolyte balance can be restored as the result of osmotic and concentration gradients between the dialysate and the blood. Other substances can be removed from the blood as the result of ultrafiltration and solvent drag (movement of

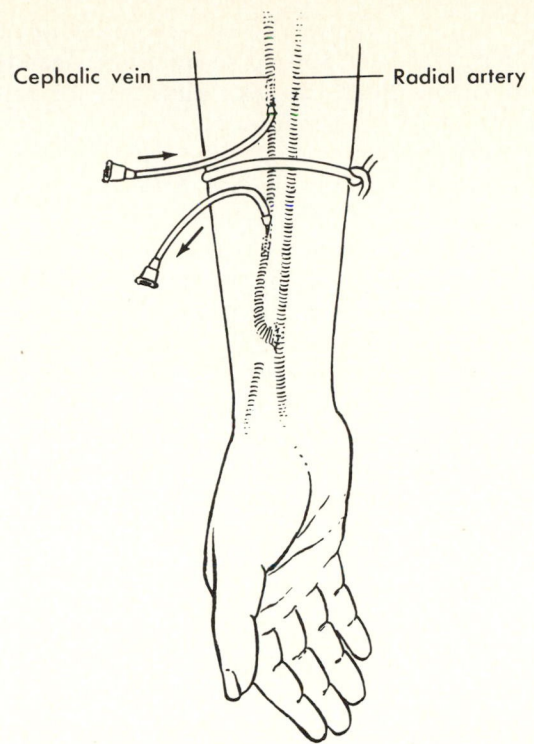

Cephalic vein — Radial artery

Fig. 7-13 Circulatory access for hemodialysis: internal arteriovenous fistula. Needles can be inserted into arterialized vein to initiate dialysis.

From Brundage, D.J.: *Nursing management of renal problems,* ed. 2, St. Louis, 1980, The C.V. Mosby Co.

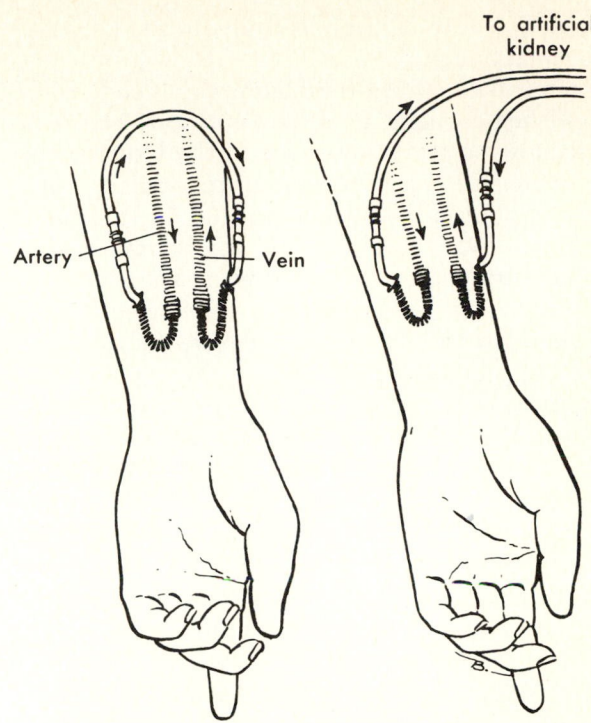

To artificial kidney

Artery — Vein

Fig. 7-14 Circulatory access for hemodialysis: external arteriovenous cannula. Cannula shown on left is closed, as it should be between hemodialysis treatments. Cannula on right is open and is attached to hemodialysis tubing.

From Brundage, D.J.: *Nursing management of renal problems,* ed. 2, St. Louis, 1980, The C.V. Mosby Co.

solutes as the result of movement of large amounts of water or solvent). Once the blood has passed through the dialyzer, it is returned to the body.

Since the dialyzer must draw blood from the body and return blood to the body, some pumps are required. In addition, the dialyzer and tubing must be "primed" with fluid or blood before the dialysis begins. Since the circulating blood volume of the infant or child is so small, it is important that the dialyzer and pump lines require a filling volume of no more than 10% of the child's circulating blood volume. Since even the smallest dialyzers require a filling volume of 60 to 75 ml, the smallest child suitable for dialysis with conventional equipment is approximately 8 to 10 kg. Though a few centers are able to successfully hemodialyze smaller infants, peritoneal dialysis is generally utilized for the infant with renal failure.

The dialyzer and blood lines are primed with either isotonic saline or 5% albumin. In young infants the dialyzer may be primed with blood components. A portion of this prime may later be electively infused into the patient at the end of the dialysis procedure. The dialysate solution contains glu-

cose, sodium, calcium, and potassium, in concentrations that are specified by the physician. The dialysate usually contains very little potassium (between 0 and 4 mEq/L) and no urea, so high concentration gradients between the dialysate and the blood will hasten removal of these solutes from the blood. The presence of glucose in the dialysate at levels of 200 to 250 mg/dl creates a high osmotic pressure in the dialysate; this favors the movement of water from the blood to the dialysate.

The blood and the dialysate are usually pumped through the dialyzer in opposite directions. This maximizes the concentration and osmotic gradients between the dialysate and the blood, so dialysis can be accomplished within a short period of time (approximately 6-hour exchange time).

Just before hemodialysis is initiated, the patient or the blood entering the dialyzer must be *heparinized* to prevent clot formation within the dialyzer or dialysis tubing. Intermittent heparinization is accomplished up to the time of dialysis; then continuous or intermittent intravenous heparinization can be provided during the dialysis procedure itself. The Lee-White clotting time or the Activated Clotting

Time (ACT) can be utilized to evaluate the adequacy of heparinization.

Removal of excess fluid from the blood can be accomplished during dialysis in two ways. The resistance to flow on the venous side of the blood circuit can be increased. This increase in resistance is usually accomplished by placement of an adjustable clamp on the venous blood line; the clamp is then tightened until the desired pressure in the blood line is reached. This application of resistance to the venous portion of the dialyzer is referred to as the application of *positive pressure.*

Removal of excess fluid from the blood can also be accomplished by application of suction to the dialysate. This *negative pressure* is transmitted to the blood compartment, and free water and small particles are drawn from the blood, across the semipermeable membrane, and into the dialysate. The use of either positive or negative pressure or both will determine the rate of fluid removal from the blood. The dialysis nurse and the bedside nurse will be responsible for continuously evaluating the effect of fluid removal on the patient's systemic perfusion. If the patient's clinical condition deteriorates, some adjustment often must be made in the rate of fluid removal.

■ Complications

Though hemodialysis is efficient, it is extremely expensive, and it may produce some complications that do not develop during peritoneal dialysis. These complications are largely related to hypovolemia and resultant hypotension, fluid shifts (also known as dysequilibrium), hypervolemia, bleeding, anemia, infection, malfunction of the vascular access site, or continued complications of renal failure and uremia. Each of these will be discussed separately below.

Hypotension/hypovolemia. Hypotension can develop as the result of removal of a large amount of intravascular water (and resultant hypovolemia) or as the result of circulatory instability. The patients most at risk for the development of hypotensive crises during dialysis are patients with vasomotor instability (including patients with paraplegia or quadriplegia), those with low cardiac output or myocardial dysfunction, patients treated with vasodilators,[88] or those patients with a history of hypotensive episodes during dialysis.

If the child develops hypotension during dialysis the dialysis nurse must reduce any positive venous pressure or negative dialysate pressure that may be present within the dialyzer, since these factors enhance water removal from the blood. In addition, the bedside nurse may be required to administer albumin or other volume expanders (per unit policy or physician order), place the patient in modified Trendelenberg's position (head flat, feet elevated), or initiate cardiopulmonary resuscitation.

To avoid hypotension, any existing hypovolemia should be corrected before dialysis is begun. In addition, the patient's blood should be *slowly* drawn into the dialyzer, so the patient does not experience an acute loss of intravascular volume. If excess intravascular water is to be removed during dialysis, venous positive pressure or dialysate negative pressure should be applied very slowly. The dialysis nurse *and* the bedside nurse are both responsible for monitoring the child's systemic arterial blood pressure and systemic perfusion. Deterioration in clinical status should be reported immediately to a physician.

Fluid shifts and dysequilibrium. If many osmotically active particles, such as sodium or urea, are rapidly removed from the patient's blood, the patient's serum osmolality will quickly fall. As a result, water may shift from the intravascular to the intracellular space, and the brain tissue and other tissues will swell. This tissue swelling following dialysis has been called the dialysis dysequilibrium syndrome. The child may complain of severe headaches or may demonstrate nausea, vomiting, confusion, irritability, or seizures.[17] To prevent dysequilibrium, the rate of solute removal from the blood must be gradual. Peritoneal dialysis may be performed initially to reduce the blood urea nitrogen concentration gradually. In addition, the efficiency of the hemodialysis can be reduced; the blood flow through the dialyzer can be slowed, the dialysate can be run in the same direction of flow as the blood, the duration of the dialysis treatment can be shortened, or intravenous mannitol may be administered.

Hypervolemia. If too much fluid is administered to the patient during dialysis, or excessive fluid and blood is transfused to the patient from the dialyzer at the end of dialysis, the child can develop hypervolemia. This can produce significant cardiovascular problems, particularly if the child has preexisting cardiac disease. The child can quickly develop signs of congestive heart failure, including tachycardia, peripheral vasoconstriction, decreased urine output, hepatomegaly, periorbital edema, elevated central venous pressure, tachypnea, and increased respiratory effort. If severe hypervolemia is present, the child can develop pulmonary edema or hypertension.

Since most children who require dialysis are oliguric or anuric, additional dialysis is usually required to remove excess intravascular water. If the child does have adequate urine volume, spontaneous diuresis may reduce intravascular volume.

Bleeding and anemia. Since the child's blood must be heparinized during dialysis, bleeding can occur. The child can bleed from wounds, puncture sites, or into the brain, pericardium, or abdomen. To reduce the risks of such bleeding, *regional heparinization* may be performed. The heparin is injected into the dialysis blood line, which carries blood from the patient to the dialyzer. As a result of the heparin injection, blood passing through the dialyzer will be heparinized. To prevent large amounts of heparin from returning to the patient, protamine sulfate will be administered into the venous blood line returning blood from the dialyzer to the patient. Protamine sulfate neutralizes heparin but can produce a coagulopathy or hypotension if it is administered separate from or in excess of heparin,[77] or if the patient inadvertently receives a bolus of the protamine.

The patient with chronic renal failure who requires dialysis is often anemic. This anemia can result from loss of blood within the dialysis system (through blood leaks, loose connections, clot formation, sampling, or dilution of blood with dialysis tubing "prime"), from hemorrhage, or from the effects of uremia). Levels of erythropoietin are low among uremic patients, so red blood cell production and survival are both reduced.

To prevent anemia, blood sampling should be minimized. Whenever blood is drawn, the amount should be recorded on the child's flow sheet, and replacement should be provided whenever the blood loss totals 5% to 7% of the child's circulating blood volume (see Chapter 3, Table 3-9, for calculation of circulating blood volume). Since hemodialysis is often accomplished through use of an arterial access catheter, laboratory sampling of blood can be accomplished while the patient is dialyzed. This not only reduces the number of venipunctures the child requires, it also allows immediate replacement of the sample amount through the dialyzer. Transfusions of packed red blood cells are usually administered to replace blood lost, since they provide red blood cells without excessive fluid volume. Iron therapy may also help treat the anemia. Anemia is to be particularly avoided in children with associated cardiovascular disease, since anemia increases cardiac output requirements.

Infection/febrile reactions. The patient who receives hemodialysis is at risk for the development of infection because of multiple invasive lines or cannulas, compromised nutritional status, frequent handling by a variety of hospital personnel, and frequent transfusions. The risk of infection can be minimized among dialysis patients if good handwashing technique and strict asepsis are practiced, good nutrition is provided, and hepatitis screening is performed by the blood bank (for further discussion of hepatitis see Chapter 8).

The nurse should assess all of the patient's wounds and vascular access sites daily and report any areas of inflammation to a physician. All wounds should be dressed according to unit policy or physician order.

Patients receiving hemodialysis may experience a sudden increase in temperature, known as a febrile reaction. This fever may be the result of an allergic reaction to the dialyzer membrane materials or to a blood transfusion administered during dialysis, from systemic seeding from an infected shunt, or from improperly sterilized dialysis equipment. A preexisting fever may suddenly become manifest when the patient's serum urea, which may act as an antipyretic, is lowered.

When the fever is reported to a physician, blood cultures may be requested from two different collection points; one set of cultures is usually collected from the dialysis tubing by the dialysis nurse after a 3-minute povidone-iodine (Betadine) scrub. The second culture is usually obtained from a peripheral vein. Cultures may also be collected from the dialysate. If a transfusion reaction is suspected, specimens are collected from the transfusion bag, the patient, and the infusion port and sent to the laboratory to check for hemolysis and incompatibility. If hemolysis is present, the child's serum potassium concentration should be monitored closely, since hyperkalemia can occur.

Malfunction of the hemodialysis access. The establishment and maintenance of vascular access in small children is one of the major problems associated with pediatric hemodialysis. Frequently, prosthetic materials such as polytetrafluoroethylene (Goretex or Impra) are utilized to provide shunts in children. Once the shunt is constructed, only personnel familiar with care of the shunts should handle them. Dressing changes and cleaning of the shunt exit wound is done so as to avoid compression or twisting of the shunt. Sterile Q-tip cotton applicators are used to gently remove debris from the wound; antibiotic ointment and then sterile dressings are applied. The ends of tapes placed over the dressings are tabbed for ease of removal. The ends of an external shunt are bridged by a double length of plastic tape, also tabbed on the ends for ease of removal. The bridge is then wrapped once around with another length of plastic tape. Sharp instruments are never used around the shunt. Special shunt clamps are maintained continually at hand for use in clamping the external shunt should the ends become disconnected. (See the procedure for arteriovenous shunt care in the following box).

A-V SHUNT CARE

Supplies

1 blue pad	Cotton-tip applicators	1" paper tape
1 pkg 4 × 3s	Betadine	Betadine ointment
1 pkg Kling	Hydrogen peroxide (H$_2$O$_2$)	

When to clean shunt

Daily on off-dialysis days; before and after dialysis on those days; whenever bandage is soiled and/or wet.

Purpose

To keep clean, to prevent infection by keeping normal skin bacteria to a minimum; to remove crusts and drainage that leave paths for bacteria to enter tissues; to check for redness and tenderness and pus that are signs of infection; to check for bleeding; to check for fibrin that can indicate imminent clotting or actual separation of the blood within the shunt indicating clotting has occurred.

Procedure	Rational
1. Assemble supplies.	
2. Wash hands before proceeding and after handling old dressing, e.g., with pHisoHex or Betadine scrub.	Clean hands, cut down on transmission of bacteria to shunt sites.
3. Place blue pad under extremity.	Protective covering and clean field.
4. Remove dressing and lay cannula out flat; wash hands. Have cannula clips handy. Check to make sure the shunt is bridged with tape at the separation to prevent the cannulas from coming apart.	Need clips nearby in case of accidental shunt separation.
5. Clean each exit site separately; if stitches are still in, clean each stitch separately. After stitches are removed, continue to clean area until it is healed. Clean first with hydrogen peroxide to remove crusting and any old drainage. If drainage looks like pus and exit sites or stitches are red and tender, obtain a culture before cleaning. After cleaning with H$_2$O$_2$ clean with Betadine using same procedure. Use applicator and clean from inside out, (discarding before moving on to next site). If necessary, remove H$_2$O$_2$ foam with dry Q-tip and repeat cleaning until old blood, drainage, or crusts are removed, then apply Betadine generously.	Do not go from exit site to exit site or stitch to stitch with same applicator because of possibility of transmitting bacteria from one area to another. Do not clean outside and then move in around site because of same reason. Obtain culture before cleaning to ascertain what bacteria if any are growing and consult physician immediately for antibiotic orders. Remove old crusts and drainage, which can act as bacteria traps. Infections will lead to clotting or loss of cannula because of breakdown of vessels, bleeding, or sepsis.
6. Apply Betadine ointment around exit sites.	Acts as sealant against bacteria but still allows any drainage to leave exit site.
7. Apply 4 × 3 gauze sterile side down around exit sites and stitches making sure they are completely covered and making sure wings are lying flat.	Exit sites and stitches should be covered at all times during cleaning.
8. Fold cannula back over the 4 × 3 and tape down so there are no kinks. Double check for kinks.	Kinking will cause clotting by reducing blood flow.
9. Wrap Kling around shunt allowing a little of the cannula to show at either end to check for clotting.	Instruct patient to check shunt often for red color (whiteness indicating separation) and to check for warmth (cold indicates clotting).
10. Attach clips to bandage or to clothing within easy access.	Cannula clips must be near cannula at all times in case of accidental shunt separation.
11. If area around exit sites is dirty or Betadine stained, wash with pHisoHex and rinse off thoroughly with sterile saline. Dry with sterile 4 × 3 gauzes—one for each exit site. Never use alcohol because it dries the skin. Never use lotion directly around sites because it contains bacteria.	Do not use water to rinse off the pHisoHex because it contains bacteria.

Continued problems of uremia. The patient requiring hemodialysis is still susceptible to problems associated with renal failure and resultant uremia. Though temporary relief of hypervolemia, hyperkalemia, uremia, and acidosis is often achieved during dialysis, anemia, hypertension, infection, osteodystrophy, endocrine imbalance, pruritis, anorexia, nausea, vomiting, fatigue, ulcers, and depression can persist (see the section on chronic renal failure later in this chapter).

Throughout the care of the child with renal failure, the nurse should gather the support personnel to assist in the psychosocial care of the child and family as well as the physical care of the child. As appropriate, the bedside nurse should begin to plan for the child's discharge to home or to another unit.

Whenever the critically ill child requires dialysis, the bedside nurse remains responsible for coordinating the care of the child and family. Though a dialysis nurse may be present and responsible for the use of the dialyzer, the bedside nurse still must keep track of the child's fluid balance and must be able to assess the child's systemic perfusion. The dialysis nurse and the bedside nurse should coordinate efforts. It will be important to time administration of medications, blood products, and fluid according to the timing and effectiveness of the dialysis. Both the dialysis nurse and the bedside nurse must provide the child and family with support, warmth, and compassion.

■ Specific Diseases

■ NEPHROTIC SYNDROME
■ Etiology

Nephrotic syndrome is an association of clinical signs and biochemical abnormalities that may develop during the course of several different types of renal diseases. It is described as the simultaneous presence of proteinuria (in excess of 0.1 gm/kg/day or 2.0 gm/m²/day), hypoalbuminemia, hyperlipidemia, and edema.[58]

Nephrotic syndrome may be classified according to either etiology or the histologic changes present in the glomerulus. The nephrotic syndrome without evidence of systemic disease is classified as primary (or idiopathic) nephrotic syndrome if no apparent causative agent is found. This is the most common form of nephrotic syndrome. The glomerulonephritis (GN) associated with primary nephrotic syndrome is classified as (1) minimal change GN, (2) membranous GN, (3) membranoproliferative GN, and (4) chronic or focal GN. The glomerular lesions have also been classified as (1) minimal change disease, (2) focal sclerosing, and (3) proliferative types.

Primary nephrotic syndrome. *Minimal change nephrotic syndrome* is present in 52% to 78% of all children with nephrotic syndrome.[58] These children all have uncomplicated idiopathic (or primary) nephrotic syndrome and no glomerular changes seen with light microscopy. The term, "minimal change nephrotic syndrome" has repaced other descriptive terms for the same disease, including "lipoid nephrosis" and "idiopathic nephrotic syndrome of childhood."

Approximately 9% to 15% of children who develop nephrotic syndrome have *mesangial proliferation* or *focal glomerulosclerosis*. These children have signs and symptoms identical to children with minimal change nephrotic syndrome; however, they do not respond to the initial course of steroid treatment.

Primary nephrotic syndrome can also occur as the result of recessive gene transmission. These children have clinical signs and symptoms identical to children with minimal change nephrotic syndrome. However, differences in biopsy findings as well as in response to steroid treatment separate these children from those with minimal change nephrotic syndrome. The common element in these diseases is damage to the glomerular basement membrane, which results in increased glomerular permeability to protein.

Secondary nephrotic syndrome. Nephrotic syndrome can also occur as the result of secondary renal involvement associated with systemic diseases. Most commonly, the primary causes include infections, poisons or toxins, sickle cell disease, renal vein thrombosis, Hodgkin's disease, systemic lupus erythematosus, or Henoch-Schönlein purpura.[58]

■ Pathophysiology

While nephrotic syndrome can occur at any age, most children develop their initial onset of the disease between 2 and 7 years. Nephrotic syndrome is seen approximately twice as often in boys as in girls in this age-group.[58]

Since the pathophysiology of minimal change nephrotic syndrome is somewhat different from that of other types of glomerulonephritis, it will be discussed separately below.

Minimal change nephrotic syndrome. The pathogenesis of minimal change nephrotic syndrome is unclear. There is no direct evidence that immunologic mechanisms are involved, although relapses are associated with upper respiratory illnesses. The permeability of the glomerular basement membrane is increased, despite the lack of evidence of structural glomerular changes. This increase in permeability may be related to a change in electrostatic charge of the membrane. As a result, large proteins pass through the glomerular membrane, resulting in severe proteinuria.[58]

Membranoproliferative glomerulonephritis—focal glomerulosclerosis—mesangial proliferation. The patients with membranoproliferative glomerulonephritis develop thickening or proliferative changes in the glomeruli. Children with focal glomerulosclerosis have some partially or totally sclerotic glomeruli. The common element in these diseases is damage of the glomerular basement membrane, which results in increased glomerular permeability and proteinuria.

Common elements. Regardless of the type of the nephrotic syndrome, the proteinuria causes a fall in serum albumin levels, which in turn results in a decrease in intravascular osmotic pressure. This allows movement of fluid from the intravascular to the extravascular spaces, producing edema and decreased intravascular volume. The glomerular filtration rate will fall as a result of the fall in intravascular volume, and aldosterone and antidiuretic hormone release will be stimulated. This produces an increase in sodium and water reabsorption, which can further reduce intravascular osmolality and enhance movement of fluid into the tissues. Generalized edema is likely to develop once the serum albumin concentration falls below 2 gm/dl.

■ Clinical signs and symptoms

Periorbital edema is often the first sign noted by parents of children with nephrotic syndrome. Initially, the eyes are only puffy in the morning, and they appear normal later in the day. Soon, however, the child may develop a dependent edema; if the child is ambulatory, the edema will first become apparent in the ankles and feet. As the edema becomes more generalized, it will be noted in the abdomen (ascites). The development of abdominal distention may accentuate inguinal and umbilical hernias, and labial and scrotal edema may be excessive. Moderate hepatomegaly is often noted. If ascites becomes severe, respiratory distress may develop as the result of decreased diaphragmatic excursion.

Generalized edema may also produce diarrhea, vomiting, and anorexia. These gastrointestinal symptoms and the presence of generalized catabolic state further deplete body protein sources; malnutrition and loss of muscle mass may become quite severe but may not become apparent until the edema resolves. During the edematous phase, fever may be absent even if a severe infection is present.

The patient with active nephrosis is oliguric; the urine has an acid pH, contains large quantities of proteins (so it foams excessively), it may be tinted pink or red from microscopic hematuria, and it may contain granular and cellular casts. Lipoid bodies are also present; significant pyuria is not common among patients with primary nephrotic syndrome.

Severe hypoalbuminemia is generally present among children with nephrotic syndrome, and most have albumin levels less than 2.5 gm/dl. Serum complement levels in patients with nephrotic syndrome associated with some glomerular disease are low (see membranoproliferative glomerulonephritis or systemic lupus erythematosus nephritis), though complement levels in minimal change nephrotic syndrome are normal. Total serum calcium levels may be falsely low; since hypoalbuminemia is present, the fraction of the total calcium bound to protein is reduced, so serum ionized calcium concentration is often normal. The patient with chronic nephrotic syndrome, however, may demonstrate genuine hypocalcemia because of loss of vitamin products in the urine and resultant drop in serum vitamin D levels.[58] In most children with nephrotic syndrome, the remaining serum electrolytes, creatinine, and BUN are normal. However, approximately one fourth of children with minimal change nephrotic syndrome may demonstrate an increase in serum creatinine and blood urea nitrogen. Children who have focal glomerulosclerosis may have glycosuria and bicarbonaturia, with only moderate reduction of creatinine clearance.[58]

A secondary anemia may be present and may be severe when significant glomerular disease is associated with renal failure. Since the patient's skin is edematous, the pallor of anemia may be more pronounced. If the child's intravascular volume is reduced as the result of edema, the child's hematocrit may be falsely elevated as a result of hemoconcentration.

The risk of thromboembolism is high among patients with nephrotic syndrome. These children seem to have a hypercoagulability that may be related to increased platelet aggregation and increased levels of β-thromboglobulin,[58] as well as decreased fibrinolytic activity. As a result, the nurse should monitor for signs of thromboembolic events, and performance of venipunctures or use of long-standing central venous or arterial lines should be avoided.

During nephrotic syndrome relapse, edema can accumulate rapidly in the tissues, depleting the intravascular volume. If this fluid shift from the intravascular space is accompanied by sodium restriction and diuretic therapy, intravascular volume can be severely depleted, resulting in circulatory collapse.

Children with nephrotic syndrome usually demonstrate growth failure. The administration of steroids and immunosuppressive agents can further compromise the child's growth. In addition, the steroids and immunosuppressive agents increase the child's risk of infection. Sepsis, especially gram-positive sepsis, frequently occurs among children with nephrotic syndrome in relapse.

Though a renal biopsy is necessary to firmly establish the degree of glomerular damage associated with nephrotic syndrome, not all children with nephrotic syndrome are subjected to a renal biopsy as part of their initial workup. Since minimal change nephrosis is the most common form of nephrotic syndrome occurring in children, a 4-week course of corticosteroid therapy abolishes symptoms in approximately 93% of children with nephrotic syndrome who are more than 1 year and less than 6 years of age.[42]

If the child with nephrotic syndrome does not respond to the initial steroid therapy, a renal biopsy is often indicated. The biopsy specimen is examined using both electron and light microscopy techniques. Identification of the degree of glomerular involvement will enable better evaluation of therapy and establishment of prognosis.

■ **Medical treatment and nursing intervention**

Treatment of the child with nephrotic syndrome is aimed at restoration or maintenance of adequate circulating blood volume, minimization of glomerular damage and maximization of renal function, maintenance of fluid and electrolyte balance, maximization of patient comfort, and prevention of infection.

If the child with nephrotic syndrome has signs of poor systemic perfusion (e.g., tachycardia, cool, clammy extremities, and decreased intensity of peripheral pulses) as the result of a fluid shift from the intravascular space, a large bore central venous catheter should be inserted. This catheter will enable assessment of central venous pressure and infusion of intravenous fluids. Usually, a bolus administration of 10 to 20 ml/kg of saline, lactated Ringer's solution, albumin, or a mixture of saline and albumin (80 ml of saline plus 20 ml of 25% albumin) will reestablish adequate intravascular volume (see the section on medical treatment and nursing interventions, low cardiac output in Chapter 3). If the child is oliguric, fluid administration should probably be curtailed as soon as intravascular volume is adequate (as evidenced by a central venous pressure [CVP] of ≥5 mm Hg, with good systemic perfusion and a heart rate that is appropriate for age and clinical condition).

Once the child is stable, laboratory studies should be performed, including complete blood count, serum electrolytes, calcium, phosphorus, blood urea nitrogen, creatinine, total protein, albumin, globulin, cholesterol, triglycerides, complement (C_3), and urinalysis. Each time the child voids, the urine should be measured and tested for proteins. The urine specific gravity will be falsely elevated in the presence of proteinuria or osmotic diuretics. The urine osmolality is the best indicator of renal function, since it reflects renal concentrating ability and is not affected by the presence of large molecules in the urine.

Collection of urine samples from the infant or child with nephrotic syndrome may be difficult. Catheterization should be avoided, if possible, because of the risk of infection. Urine collection bags should also be avoided, since the adhesive rim of the collecting bag can be extremely irritating to edematous skin. Small children may be allowed to void on *nonabsorbant* surfaces (such as the *outside* of a disposable diaper) so that some urine can be collected for analysis. Though some urine can be squeezed into a syringe from the absorbant side of a diaper, the fluid obtained in this matter may have a falsely low osmolality, since solutes may be trapped within the absorbant diaper.

The child with nephrotic syndrome requires careful measurement of all sources of fluid intake and output. The child's daily weight should be measured using the same scale, at the same time of day. Frequent (although rough) estimates of the degree of edema present should be made. If ascites is present, the child's abdominal girth should be measured at least once every day.

Usually, children with nephrotic syndrome are asymptomatic except for the discomfort caused by their edema. Bed rest is necessary only during acute infections or when severe incapacitating edema is present. Because bed rest is associated with problems of large vessel venous stasis, possible decubitus, and possible development of contractures, mobility is encouraged as soon as it is feasible.

Salt restriction, albumin infusion, or diuretics may be necessary to reduce edema. All of these methods of reducing edema can also result in intravascular volume depletion, so they should be pursued with caution. In addition, the hemoconcentration produced by edema and vigorous diuresis can aggravate the hypercoagulability, resulting in thromboembolic events. If a diuretic is prescribed, the nurse should carefully assess the child's systemic perfusion before administering the drug and then during and after diuresis. Loop diuretics seem to be the most effective in promoting diuresis in nephrotic patients (see Table

7-2 in this chapter for diuretic dosages). Furosemide (1 to 2 mg/kg/IV dose) may be prescribed; this dosage can be increased each time the drug is given until a maximum of 4 to 5 mg/kg/12 hours is reached. If an additional diuretic such as spironolactone (an aldosterone antagonist) is added (at a dose of 1.5 to 3.3 mg/kg/day), potassium loss in the urine is reduced.

For maximal diuretic effect, the infusion of salt-poor albumin may be ordered, to be followed within 30 minutes by intravenous administration of furosemide (1 to 2 mg/kg). The administration of 0.5 to 1.0 gm/kg of human albumin over 60 minutes ensures that the child's circulating blood volume is adequate.[50] However, the nurse should also monitor for signs of hypervolemia, including tachycardia, hypertension, or congestive heart failure. The increase in intravascular volume is usually only transient, while the albumin remains in the vascular space. Since the treatment of choice for the child with nephrotic syndrome is use of steroids, diuretics are infrequently required beyond the first 7 to 14 days of therapy.

If the child with nephrotic syndrome is over the age of 1 year but is younger than 7 years, with a normal complement (C_3) concentration and minimal hematuria, minimal change nephrotic syndrome is the most likely diagnosis, and steroid therapy is the treatment of choice.[58] Prednisone is given in a dose of 2 mg/kg/24 hours (to a maximum of 80 mg) in divided doses.[58] Proteinuria should disappear within the first weeks of therapy in most children with minimal change nephrotic syndrome. Once the child does respond to the prednisone, it can be tapered over a period of several months, while the child or parents continue to test the child's urine for the presence of proteinuria.

If the child continues to demonstrate proteinuria after 28 days of continuous prednisone therapy, a renal biopsy is usually planned to determine the etiology of the nephrotic syndrome. The child who does not respond to prednisone may still have minimal change nephrotic syndrome or may have mesangial proliferation or focal glomerulosclerosis.

If the child does not respond to prednisone, or if the child relapses unless prednisone therapy is continued, use of alkylating agents, such as cyclophosphamide or chlorambucil, may be indicated. These drugs can produce alopecia, leukopenia, and increased susceptibility to infection, so the child and the parents require careful evaluation and preparation before such drugs are prescribed.

The child with nephrotic syndrome will be extremely uncomfortable if severe edema is present. Measures should be taken to avoid friction between adjacent skin surfaces (such as between the inner leg and the scrotum or between the chest and under-arm areas). Rolls of cotton can be placed in these areas, or nonperfumed talc or cornstarch can be placed over friction points. Since the skin is very fragile, most types of hospital tape should be avoided. When the child is in bed, frequent turning will be necessary to avoid pressure sores over bony prominences.

Children with nephrotic syndrome often have poor resistance to infection as a result of the compromised circulation, steroid and/or immunosuppressive therapy, poor nutrition, and appetite loss. The nurse and dietician should make every effort to provide the child with small, frequent, nutritious meals that are appetizing. The development of large abdominal effusions may increase the risk of peritonitis, causing unexplained fever and ascites. Administration of prophylactic antibiotics is not usually indicated, since it may only foster the growth of resistant organisms.

The prognosis for children with minimal change nephrotic syndrome is best if the child has only signs of proteinuria and if the child responds immediately to prednisone therapy. If the child has nonresponsive or steroid-dependent nephrotic syndrome, recovery is less complete, and the child may develop frequent relapses. If the child is unresponsive to both steroids and alkylating agents, the prognosis is poor, since many of these patients develop progressive renal failure.[58] Those patients who have severe glomerular sclerosis that is resistant to treatment often have a fulminant and fatal course.[26]

Since the child's illness is often sudden and the prognosis is usually uncertain for several weeks, it is imperative that the child and family receive adequate support and consistent information from all members of the health care team.

■ **ACUTE GLOMERULONEPHRITIS**
■ **Etiology**

Glomerulonephritis is a form of injury to the glomerulus that results in hematuria, mild proteinuria, edema, hypertension, and oliguria. The injury to the glomerulus seems to be related to the formation of antigen-antibody complexes, and their deposition within the glomeruli. Nephritogenic forms of streptococcus have been linked with the most common form of glomerulonephritis in children, though other bacterial, viral, parasitic, pharmacologic, and toxic agents have been linked to the development of glomerulonephritis.[43,44]

■ **Pathophysiology**

Though the pathophysiology of glomerulonephritis is not certain, it does seem that antigen-antibody complexes become fixed to the glomerular basement membrane. The glomerular membrane endothelial cells proliferate, and the area is invaded by white blood cells. This can cause temporary or permanent changes in the glomerular membrane structure or permeability.[7,37,44]

■ Clinical signs and symptoms

The onset of glomerulonephritis is usually abrupt. If it is related to a nephritogenic streptococcal infection, the onset of symptoms is usually 8 to 14 days after group A beta-hemolytic streptococcal pharyngitis and 14 to 21 days following streptococcal pyoderma (impetigo).

The child usually has hematuria, which can be macroscopic (causing rusty-colored urine) or microscopic. The child usually develops edema; periorbital edema may be noted initially, although generalized edema is often present. Proteinuria is often present, although usually not to the degree (2 gm/m²/day) seen in children with nephrotic syndrome. Hypertension may be present and severe, and signs of hypertensive encephalopathy can develop. The child is usually oliguric but rarely anuric. The glomerular filtration rate is decreased, and sodium and water retention are increased. Signs of circulatory congestion may develop as the result of sodium and water retention; these include tachycardia, hepatomegaly, rising central venous pressure, tachypnea, increased respiratory effort, and radiologic evidence of pulmonary congestion.

A urinalysis reveals hematuria in nearly all affected patients and proteinuria in most patients. The renal concentrating ability may be unaffected, although the fractional excretion of sodium is often reduced (see the section on acute renal failure earlier in this chapter for further information about fractional excretion of sodium).

The child's creatinine is often normal, but the BUN is usually elevated. The child may demonstrate dilutional hyponatremia, and the serum albumin concentration may be low. Serum hyperkalemia may also develop.

The child with poststreptococcal glomerulonephritis usually will have antibodies to streptococcal products (such as antistreptolysin-O) that will confirm the presence of a precedent streptococcal infection. Children with acute glomerulonephritis also will have depression of hemolytic complement activity and C_3 levels.[44]

Anemia may also be present as the result of hemodilution.

Renal biopsy is rarely indicated to confirm the diagnosis of glomerulonephritis.

■ Medical treatment and nursing intervention

Most children with acute glomerulonephritis will recover completely if complications of their renal disease can be prevented.[57] If the child develops acute renal failure, fluid restriction will be required, and treatment of electrolyte and acid-base imbalances will be necessary (see the section on acute renal failure earlier in this chapter).

If the child develops hypertension, the nurse should notify the physician and perform frequent neurologic examinations to detect any deterioration in the child's level of consciousness. The child with significant hypertension may develop headaches and signs of encephalopathy, including nausea, vomiting, irritability, lethargy, seizures, coma, and increased intracranial pressure (see the section on increased intracranial pressure in Chapter 6). If hypertension is thought to be producing encephalopathy, treatment with diazoxide (5 mg/kg intravenous push, or drip over 30 minutes) and furosemide (1 to 2 mg/kg intravenously) is the treatment of choice.[44] In the absence of encephalopathy, hydralazine (0.15 to 0.30 mg/kg intravenously or intramuscularly every 4 to 6 hours) may be given with the furosemide. Alternative antihypertensive medications include oral prazosin (25 µg/kg/dose every 6 hours), propranolol (0.5 to 1.0 mg/kg/day in 4 divided doses), or reserpine (0.04 to 0.07 mg/kg intramuscularly, maximum dose: 1 mg).

If the child develops hyperkalemia, administration of calcium, glucose, glucose and insulin, or sodium polystyrene sulfonate (Kayexalate) enema may be required (see the sections on hyperkalemia and acute renal failure earlier in this chapter).

If signs of congestive heart failure are present, the child will require treatment with fluid restriction and diuretics. Intravenous vasodilators such as nitroglycerin (0.1 to 10 µg/kg/minute) or sodium nitroprusside (0.5 to 8.0 µg/kg/minute) may also be prescribed if evidence of low cardiac output is present (see the section on treatment of low cardiac output in Chapter 3).

Since antibiotic administration does not influence the recovery of children with glomerulonephritis, antibiotic administration is only indicated if the child has positive bacterial cultures.[44]

■ SYSTEMIC LUPUS ERYTHEMATOSUS (SLE): RENAL INVOLVEMENT

The glomerular lesions in patients with SLE result from the deposition of complexes of anti-DNA antibodies and DNA. The biopsy material of a patient with SLE has some features that are typical to SLE, but it also has the characteristic "humps" of granular densities at irregular intervals and large polymorphonuclear infiltrates that are present in antigen-antibody glomerulonephritis. There are three types of renal involvement of SLE: focal lupus nephritis, diffuse lupus nephritis, and membranous lupus nephritis.

Focal lupus nephritis is rarely manifested by nephrotic syndrome, since most glomeruli appear histologically normal or minimally abnormal. This form of lupus nephritis almost always resolves completely with adrenal corticosteroid therapy.

Diffuse lupus nephritis is characterized by severe proteinuria, hypertension, and renal insufficiency. Remissions may occur, but are incomplete with frequent relapses. The prognosis for this form of lupus nephritis is poor, and death usually occurs within 3 to 5 years.

In *membranous lupus nephritis*, the renal biopsy is characterized by widespread glomerular involvement with many cellular changes. Membranous lupus nephritis is manifested by diffuse and fairly uniform thickening of glomerular capillary walls. The patient has proteinuria and, less commonly, hematuria, renal insufficiency, and hypertension. Remission with treatment is observed in some cases, but proteinuria usually persists. Progression to uremia or death is uncommon.

■ ANAPHYLACTOID (HENOCH-SCHÖNLEIN PURPURA) NEPHRITIS

Anaphylactoid purpura is a disease of childhood with the greatest incidence between 2 to 8 years of age. It is a disease of unknown etiology manifested by nonthrombocytopenic purpura on the lower extremities and buttocks, pain, joint swelling, and signs of glomerular disease. It effects boys more commonly than girls, and recurrent episodes are not uncommon. Serum complement levels are normal and microscopic hematuria may be present. Attempts to relate this disease to previous bacterial or viral infections or food allergies have been unsuccessful. The renal biopsy shows antibody-antigen complexes with fibrin. Patients with the worst prognosis include those who have nephrotic syndrome or an acute nephrotic syndrome associated with oliguria and hypertension, those who are over 7 years of age, or those who developed nephritis after 4 weeks of illness. These patients tend to develop renal failure and have the highest mortality (see the section on acute renal failure earlier in this chapter).

■ HEMOLYTIC-UREMIC SYNDROME (HUS)
■ Etiology

Hemolytic-uremic syndrome is the association of an acute hemolytic anemia, thrombocytopenia, and acute renal failure. This syndrome is one of the most common causes of acute renal failure in children.[40] It affects both sexes equally and 90% of the cases occur in children less than 4 years of age. HUS occurs more frequently during the summer and fall in the northern hemisphere.[38] It often follows a mild gastrointestinal illness or, in older children, an upper respiratory illness. Though coxsackieviruses have been isolated from HUS patients, the specific infectious etiologic agent is unknown.[40]

■ Pathophysiology

The primary sites of injury with hemolytic-uremic syndrome are presumed to be the endothelial lining of the small arteries and arterioles, particularly in the kidney. This microangiopathic process results in the intravascular deposition of platelets and fibrin, resulting in partial or complete occlusion of small arterioles and capillaries in the kidney. As erythrocytes and platelets traverse these partially occluded vessels, they are thought to be fragmented by the narrowed vessels and the fibrin strands.[28,40] The damaged erythrocytes are removed from the circulation by the spleen, and the life span of the erythrocytes is reduced; this results in a severe and often rapidly progressing anemia. Although this theory of erythrocyte damage is probably accurate, recent evidence suggests that the red blood cells of patients with HUS may be more susceptible to injury than the erythrocytes of normal patients, so this may contribute to the magnitude of the hemolytic anemia.[28]

Most patients with HUS also demonstrate thrombocytopenia for 1 to 2 weeks. It is not clear if this thrombocytopenia results from destruction of the platelets, consumption of the platelets, or aggregation of the platelets within the kidney. It is clear that platelet survival time is drastically reduced (from a normal survival of 7 to 10 days to approximately 1.5 to 5 days), that platelet antigen has been found in the kidneys of affected patients, that HUS patients often demonstrate a thrombocytopathia, and that there is evidence of peripheral platelet destruction.[28]

As noted above, patients with HUS develop damage to the glomerular endothelial cells. The cells tend to swell and detach from the glomerular basement membrane, and the space between the cells and the membrane becomes filled with lipid, fibrin strands, platelets, and cell fragments. The glomerular capillary lumen itself is often occluded by fibrin, thrombi, and platelets.[28] As a result, renal blood flow and glomerular filtration rate can be reduced to a degree proportional to the glomerular injury. Renal ischemia may produce cortical necrosis, and renal tubular injury may also be seen. While much of this damage is reversible, recurrences can occur, or progressive renal failure can develop.[28]

Children with HUS may also demonstrate gastrointestinal or central nervous system involvement. Young children often have a mild gastroenteritis, which may progress to bloody diarrhea. The severity of the neurologic symptoms do not seem to be related to the severity of the HUS. The patient may develop irritability, seizures, abnormal posturing, hemiparesis, or hypertensive encephalopathy.[28,40]

■ **Clinical signs and symptoms**

The appearance of HUS closely follows or is coincident with an episode of mild gastroenteritis which may include bloody stools. HUS may also follow upper respiratory infections, urinary tract infections, measles, or varicella.[28] Within 1 to 2 days, the child demonstrates a notable pallor, often purpura, rectal bleeding, or other signs of hemorrhage (including bleeding, petechiae, or ecchymoses). The child's peripheral blood smear shows fragmented red blood cells (a microangiopathic hemolytic anemia), fibrin split products, and a decreased platelet count (thrombocytopenia).[43] Within a few days of the onset of anemia, the reticulocyte count will be high. The serum bilirubin level is usually not elevated, though hepatosplenomegaly is often present.

The child may be oliguric or anuric. As a result, serum levels of creatinine, blood urea nitrogen, phosphorus, and potassium are elevated. Hyperkalemia is more likely to develop rapidly if gastrointestinal bleeding (with gastrointestinal reabsorption of blood products) is present. Congestive heart failure, pulmonary edema, and hypertension may all develop as a result of decreased renal function, hypervolemia, and increased plasma renin activity.

Examination of the child's urine reveals the presence of fibrin, proteinuria, micro- or macroscopic hematuria, and urinary cell casts.

There are no irregularities in immunoglobulins and complement studies are normal.[38] There are no antibodies, no abnormal hemoglobin, and no abnormal erythrocyte enzymes, and the Coombs' test is negative. Evidence of consumptive coagulopathy (decreased levels of fibrinogen, factor V and factor VIII) is not found.[43] Attempts to detect circulating or fixed bacterial endotoxin or virus particles have also been unsuccessful. HUS seems to be related to a localized renal intravascular coagulation.[28]

The majority of children under the age of 2 years have less severe hemolytic anemia and renal involvement and a tendency for the disease to run a short course. Recent mortality has declined to approximately 4% to 10%.[28] A small number of patients recover renal function slowly, while some will continue with renal failure and will require chronic renal failure management and dialysis until transplantation is available. Recurrence of HUS has been reported following renal transplantation.[28]

■ **Medical treatment and nursing interventions**

The management of the child with hemolytic uremic syndrome requires attention to fluid and electrolyte balance, administration of red blood cells as needed, management of hypertension, and minimization of neurologic complications.

If the child becomes anuric or develops oliguric renal failure, fluid and electrolyte therapy must be adjusted accordingly (see the section on acute renal failure earlier in this chapter). Peritoneal or hemodialysis may be necessary if hypervolemia, hypertensive encephalopathy, severe bleeding, hyperkalemia, metabolic acidosis (unresponsive to therapy), severe uremia, hypernatremia, or hypercalcemia develop (see the section on dialysis earlier in this chapter).

The child's anemia should be treated through careful administration of packed red blood cells whenever the child becomes symptomatic or the hematocrit falls below 20%.[40] Frequent transfusions may be required since the life span of even transfused erythrocytes is shortened in the presence of HUS.[28] Only small amounts (3 to 5 ml/kg) of blood should be administered at any one time if the child has hypervolemia, hypertension, or hyperkalemia as the result of renal failure. Often, transfusions will be planned immediately after several exchanges of peritoneal dialysis have been performed or following hemodialysis. Fresh packed red blood cells are desirable to reduce the transfusion potassium content, and leukocyte-poor packed red blood cells are indicated if irreversible renal failure (and ultimate renal transplantation) is anticipated.[40]

Platelet transfusions are often avoided unless severe thrombocytopenia (platelet count less than 10,000/mm^3) develops, since administered platelets may contribute to the thrombotic glomerular events.

Hypertension should be managed with dialysis or with pharmacologic agents, including nitroglycerin (0.5 to 10 μg/kg/minute continuous infusion), sodium nitroprusside (0.5 to 8 μg/kg/minute continuous infusion), or diazoxide (5 mg/kg intravenous push, or drip over 30 minutes). These drugs may be given in conjunction with furosemide (1 to 2 mg/kg intravenously). If encephalopathy is not present, the hypertension can be controlled with hydralazine (0.15 to 0.30 mg/kg intravenously every 4 to 6 hours), prazosin (25 μg/kg/dose every 6 hours), propranolol (0.5 to 1.0 mg/kg/day in 4 divided doses), or reserpine (0.04 to 0.07 mg/kg intramuscular dose, to a maximum dose of 1 mg).[44] It is important that *dosages of these and any other drugs that the child is receiving be evaluated in the presence of oliguria and decreased renal function.*

The nurse should perform a careful neurologic assessment at least every hour. Signs of irritability, lethargy, seizures, posturing, or hemiparesis should be reported to a physician. If the child develops signs of neurologic deterioration, refer to the section on increased intracranial pressure in Chapter 6.

If the child continues to have bloody diarrhea or abdominal distension with decreased intestinal motility, the child should receive nothing by mouth, and plans should be made to provide the child's caloric requirements through parenteral alimentation (see Chapter 8). These calories should be provided utilizing more glucose and less protein than would be used in patients without renal failure, and they must be provided within the fluid restrictions necessary to prevent hypervolemia.

The parents of the child with hemolytic uremic syndrome will require a great deal of support. They will require reassurance that there was no way to anticipate that the child's prodromal illness was unusual. It is imperative that all members of the health care team utilize consistent terminology and provide a consistent prognosis, so that confusion is minimized.

■ DIABETES INSIPIDUS (DI)
■ Etiology

Diabetes insipidus ultimately results in the inability of the kidney to concentrate urine; as a result, large amounts of water are lost in the urine. Diabetes insipidus can result from decreased hypothalamic production of vasopressin (antidiuretic hormone, or ADH) or from decreased renal response to vasopressin.

A deficit in hypothalamic secretion of vasopressin, termed *central (or neurogenic) diabetes insipidus*, may often be seen in pediatric patients following neurosurgical procedures, severe head trauma, infections of the central nervous system, intraventricular hemorrhage (IVH), or hypoxic encephalopathy. In central DI, the circulating vasopressin levels are low or absent. When exogenous vasopressin is administered, the appropriate renal response of increased water reabsorption is elicited.

Nephrogenic diabetes insipidus (NDI) involves a defect in the kidneys' ability to respond to antidiuretic hormone. In its purest and most severe form, it occurs as a hereditary disorder transmitted to male infants as a sex-linked recessive trait (female children are heterozygous, hence they carry the gene but are without disease). Nephrogenic diabetes insipidus does not respond to vasopressin administration.

■ Pathophysiology

The kidney regulates serum osmolality through adjustment in the water permeability of the collecting duct and distal tubule. When the serum becomes too concentrated, centrally-located osmoreceptors cause the hypothalamus to synthesize vasopressin; this increases renal water reabsorption, results in a fall in serum osmolality, and eliminates the stimulus to the hypothalamus (see Fig. 7-9). If vasopressin is absent, or if the kidney is structurally unable to respond to vasopressin, volumes of water that should be reabsorbed are lost into the urine. This increased urinary water loss concentrates the serum electrolytes, producing a profound hypernatremia. The increasing osmolality of the plasma draws interstitial and intracellular water into the vascular compartment, where it will be filtered by the glomerulus and then lost into the urine. Volume-sensitive receptors respond to the decrease in circulating volume; this results in an increase in aldosterone secretion and an increase in sodium and water reabsorption by the proximal tubule. This further increases the serum sodium concentration, producing serum sodium levels greater than 160 to 200 mEq/L. If this cycle is uninterrupted, shock will lead to the patient's demise.

The otherwise healthy child older than 2 to 3 years with DI can adapt to the polyuria by consuming large quantities of fluid, often selectively water, and by the development of a large bladder. Interference with the child's ability to consume water will quickly lead to hyperosmolality, hypernatremia, and circulatory compromise. Situations as minor as a mild upper respiratory infection may alter drinking habits and require hospitalization for intravenous fluid replacement.

■ Clinical signs and symptoms

The cardinal signs of diabetes insipidus in the ambulatory pediatric patient include polydipsia and polyuria. If the critically ill child is sedated or comatose, the chief indication of diabetes insipidus is polyuria, with a high serum osmolality. The child's urine output may be as high as 200 to 300 ml urine/m²/hour. The presence of a low urine sodium and low urine osmolality will help differentiate DI from nonoliguric acute tubular necrosis (ATN); both urine sodium and osmolality are high when ATN is present.

If the excessive urine fluid losses are not replaced, hypovolemic shock can quickly develop. As the child's intravascular volume is depleted, the central venous pressure will fall, mucous membranes will be dry, and the patient may act irritable. In the infant, the anterior fontanelle may become depressed. The child will be tachycardic, and extremities will be cool. As hypovolemia becomes worse, poor capillary refill, decreased intensity of peripheral pulses, hypotension, and metabolic acidosis will develop.

Children with nephrogenic DI usually exhibit polyuria and polydipsia from birth. The polyuria becomes especially noticeable when breast milk feedings are discontinued and commercial newborn formula, with a higher osmotic load, is substituted. Hypernatremia with dehydration, fever, vomiting, and failure to thrive are often initially attributed to infectious gastroenteritis. Only when urinalysis with urine specific gravity and osmolality are obtained is the diagnosis of DI clear. The urine specific gravity is consistently below 1.010, and the urine osmolality is always below 280 mOsm/ml. A family history of male babies with failure to thrive, seizures, and mental retardation should provide further support for the diagnosis of nephrogenic diabetes insipidus.

■ **Medical treatment and nursing interventions**

Acute management of the critically ill child with diabetes insipidus requires the replacement of urinary water losses with intravenous fluids of equal volume and electrolyte content. In addition, vasopressin (Pitressin) is administered to those patients with vasopressin-sensitive diabetes insipidus.

When the child develops diabetes insipidus, insertion of two large-bore venous catheters is advisable. One catheter should be a central venous catheter, to be used for CVP measurements, administration of medications, and replacement of normal insensible fluid loss. The second venous line is utilized for replacement of the volume of urinary fluid losses. For this replacement, low concentrations of sodium (1/16 to 1/8 normal saline) and glucose (2½% glucose) are usually utilized. If hypovolemic shock is present, the child should receive a bolus of 10 ml/kg of 2½% glucose and 0.45 normal saline over 15 to 30 minutes. This bolus may be repeated until the child's CVP reaches 3 to 5 mm Hg and systemic perfusion improves.

The child's urine losses should be totaled at least hourly; if urine output is large, half-hourly totals may be required. The volume of urine loss is then replaced over the next hour (or half hour if half hour totaling is performed) through the replacement intravenous line. Throughout replacement therapy, the nurse should assess the child carefully for signs of hypovolemia; these signs should be reported to a physician as soon as they occur (see the preceding section on clinical signs and symptoms). To monitor the effectiveness of volume replacement, simultaneous urine and serum sodium, potassium, chloride, and osmolalities should be measured as often as every hour.[54] The urine specific gravity should also be recorded at least every hour.

If the child has vasopressin-sensitive (central) DI, administration of vasopressin is indicated. This vasopressin can be given as an intramuscular injection of vasopressin tannate (Pitressin Tannate) in oil, or as intravenous or subcutaneous infusion of aqueous vasopressin. If the vasopressin is administered intramuscularly (0.2 ml/dose IM every 1 to 3 days) or subcutaneously (1 to 3 ml/day divided in 3 doses), the absorption may be slow and inconsistent, and the injection site may remain painful for several days. Therefore intravenous administration of aqueous vasopressin is often preferred. The vasopressin may be administered in a single dose (1 to 3 ml/day of the 20 unit/ml aqueous solution, divided into 3 doses) *slowly*, or a continuous drip infusion totalling 15 mU/hour. To prepare this infusion, a dilution of 2 mU/ml is *carefully* prepared from the original ampule containing 20 units/ml.[54] Once the infusion is started, the child's urine volume and specific gravity should be measured every 15 minutes, and urine and serum sodium, potassium, chloride, and osmolality should be measured every hour.

A positive response to any vasopressin administration will be a decrease in urine volume (to less than or equal to 1 ml/kg/hour) and a rise in urine specific gravity (to greater than 1.010) and osmolality (to 280 to 300 mOsm/ml). If there is no response to an intramuscular, subcutaneous, or intravenous vasopressin dose, the dose may be repeated on the order of a physician. If there is no response to a continuous infusion of 15 mU/hour, the dose can be doubled to total 30 mU/hour or up to 60 mU/hour as needed. *Throughout any administration of vasopressin, the nurse should observe the patient closely for evidence of tachycardia, bradycardia, hypertension, hypotension, or other signs of hypersensitivity.* Abdominal cramping may also follow vasopressin administration.

A synthetic analogue of vasopressin, 1-deamino-8-d-arginine-vasopressin (DDAVP) has been developed, which can be administered via a nasal spray. This form of vasopressin has fewer systemic effects than other forms of vasopressin and has reduced the need for subcutaneous, intravenous, or intramuscular vasopressin administration. The initial dose of DDAVP in a child with DI is usually between 1 to 5 mg. The dose must be administered into the posterior nasal area rather than to the nasal pharynx. The most effective dose of DDAVP is only roughly dependent on the weight or age of the patient; each patient will set his own pattern for duration of response, varying from 8 to 20 hours.[12] A positive response to DDAVP administration is a decrease in urine volume and an increase in urine osmolality (as noted above).

If the patient is vasopressin-responsive after any form of vasopressin therapy, the urine volume will rapidly decline and the rate of the replacement intravenous fluids will require adjustment to prevent water intoxication.

Treatment of *vasopressin-resistant diabetes insipidus* also requires provision of adequate replacement for urinary water losses at all times. A low sodium and low protein diet is combined with the use of a thiazide diuretic to treat vasopressin-resistant DI. The diuretic most frequently used is hydrochlorothiazide, in doses of 1 to 2 mg/kg/day.[75] The thiazide *antidiuretic* effect results in part from its effect in reducing body sodium levels, thereby reducing GFR. Proximal tubule sodium reabsorption then results in an increase in water reabsorption. Thiazide diuretics can reduce the water requirement of the child with DI by 30% to 50%. However, these drugs can cause potassium depletion, so potassium supplements may be required. Other side effects of thiazide diuretics include hyperuricemia and hypercalcemia.[24]

It is difficult to supply enough calories for growth when the child has polydipsia. A diet low in sodium and potassium and low in protein is important to reduce renal solute load. Starch, butter, oil, and vitamins are important food sources, while fruits and vegetables rich in mineral salts are avoided. Growth for the child with nephrogenic DI is often less than normal, and if the diagnosis has not been made until after multiple episodes of dehydration and hypernatremia, developmental and growth retardation may be permanent.

The parents of a child with nephrogenic diabetes insipidus often have tremendous feelings of guilt associated with the inherited nature of the disease. They may be angry at the physicians and nurses if identification of the DI was not made after repeated hospitalizations. Whether the parents are passive or overtly angry, they will require consistent information and compassionate support.

■ DIABETES MELLITUS/DIABETIC KETOACIDOSIS
■ Etiology

Diabetes mellitus is a disease of impaired glucose utilization caused by a relative lack of insulin. Since most patients with diabetes mellitus do not require intensive care, the following discussion will confine itself to the development and potential complications of ketoacidosis.

■ Pathophysiology

Because of a lack of insulin, glucose is unable to enter the cells to provide substrate for cellular metabolism. Metabolic processes utilize lipids as a source of energy. These lipids, however, are only partially oxidized into free fatty acids and acetoacetic acid. Free fatty acids accumulate at a rate faster than the kidneys can excrete them. The acetoacetic acid is converted into ketones. Metabolism of the fats and the accumulation of their by-products result in the development of a metabolic acidosis. As a compensatory mechanism for the metabolic acidosis and ketosis, the patient usually demonstrates deep, rapid respirations (*Kussmaul* respirations), which result in an increase in carbon dioxide exhalation and a fall in intravascular bicarbonate ion concentration and arterial carbon dioxide tension.

The patient with diabetic ketoacidosis is usually hyperglycemic because intravascular glucose is not utilized, and because gluconeogenesis and glycogen breakdown are stimulated by the relative lack of intracellular glucose. The hyperglycemia produces an increase in intravascular osmolality and may draw fluid from cells into the vascular space. Once the serum glucose concentration exceeds the renal threshold for glucose (approximately 180 mg/dl), glycosuria develops; this produces an osmotic diuresis that can further increase the serum osmolality. Urinary excretion of ketoacids enhances urine sodium and potassium losses, though the patient's serum potassium concentration may initially be normal because of the intravascular shift of potassium ions with acidosis.

With severe hyperglycemia and acidosis, the patient will become lethargic and then unresponsive, and coma can develop. Rarely, but tragically, some patients can develop fatal cerebral edema.[73]

■ Clinical signs and symptoms

The classic signs of diabetes mellitus include polyuria, polydipsia, and polyphagia. The polyuria results from the osmotic diuresis from the hyperglycemia and glycosuria. The polydipsia occurs because the patient is attempting to compensate for urinary fluid losses, and the polyphagia results from a relative lack of adequate intracellular glucose energy stores. The diabetic patient often demonstrates weight loss.

When the patient develops ketoacidosis, a metabolic acidosis is present, with a respiratory compensation. As a result, the serum bicarbonate will be low. The patient's serum sodium and chloride concentrations are often low, and total body potassium is usually reduced, though the serum potassium concentration may initially be normal (until the acidosis is corrected). Serum glucose and acetoacetate levels will be elevated.

The child may complain of abdominal pain and may vomit. Gastroenteritis and resultant vomiting or the development of an infection can be complicating factors that have triggered the ketoacidosis.

Patients with ketoacidosis may develop lethargy and decreased response to stimuli as they become progressively hyperglycemic and acidotic. This low level of responsiveness should improve, however, as the patient is treated.

Thus far, no markers have been found that identify those children at risk for the development of cerebral edema. There is no apparent correlation between level of hyperglycemia, degree of acidosis, rate of blood glucose correction, or speed of rehydration with the development of cerebral edema.[73] Signs of cerebral edema in the diabetic patient with ketoacidosis include a sudden change in responsiveness, incontinence, sudden change in respiratory rate or pattern, and finally, respiratory or cardiorespiratory arrest (see the section on clinical signs and symptoms of increased intracranial pressure in Chapter 6).

With the development of severe ketoacidosis and hyperglycemia, severe dehydration can result in prerenal azotemia.[20] These patients may demonstrate oliguric or nonoliguric renal failure (see the section on acute renal failure earlier in this chapter).

■ Medical treatment and nursing interventions

The goals of treatment of the child with diabetic ketoacidosis include rehydration, administration of insulin, restoration and maintenance of serum electrolyte and acid-base balance, and prevention or early detection of complications such as cerebral edema or prerenal failure.

When the child is admitted with ketoacidosis, initial laboratory studies should include a complete blood count (with white blood cell differential), serum glucose and acetone (or acetoacetone or ketone bodies), arterial blood gases (or at least a pH), serum elec-

trolytes and BUN, serum osmolality, and urine sample for testing of glucose, acetones, and osmolality.

The child with ketoacidosis usually receives 0.9% sodium chloride or lactated Ringer's solution to restore intravascular volume and sodium concentration and to reduce intravascular osmolality. If the child demonstrates signs of poor systemic perfusion, the physician may order that a fluid bolus of 10 to 20 ml/kg of isotonic fluid be administered. Administration of additional 5% albumin or other plasma expanders may also be needed if shock is present. Such boluses should be administered carefully, however, because of the risk of cerebral edema.

The rate of fluid administration is usually calculated to provide the child with 1½ to 2 times maintenance fluid requirements during the first 24 hours of therapy, because the fluid deficit is usually calculated at 10% to 15% of body weight. Half of the deficit is replaced in the first 12 hours and half in the second 12 hours of therapy. This fluid administration plan should be evaluated constantly, however, in light of the patient's clinical status. If evidence of hypervolemia, increased intracranial pressure, or oliguria develops, a physician should be notified immediately and fluid administration should probably be curtailed (see Chapter 6 on increased intracranial pressure and p. 487 for acute renal failure).

Usually, intravenous solutions are free of glucose until the child's serum glucose concentration falls below 300 mg/dl[20,78]; then 5% glucose with half-normal or normal saline is utilized. Potassium chloride is usually not added to the intravenous solutions until the child has demonstrated adequate urine output. Then 40 mEq/L (or more, per hospital protocol) or the equivalent of 2 to 4 mEq/kg/24 hours of potassium chloride (to a maximum of 40 to 60 mEq/L) can be added to the intravenous fluids.[20,78,83] Occasionally some potassium phosphate is utilized for the daily supplement. The potassium replacement should constantly be reevaluated in light of the child's urine output, serum potassium concentration, and acid-base status. If the serum potassium concentration remains 3.5 to 4.5 mEq/L after the child's acidosis is corrected, the potassium supplement may be reduced.

If the child's serum pH is less than 7.15, sodium bicarbonate may be administered in doses of 1 to 2 mEq/kg. The sodium bicarbonate dose may also be calculated from the base deficit (see the section on metabolic acidosis, under acute renal failure earlier in this chapter); generally, only 25% to 50% of the calculated dose is administered slowly over several hours, since the ketoacidosis should also be corrected with administration of fluids and insulin.

#71800
Rev. 5/77

ADM TIME. _____

ADM. DATE _____

ADM. WGHT _____

DIABETIC SUMMARY
KETOACIDOSIS AND/OR 6° MANAGEMENT

NAME _____

ROOM _____

HOSP. # _____

PLASMA GLUCOSE mg/dl															
1, 000															
900															
800															
700															
600															
500															
400															
300															
200															
100															

INSULIN DOSE

INF. RATE															
IV BOLUS															
SC/IM															

TIME															
CLOCK TIME															

URINE

GLUCOSE															
KETONES															
VOLUME															

PLASMA

GLUCOSE															
Na															
K															
CO_2															
pH															

FLUID TYPE															
FLUID VOLUME															
DIET-G'S															

Fig. 7-15 Sample flow sheet for use in care of patient in diabetic ketoacidosis. Top portion of sheet is utilized to graphically depict patient's plasma glucose concentration. Remainder of sheet is used to record administration of fluid and medications, fluid output, and concentrations of urine and plasma electrolytes and ketones.

From The Children's Memorial Hospital, Chicago, 1983.

Children with diabetic ketoacidosis require administration of insulin; this may be given subcutaneously or intravenously. An initial combination of regular insulin can be given: 0.5 to 2 units/kg, divided equally, so that half of the dose is administered intravenously and half of the dose is administered subcutaneously.

Since absorption of subcutaneous insulin may be slow and unpredictable in the presence of acidosis and dehydration, some physicians prefer to correct ketoacidosis through the continuous infusion of low-dose insulin.[20,47,83] To begin the infusion, the child receives 0.1 unit of regular insulin/kg by intravenous push. Then a continuous infusion of 0.1 unit/kg/hour is administered intravenously, controlled by a reliable intravenous infusion pump. The solution of insulin and saline can be mixed in three ways.[20,47,78,83]

1. 5 units regular insulin/kg body weight in 250 ml of normal saline; if solution is run at 5 ml/hour, 0.1 unit/kg/hour will be administered.
2. 50 units of regular insulin can be added to a 250 ml bottle of normal saline; if the solution is run at 0.5 times the child's body weight (as ml/hour), 0.1 unit/kg/hour will be administered.
3. Either of the above solutions may be mixed with 3 ml of 25% albumin to prevent adherence of insulin to the glass bottle and/or plastic bag and tubing. However, the amount of insulin adsorbed may not be sufficient to warrant the addition of the albumin, so many units dispense with it.

Once the child's serum glucose level falls below 250 mg/dl, subcutaneous insulin is given (0.25 to 0.5 unit/kg). The intravenous insulin infusion is then discontinued when the serum pH reaches 7.35.[83] From that point, the serum glucose concentration

---

MANAGEMENT OF THE CHILD WITH DIABETIC KETOACIDOSIS

1. Emergency room
   If the diagnosis of diabetic ketoacidosis is established in the emergency room, serum glucose and electrolytes are drawn, an IV of normal saline is started, and the first dose of regular insulin is given. This dosage is determined jointly by the emergency room resident and the house staff taking responsibility for the patient on the floor. If the patient is in shock, 5% albumin or plasma expander may be needed.

2. First hour after admission
   Ideally a special nurse experienced in care of the patient with diabetic ketoacidosis should be assigned to the patient for the first few hours, as diabetic ketoacidosis is a grave medical emergency.

   I. Assessment
      A. Clinical
         1. Level of consciousness
         2. Degree of dehydration
         3. Vital signs
      B. Laboratory
         1. Urine: glucose, ketone bodies, albumin, and white cells
         2. Blood: glucose, ketone bodies, electrolytes, CBC, BUN, calcium, creatinine, phosphorus, and blood gases.
            Serum amylase may also be helpful.
      C. History
         Concentrate on recent insulin requirements, urine tests, food intake, and pertinent symptoms.

   II. Therapy
      A. Insulin
         1. Traditional method: One-half to two units of regular (unmodified) insulin per kilogram of body weight is given, one-half the dose IV and one-half the dose subcutaneously. The dose varies according to the degree of acidosis and is based on the physician's clinical judgment.
         2. Constant Insulin Infusion Method: Loading dose of 0.1 unit per kilogram of body weight is given IV push, followed immediately by constant infusion of 0.1 unit per kilogram per hour in a normal saline solution via a reliable infusion pump.

Modified from Nursing Procedures, Critical and Intermediate Care, The Children's Memorial Hospital, Chicago, Illinois, 1983.

Continued.

MANAGEMENT OF THE CHILD WITH DIABETIC KETOACIDOSIS—cont'd

    B. Fluids

       Over the first hour a bolus of 20 cc per kilogram of normal saline is often given IV, especially if the patient is in shock or hypotensive. For severe hypotension 5% albumin or whole blood (if anemic) may be used.

    C. Bicarbonate—*used at the physician's discretion*

       1. One suggested criteria for administration

          a. If pH >7.2—NO

          b. If pH <7.1—YES

       2. Dosage

          25-50% of calculated base deficit, given as an IV drip over 1 to 3 hours (usual dose is in a range of 2.0 to 2.5 mEq/Kg)

          Bicarbonate is *not* given by IV push.

3. Second to twelfth hour

   NOTE: Close observation of the patient by both nurses and residents is essential during this time, to evaluate the effectiveness of the therapy given.

  I. Assessment

    A. Clinical

       1. Level of consciousness—monitor closely. If the clinical state does not improve as the blood values return to normal, the resident should be notified.

       2. Vital signs—hourly.

       3. Degree of dehydration—hourly intake and output is especially important. If the patient cannot void on demand, catheterization may be necessary.

       4. Infection—Because infection is a common precipitating factor in either a new or old diabetic with acidosis, it should be searched for, cultures taken, and proper antimicrobial therapy started. Do not give sulfa drugs.

       5. Cardiac status—EKG rhythm strips may be helpful.

    B. Laboratory

       1. Urine: glucose and ketones hourly if possible. Chart on ketoacidosis flowsheets (see Fig. 7-15).

       2. Blood: glucose, ketones every 1-2 hours. BUN, creatinine, and blood gases may be helpful every 2-4 hours.

  II. Therapy

    A. Insulin

       1. Traditional method: Until blood glucose and CO_2 improve, ¼-1 unit of regular insulin per kilogram of body weight may be given SQ every 3-6 hours.

       2. Constant Insulin Infusion method: Infusion continues until glucose falls below 250 mg%. At this point 0.25 units per kilogram of regular insulin is given subcutaneously. Infusion may be discontinued in 2-3 hours, depending on serum glucose.

    B. Fluids

       1. Normal saline—10-20 cc per kilogram is given IV in the first hour depending upon the degree of dehydration. When adequate urine flow is established, a phosphate salt of potassium is added to the IV in a dose of 2-4 mEq/Kg body weight/24 hours. (Do not exceed 40-60 mEq/L)

       2. D_5/NS—begin when blood sugar is below 250 to 300, and the urine no longer has 5% glucose with large amounts of ketones.

       3. Ice chips may be given PO if nausea is absent.

    C. Saline enema—may be necessary for cleansing and relief of constipation.

4. Post twelfth hour

   Previous regime continues until the patient's blood glucose and electrolytes return to normal. Six-hour management is then begun.

should be managed utilizing subcutaneous insulin injections.

Generally, patients with diabetic ketoacidosis should receive nothing by mouth until the acidosis is corrected and the hyperglycemia is controlled. Many of these children can develop nausea and vomiting or decreased intestinal motility during the ketoacidosis, so it is usually wise to restrict oral intake (with the possible exception of small amounts of ice chips).

Throughout the child's care, careful records of fluid intake and output and urine and serum chemistries should be kept (see Fig. 7-15). In addition, the hospital protocol for management of ketoacidosis should be readily available for reference (see the box on management of the child with diabetic ketoacidosis).

■ CHRONIC RENAL FAILURE (CRF)
■ Etiology

The state of chronic renal failure results when the normal concentrations of body substances cannot be maintained by the kidney under the conditions of normal living. The reserve of the kidney is such that more than 50% of renal capacity must be lost before imbalances occur. There are varying degrees of the manifestations of renal insufficiency. Chronic dialysis will be necessary for the patient with severe renal insufficiency, while the patient with moderate renal impairment responds to careful medical and dietary management. Functional disturbances associated with CRF will involve not only the impaired removal of metabolic by-products but fluid excesses and electrolyte and acid-base imbalances. Renal dysfunction will affect the growth and formation of bones, red cell formation, and general body growth and can greatly alter the child's daily life.

■ Pathophysiology

Situations leading to chronic renal failure may result from malformation of the renal system, infections, inherited renal disorders, severe trauma, or glomerular disease. Glomerular nephropathy is the chief cause of CRF.[75]

Chronic renal failure occurs when renal function is reduced below 25% to 30% of normal as reflected in a creatinine clearance of 30 to 40 ml/min/1.73 m². At this level, the serum urea is increased to greater than 20 mg/dl and serum creatinine is elevated to greater than 1.5 mg/dl. (Normal creatinine level in infants and small children is approximately 0.3 to 0.8 mg/dl; the creatinine level in larger children and adults is approximately 0.7 to 1.5 mg/dl.)

Uremia. Uremia (or uremic syndrome) refers to the cluster of symptoms, clinical signs, and biochemical changes that occur as the result of the accumulation of waste products and the fluid and electrolyte imbalances that occur in patients with chronic renal failure. These changes can include hypervolemia, electrolyte and acid-base imbalances, anemia, hypertension, renal osteodystrophy, metastatic calcification, and accumulation of uremic toxins.[50]

Sodium and water balance. In the initial stage of renal insufficiency, the principal feature is a defect in renal ability to concentrate urine. This defect leads to production of urine with a fixed osmolality. These patients may maintain relatively normal serum sodium concentrations despite marked reductions in GFR because the remaining functioning nephrons handle more sodium. Most patients with chronic renal failure are able to excrete reasonable quantities of sodium and maintain normal serum sodium concentrations, provided that acute increases in sodium intake are avoided.

Severe sodium and water restriction may result in hyponatremia because the diseased kidneys are unable to conserve sodium. The resultant urinary loss of sodium and water can result in volume depletion, further reductions in the GFR, and a greater increase in BUN. Prolonged administration of diuretics may also lead to sodium depletion.

A difference in sodium balance is seen with severe (end-stage) renal failure. In these patients, the very low glomerular filtration rate is inadequate to excrete the amounts of sodium and water normally ingested. Retention of sodium and water produce edema and vascular congestion, often with resultant hypertension, pulmonary edema, and heart failure. These complications must often be treated with dialysis.

Potassium balance. Since the entire quantity of potassium filtered by the glomerulus is reabsorbed by the proximal tubule, the urinary potassium is dependent upon the secretion of that ion by the distal tubules. When renal damage is present, undamaged nephrons have the ability to increase potassium secretion by 600%. Patients with chronic renal failure (and chronically low GFR) may generate a urine containing a secreted potassium concentration in excess of the amount present in the filtrate. For this reason, it is usually not necessary to restrict dietary potassium for a patient with chronic renal failure unless or until the GFR is at very low levels. The patient with chronic renal insufficiency does require a longer period of time to rid the body of excess potassium, however. As a result, acute hyperkalemia may result from the ingestions of a large potassium load, from hemolysis, acidosis, or from a catabolic state associated with fever. If the resultant hyperkalemia is not severe, treatment may focus on elimination of the cause of the elevation. If the hyperkalemia is severe, however, and ECG changes develop, urgent treatment with calcium, glucose, insulin, or sodium polystyrene sulfonate is indicated (see the section on hyperkalemia under acute renal failure earlier in this chapter).

Hypokalemia occasionally develops as a result of a decreased potassium intake or diuretic therapy.

Acidosis. One of the primary functions of the kidney is the excretion of metabolic acids. This involves three aspects of tubular function: reabsorption of bicarbonate, secretion of ammonium ion, and secretion of titratable acids (acidification of urinary buffers). Patients with chronic renal failure generally develop metabolic acidosis as the result of bicarbonate wasting and decreased distal tubule ability to produce ammonia. The rate of ammonia production decreases in proportion to the fall in glomerular filtration rate. The ability of the kidney to form titratable acids, however, seems to remain nearly normal.

The loss of bicarbonate in the urine may negate any attempts to correct the acidosis with bicarbonate administration.

Calcium, phosphorus, and bone. Patients with chronic renal failure have reduced intestinal absorption of calcium. This reduced absorption may result from the deficiency of the active form of vitamin D, which is produced by the kidney.

When the GFR falls below 25% of normal, the plasma phosphate concentration begins to rise. Under normal conditions, a reciprocal fall in the serum level of ionized calcium follows the phosphate retention, as a result of calcium-phosphate precipitation. This lowering of the ionized calcium stimulates release of parathyroid hormone (PTH). The increased PTH level promotes bone breakdown, liberating calcium and phosphate ions. It simultaneously reduces renal phosphate reabsorption. PTH also assists the kidney in formation of active vitamin D, which will increase intestinal calcium absorption and bone reabsorption. Increased renal excretion of phosphate lowers the serum phosphate, and the serum calcium level returns to normal, removing the stimulus for PTH secretion. When renal disease is present, the rise in phosphate concentration results in a fall in serum ionized calcium. The lower serum calcium level stimulates PTH release. Since the kidneys are impaired, they are unable to excrete more phosphate, and cannot synthesize vitamin D to increase intestinal calcium absorption. The serum calcium remains low, the PTH stimulus continues, and chronic bone reabsorption occurs (called renal osteodystrophy). A secondary hyperparathyroidism also results.

Anemia. Chronic renal failure affects both red cells and platelets. Red cell production is impaired, and the life span of the red blood cell is shortened because of uremia. Though the platelet count is normal, the platelet function is reduced (a thrombocytopathia is present).

Uremic encephalopathy and neuropathy. The cause of uremic encephalopathy occurring in patients with CRF is unknown. It seems to be related to changes in the fluid and electrolyte balance, serum osmolality, and accumulation of uremic toxins. Ultimately, these abnormalities can affect the brain cell membrane permeability, the sodium-potassium pump, and the cerebral uptake of glucose.[46]

Chronic renal failure can also be associated with the development of a peripheral neuropathy. With this neuropathy, demyelination of distal portions of the nerves can occur, resulting in decreased nerve conduction.[46]

■ Clinical signs and symptoms

Patients with chronic renal failure often develop vague complaints of fatigue, weakness, anorexia, nausea, abdominal pain, headaches, and failure to grow. Specific symptoms include an initial polyuria and polydipsia, mild edema, especially about the eyes, or oliguria. The child's complexion may be sallow or pale with a faint uremic tint. Skin rashes or arthritis may also be present. The child usually has a history of previous kidney or urologic disease or of an episode of renal injury.

Serum electrolytes, phosphate, pH, bicarbonate, BUN, creatinine, P_{CO_2} and base excess, as well as hematocrit and hemoglobin, white cell count, and blood culture are obtained. Urine is collected and sent for culture, sediment, pH, osmolality, and sodium. A 24-hour urine collection is performed to quantify urine volume and creatinine and protein excretion.

The child with chronic renal failure usually demonstrates a normal serum sodium and potassium concentration (unless chronic diuretic therapy is utilized, then hypokalemia may be present), a high serum phosphate and low serum calcium concentration, a high BUN, high uric acid, and an elevated serum creatinine concentration. Metabolic acidosis may be present, and serum bicarbonate ion concentrations are low. If an infection is present, the child's white blood cell count may be elevated. In addition, the child is usually anemic, with a prolonged bleeding time (resulting from thrombocytopathia). The child with CRF often demonstrates growth failure.

If uremic encephalopathy develops, the child may demonstrate signs of increased intracranial pressure (see the section on increased intracranial pressure in Chapter 6), irritability, lethargy, or seizures. If a uremic neuropathy is present, the child may develop muscle cramps, tetany, weakness, or muscle wasting.[46]

■ Medical treatment and nursing interventions

The care of the hospitalized child with chronic renal failure requires careful fluid and electrolyte therapy. Most of the parents of children with CRF will be valuable resources regarding the child's food preferences and feeding techniques. The dietician will assist by helping plan menus on an individual basis.

Children with CRF are more susceptible to infections and need careful skin and wound attention. The staff must be extremely careful to utilize good handwashing techniques before and after examination of the child.

Once the child develops any form of renal failure, dosages of medications must be reduced accordingly (see the section on adjustment of medication dosages in the discussion of acute renal failure earlier in this chapter).

Treatment of uremia in the child with chronic renal failure may be accomplished through dietary restrictions and/or dialysis. The indications for dialysis in the child with chronic renal failure are generally the same as for the child with acute renal failure and include: hypervolemia or congestive heart failure, deterioration in neurologic status, severe bleeding, metastatic calcification as a result of calcium phosphate precipitation, severe hyperkalemia, acidosis, a BUN greater than 125 to 150 mg/dl, a serum sodium concentration above 160 mEq/L, or a serum calcium concentration above 12 mg/dl. Generally, once the child with CRF has stabilized, regular intervals for dialysis are established. Then hemodialysis or CAPD can be utilized to maintain fluid and electrolyte balance (see the section on dialysis in children earlier in this chapter).

Whenever possible, the child with CRF is prepared for renal transplantation.

■ Diagnostic Tests

Most of the tests used to evaluate renal function, including creatinine clearance, fractional excretion of sodium, and measurement of urine osmolality, have been discussed in previous sections of this chapter (see the sections on essential anatomy and physiology and on acute renal failure). For further information regarding clinical assessment of renal function in children, the reader is referred to a very comprehensive chapter by Barratt and Chantler[9] and one by Greenhill and Gruskin.[32]

Since many techniques utilized for clinical evaluation of renal function require an accurately timed collection of a urine specimen, the technique for collection of a 24-hour urine specimen is reviewed briefly here.

Whenever timed collection of a urine specimen is planned, the child, family, and other nursing staff should receive specific instructions about the collection (and these should be recorded in the patient's care plan).

A timed urine collection begins when the first urine specimen is collected and discarded. Following that discard, all urine is saved in appropriate containers until the end of the collection period. At the time that the collection is to end, the patient is encouraged to void (or the Foley catheter tubing and urinometer are emptied), and the collection bottle is labeled with the patient's name, hospital number, the time the collection was begun, and the time the collection ended.

It is important that the nurses discuss "contingency plans" with a physician for use in the event that a portion of the collection is lost or inadvertently discarded. If the continuous collection is interrupted, it may be possible to perform studies on the collection amount and duration up to the time of the specimen loss (e.g., instead of a 24-hour creatinine clearance study, a 12- or 16-hour one may be performed). If estimates of the quantity of urine lost are available, the collection may continue, with special note made of the quantity and timing of specimen loss. Whatever the contingency plans are, they should be discussed with the nursing staff and the specimen laboratory *before* the collection is begun. The plans should also be carefully documented in the nursing care plan, so that there is no confusion about appropriate response to specimen loss.

Finally, some timed urine collections require use of specially prepared containers and refrigeration of the urine sample during the collection period. These specifications should be strictly followed, or the sampling results may be inaccurate.

If the child has acute renal failure and oliguria, it is important to know that long urine collections are not necessary to evaluate renal function. Fractional excretion of sodium, creatinine clearance, and urine osmolality can usually be calculated from even small quantities of urine. Many of these calculations will, however, require simultaneous collection of blood samples for measurement of serum sodium or creatinine concentrations or serum osmolality.

REFERENCES

1. Abel, R.M., and others: Improved survival from acute renal failure after treatment with intravenous essential L-amino acids and glucose, N. Engl. J. Med. **288:**695, Apr. 5, 1973.
2. Abel, R.M., and others: Etiology, incidence, and prognosis of renal failure following cardiac operations: results of a prospective analysis of 500 consecutive patients, J. Thorac. Cardiovasc. Surg. **71**(3):323, 1976.
3. Alexander, S.R.: Pediatric CAPD update, Presented at the Third Annual Conference on CAPD, Kansas City, Mo., Feb., 1983.
4. Alexander, S.R., and others: Clinical parameters in CAPD for infants and children. In Moncrief, J.W., and Popvich, R.P., editors: CAPD update, New York, 1981, Masson Publishing USA, Inc.
5. Amair, P., and others: Continuous ambulatory peritoneal dialysis in diabetics with end-stage renal disease, N. Engl. J. Med. **306**(11):625, 1982.
6. Anand, S.R.: Acute renal failure in the neonate, Pediatr. Clin. North Am. **29**(4):791, 1982.
7. Andres, G., Supulvada, M., and McClusky, R.: Immunopathology of glomerulonephritis. In Rubin, M.I., editor: Pediatric nephrology, Baltimore, 1975, Williams & Wilkins.
8. Barratt, T.M.: Renal failure in infancy. In Rubin, M.I., editor: Pediatric nephrology, Baltimore, 1975, Williams & Wilkins.
9. Barratt, T.M., and Chantler, C.: Clinical assessment of renal function. In Rubin, M.I., editor: Pediatric nephrology, Baltimore, 1975, Williams & Wilkins.
10. Bates, J., Newberger, E.H., and Mandell, F.: Emergencies, child abuse, and sudden infant death syndrome. In Graef, J.R., and Cone, T.E., editors: Manual of pediatric therapeutics, ed. 2, Boston, 1980, Little, Brown & Co.
11. Baum, M., and others: Continuous ambulatory peritoneal dialysis in children, N. Engl. J. Med. **307:**1537, 1982.
12. Becker, D., and Foley, T.: 1-Deamino-8-D-arginine vasopressin in the treatment of central diabetes insipidus in childhood, J. Pediatr. **92**(6):1011, 1978.
13. Bennett, W.M., and others: Guidelines for drug therapy in renal failure, Ann. Intern. Med. **86**(6):754, 1977.
14. Betkurer, M.V., and others: Indomethacin and its effect on renal function and urinary kallikrein excretion in premature infants with patent ductus arteriosus, Pediatrics **68**(1):99, 1981.
15. Biller, J.A., and Yaeger, A.M.: Fluid and electrolyte therapy. In: The Harriet Lane handbook, ed. 9, Chicago, 1981, Year Book Medical Publishers, Inc.
16. Brown, J.J., and others: Renin and acute renal failure in man: studies in man, Br. Med. J. **1:**253, Jan. 31, 1970.
17. Brundage, D.J.: Hemodialysis. In: Nursing management of renal problems, ed. 2, St. Louis, 1980, The C.V. Mosby Co.
18. Brundage, D.J.: Peritoneal dialysis. In: Nursing management of renal problems, ed. 2, St. Louis, 1980, The C.V. Mosby Co.
19. Cannon, P.: Diuretic therapy in patients with renal disease. In Winters, R., editor: The body fluids in pediatrics, Boston, 1973, Little, Brown, & Co.
20. Chipman, J., and Marks, J.K.: Diabetic ketoacidosis. In Levin, D.L., Morriss, F.C., and Moore, G.C., editors: A practical guide to pediatric intensive care, ed. 2, St. Louis, 1984, The C.V. Mosby Co.
21. Clark, D.A.: Times of first void and first stool in 500 newborns, Pediatrics **60**(4):457, 1977.
22. Dell, R.: Pathophysiology of dehydration. In Winters, R., editor: The body fluids in pediatrics, Boston, 1973, Little, Brown, & Co.
23. Dobrin, R., and Kjellstrand, C.: The management of acute renal failure in pediatrics. In Chapman, A., editor: Acute renal failure, New York, 1980, Churchill Livingstone, Inc.
24. Donckerwolcke, R.A.: Diagnosis and management of renal tubular disorders in children, Pediatr. Clin. North Am. **29:**895, 1982.
25. Ellis, D., Gartner, J.C., and Galvis, A.G.: Acute renal failure in infants and children: diagnosis, complications, and treatment, Crit. Care Med. **9:**607, 1981.
26. Ellis, D., and others: Focal glomerular sclerosis in children: correlation of histology with prognosis, J. Pediatr. **93**(5):762, 1978.
27. Fine, R.N.: Peritoneal dialysis update, J. Pediatr. **100:**1, 1982.
28. Fong, J.S.C., de Chadarevian, J.P., and Kaplan, B.S.: Hemolytic-uremic syndrome: current concepts and management, Pediatr. Clin. North Am. **29:**835, 1982.
29. Friedman, A.L., and Segar, W.E.: Antidiuretic hormone excess, J. Pediatr. **94**(4):521, 1979.
30. Gabow, P.: Disorders of potassium metabolism. In Schrier, R.W., editor: Renal and electrolyte disorders, Boston, 1976, Little, Brown, & Co.
31. Gordillo-Paniagua, G., and Velasquez-Jones, L.: Acute renal failure, Pediatr. Clin. North Am. **23:**817, 1976.
32. Greenhill, A., and Gruskin, A.: Laboratory evaluation of renal function, Pediatr. Clin. North Am. **23:**661, 1976.
33. Grupe, W.: The kidney. In Klaus, M., editor: Care of the high-risk neonate, Philadelphia, 1973, W.B. Saunders Co.
34. Gruskin, A.B., and others: Serum sodium abnormalities in children, Pediatr. Clin. North Am. **29:**907, 1982.
35. Guignard, J.P.: Renal function in the newborn infant, Pediatr. Clin. North Am. **29:**777, 1982.
36. Guyton, A.C.: Micturation, renal disease, and diuresis. In Textbook of medical physiology, ed. 5, Philadelphia, 1976, W.B. Saunders Co.
37. Heird, W.C., and Winters, R.W.: Fluid therapy for the pediatric surgical patient. In Winters, R., editor: The body fluids in pediatrics, Boston, 1973, Little, Brown, & Co.
38. Herdman, R., and Urizar, R.: Coagulopathy in renal disease—including hemolytic-uremic syndrome. In Rubin, M., editor: Pediatric nephrology, Baltimore, 1975, Williams & Wilkins.

39. Hogg, R.J.: Acute renal failure. In Levin, D.L., Morriss, F.C., and Moore, G.C., editors: A practical guide to pediatric intensive care, ed. 2, St. Louis, 1984, The C.V. Mosby Co.

40. Hogg, R.J., and Buchanan, G.R.: Hemolytic-uremic syndrome. In Levin, D.L., Morriss, F.C., and Moore, G.C., editors: A practical guide to pediatric intensive care, ed. 2, St. Louis, 1984, The C.V. Mosby Co.

41. Hogg, R.J., and Stein, P.: Acute peritoneal dialysis. In Levin, D.L., Morriss, F.C., and Moore, G.C., editors: A practical guide to pediatric intensive care, ed. 2, St. Louis, 1984, The C.V. Mosby Co.

42. International Study of Kidney Disease in Children: The primary nephrotic syndrome in children; identification of patients with minimal change nephrotic syndrome from initial response to prednisone, J. Pediatr. **98**(4): 561, 1981.

43. James, J.A.: Renal disease in childhood, ed. 3, St. Louis, 1976, The C.V. Mosby Co.

44. Jordan, S.C., and Lemire, J.M.: Acute glomerulonephritis: diagnosis and treatment, Pediatr. Clin. North Am. **29**:857, 1982.

45. Kaplan, B.S., and Drummond, K.N.: Acute renal failure. In Rubin, M.I., editor: Pediatric nephrology, Baltimore, 1975, Williams & Wilkins.

46. Kaplan, B.S., and Drummond, K.N.: Chronic renal failure. In Rubin, M.I., editor: Pediatric nephrology, Baltimore, 1975, Williams & Wilkins.

47. Kaufman, I.A., Keller, M.A., and Nyhan, W.L.: Diabetic ketosis and acidosis: the continuous infusion of low doses of insulin, J. Pediatr. **87**:846, 1975.

48. Kleeman, C.R., and Fichman, M.P.: The clinical physiology of water metabolism, N. Engl. J. Med. **277**:1300, 1967.

49. Klenk, E.L., and Winters, R.: Disorders of antidiuretic hormone secretion. In Winters, R., editor: The body fluids in pediatrics, Boston, 1973, Little, Brown & Co.

50. Lancaster, L.: Renal failure: pathophysiology, assessment, and intervention, Nephrol. Nurse **4**:38, March-April, 1983.

51. Levin, D.L.: Abnormalities in fluids, minerals, and glucose. In Levin, D.L., Morriss, F.C., and Moore, G.C., editors: A practical guide to pediatric intensive care, ed. 2, St. Louis, 1984, The C.V. Mosby Co.

52. Levinsky, N.G.: Pathophysiology of acute renal failure, N. Engl. J. Med. **296**:1453, 1977.

53. Linton, A.L.: Diagnostic criteria and clinical course of acute renal failure. In Chapman, A., editor: Acute renal failure, New York, 1980, Churchill Livingstone, Inc.

54. Marks, J.F.: Central diabetes insipidus. In Levin, D.L., Morriss, F.C., and Moore, G.C., editors: A practical guide to pediatric intensive care, ed. 2, St. Louis, 1984, The C.V. Mosby Co.

55. Marks, J.F.: Inappropriate secretion of antidiuretic hormone. In Levin, D.L., Morriss, F.C., and Moore, G.C., editors: A practical guide to pediatric intensive care, ed. 2, St. Louis, 1984, The C.V. Mosby Co.

56. Mathew, O.P., and others: Neonatal renal failure: usefulness of diagnostic indices, Pediatrics **65**:57, 1980.

57. McDonald, B.M., and McEnery, P.T.: Glomerulonephritis in children: clinical and morphologic characteristics and mechanisms of glomerular injury, Pediatr. Clin. North Am. **23**:691, 1976.

58. McEnery, P.T., and Strife, C.F.: Nephrotic syndrome in childhood, Pediatr. Clin. North Am. **89**:875, 1982.

59. McEvoy, G., editor: Cardiac drugs. In: The American hospital formulary service, Bethesda, Md., 1983, The American Society of Hospital Pharmacists.

60. Mendoza, S.: Syndrome of inappropriate antidiuretic hormone secretion (SIADH), Pediatr. Clin. North Am. **23**:681, 1976.

61. Metheny, N.M., and Snively, W.D.: The role of nursing observations in the diagnosis of body fluid disturbances. In: Nurses' handbook of fluid balance, ed. 3, Philadelphia, 1978, J.B. Lippincott Co.

62. Orloff, S., Potter, D., and Holliday, M.: Acute renal failure. In Smith, C., editor: The critically ill child, ed. 2, Philadelphia, 1977, W.B. Saunders Co.

63. Papadopoulou, Z.L., and Novello, A.C.: The use of hemoperfusion in children, Pediatr. Clin. North Am. **29**:1039, 1982.

64. Phibbs, R.H.: Resuscitation of the asphyxiated infant. In Avery, G.B., editor: Neonatology: pathophysiology and management of the newborn, ed. 2, Philadelphia, 1981, J.B. Lippincott Co.

65. Pitts, R.F.: Anatomy of the kidney. In: Physiology of the kidney and body fluids, ed. 3, Chicago, 1974, Year Book Medical Publishers, Inc.

66. Pitts, R.F.: Reabsorption and excretion of ions and water. In: Physiology of the kidney and body fluids, ed. 3, Chicago, 1974, Year Book Medical Publishers, Inc.

67. Pitts, R.F.: Renal circulation. In: Physiology of the kidney and body fluids, ed. 3, Chicago, 1974, Year Book Medical Publishers, Inc.

68. Pitts, R.F.: Renal regulation of acid-base balance. In: Physiology of the kidney and body fluids, ed. 3, Chicago, 1974, Year Book Medical Publishers, Inc.

69. Pitts, R.F.: Tubular reabsorption. In: Physiology of the kidney and body fluids, ed. 3, Chicago, 1974, Year Book Medical Publishers, Inc.

70. Rahill, W.F.: Renal physiology—clinical variations. In Rubin, M.I., editor: Pediatric nephrology, Baltimore, 1975, Williams & Wilkins.

71. Robertson, G., Athar, S., and Shelton, R.L.: Osmotic control of vasopressin function. In Adreoli, T., editor: Disturbances in body fluid osmolality, Bethesda, Md., 1977, American Physiological Society.

72. Robson, A.M.: Parenteral fluid therapy. In Behrman, R.E., and others, editors: Nelson textbook of pediatrics, ed. 12, Philadelphia, 1983, W.B. Saunders Co.

73. Rosenbloom, A.L., and others: Cerebral edema complicating diabetic ketoacidosis in childhood, J. Pediatr. **93**(3):357, 1980.

74. Royer, P., and others: Pediatric nephrology, Philadelphia, 1974, W.B. Saunders Co.

75. Royer, P., and others: Parenteral fluid therapy. In Behrman, R.E., and others, editors: Nelson textbook of pediatrics, ed. 12, Philadelphia, 1983, W.B. Saunders Co.

76. Salusky, I.B., and others: Continuous ambulatory peritoneal dialysis in children, Pediatr. Clin. North Am. **29:**1005, 1982.
77. Shapira, N., and others: Cardiovascular effects of protamine sulfate in man, J. Thorac. Cardiovasc. Surg. **84:** 505, 1982.
78. Spack, N.P.: Diabetes mellitus. In Graef, J.W., and Cone, T.E., Jr., editors: Manual of pediatric therapeutics, ed. 2, Boston, 1980, Little, Brown, & Co.
79. Spann, J.F., and Hurst, J.W.: The recognition and management of heart failure—diuretics. In Hurst, J.W., editor-in-chief: The heart, arteries, and veins, ed. 5, New York, 1982, McGraw-Hill Book Co.
80. Stefanidis, C.J., Hewitt, I.K., and Balfe, J.W.: Growth in children receiving continuous ambulatory peritoneal dialysis, J. Pediatr. **102**(5):681, 1983.
81. Strauss, J., Daniel, S.S., and James, L.S.: Postnatal adjustment in renal function, Pediatrics **68:**802, 1981.
82. Vander, A.J.: Renal physiology, New York, 1975, McGraw-Hill Book Co.
83. Veeser, T.E., and others: Low-dose intravenous insulin therapy for diabetic ketoacidosis in children, Am. J. Dis. Child. **131:**308, 1977.
84. Waterhouse, K.: Pediatric urology (surgical aspects). In Rubin, M.I., editor: Pediatric nephrology, Baltimore, 1975, Williams & Wilkins Co.

85. Weil, W., and Bailie, M.: Fluid and electrolyte metabolism in infants and children, New York, 1977, Grune & Stratton, Inc.
86. Weisfeldt, M.L., and Chandra, N.: Cardiopulmonary resuscitation and subsequent management of the patient. In Hurst, J.W., editor-in-chief: The heart, arteries, and veins, ed. 5, New York, 1982, McGraw-Hill Book Co.
87. Williams, G., Klenk, E., and Winters, R.: Acute renal failure in pediatrics, Boston, 1973, Little, Brown, & Co.
88. Williams, J.A.: Hypotensive crises: identifying the high-risk patient on hemodialysis, Heart Lung **10**(2): 309, 1981.
89. Winters, R.: Regulation of normal water and electrolyte metabolism. In Winters, R., editor: The body fluids in pediatrics, Boston, 1973, Little, Brown, & Co.
90. Winters, R.W.: Restoration of body potassium deficits. In: Principles of pediatric fluid therapy, ed. 2, Boston, 1982, Little, Brown & Co.
91. Yaffe, S.J., and Chudzih, G.: Drugs and the kidney. In Rubin, M.I., editor: Pediatric nephrology, Baltimore, 1975, Williams & Wilkins Co.

CHAPTER EIGHT

Gastrointestinal Disorders

DEBORAH RIFFEE MILLER*

This discussion of the intensive care of children with gastrointestinal disorders does not attempt to cover all disorders of the gastrointestinal tract, nor does it cover neonatal gastrointestinal problems in as great detail as those occurring in infants and children. (Other sources are suggested for an in-depth discussion of neonatal disorders.[7,47,48,55])

Instead, this chapter is designed to provide the bedside nurse with information on physiology and assessment to enable her to make sound clinical judgments and to provide skilled nursing care for common pediatric gastrointestinal conditions requiring intensive care. It begins with a review of normal anatomy and physiology of the gastrointestinal tract and a discussion of nutrition.

■ Essential Anatomy and Physiology

■ FUNCTIONS OF GASTROINTESTINAL ORGANS

A description of basic digestive and absorptive functions of each organ follows (the major body organs included in the gastrointestinal tract are reviewed in Fig. 8-1).

Esophagus. Channel for passage of food from mouth to stomach; distal 3 to 5 cm functions as a sphincter protecting the esophageal mucosa from reflux of gastric acid secretions

Stomach. Reservoir for ingested food; renders ingested food isotonic by secretory and mechanical breakdown; secretes intrinsic factor necessary in vitamin B_{12} absorption

*Susan DeJong contributed initial material for the sections on acute abdomen, gastrointestinal bleeding, and infant botulism and for Table 8-19. The author gratefully acknowledges this contribution.

Duodenum. Primary site of intestinal secretion and absorption

Jejunum. Additional site of intestinal secretion and absorption

Ileum. Specific site of absorption of vitamin B_{12} and reabsorption of bile salts

Colon. Secretes mucus; reabsorbs water and electrolytes; propels fecal mass for elimination

Pancreas. Secretes hormones essential for digestion of carbohydrates; secretes enzymes vital for digestion of fats and proteins; secretes bicarbonate, other electrolytes, and water, which neutralize gastric acid secretions in the duodenum

Biliary tract. Transports and provides storage mechanism for bile from liver to duodenum

Liver. Secretes bile, which is essential for the utilization of fats; is the primary site of glycogenesis and glycolysis with subsequent production of glycogen intermediates (uridine triphosphate and cytidine triphosphate); metabolizes proteins into amino acids and subsequently synthesizes them into needed proteins (e.g., albumin and clotting factors); metabolizes steroids, causing catabolism of hormones and glucocorticoids; stores fat-soluble vitamins; detoxifies foreign or toxic substances, including many medications

■ GASTROINTESTINAL—PORTAL CIRCULATION

Unlike other organ systems within the body, the venous return from organs of the gastrointestinal tract drains first into the portal venous system before passing into the inferior vena cava and returning to the heart (Fig. 8-2).

The liver receives blood from two major sources,

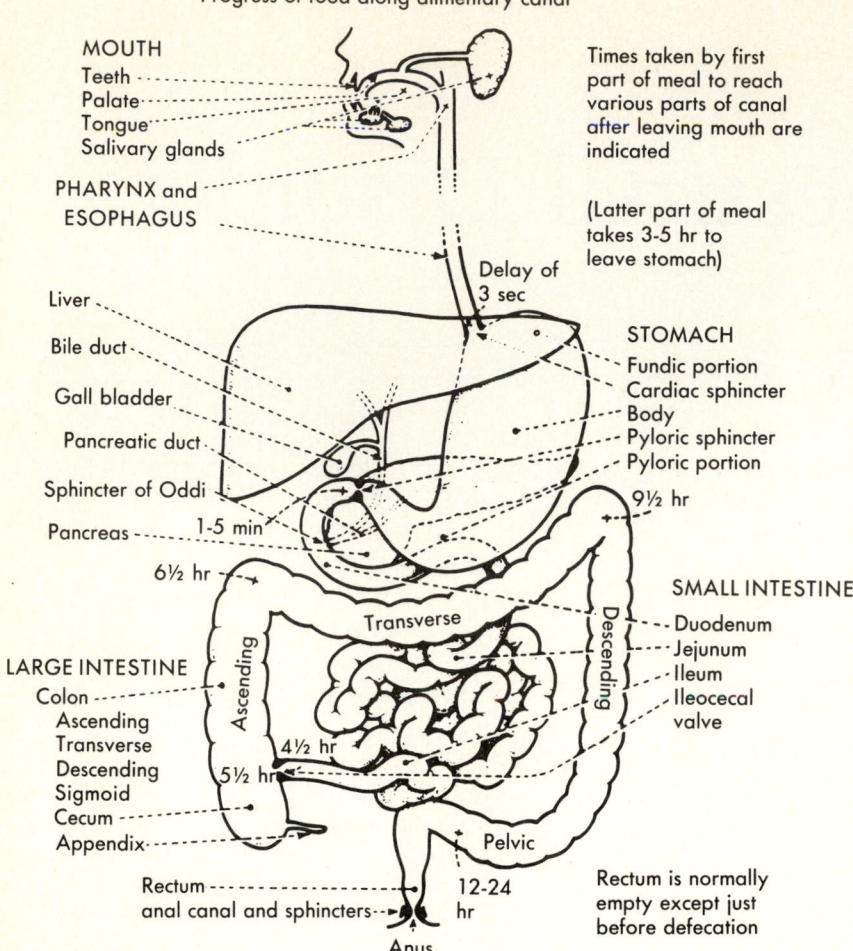

Progress of food along alimentary canal

MOUTH
  Teeth
  Palate
  Tongue
  Salivary glands

PHARYNX and
ESOPHAGUS

Times taken by first
part of meal to reach
various parts of canal
after leaving mouth are
indicated

(Latter part of meal
takes 3-5 hr to
leave stomach)

Delay of
3 sec

Liver

Bile duct

Gall bladder

Pancreatic duct

Sphincter of Oddi

Pancreas   1-5 min

6½ hr

STOMACH
  Fundic portion
  Cardiac sphincter
  Body
  Pyloric sphincter
  Pyloric portion

9½ hr

SMALL INTESTINE
  Duodenum
  Jejunum
  Ileum
  Ileocecal
  valve

Transverse

Ascending   Descending

LARGE INTESTINE
  Colon
    Ascending
    Transverse
    Descending
    Sigmoid
    Cecum
  Appendix

4½ hr

5½ hr

Pelvic

Rectum
anal canal and sphincters

12-24
hr

Rectum is normally
empty except just
before defecation

Anus

Fig. 8-1 The gastrointestinal tract.

Modified from McNaught, A., and Callender, R.: Illustrated
physiology, ed. 4, New York, 1979, Churchill Livingstone, Inc.

the portal vein and the hepatic artery. The *portal vein* receives blood rich in nutrients from the gastrointestinal tract, and the *hepatic artery* supplies oxygenated blood. In the adult the hepatic artery and the portal vein carry approximately 13% to 25% of cardiac output (800 to 1500 ml) to the liver per minute, 75% of which is supplied by the portal vein.[40] After this blood is filtered through the liver, all of it normally passes into the hepatic vein and is returned to the heart.

■ **FLUIDS OF THE
GASTROINTESTINAL TRACT**

Large volumes of fluid are secreted and reabsorbed throughout the length of the gastrointestinal tract. An average of 7 to 9 L enters the gastrointestinal tract daily in an 8-year-old child, yet the stool water content is approximately only 100 to 200 ml.[76] Both the small bowel and colon reabsorb the majority of these nonexcreted fluids. Gastrointestinal fluids are composed of water, electrolytes, and nonelectrolytes. Table 8-1 shows the concentrations of the major electrolytes in gastrointestinal secretions.

Fluids and electrolytes can be lost from the gastrointestinal tract by vomiting, diarrhea, gastrointestinal suction, wound drainage, obstruction, fistulas, hemorrhage, infection, surgery, and prolonged use of enemas or laxatives. Whenever the patient has a known source of gastrointestinal fluid loss, it is important to record both the volume and composition, since each type of fluid has a specific chemical composition that must be considered when replacing lost fluids and anticipating complications. Estimated

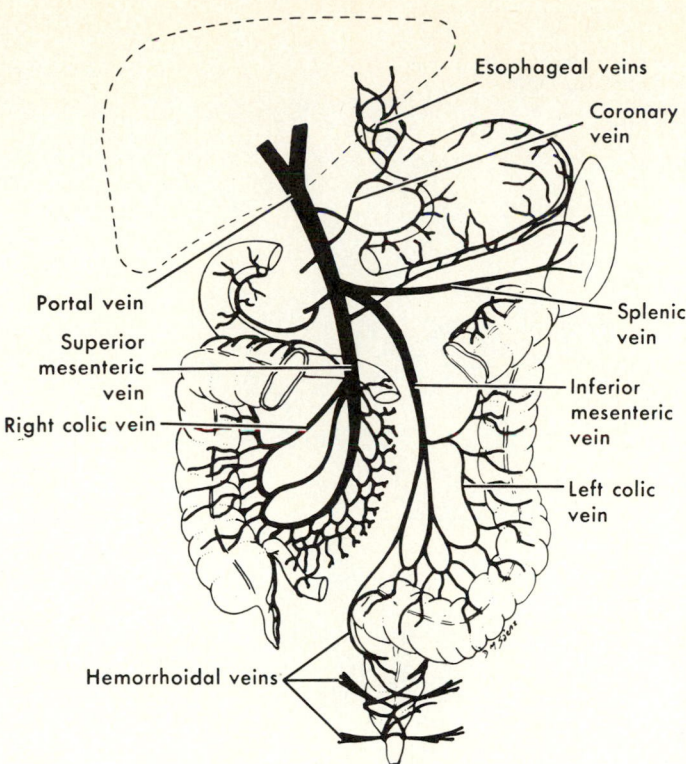

Fig. 8-2 Portal circulation.

From Given, B., and Simmons, S.: Gastroenterology in clinical
nursing, ed. 4, St. Louis, 1984, The C.V. Mosby Co.

daily insensible water losses in children beyond the
neonatal period are approximately 300 ml/m² body surface area per day. Approximate specific losses are
further divided in Table 8-2. Guidelines for calculating required daily maintenance fluid intake and electrolytes in children are listed in Table 8-3.

The nurse must obtain information about fluid
and electrolyte balance as soon as the child is admitted to the intensive-care unit (ICU). Recent
sources and quantity of fluid intake, medications the
patient has been taking that may affect fluid and electrolyte balance, and any history of vomiting, diarrhea,
ascites, or decreased or increased urine output must
be determined. The most common imbalance of
fluids and electrolytes caused by gastrointestinal disease are those resulting in excesses or deficits of chloride, magnesium, sodium, potassium, bicarbonate,
calcium, or hydrogen ions (Table 8-4 lists clinical
signs and symptoms of these imbalances).

■ **DIGESTION AND ABSORPTION**

The ingestion of food initiates many physical
and chemical processes that allow the body to use the
ingested nutrients for maintenance of body temperature and function of its vital organ systems, construction of new tissue for growth or repair, and performance of work. These processes are generally known
as digestion, absorption, and metabolism of nutrients.

There is strong popular conviction but very little data regarding the "digestibility" of specific foods
and their effect on the physiology of the gastrointestinal tract. Foods are said to be "hard to digest" or,
conversely, "easy to digest." "Digestibility" of a food
has been equated with the rate at which it leaves the
stomach. Because fat remains longest in the stomach,
it is thought to be more difficult to digest than protein
and carbohydrate foods. Fried foods are said to be "irritating" to the gastrointestinal tract although there
is little scientific evidence to support these statements.

In medical usage, the term "digestibility" refers
to the portion of food that becomes available to the
body as absorbed nutrients; the indigestible portion is
excreted in the feces. Under normal conditions the
bulk of the indigestible residue consists of cellulose,
pectins, and other complex carbohydrates found in
foods of plant origin, which cannot be degraded by the
Text continued on p. 554.

Table 8-1 Approximate composition of gastrointestinal secretions[17,26,62,66,77] (electrolyte values are mEq/L)

Fluid	Fasting				Fed			
	Newborn	Infant	Child	Adult	Newborn	Infant	Child	Adult
Saliva								
pH	7.0	7.3	7.3	6.4	7.3	7.3	7.3	6.4
Na	10-15	10-15	10-15	5-12	70-90	70-90	70-90	60-80
Cl	10-20	10-20	7-15	10-20	30-45	30-45	20-30	30-45
K	24-30	24-30	24-30	20-26	20-25	20-25	20-25	16-20
HCO$_3$	15-20	15-20	15-20	15-20	40-60	40-60	40-60	40-60
Gastric								
pH	2.5	3.2	3.2	1.0	6.8	7.0	7.0	5.0
Na	80-100	80-100	80-100	80-100	20-30	20-30	20-30	20-30
Cl	100-130	100-130	100-130	100-130	120-150	120-150	120-150	120-150
K	5-15	5-15	5-15	5-15	5-15	5-15	5-15	5-15
HCO$_3$	0	0	0	0	0	0	0	0
Biliary								
pH	7.2	7.2	7.2	7.2	7.8	7.8	7.8	7.8
Na	140-180	140-180	140-180	140-180	140-180	140-180	140-180	140-180
Cl	60-80	60-80	60-80	60-80	90-120	90-120	90-120	90-120
K	3-12	3-12	3-12	3-12	3-12	3-12	3-12	3-12
HCO$_3$	20-30	20-30	20-30	20-30	40-50	40-50	40-50	40-50
Pancreatic								
pH	8.0	8.0	8.0	8.0	8.0	8.0	8.0	8.0
Na	125-135	125-135	135-150	135-150	125-135	125-135	135-150	135-150
Cl	90-110	90-110	85-95	85-95	20-40	20-40	20-40	20-40

K	7-15	7-15	3-8	3-8	7-15	7-15	3-8	3-8
HCO₃	25-60	25-60	25-60	25-60	110-130	110-130	110-130	110-130
Jejunal								
pH	7.5	7.5	7.5	7.5	7.5	7.5	7.5	7.5
Na	125-135	125-135	135-150	135-150	125-135	125-135	135-150	135-150
Cl	120-145	120-145	120-145	120-145	120-145	120-145	120-145	120-145
K	7-15	7-15	3-8	3-8	7-15	7-15	3-8	3-8
HCO₃	20	20	20	20	20	20	20	20
Ileal								
pH	8.0	8.0	8.0	8.0	8.0	8.0	8.0	8.0
Na	125-135	125-135	135-150	135-150	125-135	125-135	135-150	135-150
Cl	70-85	70-85	70-85	70-85	70-85	70-85	70-85	70-85
K	7-15	7-15	3-8	3-8	7-15	7-15	3-8	3-8
HCO₃	40	40	40	40	40	40	40	40
Fecal excretion								
pH	—	—	—	—	6.1	*7.5 †4.9	7.2	7.2
Na (mEq/kg)	—	—	—	—	100-150	*50-100 †100-200	20-40	13-27
Cl (mEq/kg)	—	—	—	—	15-25	*30-50 †60-100	10-25	7-15
K (mEq/kg)	—	—	—	—	12-50	*125-375 †250-750	50-150	35-100
HCO₃	—	—	—	—	30	30	30	30
Amount (kg/24 hr)	—	—	—	—	.07-.09	*0.03-0.05 †.015-.025	.08-.12	.10-.20

*Bottle-fed.
†Breast-fed.

Table 8-2 Estimation of daily insensible water loss in children consuming maintenance caloric intake*

Source	Infant	1-2 yr	2-6 yr	7-9 yr	10-12 yr
Lungs	18-22.5 ml/kg	13.5-15 ml/kg	12-13.5 ml/kg	10.5-12 ml/kg	7.5-9 ml/kg
Skin	48-60 ml/kg	36-40 ml/kg	32-36 ml/kg	28-32 ml/kg	20-24 ml/kg
Stool	6-7.5 ml/kg	4.5-5 ml/kg	4-4.5 ml/kg	3.5-4 ml/kg	2.5-3 ml/kg
TOTAL	72-90 ml/kg	54-60 ml/kg	48-54 ml/kg	42-48 ml/kg	30-36 ml/kg

Based on standard pediatric caloric maintenance tables and water expenditure per 100 calories metabolized per 24 hours as listed in Biller, J.A., and Yeager, A.M.: The Harriet Lane handbook, ed. 9, Chicago, 1981, Year Book Medical Publishers, Inc.
*Insensible water losses/m^2 body surface area (BSA): approximately 300 ml/m^2/BSA daily.

Table 8-3 Calculation of daily maintenance fluid and electrolyte requirements for children

Child's weight	Kilogram body weight formula
Fluids	
Newborn (up to 72 hr after birth)	60-100 ml/kg
Up to 10 kg	100 ml/kg (may increase up to 150 ml/kg to provide caloric requirements if renal and cardiac function adequate)
11-20 kg	1000 ml for the first 10 kg + 50 ml/kg for each kg over 10 kg
21-30 kg	1500 ml for the first 20 kg + 25 ml/kg for each kg over 20 kg
Body surface area (BSA) formula: 1500 ml/m^2 BSA/day	
Electrolytes	
Sodium (Na^+)	3-4 mEq/kg/24 hr
Potassium (K^+)	2-3 mEq/kg/24 hr
Calcium (Ca^+)	50-100 mg/kg/24 hr
Magnesium (Mg^{++})	0.4-0.9 mEq/kg/day

Table 8-4 Causes and symptoms of common gastrointestinal electrolyte imbalances

Imbalance	Cause	Symptoms	Diagnostic tests
Sodium deficit (hyponatremia)	Excessive diaphoresis (e.g., cystic fibrosis), gastrointestinal suction or vomiting, water enemas and irrigations, ileostomy drainage, GI fistula drainage, biliary drainage, potent diuretics, excessive infusion of carbohydrate solution without electrolytes, obstruction, peritonitis, pancreatitis, diarrhea NOTE: Hyperglycemia may result in an artificially reduced serum sodium value that reverses as serum glucose is reduced	Apprehension, abdominal cramps, convulsions, oliguria or anuria, diarrhea, fingerprinting on sternum, muscle twitching, salivation, increased deep tendon reflexes, lethargy or confusion, vasomotor collapse: hypotension, tachycardia, cold, clammy skin, cyanosis	Decreased serum sodium, decreased serum chloride, decreased urine specific gravity, increased Hct, increased serum proteins, BUN, and creatinine
Sodium excess (hypernatremia)	Excessive ingestion of salt, watery diarrhea, inadequate water intake with milk and cream NOTE: With severe dehydration, serum sodium values may be elevated due to hemoconcentration; as the patient is rehydrated, serum sodium values may decrease	Dry, sticky mucous membranes, flushed skin, intense thirst, rough and dry tongue, oliguria or anuria, increase in temperature, firm tissue turgor, pitting edema, elevated blood pressure, weight gain (if fluid intake is normal), excitement, mania, convulsions	Increased serum sodium, increased serum chloride, increased urine specific gravity, increased RBC, Hct
Potassium deficit (hypokalemia)	Potent diuretics, vomiting, ulcerative colitis, diarrhea, fistulas of small intestine or colon, starvation or wasting disease, low sodium diet, GI suction, hemorrhage, chronic laxative use, water enema, peritonitis, pancreatitis, prolonged parenteral nutrition, acid-base imbalance	Thirst, malaise or muscle weakness, apathy or drowsiness, tremors, diminished reflexes, flaccid paralysis, tachycardia, hypotension, vomiting, diminished or absent bowel sounds, shallow respirations, anorexia, myocardial irritability	Decreased serum potassium, decreased serum chloride, increased serum HCO_3, acidic urine, ECG changes (see Chapter 3), cardiac arrhythmias: heart block, cardiac arrest, prolonged QT interval, ventricular irritability

Modified from Given, B., and Simmons, S.: Gastroenterology in clinical nursing, ed. 4, St. Louis, 1984, The C.V. Mosby Co.

Continued.

Table 8-4 Causes and symptoms of common gastrointestinal electrolyte imbalances—cont'd

Imbalance	Cause	Symptoms	Diagnostic tests
Metabolic alkalosis	Potent diuretics, vomiting (excess), ingestion of alkali (soluble antacids), GI suction, administration of adrenocortical hormones, potassium depletion, increased loss of chloride, intestinal obstruction, peritonitis, pancreatitis, prolonged hypercalcemia	Diminished or absent bowel sounds, irregular pulse, shallow, slow respiration, cyanosis, hypoxia: tremors, muscle twitching, confusion, irritability, muscle weakness, paresthesia, muscle cramps, tetany	Urine pH >7.0, serum pH >7.45, increased serum bicarbonate, decreased serum potassium, increased serum carbon dioxide, decreased serum chloride, decreased calcium ionization
Metabolic acidosis	Diabetes mellitus, systemic infections, malnutrition, excessive vomiting or diarrhea, pancreatitis, obstruction, lactic acidosis, increased loss of pancreatic juice, bile, intestinal juice	Shortness of breath, deep, rapid respirations (Kussmaul), anorexia, stupor → coma, weakness or malaise, flushed skin, soft eyeballs, decreased tissue turgor, restlessness, gastric dilation, headache, nausea or vomiting, asterixis	Urine pH <6.0, serum pH <7.35, decreased serum bicarbonate, decreased serum carbon dioxide, decreased serum chloride, decreased serum sodium, decreased serum potassium
Calcium deficit (hypocalcemia)	Acute pancreatitis, generalized peritonitis, excessive infusion of citrated blood, sprue, fistulas of pancreas or small intestine, malabsorption, diarrhea	Tingling of fingers and toes, tetany, abdominal cramps, muscle cramps and twitching, carpopedal spasm, convulsions	Decreased serum calcium, ECG changes (see Chapter 3)
Magnesium deficit	Malabsorption syndrome, diarrhea, bowel resection, alcoholism, hypercalcemia, diuretic therapy, diabetic acidosis, prolonged nasogastric suction	Insomnia, twitching, tremors, seizures, muscle weakness, leg or foot cramps, hypotension, arrhythmias, disorientation, convulsions	Decreased serum magnesium, normal serum calcium

digestive enzymes in humans. Some of the protein, fat, and carbohydrates of foods is also passed in the feces. In healthy individuals without malabsorptive disease, 92% of protein, 95% of fat, and 98% of carbohydrates ingested are absorbed.[38]

Digestion and absorption are a series of four sequential phases: the intraluminal phase, the mucosal (brush border) phase, the intracellular phase, and the removal or delivery phase (Fig. 8-3).

The intraluminal phase involves aspects of digestion that occur within the lumen of the stomach or small intestine. Secretion of digestive enzymes and bile is part of the intraluminal phase. The mucosal phase includes the parts of digestion that occur along the brush border of the intestinal villi, and the intracellular phase occurs within the intestinal cell. The removal phase indicates the transportation of the final products from the intestinal cell to other organs for storage or metabolism.

Absorption consists primarily of the transfer of

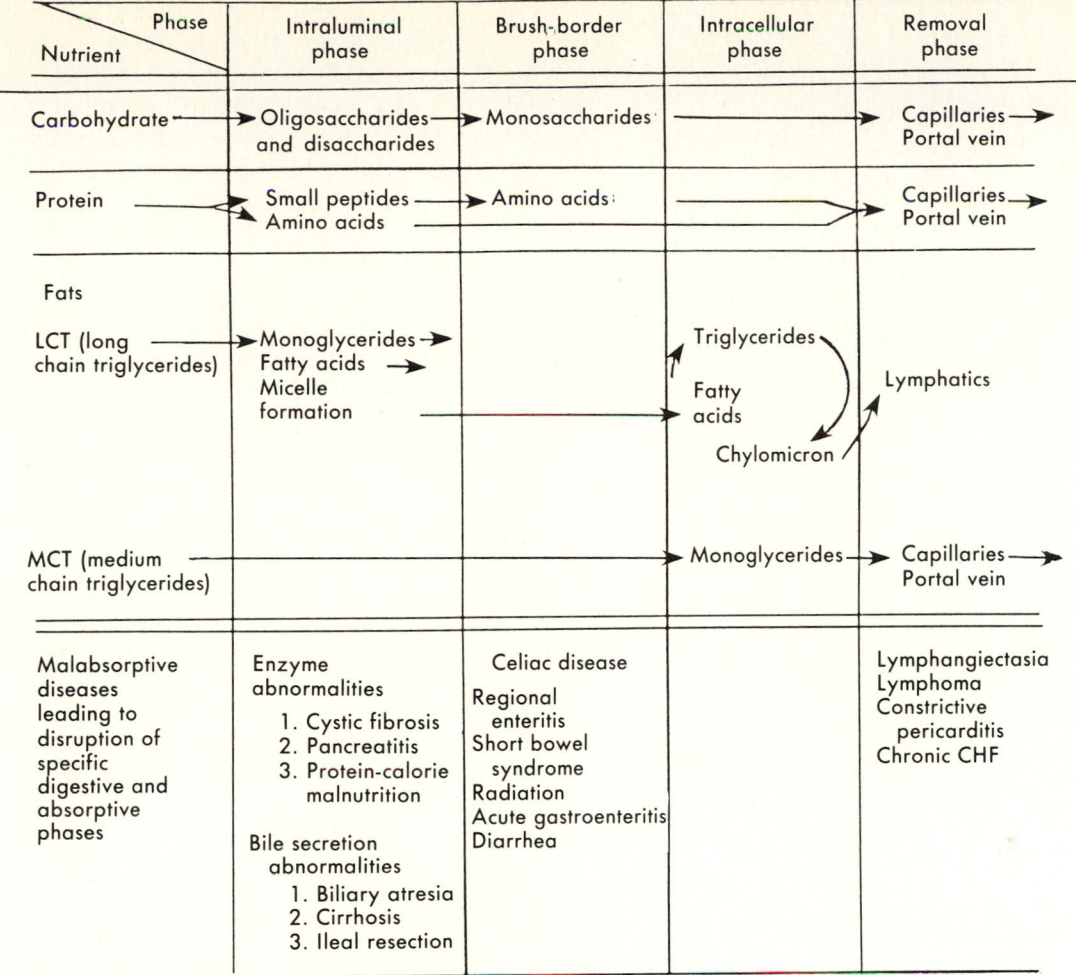

Nutrient \ Phase	Intraluminal phase	Brush-border phase	Intracellular phase	Removal phase
Carbohydrate	Oligosaccharides and disaccharides →	Monosaccharides		Capillaries Portal vein →
Protein	Small peptides — Amino acids	Amino acids		Capillaries Portal vein →
Fats				
LCT (long chain triglycerides)	Monoglycerides → Fatty acids → Micelle formation		Triglycerides ↗ Fatty acids Chylomicron ↗	Lymphatics
MCT (medium chain triglycerides)			Monoglycerides →	Capillaries Portal vein →
Malabsorptive diseases leading to disruption of specific digestive and absorptive phases	Enzyme abnormalities 1. Cystic fibrosis 2. Pancreatitis 3. Protein-calorie malnutrition Bile secretion abnormalities 1. Biliary atresia 2. Cirrhosis 3. Ileal resection	Celiac disease Regional enteritis Short bowel syndrome Radiation Acute gastroenteritis Diarrhea		Lymphangiectasia Lymphoma Constrictive pericarditis Chronic CHF

Fig. 8-3 Phases of digestion and absorption. Note that some digestive or absorptive phases are necessary for nutrient breakdown, and others are not. The brush-border phase is essential for carbohydrate digestion and absorption whereas it is not necessary for fat. Injury to mucosal brush border secondary to diarrhea leads to acute carbohydrate malabsorption.

Modified from Gray, G.M.: Mechanism of digestion and absorption of food. In Sleisinger, M.H., and Fordtran, J.S., editors: Gastrointestinal disease, ed. 2, Philadelphia, 1978, W.B. Saunders Co.

nutrients from the lumen of the small intestine through the intestinal brush border into the intestinal cell, where the nutrients enter the blood and lymph vessels. Limited amounts of water, alcohol, simple salts, and glucose are absorbed through the gastric mucosa; the small intestine is by far the most important organ for absorption. The most active absorptive areas in the small intestine are the initial third of the duodenum and the first portion of the jejunum (Table 8-5).

■ METABOLISM

Nutrients pass from the blood into the cells. *Metabolism* is defined as the processes by which cells convert the nutrients into energy that can be utilized for performance of work and for synthesis of new compounds vital for cellular structure and function.[43] The process by which nutrient molecules are degraded, with concurrent release of energy and subsequent elimination of waste products, is generally

Table 8-5 Sites of absorption of nutrients within the gastrointestinal tract[6]

Nutrient	Site of absorption
Glucose	Lower duodenum, upper jejunum
Amino acids	Lower duodenum, jejunum
Fats	Lower duodenum, upper jejunum
Iron	Duodenum
Calcium	Duodenum
Sucrose	Jejunum, ileum
Lactose	Jejunum, upper ileum
Vitamin D	Jejunum, ileum
Vitamin B_{12}	Terminal ileum

known as *catabolism. Anabolism* refers to the synthesis of new compounds. The anabolic processes depend on energy derived from the catabolic processes. Metabolism is an ongoing process in every cell of the body, requiring a continuous supply of nutrients.

In the period immediately following ingestion of food, the levels of most nutrients in the blood available for metabolic processes rise because of absorption of these nutrients from the intestine. The rate of absorption varies with the specific nutrient, the quantity ingested, and the individual. In general, the peak blood level for carbohydrates (glucose) is reached in 1 hour, and for fats (chylomicron triglycerides) in 4 to 6 hours after ingestion. The peak blood level of protein (amino acid) is reached between 1 and 4 hours after eating.[38] After absorption, the uptake of nutrients from the blood by the tissues is rapid and eventually results in a gradual return in the blood levels of the nutrients to fasting levels. In most individuals, fasting blood levels for glucose are reached 2 to 3 hours after eating, and fasting levels of triglycerides are attained by 8 to 12 hours after eating. The removal of some amino acids by the tissues is so rapid that only small increases in blood levels occur for only a short time during absorption.

Many nutrients enter the cellular catabolic pathways immediately. The remaining nutrients are converted to various storage forms in liver, muscle, and fat; they can be utilized from these stores when needed. Some glucose is converted to glycogen to replenish tissue stores; however, since the body has a limited ability to store glycogen, most of the remaining glucose is converted to fat and stored as triglycerides in the adipose tissue and in the liver and muscle. Excess dietary fatty acids also are stored as triglycerides. Protein synthesis occurs in the tissue after ingestion of a balanced mixture of amino acids; excess amino acids are oxidized to provide energy, or they are converted to glucose or fat.

■ NUTRITIONAL (ENERGY) REQUIREMENTS

A principle function of the gastrointestinal tract is to provide a means for nourishing the body. Nutrition is the mechanism by which the human body maintains its energy balance. To maintain a steady state, the energy content of food must equal the energy expenditure by the body. The body's basic energy requirement is called the basal metabolic rate (BMR). BMR is the energy required for the maintenance of fundamental cellular activities essential to the maintenance of life, particularly maintenance of active transport in the cells. Also included in this basal energy requirement are activities of the brain, muscle, kidneys, liver, and other tissues; the mechanical work performed by the contraction of the respiratory, cardiac, and gastrointestinal muscles; and the heat produced by metabolic processes.[43] The BMR is the total energy requirement of all the individual cells, tissues, and organs of the body, and it equals approximately 90% of the total energy that is expended by an individual in 24 hours.

Some factors known to affect BMR include:
1. *Age.* BMR is highest at ages up to 24 months; then the BMR decreases as age increases.
2. *Nutritional status.* The BMR decreases with extreme starvation and chronic obesity.
3. *Temperature.* Each degree centigrade of temperature elevation increases BMR by 12%.
4. *Pathologic states* such as trauma, infection, and disease. The presence of a malignancy has been reported to increase the patient's BMR by as much as 120%; surgical procedures increase the BMR by as much as 80%.[14]

In children the BMR must also include the requirement for growth. Physical growth is defined as an increase in the size of an individual as measured by changes in height or weight. Growth occurs continuously from conception to full maturity, but it is not a uniform process. It consists of two periods of rapid growth—infancy and adolescence—separated by a period of uniform but slower increase in size. Infants normally double their birth weight by 5 to 6 months of age and triple it by the end of the first year. Growth during the second year of life slows down, and a weight gain of only 8 to 10 pounds is considered average.[14] Thus infants who tripled their weight during the first year will be approximately four times their birth weight at the end of 2 years. From 2 to 9 years of age, annual weight gain is approximately 5 pounds.[80]

As a rule, annual height increments are highest during infancy, then gradually decrease until the period of the adolescent growth spurt. These annual increments in height usually average 2½ inches per year until adolescence. Birth length is usually doubled by 4 years.

It is important to graph height and weight measurements on standard growth charts to obtain information about the child's nutritional needs and to assess the effects of an illness on growth. The child with an acute weight loss will need additional calories to achieve "catch-up" growth as well as to maintain daily caloric requirements.[80]

When daily nutritional requirements for hospitalized children are calculated (Table 8-6), consideration must be given to the distribution of the caloric requirement (Table 8-7). If a child is comatose, caloric intake may be reduced because of absence of physical activity. If the child is febrile, caloric requirements are increased because of increased BMR requirements. The presence of gastrointestinal disease, which impairs nutrition, must also be considered (see the box on p. 558). Specific daily requirements for nutrients and major vitamins in infants and children are listed in Appendix E.

■ Common Clinical Conditions

■ DEHYDRATION
■ Etiology

Dehydration occurs when the total output of all fluids and electrolytes exceeds the individual's total fluid intake. The fluid deficit in dehydration can range from mild to very severe. Three important factors in evaluating the degree of dehydration in infants are that (1) 75% to 80% of the infant's body weight is water,[86] (2) the infant's high metabolic and respiratory rate demands a large water volume, and (3) the infant's immature kidneys are not able to readily concentrate urine.[39]

Table 8-6 Nutritional requirements for infants and children[23,33]

Age	Calories/kg/24 hr
Up to 6 mo	120
6-12 mo	100
12-36 mo	90-95
4 yr-10 yr	80
>10 yr, male	45
>10 yr, female	38

Nutrient	Percent of total calories	
Carbohydrates	40%-45%	combined 85%-88%
Fat	40%	
Protein	20%	

Table 8-7 Distribution of energy requirements for infants and children[9,33]

	Percent of caloric requirements*	
	Infant	Child
BMR	50%	50%
Activity	20%	Combined 48%†
Growth	25%	
Loss in stools	5%	2%

*An additional 12% is added to BMR for each degree centigrade elevation of body temperature.
†Fluctuates with age and activity level.

GASTROINTESTINAL FACTORS THAT IMPAIR GENERAL NUTRITION

Factors that interfere with intake

Impaired appetite, nausea, vomiting, anorexia, pain, medications, infections, depression

Disease: ulcers, diarrhea, biliary or liver disease, obstruction, malignancy

Medical therapy, diagnostic tests

Factors that increase tissue destruction

Malignancy

Tissue ulceration or necrosis

Factors that interfere with absorption

Absence of normal digestive secretions: achlorhydria, biliary obstruction, pancreatic insufficiency, cystic fibrosis

Intestinal hypermotility: diarrhea, inflammatory bowel disease

Decreased absorbing surface: resection of small bowel

Impaired mucosal intrinsic mechanics of absorption: celiac sprue, Crohn's disease, *Salmonella* species

Drugs preventing absorption

Decreased bile salts: parenchymal liver disease, Crohn's disease, drugs (neomycin or cholestyramine)

Endocrine and metabolic disorders: diabetes mellitus

Factors that interfere with utilization and storage

Impaired liver function: hepatitis, cirrhosis

Neoplasms of gastrointestinal tract; pancreatitis

Factors that increase excretion or loss

Serous exudate, pancreatitis, ascites, wound drainage

Hemorrhage

Abscesses and fistulas

Nasogastric or intestinal suction, nausea, vomiting

Glycosuria and albuminuria

Surgery: vagotomy, gastric resection with gastrojejunal anastomosis

Diarrhea: inflammatory bowel disease

Protein loss: gastritis, colitis, megacolon, inflammatory bowel disease, malignancy

Factors that increase nutritional requirements

Increased metabolism: fever, chronic infection, maligiancy

Rise in physical activity

Rapid growth

Insulin, high-carbohydrate diet

Modified from Given, B.A., and Simmons, S.J.: Gastroenterology in clinical nursing, ed. 4, St. Louis, 1984, The C.V. Mosby Co.

Table 8-8   Types of dehydration

Type	Deficit	Serum Na+ concentration (mEq/L)	Water loss (ml/kg)
Isotonic	5%-10% loss of body weight; water loss is from intravascular (extracellular) fluid	130-150	50-150
Hypotonic	High electrolyte loss or excessive solute-poor fluid intake; osmotic electrolyte shifts cause Na+ loss in stools and water shifts to intracellular fluid, resulting in decreased intravascular volume and shock	130	40-80
Hypertonic	Greater water loss than electrolyte loss or greater intake of electrolytes than water, and osmotic shifts cause water to move from the cells to the vascular space (so intravascular volume may be maintained at the expense of the cells); signs and symptoms develop more slowly	150	60-170

■ Pathophysiology

Dehydration may be classified as isotonic, hypotonic, or hypertonic. In addition, the degree of dehydration may be indicated as a percent of total body weight loss. If the child's normal weight (before dehydration) is not available, the degree of dehydration must be determined by clinical assessment. (Table 8-8 defines degrees of dehydration and associated changes in water and serum electrolyte concentrations.) For infants and young children with isotonic dehydration, the fluid deficit is evaluated as 5%, 10%, or 15% dehydration:

Mild deficit: 5% dehydration, or a loss of body weight up to 50 ml per kilogram body weight

Moderate deficit: 5% to 10% dehydration, or a loss of body weight up to 100 ml per kilogram body weight

Severe deficit: 10% to 15% dehydration, or a loss of body weight up to 150 ml per kilogram body weight[75]

Total body water and extracellular fluid volume represent a smaller percentage of body weight in older children and adults than in infants. Any percentage loss of body weight resulting from fluid and electrolyte deficits indicates a more severe depletion of fluid compartments in the older age-groups. Therefore isotonic dehydration for the older child is classified as mild if 3% of body weight is lost, moderate if 6% of body weight is lost, and severe if 9% of body weight is lost.

Fluid loss with *hypotonic* dehydration is from *extracellular* fluid, causing the clinical signs of dehydration to be more severe, although the quantity of fluid loss is smaller than with hypertonic dehydration. With this form of dehydration the loss of body sodium is greater than the loss of body water. With *hypertonic* dehydration, the source of fluid loss is *intracellular*. The clinical signs of hypertonic dehydration are generally not as severe as those with hypotonic dehydration; however, the quantity of fluid loss is greater. With hypertonic dehydration, the loss of body fluid is greater than the loss of body sodium[75] (see Chapter 7 for further discussion of dehydration).

In children, dehydration is most often the result of an acute viral or bacterial infection or gastroenteritis and resultant diarrhea. Table 8-9 lists characteristics of infectious diarrhea.

■ Clinical signs and symptoms

The clinical signs and symptoms of dehydration may include changes in vital signs and physical appearance. Severity of these changes is related to the degree of dehydration. Fig. 8-4 illustrates the degree of dehydration according to clinical assessment in infants with isotonic dehydration (see also Chapter 7).

Table 8-9 Characteristics of acute infectious diarrhea

	Rotavirus	Norwalk agent	*Shigella*
Site of infection	Small intestine	Small intestine	Distal ileum and colon
Pathogenic mechanism	Cell damage and inflammation	Cell damage and inflammation	Epithelial penetration
Stool character			
Volume	Moderate	Moderate	Low
Frequency	Up to 10/day		Great
Consistency	Watery		Viscous
Mucus	Rarely		Frequently
Blood	Absent		Frequently
Odor	Odorless		Relatively odorless
Color	Green, yellow, or colorless		Bloody/green
Leukocytes	Absent		Present
Nausea and vomiting	At onset	Present	Rare
Fever	Present	Low grade	Frequent
Pain	Tenesmus	Abdominal cramps Myalgia Headache	Tenesmus Cramps Headache
Miscellaneous		Malaise Anorexia	Convulsions, onset often abrupt
Duration (untreated)	5-7 days	Self-limiting 24 hours	>7 days
Treatment*			Ampicillin when susceptible

Courtesy Ross Laboratories: Acute diarrhea in infants and children, Pamphlet F180, Columbus, Ohio, Jan. 1979, Ross Laboratories.
*Immediate treatment aimed at relieving dehydration in all gastroenteritis.

Salmonella	Enteroinvasive *E. coli*	Enterotoxigenic *E. coli*	Cholera
Ileum and colon	Colon and distal small bowel	Small bowel	Small bowel
Epithelial penetration	Epithelial penetration	Enterotoxin production	Enterotoxin production
Small	Small	Profuse	Copious
Frequent	Frequent	Frequent	Almost continuous
Slimy	Viscous	Watery	Watery
Present	Present	Present	Flecks
Sometimes	Present	Absent	
Foul (rotten eggs)	Not specific	Strongly fecal	Fish-like
Green	Bloody/green	Colorless	
Present	Present		
Present		None	Rare
Common	Present	None	
Tenesmus	Tenesmus	Sometimes	Cramping
Colic	Cramping		
Headache			
Bacteremia	Urgency	Urgency	
Focal infections may occur	Hypotension	Occasional abdominal distention	
	Systemic toxemia		
3-7 days	Variable	Brief	
Ampicillin or chloramphenicol only with sepsis and focal suppurative disease	Colistin	Neomycin	Tetracycline

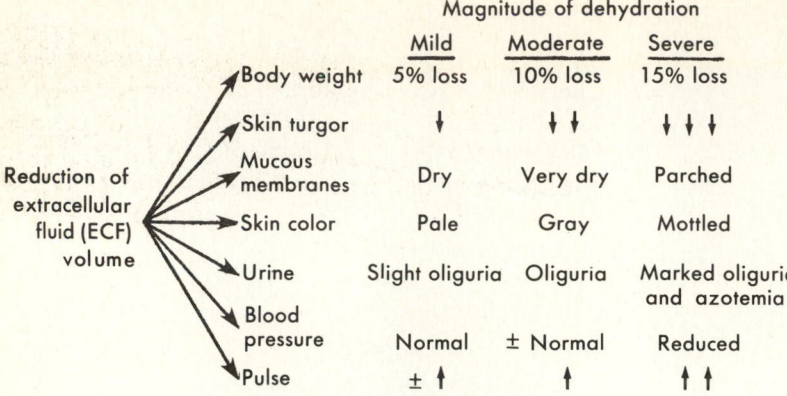

Fig. 8-4 Clinical signs of *isotonic* dehydration in an infant. Correlation of the intensity of clinical signs with the magnitude of dehydration.

From Winters, R.: The body fluids in pediatrics, Boston, 1973, Little, Brown & Co.

On physical examination, the child's eyes appear sunken and dark. Dehydrated infants less than 16 to 18 months of age often have marked depression of the anterior fontanelle. The skin turgor is a good indicator of level of hydration. Normally, when the skin and subcutaneous tissue are pinched between the thumb and the first finger and then released, they return to their former position immediately. Delay in this return is called *tenting* of the skin. Tenting is indicative of severe dehydration. Skin and mucous membranes may feel dry or clammy, depending on the type of dehydration present. Urine volume is decreased, and urine specific gravity and osmolality are increased.

Dry skin and mucous membranes and poor skin turgor are observed when the child has mild (5%) dehydration. The child's temperature may be low and the heart rate rapid, but the blood pressure and respiratory rate are usually normal. With moderate dehydration (approximately 10%), the child looks ill and has dry mucous membranes, poor skin turgor, and a depressed fontanelle. Gross (approximately 15%) dehydration is associated with signs of peripheral circulatory failure. The child is tachycardic and tachypneic, skin perfusion is decreased, extremities are cool and clammy, nail beds and mucous membranes are pale, urine output is dramatically reduced or absent, peripheral pulses are weak, and blood pressure may be lower than the patient's normal blood pressure. With hypovolemic shock (usually approximately 15% dehydration), the child appears moribund. Severe hypotension and signs of circulatory failure (including metabolic acidosis) are present. Rapid, shallow respirations may be seen with respira-

tory compensation for metabolic acidosis.

Evaluation of the child's responsiveness may provide further information regarding his fluid balance. Irritability and lethargy are present in the infant with dehydration. The child becomes restless and agitated, then becomes confused and disoriented. Mental irritability may be an early indication of shifts of fluid from the extracellular to the intracellular space and should be particularly noted during the administration of parenteral fluid.[19]

Dehydration causes imbalances in sodium and potassium levels. Fluid loss from excessive sweating, diarrhea, or vomiting can cause sodium depletion. In fact, *total body* sodium is depleted in all three forms of dehydration.[75] With hypotonic dehydration, serum sodium concentration is usually low. When hypertonic dehydration is present, serum sodium concentration is high, because of relatively greater water loss and hemoconcentration. In all forms of dehydration, some sodium will need to be replaced. Potassium depletion occurs with increased urine output or poor potassium intake. Serum potassium values may rise in the presence of metabolic acidosis (they may fall with correction of the acidosis).

■ **Medical treatment and nursing interventions**

Acute medical management is aimed at correcting the fluid deficit rather than the cause of the deficit. The treatment of dehydration is threefold: (1) to treat and correct hypovolemia, (2) to replace excessive ongoing fluid losses, and (3) to supply maintenance fluids and electrolytes.

Treatment of hypovolemia is aimed at expanding intravascular fluid volume to improve cardiovascular and renal function. Since intravenous (IV) access may be difficult to obtain in the poorly perfused child, an IV cutdown or insertion of a central venous catheter may be required. To restore circulation, bolus administration (10-20 ml/kg body weight) of normal saline or lactated Ringer's solution is given. This bolus of fluid can be repeated two or three times if necessary to restore circulation. During this infusion the nurse must monitor changes in the child's central venous pressure (CVP) and systemic perfusion. A CVP of less than 5 mm Hg is usually noted when the patient is hypovolemic, unless congestive heart failure is also present. During fluid administration, the CVP and blood pressure should rise and the child's heart rate should fall to approximately normal levels. Once these have reached acceptable values (in light of the child's previous and current clinical condition), the fluid therapy is tapered. Fluid therapy is then directed toward replacement of the quantity and composition of the deficit and any ongoing losses. Potassium supplements are usually not given until adequate urine output is demonstrated, since hyperkalemia can quickly develop in the presence of oliguria or anuria.

Calculation of fluids for rehydration is based on the child's degree and type of dehydration. Table 8-10 provides guidelines for fluid and electrolyte replacement with various types of dehydration. If the child's preillness weight and present weight are known, the absolute amount of fluid deficit can be calculated; if, however, such weights are unknown, fluid replacement will have to be estimated by the table. In general, if isotonic or hypotonic dehydration is present, *in addition to normal maintenance fluids* the child's fluid deficit is replaced within the initial 24 hours of therapy. Half of the deficit is replaced during the first 8 hours, and the remaining half of the deficit is replaced during the second 16 hours of therapy. It is important that the nurse ensure that the child be given replacement fluids in addition to his normal maintenance fluids. Correction of fluid deficit in the infant or child with *hypertonic dehydration* is accomplished more slowly (see the section on dehydration in Chapter 7). The following case study is provided to demonstrate appropriate fluid therapy calculations for a child with isotonic or hypotonic dehydration (see Chapter 7 for a case study pertaining to fluid replacement for *hypernatremic dehydration*).

CASE STUDY

A 9 kg, 10-month-old infant is admitted with a history of vomiting and diarrhea. His weight before the illness was 10 kg. He demonstrates a sunken fontanelle, dry and pale mucous membranes, skin tenting, cool, clammy extremities, slow peripheral capillary filling, oliguria, and weak peripheral pulses. Blood pressure and serum electrolytes are normal. This child's hourly IV fluid requirements for the first 8 hours and the second 16 hours are calculated thus:

Degree of deficit:	1 of 10 kg (or 10%)
Fluid deficit:	1 kg (1000 ml)
Replacement during initial 8 hours:	½ of fluid deficit or 500 ml over 8 hours, or 62.5 ml/hour for 8 hours
Normal daily maintenance fluid requirement:	100 ml/kg/24 hours or 1000 ml/24 hours, or 41.7 ml/hour for 24 hours

Therefore the IV fluid rate during the initial 8 hours of therapy will total 62.5 ml + 41.7 ml per hour, or 104.2 ml per hour for 8 hours.

Replacement during next 16 hours:	½ of fluid deficit or 500 ml over 16 hours, or 31.25 ml/hour for 16 hours

Therefore the IV fluid rate during the next 16 hours of therapy will total 31.25 ml per hour + 41.7 ml per hour, or 72.95 ml per hour for 16 hours.

Summary. In the first 24 hours of therapy, the infant will receive a total of 2098.4 ml. If there are additional ongoing sources of fluid loss, additional fluids may be required. The type of IV fluids administered will depend on the child's electrolyte status and composition of the fluid losses. Normal or half-normal saline is usually prescribed for rehydration.

Restoration of normal fluid and electrolyte balance in the dehydrated child requires careful observation and regulation of fluid therapy. Assessment includes observation of indirect evidence of systemic perfusion (color, warmth, and pulses of extremities; quantity and specific gravity of urine output; and blood pressure), respiratory rate and effort, and skin color and turgor.

Accurate measurement of the child's daily weight provides a consistent parameter for evaluation of fluid therapy. The child should be weighed at the same time of day on the same scale, and the specific scale used for the child's daily weight is noted on the nursing-care plan. Meticulous measurement of all intake and output (urine, stool, nasogastric drainage, and emesis) is imperative. Rehydration is often achieved during the first 24-48 hours of therapy, and the child's clinical appearance should gradually improve during that time. Once adequate intravascular volume has been restored, systemic perfusion usu-

Table 8-10 Correction of deficits of fluids, minerals, and glucose

Component	Deficit	Dose			Example (5-kg infant)		
Water*	5% (mild)	Maintenance plus maintenance × 0.5			500 ml + 250 ml = 750 ml		
	10% (moderate)	Maintenance plus maintenance × 1.0			500 ml + 500 ml = 1,000 ml		
	15% (severe)	Maintenance plus maintenance × 1.5			500 ml + 750 ml = 1,250 ml		
Electrolytes		Hypotonic	Isotonic	Hypertonic†	Hypotonic	Isotonic	Hypertonic
		(mEq/kg/24 hr)			(mEq/kg/24 hr)		
Sodium (Na)		10-12	8-10	2-4	55	45	15
Potassium (K)‡		8-10	8-10	0-4	45	45	10
Chloride (Cl)		10-12	8-10	2-6§	55	45	0-15
Calcium (Ca)		200 mg/kg/24 hr divided, by slow IV push every 3-4 hr (as gluconate)			≈ 150 mg every 4 hr		
Magnesium (Mg)		1 mEq/kg/24 hr in 3 divided doses, by slow IV push			≈ 1.5 mEq every 8 hr		
Phosphate (PO₄)		5-10 mg/kg (0.15-0.33 mmol/kg) IV over 6 hr (initial dose, then repeat measurement)			≈ 3.75 mg over 6 hr		
Glucose		Increase by 100 mg/kg/hr repeatedly until serum glucose is 90 mg/dl (may desire higher concentrations, e.g., in Reye's syndrome)					

From Levin, D.L.: Abnormalities in fluids, minerals, and glucose. In Levin, D.L., Morriss, F.C., and Moore, G.C., editors: A practical guide to pediatric intensive, ed. 2, St. Louis, 1984, The C.V. Mosby Co.
*Usually the first half of correction is carried out in the first 8 hours, and the second half of correction is carried out over the next 16 hours. If the patient is hypotensive or in shock, immediately give 0.9% sodium chloride or lactated Ringer's solution, 20 ml/kg. Repeat this until arterial blood pressure, capillary filling, and urinary output are restored.
†Patients with hypertonic dehydration may develop cerebral edema and seizures with rapid correction of water deficit. Correct such patients slowly over 48 to 72 hours. Never give such a patient fluid without some salt content (usually these patients are acidotic, and sodium bicarbonate can be added to D₅W to correct acidosis and provide some salt). This will help prevent the development of cerebral edema.
‡Potassium at a concentration ≤80 mEq/L at a rate ≤0.3 mEq/kg/hr.
§Balance indicates excess at the beginning of treatment.

ally improves. Urine specific gravity and osmolality should be measured and recorded at least every 8 hours to evaluate the effectiveness of rehydration and the kidney's ability to concentrate urine. With rehydration and normal kidney function, urine volume will increase and the specific gravity should fall. The nurse must monitor the child's urine volume and tolerance of fluid therapy. If the child's CVP continues to rise (above 5 mm Hg) with no urine output beyond the first 24 hours of therapy, the child's kidney function (including analysis of serum and urine creatinine and serum blood urea nitrogen, or BUN) should be checked. Reevaluation of fluid therapy is necessary if anuria persists, or fluid overload may result. The child's serum potassium concentration must be monitored closely as the child's acid-base status and urine volume change. The electrolyte content of any ongoing fluid losses should be checked so that appropriate electrolyte replacement can be given.

Restoration of adequate fluid volume depends on uninterrupted administration of appropriate parenteral fluids. This, in turn, requires insertion of a reliable IV catheter. If the nurse thinks that the catheter is tenuous, she must ensure that it is replaced with a more secure catheter (or personally replace it, as hospital policy allows). The IV line must be taped securely so that even if the child moves vigorously, the line will not be dislodged. The child's hands should be mittened, and the catheterized extremity may need to be restrained.

Children with diarrhea often require isolation until the cause of the diarrhea is determined. Enteric isolation must be enforced with meticulous attention to hand washing. On the child's admission and 24 hours later, stool cultures are obtained. If a nonlactose fermenter is identified in the stool, the child remains in isolation until repeated cultures reveal normal stool flora.

As the gastrointestinal infection resolves, treatment becomes supportive. Initially (when stools are frequent and watery), the child receives nothing by mouth and maintenance fluid requirements are provided by IV fluids. The irritated gastrointestinal tract requires a period of rest, followed by gradual resumption of oral feedings. Dextrose water, Pedialyte, or Jell-O water is initially introduced. If these fluids are tolerated, the infant's regular formula is offered in gradually increased concentrations (i.e., quarter strength, half strength, three-quarters strength, and full strength). If diarrhea resumes during the advancement of formula concentration, the child is placed back on the last-tolerated formula concentration.

If diarrhea is noted following feeding, the nurse should check the stool for the presence of *reducing*

sugars. To perform this test, a small amount of stool is mixed with approximately 10 drops of water, and a Clinitest is performed on the resulting suspension. When the Clinitest is positive, simple reducing sugars are present in the stool; these sugars are derived from bacterial metabolism of nonabsorbed complex sugars. This means that malabsorption is occurring. If reducing sugars are present, a physician should be notified, and oral feedings may be discontinued temporarily to allow the gastrointestinal tract further rest.

Since intestinal mucosal injury results in a temporary lactase enzyme deficiency, use of a lactose-free formula and elimination of dietary milk and milk products may be necessary during the recovery phase of diarrhea.

■ ACUTE ABDOMEN
■ Etiology

The term "acute abdomen" is used to describe any abdominal condition for which urgent surgical intervention must be considered. Patients may also be said to have an acute abdomen when they complain of the sudden onset of abdominal pain or tenderness. An acute abdomen usually results from abdominal inflammation, obstruction, perforation, hemorrhage, or blunt trauma. In infants, an acute abdomen may result from gastrointestinal perforation (organ rupture) because of intestinal obstruction, ischemia, gangrenous volvulus, necrotizing enterocolitis, or iatrogenic perforations.[69] An acute abdomen is characteristically seen with a perforated appendix, intestinal disease, trauma, or severe inflammatory bowel disease. Since peritonitis may cause or complicate the development of the acute abdomen, the need for urgent surgery is always considered.

Acute abdomen caused by blunt trauma may result from motor vehicle accidents, fights, falls from windows, bicycles, or sleds, or trauma resulting from child abuse. Blunt trauma is deceptive and difficult to diagnose because signs and symptoms can be masked or delayed for several hours or days. Untreated visceral perforation or gastrointestinal hemorrhage following blunt trauma will result in peritonitis or hypovolemic shock. Indications for emergency surgery after blunt trauma include persistent decline in hematocrit and evidence of progressive hypovolemia (hemorrhage) despite adequate fluid intake and absence of other bleeding sites, severe abdominal tenderness with rigidity, development of peritonitis, or evidence of visceral rupture or peritoneal perforation.

Penetrating abdominal trauma is less common in children but can occur from motor vehicle accidents, gunshot wounds, or stab wounds. These injuries require emergency surgical intervention.

Appendiceal obstruction and infection may cause appendicitis. Appendiceal perforation with appendicitis is more likely in school-age children or adolescents and usually results in development of peritonitis.

■ Pathophysiology

Bowel perforation or rupture may result from progressive inflammation or trauma. This perforation causes leakage of gastrointestinal content into the peritoneum. If the peritoneal defenses are successful in containing the inflammation, the area of peritoneal insult may remain localized and an abscess may form. However, if local responses are unsuccessful, diffuse peritonitis may result.

Upper gastrointestinal perforation will result in leakage of hydrochloric acid, digestive enzymes, or bile, causing chemical irritation of the peritoneum, and a chemical (aseptic) peritonitis may follow. Leakage of fecal material from the lower gastrointestinal tract not only releases aerobic and anaerobic bacteria into the peritoneum, but it may release endotoxins from the cell walls of aerobic gram-negative bacteria (such as *Escherichia coli*). Bacteria and endotoxins may cause a suppurative bacterial peritonitis, and they may be absorbed through the peritoneal surface to cause sepsis.[78]

Hemoperitoneum from blunt or penetrating abdominal injury or from vascular injury may not produce peritonitis, since whole blood does not act as a chemical irritant. If the red blood cells lyse, however, the hemoglobin and iron will cause peritoneal irritation, producing chemical peritonitis. A secondary bacterial infection may also occur.[78]

Peritoneal contamination or irritation produces increased blood flow to and capillary permeability in the affected area. This causes transudation of fluid into the peritoneal cavity. Children with an acute abdomen may demonstrate shifting of body fluids, known as "third spacing." *Third spacing* is internal redistribution of intracellular and intravascular fluid into nonfunctional, extravascular compartments, especially into the peritoneum, bowel wall, and other tissues. As a result of this large amount of intravascular fluid loss, the patient may demonstrate evidence of hypovolemia and low cardiac output.[78]

With peritoneal irritation or injury, bowel motility is depressed, and an ileus usually results. The bowel lumen fills with air and fluid, and abdominal distention is noted.

■ Clinical signs and symptoms

The most common symptom of an acute abdomen is pain. The pain secondary to peritonitis characteristically increases with any movement, including breathing, so that the patient's respirations are usually rapid and shallow. Voluntary, then involuntary, abdominal wall contraction (guarding) is noted before the examination, and the abdomen is tender to palpation. Following release of slight pressure on the abdominal wall, *rebound tenderness* is also noted. Bowel sounds may be decreased or absent. Anorexia, nausea, vomiting, and a low-grade fever may also be noted. The child usually is tachycardic (because of pain, hypovolemia, or fever); he lies very still and appears to be ill. In children under 5 years of age, the cause of abdominal pain may be difficult to discern, since the child has difficulty localizing and expressing pain, and crying produces abdominal rigidity.[68]

Appendicitis characteristically causes abrupt, persistent pain, localized to the right lower quadrant. This pain may be accompanied by nausea and vomiting. Abdominal guarding and rebound tenderness are often present. In children, appendiceal perforation may occur more readily because the wall of the appendix is very thin and the immature omentum may not provide protection against peritonitis.[32,68] The vast majority of those under 4 years have a perforated appendix by the time the diagnosis is made.[68]

In young children, visceral perforation causes signs and symptoms of an acute illness and third spacing of fluids. The child has a fever, soon begins to appear septic and dehydrated, and demonstrates signs of hypovolemia. When perforation occurs, children over 5 years of age may feel relieved of pain. This frequently encourages the child not to complain; thus medical treatment may be postponed. However, the child often will continue to vomit or will have diarrhea, causing further loss of fluid and electrolytes. If large amounts of intravascular fluid are lost to the peritoneal cavity, increasing abdominal girth, abdominal distention, evidence of systemic hypovolemia (tachycardia, decreased urine output, low CVP), and, finally, decreased peripheral pulses, poor peripheral perfusion, hypotension, and metabolic acidosis will result. Untreated visceral perforation can lead to decreased blood flow to the remaining bowel, subsequent bowel necrosis, and, possibly, death.

Severe abdominal pain, tenderness, and distention can compromise diaphragmatic excursion, resulting in decreased effective ventilation (hypoventilation). Mild hypoxemia or hypercapnia may be noted. Atelectasis (especially in the lung bases) may be noted on a chest radiograph.

If visceral perforation has occurred, free air in the abdominal cavity may be seen on an abdominal x-ray film. In addition, edema of the bowel wall and intraluminal bowel air will be visualized. Radionuclide imaging of the liver and spleen will not only help determine their size, position, and shape, but it will demonstrate the presence of rupture or laceration of these organs.[72]

■ **Medical treatment and nursing interventions**

Medical management of the child with an acute abdomen begins with expansion of the child's intravascular volume to correct hypovolemia and shock. Frequently, a peritoneal lavage is necessary to determine if abdominal bleeding has occurred. A nasogastric tube is inserted to decompress the stomach, and any drainage obtained is checked for the presence of blood. A urinary catheter is also inserted to check for hematuria (which may occur with kidney, ureter, or bladder trauma) and to enable accurate measurement of urine output. If significant bleeding or clinical deterioration are present, urgent surgical intervention is necessary.

The nurse is primarily responsible for careful assessment of the child's condition. Often, the child with an acute abdomen is admitted to the pediatric critical-care unit for skilled, continuous observation; thus it is imperative that the nurse be able to recognize early signs of clinical deterioration in the child, which include:

1. *Signs of peritonitis.* Fever, abdominal tenderness, rigidity, and distention; diffuse pain, nausea, vomiting, and decreased bowel motility
2. *Signs of third spacing of fluid.* Increasing abdominal girth, electrolyte imbalances, and evidence of hypovolemia (tachycardia, decreased urine volume, with increased urine specific gravity, low CVP, decreased intensity of peripheral pulses, cool extremities with decreased capillary refill, and, ultimately, hypotension and metabolic acidosis)
3. *Persistent pain.* Irritability, restlessness, elevated heart and respiratory rates, and possible increased systolic blood pressure
4. *Signs of abdominal obstruction.* Abdominal distention, vomiting (particularly projectile vomiting or vomiting of bile or fecal material), fever, absence of bowel sounds
5. *Signs of gastrointestinal hemorrhage.* Tachycardia; cool, clammy extremities; hematemesis, melena, and hematochezia (bloody

stools); signs of hypovolemia; and falling hemoglobin and hematocrit
6. *Signs of respiratory compromise secondary to increased abdominal tenderness and decreased diaphragmatic excursion.* Tachypnea, increased respiratory effort (retractions, nasal flaring, use of other accessory muscles of respiration, grunting), cyanosis, and hypoxemia or hypercapnia (if blood gases obtained)

Identification of the signs and symptoms of clinical deterioration should be promptly reported to the physician to avoid progressive deterioration, shock, and possibly, death.

Once the child develops abdominal distention, the head of the bed should be elevated 30 to 45 degrees to allow maximum diaphragmatic excursion. Emergency intubation and ventilation equipment should be readily available. Strict recording of all fluid intake and all output, including all emesis, stool, and urine and nasogastric secretion is important to assess the child's fluid balance. No oral fluid or food is provided since surgery may be necessary. Administration of IV fluids, with peripheral or central venous parenteral nutrition, may be necessary if oral intake is to be prohibited for several days.

■ **GASTROINTESTINAL BLEEDING**
■ **Etiology**

Gastrointestinal bleeding in children may result from inflammation or perforation of abdominal viscera, congenital visceral or vascular anomalies, trauma, esophageal varices secondary to portal hypertension, or coagulopathies (Table 8-11). Microscopic bleeding may cause no symptoms and may be detectable only through analysis of gastrointestinal secretions or feces. Significant gastrointestinal bleeding may result in hypovolemia and low cardiac output, shock, and death.

■ **Pathophysiology**

The physiologic response to gastrointestinal bleeding depends on the rate and duration of blood loss and on the patient's individual capacity to respond to volume depletion; this capacity is affected by the child's age, presence of other diseases, and state of hydration.

The most striking physiologic response follows acute massive gastrointestinal bleeding, with loss of greater than 15% of the patient's intravascular blood volume within a few minutes or hours. When this

Table 8-11 Etiology of gastrointestinal bleeding in children (based on age)[12,24,72]

Age-group	Upper GI bleeding	Lower GI bleeding
Neonatal period		
Well neonate	Swallowed maternal blood, hemorrhagic disease of the newborn, esophagitis, gastric duplication	Swallowed maternal blood, infectious colitis, milk allergy, hemorrhagic disease of the newborn, duplication of the bowel, Meckel's diverticulum
Sick neonate	Stress ulcer, gastritis, esophageal varices, esophagitis	Necrotizing enterocolitis, infectious colitis, disseminated coagulopathy, mid-gut volvulus, intussusception, congestive heart failure
Infancy		
	Chalasia with reflux, esophagitis, gastritis, gastric duplication or web, portal hypertension, trauma, pyloric stenosis	Anal fissure, infectious colitis, milk allergy, nonspecific colitis, juvenile polyps, intussusception, Meckel's diverticulum, hemolytic-uremic syndrome
Preschool age		
	Esophagitis, gastritis, peptic ulcer disease, foreign body, caustic ingestion, vascular disease (Rendu-Osler-Weber disease; hemophilia), trauma, portal hypertension, nasopharyngeal lesion	Infectious colitis, juvenile polyps, anal fissure, intussusception, Meckel's diverticulum, angiodysplasia, Henoch-Schönlein purpura, hemolytic-uremic syndrome, inflammatory bowel disease
School-age and adolescence		
	Esophagitis, gastritis, stress ulcer, peptic ulcer disease, portal hypertension, trauma, nasopharyngeal lesion	Infectious colitis, inflammatory bowel disease, polyps, angiodysplasia, Henoch-Schönlein purpura, hemolytic-uremic syndrome, hemorrhoids, rectal trauma

occurs, a series of autonomic cardiovascular responses are initiated in an attempt to maintain adequate blood pressure and systemic perfusion. As the blood volume falls, adrenergic secretion produces tachypnea, tachycardia, and arterial and venous constriction. Initially, these measures may maintain the child's cardiac output and blood pressure at or near normal levels. Venous constriction increases venous return to the heart, and arterial constriction may initially maintain the systolic blood pressure at adequate levels. Systemic vasoconstriction will, however, result in decreased renal perfusion (and a fall in urine output) and decreased gastrointestinal and peripheral perfusion. With continued hemorrhage, cardiac output and systemic perfusion will fall significantly.

During the early stages of gastrointestinal hemorrhage, blood pressure changes may be minimal while the patient is in the recumbent position. The systolic blood pressure may remain normal, and the diastolic blood pressure may be normal or decreased. Movement of the patient to an upright or sitting position may demonstrate a drop in systolic blood pressure; this drop in pressure with change from recumbent to an upright position is called *orthostatic hypotension.*

When continued unreplaced blood loss totals 15% to 20% of the child's circulating blood volume (or approximately 11 to 16 ml per kg body weight), the child's systolic and mean arterial blood pressures fall. Tissue hypoxemia and metabolic acidosis result from inadequate cardiac output and poor systemic perfusion. If the patient does not receive skilled resuscitation with rapid replacement of lost blood and intravascular volume, cardiovascular collapse and death will occur.

With severe hemorrhage and reduced renal blood flow and perfusion pressure, acute renal tubular necrosis may result (see Chapter 7). Rarely, prolonged mesenteric vascular insufficiency results in acute ischemic disease of the bowel or central lobular necrosis of the liver.

■ **Clinical signs and symptoms**

The appearance of the child with gastrointestinal bleeding varies considerably, depending on the amount and rapidity of blood loss. Usually, the child is brought to the physician or emergency room for treatment after vomiting blood, passing black, tarry stools *(melena)*, or passing bright red blood per rectum *(hematochezia)*. Bright red vomitus indicates recent or ongoing upper gastrointestinal hemorrhage, while coffee-ground vomitus indicates that there has been partial digestion of blood. The patient who develops sudden, significant bleeding is more likely to demonstrate faintness, pallor, tachycardia, thready pulses, diaphoresis, thirst, apprehension, and other signs of acute blood loss. The child with gradual bleeding, however, may experience only weakness and faintness; this patient may be aware of passing black stools but may not know that they usually signify blood loss.

It is important that the nurse remember that the child *may have a normal systolic blood pressure,* particularly in the recumbent position, *despite significant intravascular volume loss.* Signs of decreased peripheral perfusion are usually the earliest signs of severe hemorrhage. The skin is cool, peripheral pulses are decreased in quality, and oliguria or anuria are present (urine output averaging less than 0.5 to 1.0 ml/kg body weight/hour). The skin color is pale or mottled. Arterial constriction makes blood pressure measurement by cuff difficult or impossible since Korotkoff's sounds are muffled. The arterial waveform displayed from an indwelling arterial line is usually dampened in appearance, with a narrow pulse pressure. Metabolic acidosis may be noted when arterial blood gases are obtained, and arterial hypoxemia may also be present. If simultaneous venous blood gases are obtained, a large arterial-venous oxygen content difference (Av O_2) is often noted, signifying low cardiac output. The nurse should notify the physician immediately of these findings, since the patient's status is critical (see Chapter 3 for further discussion of the treatment of low cardiac output).

Digested blood has a specific odor that may be noted on the patient's breath even before the onset of melena or the first expulsion of hematemesis. This odor is qualitatively the same as that of melena, but it is usually fainter.

■ **Medical treatment and nursing interventions**

The three phases of critical management of the child with gastrointestinal bleeding are (1) resuscitation, (2) specific diagnosis, and (3) specific treatment. Fig. 8-5 presents details of these phases.

During resuscitation and replacement of intravascular volume, observations are made that may help determine the source of the child's bleeding. If iced saline lavage reveals grossly bloody or red-tinged aspirate, ongoing upper intestinal bleeding is present. A coagulation panel is usually obtained to rule out coagulopathy. To determine the source of the bleeding, endoscopy is performed once the child is stabilized. Vasopressin may be administered if the bleeding is due to esophageal varices (see the section on portal hypertension later in this chapter).

The color and the source of the bleeding also provide clues to the location of the bleeding. Bright red vomitus usually is from esophageal or gastric bleeding, and bright red blood in the stool results almost exclusively from rectal bleeding. Coffee-ground stool often indicates the presence of upper gastrointestinal bleeding (perhaps even from the stomach), which has been partially digested during passage through the intestines.

Nursing interventions during the resuscitation phase include the following.

1. Ensure placement of at least one large bore venous catheter. Two venous catheters are often inserted to allow one line to be used for rapid volume expansion, while the other line is used for frequent or continuous measurement of the child's CVP. An arterial line is also often inserted, and a urinary catheter should be placed.
2. Measure arterial and central venous pressure.
   a. Record arterial cuff pressure or continuous waveform display and analysis.
   b. Note venous pressure.
   c. Recalibrate and "zero" measurement equipment as needed to ensure accuracy.
   d. Palpate peripheral pulses and record quality of peripheral pulses and peripheral perfusion on nursing flow sheet with vital signs.
3. Obtain samples for frequent (at least every 2 to 4 hours) measurement of hematocrit; notify physician of a fall in values. Transfusion is generally indicated with a drop in hematocrit to 40%-45% in infants and 30%-35% in children over 1 year (this is often determined by hospital protocol).

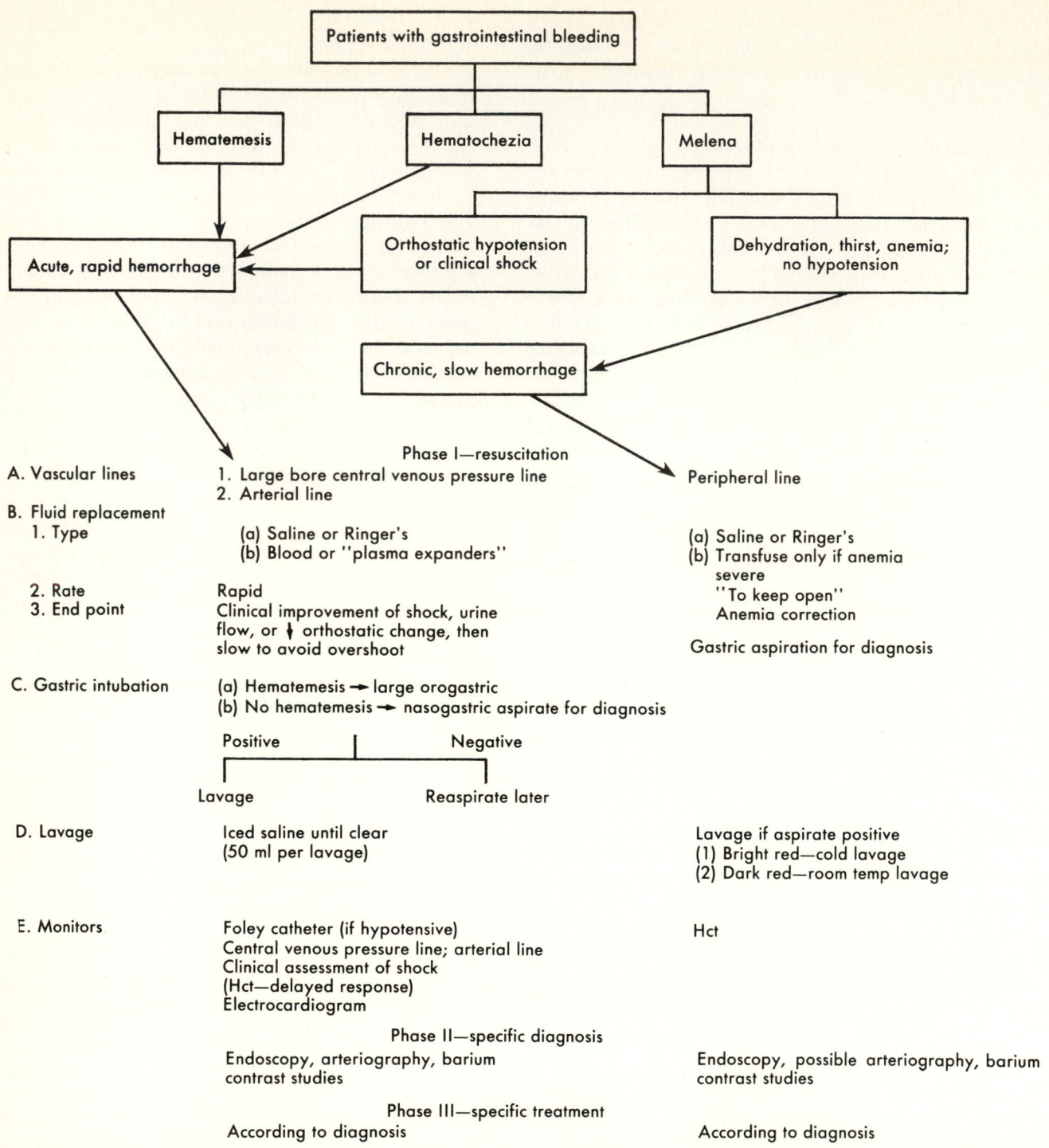

Fig. 8-5 Critical management of acute gastrointestinal bleeding.

Modified from Law, D.H.: Gastrointestinal bleeding. In Sleisenger, M., and Fordtran, J., editors: Gastrointestinal disease, Philadelphia, 1973, W.B. Saunders Co.

4. Administer parenteral fluids, including blood volume expanders, whole blood, or packed red blood cells as ordered. Warm blood products before transfusion in infants and small children (according to hospital policy) to prevent cold stress.

5. Observe for signs of transfusion reaction during administration of blood products (fever, tachycardia, pruritus, rash, hives).

6. Assess for signs of further hemorrhage (cool, clammy extremities, decreased peripheral perfusion, oliguria or anuria, restlessness,

abdominal pain or tenderness, changes in bowel sounds, hematemesis, or hematochezia).

7. Assess for signs of hypervolemia secondary to excessive fluid administration (tachypnea, dyspnea, tachycardia, increased respiratory effort, decreased urine output, increased weight, possible hypertension or hepatomegaly).

8. Observe for signs of hypocalcemia following transfusion with large amounts of citrate prepared blood (since the phosphate in this blood may precipitate with calcium, resulting in decreased ionized calcium concentration).

9. Assess for signs of gastric or intestinal perforation (severe, persistent pain, abdominal tenderness and rigidity, fever).

10. If iced saline lavage is necessary to reduce upper gastrointestinal bleeding, monitor the child's temperature closely, since cold stress increases oxygen consumption.

11. If vasopressin is administered, monitor for potential side effects such as chest pain, hyponatremia, decreased urine output, and decreased peripheral perfusion (see the section on portal hypertension later in this chapter).

12. Assess the child's need for supplemental oxygen therapy in the presence of hypoxemia and reduced intravascular oxygen-carrying capacity (caused by reduced hemoglobin concentration).

13. Use aseptic technique with all procedures to decrease the risk of nosocomial infection.

14. Provide careful, sensitive explanations of all procedures in language and approach appropriate for the child's cognitive and emotional development. Allow for visitors and diversional activities as possible to allay the child's anxiety. Provide explanations and support for the parents.

If esophageal varices are identified as the source of upper gastrointestinal bleeding, a Sengstaken-Blakemore tube (discussed in the portal hypertension section of this chapter) may be inserted.

■ **HYPERBILIRUBINEMIA**
■ **Etiology**

Bilirubin is the major product of hemoglobin breakdown. It results from oxygenation of the heme portion of hemoglobin when red-cell lysis occurs. Hyperbilirubinemia and jaundice are signs of hepatobiliary or hematologic disease. Jaundice, also known as *icterus,* is characterized by accumulation of yellow pigment in the skin and other tissues. *Kernicterus* is the presence of yellow pigment in the nuclear areas of the brain; it is caused by high concentrations of *unconjugated* bilirubin during the neonatal period and results in encephalopathy, with permanent brain damage.

■ **Pathophysiology**

When red blood cells reach the end of their 120-day life span, they are normally sequestered in the spleen. The cells are destroyed, the heme portion of the hemoglobin molecule is oxidized, and bilirubin is made. Bilirubin is bound to albumin in the plasma; in the liver it is combined with a sugar residue, called a glucuronate. Bilirubin that is attached to the glucuronate is called *conjugated* bilirubin; it is water soluble and is normally excreted in bile (Fig. 8-6 summarizes this process). "Free" bilirubin, called *unconjugated* bilirubin, is *not* attached to a sugar residue; it is lipid soluble (not water soluble). Since unconjugated bilirubin is thought to diffuse most freely into brain and liver tissue, high concentrations of this form of bilirubin are dangerous to neonates.

Increased serum bilirubin concentrations may result from an elevation in conjugated bilirubin (that attaches to glucuronates) or unconjugated bilirubin ("free" bilirubin). An elevation in the level of conjugated bilirubin is known as *direct hyperbilirubinemia.* It most commonly results from biliary tree obstruction, liver disease, or bowel obstruction, although it may also occur with metabolic disorders such as sepsis, drug sensitivities, pyelonephritis, meningitis, or gram-negative gastroenteritis. Neonatal hepatitis may cause hepatocellular damage and increased (direct) bilirubin clearance. Some genetic disorders (including Rotor's syndrome and Dubin-Johnson syndrome) are also associated with direct hyperbilirubinemia.[20]

Elevation of unconjugated bilirubin levels is known as *indirect hyperbilirubinemia.* It most commonly occurs as a result of excessive bilirubin production. In addition, it may result from impaired transport of bilirubin caused by hypoxia, acidosis, or administration of albumin-binding drugs (that displace bilirubin from the albumin). Impaired hepatic uptake of bilirubin may also cause indirect hyperbilirubinemia.

■ **Clinical signs and symptoms**

Jaundice (icterus) can usually be detected when the child's serum level of total bilirubin exceeds 3.0

Metabolic step   Location

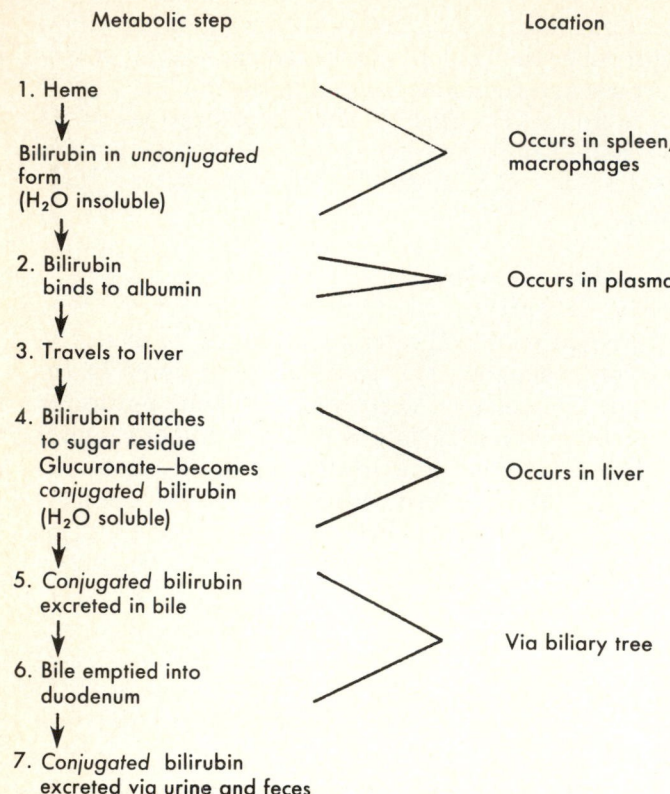

1. Heme
   ↓
   Bilirubin in *unconjugated*
   form
   (H_2O insoluble)   Occurs in spleen,
                                                   macrophages
   ↓
2. Bilirubin
   binds to albumin   Occurs in plasma
   ↓
3. Travels to liver
   ↓
4. Bilirubin attaches
   to sugar residue
   Glucuronate—becomes   Occurs in liver
   conjugated bilirubin
   (H_2O soluble)
   ↓
5. *Conjugated* bilirubin
   excreted in bile
   ↓   Via biliary tree
6. Bile emptied into
   duodenum
   ↓
7. *Conjugated* bilirubin
   excreted via urine and feces

Fig. 8-6 Normal metabolism of bilirubin.

Modified from Gray, G.M.: Mechanism of digestion and absorption of food. In Sleisinger, M.H., and Fordtran, J.S., editors: Gastrointestinal disease, ed. 2, Philadelphia, 1978, W.B. Saunders Co.

mg/dl (normal is less than 1.5 mg/ml). Jaundice is usually most readily detected in the sclera and soft palate, and it may be visible in the skin. The urine may darken because of the urinary excretion of conjugated bilirubin, and the stools may become gray, indicating absence of normal fecal elimination of bilirubin.

It is possible to measure serum levels of *total* bilirubin and *direct* (or conjugated) bilirubin (normal: 0.2-0.4 mg/dl). Most hospitals are not equipped to measure serum *indirect* (or unconjugated) bilirubin levels. As a result, the level of *indirect* bilirubin is inferred from the difference between the *total* bilirubin level and the *direct* bilirubin level. If the child with a high serum total bilirubin level has a normal or only slightly elevated direct bilirubin level, the indirect bilirubin level must be high. The higher the amount of indirect or unconjugated bilirubin in the serum, the greater is the neonate's risk of developing kernicterus.

The serum levels of total and direct bilirubin provide information about the cause of the hyperbilirubinemia. The child with hepatobiliary obstruction has, primarily, elevation of total and direct bilirubin levels. Occasionally, the indirect bilirubin level is also increased. Although this child would also demonstrate an elevation in serum alkaline phosphatase, serum liver enzymes would be normal or only slightly increased (Table 8-12).

The child with hemolytic disease has indirect hyperbilirubinemia; total and indirect bilirubin levels are elevated, but the direct bilirubin level may be normal. Serum alkaline phosphatase levels and serum liver enzyme concentrations are normal. If the child has hepatic disease, indirect hyperbilirubinemia is present and the direct bilirubin level is lower than normal, since the liver is not able to conjugate normal amounts of bilirubin. Serum liver enzyme concentrations—including serum glutamic-oxalocetic transaminase (SGOT), serum glutamic-pyruvic transaminase (SGPT), lactate dehydrogenase (LDH), and alkaline phosphatase—would be elevated, and coagulopathies may also be present (see Table 8-12).

If the infant with hyperbilirubinemia is receiving phototherapy treatment, the phototherapy light is turned off while blood specimens are obtained. If the blood specimens are exposed to light (especially phototherapy), the bilirubin may be oxidized, altering the measured serum bilirubin levels in the samples.

The child's urine may be tested for the presence of conjugated bilirubin. These urine specimens must be collected in dark (light-resistant) containers to avoid conversion of the urine bilirubin and alteration of measured urine bilirubin levels.

Biliary nuclear scans may be ordered to evaluate bile excretion, and a liver biopsy may be performed to determine the etiology of the disorder.

A clinical symptom of hyperbilirubinemia that may be present is pruritus resulting from irritation of cutaneous nerves by the bile salts.[37]

■ **Medical treatment and nursing interventions**

If *direct hyperbilirubinemia* is present, the nurse should be alert for the appearance of additional signs of liver disease or decreased hepatic function. These signs include edema or ascites (secondary to hypoalbuminemia), prolonged bleeding because of coagulopathy, pruritus, and encephalopathy. If coagulopathies are present, the child's hematocrit and platelet count are monitored closely. The nurse should also monitor for signs of hemolytic anemia, including pallor and fatigue. Appropriate blood component therapy for anemia or thrombocytopenia is administered (see Table 3-10). If the child develops encephalopathy, the nurse must monitor for signs of increased intracranial pressure, and seizure precau-

Table 8-12   Diagnostic tests used in differential diagnosis of jaundice

	Normal	Hemolytic	Liver disease	Biliary tract obstruction secondary to atresia or stone
Serum tests				
Alkaline phosphatase	4.0-13.0 King-Armstrong units	Normal	Increased 1 to 3 times; urine dark (late); skin yellow, orange, green	Increased three to eight times; urine dark yellow; skin orange or green
Bilirubin				
Total	0.5-1.4 mg/dl	5-20 mg/dl	Over 15 mg/dl	Normal to 25 mg/dl
Direct	0.2-0.4 mg/dl	Normal or increased	Decreased	Increased
Indirect	0.4-0.8 mg/dl	Increased	Increased	Increased
Cholesterol (total)	150-250 mg/dl	Normal	Normal or decreased	Increased
SGOT	12-36 U	Normal	300-5000 U	300 U or less
SGPT	6-25 U	Normal	300-5000 U	300 U or less
Protein				
Total	6.0-7.8 g/dl	Decreased	Decreased	Normal or slight increase
Albumin	3.9-4.6 g/dl	Decreased	Decreased	Normal or slight increase
Globulin	2.3-3.5 g/dl	Normal	Moderate increase	Normal or slight increase
Prothrombin time	11.0-17.0 sec	Normal	Often abnormal despite vitamin K administration	Normal or returns to normal following vitamin K administration
Urine tests				
Bilirubin	0	0	Positive	Positive
Urobilinogen	1-4 mg/24 hr	Increased	Increased	Normal
Stool tests				
Urobilinogen	40-280 mg/24 hr	Over 250 mg/24 hr; normal color	Normal or decreased; normal color	Acholic (0-5 mg/24 hr); clay-colored stool

Modified from Jaundice-Biochemical Differential Diagnosis, Warner-Teed Pharmaceuticals, Inc., Columbus, Ohio, 1970. In Given, B.A., and Simmons, S.J.: Gastroenterology in clinical nursing, ed. 4, St. Louis, 1984, The C.V. Mosby Co.

tions should be taken (see Chapter 6). Antibiotic therapy is indicated if infection or sepsis is present.

If liver function is impaired, supportive therapy including administration of an elementary diet (with medium-chain triglycerides), or parenteral alimentation may be indicated. However, parenteral intralipid therapy is often contraindicated, since the free fatty acids may displace bilirubin from albumin. Any medications prescribed for the child must be reviewed; if any of the medications are metabolized by the liver, the dosages must be adjusted to prevent toxic accumulation of the drugs.

The child with direct hyperbilirubinemia must be kept well-hydrated, since dehydration results in decreased excretion of conjugated bilirubin. However, if hypoalbuminemia is also present, it may be accompanied by significant edema and ascites, which may necessitate careful diuresis.

Occasionally, the child with direct hyperbili-

rubinemia will require surgical repair of biliary atresia or a liver transplant.[60] *Indirect hyperbilirubinemia* is most commonly seen during the neonatal period, and it often complicates the care of premature infants. Neonatal indirect hyperbilirubinemia is treated with phototherapy, exchange transfusions, or pharmacologic agents to avoid kernicterus (Fig. 8-7 summarizes these treatment modalities). Drugs that bind with serum albumin are avoided, if possible, since they may displace serum bilirubin from albumin, increasing the concentration of "free" bilirubin and the risk of bilirubin diffusion into brain tissue (kernicterus).

Phototherapy with blue or ultraviolet light during the neonatal period causes bilirubin oxidation and destruction. The infant receiving phototherapy is kept unclothed for maximum light exposure. Protective patches are placed over the infant's closed eyes. A hat, made of stockinette material (knotted at one

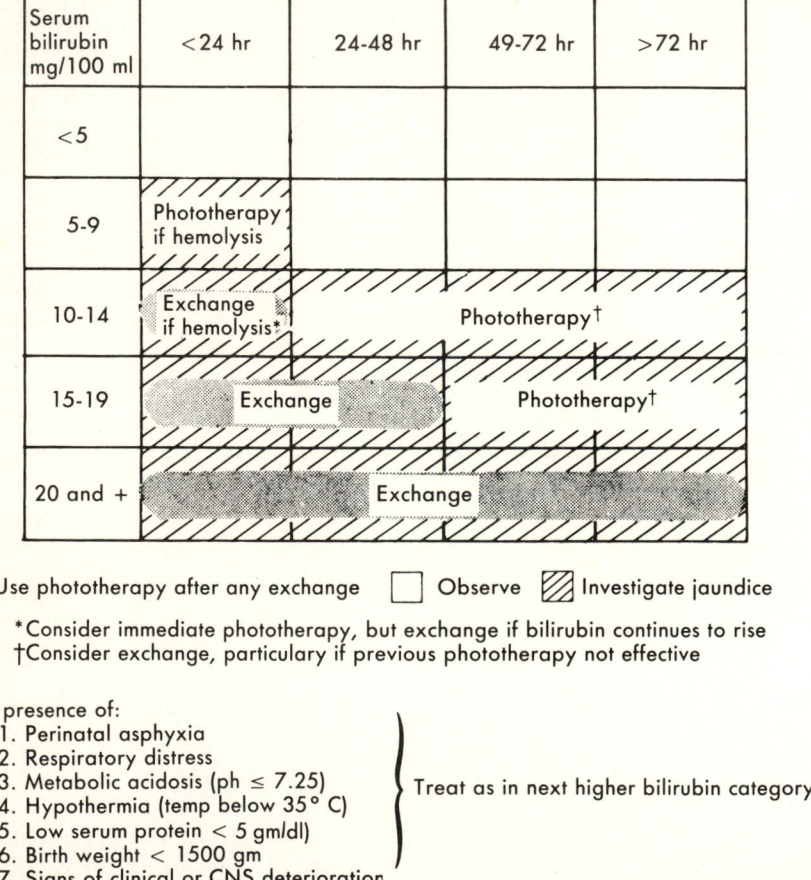

Use phototherapy after any exchange   ☐ Observe   ▨ Investigate jaundice

*Consider immediate phototherapy, but exchange if bilirubin continues to rise
†Consider exchange, particulary if previous phototherapy not effective

In presence of:
1. Perinatal asphyxia
2. Respiratory distress
3. Metabolic acidosis (ph ≤ 7.25)
4. Hypothermia (temp below 35° C)   } Treat as in next higher bilirubin category
5. Low serum protein < 5 gm/dl)
6. Birth weight < 1500 gm
7. Signs of clinical or CNS deterioration

Fig. 8-7 General guidelines for the management of hyperbilirubinemia.

From Brown, A.K.: Jaundice. In Behrman, R.E., editor: Neonatology; diseases of the fetus and infant, St. Louis, 1973, The C.V. Mosby Co.

end), may be used to keep the patches in place without exerting pressure on the eyes since such pressure could cause retinal detachment. Unless serum bilirubin levels are critically elevated, phototherapy should be briefly interrupted several times each day. During these interruptions the eye patches should be removed, and the infant should be wrapped and held to provide comforting tactile and visual stimulation.

Because the infant's insensible water loss is increased during phototherapy, accurate measurement of fluid intake and output and twice-daily weights should be kept. Evidence of excessive fluid loss or inadequate fluid intake should be discussed with the physician immediately. Neonates receiving phototherapy often develop diarrhea, which may result from damage to intestinal mucosa by excretion of the photobilirubin. This diarrhea may cause excessive fluid and nutritional loss in these infants.[87]

The skin of black infants may darken or lighten during phototherapy; these effects usually disappear after the therapy is discontinued. Occasionally, bile pigments may be reabsorbed from the duodenum, causing a direct hyperbilirubinemia. This phenomenon, known as the "bronze baby" syndrome, should be suspected if the neonate receiving phototherapy develops a dark-brown discoloration of the skin, serum, and urine. This syndrome usually resolves after phototherapy is discontinued.

If the child with hyperbilirubinemia develops pruritus, good skin care is very important. Mild soaps should be used for cleansing, and abrasive solutions should be avoided. The child should turn or be turned frequently. Gentle massage may relieve the pruritus, particularly if soothing lotions are used.

■ **ASCITES**
■ **Etiology**

Ascites is the accumulation of free fluid in the peritoneal cavity. It may result from diffuse inflammation of the peritoneal surface because of peritonitis or because of increased portal capillary pressure as the result of cirrhosis, severe congestive heart failure, or other constrictive vascular conditions. Ascites is also associated with diseases that result in sodium and water retention with decreased plasma colloid osmotic pressure (e.g., nephrotic syndrome). In children, significant ascites is most often caused by liver disease or severe congestive heart failure.

■ **Pathophysiology**

Ascites results from exudation of fluid from the surface of the liver or bowel. This fluid enters the abdominal cavity instead of the mesenteric or portal venous system if there is obstruction to flow between the mesenteric or portal vein and the inferior vena cava; if the CVP is extremely high; if serum albumin content is low; or if proteinaceous fluid is present in the peritoneal cavity.

When blood passes through any capillary bed, the amount of fluid filtered out of the capillaries (the vascular space) depends on pressure gradients across the capillary bed (from the arterial to the venous end and between the intravascular and the extravascular or interstitial space) and the difference in oncotic pressure between the intravascular and extravascular spaces. Under normal circumstances these factors, known as Starling's capillary forces, favor fluid *filtration* (flow into the interstitial space) at the arterial end of the capillary bed and fluid *reabsorption* (flow back into the capillary) at the venous end of the capillary bed, so that an equilibrium exists between fluid filtration and reabsorption. A rise in venous hydrostatic pressure, an increase in extravascular (interstitial) oncotic pressure, or a fall in intravascular oncotic pressure can destroy the capillary equilibrium and result in a net loss of fluid from the vascular space to the extravascular space. This net loss of fluid to the extravascular space occurs with ascites.

When hepatic and portal venous blood flow is obstructed (such as occurs with cirrhosis of the liver), venous capillary and hepatic sinusoidal pressures rise. Initially, the veins and sinusoids expand to accommodate larger quantities of blood. Eventually, however, fluid begins to exudate from the surface of the liver into the peritoneal cavity, caused by the high capillary venous hydrostatic pressure. Since liver sinusoids are far more permeable than normal capillaries, both fluid and protein leak into the abdominal cavity. The presence of proteins in the abdominal cavity creates an increase in colloidal oncotic pressure in the ascitic fluid; this draws even more fluid into the abdominal cavity (Fig. 8-8).

When the child develops congestive heart failure, the CVP rises. Initially, hepatic venous and sinusoidal pressures rise, and the veins and sinusoids expand to accommodate a greater blood volume. This causes one of the earliest signs of congestive heart failure in children, hepatomegaly (see Chapter 3). If the CVP continues to rise, the liver's storage capacity is exceeded, and fluid and protein will exude into the abdominal cavity, causing ascites.

Children with nephrotic syndrome or hypoalbuminemia resulting from other causes have a low plasma oncotic pressure, which produces generalized edema, including ascites.

Peritoneal inflammation may also cause abdom-

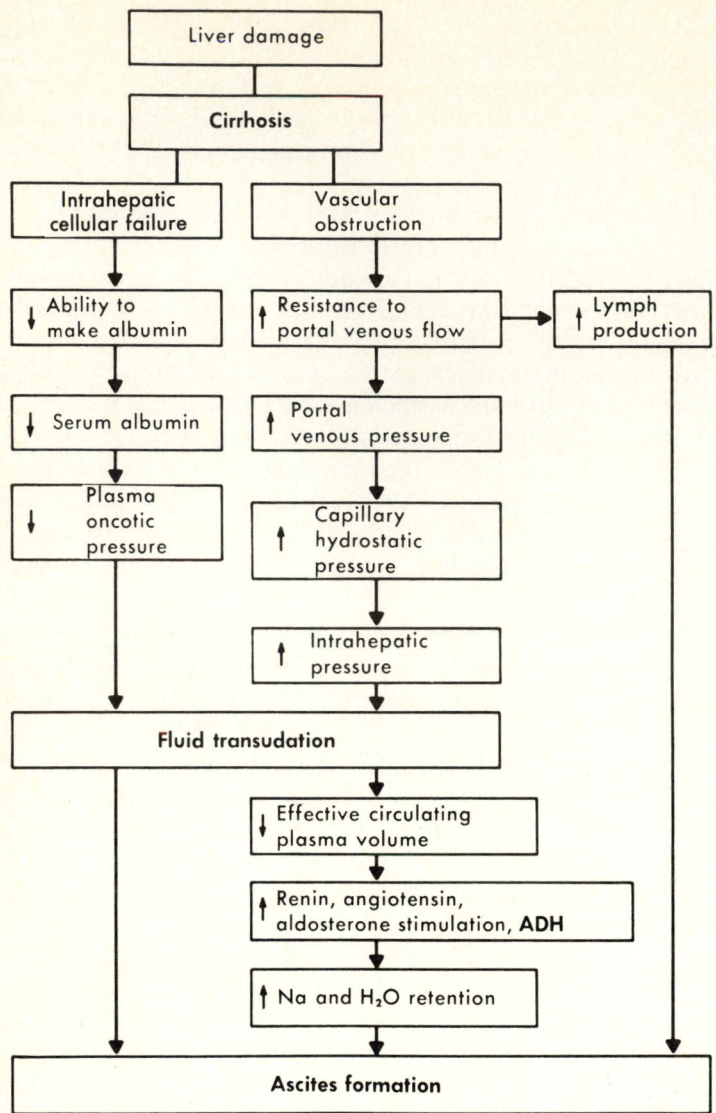

Fig. 8-8 Pathogenesis of ascites.

From Given, B., and Simmons, S.: Gastroenterology in clinical nursing, ed. 4, St. Louis, 1984, The C.V. Mosby Co.

inal fluid exudate. If this fluid contains proteins, it will create increased colloidal osmotic pressure in the peritoneal cavity, drawing more fluid from the vascular space into the abdominal cavity (ascites).

■ **Clinical signs and symptoms**

Early development of ascites frequently is unnoticed by the child or parents unless there are other symptoms of the primary disease. Clothing may be perceived as too tight around the waist, and belts must be loosened as weight gain occurs and abdominal girth increases. Peripheral, ankle, and presacral edema may not be present unless or until hypoalbuminemia occurs. If the ascites results from inferior

vena caval, portal, or abdominal venous obstruction or high CVP, superficial abdominal veins will be distended (this is called *caput medusae*).

On examination the child's abdomen appears distended. The abdominal girth is measured at this time and then every 2 to 4 hours (or more often if the patient's condition changes) to allow comparison of measurements. The abdomen is generally dull to percussion, indicating the presence of fluid. The location of the area of dullness may change when the patient changes position; this is called *shifting dullness*, and it is often observed when the child has ascites. Note that because of effects of gravity, the fluid will usually be located in the dependent areas of the abdominal cavity.

If the child is cooperative and a second observer is present, a *fluid wave* may be elicited as a result of the ascites. The first observer places a hand firmly on the midline of the child's abdomen. The second observer places one hand along one side of the child's abdomen and, with the second hand, sharply taps the other side of the child's abdomen. If significant amounts of peritoneal fluid are present, the first observer should feel the "wave" of fluid strike the anterior wall of the abdomen, along the midline.[3,8]

Patients with ascites may demonstrate hypoalbuminemia. This may occur as a result of the primary disease or as a result of loss of protein into the ascitic fluid. Protein synthesis is also decreased if liver function is impaired. If the child has cirrhosis, antidiuretic hormone (ADH) levels are elevated, since the liver does not inactivate the ADH; this causes water retention and may produce a dilutional serum hyponatremia. In addition, aldosterone is not inactivated by the cirrhotic liver, which can produce both water and sodium retention. Hypokalemia may result from aldosterone excess or from potassium loss with vigorous pharmacologic diuresis.[63]

If significant fluid accumulates in the child's abdomen, diaphragmatic excursion during respiration may be impaired; this may cause the child to breathe rapidly and shallowly. It is important that the nurse watch these children closely for signs of respiratory distress. With accumulation of large amounts of ascitic fluid, the child may develop a *hydrothorax*, or accumulation of fluid in the thorax. This fluid most commonly enters the right chest, although bilateral pleural effusion may be seen. The child with a hydrothorax demonstrates dyspnea, increased respiratory effort (retractions and nasal flaring), and tachypnea. Breath sounds over the area of effusion are usually decreased (in infants, however, breath sounds may be referred from other areas of the lung; thus breath sounds may be present bilaterally, though they will differ in quality or pitch).

If the ascites is secondary to liver, cardiovascular, or genitourinary disease, signs of the primary disease are noted (see discussion of these diseases in this chapter or in Chapter 3 or Chapter 7).

The child with ascites may be extremely self-conscious about the abdominal distention. These children often complain of a sensation of "fullness" in the abdomen, and they may be anorexic. Nutritional weight loss may be masked by the weight of the ascites.

■ **Medical treatment and nursing interventions**

It is important that the development of ascites be recognized before respiratory compromise or significant fluid shift occurs. The child at risk for the development of ascites requires careful measurement of fluid intake and output and daily or twice-daily weights. The child should be weighed at exactly the same time(s) of the day on the same scale each time to ensure consistency, so that even small changes in weight can be recognized. Abdominal girth is measured every 2 to 4 hours or as frequently as the child's condition warrants.

Frequently, strict fluid and possibly sodium restriction is necessary in the management of severe ascites. If diuresis is required, the nurse should assess the child carefully to ensure that the intravascular volume remains adequate. Signs of hypovolemia include tachycardia, tachypnea, peripheral vasoconstriction, low CVP,* decreased or absent urine output, and high urine specific gravity (see the discussion of low cardiac output in Chapter 3). Fluid and electrolyte balance must be monitored closely.

If the child is allowed oral feedings and is of school age or older, hard candy may be given to assuage thirst and provide caloric intake while the child's fluid intake is restricted. An effort must be made to make meals palatable. Small, frequent feedings are usually better tolerated than infrequent, larger ones, since gastric distention only increases the sensation of abdominal fullness.

The child should be encouraged to cough and take deep breaths to prevent the development of lower lobe atelectasis (from pressure of abdominal fluid on the diaphragm and resultant shallow breathing). Rib-springing exercises will also promote deep breathing (see Chapter 4). If the child develops signs of respiratory distress, elevate the head of the bed or place the child in a semi-Fowler's position to maximize diaphragmatic movement. Infants may be placed in an infant seat, and older children may prefer to dangle at the side of the bed, leaning forward over a bedside table. If development of a hydrothorax is suspected, a physician should be notified immediately, and a chest radiograph will be obtained. A standard anterior-posterior and lateral set of chest films will reveal the presence of large amounts of fluid in the pleural space, and a lateral decubitus film may be ordered to detect smaller amounts of fluids (see Fig. 5-4). If the presence of a hydrothorax is confirmed, a thoracentesis is performed or a chest tube is inserted (see Appendix A). Occasionally, if severe respiratory distress is present, oxygen administration or mechanical ventilatory support will be required until the

---

*If the tip of the central venous line is in the inferior vena cava (rather than the right atrium) and vena caval obstruction is present, the measured pressure from that line may be high because of the obstruction, although the right atrial pressure may be very low.

child's gastrointestinal problem resolves. Pericentesis may also be indicated to remove some of the abdominal fluid.

Peritonitis or gastrointestinal bleeding may complicate the condition of the child with ascites and cirrhosis (see discussions of these topics earlier in this chapter).

Any child with ascites requires good skin care. The child must turn or be turned frequently to prevent development of pressure sores, particularly on skin covering bony prominences.

■ **PORTAL HYPERTENSION**
■ **Etiology**

Portal hypertension is an increase in portal venous pressure above 5 to 10 mm Hg. It is caused by obstruction to the normal flow of blood through the portal venous system, the liver sinusoids, or the hepatic vein. It may be caused by (1) obstruction of the portal vein or its immediate tributaries (this is a form of *extrahepatic* portal hypertension), (2) an increase in vascular resistance within the liver that occurs secondary to fibrosis of the liver (this form is called *intrahepatic* portal hypertension), or (3) obstruction of hepatic venous outflow into the inferior vena cava (this is a form of *suprahepatic* portal hypertension). These major forms of portal hypertension are depicted in Fig. 8-9.

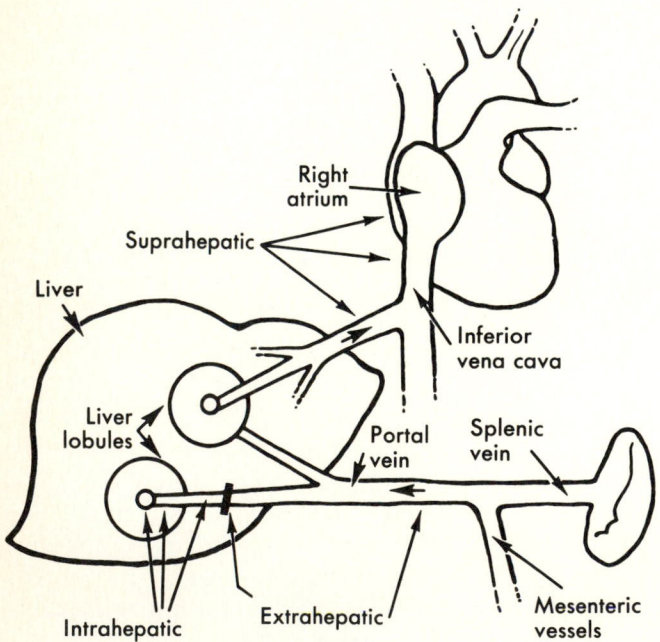

Fig. 8-9 Location of obstruction in portal hypertension.

From Wyllie, R., and others: Location of obstruction in portal hypertension, J. Pediatr. **97**:172, 1980.

Children may develop extrahepatic portal hypertension as a result of thrombosis of the portal vein. This thrombosis may be congenital, or it may result from the use of umbilical venous catheters during the newborn period. Intrahepatic portal hypertension may complicate any form of chronic liver disease, including neonatal or childhood hepatitis, or liver disease secondary to infection or metabolic diseases. Inferior vena caval obstruction or hepatic vein occlusion or thrombosis may be responsible for suprahepatic portal hypertension.

■ **Pathophysiology**

Portal venous blood flows into liver sinusoids (see Fig. 8-2). Since these sinusoids offer more resistance to blood flow than normal capillaries, pressure in the portal vein is normally higher than the CVP. If this flow is obstructed, pressure in the portal vein (and circulation emptying into it) may rapidly become very high.

Anything that obstructs blood flow within the portal venous system, liver, or inferior vena cava can produce portal hypertension. Thrombosis of the portal vein will cause a significant rise in pressure in the portal vein proximal to the clot. Fibrosis of the liver compresses and distorts liver architecture and blood vessels, which increases resistance to blood flow through the liver and portal venous pressure. Any obstruction to flow of blood through the hepatic vein and into the inferior vena cava can increase sinusoidal pressure and distend the liver sinusoids with blood. If this obstruction is severe or chronic, resistance to flow of blood into those sinusoids will increase and portal hypertension will result. Three major physiologic complications of portal hypertension are congestion of the splenic and mesenteric circulations, development of collateral vessels, and sequestration of blood in the splanchnic circulation (the blood vessels from the gut and spleen that normally drain into the portal vein).

When portal vein pressure increases, blood flow from the splanchnic circulation is impeded; this results in pooling of blood in the splanchnic circulation, called *sequestration*. When a large amount of blood is sequestered and is unable to return to the inferior vena cava (and back into the general circulation), the heart, adrenal cortex, and kidneys perceive a decrease in circulating blood volume; thus sodium and water are retained by the kidneys (because of hyperaldosteronism), causing an increase in total circulating blood volume. Although the total amount of blood in the body is increased, the pooled blood in the splanchnic circulation is effectively trapped and cannot be mobilized during circulatory crises (such as hemorrhage).

The pooling of blood in the splanchnic circulation causes splenic congestion. Hypersplenism and stasis of blood in the spleen cause damage to the formed elements of the blood, producing anemia, thrombocytopenia, and neutropenia. Engorgement of mesenteric vessels may cause mesenteric vein thrombosis or mesenteric infarction.

Impedance to portal blood flow and the hypertension in the portal and splanchnic circulation promote the formation of collateral vessels between the splanchnic and portal circulations and the inferior vena cava or other major central veins. Major collateral vessels form from the portal vein, along the stomach and esophagus to the intercostal veins, in the paraumbilical veins (causing enlarged abdominal wall vessels), and around the rectum and anus (in the hemorrhoidal veins). Submucosal veins of the esophagus often enlarge and form collateral vessels between the portal venous system and the vena cavae. These enlarged veins often protrude into the esophagus and are known as *esophageal varices.*

Cavernous transformation of the portal vein occurs when there is thrombosis of the portal vein with subsequent development of multiple collateral vessels around the thrombosed vein.

■ Clinical signs and symptoms

Splenomegaly is one of the first clinical signs of portal hypertension in children. The presence of hemorrhoids, dilated abdominal veins, and esophageal varices are additional clinical findings. Children with extrahepatic portal hypertension secondary to cavernous transformation of the portal vein may suddenly develop acute upper gastrointestinal bleeding without any previous history of clinical symptoms or problems.[70]

Children with portal hypertension often have ascites, markedly dilated superficial abdominal veins (caput medusae), and hypoalbuminemia. If cirrhosis is present, the child often appears emaciated. Anemia, thrombocytopenia, and leukopenia are present because of hypersplenism.

If the child has esophageal varices, sudden, severe esophageal and gastrointestinal bleeding may occur without warning (see the discussion of acute gastrointestinal bleeding) with the onset of hematemesis, melena, or rectal bleeding. The bleeding from esophageal varices is particularly difficult to stop because the pressure in the vessels is usually high and because these children often have thrombocytopenia. Bleeding episodes are frequently precipitated by a fe-

brile illness (such as an upper respiratory infection) and administration of aspirin,[70] which can depress the function of existing platelets. The mortality rate for patients with these bleeding episodes was previously high.[15] However, current treatment with balloon tamponade (Sengstaken-Blakemore tube) or vasopressin are generally effective in controlling bleeding in children.[5]

The diagnosis of portal hypertension can be confirmed with splenic or hepatic vein pressure measurements. Liver function tests and a liver biopsy may be performed to determine the cause or extent of the primary disease. A barium swallow may be ordered to look for compression of the esophageal barium by dilated varices, and contrast material may be injected into the spleen or umbilical vein (called splenoportography) to depict the portal venous structures and to localize the exact site of venous obstruction.

■ Medical treatment and nursing interventions

Nursing interventions in acute episodes of gastrointestinal bleeding secondary to portal hypertension have already been discussed. Additional nursing interventions in the care of children with portal hypertension include the following.
1. Avoid rectal temperature measurement because it may traumatize internal and external hemorrhoids, causing rectal bleeding.
2. Prevent prolonged and vigorous crying episodes, since they can increase esophageal variceal pressure; sedation may be required (with physician's order).
3. Closely monitor stool consistency and frequency; constipation and straining can cause increased abdominal pressure, which can precipitate bleeding of esophageal or gastric varices.
4. Avoid other factors that may lead to increased abdominal pressure (such as use of inspirometers or other respiratory care equipment that requires prolonged periods of breath holding or Valsalva's maneuver).
5. When oral intake is resumed, initially avoid foods with rough, sharp consistencies that may cause esophageal irritation (e.g., raw carrots and potato chips).
6. Perform a guaiac test or hematest any gastrointestinal fluids or stool.
7. Ensure that adequate amounts of blood and blood components (as ordered) are available in the blood bank.

Medical treatment of an acute bleeding episode

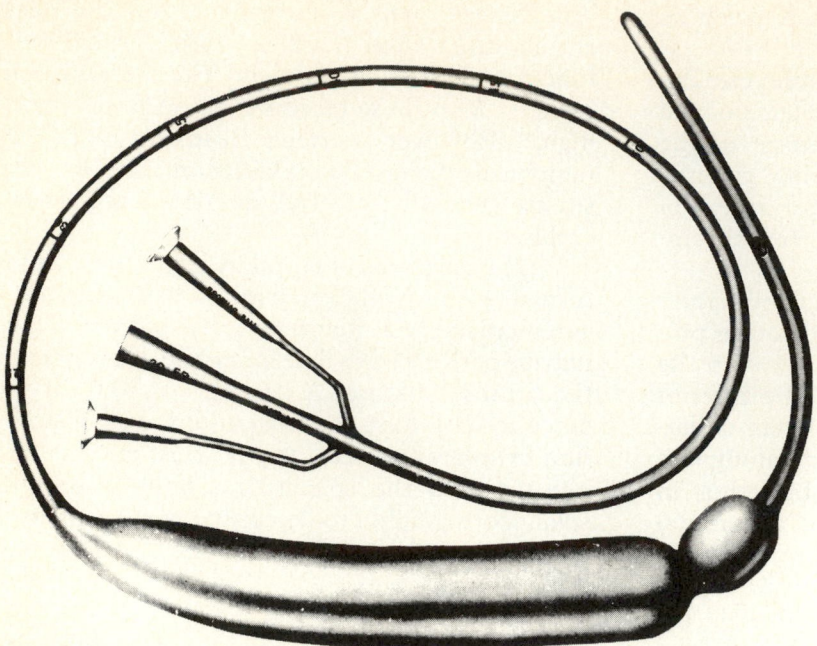

Fig. 8-10 Sengstaken-Blakemore tube. Used to control bleeding from esophageal varices in children and adolescents. The tube has three lumens: one allows use of gastric suction, one allows inflation of the esophageal balloon, and one allows inflation of the gastric balloon.

Courtesy Davol, Inc., Providence, R.I. In Given, B., and Simmons, S.: Gastroenterology in clinical nursing, ed. 4, St. Louis, 1984, The C.V. Mosby Co.

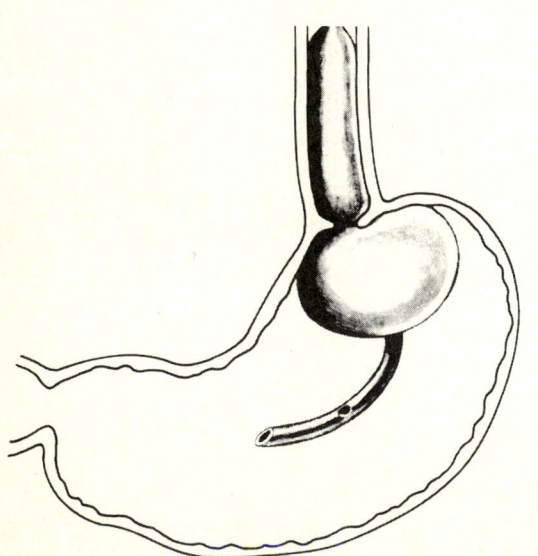

Fig. 8-11 Positioning of the Sengstaken-Blakemore tube.

From Given, B., and Simmons, S.: Gastroenterology in clinical nursing, ed. 4, St. Louis, 1984, The C.V. Mosby Co.

secondary to portal hypertension is directed toward the stabilization of the patient's vital signs and blood volume. Bleeding from esophageal varices is usually stopped by irrigation with iced 1% sodium bicarbonate or iced saline via nasogastric tube.[70] If the bleeding is not quickly stopped, mechanical occlusion of the bleeding varices is necessary. A child-size Sengstaken-Blakemore tube, which has two balloons and three lumens (Fig. 8-10), is inserted as a mechanical means to stop bleeding. The child should have nothing by mouth before balloon insertion, and the stomach should be emptied to prevent aspiration of vomitus while the tube is passed. The lubricated tube is inserted through the nose into the stomach, and the gastric balloon is inflated to keep the tube in place. After radiographic confirmation of proper tube placement, the balloon remaining in the esophagus is inflated to a pressure of 20 to 40 mm Hg. The esophageal balloon applies direct pressure to the esophageal veins, while the inflated gastric balloon supplies pressure at the esophagogastric junction (Fig. 8-11).[70]

Traction is often applied to the outer portion of the Sengstaken-Blakemore tube to prevent the gastric balloon from slipping into the antrum. The traction and the inflation pressures are usually maintained up to 48 hours; then after all bleeding has stopped the balloons are deflated gradually during a 24-hour period. Too much balloon pressure can cause discomfort and may lead to ulceration or necrosis of the esophageal and gastric mucosa. The tube is generally not withdrawn until 48 hours after bleeding has ceased.[70]

Vasopressin may be administered to control the hemorrhage. It is thought to act by causing constriction of the vascular bed, which reduces splanchnic circulation and, thus, blood flow to the esophageal varices. The drug is usually given intravenously when acute hemorrhage is present. The side effects include hypertension, arrhythmias (including bradycardia), abdominal pain and cramping, defecation, and decreased urine output. The child's vital signs should be watched during and immediately following IV drip infusion of this drug, and careful monitoring of fluid intake and output is mandatory.

The child's serum potassium must be monitored closely, since hyperaldosteronism (caused by renal response to blood sequestration in the splanchnic circulation) causes increased urinary potassium excretion. As a result, most of these children demonstrate significant hypokalemia. In addition, hyponatremia and a metabolic alkalosis may result from the hyperaldostronism.

Nursing responsibilities during care of patients requiring the Sengstaken-Blakemore tube include the following.

1. Check integrity and patency of the two balloons and three lumens before passage of tube.
2. Check desired pressure of inflation and pounds of traction with the physician, and record them on patient's care plan and at bedside.
3. Ensure patency of the third lumen of the tube (which is used to suction blood) by irrigating frequently.
4. Carefully label each lumen of the tube to prevent accidental deflation of the balloons.
5. Assess for signs of pulmonary aspiration of secretions; airway obstruction from emesis or bronchial secretions may occur (it is difficult for vomitus to pass around the esophageal tube).
6. To prevent inconsistent esophageal or gastric pressure or dislodgement of the tube, maintain proper positioning of patient when traction is used.
7. To prevent confusion and inadvertent pro-

longed balloon inflation and development of esophageal or gastric necrosis, carefully record times the balloons are inflated and the exact inflation pressures used.
8. Provide the child with calm, supportive care; the sight of massive hematemesis and the urgency of the intensive-care treatment will probably be frightening to the child and family.
9. In an attempt to avoid or reduce the frequency of additional bleeding episodes, provide the child and parents with appropriate instruction. Contact sports, aspirin, and prolonged Valsalva's maneuver should be avoided. A bland diet may also be recommended to prevent any friction along the esophagus.

Surgery to decompress the hypertensive portal system is necessary if life-threatening variceal bleeding frequently recurs, although these procedures are most successful when performed in children over 10 years of age (when veins are of larger size).[70] The surgical procedures require diversion (shunting) of portal blood flow directly into the inferior vena cava; this bypasses the scarred liver or thombosed portal vein. The shunting procedures most frequently used in children are the splenorenal shunt and the portacaval shunt (Fig. 8-12 illustrates the various shunting procedures). The splenorenal shunt requires anastomosis of the splenic vein to the left renal vein; the portacaval shunt requires anastomosis of the portal vein to the inferior vena cava.

A major postoperative complication includes thrombosis of the anastomotic vessel and resultant recurrence of the portal hypertension. An additional serious complication is gastrointestinal hemorrhage from the newly anastomosed vessels; this bleeding occurs most frequently if the portal diversion shunt is performed on a child under 10 years of age or if a splenectomy has also been performed. In addition, risk of postoperative bleeding is increased if the child has significant preoperative coagulopathies because of primary liver disease.[70] Since the surgical shunts allow blood from the splanchnic circulation to bypass the liver, liver detoxification of certain circulating toxins (such as nitrogenous substances) is prevented; therefore the nurse must monitor for the development of hepatic encephalopathy (see the following section). Additional nursing interventions are outlined in the postlaparotomy care plan (postoperative care is discussed later in this chapter).

The child with esophageal varices and the parents will require the support of each nurse and physician involved in their care. The risk of sudden, mas-

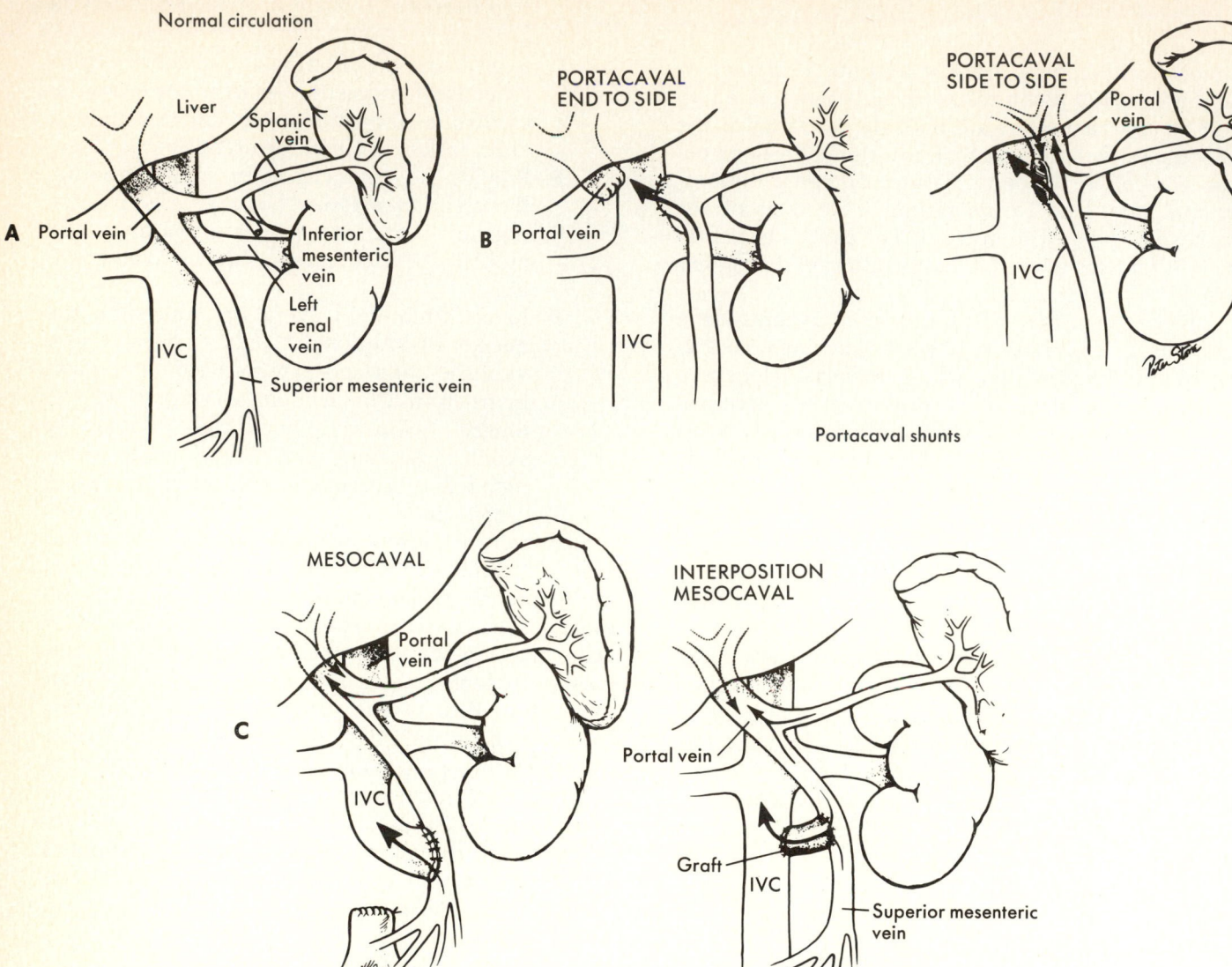

Fig. 8-12 Surgical shunt procedures for decompression of portal hypertension. **A,** Normal portal venous blood flow consists of visceral venous blood, carried by the superior mesenteric vein, and splenic venous blood. This portal venous blood normally passes through the liver, then into the hepatic vein. It enters the systemic venous circulation through the inferior vena cava. **B,** Portacaval shunts. In these shunts the portal vein is sewn to the inferior vena cava so that some or all of portal venous blood enters the inferior vena cava without passing through the liver. In the *end-to-side* portacaval shunt, the portal vein is tied off just before it enters the liver. The remaining portion of the portal vein is sewn to the side of the inferior vena cava. As a result all portal blood flow is diverted directly into the inferior vena cava, and none passes into the liver. In the *side-to-side* portacaval shunt, the side of the portal vein is sewn to the side of the inferior vena cava. As a result some of the portal venous blood can flow into the liver if resistance to flow is low; however, most portal blood flow enters the inferior vena cava directly. **C,** Mesocaval shunts. With these shunts the superior mesenteric vein is sewn to the inferior vena cava so that some or all of visceral venous

blood flow from the superior mesenteric vein is diverted into the inferior vena cava. When the standard mesocaval shunt is constructed, the inferior vena cava is transected below the level of the renal veins and the proximal portion of the inferior vena cava is sewn to the side of the mesenteric vein. As a result the major direction of visceral venous blood flow is into the inferior vena cava (bypassing the liver). Some of the superior mesenteric venous flow can pass into the liver, however, if resistance to blood flow is low. Splenic venous blood flow can also continue into the liver. An *interposition mesocaval shunt* is hemodynamically similar to the standard mesocaval shunt, but it does not involve transection of the inferior vena cava. Instead, an autogenous vein graft is used to create a route of blood flow between the inferior vena cava and the superior mesenteric vein. As a result visceral venous blood flow can pass through the graft into the inferior vena cava, or it can continue into the portal venous circulation and into the liver if resistance to flow is low.

Reproduced with permission from Altman, R.P.: Portal hypertension. In Ravitch, M.M., et al. editors: Pediatric surgery, ed. 3. Copyright © 1979 by Year Book Medical Publishers, Inc., Chicago.

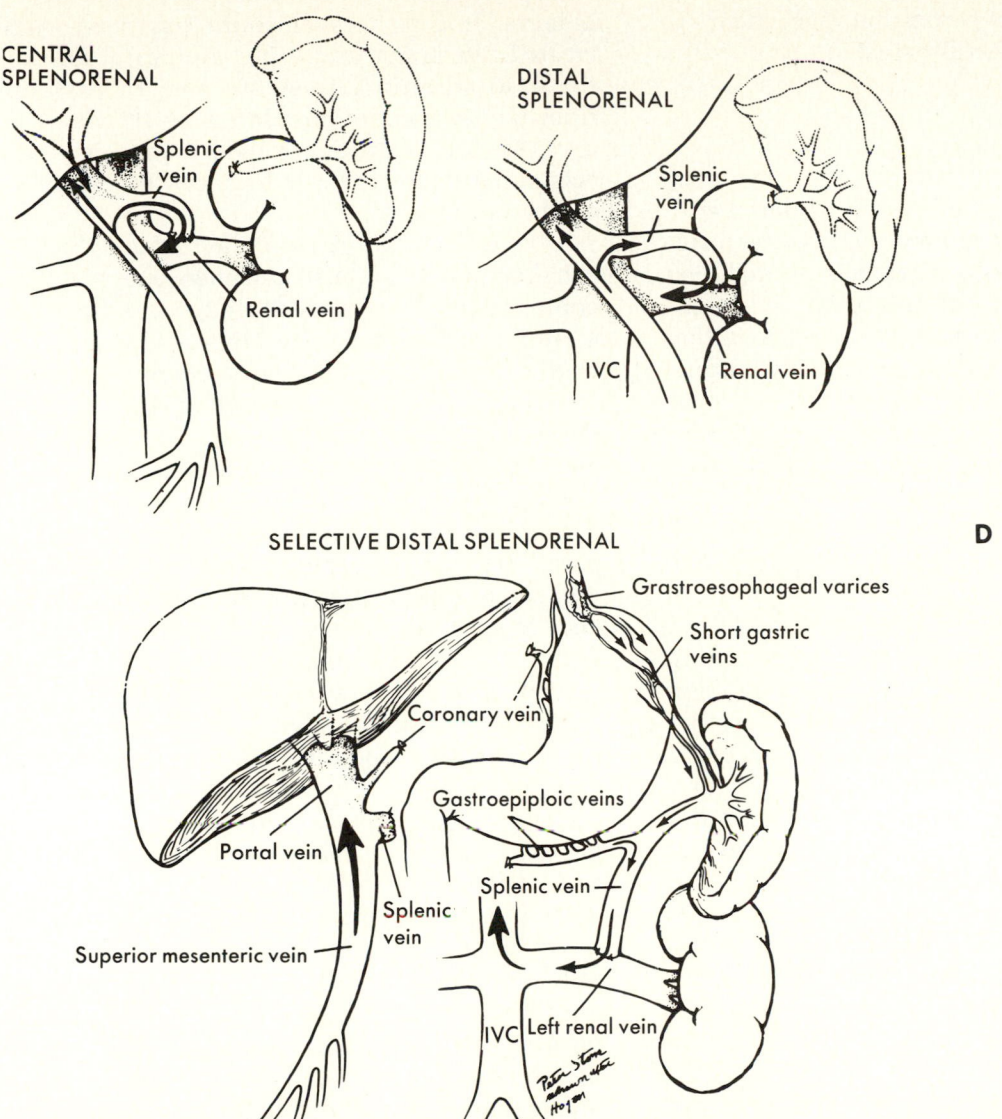

CENTRAL SPLENORENAL

Splenic vein

Renal vein

DISTAL SPLENORENAL

Splenic vein

IVC

Renal vein

SELECTIVE DISTAL SPLENORENAL

Grastroesophageal varices

Short gastric veins

Coronary vein

Gastroepiploic veins

Portal vein

Splenic vein

Splenic vein

Superior mesenteric vein

IVC Left renal vein

D

Fig. 8-12, cont'd D, Splenorenal shunts. These shunts use a portion of the splenic vein to provide a pathway to divert some of the portal venous blood into the renal vein. From there, the diverted blood passes into the systemic venous circulation via the inferior vena cava. When the *central splenorenal shunt* is created, the spleen is removed and the remaining splenic vein is used to divert some portal venous blood into the renal vein (and thus it will flow into the systemic venous circulation through the inferior vena cava). This shunt is labeled a central shunt because the splenic vein segment is sewn to the renal vein near the junction of the renal vein and the inferior vena cava. When the *distal splenorenal shunt* is created, the spleen is also removed. This shunt is similar to the central splenorenal shunt, although the splenic vein segment is sewn to the renal vein nearer the kidney (and farther from the junction of the renal vein and the inferior vena cava). In a *selective distal splenorenal shunt* the portal venous flow is partitioned. Visceral venous blood from the superior mesenteric vein continues to flow into the portal vein, then into the liver. The splenic vein is separated from the portal venous circulation, and it is sewn into the renal vein. Thus splenic venous circulation is diverted into the renal vein, and it passes into the systemic venous circulation through the inferior vena cava. Gastroesophageal varices are successfully decompressed through short gastric veins. They flow with splenic venous blood into the renal vein.

sive, life-threatening gastrointestinal bleeding is terrifying. The parents may require genetic counseling, particularly if the portal hypertension is secondary to inherited liver or metabolic disease.

■ **LIVER FAILURE**
■ **Etiology**

Liver failure is most often seen in children with chronic liver disease. Less commonly, it is the result of acute massive necrosis of a previously normal liver (fulminant hepatic failure); this more acute liver failure usually occurs as the result of a viral illness. Other causes of acute liver failure in previously normal children include idiosyncratic reactions to anesthetics, antibiotics, and chemotherapeutic agents. Accidental ingestion of drugs or toxins such as acetaminophen, pesticides, cleaning compounds, or some plant alkaloids may also produce acute hepatic failure.[64] Liver failure not only produces clinical and biochemical evidence of failing liver function, but it can result in development of hepatic encephalopathy.

Hepatic encephalopathy in children with chronic liver disease is usually precipitated by such complicating events as gastrointestinal bleeding, large ingestion of protein, excessive use of diuretics, sepsis, or the administration of sedatives. It is not uncommon after surgical creation of portacaval shunts (for the control of gastrointestinal bleeding secondary to portal hypertension), since the portacaval shunt carries blood from the gut directly into the inferior vena cava. Successful prompt correction of the precipitating events will usually relieve the symptoms of encephalopathy.

■ **Pathophysiology**

Liver failure produces both an accumulation of substances normally removed by the liver and a lack of substances normally manufactured by the liver. Hepatic encephalopathy is thought to result from failure of the liver either to remove toxic substances (such as ammonia or amino acids) from the circulation or to contribute essential elements of cerebral metabolism (such as uridine triphosphate and cytidine triphosphate).

One factor commonly thought to contribute to hepatic encephalopathy is hyperammonemia. Often the child's serum ammonia levels inversely parallel the child's level of consciousness during development of hepatic encephalopathy. Ammonia is formed in the gastrointestinal tract from amino acids following bacterial and enzymatic breakdown of proteins. The ammonia created is normally absorbed into the splanchnic and portal venous systems, converted to nontoxic urea (by the liver), and ultimately excreted by the kidneys. If a portacaval shunt has been surgically created, ammonia and other amines absorbed from the gastrointestinal tract are able to pass directly from the splanchnic circulation to the inferior vena cava. Thus liver failure or liver bypass may result in accumulation of toxic substances that may impair cerebral function.

With liver failure the child's serum glucose level can drop rapidly because gluconeogenesis is no longer completed by the liver. Since glucose is the major substrate metabolized by the brain for energy, hypoglycemia can further compromise cerebral function.

The child with liver failure will also demonstrate coagulopathies. The liver will no longer produce normal amounts of prothrombin, and it will not remove the activated clotting factors from the circulation. In addition, if the child with liver failure has portal hypertension, the resultant hypersplenism can produce thrombocytopenia, anemia, and leukopenia, and esophageal varices will further increase the child's risk of hemorrhage.

When the child with liver failure has significant intravascular fluid loss because of ascites or splanchnic sequestration because of portal hypertension, an apparent decrease in circulating blood volume is perceived by the heart, the adrenal cortex, and the kidneys, so that more aldosterone is secreted, causing retention of renal sodium and water. With hyperaldosteronism more potassium and magnesium are lost in the urine, and more hydrogen ion is excreted (the kidneys excrete hydrogen ion in exchange for the sodium that is saved). The excess loss of hydrogen can produce a mild metabolic alkalosis, which can further increase renal potassium loss. Excess excretion of hydrogen ion by the kidney increases the renal production of ammonia; when large amounts of ammonia are produced, some of the ammonia can enter the renal venous blood, further increasing serum ammonia levels.

Children with end-stage cirrhosis, severe hepatic failure, or ascites refractory to diuretic therapy may develop hepatorenal syndrome, a progressive, functional renal failure of unknown cause. These children demonstrate a decrease in glomerular filtration rate, oliguria, and azotemia.

Many alterations in acid-base and electrolyte balance are possible when liver failure develops. As already mentioned, chronic hyperaldosteronism may cause a metabolic alkalosis and prevent the kidneys from retaining potassium. Gastrointestinal disturbances (such as diarrhea and vomiting) can result in further potassium loss and development of metabolic acidosis or alkalosis. Some children with chronic liver disease and ascites demonstrate intrapulmonary right-to-left shunting (some blood passes through unaerated areas of the lung so that it returns to the left heart desaturated) and a lowered arterial oxygen tension (Pao_2); this hypoxemia may improve with administration of oxygen.[42] Fig. 8-13 further describes the pathophysiology of liver failure and the resulting clinical signs and symptoms.

■ Clinical signs and symptoms

Signs of chronic liver disease include ascites with dilation of superficial abdominal veins (caput medusae), xanthoma formation, clubbing of nails, gynecomastia, skin ecchymosis, palmar erythema, and spider angiomas. Jaundice is often present. The child frequently appears malnourished, and ascites may be present. Early signs of hepatic encephalopathy and liver failure include malaise, extreme irritability or lethargy, inappropriate laughter or tears, forgetfulness, mild tremors, slurred speech, and reversal of day-night sleep patterns. Advanced stages include deep coma.

Neurologic signs of hepatic encephalopathy include tremors, incoordination, muscle twitching, and violent movements. The classic early finding is a peculiar flapping tremor known as *asterixis*. It can be elicited in an older child by having the youngster outstretch the arms and dorsiflex the hand. The patient will be unable to maintain the hyperextended position of the hand, and coarse bursts of twitching movements will appear at the wrist (see Chapter 6 for further discussion of neurologic aspects of hepatic encephalopathy).

Decreased production of serum clotting factors by the liver causes a prolonged prothrombin time (PT), manifested by ecchymosis or petechiae and increased bleeding from puncture sites or from mucosal irritation. Clotting factors VII and VIII may also be reduced. Serum-direct bilirubin, transaminases, alkaline phosphatase, and ammonia are usually elevated. Hepatic enzymes—SGOT, SGPT, LDH, and creatine phosphokinase (CPK)—and serum bilirubin will also be higher than normal; serum albumin is usually low. Anemia, leukopenia, hypoglycemia, hypokalemia, and hypocalcemia will develop in the presence of significant hepatic necrosis.

Clinical signs of hepatorenal syndrome include abrupt oliguria and azotemia, often apparently without precipitating factors. Laboratory findings include a normal urinalysis, serum hyponatremia (even

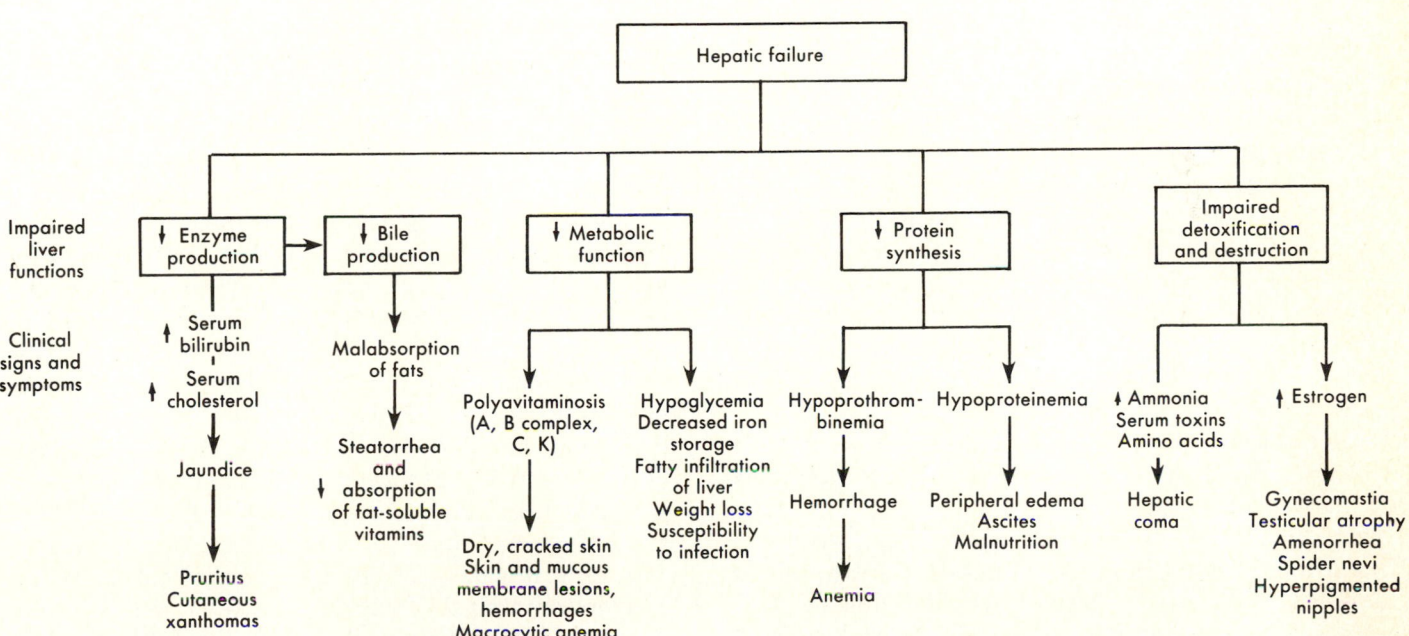

Fig. 8-13 Pathophysiology of hepatic failure.

Modified from Whaley, L., and Wong, D.: Nursing care of infants and children, ed. 2, St. Louis, 1983, The C.V. Mosby Co.

though the kidneys attempt to retain sodium, serum sodium drops because of dilution from relatively greater absorption of water), hypokalemia, and azotemia. The serum creatinine will rise and urine creatinine will fall, with significant impairment of renal function (see the discussion of renal failure in Chapter 7).

Cyanosis will be noted if intrapulmonary shunting is present. Children with liver disease and chronic hypoxemia may develop clubbing of digits and polycythemia (see Chapter 3 for discussion of potential systemic consequences of polycythemia). Arterial blood gases should be obtained if cyanosis is present, since administration of supplemental oxygen may be required.

If the cause of the hepatic failure is uncertain, diagnostic studies will be performed immediately. These studies include extensive toxicology screening (for evidence of alcohol, drug, or chemical ingestion), liver function studies, liver-spleen scan, angiography, and possible liver biopsy. The liver biopsy cannot be performed in the presence of significant coagulopathy; thus a coagulation profile should be obtained before biopsy is planned. Viral, bacteriologic, and fungal blood cultures may also be ordered.

If Reye's syndrome (discussed later in this chapter) is the cause of liver failure, hepatic encephalopathy, hyperammonemia, elevation of serum enzymes, and hypoglycemia may be present without jaundice.

■ **Medical treatment and nursing interventions**

All children who are critically ill require planned nursing assessments and interventions for all body systems; the child with liver failure is no exception. Careful monitoring for evidence of sepsis or infection and assessment of cardiac, respiratory, neurologic, and renal function is often more important than monitoring the child's liver function (see Chapters 3, 4, 6, and 7 for further information about assessment of these body systems). The focus of the discussion here is on clinical assessment and prevention of the complications of liver failure and encephalopathy.

The principal problems of the child with liver failure include any or all of the following: alteration in neurologic function, blood loss, changes in intravascular and interstitial fluid balance, compromised nutritional status, renal dysfunction, electrolyte or acid-base imbalance, respiratory insufficiency, increased risk of infection, decreased activity level, and patient and family anxiety.

Until liver function returns, treatment of the child with liver failure is primarily supportive. During the acute phase the most important goal of therapy is prevention of major complications such as increased intracranial pressure, hemorrhage, fluid and electrolyte imbalances, and renal failure. If the child's liver function does not return quickly, nutritional support and prevention of complications of chronic liver failure (such as portal hypertension) becomes important.

The child with hepatic failure may develop encephalopathy and resultant increased intracranial pressure. As a result it is imperative that the nurse be able to detect early signs of neurologic compromise. A brief but careful neurologic evaluation should be performed when vital signs are measured; pupil size and constriction to light should be noted, and any pupil sluggishness or inequality should be reported to a physician. The child's voluntary movements should be observed, and any decreased movement, decreased sensation, abnormal posturing, asterixis, or seizure activity should be reported to a physician immediately. Assessment of the child's level of consciousness is extremely important. The presence of unusual irritability or lethargy may indicate the development of increased intracranial pressure. To enable consistent objective evaluation of the older child's level of consciousness, the nurse may wish to use a short standard questionnaire (such as the numbers' connection exercise designed by Merrell National Laboratories[65]). The child may also be asked to write his name or identify common objects in the room. The names of the child's siblings and household pets should be noted in the nursing-care plan, since conversation about them may be used to evaluate the child's short- and long-term memory. Whatever the method of evaluation, the specific questions asked should be noted on the nursing-care plan in order to make the evaluation as consistent as possible.

If the child does develop encephalopathy or if a significant intrapulmonary (right-to-left) shunt develops, initiation of mechanical ventilation may be required to ensure effective gas exchange. In addition, mechanical ventilation will enable more direct manipulation of the child's arterial carbon dioxide tension (Pa_{CO_2}), which is often a crucial component of the management of increased intracranial pressure. Since hypercapnia produces cerebral vasodilation (and enhances cerebral blood flow), it can contribute to the development of increased intracranial pressure; as a result it is desirable to maintain the child's Pa_{CO_2} at approximately 25 to 29 torr if intracranial pressure is elevated (see Chapter 6). Since hypoxemia and hypoglycemia can also contribute to neurologic compromise, they should be prevented.

High serum ammonia levels may contribute to the development of hepatic encephalopathy; thus attempts are usually made to decrease the child's ammonia production and absorption. Since ammonia is produced in the gastrointestinal tract during bacterial and enzymatic breakdown of proteins, the child's protein intake is often reduced to 0.5 gm/kg/day.[21] Blood also contains proteins. Consequently, any blood in the stomach (such as occurs with nosebleeds or stress ulcers) should be removed with nasogastric drainage, using a soft nasogastric tube. Nonabsorbable antibiotics (such as neomycin, 4 to 8 gm/m²/day) may be administered to eliminate gastrointestinal bacteria. Antacids may be prescribed to prevent ammonia absorption, and lactobacillus may be given to acidify colonic content, promoting ammonium ion excretion. Finally, colonic lavage may also be prescribed to decrease ammonia absorption.

If the child has any clinical or laboratory (serologic) evidence of coagulopathies, blood components are administered (see Table 3-10). The child's total circulating blood volume should be calculated and any blood loss considered a percentage of this blood volume; blood loss totaling 7% to 10% of the child's blood volume should be replaced to prevent hemodynamic compromise. If a severe gastrointestinal hemorrhage occurs, prompt treatment is required to prevent shock (see the discussion earlier in this chapter). Blood and blood components should be available (typed and cross-matched) in the blood bank for use during sudden bleeding episodes. All efforts must be made to prevent oral, tracheal, and gastrointestinal trauma during intubation, suctioning, and mouth care.

Anemia should be prevented, since it reduces the child's oxygen-carrying capacity and may contribute to increased cardiac work and hypoxemia.

The child with hepatic failure can develop fluid shifts and fluid imbalance because of hyperaldosteronism (and increased sodium and water retention), hypoalbuminemia, portal hypertension and resultant splanchnic sequestration (see discussion of portal hypertension), or hepatorenal syndrome. All sources of the child's fluid intake and output must be measured, and accurate body weights are obtained at least once a day. The nurse can evaluate the child's level of hydration by assessing moistness of mucous membranes, presence of tearing, fullness of the fontanelle (in infants less than 16 to 18 months of age), skin turgor, and urine output. To enable more precise evaluation of the child's intravascular volume, it is desirable that a central venous catheter also be placed to provide direct measurement of the child's CVP. The presence of a high CVP is undesirable, since it may contribute to an increase in intracranial pressure and may increase esophageal variceal pressure (and promote

bleeding). As a result, when blood component administration is necessary, constant assessment of the child's response is required. Diuretics may be prescribed to promote diuresis; the child's response to therapy should be monitored, and the physician should be notified of inadequate urine response.

To prevent shock hypovolemia requires prompt treatment. Administration of blood components and albumin is usually required during the course of therapy.

The child's urine output must be monitored closely. If urine volume is less than 0.5-1.0 ml/kg/hour despite adequate fluid intake, the physician should be notified. While a decrease in urine output may be appropriate in the face of ascites and decreased intravascular volume, oliguria accompanied by azotemia usually indicates the development of renal failure.

Electrolyte imbalance may result from fluid shifts, hyperaldosteronism, or diuretic therapy. Serum electrolyte concentrations should be checked frequently, and electrolyte replacement therapy will often be required. Hypoglycemia can develop rapidly, especially in infants, so the child's serum glucose (or the infant's heelstick glucose) should be frequently checked and supplemental glucose administered (with the physician's order) as needed.

The child's abdominal girth should be measured and recorded at least every 4 hours. If the child develops ascites, the nurse should monitor particularly for the development of decreased intravascular volume, hypoventilation and respiratory distress (because of decreased diaphragmatic excursion secondary to abdominal distention), and the development of hydrothorax.

Nutritional compromise can rapidly develop when the child has hepatic failure. Parenteral nutrition will be required if the child is unable to tolerate oral or tube feedings. The child's daily caloric requirements should be calculated and the physician consulted if the child is not receiving them with current therapy. Administration of vitamin supplements (especially A, B complex, C, D, E, and K) is usually necessary. If the child is receiving any medications normally metabolized by the liver, the dosages of these medications should be reviewed and adjusted as necessary (to prevent development of toxic drug levels).

Steroids may be prescribed, particularly if the child develops hepatic encephalopathy. Hemodialysis or exchange transfusion may be ordered to reduce serum ammonia levels and eliminate some accumulated toxins. Table 8-13 details nursing interventions appropriate for care of the child with hepatic failure (note that it assumes that all of the diagnostic studies have been performed).

Text continued on p. 596.

Table 8-13   Nursing care of the child with liver failure

Nursing diagnosis	Expected outcome	Nursing actions
A. *Potential alteration in neurologic function/ orientation* secondary to decreased ammonia excretion, decreased liver detoxification of nitrogenous wastes, decreased liver secretion of important substrates, hypoglycemia, and possible cerebral edema	1. Patient will be oriented to time, place, and person 2. Patient will regain prefailure level of speech and neuromuscular function 3. Patient will have serum ammonia, glucose, and BUN levels within normal range	1. Assess for signs of neurologic deterioration (irritability or lethargy, inappropriate laughter or tears, forgetfulness, mild tremors, slurred speech, reversal of day/night sleep patterns, decreased response to verbal or tactile stimulation) 2. Monitor for signs of increased intracranial pressure: irritability, lethargy, sluggish or unequal pupil response to light, headache, vomiting, alteration in respiratory rate or rhythm, apnea, systolic hypertension, bradycardia, abnormal posturing, ataxia, tense fontanelle in infants <18 months of age (see Chapter 6 for details of increased intracranial pressure) 3. Perform frequent age-appropriate mental status examinations (every 1-2 hr, and as indicated by patient status) with reorientation to time/ person/place as needed; immediately notify physician of inappropriate response 4. When possible, ask patient to daily write his or her name; comparison from day to day often reflects neuromuscular changes 5. Daily use of a numbers-connection exercise, such as the tool designed by Merrell National Laboratories,[65] is useful for school-age children and adolescents 6. Remove any gastrointestinal blood by nasogastric drainage (since the blood may enhance ammonia formation) 7. Promote ammonia excretion by administration of lactulose (given by mouth, nasogastric tube, or enema), which acidifies colonic content and promotes ammonium ion excretion in stool 8. Decrease nitrogen- and ammonia-forming intestinal bacteria by administering non-absorbable oral antibiotics as ordered (neomycin, kanamycin, tetracycline)

Table 8-13 Nursing care of the child with liver failure—cont'd

Nursing diagnosis	Expected outcome	Nursing actions
A. *Potential alteration in neurologic function/orientation* secondary to decreased ammonia excretion, decreased liver detoxification of nitrogenous wastes, decreased liver secretion of important substrates, hypoglycemia, and possible cerebral edema —cont'd		9. Assess for and ensure prompt treatment of potential causes of hepatic encephalopathy. Potentially preventable causes include gastrointestinal bleeding, uremia, hypoglycemia and administration or patient ingestion of high protein load 10. Monitor tolerance to all prescribed medications that require liver clearance or detoxification; signs of toxic effects may become evident following even small dosages 11. Avoid use of opiates, sedatives, tranquilizers, and antihistamines as possible; if sedation is needed, phenobarbital or chloral hydrate is preferred 12. Monitor serum albumin, BUN, ammonia, and glucose; monitor capillary glucose by heelsticks as needed in infants; notify physician of abnormalities 13. Maintain protein restrictions as ordered; begin low protein diet when oral intake is resumed (because the liver has decreased ability to metabolize a high protein load)
B. *Blood loss* (and hypovolemia) secondary to 1. Portal hypertension and resultant esophageal varices and splenic congestion or 2. Alteration in blood-clotting mechanism secondary to decreased hepatic synthesis of necessary clotting factors and decreased absorption of fat-soluble vitamin K	1. Patient will be protected from trauma and injury 2. Patient will not experience hemodynamic compromise from bleeding episodes (they will be prevented or treated promptly) 3. Patient's Hct will be maintained at satisfactory levels (determined by medical team): Hct >40%-45% (infants) Hct >30%-35% (children) NOTE: These values should be individualized for *each* patient based on hemodynamic status, body weight, and admission Hct	1. Monitor laboratory results of Hct and coagulation profile (PT/PTT, platelet count); notify physician of any abnormalities 2. Monitor for clinical signs of coagulopathy (presence of petechiae, ecchymosis, prolonged or spontaneous bleeding from venipuncture sites or mucous membranes) 3. Assess location of blood loss or presence of gastrointestinal bleeding (hematest or guaiac for all emesis, nasogastric secretions, or stool); monitor heart rate, blood pressure, and systemic perfusion closely 4. Instruct patient to avoid excessive straining during bowel movements, which could cause bleeding from rectal mucosa or hemorrhoids; administer stool softeners as prescribed

Continued.

Table 8-13 Nursing care of the child with liver failure—cont'd

Nursing diagnosis	Expected outcome	Nursing actions
B. *Blood loss* (and hypovolemia) secondary to—cont'd		5. Clip child's fingernails to prevent injury from scratches
		6. Prevent bleeding by using small-gauge needles when possible for venipuncture or intramuscular injections; maintain indwelling catheters for routine collection of blood samples. Use foam toothbrush and gentle mouth care to prevent oral bleeding
		7. If bleeding occurs, notify physician, administer therapy as ordered, including iced saline lavage, use of Sengstaken-Blakemore tube, or administration of fresh whole blood, fresh frozen plasma, clotting factors, or platelets (see discussion of gastrointestinal bleeding). Blood loss totaling 5%-10% of patient's total circulating blood volume should be promptly replaced (refer to Table 3-10)
		8. Monitor for signs of transfusion reaction (fever, rash, hives, pruritus)
		9. Restrict child's activities as needed to prevent injury; pad side rails if child demonstrates vigorous movements that could cause injury
C. *Potential alteration in intravascular and interstitial fluid balance* secondary to hypoalbuminemia, ascites, and possible hemorrhage	1. Patient will maintain adequate intravascular volume as measured by blood pressure, heart rate, CVP, urine output, and indirect evidence of systemic perfusion	1. Calculate daily fluid requirements (see Table 8-3)
		2. Measure all forms of fluid loss (such as GI secretions, urine, and diarrhea)
		3. Monitor for signs of increasing ascites (increase in daily weight or abdominal girth or development of anasarca or edema); notify physician if these occur
		4. Administer plasma or colloids as ordered to maintain intravascular oncotic pressure; monitor patient serum osmolality
		5. Administer diuretics as ordered; monitor patient response, and discuss inadequate or excessive diuresis with physician

Table 8-13 Nursing care of the child with liver failure—cont'd

Nursing diagnosis	Expected outcome	Nursing actions

C. *Potential alteration in intravascular and interstitial fluid balance* secondary to hypoalbuminemia, ascites, and possible hemorrhage—cont'd	2. Patient will gain minimum fluid weight; significant weight gain or loss will be discussed with physician. "Significant" weight changes are approximately:
	  ≥50 gm/24 hr (infants)
	  ≥200 gm/24 hr (children)
	NOTE: These weight changes should be individualized for each patient, with agreement among the medical team
	
	3. Patient will demonstrate adequate hydration: adequate tearing (if >6 wk of age), good skin turgor, non-depressed fontanelle if <18 mo of age
	
	4. Patient's abdominal girth will remain stable or decrease in size
	
	5. Patient will not demonstrate respiratory compromise secondary to compromised diaphragmatic excursion or hydrothorax
	
	6. Patient will maintain serum albumin levels within normal range
		6. Monitor for signs of adequate intravascular volume (tachycardia, peripheral vasoconstriction, dry mucous membranes, hypotension, low CVP) especially after diuresis; notify physician if these are noted
		
		7. Monitor Hct and electrolyte values, particularly serum sodium and potassium; discuss any abnormalities with physician
		
		8. Monitor for signs of electrolyte loss associated with diuretic therapy (decreased potassium, chloride, phosphate, and sodium)
		
		9. Maintain fluid and sodium restrictions as ordered
		
		10. Maintain strict record of intake and output, including all medications, IV solutions, blood products, nasogastric replacement and oral intake; discuss significant imbalances or sources of excessive fluid loss with physician
		
		11. Monitor for signs of respiratory distress (tachypnea, retractions, nasal flaring, cyanosis) or change in quality or pitch of breath sounds; this may indicate hypoventilation or the development of a hydrothorax (see problem G)
		
		12. Assist with paracentesis if significant hydrothorax develops. Ensure sterile field and technique; monitor for signs of inadequate intravascular volume after procedure
		
		13. Monitor for signs of hepatorenal syndrome (oliguria and azotemia)

Continued.

Table 8-13 Nursing care of the child with liver failure—cont'd

Nursing diagnosis	Expected outcome	Nursing actions
D. *Potential alteration in nutritional status* secondary to fluid or protein restriction, increased catabolic state, anemia, impaired liver digestive functions, or impaired absorption of fat-soluble vitamins	1. Patient will receive adequate calories to promote healing and eliminate catabolic state. Adequacy of caloric intake should be determined by assessment of patient skin turgor and wound healing, liver function studies (these should reveal liver healing), coagulation profile, electrolyte status 2. Patient will progress to oral alimentation, tolerating low-protein diet and receiving adequate calories for age and metabolic needs	1. When patient is unable to tolerate oral feedings, tube feedings or peripheral or central parenteral nutrition with reduced amino acid concentration should be considered (see discussion of parenteral nutrition) 2. Monitor serum (or heelstick) glucose levels, and report hypoglycemia immediately to physician 3. When nasogastric or oral feedings progress, calculate protein intake per physician's recommendation. Number of grams of protein provided per day will vary with age, weight, and clinical condition of the patient 4. Calculate patient's daily caloric energy requirement (see Table 8-6). Report any deficiency in intake to physician; develop strategies for providing optimum caloric requirements within the fluid restriction 5. Administer vitamins (especially A, B complex, C, D, E, and K) as ordered orally or via parenteral solution 6. Allow for adequate rest and maintain stable environmental temperature to promote optimum use of calories

E. *Potential alteration in renal function* resulting from chronic liver disease and resultant hyperaldosteronism and possible development of hepatorenal syndrome	1. Patient's urine output will remain ≥0.5-1.0 ml/kg/hr average (if fluid intake is adequate)
	
	2. Patient will gain minimum fluid weight
	Weight gain
	  ≥50 gm/24 hr (infants)
	  ≥200 gm/24 hr (children)
	will be discussed with physician
	
	3. Patient's urinary creatinine clearance and serum BUN and creatinine will remain or return to normal
		1. Carefully measure all sources of fluid intake and output. Measure urine specific gravity at least every 4-8 hr. Notify physician of urine output <0.5-1.0 ml/kg/hr
		
		2. Weigh patient daily or twice daily at same time(s) of the day on same scale; discuss excessive weight gain with physician
		
		3. Monitor for signs of fluid retention (increased abdominal girth, periorbital edema, positive calculated fluid balance), and discuss these with physician
		
		4. Administer diuretics as ordered; monitor patient response and report inadequate or excessive diuresis immediately to physician

Table 8-13 Nursing care of the child with liver failure—cont'd

Nursing diagnosis	Expected outcome	Nursing actions
E. *Potential alteration in renal function* resulting from chronic liver disease and resultant hyperaldosteronism and possible development of hepatorenal syndrome—cont'd	4. Patient will not demonstrate evidence of cardiovascular compromise (tachycardia, hypotension, poor systemic perfusion) secondary to renal failure	5. Monitor serum electrolyte levels (especially serum potassium, sodium, and chloride, since these can be altered by diuretic therapy and renal failure), BUN, and creatinine; discuss abnormalities with physician 6. Assist with paracentesis, exchange transfusion, or hemodialysis as ordered 7. Collect urine samples for laboratory analysis (e.g., electrolytes and creatinine clearance) as ordered 8. Report evidence of circulatory compromise (tachycardia, hypotension, poor systemic perfusion) immediately to physician (see discussion of low cardiac output in Chapter 3) 9. Administer corticosteroids as ordered to enhance diuresis
F. *Potential alteration in serum electrolyte concentrations and acid-base balance* secondary to hyperaldosteronism, renal dysfunction, diuretic therapy, gastrointestinal fluid loss, hemorrhage, liver dysfunction, and acid-base imbalance	1. Patient's serum electrolyte concentrations will remain at or return to normal 2. Patient will not demonstrate cardiovascular compromise (hypotension, arrhythmias, poor systemic perfusion, tachycardia) secondary to electrolyte imbalance 3. Patient's arterial pH, bicarbonate, and CO_2 values will remain or return to normal	1. Monitor serum electrolyte values (particularly check for hypokalemia, hyponatremia, hypoglycemia, hypocalcemia), and discuss abnormalities with physician. Particularly note effects of administration of diuretics on potassium and sodium concentration 2. Monitor for clinical signs of electrolyte or acid-base imbalance (see Table 8-4) 3. Monitor arterial pH and serum bicarbonate and CO_2 concentrations. Discuss evidence of acidosis or alkalosis with physician 4. Administer electrolyte supplements or bicarbonate as ordered 5. See discussion of renal failure in Chapter 7
G. *Potential respiratory insufficiency* related to compromise of diaphragmatic excursion, ventilation-perfusion abnormalities (pulmonary right-to-left shunt), encephalopathy, and possible hydrothorax	1. Patient will demonstrate normal respiratory rate (determination of individual patient's "normal" range requires consideration of that patient's age, clinical condition, and preillness respiratory rate)	1. Monitor patient's ABG and discuss abnormalities with physician 2. Monitor for cyanosis; notify physician if this is present 3. Administer supplemental oxygen as ordered, and monitor its effect on patient's ABG and color

Continued.

Table 8-13 Nursing care of the child with liver failure—cont'd

Nursing diagnosis	Expected outcome	Nursing actions
G. *Potential respiratory insufficiency* related to compromise of diaphragmatic excursion, ventilation-perfusion abnormalities (pulmonary right-to-left shunt), encephalopathy, and possible hydrothorax—cont'd	2. Patient will demonstrate no evidence of increased respiratory effort (retractions, nasal flaring, grunting) 3. Patient's arterial blood gas (ABG) values will remain at or return to normal	4. Assess patient's breath sounds and chest expansion bilaterally; notify physician of significant change in breath sounds (monitor especially for evidence of atelectasis or hydrothorax) 5. If significant deterioration in patient respiratory function develops (as evidenced by tachypnea, increased respiratory effort, a fall in Pa_{O_2} or pH, a rise in Pa_{CO_2}, or a deterioration in the patient's color), notify physician immediately. A chest film will be ordered. Prepare for emergency thoracentesis, chest-tube insertion, or intubation 6. Be prepared to provide ventilatory support as needed 7. Encourage the patient to cough and take deep breaths every 2-4 hr to prevent atelectasis and minimize ventilation-perfusion mismatch. Perform "rib-springing" exercises in infants and small children to promote deep breathing 8. Administer analgesics and sedatives with caution, and monitor their effect on respiratory function 9. If encephalopathy is present, monitor for changes in respiratory rhythm or apnea as a result of increased intracranial pressure; be prepared to institute emergency resuscitative measures
H. *Potential development of contractures or skin breakdown* as the result of immobilization	1. Patient will maintain full range of motion of all extremities 2. Patient will not demonstrate skin breakdown or contractures	1. Provide active or passive range of motion to all extremities every 2-4 hr 2. Turn patient frequently (every 1-2 hr), or change position 3. Promote optimum pulmonary hygiene by encouraging patient coughing and deep breathing, or suction every 2 hr (and as needed) 4. Pad pressure points of skin as needed 5. Use sheepskin or air mattress as needed 6. As soon as possible, provide for activity progression (dangling feet over bedside, out of bed to chair, short ambulation)

Table 8-13 Nursing care of the child with liver failure—cont'd

Nursing diagnosis	Expected outcome	Nursing actions
H. *Potential development of contractures or skin breakdown* as the result of immobilization—cont'd		7. Apply supportive stockings to lower extremities as needed to prevent venous stasis 8. Monitor for signs of thrombophlebitis and pulmonary embolism
I. *Potential patient or family anxiety* secondary to child's altered neurologic function, the gravity of the child's illness and prognosis	1. When alert, patient will express anxiety through verbalization or projective play 2. Patient will communicate with family members as often as possible 3. Family will demonstrate comprehension of child's basic disease process and treatment plan and realistic appraisal of child's prognosis	1. Assess child's (as appropriate) and family's comprehension of child's illness, prognosis, and treatment plan 2. Explain all procedures, movements, sounds to child *before* initiating procedures, regardless of child's level of consciousness 3. Place familiar object(s) near child (blanket, toy, book, tape recording of family or friends, pictures) 4. Keep parents and significant others aware of child's condition; keep child informed of parents' location (when they are not with the child) 5. Provide consistent explanations and information 6. Provide opportunities for projective play when possible. Supervise syringe and needle play with doll; offer water play 7. Provide diversional activities as possible (television, radio) 8. Encourage visitation of hospital play therapist or child-life worker, if available 9. Request involvement of the unit social worker if additional family financial or emotional support is needed
J. *Increased risk of infection* because of leukopenia, hypoalbuminemia, multiple invasive monitoring lines, invasive diagnostic tests, and poor nutritional status	1. Patient will demonstrate no new evidence of infection (fever, localized inflammation, leukocytosis)	1. Monitor patient temperature, and notify physician of temperature above 38.5° C 2. Since acetaminophen is contraindicated in patient with hepatic failure and aspirin would further depress platelet function, a cooling blanket or sponge baths may be ordered to reduce fever

Continued.

Table 8-13 Nursing care of the child with liver failure—cont'd

Nursing diagnosis	Expected outcome	Nursing actions
J. *Increased risk of infection* because of leukopenia, hypoalbuminemia, multiple invasive monitoring lines, invasive diagnostic tests, and poor nutritional status—cont'd		3. Maintain strict hand-washing technique before and after each patient contact. Monitor hand-washing technique of other medical personnel
		4. Obtain blood cultures and complete blood count as ordered
		5. Monitor appearance of wounds and intravascular catheter entrance sites for signs of erythema or exudate; notify physician if these appear, and obtain cultures as ordered

■ DISSEMINATED INTRAVASCULAR COAGULATION

■ Etiology

Disseminated intravascular coagulation (DIC) is a syndrome caused by abnormal activation of the clotting mechanism. This abnormal activation of blood coagulation can be triggered by a variety of circumstances, including overwhelming sepsis, shock, hypoxia, trauma, or liver disease. Widespread clotting activation causes rapid consumption of coagulation factors, with resultant coagulopathy.

■ Pathophysiology

Abnormal activation of the clotting mechanism leads to rapid depletion of platelets, prothrombin, fibrinogen, and specific clotting factors, hemorrhage, and deposition of fibrin plugs in vessels of all sizes. Subsequent thromboembolic formation may be apparent in large vessels such as the femoral artery, and it may produce tissue ischemia and necrosis in the brain, lungs, kidneys, liver, or gastrointestinal tract. Hemolytic anemia often results from red blood cell fragmentation. Further illustration of the pathophysiology of DIC is presented in Fig. 8-14.

■ Clinical signs and symptoms

Classic signs of DIC are those resulting from the coagulopathy, and they are usually evidenced by a petechial or purpuric rash over much of the body. There is diffuse bleeding from any venipuncture or access site. Organs most vulnerable to bleeding are the skin, lungs, kidney, and brain. The intensity of bleeding corresponds closely to levels of fibrinogen and the child's platelet count. Neonates with DIC are more vulnerable to intracranial hemorrhage.

Hypoxemia and hemoptysis may occur with pulmonary involvement. Oliguria, hematuria, or renal failure may also be seen (see Chapter 7 for further discussion of renal failure), and signs of liver failure may develop (see the section in this chapter on liver failure). Shock will occur with significant hemorrhage (see Chapter 3 for details of low cardiac output). Laboratory studies confirm the presence of prolonged PT and partial thromboplastin time (PTT) and a decrease in platelet count, fibrinogen, and clotting factors II, V, and VIII. Fibrin split products (FSP) are present, anemia is noted, and red blood cell fragments are visible on peripheral blood smear.

■ Medical treatment and nursing interventions

Effective treatment of DIC requires correction of the precipitating condition. Replacement of depleted clotting factors is necessary when there is uncontrollable hemorrhage or grossly abnormal coagulation values that place the patient at risk for serious bleeding episodes (e.g., platelet count less than 20,000/ml, PT and PTT greater than twice normal, fibrinogen less than 75 mg/dl). Platelet transfusions (1 U/5 kg) are administered as needed to decrease active bleeding and maintain adequate platelet concentration. Fresh frozen plasma (10 to 15 ml/kg body weight) is administered as often as necessary to replace fibrinogen, prothrombin, and clotting factors V and VIII (for further information regarding blood

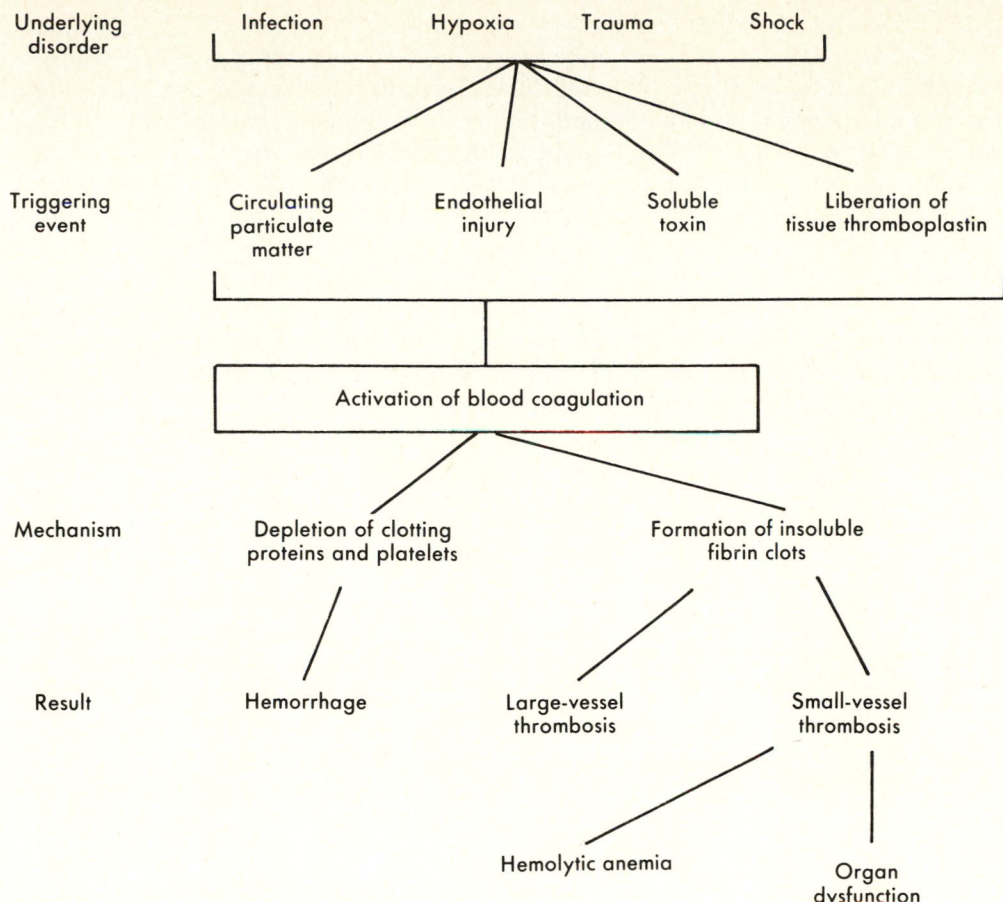

| Underlying disorder | Infection | Hypoxia | Trauma | Shock |

Fig. 8-14 Pathophysiology of disseminated intravascular coagulation.

From Levin, D., Morriss, F.C., and Moore, G.C.: A practical guide to pediatric intensive care, ed. 2, St. Louis, 1984, The C.V. Mosby Co.

component therapy, see Table 3-10). Whole blood or packed red blood cells are often required to maintain an adequate hemoglobin concentration and circulating blood volume, and intramuscular vitamin K injections are often administered.

The treatment of DIC with heparin is controversial. Heparin prevents coagulation and thus should prevent further thrombosis and eliminate the consumptive coagulopathy. However, heparin can also worsen any existing bleeding, and it has not been shown to improve patient survival.[22] Heparin therapy is contraindicated in patients with diffuse vasculitis or severe thrombocytopenia and those who are prone to intracranial bleeding. If heparin therapy is ordered, a loading dose (50 U/kg body weight) is often prescribed initially. Heparin therapy may then be accomplished through continuous IV infusion (10 to 20 U/kg/hour) or with intermittent IV doses (50 to 75 U/kg every 4 hours; see Table 3-10). Since heparin

therapy prolongs the PTT and clotting time, measurements of these values will no longer provide information about the progression of the DIC. Response to therapy will be evident by a rise in the child's fibrinogen levels.[22]

Since the neonate often cannot tolerate large infusions of platelets, plasma, or blood products, exchange transfusion may be required to control the coagulopathy.

During therapy the nurse should closely assess the patient for evidence of bleeding. All venipuncture sites should be watched closely, and a guaiac test should be performed on any secretions or drainage to document the presence of blood. Generalized bleeding can occur from the lung, the gastrointestinal tract, and the mucous membranes of the critically ill child (see the discussion of gastrointestinal bleeding for specific nursing interventions). A pressure dressing should be applied to active bleeding sites. All venipunctures will require application of pressure for several minutes.

The patient's hemoglobin, hematocrit, and coagulation profile should be monitored frequently. A sudden fall in hematocrit or an increase in PT and PTT can reflect activation or exacerbation of the DIC.

Frequent measurement of the patient's vital signs is necessary, since tachycardia and hypotension can occur as the result of the underlying disorder or in response to hemorrhage. The nurse should especially watch for signs of decreased systemic perfusion and hypovolemic shock (see the discussion of low cardiac output in Chapter 3). Since hypoxemia and acidosis can precipitate DIC, it is imperative that effective ventilation be established and maintained. If sepsis is present or strongly suspected, prompt antimicrobial therapy is indicated.

■ Postoperative/Postprocedure Care—Abdominal Surgery

Abdominal surgery in children is indicated to explore the cause of an acute abdomen or the source of a major gastrointestinal hemorrhage; it is also indicated for correction of known anomalies, including mechanical obstructions and deformities, organ malfunction, inflammation, or malignancies. Postoperative complications of abdominal surgery include dehydration, third spacing of extracellular fluid, infection, paralytic ileus, bowel obstruction, diarrhea, electrolyte imbalance, hemorrhage, malnutrition, and respiratory problems secondary to immobility.

■ POSTOPERATIVE COMPLICATIONS

Dehydration can occur in the immediate postoperative period if perioperative fluid and blood losses are not corrected. Adequate replacement of colloids and electrolytes is necessary. The child with dehydration (or inadequate fluid administration) will demonstrate dry mucous membranes, decreased urine output (with high specific gravity), flat or sunken fontanelle, and a low CVP.

After abdominal surgery, patients may have major shifts of fluid from intracellular and intravascular spaces into nonfunctional compartments such as the peritoneum and bowel wall. This is known as *third spacing* of fluids. Third spacing occurs from injury or infection, which causes increased capillary permeability, thereby allowing plasma protein to diffuse into nonfunctional body compartments. Frequently, third spacing of fluids is difficult to detect. Third spacing initially causes signs of decreased in-

travascular volume, evidenced by increased heart rate, peripheral vasoconstriction, low urine output, high urine specific gravity and osmolality, low CVP, and, finally, hypotension. Treatment of third spacing requires maintenance of intravascular volume with appropriate fluids and colloids. Colloid administration helps to increase the intravascular osmotic pressure, which should reduce further fluid loss from the vascular compartment. Often, administration of a diuretic (furosemide, 1 to 2 mg/kg/dose) is ordered immediately after the administration of the colloid to promote diuresis of excess fluid that returns to the vascular space.

As postoperative inflammation or infection decreases, the patient begins to rebound from the third-spacing phenomenon. As the tissues and injured areas heal, the capillaries also heal and regain their normal permeability and osmotic pressure, and fluids in the nonfunctional compartments shift back into the vascular space. This recovery phase is identified by a sudden marked diuresis with low urine specific gravity and osmolality. Fluid administration during this time should be reevaluated, since the increase in the intravascular volume may cause circulatory overload. Frequently, parenteral fluid administration rate is tapered until the fluid shift and diuresis have occurred.

The development of a paralytic ileus will delay the return of normal gastrointestinal motility. Oral feedings are held, and a nasogastric tube is often inserted to remove air and gastric secretions. Return of normal bowel activity will produce active bowel sounds, and the child will begin to pass flatus and stool. If the patient is given nothing by mouth for longer than a few days, peripheral parenteral nutrition should be considered. This nutritional support supplies the patient with the appropriate calories, amino acids, glucose, electrolytes, and minerals needed for tissue healing (see discussion of total parenteral nutrition).

If bowel rupture occurs preoperatively or during surgery, the peritoneum has been contaminated by the nonsterile gastrointestinal contents. This increases the child's risk of postoperative infection, most commonly gram-negative infection. The risk of postoperative gram-negative sepsis is particularly high in neonates.

Healing of any surgical anastomoses may produce scarring, constriction, and ultimate obstruction of the intestinal lumen. In addition, perioperative infection or inflammation can produce adhesions, which may also cause bowel obstruction. Signs of obstruction include nausea; abdominal distention, rigidity, and tenderness; an increase in nasogastric aspirate; or vomiting (particularly—but not exclusively—if vomiting is projectile or contains bilious material).

Diarrhea may occur in the immediate postoperative period and may be responsible for increased fluid losses during this time. Once oral feedings are resumed, diarrhea and malabsorption because of lactose or sucrose intolerance is often observed (see the section on diarrhea). If diarrhea is severe following resumption of oral diet, the oral feedings may have to be suspended to allow longer time for healing of bowel mucosa. When feedings are resumed, food should be introduced gradually, with gradual increase in osmolality. Postoperative lactose intolerance should be anticipated, and an alternative, lactose-free diet should be planned. If diarrhea persists, lactose- and sucrose-free feedings are often ordered. Elemental diets, including medium-chain triglycerides (instead of more complex fats) and amino acids may also be offered. If severe diarrhea persists with evidence of malabsorption (evidence of reducing substances in the stool), oral feedings should again be discontinued, and parenteral alimentation planned for several more days to allow bowel healing.

Vomiting, diarrhea, and third spacing of fluids can all contribute to electrolyte imbalances during the postoperative period. Hydrogen, chloride, and potassium ions are lost in vomitus and nasogastric aspirate; bicarbonate and potassium ions are lost when diarrhea occurs. If the patient requires a temporary gastrostomy, jejunostomy, ileostomy, or colostomy, specific electrolytes lost through these stomas will correspond to the electrolyte content of fluids in each of these portions of the bowel (see Table 8-1). Gastric losses are replaced with half-normal (0.45%) saline with potassium chloride supplement (20 to 40 mEq/L), and gastric and duodenal secretions are replaced with lactated Ringer's solution and potassium chloride supplement (20 to 40 mEq/L). Ileostomy drainage is replaced with lactated Ringer's solution. Excessive fluid loss from diarrhea is replaced with half-normal (0.45%) saline or lactated Ringer's solution with potassium chloride supplement (20 to 40 mEq/L).[56]

Hemorrhage can occur from breakdown or rupture of the gastrointestinal anastomoses or from DIC. To maintain intravascular volume and prevent the development of shock, early recognition and prompt replacement of excessive blood loss is imperative (see the discussion on gastrointestinal bleeding).

If nutritional needs are not met by administration of parenteral alimentation during bowel healing, the patient may develop a catabolic state, which can prevent wound healing and increase the risk of suture-line dehiscence.

■ NURSING INTERVENTIONS

Postoperative care of the child recovering from abdominal surgery requires prevention of respiratory complications, meticulous attention to the child's fluid and electrolyte balance and nutrition, and prevention of infection (Table 8-14).

During the immediate postoperative period, prevention of respiratory compromise is mandatory. Since abdominal distention or ascites can compromise diaphragmatic excursion and produce hypoventilation, postoperative ventilatory assistance may be planned for the child who requires major gastrointestinal manipulation or resection (see Table 4-15 for nursing care of the child requiring mechanical ventilation).

While the child is recovering from abdominal surgery, the head of the bed should be elevated 30 to 45 degrees to promote optimum diaphragmatic excursion. The child is encouraged to cough and breathe deeply; spirometry, chest physical therapy, and rib-springing exercises may be ordered to prevent atelectasis.

The nurse is responsible for strict measurement and recording of all fluid intake and output. Third spacing of fluids should be anticipated postoperatively, and the nurse should monitor for evidence of inadequate intravascular volume (hypovolemia).

A nasogastric tube is inserted postoperatively to prevent abdominal distention, discomfort, and excessive tension to the suture line. Nasogastric tubes should be irrigated and aspirated every 2 to 4 hours (per hospital routine and physician's order) with normal saline or small amounts of air. The child's loss of sodium, potassium, chloride, and hydrogen ions will be increased if mechanical intermittent suction is applied to the tube. All nasogastric drainage should be totaled every 4 to 8 hours; this fluid loss is usually replaced milliliter for milliliter with half-strength (0.45 percent) saline or lactated Ringer's solution[56]; the specific IV solution for replacement will be determined by the physician. Continuous nasogastric suction can cause irritation to the gastric mucosa and may cause gastrointestinal bleeding (see the section on gastrointestinal bleeding). Unreplaced loss of potassium and hydrogen ions can cause the development of metabolic alkalosis and consequences of hypokalemia (see Table 8-3).

The nurse should auscultate for bowel sounds every time vital signs are taken. Initially, bowel sounds are usually absent (an ileus is present); as the bowel recovers, bowel sounds will gradually return, and the child will begin to pass flatus or stool. The nasogastric tube is usually left in place until bowel sounds return. It may then be clamped for 4 to 6 hours; if the child does not develop abdominal distention, nausea, or vomiting, the tube may be removed. Oral feedings are not resumed until bowel sounds are present.

If the child has an acute abdomen preoperatively, pain medication is often withheld during that time to prevent masking of clinical signs and symptoms. Postoperatively, however, the child should receive adequate pain medication to prevent splinting of the abdominal incision, with resulting hypoventilation and immobility. The analgesic frequently administered is intravenous morphine (at a dose of 0.1 mg/kg body weight) or intravenous or intramuscular meperidine (at a dose of 1 mg/kg/body weight) every 3 to 4 hours. It is important to remember that most narcotics (especially morphine and meperidine) will decrease gastrointestinal motility; therefore bowel sounds may be decreased while the child is receiving narcotics.

Administration of intravenous antibiotics is in-dicated when peritonitis is present. Broad-spectrum antimicrobials are often ordered initially until specific infecting organisms are identified.

If abdominal drains are placed intraoperatively, the patient requires wound and skin isolation. The amount, consistency, odor, and color of wound drainage should be monitored closely, and wound and blood cultures are usually ordered if wound drainage becomes purulent or the patient becomes febrile (see Table 8-14).

All procedures and treatments should be carefully explained to the child and family. The child should be given the opportunity to discuss his response to therapy and offered diversional activities, as they are feasible. Surgical incisions may be frightening and threatening to the child's body image and sense of body integrity. The nurse can provide reassurance that the child's body is intact and that it will heal. Therapeutic play may offer the child the opportunity to express concerns or anger about the surgery.

Text continued on p. 606.

Table 8-14 Postoperative laparotomy nursing-care plan

Nursing diagnosis	Expected outcome	Nursing actions
A. Potential bowel obstruction secondary to structural defect or paralytic ileus related to operative manipulation	1. Patient will demonstrate patent GI tract as measured by passage of flatus and stool, absence of vomiting, and presence of normal bowel sounds 2. Patient will tolerate regular diet for age with consistent, gradual weight gain (appropriate for age and height)	1. Observe for signs of paralytic ileus (increasing NG output via NG tube, absent or diminished bowel sounds, increasing abdominal girth) 2. Maintain "NPO" until bowel function returns 3. Maintain patency of NG tube (irrigate and aspirate every 2-4 hr as needed with 5-20 cc of saline or air, according to hospital policy and physician's order) 4. Ensure proper position of NG tube; note color, amount and consistency of drainage, and listen for "whoosh" of air over stomach when small amounts of air are injected into NG tube 5. Monitor for return of bowel function (presence of bowel sounds, passage of flatus and stool, stable abdominal girth, soft, nontender abdomen) 6. Graph patient height and weight on growth chart to monitor weight gain or loss; discuss inadequate weight gain with physician

Table 8-14 Postoperative laparotomy nursing-care plan—cont'd

Nursing diagnosis	Expected outcome	Nursing actions
B. Potential alteration in electrolyte status secondary to fluid loss from the gastrointestinal tract, medications, or third spacing of fluids	1. Patient will be adequately hydrated with fluid intake and output (I and O) in balance 2. Patient will demonstrate no clinical signs of electrolyte imbalance (see Table 8-3), and serum electrolytes will remain within normal range	1. Measure and record fluid I and O every 1-2 hr (include losses from wounds, ostomies, NG tube) 2. Monitor serum electrolytes every 6-12 hr (or per unit policy or physician order) when NG tube is connected to suction 3. Monitor for signs of third spacing of fluids (including increased abdominal girth, abdominal distention, evidence of intravascular hypovolemia, including hypotension, tachycardia, and peripheral vasoconstriction) 4. Replace NG drainage with appropriate IV fluid ml for ml per physician's order 5. Monitor serum electrolyte concentrations for evidence of electrolyte losses associated with diuretic therapy (decreased potassium, chloride, phosphate, and sodium). Monitor for clinical evidence of electrolyte imbalance (see Table 8-4) 6. Administer electrolyte replacement as ordered; monitor patient's response
C. Potential alteration in intravascular and extracellular fluid balance secondary to hemorrhage and/or third spacing of fluids	1. Patient will maintain adequate intravascular volume as measured by normal blood pressure and heart rate for that patient, a CVP of 3-5 mm Hg or a mean pulmonary artery pressure of 6-18 mm Hg, and an average urine output of 0.5-1.0 ml/kg/hr 2. Patient will demonstrate strong peripheral pulses, pink nail beds, and warm extremities (good peripheral perfusion)	1. Measure and record I and O, including all medications, IV solutions, blood products, NG replacement, and oral intake; notify physician if urine output is <0.5-1.0 ml/kg/hr or if fluid losses exceed intake 2. Calculate daily fluid requirements (see Table 8-3); if patient is receiving inadequate or excessive fluids, discuss with physician 3. Monitor for signs of third spacing of fluids and ascites (increasing weight, increased abdominal girth, anasarca, edema, peripheral vasoconstriction, tachycardia, and hypotension) 4. Assess hydration (measure urine specific gravity; assess skin turgor)

Continued.

Table 8-14 Postoperative laparotomy nursing-care plan—cont'd

Nursing diagnosis	Expected outcome	Nursing actions
C. Potential alteration in intravascular and extracellular fluid balance secondary to hemorrhage and/or third spacing of fluids—cont'd	3. Patient will gain minimum fluid weight. Significant weight gain or loss (>50 gm/day in infants or >200 gm/day in children) will be discussed with physician	5. Administer plasma or colloids as ordered to maintain intravascular oncotic pressure; monitor for evidence of transfusion reaction 6. Administer diuretics as ordered; note patient response, and notify physician of inadequate or excessive urine output 7. Monitor for signs of hemorrhage (change in vital signs, including tachycardia, hypotension, cool extremities, pallor) 8. Monitor for development of gastrointestinal bleeding (perform hematest or guaiac test all emesis, NG secretions, and stool) 9. Monitor hemoglobin and Hct; notify physician if either is abnormal 10. If bleeding occurs, notify physician; administer therapy as ordered, including fresh whole blood, packed RBCs (see section on gastrointestinal bleeding)
D. Potential infection (peritonitis, abscess, and wound infection) secondary to bacterial invasion or wound contamination	1. Patient will be protected from contamination of or infection in operative site 2. Patient will demonstrate wound healing with clean, dry, intact surgical incision (and absence of erythema or purulent exudate) 3. Patient will be afebrile without signs of leukocytosis, peritonitis, sepsis, or abscess	1. Monitor dressings for drainage. Note color, amount, and consistency; obtain wound culture if purulent drainage is noted 2. Observe incision; report evidence of erythema, heat, purulent drainage, or wound fluctuance to physician 3. Change dressing, using aseptic technique 4. Wound may be left open to allow drainage; pack and redress per physician's order, using aseptic technique 5. If wound is contaminated, maintain wound and skin isolation (use of gowns, gloves, and strict hand washing when caring for patients) 6. Administer antibiotic therapy as ordered 7. Monitor CBC for evidence of leukocytosis; report to physician

Table 8-14 Postoperative laparotomy nursing-care plan—cont'd

Nursing diagnosis	Expected outcome	Nursing actions
D. Potential infection (peritonitis, abscess, and wound infection) secondary to bacterial invasion or wound contamination—cont'd		8. Observe for signs of peritonitis (abdominal distention progressing to rigidity, diffuse pain, tenderness to palpation, fever, tachycardia, nausea, vomiting—see section on acute abdomen)
		9. Observe for signs of abscess (localized abdominal pain, fever, leukocytosis)
		10. Observe for signs of sepsis (in older child: fever, localized rash, tachycardia, tachypnea, diarrhea, malaise; in neonate: hypothermia or fever, increased gastric residuals, lethargy or irritability, systemic rash, apnea, bradycardia, watery stools); report evidence of sepsis to physician immediately
E. Potential pain secondary to operative procedure and incision	1. Patient will be comfortable after administration of narcotic analgesics in first 72 hr postoperatively and after administration of nonnarcotic analgesics beyond 72 hr postoperatively	1. Assess for signs of pain (subjective complaints, restlessness, increased systolic blood pressure, tachycardia, abdominal guarding and splinting with movements). NOTE: The nurse must be extremely sensitive to evidence of discomfort or pain in the infant or small (less verbal) child
		2. Medicate with narcotic analgesics every 4-6 hr in first 48 hr as needed (and per physician order) to promote optimum comfort and to avoid respiratory depression
		3. Medicate with nonnarcotic analgesics as needed (and per physician order) after first 72 hr; assess patient response and relief
		4. Position infant or child with head of bed elevated and body supported with pillows or linen rolls to maximize comfort
		5. Provide soothing, gentle, comforting care
F. Potential nutritional compromise secondary to decreased caloric intake and fluid restrictions	1. Patient will receive maximum calories within allotted fluid restriction	1. Calculate daily caloric requirement. Report inadequate caloric intake to physician; develop strategies to provide optimum caloric content in fluids administered

Continued.

Table 8-14 Postoperative laparotomy nursing-care plan—cont'd

Nursing diagnosis	Expected outcome	Nursing actions
F. Potential nutritional compromise secondary to decreased caloric intake and fluid restrictions—cont'd	2. Patient will receive daily caloric requirements for age through IV fluids, TPN, or oral alimentation	2. When patient is NPO, provide peripheral or central parenteral nutrition (see Table 8-18 for nursing care of the patient receiving parenteral nutrition) 3. Allow for periods of adequate rest, and provide warm environment to promote optimum use of calories (cold or heat stress increases caloric requirements in infants; fever increases caloric requirements in all children) 4. When oral intake is resumed, monitor progression from clear liquids to regular diet. Maintain calorie count. Notify physician immediately (and halt feeding as necessary) if vomiting, diarrhea, or abdominal distention occurs 5. When oral intake is resumed, provide for minimum distractions during mealtimes to encourage optimum intake
G. Potential complications of immobilization (skin breakdown, decreased respiratory function, venous stasis, decreased range of motion in extremities)	1. Patient will not demonstrate skin breakdown or contractures 2. Patient will demonstrate adequate respiratory function as evidenced by respiratory rate within normal limits, Pao_2 and $Paco_2$ within normal limits and absence of retractions, nasal flaring, and grunting 3. Patient will maintain full range of motion to all extremities 4. Patient will progress in activity level daily until ambulatory	1. Pad pressure points of skin as needed to prevent breakdown 2. Use sheepskin or air mattress as needed to prevent skin breakdown 3. Provide active or passive range of motion to all extremities every 2-4 hr 4. Turn the patient every 1-2 hr, changing patient position 5. Assess respiratory status; evaluate breath sounds, noting any areas of decreased aeration or congestion or increased respiratory rate secondary to pain and splinting of incision; notify physician if these develop 6. Promote optimum pulmonary hygiene by encouraging coughing and deep breathing (as age-appropriate) 7. Provide rib-springing, percussion, and vibration for small children to encourage deep breathing

Table 8-14 Postoperative laparotomy nursing-care plan—cont'd

Nursing diagnosis	Expected outcome	Nursing actions
G. Potential complications of immobilization (skin breakdown, decreased respiratory function, venous stasis, decreased range of motion in extremities)—cont'd		8. As soon as possible, provide for activity progression (dangling feet over bedside, out of bed to chair, short periods of ambulation) 9. Use supportive stockings to prevent venous stasis in lower extremities 10. In older children, monitor for signs of thrombophlebitis in lower extremities (tenderness, erythema, heat over calves)
H. Potential anxiety secondary to immobility, pain, surgical scar, multiple tubes, and environment of ICU	1. When alert, patient will express anxiety through conversation or projective play 2. Patient will communicate with family members as often as possible 3. Patient and family will demonstrate comprehension of patient condition, procedures, and policies of the ICU	1. Explain all procedures, movements, and sound to child before initiating treatment, regardless of child's level of consciousness 2. Place familiar object(s) near child (blanket, toy, book, tape recording of family or friends, pictures) 3. Keep parents and significant others aware of child's condition; keep child informed of parents' location when they are not with him 4. Provide opportunities for projective play when possible. Supervise syringe and needle play with doll; provide water play 5. Provide diversional activities as possible (television, radio) 6. Encourage visitation of hospital play therapist or child-life worker if available 7. Assess patient and family's understanding of postoperative management and procedures. Explain all treatments and time schedule for procedures

■ PARENTERAL NUTRITION

When a patient is unable to eat by mouth or absorb nutrients through the gastrointestinal tract, total parenteral nutrition (TPN) is indicated. First demonstrated as a practical mode of nutritional therapy in 1968 by Dudrick, TPN is now widely accepted as therapeutically beneficial to nutritionally compromised patients.[27]

Parenteral nutrition is defined as administration of nutrients via the intravascular route. This technique of nutritional support has frequently been referred to in medical and nursing texts as "hyperalimentation." That term is actually a misnomer because the technique in most cases does not provide greater nutrition than oral forms of alimentation, nor is it a form of alimentation, since that term implies use of the gastrointestinal tract. A more accurate term is parenteral nutrition, which may be regarded as either partial or total.[30]

■ Indications for parenteral nutrition

Parenteral nutrition is most often used as a supportive rather than curative therapy for infants and children with complex illnesses and structural gastrointestinal anomalies. Indications for supportive use of TPN in the neonatal period include congenital anomalies requiring major resection of the small bowel, intestinal obstruction, gastroschisis, necrotiz-

ing enterocolitis, and intractable diarrhea. Beyond infancy, pediatric patients requiring supportive parenteral nutrition include those with severe malnutrition, preoperative weight loss, inadequate postoperative nutrition, acute pancreatitis, fulminant hepatitis, ulcer disease, inflammatory bowel disease, extensive burns, malabsorption syndromes, refractory anorexia nervosa, and malignancy.

Parenteral nutrition may be used over a long period to allow the inflamed or diseased gastrointestinal tract to rest while healing is enhanced by provision of adequate IV nutrition. TPN can be used for long periods in diseases like enterocutaneous fistulas[58] (e.g., those occurring in Crohn's disease), growth failure secondary to inflammatory bowel disease,[46] acute renal failure,[1] cardiac failure,[2] and hepatic failure.[31]

■ Routes of administration

Central venous administration. Concentrated (20% to 30%) solutions of glucose and amino acids can cause vein sclerosis if they are given through short catheters in peripheral veins. Long plastic catheters, threaded through antecubital veins into the superior vena cava, may cause thrombophlebitis.

Direct catheterization of the subclavian or other large veins allows the infusion of high-osmolarity solutions into a high-flow venous system, deceasing the likelihood of thrombophlebitis and sclerosis.[27] The original catheters used for subclavian vein cath-

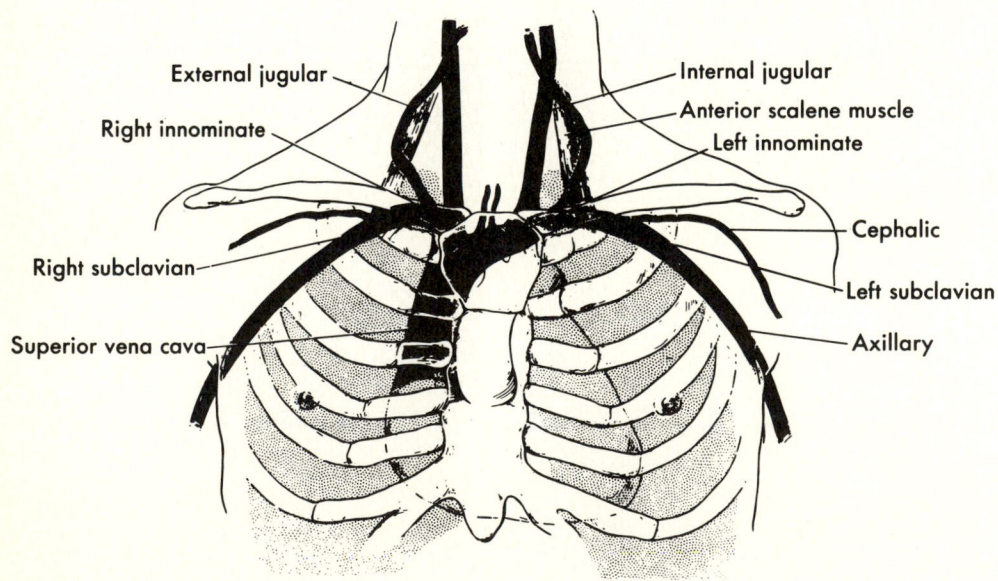

Fig. 8-15 Venous anatomy of central venous catheter insertion sites.

From Fisher, J.: Total parenteral nutrition, Boston, 1976, Little, Brown & Co.

eterization were polyethylene and polyvinyl; more recently, Teflon and Silastic catheters have been used. Central venous catheters may also be inserted into the superior vena cava through the subclavian vein, innominate vein, jugular vein, and axillary vein (Fig. 8-15). Insertion of central venous catheters for parenteral nutrition is performed in the operating room or in the intensive care unit (ICU) using sterile technique. Complications of surgical insertion of central venous catheters are listed in Table 8-15, and they include bleeding, cardiac arrhythmias, thrombosis, embolism, and pneumothorax, hydrothorax, and hemothorax.

Peripheral venous administration. Parenteral nutrition can be administered for a short time through peripheral veins; this mode of administration avoids possible complications of central venous catheterization. Peripheral veins of the scalp and extremities may be used, and insertion does not require use of the operative room or sterile technique.

The principal disadvantage of peripheral administration of parenteral nutrition is that the maximum glucose concentration of the solution is limited to 10% to 15%; higher concentrations can cause vein sclerosis or burns. If the high-osmolarity solution infiltrates into surrounding tissues, it can possibly cause sclerosis, thrombosis, or skin sloughing. As a result peripheral nutrition infusion sites must frequently be changed; thus the child is subjected to frequent venipunctures.

■ Parenteral nutrition solutions

Parenteral nutrition solutions consist primarily of glucose as a source of calories and amino acids (protein hydrolysates) as a source of nitrogen for protein synthesis. Electrolytes, vitamins, minerals, and trace elements are also added to solutions to meet all of the child's known nutritional energy requirements (Table 8-16). Fat emulsions (Intralipid or Liposyn) may be administered as a separate solution to provide a major source of calories and to prevent essential fatty acid deficiency states.

■ Nursing interventions

Careful assessment of pediatric patients receiving parenteral nutrition is necessary for early detection and avoidance of complications. This requires documentation of the quantity and content of the child's fluid intake and output and evaluation of the child's fluid and electrolyte status (Fig. 8-16 provides an example of a nursing flow sheet designed for documentation of assessment required for patients receiving parenteral nutrition). Many hospitals design guidelines for use of specific tests to monitor patient status during TPN (Table 8-17).

Whenever the child receives concentrated glucose solutions, the nurse must verify that the fluid content is appropriate for the child. Daily caloric requirements can be calculated (see Tables 8-6 and 8-

Table 8-15 Complications of central venous catheterization for total parenteral nutrition

Anatomic location	Complication
Pleural space	Pneumothorax, tension pneumothorax, hemothorax, hydrothorax, hydrothorax with intrapleural infusion
Mediastinum	Hemomediastinum, hydromediastinum
Neck	Arterial injury (subclavian, carotid, cervical or thoracic arteries) including hematoma, AV malformation, false aneurysm, stenosis
Nerves and lymphatics	Injury to phrenic, vagus, or brachial plexus nerves; injury to thoracic lymph duct
Veins	Laceration with hemorrhage, air embolism, catheter embolism, cardiac arrhythmia, myocardial perforation, hepatic vein thrombosis, superior vena cava thrombosis, catheter sepsis

From Fisher, J.: Total parenteral nutrition, Boston, 1976, Little, Brown & Co.

Table 8-16 Daily intravenous nutritional requirements for children[75]

	<10 kg	>10 kg
Water	100-150 ml/kg	1500-2000 ml/m²
Calories	100-120 cal/kg	2000 cal/m²
Glucose	20-30 gm/kg	25-30 gm/kg
Protein	2-3 gm/kg	1-2 gm/kg
Sodium	3-5 mEq/kg	3-5 mEq/kg
Potassium	2-4 mEq/kg	2-4 mEq/kg
Chloride	3 mEq/kg	2-3 mEq/kg
Calcium	20-40 mg/kg	20-40 mg/kg
Phosphate	2-3 mEq/kg	2-3 mEq/kg
Magnesium	0.25-0.5 mEq/kg	0.25-0.5 mEq/kg
Zinc	300 μg/kg	5 mg
Copper	20 μg/kg	300 μg
Ascorbic acid	35 mg	40 mg
Vitamin A	1400 IU	2500 IU
Vitamin D	400 IU	400 IU
Vitamin E	4 IU	9 IU
Thiamine	0.3 mg	0.9 mg
Riboflavin	0.4 mg	1.1 mg
Pyridoxine	0.3 mg	0.9 mg
Niacinamide	5 mg	12 mg
Panthenol	5 mg	10 mg
Folic acid	0.2 mg	0.3 mg
Vitamin K	1.5 mg	2.5 mg
Vitamin B_{12}	0.3 μg	1.5 μg
d-Biotin	0.3 mg	0.4 mg

Compiled from guidelines established for pediatric house staff at The Children's Hospital of Philadelphia, 1981.

16) for each patient to ensure that these substances are being provided in the parenteral fluid.

Before each new TPN solution is hung, the nurse should confirm that the appropriate solution has been prepared. This is accomplished by checking the solution content with the physician's original order.

Potential complications of TPN are summarized in the nursing-care plan (Table 8-18); they include infection, hepatic dysfunction, hyperglycemia, hypoglycemia, acidosis, hypomagnesemia, hyperlipidemia, copper deficiency, zinc deficiency, cardiac ar-rhythmias, venous thromboses, air embolus, and skin sloughing. Potential complications of intralipid therapy include ventilation-perfusion abnormalities, eosinophilia, and bilirubin displacement from albumin.[45] These complications are discussed in detail in the following paragraphs.

Since the TPN solution contains high concentrations of glucose, it provides a perfect medium for bacterial growth. When the nurse hangs the new TPN solution and tubing, it is imperative to use strict clean technique to prevent line contamination. Many hospitals require that the entire tubing system (be-

THE CHILDREN'S HOSPITAL OF PHILADELPHIA

NUTRITION SUPPORT SERVICE

PARENTERAL NUTRITION TREATMENT FLOW SHEET

(Please record Strict I and O Daily weights on
patient assessment and treatment flow sheet).

Catheter inserted ____ - __-8
(for central lines only)

TREATMENT	0700 1500	1500 2200	2200 0700	0700 1500	1500 2200	2200 0700	0700 1500	1500 2200	2200 0700	0700 1500	1500 2200	2200 0700	0700 1500	1500 2200	2200 0700	0700 1500	1500 2200	2200 0700	0700 1500	1500 2200	2200 0700
1. DATE OF THERAPY																					
2. DAY OF THERAPY																					
3. TIME-SOLUTION SET UP CHANGED																					
4. URINE SUGAR & ACETONE																					
5. URINE DIPSTICK																					
6. URINE SPECIFIC GRAVITY																					
7. DEXTROSTIX																					
8. INFANT LENGTH - q Mon.																					
9. INFANT HEAD CIRCUMFERENCE - q Mon.																					
10. SKIN INTEGRITY																					
11. MOUTH CARE																					
12. CHEST X-RAY																					
13. CENTRAL LINE CLAMP																					
TEMP. SPIKE																					
14. TIME/TEMP.																					
15. TIME SOLUTION SENT TO MICROBIOLOGY																					
16. M.D. AND NUTRITION SUPPORT SERVICE NOTIFICATION																					
17. BLOOD CULTURE PERIPHERAL/THRU CATHETER																					
18. OTHER CULTURES																					
19. CATHETER INSERTION SITE																					
20. DRESSING CHANGED																					
21. CONDITION OF SITE																					
22. SITE CULTURE																					

Nursing 2/80

Fig. 8-16 Nursing-care flow sheet for children
receiving parenteral nutrition.

Reproduced with permission from The Children's Hospital of
Philadelphia, 1980.

Table 8-17 Recommended monitoring of patients receiving parenteral nutrition

Monitoring	Frequency
General	
Vital signs	Every 4 hr (or more often as patient condition warrants)
Weight	Daily
Strict intake and output	Constant
Caloric intake	Daily
Length or height	Weekly
Head circumference	Weekly
Blood	
Glucose	Daily until stable (more often in infants)
Electrolytes	Daily until stable
BUN	Weekly
Ca, PO₄, Mg	Weekly
Alkaline phosphatase, SGOT, SGPT, total and direct bilirubin	Weekly
Creatinine	Weekly
Total protein, albumin	Weekly
CBC with differential	Weekly
Triglycerides, cholesterol	As indicated when fat infusions are increased
Zinc, copper	Monthly
Dextrostix	When TPN is abruptly discontinued or when urine is +2 for glucose
Urine	
Glucose	Every 4 hr until stable, then every 8 hr
Protein	Every 4 hr until stable, then every 8 hr
Ketone	Every 4 hr until stable, then every 8 hr
Specific gravity	Every 4 hr until stable, then every 8 hr
pH	Every 4 hr until stable, then every 8 hr

From guidelines for pediatric house staff at The Children's Hospital of Philadelphia, 1981.

tween TPN solution and the patient, including infusion-pump tubing) be changed every 12 or 24 hours to decrease the possibility of significant bacterial growth. In addition, many hospitals require that a micropore filter be placed in the IV tubing system so contaminants can be eliminated. The dressing over the catheter insertion site should be changed every 24 to 48 hours (as per hospital policy), using sterile technique and an occlusive dressing. The nurse should assess the wound for evidence of inflammation (erythema or exudate) and should report any abnormalities to a physician. Wound exudate should be cultured and sent for Gram's stain (with physician's order).

The child's temperature should be monitored at least every 2 hours (or according to hospital TPN standard-care plan). Blood cultures are usually ordered if the child's temperature rises above 38.5° C or if the child develops unexplained acidosis, lethargy, or glycosuria.[57] Hypothermia may be the first sign of sepsis in neonates. If the child with an indwelling central venous catheter becomes febrile, two sets of blood cultures are usually drawn; one set is obtained from the central line, and one set is obtained through a separate venipuncture. If only the cultures drawn through the central line are positive, the stopcock alone may be contaminated (colonized) and should be changed. The central line catheter may also be colonized. If both sets of cultures are positive and contain the same organism, the child has bacteremia. The central venous catheter is presumed to be colonized, and it may be withdrawn (per physician's order or hospital policy) so that it does not continue to provide a site of bacterial infection. If the presence of bacteremia is suspected, some hospitals require that a sample from the TPN bottle be sent for culture (to rule out TPN-solution contamination). The child will be placed on appropriate antibiotics, and the TPN may be resumed using a new solution and a new peripheral venous line until the blood cultures are negative.

When TPN is begun, the glucose concentration and the rate of solution infusion must be begun at low levels and increased gradually, so that the child's insulin production can accommodate the continuous glucose load. Once the TPN is begun, the infusion should be maintained at a uniform rate; it should not be decreased or increased, since hypoglycemia or hyperglycemia can result. When TPN is to be discontinued, the glucose concentration and the rate are gradually weaned.

When TPN infusions are begun, serum glucose measurements may be performed several times a day. Heelstick glucose measurements (using Dextrostix) may be performed every 2 to 4 hours in infants. Urine specimens should be checked at least every 4 hours (some hospitals require testing of urine from every void) for the presence of sugar or ketones. The presence of either glucosuria or ketonuria should be reported to a physician and the child's serum glucose level should be checked (with physician's order). Glucosuria usually indicates the presence of high serum glucose levels (exceeding the renal threshold of 150 to 200 mg/dl blood). In addition, bacterial and fungal infections can produce glucosuria. Ketonuria in a non-diabetic child usually indicates the presence of low serum glucose levels and resultant breakdown of triglycerides.

If the TPN IV line infiltrates or becomes occluded, it is important that a new line be inserted promptly, so that the child will not experience a sudden cessation of glucose infusion and subsequent hypoglycemia; the child should be monitored closely for clinical evidence of hypoglycemia (lethargy, irritability, tremors, diaphoresis, tachycardia, headache, vomiting, dizziness, blurring of vision) until the TPN infusion has been resumed. Heelstick glucose measurements may be obtained from infants to rule out hypoglycemia.

Acidosis may occur in the premature infant or in children with renal failure if large (greater than 4 gm/kg/day) protein loads are administered.[45] This can occur because the kidneys are not able to excrete all of the ammonia resulting from amino acid breakdown; thus some ammonia (with hydrogen ion) is reabsorbed, and serum levels of hydrogen ion rise. Serum and urine pH should be monitored daily (see Table 8-17) or more frequently if indicated by patient condition.

Since serum magnesium, phosphate, and calcium levels may fall during parenteral nutrition, they should be monitored at least weekly. Trace element deficiencies are more likely to develop with long-term TPN therapy or when TPN therapy is used in premature infants.[57] Signs and symptoms of copper deficiency include anemia, neutropenia, loss of taste, and rash. Zinc deficiency may produce an erythematous maculopapular rash (called *acrodermatitis enteropathica*) over the face, trunk, and digits; poor wound healing; hair loss and loss of taste; and a fall in serum alkaline phosphatase.[44,45,57]

Cardiac arrhythmias may occur if the central venous catheter migrates into the heart, particularly into the right ventricle. Venous thrombosis can occur if a clot is allowed to form at the catheter tip; thrombosis of the superior vena cava has been reported; it occurs more often in infants who require prolonged TPN therapy. Air embolus can be caused by careless coupling of the IV line or stopcock. Since the central venous TPN catheter is inserted into a relatively large vein, a loose or cracked tubing connection can rapidly result in significant loss of blood (hemorrhage). It is important that the nurse check all tubing and catheter connections at least every hour. Since insertion of a central venous catheter involves risk of significant complications, the nurse must ensure that the catheter is secured in place, with no possibility of dislodgement.

The peripheral infusion site should be inspected at least every 30 minutes to 1 hour for signs of erythema or edema, and a physician should be notified immediately if these are observed. A temporary phlebitis may develop when parenteral nutrition is administered through small veins. If phlebitis develops, the venous administration site should be changed, and warm packs should be applied over the inflamed area. Tissue slough can occur if the parenteral nutrition solution infiltrates into surrounding tissue. As soon as any infiltration is observed, the infusion is discontinued (and begun at another site). Some physicians inject hyaluronidase into the area of infiltration[57] to promote dispersion and absorption of the high osmolarity solution. Infiltration of parenteral nutrition occasionally produces sufficient skin scarring to require later skin grafting.[57]

Intralipids are usually "piggybacked" into the TPN line at the last T connector or stopcock just before the solution enters the vein. This practice has been adopted because of the fear that prolonged contact between the TPN amino acids and the lipids will cause emulsification of the fat and result in production of fat emboli. Combination of TPN and intralipid solutions should be accomplished according to hospital procedure.

Children may develop adverse reactions to lipid infusion, demonstrated by dyspnea, flushing, nausea, headache, dizziness, or chest and back pain. Evidence of respiratory distress may also indicate the development of ventilation-perfusion abnormalities or development of a hemothorax, hydrothorax or pneumothorax secondary to subclavian catheter insertion or central venous catheter migration. The physician should be notified immediately if the patient develops respiratory distress, and arterial blood gases and a portable chest film should be obtained (with physician's order).

Since lipid binds with albumin, it will displace bilirubin and result in an increased risk of kernicterus; thus lipid administration is contraindicated in neonates with jaundice. Intralipid infusion is also contraindicated in patients with significant liver disease.

Children who receive parenteral nutrition frequently demonstrate abnormalities in liver function studies and elevations in serum levels of liver enzymes. Many of these abnormalities are transient and resolve shortly after parenteral nutrition is discontinued. Cholestatic jaundice is a more serious complication. It produces periportal fibrosis, bile duct proliferation, and bile stasis. The child initially has jaundice, and laboratory analysis reveals an elevation in serum conjugated bilirubin, alkaline phosphatase, SGPT, and SGOT. Usually, the jaundice disappears and liver function studies return to normal soon after TPN therapy is discontinued. However, some degree of fibrosis may persist, and some infants may develop progressive liver failure.[57]

Table 8-18 provides a detailed summary of nurs-

Text continued on p. 617.

Table 8-18 Nursing care of the child receiving parenteral nutrition

Nursing diagnosis	Expected outcome	Nursing actions
A. Potential infection secondary to break in aseptic technique during 1. Catheter insertion 2. Maintenance of catheter entrance site 3. Maintenance of infusion system	1. Patient will be protected from infection or trauma to catheter insertion site 2. Septic or infectious complications will be immediately recognized and reported	1. Ensure strict adherence to aseptic technique during catheter insertion and care 2. Maintain a continual closed delivery system 3. Perform no blood sampling and administer no medication through the catheter (to minimize possibility of contamination) if at all possible

Table 8-18 Nursing care of the child receiving parenteral nutrition—cont'd

Nursing diagnosis	Expected outcome	Nursing actions
A. Potential infection secondary to break in aseptic technique during—cont'd 4. Preparation of solution		4. Change delivery system tubing every 24 hr (or per unit policy) 5. Observe dressing for any drainage from site or leakage of fluid 6. Assess for signs of infection: elevation of temperature, chills, lethargy, restlessness, glycosuria, thrombocytopenia, leukocytosis, or hypothermia (in neonates). Notify physician if these develop, and obtain cultures as ordered 7. Date all bottles and tubing when they are hung; discard any solution that is cloudy, that contains sediment, or that is older than hospital policy allows 8. Change dressing at least three times weekly (or per hospital policy). *Procedure for dressing change:* remove old dressing using aseptic technique and then put on sterile gloves. Clean area around catheter insertion site with acetone. This defats the area and removes debris and bacteria from the skin. Swab catheter tip with povidone-iodine (Betadine), circling outward. Place drop of iodine ointment on catheter insertion site. Place sterile 2 × 2 gauze over site. Cover area with nonporous tape or material forming an occlusive dressing. Ensure that all tubing can be changed without infringement on the catheter insertion site dressing 9. Change peripheral catheters every 72 hr (or per hospital policy) 10. Swab delivery system connections with alcohol or an iodine solution before opening
B. Potential central venous catheter complications	1. Patient will be mobile without tension to catheter insertion site	1. Notify physician if sutures are not secure 2. Tape the catheter securely

Continued.

Table 8-18 Nursing care of the child receiving parenteral nutrition—cont'd

Nursing diagnosis	Expected outcome	Nursing actions
1. Dislodgement of the catheter secondary to inadequate placement of securing sutures; improper taping of the exit site dressing; movement of the patient, causing tension on the catheter	2. Patient will have equal and adequate aeration in all lobes of lungs	3. Make sure the child is not able to pull on the catheter. Pay strict attention to the catheter when changing the patient's position. The entire length of tubing should be positioned so it is visible to the nurse
2. Thrombosis of vena cava secondary to fibrin sleeve formation around the catheter, causing partial or total occlusion of the vessel. The incidence of this complication is increased with (a) extended length of therapy, (b) sepsis, (c) very high concentrations of glucose (>20%) infusion, and (d) the use of polyethylene catheters	3. Listed complications will be recognized immediately and reported	4. Obtain radiologic confirmation of central venous catheter tip placement before delivery of TPN solution (through chest radiograph)
		5. *Always* clamp the catheter when the delivery system is opened
		6. Keep padded hemostat with infusion set up at all times in case of emergency
		7. Infuse TPN via a pump equipped with alarm indicating air in the line, disconnection, and occlusion
3. Pneumothorax, hemothorax, or hydrothorax secondary to improper placement of the catheter into the pleural cavity, which may cause air, blood, or fluid (respectively) to enter the pleural cavity		8. Assess for signs of intrathoracic fluid infiltration: chest pain, leakage of solution onto dressing, edema or erythema of chest or face, increased arm circumference on affected side if subclavian vein is used, diminished breath sounds on affected side
4. Embolism secondary to air entering the venous system during catheter insertion or maintenance		9. Assess for signs of air embolism: dyspnea, tachycardia, chest pain, cyanosis, confusion or disorientation
5. Hemorrhage		10. Monitor for any fluid or blood drainage at catheter connections. If significant blood is lost from catheter leak, connection crack, or inadvertent tubing disconnection, assess patient for evidence of hypovolemia (tachycardia, tachypnea, hypotension, peripheral vasoconstriction, decreased urine output, poor color), and notify physician immediately. An Hct should be ordered and the child may require colloid or blood replacement of fluid lost
C. Potential complications of peripheral venous catheter	1. Patient will not develop phlebitis or skin sloughing	1. Check peripheral catheter site every half hour for signs of inflammation, infiltration, or phlebitis
1. Phlebitis secondary to delivery of hypertonic solution		2. Report signs of phlebitis to IV team, nutrition support nurse, or physician

Table 8-18 Nursing care of the child receiving parenteral nutrition—cont'd

Nursing diagnosis	Expected outcome	Nursing actions
C. Potential complications of peripheral venous catheter—cont'd 2. Sloughing or swelling of subcutaneous tissue secondary to continual infusion of solution after catheter has been displaced from the vein (there is a high association of this with the use of infusion pumps)		3. Discontinue infusion if signs of significant erythema, sloughing, or subcutaneous tissue swelling is noted. Notify physician
D. Potential serum glucose imbalance 1. Hyperglycemia, glycosuria, osmotic diuresis, or dehydration can develop if glucose infusion is too rapid, particularly in stressed or septic patients or in infants with low birth weight 2. Hypoglycemia may develop secondary to sudden cessation of infusion	1. Patient will maintain serum glucose within normal limits and will not demonstrate glucosuria	1. Begin infusion at a slow constant rate 2. Check blood glucose and urine every 4-8 hr until stable (or per hospital protocol) 3. Monitor for signs of hypoglycemia (irritability, lethargy, tachycardia, tremors, headache, dizziness, vomiting, blurring of vision) 4. Assess for intolerance of concentrated glucose solution, including signs of hyperglycemia, or glycosuria 5. Maintain infusion at constant rate; if peripheral TPN infusion must be discontinued (because of infiltration or occlusion), ensure that new catheter is immediately inserted so that glucose infusion is not interrupted 6. When TPN is to be discontinued, ensure that glucose concentration and infusion rate are gradually weaned, and monitor for signs of hypoglycemia
E. Potential electrolyte disorders 1. Hypernatremia or hyponatremia secondary to inappropriate sodium intake in relation to water intake, particularly in the presence of abnormal fluid losses (e.g., gastrointestinal losses and osmotic diuresis)	1. Patient will maintain serum sodium, potassium, phosphorus, and magnesium within normal range 2. Signs of electrolyte imbalance will be recognized immediately and reported to physician	1. Monitor serum electrolytes daily until stable 2. Monitor fluid and electrolyte losses from GI tract, and replace (discuss with physician) 3. Assess for hypo-/hyper-conditions of electrolytes (see Table 8-4)

Continued.

Table 8-18 Nursing care of the child receiving parenteral nutrition—cont'd

Nursing diagnosis	Expected outcome	Nursing actions

E. Potential electrolyte disorders—cont'd
  2. Hypokalemia secondary to insufficient potassium intake associated with protein anabolism
  3. Hyperkalemia secondary to excessive potassium administration, particularly with presence of acidosis
  4. Hypophosphatemia secondary to insufficient inorganic phosphate intake
  5. Hypomagnesemia secondary to inadequate intake of magnesium		

F. Potential hepatic dysfunction; cholestatic jaundice secondary to hepatotoxicity may develop because of unknown factors or amino acid imbalance, prolonged use of parenteral nutrition, extreme prematurity	1. Patient will maintain normal serum bilirubin and serum transaminases and will be jaundice-free	1. Assess for signs of cholestasis: pruritus, jaundice, dark urine 2. Monitor serum SGOT, SGPT, alkaline phosphatase, and bilirubin weekly (or per hospital policy) 3. Palpate liver size; notify physician of increased liver size or tenderness, or increased abdominal girth

G. Potential disorder in fat metabolism
  1. Hyperlipemia secondary to intravenous fat emulsion
  2. Decreased pulmonary diffusion secondary to fat embolism
  3. Eosinophilia secondary to fat emulsion infusion
  4. Essential fatty acid deficiency secondary to fat-free TPN for prolonged periods
	1. Patient will maintain adequate pulmonary function
	2. Patient will not demonstrate signs of essential fatty-acid deficiency
		1. Assess pulmonary function; notify physician of increased congestion, respiratory distress, or cyanosis
		2. Administer test dose of fat infusion before full dose administration; monitor for signs of reaction
		3. Assess for essential fatty acid deficiency: poor wound healing, alopecia, thrombocytopenia, increased capillary fragility, and dry, scaly skin

Table 8-18 Nursing care of the child receiving parenteral nutrition—cont'd

Nursing diagnosis	Expected outcome	Nursing actions
H. Potential bleeding secondary to vitamin K deficiency or liver dysfunction	1. Patient will maintain PT and PTT within normal limits 2. Patient will not bleed excessively from venipuncture sites nor develop petechiae and ecchymosis	1. Administer IM vitamin K doses weekly as ordered 2. Assess for excessive bleeding from venipuncture sites, mucous membranes, petechiae, or ecchymoses 3. Provide gentle mouth care every 4 hr 4. Monitor serum PT and PTT as ordered
I. Potential demineralization of bones or rickets secondary to vitamin D deficiency	1. Patient will maintain normal serum calcium and phosphorus 2. Patient will be protected from injury during positioning and movement	1. Assess for bone pain while positioning and handling patient and while he is ambulating 2. Observe for the development of rickets (late sign) in infants and small children

ing assessment and interventions required when the child is receiving TPN.

■ Specific Diseases

■ CONGENITAL GASTROINTESTINAL ABNORMALITIES

The most important aspects of managing neonatal congenital anomalies are early diagnosis, adequate surgical repair, and prevention or treatment of postoperative complications. One early sign of several fetal gastrointestinal anomalies is maternal polyhydramnios, or excessive amniotic fluid during pregnancy. When intestinal blockage prevents normal passage and reabsorption of amniotic fluid in the fetus, there is an increase in amniotic fluid.

Another sign of congenital gastrointestinal anomalies is the failure of air to pass through the gastrointestinal tract immediately after birth. As the neonate's lungs fill with air for the first time, air should also enter the stomach. This air is normally passed through the gastrointestinal tract in a predictable sequence: with the second breath, air reaches the duodenum; at 6 hours of life, air reaches the cecum; and at 24 hours of life, air reaches the rectum.[28]

Abnormal abdominal radiographs after the first 12 hours of life are most often diagnostic of gastrointestinal abnormalities. In addition, failure to pass meconium in the first 24 hours of life is a strong clinical indicator of gastrointestinal malfunction.

Congenital anomalies of the gastrointestinal tract are presented in Table 8-19. Since neonatal intensive care is not specifically addressed in this text, nursing care of the newborn with these anomalies will not be elaborated.

■ NECROTIZING ENTEROCOLITIS
■ Etiology

Necrotizing enterocolitis (NEC) is an acquired disorder of the gastrointestinal tract, which occurs most frequently in stressed premature infants. Several epidemiologic factors have been associated with this condition; however, the precise cause is unknown. Identified associated factors include (1) gastrointestinal vasoconstriction in response to stress (the "diving reflex"), (2) sepsis, (3) mucosal injury as a result of use of hyperosmolar oral feedings, (4) insufficient host immunologic protection, (5) use of umbilical arterial or venous catheters (which may produce mesenteric thromboembolus), (6) asphyxia or significant hypoxemia, (7) low cardiac output, (8) polycythemia, (9) acidosis, and (10) hypoglycemia.[41]

High-risk factors associated with the development of necrotizing enterocolitis are summarized in Table 8-20.

Text continued on p. 622.

Table 8-19 Congenital gastrointestinal anomalies

Disease	Etiology	Pathophysiology	Clinical signs and symptoms	Nursing interventions
Congenital gastrointestinal anomalies associated with respiratory distress				
Diaphragmatic hernia	Incomplete fusion of diaphragm at 10 wk gestation; usually left side is involved	Abnormal opening between abdomen and thorax; allows stomach and intestines to enter chest; the left lung fails to develop and is hypoplastic; heart is displaced to right thorax	Abdomen appears flat; severe respiratory distress develops, including severe respiratory acidosis; heart sounds shifted; a R → L shunt is present through the patent ductus arteriosus or foramen ovale, since pulmonary vascular resistance is high	Insert NG tube to decompress stomach; Position on right side to increase perfusion of right lung; Provide skilled respiratory support; Monitor ABG; If R → L shunt exists, use β_2 blocker to dilate pulmonary bed (tolazoline); Prepare for surgical correction
Tracheoesophageal fistula	Abnormal separation of esophagus from the trachea (develops after 24 days of gestation)	Upper segment of esophagus ends in blind pouch above bifurcation of trachea; fistula to stomach is present	Respiratory distress; Dysphagia; Excessive salivation; Abdominal distention; Inability to pass NG tube; X-ray film reveals air in stomach, intestines, and upper mediastinal pouch if esophageal atresia is present	Elevate head of bed 45 degrees; IV fluids; NPO; Respiratory support; Prepare for surgical correction or palliative procedure and insertion of gastrostomy tube
Congenital gastrointestinal anomalies associated with obstructive or bleeding symptoms				
Malrotation with volvulus	Abnormal movement of the intestines around the superior mesenteric artery during week 10 of gestation	Malrotation obstructs the duodenum in various degrees; strangulation of the superior mesenteric artery results from volvulus of the small intestine	Vomiting bilious material after first 24-48 hr of life; Abdominal distention; Visible peristalsis; Melena or currant-jelly stools; Barium x-ray: abnormal rotation of bowel	Measure abdominal girth q 4 hr; notify physician if girth increases 1-2 cm; IV fluids; NPO; Prepare for surgical correction

Hirschsprung's disease	Failure of innervation of GI tract at 5-12 wk of gestation	With this interruption of peristalsis in the lower GI tract, fecal contents are not eliminated; internal sphincter fails to relax	Newborns: failure to pass meconium within 24-48 hr after birth; bilious vomiting; abdominal distention; explosive diarrhea; enterocolitis Child: constipation; ribbon-like, foul-smelling stool; abdominal distention; visible peristalsis; malnutrition; anemia; malabsorption Barium x-ray—transition zone of aganglionic segment	Newborn • IV fluids • NG tube • Prepare for surgical re-anastomosis, pull though, and temporary colostomy Child • Low-residue, high-calorie, high-protein diet • Enemas when needed or stool softeners • Prepare for surgical correction; pull through primary consideration
Imperforate anus and intestinal atresia	Abnormal partitioning between cloaca and urorectal septum at 8 weeks of gestation	Single membrane covering anus or anal agenesis or intestinal atresia; lack of patency of any segment of bowel because of poor vascular supply to that area of bowel	Abdominal distention; vomiting *High atresia* • X-ray—shows lack of progression of air through bowel • May pass meconium *Low atresia* • Abdominal distention; lack of stools; vomiting • X-ray—obstructed pattern with dilated, air-filled bowel	Measure abdominal girth q 4 hr; notify physician if girth increases 1-2 cm Note absence or presence of meconium or stools Note color of vomitus IV fluids NG tube Prepare for surgical correction
Intussusception	Occurs in otherwise healthy infants ages 3-11 mo; three times more common in boys than girls; some correlation with adenovirus	Slipping or telescoping of one intestinal segment into another, thereby compromising blood supply and intestinal patency	Acute paraxysmal abdominal pain (infant draws knees to chest); vomiting that increases as condition worsens; stools become red (like currant jelly); abdominal tenderness; URQ may have sausage-shaped mass; LRQ may feel empty	Provide appropriate IV replacement fluid and electrolytes as ordered Monitor stools Insert NG tube NPO VS Observe for shock, secondary to perforation Prepare for barium enema reduction

Continued.

Table 8-19 Congenital gastrointestinal anomalies—cont'd

Disease	Etiology	Pathophysiology	Clinical signs and symptoms	Nursing interventions
Congenital gastrointestinal anomalies associated with obstructive or bleeding symptoms—cont'd				
Intussusception—cont'd				Prepare for surgical correction if barium enema reduction is unsuccessful
Meckel's diverticulum	Outpouching of the ileum containing ectopic gastric mucosa; results from incomplete obliteration of the omphalomesenteric duct during embryonic development	Irritation and ulceration of the ectopic gastric mucosa leads to painless lower GI bleeding	Bright red or dark red rectal bleeding is more common than black, tarry stools and represents acute hemorrhage, and may result in severe anemia and shock	Observation and treatments necessary for stabilization of hypovolemic shock (see Chapter 3) Prepare for surgical resection of diverticulum
Congenital gastrointestinal anomalies associated with abdominal wall defect				
Omphalocele	Failure of GI tract to return to abdominal cavity by 10-11 weeks' gestation; high incidence of other anomalies	Abdominal organs herniate into umbilicus and are covered by a protective sac; defect is variable in size	Temperature instability; dehydration from free water loss; protein loss; hypoglycemia from ↑ caloric expenditure; respiratory distress; all leading to shock	NPO Insert NG tube and attach to low suction Provide IV fluids or TPN. Calculate caloric intake and discuss with physician if inadequate

	Etiology	Clinical Manifestations		Nursing Interventions
				Provide neutral thermal environment
				Keep sac covered with moist sterile gauze preoperatively
				Dextrostix q 4-6 hr
				Prepare for surgical correction
Gastroschisis	Failure of mesoderm to completely invade embryonic abdominal wall at week 5 of gestation	Abdominal wall defect of 1-2 inches in diameter, usually located to the right of the umbilical cord, without a protective sac, abdominal organs herniate	Temperature instability; dehydration; protein loss; hypoglycemia from ↑ caloric expenditure; respiratory distress; all leading to shock	NPO
				Insert NG tube and attach to low suction
				Provide IV fluids or TPN. Calculate caloric intake and discuss with physician if inadequate
				Provide neutral thermal environment
				Cover sac with warm sterile saline sponges and cover with plastic bag or wrap
				Dextrostix q 4-6 hr
				Prepare for surgical correction

Table 8-20   High-risk factors associated with the development of necrotizing enterocolitis[34,82]

High-risk factors	Frequency among involved patients
Prenatal	
Premature birth (<2000 gm)	68%-80%
Premature rupture of membranes	25%-35%
Placenta previa	15%-30%
Septicemia	8%
Neonatal	
Apneic spells	13%-50%
Respiratory distress syndrome (RDS)	50%-60%
Temperature instability	35%-87%
Sepsis	30%-43%
Patent ductus arteriosus	10%-30%
Umbilical artery catheterization	25%-60%
Exchange transfusion	18%-45%

■   **Pathophysiology**

Although the specific pathogenesis of NEC is not clear, three factors are consistently present before NEC develops: mucosal injury (direct or indirect), the presence of enteric bacteria, and availability of a metabolic substrate (enteral feeding).

One example of indirect mucosal injury is injury resulting from decreased mesenteric perfusion in response to hypoxic stress. This "diving reflex" causes a redistribution of blood away from mesenteric, renal, and peripheral vascular beds to the heart and brain. If mesenteric vasoconstriction is prolonged or profound, intestinal ischemia and destruction of the intestinal mucosal layer result.[41] Without normal mu-

cosal protection, the bowel wall is injured by the intraluminal proteolytic enzymes. The bowel becomes increasingly distended, microperforations develop in the bowel wall, and gas-producing bacteria can invade the affected bowel wall. The invasion of bacteria can produce air in the liver and portal system or gut wall. The presence of subserous or intramural air is called *pneumatosis intestinales*,[54,83] and it is the pathognomonic radiographic finding with NEC.[41]

The use of hyperosmolar feedings in the premature infant has been associated with direct mucosal injury and the development of NEC. Although the precise mechanism remains unclear, the concentrated carbohydrate formula may "overwhelm" the immature small intestinal villi, leading to carbohydrate malabsorption and subsequent mucosal injury. Newborns, particularly premature infants, have decreased amount of protective gastrointestinal immunoglobins (particularly IgA); this impedes active repair of damaged mucosa. The role of breast milk, which contains active immunoglobins, macrophages, and specific antibodies, as a protection against NEC has been demonstrated in laboratory animals and is being investigated for use in the neonatal intensive ICU.[16,67] Fig. 8-17 further illustrates the proposed pathophysiology of NEC.

■   **Clinical signs and symptoms**

The classic clinical presentation of the infant with NEC includes the symptom triad of abdominal distention, guaiac- or hematest-positive stools (or other gross or occult gastrointestinal bleeding), and increased gastric residuals, with or without bilious vomiting after feeding. Signs of clinical deterioration include apnea and bradycardic episodes, lethargy, temperature instability, decreased urine output, further abdominal distention, and decreased blood pressure. If this condition is not treated, massive abdominal distention with perforation, acidosis, sepsis, shock, and death may occur.

The wide range of symptoms in NEC have lead to a clinical categorization or staging of the condition. Characteristics of three stages of NEC[11] are:
1. NEC scare
   a. History of perinatal stress
   b. Nonspecific systemic manifestations: apnea, bradycardia, lethargy, temperature instability
   c. Gastrointestinal manifestations: poor feeding, increased residuals, emesis, mild distention
   d. Radiographs: intestinal distention with mild ileus

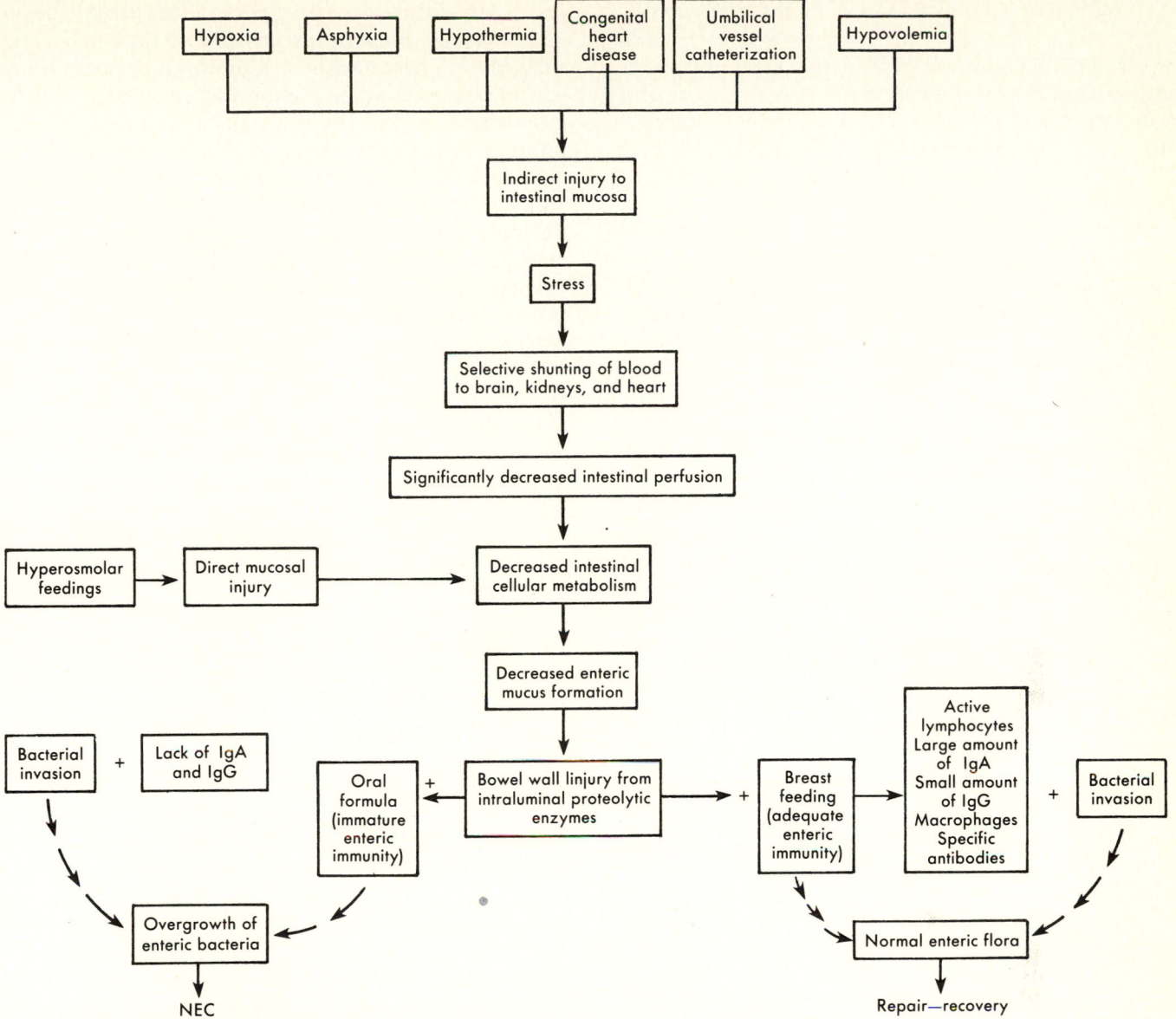

Fig. 8-17 Proposed pathophysiology of necrotizing enterocolitis.

2. Definite NEC
   a. Persistent occult or gross gastrointestinal bleeding
   b. Marked abdominal distention
   c. Radiographs: significant intestinal distention with ileus; small bowel separation; pneumatosis intestinalis
3. Advanced NEC
   a. Deterioration of vital signs
   b. Evidence of septic shock or marked gastrointestinal hemorrhage

   c. Radiographs: pneumoperitoneum
Indications for immediate surgical intervention in NEC[51] include:
1. Free intraperitoneal air
2. Cellulitis of anterior abdominal wall
3. Radiographic evidence of peritonitis
   a. Increased free peritoneal fluid
   b. Increased bowel wall edema
4. Clinical deterioration during medical therapy
   a. Irreversible metabolic acidosis
   b. Respiratory failure

If NEC is identified in its early stages and treatment is begun promptly to prevent perforation, the infant often will improve without surgical intervention. Once the diagnosis of NEC is suspected, oral feedings are discontinued and a nasogastric tube is passed to provide continuous gastric drainage and decompression.[41] Umbilical artery or vein catheters are discontinued. IV fluid therapy, including parenteral nutrition, is administered, and appropriate IV antibiotics for both gram-negative and gram-positive organisms are begun (sensitivity patterns of infections found in the nursery should be reviewed). During the early stages nursing interventions include careful measurement of abdominal girth and fluid intake and output (including all stools); measurement of temperature, vital signs (including blood pressure), and daily weight; and testing of all stools for blood (hematest or guaiac) and presence of reducing substances indicating carbohydrate malabsorption (Clinitest). The physician should be notified of any changes in the infant's condition.

If, however, acidemia persists, the infant's platelet count continues to decrease, and cardiovascular perfusion and urine output deteriorate despite adequate fluid therapy, surgical intervention is indicated. Signs of decreased systemic perfusion include tachycardia, tachypnea, hypotension, decreased intensity of peripheral pulses, coolness of extremities, pallor or cyanosis of nail beds, and urine output of less than 0.5-1.0 ml/kg body weight per hour. If the child has also developed gram-negative sepsis, extremities may be very warm and appear plethoric. The infant with sepsis may demonstrate hypothermia and lethargy rather than hyperthermia. If significant bowel edema or free peritoneal fluid is present, the infant may demonstrate evidence of third spacing of fluid, including signs of hypovolemia (inadequate circulating blood volume because of loss of fluid into the bowel wall or peritoneum). Tachycardia, decreased peripheral pulses, hypotension, peripheral vasoconstriction, lowered CVP, oliguria, or anuria may be present.

If signs of poor systemic perfusion persist, dopamine may be administered in very low doses (1 to 4 μg/kg body weight/minute continuous infusion), since this dose of dopamine is thought to produce selective ("dopaminergic") dilation of the splanchnic, renal, and mesenteric vessels.

Surgery is required if the child demonstrates evidence of bowel perforation, severe peritonitis, or clinical deterioration unresponsive to vigorous medical management. Resection of the involved bowel is necessary, although attempts are made to salvage as much viable intestine as possible. Following resection, direct anastomosis of remaining bowel is often contraindicated, since remaining segments may be ischemic. The creation of an ileostomy or a jejunostomy permits the minimum possible amount of bowel resection and allows the distal, involved intestine a period of rest. If portions of the intestine are exteriorized, closure of the stoma and direct reanastomosis are accomplished 1 to 2 months later.[41] Perioperative mortality remains high, since only the severely ill infants require surgery. Postoperative complications include temporary malabsorption and development of intestinal obstruction secondary to stricture of ischemic portions of the bowel. These infants often require provision of temporary mechanical ventilatory support postoperatively. Parenteral nutrition is also necessary until oral feedings are resumed (see section on postoperative care).

■ **INFANT BOTULISM**
■ **Etiology**

Infant botulism is a recently recognized infectious disease. It is an acute neuromuscular disease produced by the spores of *Clostridium botulinum*. The sources of these spores have not been determined. Some cases of infant botulism have been positively linked to spore contained in honey. Other possible sources presently being investigated are fresh or home-canned fruits and vegetables, topsoil, household dust, and breast milk.

■ **Pathophysiology**

Infant botulism is different from adult botulism. With adult botulism the preformed *toxin* is ingested. In infant botulism the *C. botulinum spores* are ingested. Once these spores enter the gastrointestinal tract of the infant, they germinate, multiply, and manufacture toxins. These toxins attach to nerve endings and block the release of the neurotransmitter acetylcholine; this causes paralysis.

Age is thought to be one factor in the disease development. The infants at greatest risk are less than 6 months of age. Presumably, infants reach a level of immunologic maturity after 6 months when they are significantly less susceptible to the organism causing infant botulism.

The type of milk or formula ingested may also contribute to the development of infant botulism. Distinct differences in colonic bacterial flora exist between formula-fed infants and breast-fed infants. The different bacterial flora may change germination, multiplication, and growth of *C. botulinum* spores. Since the number of identified cases is small, specific factors that influence severity of infant botulism are not clearly understood.

■ **Clinical signs and symptoms**

Most infants who contract infant botulism have been previously healthy, with uneventful gestation and birth and normal development. Occasionally, the infant will develop acute gastrointestinal symptoms, including nausea, vomiting, diarrhea, and abdominal distention. Most often, however, constipation or a decrease in number and amount of stools are the first indicators of infant botulism. Unfortunately, these vague signs are frequently missed. A subsequent sign in early development of infant botulism is decreased appetite with sucking difficulty. Mothers of bottle-fed babies note decreased formula intake, while mothers of breast-fed babies will have breast engorgement and discomfort after feedings, since the infant is not taking normal amounts of milk. This inability to suck is followed by a loss of ability to swallow and subsequent loss of the gag reflex. As the infant's cry becomes weaker, other neurologic signs become apparent. The infant becomes weak and floppy with loss of head control. Facial expressions disappear, and eyelids droop until the infant can no longer hold them open. Older infants may be unable to vocalize. Muscle weakness can progress to respiratory arrest, the most serious complication.

The timetable for progression of these symptoms is variable. Generally, symptoms occur over 2 to 3 days, but documented cases have progressed as rapidly as 4 hours or as gradually as 2 weeks. Unfortunately, infant botulism is often unrecognized until the infant becomes critically ill.

Routine hematology and chemistry laboratory tests usually are within normal limits. Transient elevation of cerebral spinal fluid (CSF) protein has been reported. If electromyography is performed, the resulting patterns are similar to those recorded in patients with primary muscle disorders. The definitive diagnosis is made on recovery of *C. botulinum* or the botulin toxin from the infant's stool or serum.

■ **Medical treatment and nursing interventions**

Once the diagnosis of botulism is made, specific IV antitoxin, trivalent ABE, is administered as soon as possible, following testing for sensitivity to the serum. Supportive care is then the recommended treatment for the infant with infant botulism, since the short half-life of the toxins make the disease self-limiting. This frequently requires that the infant be admitted to an ICU for elective intubation and mechanical ventilation before respiratory arrest occurs. Once the child is intubated and receiving mechanical ventilation, skilled respiratory care is necessary to prevent pneumonia, atelectasis, or obstruction of the artificial airway (see Chapter 4).

Nutritional support is accomplished with parenteral nutrition by a central venous catheter. The timetable for reinstitution of oral feeding varies with each infant.

The administration of antibiotics is controversial. Selective suppression of colonic bacterial flora that occurs with antibiotic therapy may lead to proliferation of *C. botulinum*. This proliferation will increase the length of time needed for reversal of the toxic paralysis.

■ **BILIARY ATRESIA**

Biliary atresia is the absence or obstruction of the biliary tree. The atresia may involve isolated segments of the bile duct system or the entire biliary tree including the gallbladder.

■ **Etiology**

The cause of biliary atresia is not known. It is believed to be the result of a viral or another injury to the developing duct system in utero or immediately after birth. Biliary atresia is often associated with the polysplenia syndrome (including abdominal visceral transposition, intestinal malrotation, and vascular and cardiac anomalies).[4]

■ **Pathophysiology**

Because there is atresia or obstruction of the biliary tree, bile cannot drain from the liver into the intestines (for excretion in feces). Accumulation of bile in the liver causes direct (conjugated) hyperbilirubinemia. If the condition is not diagnosed and surgically corrected before 3 months of age, progression to liver cirrhosis and portal hypertension occurs. An exploratory laparotomy is often required to make the definitive diagnosis.

■ **Clinical signs and symptoms**

Persistent jaundice and direct (conjugated) hyperbilirubinemia in the newborn are the first clinical signs. Acholic or gray-colored stools represent lack of bile drainage in the gastrointestinal tract. Dark-colored urine represents increased bilirubin secretion in the urine. Pruritus secondary to the increased bile salts in the blood is sometimes present. If the condition is not detected, signs of progressive liver disease are evident within the latter part of the first year. These include ascites, poor growth secondary to malabsorption of fats and fat-soluble vitamins, rickets, hypoproteinemia, edema, and petechiae. Signs of portal hypertension are also noted (see discussion on portal hypertension).

While many laboratory studies can help differentiate biliary atresia from other causes of neonatal jaundice (see Table 8-12), no one study is diagnostic for biliary atresia. Radionuclide scanning and liver biopsy may be attempted, but positive results may occur with diseases other than biliary atresia. Therefore an exploratory laparotomy and operative cholangiography is required to make the definitive diagnosis. Corrective surgery is planned and discussed preoperatively with the parents for implementation in the event the diagnosis is confirmed.[4]

■ Surgical treatment and nursing interventions

The specific surgical procedure performed for the infant with biliary atresia is determined by the location and extent of the atretic segment. Prognosis is best when the proximal biliary tree (connected to the liver) is patent and the atretic segment is *distal* (Fig. 8-18, *A*), although this condition occurs in the minority of involved patients.[4] Surgical correction of this type of biliary atresia involves resection of the atretic segment with primary anastomosis of or conduit insertion between the patent proximal biliary tree and the duodenum.

Surgical correction of *proximal extrahepatic biliary atresia* is currently attempted through use of the Kasai procedure. In 1959 a Japanese surgeon, Dr. Kasai, reported an operation using a small section of resected jejunum as an artificial biliary tree from the liver to the duodenum. The atretic segments were first resected; then a jejunal segment was anastomosed (sewn) between the liver and the duodenum, with the hope of allowing adequate bile drainage.

Several modifications of the Kasai procedure have been developed since the original operative procedure (Fig. 8-19). These modifications require creation of a stoma, known as a portoenterostomy, from which bile drains into a collection bag. External ostomy drainage allows for visual monitoring of bile drainage and is believed to decrease the incidence of postoperative infection in the jejunal-liver connection. Refeeding of bile after its external drainage from the stoma is recommended by some physicians; however, this practice varies. The portoenterostomy is usually closed after 12 to 24 months.

When the atretic segment includes the *proximal biliary tree* as well as its connection to the liver (see Fig. 8-18, *B*), the prognosis is poor because of the association of noncorrectable intrahepatic atresia. With severe forms of biliary atresia, liver transplant may be the treatment of choice.

Nursing interventions for the child undergoing a portoenterostomy procedure include postoperative laparotomy care (see the discussion of postoperative care after abdominal surgery) and stoma observation and care. Prompt application of stoma adhesive and a collection bag after surgery is essential to prevent early skin breakdown from the irritating bile drainage. Postoperative complications may include infection (including cholangitis), ascites, portal hypertension, cirrhosis, or liver failure. The risk of postoperative liver failure is increased if significant liver damage is present at the time of surgery and if progression of liver fibrosis occurs after surgery.[4] (For additional nursing interventions see discussion of liver failure earlier in this chapter.)

Nursing interventions for infants with inoperable biliary atresia (when *intrahepatic* bile ducts are atretic) include supportive therapy directed toward control of the progressive symptoms of ascites, pruritus, fat malabsorption, and liver encephalopathy (see discussions of ascites and liver failure). High doses of the fat-soluble vitamins A, D, E, and K are often required. Cholestyramine is used to assist in the removal of bile salts from the enterohepatic circulation and to reduce itching. Phenobarbital is sometimes prescribed to promote bile drainage, since it acts as a choleretic boost to the scarred liver cells.

■ VIRAL HEPATITIS

Viral hepatitis is classified as follows:
1. Type A (infectious hepatitis)
2. Type B (serum hepatitis)
3. Non-A—non-B hepatitis
4. Neonatal hepatitis

■ Etiology

Viral hepatitis is a primary infection of the liver most commonly caused by two etiologically and immunologically distinct agents: hepatitis A virus and hepatitis B virus. Occurrence of hepatitis that is

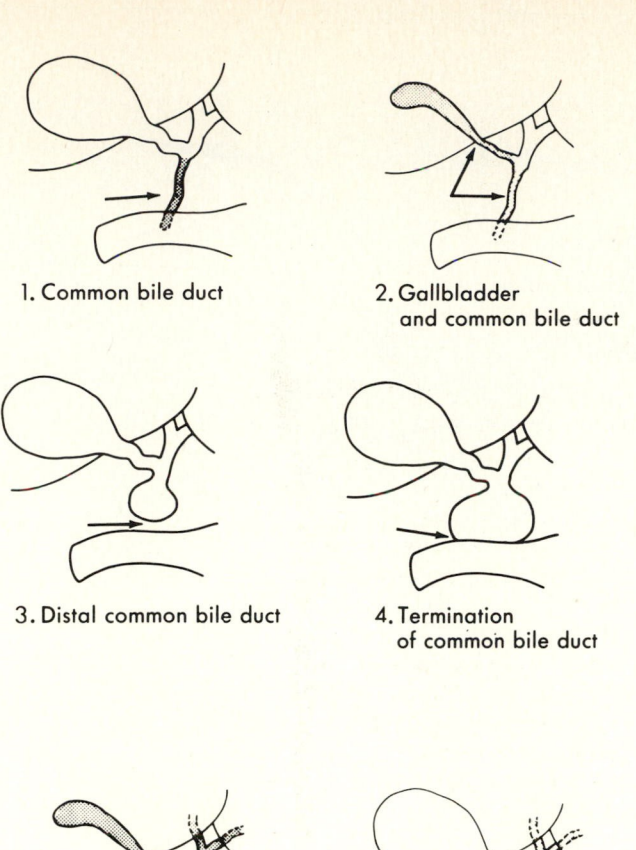

1. Common bile duct

2. Gallbladder and common bile duct

A

3. Distal common bile duct

4. Termination of common bile duct

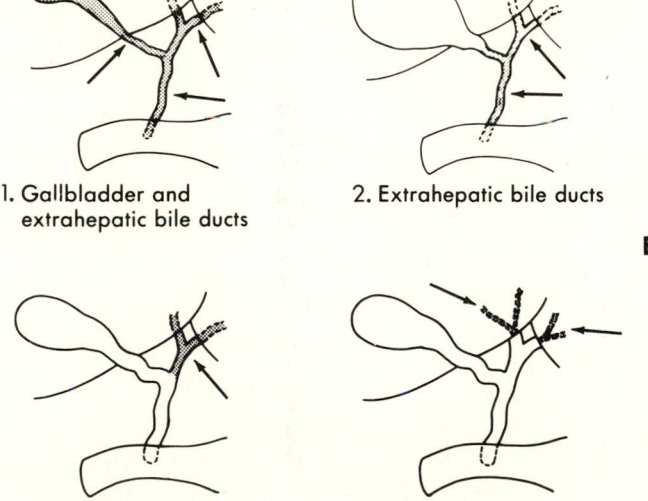

1. Gallbladder and extrahepatic bile ducts

2. Extrahepatic bile ducts

B

3. Common hepatic bile duct

4. Intrahepatic bile ducts

Fig. 8-18 Biliary atresia. **A,** Atresia of distal biliary tree (associated with proximal hepatic ductal patency). Atresia of the *1,* common bile duct; *2,* gallbladder and common bile duct; *3,* distal common bile duct; or *4,* termination of the common bile duct. These forms of biliary atresia are usually surgically corrected through insertion of a conduit between the patent hepatic ducts and the intestine or by removal of the atretic section (arrows indicate atretic areas) and direct anastomosis between the proximal and distal (patent) segments. **B,** Atresia of proximal biliary tree requires prompt diagnosis and early surgical intervention. Atresia of the extrahepatic bile ducts is present *1,* with or *2,* without gallbladder atresia, or *3,* the common bile duct or *4,* intrahepatic bile ducts are atretic. These forms of biliary atresia require biliary reconstruction.

Reproduced with permission from Lilly, J.R., and Altman, R.P.: The biliary tree. In Ravitch, M.M., et al., editors: Pediatric surgery, ed. 3. Copyright © 1979 by Year Book Medical Publishers, Inc., Chicago. (Courtesy Dr. L.K. Pickett.)

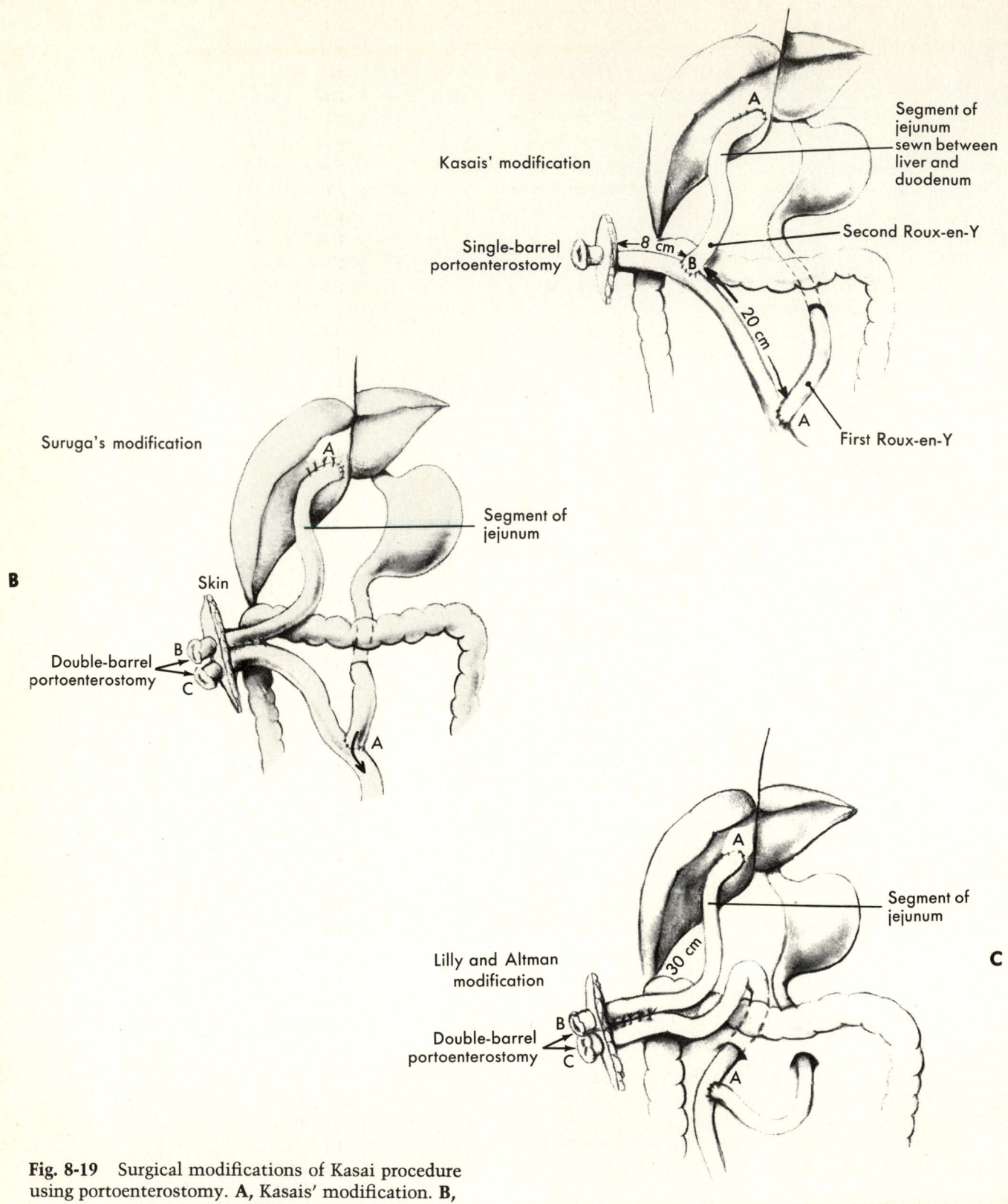

Fig. 8-19 Surgical modifications of Kasai procedure using portoenterostomy. **A,** Kasais' modification. **B,** Suruga's modification. **C.** Lilly and Altman modification.

neither type A nor type B is referred to as non-A–non-B hepatitis.[25] Neonatal hepatitis is also considered a distinct form of hepatitis.

Hepatitis A virus is present in the blood and feces during the incubation period and can be carried by persons who never develop the disease. The occupation and personal hygiene of the carrier are major factors in determining the spread of the disease. Food, water, and milk contaminated by virus-containing feces are the usual sources of hepatitis A. Outbreaks have also occurred after people ate clams or oysters obtained from polluted water. Children and younger adults are more commonly infected with hepatitis A; peak incidence in children occurs in the early school-age period. Hepatitis A usually begins as an acute illness after an incubation period of 14 to 40 days. Fever is a common symptom early in the disease, while jaundice and a prodrome of arthritis or rash are *uncommon* in children with hepatitis A.

Hepatitis B virus is transmitted via blood transfusions or other contact with secretions (including saliva, breast milk, and semen) and serum containing the B virus. This form of hepatitis is frequently preceded by a prodrome of arthritis and rash, and fever is less common. The onset of hepatitis B is usually insidious and occurs after an incubation period of 50 to 180 days.

Neonatal hepatitis occurs in the first 3 months of life and is manifested by direct hyperbilirubinemia, hepatomegaly, and jaundice. Known causes of neonatal hepatitis include a wide range of metabolic disorders and congenital infections such as rubella, cytomegalovirus (CMV), toxoplasmosis, herpes, syphilis, and other known viral agents. Extrahepatic biliary obstruction, as occurs in biliary atresia or choledolchal cyst, also causes direct hyperbilirubinemia, jaundice, and hepatomegaly and must be ruled out since prompt surgical intervention is required for these disorders (see discussion of biliary atresia). In approximately one third of the cases, neonatal hepatitis resolves with no residual liver damage. However, in the remaining two thirds of affected patients, progression of liver damage occurs and cirrhosis develops; this indicates a poor prognosis for long-term survival.[84]

■ **Pathophysiology**

Viral hepatitis causes destruction of liver cells and results in hepatic inflammation, necrosis, and autolysis. Changes occur diffusely throughout the liver, and the architectural structure may be distorted. Regeneration of cells begins as soon as damaged ones are removed by phagocytosis. In most nonneo-

natal cases there is recovery with minimum residual damage. However, chronic hepatitis and cirrhosis may develop, or fulminant hepatitis with accompanying hepatic encephalopathy may occur early in the course of the viral illness.

■ **Clinical signs and symptoms**

Viral hepatitis is characterized by three stages: the preicteric stage, the icteric stage, and the posticteric stage. Clinical signs and symptoms of the preicteric stage last approximately 1 week and include fever, chills, anorexia, malaise, epigastric distress, abdominal pain, nausea, vomiting, and joint pain. Physical examination during this stage reveals hepatomegaly and lymphadenosis.

Weakness, fatigue, pallor, jaundice of the sclera and skin, darkened urine, and gray-colored stools are beginning signs of the icteric stage. Influenza-type symptoms, persistent anorexia, pruritus, and palmar erythema occur as the icteric phase progresses, lasting from 2 to 6 weeks. The posticteric stage is marked by an initial rapid, then gradual, disappearance of jaundice, a darkening of the stools, and a return of laboratory values to normal. Anorexia and fatigue may continue for several weeks, although this is less likely in children and may be a result of the prolonged bed rest frequently prescribed.

In rare cases, for reasons not known, viral hepatitis can progress to fulminant hepatitis with massive hepatic necrosis and damage. Clinical signs of progression to fulminant hepatitis include restlessness, personality changes, lethargy, decreased level of consciousness, bleeding, and coagulopathies (see liver failure for further discussion).

The following specific laboratory serum markers of hepatitis infection have been identified: hepatitis A antigen (HA Ag) and antibody (anti-HAV), hepatitis B surface antigen (HBsAg) and antibody (anti-HBs), hepatitis B core antigen (HBcAg) and antibody (anti-HBc), and hepatitis B e antigen (HBeAg) and antibody (anti-HBe). The availability of these tests has made it possible to make a specific diagnosis of types A and B hepatitis, to identify HBV-contaminated units of blood, and to identify non-A, non-B hepatitis by ruling out other causes. If the critically ill patient is found to have any of these hepatitis serum markers, there is often confusion about possible hepatitis and contagion. Thus a brief discussion of the clinical significance of these markers follows.

The hepatitis B virion is known as a Dane particle, which consists of a DNA-containing core (HBcAg plus HBeAg), surrounded by a small filamentous surface coating (HBsAg). Presence of HBsAg, previously known as Australian antigen, indicates that hepatitis B infection exists and that the patient's blood is infectious. The infectious patient can reflect a spectrum of disease ranging from fulminant hepatic failure to an asymptomatic carrier state. The presence of HBeAg in addition to HBsAg implies an acute infectious hepatitis state. In acute hepatitis B infection, presence of serum HBsAg is present within 1 to 3 weeks of exposure to the virus and in most cases becomes undetectable by 4 months after exposure. Prolonged presence of HBsAg with concurrent normal serum liver transaminases implies a chronic carrier state, which is also infectious (the carrier is often asymptomatic but can infect others).

Anti-HBs is the neutralizing antibody, and its presence in the serum implies previous infection or previous administration of high-titer hyperimmune B globulin. After an acute hepatitis B infection, serum anti-HBs is first detectable 1 to 4 months after clearance of serum HBsAg and remains present for several years.

■ **Medical treatment and nursing interventions**

When a patient is admitted to the ICU with a diagnosis of hepatitis of undetermined type, the primary isolation precaution should be that of serum isolation. The same precautions necessary for handling feces, urine, and excretions from any other hospitalized patients should be used for patients admitted with a diagnosis of viral hepatitis. Specific precautions necessary in caring for a patient with viral hepatitis (as outlined by the Centers for Disease Control) are discussed in detail in Appendix F.

Prophylactic administration of hepatitis B immune serum globulin (ISG) is recommended for individuals exposed to hepatitis B following (1) a parenteral exposure, such as an accidental needle stick, (2) direct mucous membrane contact, such as an accidental splash, and (3) oral ingestion, such as a laboratory pipette accident—all involving HBsAg-positive blood or blood products. Since incubation period following a parenteral exposure may be short (about 1 week between time of exposure and early viral symptoms), hepatitis B ISG or gamma globulin should be administered within 48 hours of exposure. The incubation period following an oral exposure is about 2 months.[49] Since hepatitis B vaccination is now available to medical personnel, it may be recommended that nurses be screened and vaccinated against hepatitis B.

There is no cure for viral hepatitis. Medical treatment and nursing care is directed toward relief of

discomfort and maintenance of adequate nutrition and hydration. Small, frequent nutritious meals should be presented as attractively as possible. Usually the child has no dietary restrictions and so may enjoy planning favorite meals with the dietitian. Special treats such as milk shakes prepared with eggs can provide fluid, calories, and protein without appearing to be a meal, and thus they may be appetizing to a child with anorexia. Antiemetics may be required if nausea prevents adequate nutrition.

If a clinically significant coagulopathy is present, vitamin K or blood components are administered, and any evidence of bleeding should be reported to the physician.

The nurse should monitor the child closely for behavioral changes, lethargy, or irritability, which may indicate the development of hepatic coma. Nursing care of the patient with fulminant hepatitis requires careful assessment of liver function and signs of deterioration of hepatic function (see section on liver failure for further discussion).

■ **CIRRHOSIS**
■ **Etiology**

Regardless of the cause of the liver disease, if hepatic damage is sufficient and if repair does not occur, liver scarring (cirrhosis) develops. Anatomic anomalies, infection, inborn errors of metabolism, and exogenous toxins are the principle problems that cause severe liver disease and cirrhosis in infants and children (see box on causes of cirrhosis).

■ **Pathophysiology**

Cirrhosis of the liver is the result of chronic liver inflammation or disease. As liver cells are destroyed, they are replaced by new cells and by fibrotic scar tissue. If the disease is limited, hepatic regeneration can occur. With chronic liver damage, however, more and more fibrous tissue develops and the liver assumes an irregular, lobular, nodular appearance. When damage is severe and prolonged, destroyed tissue is no longer replaced by new tissue or even by fibrous tissue, but instead the tissue necroses and atrophies. This fibrous alteration in liver tissue distorts and compresses liver architecture and obstructs flow through liver sinusoids, causing portal hypertension.

Two major types of cirrhosis found in children are biliary cirrhosis and postnecrotic cirrhosis. In biliary cirrhosis, jaundice and signs of extrahepatic biliary obstruction (such as occur in biliary atresia) are present. The inflammation and scarring within the liver is concentrated around the intrahepatic bile ducts. Postnecrotic cirrhosis follows massive tissue inflammation and destruction after severe hepatitis; the scarring involves the lobular structure of the liver cells.

■ Clinical signs and symptoms

The child with cirrhosis initially demonstrates vague symptoms of gastrointestinal dysfunction, including lethargy, malaise, irritability, nausea, vomiting, anorexia, fatigue, and diarrhea or constipation; these symptoms probably result from disordered protein, glucose, and fat metabolism as a result of impaired liver function. The child may complain of epigastric or right upper quadrant pain. The liver becomes small and atrophied and is usually tender to palpation.

With liver sinusoidal obstruction, ascites and portal hypertension develop (see discussion of these problems earlier in this chapter). The child often appears cachectic, although weight loss caused by poor nutrition is often balanced by the weight gain resulting from ascites. The child's clothes will become tight as abdominal girth increases. The abdomen will feel dull to percussion, and a *fluid wave* may be elicited (see discussion of ascites). Loss of protein and fluid into the peritoneal cavity causes increased aldosterone secretion (and increased renal sodium and water retention and potassium excretion) and hypoalbuminemia. If large amounts of fluid are present in the abdomen, diaphragmatic excursion can be compromised. This causes the child to breathe rapidly and shallowly, and it may cause lower lobe atelectasis. The child is also at risk for the development of hydrothorax.

If portal hypertension is present, the child may develop splanchnic sequestration of blood, splenic congestion, and collateral circulation, including esophageal varices. Splanchnic sequestration also causes hyperaldosteronism and, as a result, increased renal excretion of potassium; this may produce a mild metabolic alkalosis. Splenic congestion produces anemia, leukopenia, and thrombocytopenia. Development of esophageal varices increases the child's risk of sudden, severe gastrointestinal bleeding (see discussion of gastrointestinal bleeding and portal hypertension).

Since the liver normally synthesizes prothrombin, fibrinogen, and factor VII and normally deactivates clotting factors, severe coagulopathies can result from cirrhosis and significant liver dysfunction.

CAUSES OF CIRRHOSIS IN CHILDREN

I. Biliary cirrhosis
  A. Extrahepatic biliary atresia
  B. Intrahepatic biliary hypoplasia
  C. Choledochal cysts
  D. Cystic fibrosis
  E. Ascending cholangitis
    1. Postoperative (atresia)
    2. Cholecystitis, cholelithiasis
    3. Tumors of the biliary tree
    4. Strictures
  F. Drugs—diphenylhydantoin (Dilantin), chlordiazepoxide (Librium), imipramine (Tofranil)
  G. Familial intrahepatic cholestasis
II. Postnecrotic cirrhosis
  A. Hepatitis virus A disease, severe
  B. Hepatitis virus B disease
  C. Neonatal hepatitis
    1. Rubella
    2. Toxoplasmosis
    3. Cytomegalovirus
    4. Syphilis
    5. Enterovirus
    6. Herpesvirus
    7. Idiopathic
  D. Chronic active hepatitis
  E. Genetic-metabolic
    1. Wilson's disease
    2. Glycogen storage, type 4
    3. Galactosemia
    4. Tyrosinemia
    5. Cystinosis
    6. Fructose intolerance
    7. Neimann-Pick disease
    8. Alpha-1-antitrypsin deficiency cirrhosis
    9. Gaucher's disease
    10. Sickle cell disease
    11. Thalassemia major, hemoglobin-S thalassemia
    12. Severe Rh isoimmunization
  F. Passive venous congestion, severe
    1. Constrictive pericarditis
    2. Ebstein's anomaly
    3. Pulmonary hypertension
    4. Severe anemia
    5. Protein malnutrition
    6. Budd-Chiari syndrome, severe
      a. Congenital abnormality of hepatic veins
      b. Tumor occlusion of hepatic veins
  G. Kwashiorkor
  H. Drugs, toxins, poisons

Modified from Roy, C.C., Silverman, A., and Cozzetto, F.J.: Pediatric clinical gastroenterology, ed. 2, St. Louis, 1975, The C.V. Mosby Co.

The child may have petechiae, prolonged bleeding from venipuncture sites, or epistaxis. The child may become jaundiced, and darkening of skin pigment may occur as a result of increased activity of melanocyte-stimulating hormone. *Spider nevi (vascular spider* or *telangiectasis)* are often present. These are spider-shaped red lesions that blanch when pressure is applied to the center. They appear most commonly on the skin of the face, upper extremities, or upper trunk.

Since most hormones secreted by the adrenal cortex and most ovarian and testicular hormones are inactivated or metabolized by the liver, children with cirrhosis may demonstrate hormone imbalance. Frequently, estrogen excess produces testicular atrophy, gynecomastia, and loss of facial, axillary, and pubic hair in the adolescent male. Girls may develop amenorrhea, and adolescents of both sexes experience loss of libido. As already discussed these children develop hyperaldosteronism and sodium and water retention, which can contribute to their ascites and generalized edema. These changes in bodily appearance caused by endocrine disorders secondary to the liver disease can be highly disturbing to an adolescent boy or girl.

■ Medical treatment and nursing interventions

The liver is responsible for carbohydrate metabolism (including storage of glycogen and gluconeogenesis), fat metabolism (secretion of bile), protein metabolism (deamination of amino acids and formation of urea and plasma proteins), storage of vitamins, deactivation of clotting factors, storage of iron, and synthesis of prothrombin, fibrinogen, and factor VII. Thus medical and nursing care is aimed at detection of alterations in these processes and prevention of their complications.

Adequate nutrition must be maintained with oral or parenteral nutrition (see discussion of TPN). The nurse must monitor for signs of hypoglycemia; these can include the development of lethargy and decreased systemic perfusion in the young infant. If these signs develop, the physician should be notified immediately, and a concentrated IV glucose solution such as 50% glucose (1.0 ml/kg body weight) is administered.

Supplementary vitamins (especially fat-soluble vitamins and vitamin K) are also usually prescribed.

If the child develops evidence of bleeding, treatment with appropriate blood components must be prompt to prevent circulatory compromise (see discussion of gastrointestinal bleeding and portal hypertension). The child's fluid intake and output must be monitored closely for evidence of increased fluid retention (ascites) and renal failure or hepatorenal syndrome (see Table 8-13). The nurse must also monitor for clinical signs and symptoms of electrolyte and acid-base imbalance (see Table 8-4). Colloids, diuretics, and corticosteroids may be administered to eliminate some of the extravascular water (see section on ascites).

The nurse must frequently check the child's

Table 8-21 Causes of acute pancreatitis in children

Trauma	Blunt, penetrating, or surgical injury
Infectious	Mumps, coxsackievirus B, hepatitis virus A or B
Obstructive	Cholelithiasis, *Ascaris*, ductal stenosis or ectasia, duplications, tumors, choledochus cysts
Drugs, toxins	Steroids (especially prednisone), chlorothiazides, salicylazosulfapyridine, alcohol, borates, tetracyclines, oral contraceptives
Systemic-endocrine-metabolic	Systemic lupus erythematosis, periarteritis nodosa, hypercholesterolemia, uremia, malnutrition, hyperparathyroidism, cystic fibrosis, peptic ulcer, vitamin A and D deficiency

Modified from Roy, C.C., Silverman, A., and Cozzetto, F.J.: Pediatric clinical gastroenterology, ed. 2, St. Louis, 1975, The C.V. Mosby Co.

neurologic status (including orientation, arousability, and alertness) since the patient is at risk for the development of hepatic encephalopathy. Extreme irritability or lethargy in an infant may indicate the development of encephalopathy (see discussion of liver failure).

■ PANCREATITIS
■ Etiology

The most frequent causes of acute pancreatitis in the pediatric age-group include drug therapy (particularly prednisone), blunt abdominal trauma, or clinical mumps (Table 8-21).

■ Pathophysiology

The characteristic feature of acute pancreatitis is the escape of pancreatic enzymes from the pancreatic cells into the blood and body fluids. The released enzymes lead to an autodigestive process of the pancreas manifested by edema, hemorrhage, or necrosis. Serum amylase levels rise sharply during the first 24 to 48 hours after the insult to the pancreas and usually return to normal by the third day. The pancreatic enzymes may alter pulmonary and peripheral capillary permeability, resulting in respiratory failure, peripheral edema, and third spacing of fluid, leading to cardiovascular failure.

■ Clinical signs and symptoms

Abdominal pain is the most consistent symptom in acute pancreatitis. The pain may develop slowly; it may be mild and of short duration or sudden in onset, severe in intensity, and of prolonged duration. The most intense pain is usually localized in the epigastrium and may radiate to the back and upper quadrants of the abdomen. The pain typically is constant and may last for 24 to 72 hours. Nausea and vomiting are common. In severe cases the patient may appear pale and sweaty and complain of dizziness.

On physical examination, the patient is quiet and prefers to lie on the side, with hips slightly flexed. In fulminating cases, shock may be present; the child's extremities are often pink and warm (because of increased capillary permeability and peripheral flow) despite intravascular hypovolemia. Mild scleral icterus may be noted. The abdomen is slightly distended and tender to palpation and percussion but not rigid. Bowel sounds are diminished in most cases. A bluish discoloration around the umbilicus (Cullen's

sign) or in the flanks (Turner's sign) signifies hemorrhagic pancreatitis with ascites. In rare cases physical findings suggest a pleural effusion. In fact, in the younger child, when localization of abdominal pain is poor, pancreatitis should always be suspected in the presence of unexplained ascites or hemorrhagic pleural effusion.

Elevation of serum amylase greater than twice normal is diagnostic of pancreatitis, but since this value often returns to normal within 72 hours, a normal serum amylase does not rule out pancreatitis. Serum lipase is also elevated and remains elevated much longer than amylase. The white blood count and differential are frequently normal, while hematocrit values reflect hemoconcentration secondary to severe dehydration. Hyperglycemia is common early in the course of pancreatitis because glucagon is released from damaged pancreatic alpha-cells. Insulin therapy may be indicated. Serum calcium is usually normal except in fulminant pancreatitis, when extensive fat necrosis produces hypocalcemia that is manifested by muscular jerking, twitching, and irritability.

■ Medical treatment and nursing interventions

Prevention, assessment, and treatment of hypovolemic shock is the primary goal in the care of the child with acute pancreatitis. Since release of pancreatic enzymes can increase capillary permeability, large amounts of fluid can be lost from the intravascular space into the peritoneal and pleural cavities. This shift of intravascular fluid into nonfunctional areas is known as *third spacing*. If a large fluid shift occurs, the child may develop signs of hypovolemic shock.

Once the diagnosis of acute pancreatitis is made, a central venous line is inserted, and fluid and electrolyte therapy is aggressive to restore or maintain vascular volume. In hypotensive patients, albumin-containing solutions, plasma, blood, or a modified plasma preparation is administered (see discussion of low cardiac output in Chapter 3).

Vital signs are checked at least every hour with careful determination of blood pressure and urine output and assessment of systemic perfusion, since these are all indirect indicators of intravascular volume. Measurement of daily weight reflects total body-fluid accumulation or loss, but because of the possibility of marked intraperitoneal shift of fluid (third spacing), increased daily weight alone cannot be interpreted as reflective of changes in intravascular volume.

Careful assessment of pain status is also important; changes in location and severity should be noted on the nursing-care plan. Duodenal perforation secondary to pancreatic compression and irritation can cause gastrointestinal bleeding and peritonitis. The use of morphine and other opiate derivatives is contraindicated in patients with pancreatitis because these medications increase spasm of the sphincter of Oddi (sheath of muscle fibers surrounding pancreas) and smooth muscles of the pancreatic ducts, causing additional pain. Intramuscular meperidine, sometimes combined with an anticholinergic drug, is the analgesic of choice. Change of position and other comfort measures are frequently necessary to provide optimum pain relief.

The child receives nothing by mouth. A nasogastric tube is placed, and continuous nasogastric suction is provided to decompress and empty the stomach. Loss of electrolytes from nasogastric suction must be calculated and replaced intravenously (per physician's order). Supportive nutritional therapy via peripheral or central parenteral nutrition is often necessary during the acute stage of pancreatitis. Careful calculation of daily caloric intake, as well as daily fluid intake, is important while oral feedings are withheld. When oral intake is resumed, a low-fat diet is usually recommended, and supplemental pancreatic enzymes are sometimes administered.

■ INFLAMMATORY BOWEL DISEASE

Inflammatory bowel disease is a general descriptive term that can be used to describe ulcerative colitis and Crohn's disease. Since inflammatory bowel disease is a chronic illness of school-age children and adolescents, it is not routinely seen by the intensive-care nurse in pediatrics. However, toxic megacolon is one complication of inflammatory bowel disease that may require the child's admission to the ICU.

■ Etiology/pathophysiology

Toxic megacolon is an acute dilation of a portion of colon secondary to severe inflammation of the bowel wall. This acute dilation may be precipitated by manipulation of the bowel during diagnostic tests required for an acute gastrointestinal illness (e.g., during barium-enema radiograph or colonoscopy). The marked dilation of the inflamed bowel causes the colon to lose its tone, and subsequent ileus and microperforations occur. The diagnosis of toxic megacolon is confirmed by the presence of marked dilation of the involved colonic segment on a single flat-plate radiograph of the abdomen.

■ Clinical signs and symptoms

Spiking fever and acute abdominal pain with distention are the primary symptoms of toxic megacolon. However, fever may not be present in patients receiving high-dose corticosteroids for severe bowel inflammation. Vomiting may or may not occur.

■ Medical treatment and nursing interventions

Observation for toxic megacolon is an important part of the care of patients with severe inflammatory bowel disease. Medical management of the patient with toxic megacolon includes discontinuation of oral intake and provision of supportive IV fluids, nasogastric suction, and systemic antibiotics. Steroid administration may be continued in patients with severe bowel inflammation.

Nutritional support through central or peripheral parenteral nutrition is necessary since oral feeding is contraindicated for several days (see discussion of TPN). Complications of high-dose systemic steroids may develop; these include leukocytosis, decreased immunologic defenses, diabetes, bone demineralization with resultant vertebral collapse or aseptic necrosis of the femoral heads, and redistribution of body fat, especially in the face (cushingoid changes), neck, and posterior shoulder area.

If toxic megacolon does not resolve with supportive medical therapy or if bowel perforation occurs, emergency surgery is required. Colectomy with ileostomy is the necessary surgical procedure. Careful preoperative preparation of the patient requiring a colectomy, including explanation and demonstration of ileostomy appliances, should be given a high priority even when time before the operative procedure is brief. When any child is admitted to the ICU with the diagnosis of toxic megacolon, the possibility and details of surgery should be explained to both patient and family. This prevents abrupt, inadequate explanations if a bowel perforation occurs and the need for surgical intervention becomes urgent.

■ REYE'S SYNDROME
■ Etiology

Reye's syndrome is a multisystem disease, characterized by a severe encephalopathy with fatty degeneration and infiltration of the viscera (especially the liver) following recovery from a viral illness. Positive confirmation of Reye's syndrome is made by a liver biopsy, reflecting the fatty degeneration. The cause of Reye's syndrome is unknown. Researchers have attempted to determine predictors of the disease or links between events occurring during the child's antecedent illness and the development and severity of Reye's syndrome. Recently, several retrospective studies have revealed an epidemiologic association between salicylate ingestion during the antecedent viral illness and later development of Reye's syndrome; children who were given aspirin during the viral illness were more likely to develop Reye's syndrome than similar children who received acetominophen or nothing.[74] While these findings are not conclusive, they were compelling enough for the American Academy of Pediatrics to recommend that aspirin not be prescribed for children with influenza or varicella.[36]

■ Pathophysiology

Liver cellular mitochondrial damage interrupts the normal pathways for detoxification of waste products; these disrupted pathways include the ornithine cycle. The ornithine cycle is responsible for the breakdown of serum ammonia to urea, which is then excreted (Fig. 8-20). As the disease progresses and this cycle remains incomplete, the serum ammonia rises (normal: 0 to 80 mg/dl or 0 to 45 mm/dl). These ammonia levels and other unknown factors become toxic to the body and contribute to the development of cerebral dysfunction (see Chapter 6). Decreased mitochondrial function triggers alternate pathways to supply the cells with needed oxygen and glucose; pyruvic acid is converted to lactic acid, and metabolic acidosis develops. The child often becomes hypoglycemic and dehydrated, particularly if vomiting develops, and hyperventilation may produce a respiratory alkalosis.

Fluid and electrolyte imbalance (including dehydration, hypoglycemia, and acidosis) and coagulopathies result from liver dysfunction. Neurologic complications result from the development of toxic encephalopathy, cerebral edema (cytotoxic edema), and increased intracranial pressure; these problems seem to be related to hyperammonemia, hypoglycemia, possible direct effects of the antecedent viral illness, and other, unknown factors.

■ Clinical signs and symptoms

Only the clinical signs and symptoms relating to the liver involvement in Reye's syndrome are discussed here (see Chapter 6 for further details about the encephalopathy encountered with this disorder).

Most often, the child with Reye's syndrome does not appear jaundiced; serum bilirubin levels are normal or mildly elevated, and hepatomegaly does not develop. Serum ammonia levels are usually elevated to 1.5 to 2 times normal for 2 to 4 days. Con-

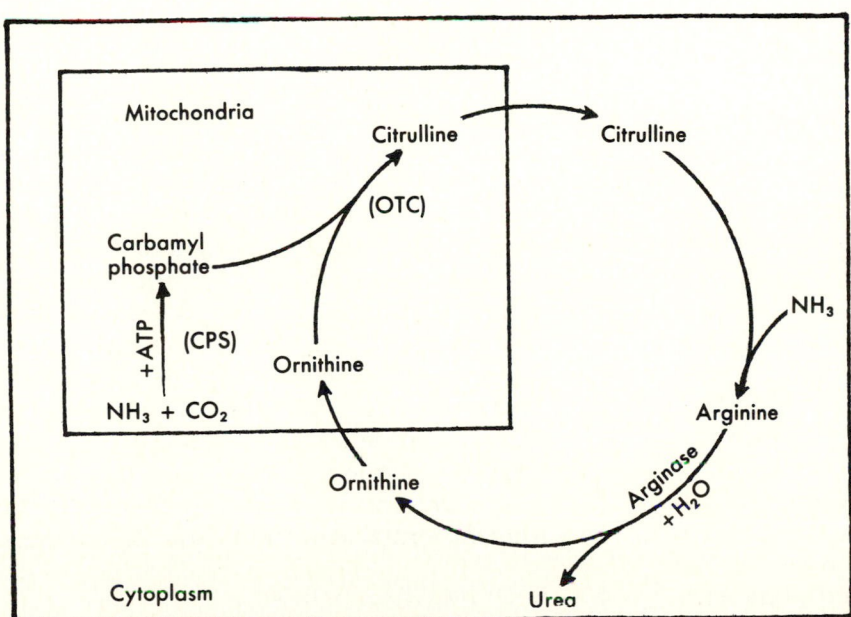

Fig. 8-20 Urea cycle and hepatic mitochondrial enzymes involved in the production of ammonia.

From Boutros, A.R.: Reye's syndrome: a predictably curable disease, Pediatr. Clin. North Am. **27**:540, Aug. 1980.

centrations of amino acids, free fatty acids, and other serum enzymes may also be elevated. Elevation of the liver transaminases SGOT and SGPT and prolonged PT and PTT are present, reflecting liver injury. Serum glucose may be normal on the child's admission but can decrease rapidly as glycogen stores are depleted. In infants and young children glycogen depletion occurs quickly, and hypoglycemia is usually noted on admission.

Reye's syndrome must be differentiated from other disorders that can produce coma and liver failure. These include severe hypoglycemia, drug ingestion (including salicylate toxicity or phenobarbital ingestion), or toxic exposure (such as lead encephalopathy).

■ Medical treatment and nursing interventions

Treatment and nursing interventions for management of the child with increased intracranial pressure are discussed in Chapter 6. If liver function is severely impaired, additional nursing concerns may be found in the discussion of liver failure in this chapter.

The child's serum glucose level should be monitored closely, since hypoglycemia can produce decreased myocardial function and poor systemic perfusion, resulting in compromise of cerebral perfusion. Hypoglycemia should be treated with continuous infusion of hypertonic glucose IV solutions (10 to 15 gm of glucose/dl or 10% to 15% glucose) and supplemental boluses of 25% glucose (1 to 2 ml/kg body weight) or D_{50} (0.5 to 1.0 ml/kg body weight) to maintain serum glucose concentrations at 200 mg/dl. Since large amounts of glucose are administered, the child will require large quantities of supplemental potassium chloride (up to 4 to 6 mEq/kg body weight/24 hours) to prevent serum hypokalemia.[52] Maintenance requirements of IV calcium (calcium gluconate: 200 mg/kg body weight/24 hours) and phosphorus (potassium phosphate: 3 to 4 mEq/kg body weight/24 hours) should also be provided. Oral neomycin (100 mg/kg body weight/24 hours) or other nonabsorbable antibiotics may be administered orally to eliminate ammonia-producing bacteria in the gut.[52]

IV fluid administration should be regulated carefully. Adequate fluid volume is necessary to maintain sufficient cardiac output and cerebral, systemic, and renal perfusion. However, excessive fluid administration may contribute to systemic edema. The child is usually given 75% of maintenance fluids (see Table 8-3). This amount is adjusted, based on the child's CVP (which should be approximately 5 mm Hg) or

pulmonary artery wedge pressure (which should be approximately 8 mm Hg) and signs of systemic perfusion (urine output should average 0.5 to 1.0 ml/kg body weight/hour, and arterial blood pressure should be normal for that patient).[52]

Fresh frozen plasma or platelets are given to correct coagulopathies or bleeding. If a liver biopsy is planned, platelets or fresh frozen plasma is infused before and possibly during the liver biopsy to prevent excessive bleeding. Vitamin K is given if needed (1.0 mg IV in one dose).

The child's temperature should be monitored continuously by skin or rectal probe or at least every hour. Hyperthermia is treated with sponge baths or a cooling mattress, since fever increases the child's oxygen requirement. Acetaminophen and aspirin are *not* administered to control fever. Significant hypothermia also increases the child's oxygen requirement and may require treatment with an over-the-bed radiant warmer or heating blanket.

The child's serum and urine osmolalities are frequently monitored during treatment. A high serum osmolality may result from dehydration or excessive administration of osmotic diuretics; a measured serum osmolality of greater than 350 mOsm for 8 or more hours in patients with increased intracranial pressure has been associated with an increased mortality.[61]

Reye's syndrome is a frightening disease for the child and family. A previously healthy child may demonstrate bizarre behavior, lapse into a coma, and die within a few hours. With the development of better supportive therapy and more sophisticated monitoring of intracranial pressure, survival rates following Reye's syndrome have improved, although the incidence of significant neurologic sequelae is still significant.[79] The child may be frightened, delirious, or comatose. The parents will require a great deal of support and time to think about all that has happened to their child. It is important that the parents be given time with their child, so that they will be able to see how sick the child is and so that the child will know his parents are near. Since the prognosis is generally guarded during the first hours or days following admission to the unit, it is imperative that the parents be given consistent information (with the use of consistent terms) about the child's condition.

■ ESOPHAGEAL BURNS
■ Etiology/pathophysiology

The most frequent cause of esophageal burns in children is ingestion of caustic agents (e.g., lye, ammonia, bleaches, or various acids). Peak incidence of these ingestions occurs between 1 and 3 years of age, since toddlers are increasingly mobile and curious.

The caustic agent produces a chemical burn in the oropharynx, esophagus, or stomach. The intensity of the burn varies from superficial esophagitis (erythema and some edema of the esophageal mucosa) to severe ulceration and necrosis of the esophagus and stomach. With severe burns esophageal perforation or gastric perforation with peritonitis can occur (see discussion of acute abdomen). A significant burn causes early mucosal ulceration, which is followed by later granulation, then fibrosis of the tissue. This fibrosis may be responsible for the later development of esophageal strictures.

■ **Clinical signs and symptoms**

After the first few sips of a caustic agent, the child is usually discouraged from further ingestion because of the intense burning and pain. The mouth, lips, and larynx become edematous and covered with an exudate. With larger volume ingestion, similar changes occur in the distal esophagus and stomach. Dysphagia occurs immediately but frequently subsides after a few days. Without early treatment severe strictures can develop and surgical intervention becomes necessary. The presence of significant esophageal damage *cannot* be determined by visual examination of the mouth and oropharynx; an esophagoscopy must be performed.

■ **Medical treatment and nursing interventions**

The child is *not* encouraged to vomit the caustic material, since this can redamage esophageal and oropharyngeal mucosa. Instead, antidotes are administered to either neutralize the ingested substance or to prevent its absorption. If the pH of the ingested substance is alkaline, large amounts of water-diluted vinegar or citrus juice are orally administered to neutralize the alkali. If the ingested substance is acidotic, milk, soap solutions, or aluminum hydroxide is administered for neutralization. Milk, egg white, or oil may be administered to sooth irritated mucous membranes following ingestion of any caustic agents.

Children with severe burns require administration of IV fluids and oral fluids and foods are withheld, since esophageal and pharyngeal burns may cause dysphagia. In addition, it may be painful for the child to swallow. If long-term therapy is anticipated, placement of a gastrostomy tube or a central venous catheter (for TPN) is indicated. Antibiotics are generally prescribed to prevent secondary infection, and corticosteroids may be given for 7 to 10 days to reduce inflammation and subsequent development of granulation and fibrotic tissue.

If severe pharyngeal edema is present, the child may develop upper airway obstruction and respiratory distress. The nurse should monitor for signs of increased respiratory effort (nasal flaring, retractions), tachypnea, restlessness, and cyanosis or signs of upper airway obstruction (stridor, decreased air movement, or prolonged inspiratory time). If significant upper airway obstruction develops, elective intubation may be performed to ensure that the child has an adequate airway until the edema subsides (see the discussion of upper airway obstruction in Chapter 4).

Esophagoscopy is often performed to allow prompt evaluation of damage. With severe burns early esophageal dilation is indicated. A regimen is often planned to slowly increase the size of the strictured esophagus over a period of months. If esophageal dilations are unsuccessful, surgical replacement of the esophagus with a segment of colon (colon interposition) is necessary to allow for return to oral alimentation.

■ **STRESS ULCERS**
■ **Etiology**

Stress ulcers, or acute stress erosions, are mucosal lesions of the upper gastrointestinal tract, which accompany physical trauma, burns, sepsis, hemorrhagic shock, and critical illness. The mucosal changes of stress ulcers are rapid in onset and lack the signs of inflammation and scarring that characterize chronic ulcer disease. The precise mechanisms leading to mucosal lesions in stress ulcers are unknown. It is clear, however, that stress ulcers cannot be reproduced experimentally without the presence of hydrochloric acid in the stomach.

■ **Pathophysiology**

Stress ulcers are usually multiple, discrete, and focal, and they are distributed primarily in the proximal portion of the stomach, although antral and duodenal involvement is not uncommon. The most widely accepted theory regarding the pathogenesis of stress ulcers is the back-diffusion of hydrogen ions through a broken gastric mucosal barrier. Disturbances in mucosal microcirculation or an acute gastric mucosal cell ischemia, or both, may also play an important role (Fig. 8-21).

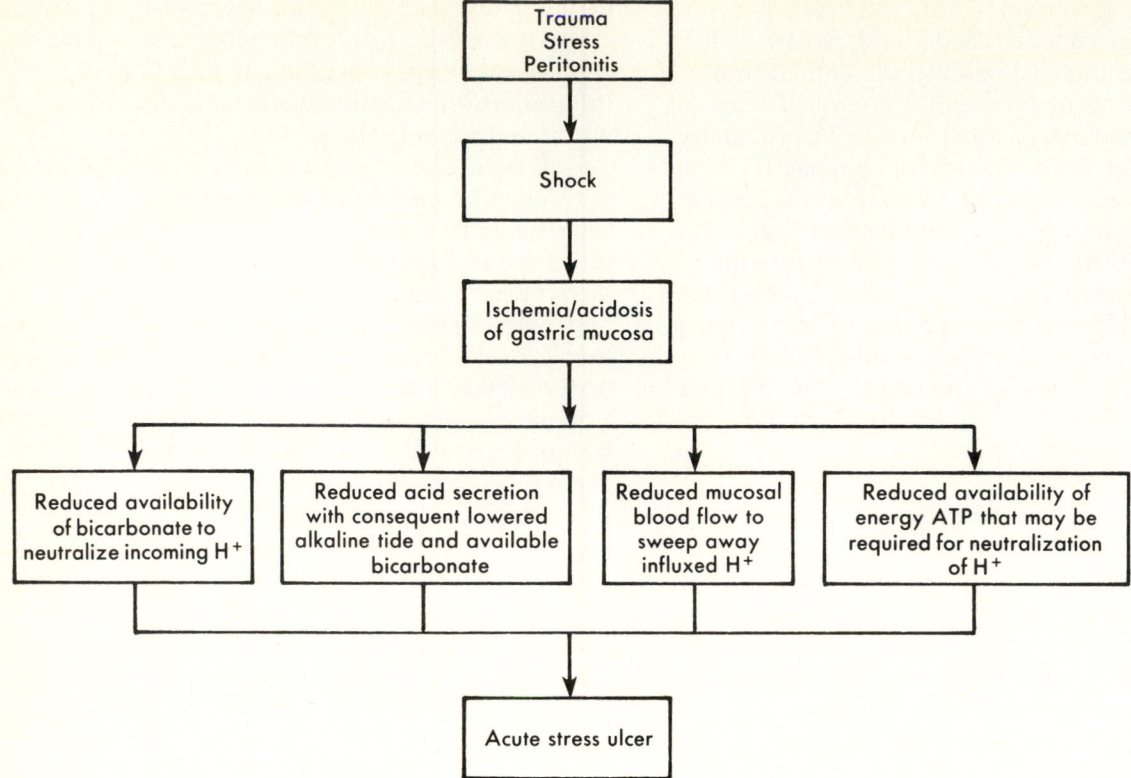

Fig. 8-21 Proposed pathophysiology of stress ulcers.

■ **Clinical signs and symptoms**

Painless gastrointestinal bleeding is the major, and often only, clinical manifestation of ulceration caused by stress. Usually, the loss of blood from multiple superficial lesions is slow. The subtle loss of blood per rectum (guaiac- or hematest-positive stools), a decline in serum hematocrit, or the appearance of flecks of blood within the nasogastric aspirate is usually the first sign of the ulcer. Occasionally, the initial gastric bleeding is rapid, and as a result, the patient may vomit or pass gross blood per rectum. This more dramatic presentation is accompanied by tachycardia, restlessness, pallor, cool moist skin, and systemic arterial hypotension—the classic signs of hemorrhagic shock (see discussion of gastrointestinal bleeding).

A chronic peptic ulcer can also be activated during periods of physical or environmental stress. Therefore, it can be difficult to distinguish between loss of blood caused by stress erosions and that resulting from activation of a chronic ulcer. The most reliable clue to the presence of stress erosions is the development of upper gastrointestinal bleeding immediately following a stress incident.

■ **Medical treatment and nursing interventions**

If severe gastric bleeding develops, the child requires immediate replacement of blood lost and may require urgent surgical intervention (for nursing interventions see the section on gastrointestinal bleeding). Current practice for prevention of stress ulcers includes the administration of antacids (Table 8-22), with concurrent monitoring of gastric pH before and after administration of the medication. If the child does not tolerate prolonged antacid therapy or if administration of antacids is contraindicated, the hydrogen (H_2) receptor antagonist, cimetadine, is sometimes prescribed* (see drug table in Appendix B) to inhibit gastric acid secretion. Use of silastic nasogastric tubes is advised in critically stressed patients to prevent additional mucosal irritation secondary to friction from the hard plastic tube.

*References 10, 18, 29, 35, 50, 53, 59, 73, 81, and 85.

Table 8-22 Antacids categorized by trade names and specific ingredients

Trade name	Calcium carbonate	Aluminum hydroxide	Magnesium hydroxide or oxide	Magnesium trisilicate	Other	Sodium content
Alka-Seltzer	—	—	—	—	Sodium bicarbonate 1.008/gm, citric acid 800 mg, potassium bicarbonate 300 mg	296 mg/tablet
Aludrox	—	307 mg/5 ml	103 mg/5 ml	—	—	1.5 mg/5 ml
Amphojel	—	320 mg/5 ml	—	—	—	6.9 mg/5 ml
Basaljel	—	400 mg/5 ml	—	—	—	1.8 mg/5 ml
Camalox	250 mg/5 ml	225 mg/5 ml	200 mg/5 ml	—	—	2.5 mg/5 ml
Di-Gel	—	—	87 mg/5 ml	—	Simethicone 25 mg/5 ml	8.5 mg/5 ml
Gelusil	—	250 mg/5 ml	—	500 mg/5 ml	Mint flavor	8.0 mg/5 ml
Kolantyl	—	150 mg/5 ml	150 mg/5 ml	—	—	—
Maalox	—	225 mg/5 ml	200 mg/5 ml	—	—	2.5 mg/5 ml
Maalox Plus	—	225 mg/5 ml	200 mg/5 ml	—	Simethicone 25 mg/5 ml	2.5 mg/5 ml
Mylanta	—	200 mg/5 ml	200 mg/5 ml	—	Simethicone 20 mg/5 ml	3.9 mg/5 ml
Mylanta-II	—	400 mg/5 ml	400 mg/5 ml	—	Simethicone 30 mg/5 ml	4-10 mg/5 ml
Phosphaljel	—	—	—	—	Aluminum phosphate 233 mg/5 ml	12.5 mg/5 ml
Riopan	—	—	—	—	Magaldrate 400 mg/5 ml	0.7 mg/5 ml
Trisogel	—	150 mg/5 ml	583 mg/5 ml	—	—	16 mg/5 ml

From American Pharmaceutical Association: Handbook of nonprescription drugs, ed. 5, Washington, D.C., 1980.

■ Diagnostic Tests

Since the critical-care nurse must often prepare the child for or accompany him to procedures or diagnostic tests to evaluate gastrointestinal function, Table 8-23 presents (for quick reference) the purpose, equipment, patient preparation, procedure, length, and postprocedure care for each of these studies.

The child who requires a treatment or procedure should receive explanations (as age-appropriate) about what he will see, hear, and feel during the procedure.

Table 8-23 Nurse's guide to selected procedures and diagnostic tests in pediatric gastroenterology

Test or procedure	General explanation/purpose	Equipment used	Patient preparation
Radiologic			
Barium swallow	Fluoroscopic x-ray exam of the esophagus by a radiologist. Diagnostic of structural abnormalities, motor disorders, and mucosal integrity	X-ray machine including fluoroscopic screen	None needed
Upper GI	Fluoroscopic x-ray exam of the esophagus, stomach, and duodenum by a radiologist. Diagnostic of structural abnormalities, motor disorders, gastroesophageal reflux, ulcerative disease, delayed gastric emptying	X-ray machine including fluoroscopic screen	Newborn-2 yr: skip last feeding before exam ≥2 yr: skip meal before exam. If scheduled in afternoon, give clear liquid breakfast that day
Upper GI with small bowel follow-through	Fluoroscopic x-ray exam by a radiologist with follow-up spot films of the esophagus, stomach, duodenum, and small intestine. Allows diagnosis of small bowel abnormalities including inflammatory bowel disease and rapid GI transit time	X-ray machine including fluoroscopic screen	Same as upper GI
Barium enema (BE)	Fluoroscopic x-ray exam of the large intestine by a radiologist. Diagnostic of structural abnormalities and mucosal integrity	X-ray machine including fluoroscopic screen	Beyond newborn period • liquids only on day of exam • cathartic may be ordered evening before exam (individualized to patient)
Air-contrast barium enema	Same as BE. Thought to be more diagnostic of mucosal integrity, especially the presence of inflammation or polyps	X-ray machine including fluoroscopic screen	Same as BE; however, an empty large bowel is essential for effective exam

The youngster should be prepared in a sequence that allows him to mobilize defenses, without providing excessive time for his imagination to increase anxiety. Small infants and toddlers benefit most from the presence of a consistent, soothing caretaker and return to their mother (or primary caretaker) as quickly as possible. Older children may benefit from more detailed explanations of the purpose of the procedure.

The child (as age-appropriate) and parents require explanations of the duration and risks of the procedure and the details of postprocedure care.

Procedure involved	Approximate length of time	Postprocedure care
Patient given small amount of liquid barium by mouth and x-ray films are taken	5-15 min	Routine postfeeding positioning of infants The nurse must ensure fecal elimination of the barium
Patient given strawberry-flavored liquid barium by mouth or tube, and x-ray films are taken	15-45 min (depends on gastric emptying time)	Same as barium swallow
Same as upper GI with added spot films at 15 min and hourly intervals until barium reaches large bowel	30 min-several hours (depends on length of time until barium reaches large bowel)	Same as barium swallow
Lubricated plastic enema tip placed in rectum; barium instilled into rectum while radiologist visualizes procedure on fluoroscopic screen	15-60 min; varies with each patient and suspected abnormality	Observe for passage of barium, abdominal distention, or bleeding If no passage of barium in 24 hr, cathartic administration is recommended If procedure performed in presence of intussusception or volvulus, monitor for evidence of bowel perforation (see *acute abdomen*)
Same as BE except less barium is instilled and air is instilled by a radiologist via a hand bulb-pump similar to that on BP cuff	15-60 min; varies with each patient and suspected abnormality	Same as BE. Patient may have gas pains and pass flatus because of air insufflation

Continued.

Table 8-23   Nurse's guide to selected procedures and diagnostic tests in pediatric gastroenterology—cont'd

Test or procedure	General explanation/purpose	Equipment used	Patient preparation
Endoscopy			
Flexible upper endoscopy (esophagoscopy, gastroscopy)	Direct visualization of the interior upper GI tract (esophagus, stomach, duodenum) for the purpose of diagnosing mucosal injury, lesions, structural abnormalities, or source of upper GI bleeding	Pediatric fiberoptic endoscope (approximately 30 Fr in diameter, the tubing is made of flexible rubber; a light source is attached to scope)	With general anesthesia, follow regular preoperative routine. If under local sedation 1. NPO 8 hr preceding procedure or gastric content is removed by NG tube before endoscopy 2. Heparin lock or IV in place 3. Oral suction at bedside 4. Consent form signed
Flexible sigmoidoscopy or colonoscopy	Direct visualization of the interior large bowel for the purpose of diagnosing mucosal injury or colonic lesions or source of lower GI bleeding. Can be advanced further than a rigid proctosigmoidoscope	Pediatric fiberoptic endoscope (approximately 30 Fr in diameter, the tubing is made of flexible rubber)	Depends on suspected abnormality; usually, either oral cathartic and clear liquid diet 24-48 hr before procedure or enema the night before procedure Consent form signed
Rigid sigmoidoscopy	Direct visualization of the lower bowel lining (rectum and sigmoid) for the purpose of diagnosing mucosal injury, polyp, or source of lower GI bleeding	Hollow metal cylindric scope with tapered end (size used varies with age and size of child)	Depends on suspected abnormality. Usually, either oral cathartic or enema the evening before the procedure
Biopsy			
Percutaneous liver biopsy	To obtain liver specimen without laparotomy	Disposable soft tissue biopsy tray or sterilized biopsy tray per hospital regimen	1. IM sedation 2. IV or heparin lock in place 3. PT and PTT results on chart 4. Consent form signed NOTE: If coagulopathy is present, blood component therapy may be required before or during the biopsy to prevent hemorrhage

Procedure involved	Approximate length of time	Post-procedure care
Patient placed on left side. Lubricated end of scope passed through mouth into esophagus by physician. Bite block is placed around tube between patient's teeth to prevent damage to tube; oral suction of secretions prn Scope is advanced under direct visualization by physician	15-45 min depending on exam required and suspected abnormality	NPO for 1 hr Clear liquids after 1 hour; advance to preprocedure diet
Patient placed on left side with knees drawn to chest; following finger rectal exam by physician, the lubricated end of scope is passed into rectum and scope is advanced under direct visualization by physician. Air and water occasionally instilled through scope to ensure optimum visualization	15-45 min depending on exam and suspected abnormality	Resume diet as before Patient may have gas pains and pass flatus or small amount of blood
Patient placed in knee-chest position or on special proctosigmoidoscopy table	5-30 min depending on abnormality suspected	May have small amount of bleeding per rectum after procedure

Patient supine with arms over head. Local anesthesia given	5-10 min	Monitor for signs of blood loss
		
		Monitor VS, with BP q 15 min × 1 hr,
		    q 30 min × 2 hr
		    q 1 hr × 4 hr
		    q 2 hr × 12 hr
		
		Do not remove pressure dressing on site for 24 hr
		
		Have patient lie on right side for 8 hr, providing additional pressure to puncture site
		
		Begin giving patient clear liquids when awake, and advance to preprocedure diet as tolerated
		
		Monitor Hct q 4 hr × 3 hr; monitor for signs of hemorrhage

Continued.

Table 8-23   Nurse's guide to selected procedures and diagnostic tests in pediatric gastroenterology—cont'd

Test or procedure	General explanation/purpose	Equipment used	Patient preparation
Nuclear medicine			
Liver-spleen scan	Scanning technique used to determine liver and spleen size or presence of mass, abscess or other abnormality in the liver or spleen. The radioactive substance used is taken up by a part of the liver cells and is then counted and imaged by the scanner. *This does not evaluate liver function*	Scanner and radioactive substance	IV or heparin lock in place. May have regular meals before test. Sedation is ordered on prn basis
Liver excretion scans (DIS-IDA, PIP-IDA and rose bengal scans)	Scanning technique used to determine liver excretory function. The radioactive substance used is taken up by the liver cells directly and excreted in the bile through the biliary tree. Lack of excretion or delayed excretion raises suspicion about extrahepatic biliary atresia	Scanner and radioactive substance	IV or heparin lock in place. May have regular meals before test. Sedation is ordered on prn basis.
Meckel's scan	Scanning technique used to identify presence of a Meckel's diverticulum. The radioactive substance administered is taken up by gastric mucosal parietal cells; if extragastric mucosa is present, it is usually detected by scan	Scanner and radioactive substance	IV or heparin lock in place. NPO 4 hr before scan

REFERENCES

1. Abel, R., Abott, W., and Fisher, J.: Acute renal failure: treatment without dialysis by total parenteral nutrition, Arch. Surg. **103:**513, 1971.
2. Abel, R., and others: Malnutrition in cardiac surgical patients, Arch. Surg. **111:**45, 1976.
3. Alexander, M.M., and Brown, M.S.: Pediatric history taking and physical diagnosis for nurses, ed. 2, New York, 1979, McGraw-Hill, Inc.
4. Altman, R.P.: Biliary atresia. In Raffensperger, J.G., editor: Swenson's pediatric surgery, ed. 4, New York, 1980, Appleton-Century-Crofts.
5. Altman, R.P., and Krug, J.: Portal hypertension: American Academy of Pediatrics Surgical Section Survey—1981, J. Pediatr. Surg. **17:**567, 1982.
6. Anderson, C., and Burke, V.: Paediatric gastroenterology, Oxford, 1975, Blackwell Scientific Publications.
7. Avery, G.B.: Neonatology: pathophysiology and management of the newborn, ed. 2, Philadelphia, 1981, J.B. Lippincott Co.
8. Barness, L.A.: Manual of pediatric physical diagnosis, ed. 5, Chicago, 1981, Year Book Medical Publishers, Inc.
9. Barness, L.A.: Nutritional requirements of the full-term neonate. In Suskind, R.M., editor: Textbook of pediatric nutrition, New York, 1981, Raven Press.

Procedure involved	Approximate length of time	Post-procedure care
Radioactive substance is injected IV Patient lies flat on table Scanner is lowered close to patient's body, and scan is taken Patient must lie still	1 hr	Radioactive linen precautions per nuclear medicine protocol
Same as liver spleen scan; repeated scans are usually done at 1-hr intervals	Initial scan: 1 hr; return for 2-, 4-, and 24-hr scans as needed	Radioactive linen precautions per nuclear medicine protocol
Same as above scans	1 hr	Radioactive linen precautions per nuclear medicine protocol

10. Behar, J., and others: Cimetidine in the treatment of symptomatic gastroesophageal reflux: a double blind controlled trial, Gastroenterology **74**:441, 1978.
11. Bell, M.J., and others: Neonatal necrotizing enterocolitis, Ann. Surg. **187**:1, 1978.
12. Berman, W.F., and Holtzapple, P.G.: Gastrointestinal hemorrhage, Pediatr. Clin. North Am. **23**:885, 1975.
13. Biller, J.A., and Yeager, A.M.: The Harriet Lane handbook, ed. 9, Chicago, 1981, Year Book Medical Publishers, Inc.
14. Blackburn, G.L., and others: Surgical nutrition. In Halpern, S.L., editor: Clinical nutrition, Philadelphia, 1979, J.B. Lippincott Co.

15. Bockus, H.L., editor: Gastroenterology, vol. 3, ed. 3, Philadelphia, 1976, W.B. Saunders Co.
16. Book, L., Herbst, J., and Jung, A.: Necrotizing enterocolitis in infants fed an elemental formula (abstract), Pediatr. Res. **8**:379, 1974.
17. Brobeck, J.R., editor: Best and Taylor's physiological basis of medical practice, ed. 10, Baltimore, 1979, The Williams & Wilkins Co.
18. Brogden, R., and others: Cimetidine: a review of its pharmacological properties and therapeutic efficacy in peptic ulcer disease, Drugs **15**:931, 1978.
19. Burgess, A.: The nurse's guide to fluid and electrolyte balance, New York, 1970, McGraw-Hill, Inc.

20. Chandra, R.K.: The liver and the biliary system. In Anderson, C.M., and Burke, V., editors: Paediatric gastroenterology, Oxford, 1975, Blackwell Scientific Publications, Inc.

21. Chandra, R.K.: Fulminant liver failure. In: The liver and biliary system in infants and children, Edinburgh, 1979, Churchill Livingstone, Inc.

22. Cohen, H.R., and Lipton, J.M.: Blood disorders. In Graef, J.W., and Cone, T.E., editors: Manual of pediatric therapeutics, ed. 2, Boston, 1980, Little, Brown & Co.

23. Committee on Nutrition, American Academy of Pediatrics: Pediatrics **57**:278, 1976.

24. Cox, K., and Ament, M.E.: Upper gastrointestinal bleeding in children and adolescents, Pediatrics **63**:408, 1979.

25. Czaja, A.J., and Davis, G.L.: Hepatitis non-A, non-B, Mayo Clin. Proc. **57**:639, 1982.

26. Diem, K., and Lentner, C.: Scientific tables, ed. 7, Basle, Switzerland, 1970, Ciba-Geigy Ltd.

27. Dudrick, S., and others: Long-term total parenteral nutrition with growth, development, and positive nitrogen balance, Surgery **64**:134, 1968.

28. Filston, H., and Izant, R.: The surgical neonate, evaluation and care, New York, 1978, Appleton-Century-Crofts.

29. Finkelstein, W., and others: Cimetidine, N. Engl. J. Med. **299**:992, 1978.

30. Fisher, J.: Total parenteral nutrition, Boston, 1976, Little, Brown & Co.

31. Fisher, J., and others: Plasma amino acids in patients with hepatic encephalopathy: effect of amino acid infusions, Am. J. Surg. **127**:40, 1974.

32. Folkman, J.: Appendicitis. In Ravich, M.M., and others, editors: Pediatric surgery, ed. 3, Chicago, 1979, Year Book Medical Publishers, Inc.

33. Fomon, S.J.: Infant nutrition, Philadelphia, 1974, W.B. Saunders Co.

34. Frantz, I., and others: Necrotizing enterocolitis, J. Pediatr. **86**:259, 1975.

35. Freston, J.: Cimetidine in the treatment of gastric ulcer: review and commentary, Gastroenterology **74**:426, 1978.

36. Fulginiti, V.A., and others: Special report from the Committee on Infectious Diseases: aspirin and Reye syndrome, Pediatrics **69**:810, 1982.

37. Given, B.A., and Simmons, S.J.: Gastroenterology in clinical nursing, ed. 4, St. Louis, 1984, The C.V. Mosby Co.

38. Gray, G.M.: Mechanism of digestion and absorption of food. In Sleisinger, M.H., and Fordtran, J.S., editors: Gastrointestinal disease, Philadelphia, 1978, W.B. Saunders Co.

39. Guignard, J.P.: Renal function in the newborn infant. Pediatr. Clin. North Am. **29**:777, 1982.

40. Healey, J.E.: Vascular anatomy of the liver, Ann. N.Y. Acad. Sci. **170**:8, 1970.

41. Hunt, C.E., and Inwood, R.: Necrotizing enterocolitis. In Raffensperger, J.G., editor: Swenson's pediatric surgery, ed. 4, New York, 1980, Appleton-Century-Crofts.

42. Iber, F.L.: Normal and pathologic physiology of the liver. In Sodeman, W.A., Jr., and Sodeman, T.M., editors: Sodeman's pathologic physiology, ed. 6, Philadelphia, 1979, W.B. Saunders Co.

43. Jensen, D.: The principles of physiology, ed. 2, New York, 1980, Appleton-Century-Crofts.

44. Johanson, B.C., and others, editors: Standards for critical care, ed. 2, St. Louis, 1984, The C.V. Mosby Co.

45. Katz, A.J., and Hyams, J.: Gastrointestinal disorders. In Graef, J.W., and Cone, T.E., editors: Manual of pediatric therapeutics, ed. 2, Boston, 1980, Little, Brown & Co.

46. Kelts, D., and others: Nutritional basis of growth failure in children and adolescents with Crohn's disease, Gastroenterology **76**:720, 1979.

47. Klaus, M.H., and Fanaroff, A.A., editors: Care of the high-risk neonate, ed. 2, Philadelphia, 1979, W.B. Saunders Co.

48. Korones, S.B., and Lancaster, J.: High-risk newborn infants: the basis for intensive nursing care, ed. 3, St. Louis, 1981, The C.V. Mosby Co.

49. Krugman, S., and others: Viral hepatitis, type B, N. Engl. J. Med. **300**:101, 1979.

50. Kruss, D., and others: Safety of cimetidine, Gastroenterology **74**:478, 1978.

51. Lake, A.M., and Walker, W.A.: Neonatal necrotizing enterocolitis: a disease of altered host defense, Clin. Gastroenterol. **6**:463, 1977.

52. Levin, D.L.: Reye's syndrome. In Levin, D.L., Morriss, F.C., and Moore, G.C., editors: A practical guide to pediatric intensive care, ed. 2, St. Louis, 1984, The C.V. Mosby Co.

53. Lilly, J., and others: Cimetidine cholestatic jaundice in children, J. Surg. Res. **24**:384, 1978.

54. Lloyd, J.: The etiology of gastrointestinal perforations in the newborn, J. Pediatr. Surg. **4**:77, 1969.

55. Lubchenco, L.: The high-risk infant, Philadelphia, 1976, W.B. Saunders Co.

56. Luck, S.R.: Fluids and electrolytes. In Raffensperger, J.G., editor: Swenson's pediatric surgery, ed. 4, New York, 1980, Appleton-Century-Crofts.

57. Luck, S.R.: Total parenteral nutrition. In Raffensperger, J.G., editor: Swenson's pediatric surgery, ed. 4, New York, 1980, Appleton-Century-Crofts.

58. MacPhayden, B., and Dudrick, S.: Management of gastrointestinal fistulae with parenteral hyperalimentation, Surgery **74**:100, 1973.

59. Mahon, W., and Kolton, M.: Hypotension after intravenous cimetidine, Lancet **1**:828, 1978.

60. Maisels, M.J.: Neonatal jaundice. In Avery, G.B., editor: Neonatology: pathophysiology and management of the newborn, Philadelphia, 1981, J.B. Lippincott Co.

61. Mattar, J.A., and others: a study of the hyperosomolar state in critically ill patients, Crit. Care Med. **1**:293, 1973.

62. Maxwell, M., and Kleeman, C.: Clinical disorders of fluid and electrolyte metabolism, ed. 3, New York, 1980, McGraw-Hill, Inc.

63. Metheny, N.M., and Snively, W.D.: Nurses' handbook of fluid balance, ed. 3, Philadelphia, 1979, J.B. Lippincott Co.

64. Mize, C.E.: Acute hepatic failure. In Levin, D.L., Morriss, F.C., and Moore, G.C., editors: A practical guide to pediatric intensive care, ed. 2, St. Louis, 1984, The C.V. Mosby Co.

65. Numbers-connection test, Merrell National Laboratories, Cincinnati, Ohio, 1975.

66. Phillips, S.: Fluid and electrolyte fluxes in the gut, Hosp. Pract. **8:**137, 1973.

67. Pitt, J., and others: Macrophages and the protective action of breast milk in necrotizing enterocolitis (abstract), Pediatr. Res. **8:**384, 1974.

68. Raffensperger, J.G.: Appendicitis. In Swenson's pediatric surgery, ed. 4, New York, 1980, Appleton-Century-Crofts.

69. Raffensperger, J.G.: Gastrointestinal perforation. In Swenson's pediatric surgery, ed. 4, New York, 1980, Appleton-Century-Crofts.

70. Raffensperger, J.G.: Portal hypertension. In Swenson's pediatric surgery, ed. 4, New York, 1980, Appleton-Century-Crofts.

71. Raffensperger, J.G., and Luck, S.R.: Gastrointestinal bleeding in children, Surg. Clin. North Am. **56:**413, 1976.

72. Raffensperger, J.G., and Pokorny, W.: Abdominal trauma. In Raffensperger, J.G., editor: Swenson's pediatric surgery, ed. 4, New York, 1980, Appleton-Century-Crofts.

73. Regal, P., and others: Cimetidine as an adjunct to oral enzymes in the treatment of malabsorption due to pancreatic insufficiency, Gastroenterology **74:**468, 1978.

74. Reye Syndrome Working Group, National Surveillance of Reye Syndrome 1981: Update, Reye syndrome and salicylate usage, Morbid. Mortal. Week. Rep. **31:**53, 1982.

75. Robson, A.M.: Parenteral fluid therapy. In Behrman, R.E., Vaughan, V.C., and Nelson, W.E., editors: Nelson textbook of pediatrics, ed. 12, Philadelphia, 1983, W.B. Saunders Co.

76. Schedl, H.P.: Water and electrolyte transport: clinical aspects, Med. Clin. North Am. **58:**1429, 1974.

77. Schwartz, S.: Principles of surgery, ed. 3, New York, 1979, McGraw-Hill, Inc.

78. Schwartz, S.I., and Sterer, E.H.: Manifestations of gastrointestinal disease. In Schwartz, S.I., editor: Principles of surgery, ed. 3, New York, 1979, McGraw-Hill, Inc.

79. Shaywitz, B.A., and others: Long-term consequences of Reye's syndrome: a sibling-matched, controlled study of neurologic, cognitive, academic, and psychiatric function, J. Pediatr. **100:**41, 1981.

80. Smith, D.W.: Growth and its disorders, Philadelphia, 1977, W.B. Saunders Co.

81. Tagamet (cimetidine): Prescribing information, Smith, Kline, & French Laboratories, Philadelphia, PA. 19101, Sept. 1977.

82. Touloukian, R.J.: Neonatal necrotizing enterocolitis: an update on etiology, diagnosis, and treatment, Surg. Clin. North Am. **56:**281, 1976.

83. Touloukian, R.J., Posch, J., and Spencer, R.: The pathogenesis of ischemic gastroenterocolitis of the neonate: selective gut mucosal ischemia in asphyxiated neonatal piglets, J. Pediatr. Surg. **7:**194, 1972.

84. Watkins, J., Katz, A., and Grand, R.: Neonatal hepatitis: a diagnostic approach, Adv. Pediatr. **24:**399, 1977.

85. Welch, R., and others: Reduction of aspirin-induced gastrointestinal bleeding with cimetidine, Gastroenterology **74:**459, 1978.

86. Wilkerson, S.A., and Adamkin, D.H.: Fluid therapy in critically ill neonates, Infusion **4:**125, 1980.

87. Wu, P.Y.: Phototherapy: in vivo side effects, Perinatol.-Neonatol. **2:**21, March-April, 1982.

CHAPTER NINE

Bioinstrumentation: Principles and Techniques

HOLLY WEEKS WEBSTER

Bioinstrumentation, as an adjunct to the care of the critically ill child, has received wide acclaim in the last decade, partly as a reflection of the rapid development of pediatric critical care as a subspecialty science. Previously, pediatric critical care suffered a developmental lag because of inadequate funding for research and educational programs and deficient technology. Instrumentation was borrowed from the adult intensive care unit (ICU) setting with few adaptations. Thus the technology lacked precision and sophistication and did not address pediatric needs.

Nursing specialists have now developed pediatric ICU orientation programs and pediatric critical-care workshops. However, one conspicuous deficiency in many critical-care educational programs is information addressing the principles of instrumentation. This chapter describes the equipment necessary for the care of critically ill children in an ICU, the principles of bioinstrumentation, and the specific uses and hazards of the devices employed in the ICU setting.

■ OVERVIEW OF PEDIATRIC BIOINSTRUMENTATION

Instrumentation in the ICU may be used to monitor, measure, or support a patient. Monitoring devices measure physiologic parameters in the patient, giving warning or advising the clinician of the status of that parameter. Measuring devices regulate components that are given to the patient, such as IV fluids. Patient support systems, such as ventilators, may both monitor and measure while they provide vital support. For the sake of brevity, all items of equipment described in this chapter are referred to as "monitoring devices." These instruments may be further subdivided into two types: those considered "invasive," which break the normal physiologic barriers (e.g., an arterial line), and those considered "noninvasive," which do not break the physiologic barriers and, in some instances, do not even touch the patient directly.

Not all instruments are necessarily useful or precise. The clinical need for and performance of each device must be ascertained by a collaborative effort between the clinicians and the bioengineers who are responsible for purchasing the unit. Karselis[34] maintains that the prime purpose of an instrument is to "extend the range and/or sensitivities of man's faculties" and, as such, should do so "with speed, reproducibility, reliability and cost-effectiveness."

The equipment discussed in this chapter is categorized according to the physiological system that is being monitored. Each type of equipment is considered separately.

■ Characteristics of children that affect instrumentation

The physical characteristics of children that influence the development and use of pediatric instruments are many. The more important considerations are listed here.

Body size of the child. Children have increased total body surface area (BSA) in proportion to body mass, which causes increased heat loss and fluid loss.

Devices requiring exposure of the child to ambient air (such as over-bed warmers) may aggravate fluid or heat loss in the child.[91] There is decreased absolute surface area in children available for skin electrodes or other contact devices, and this influences the design of some instruments.

Cardiovascular characteristics. Children have smaller arteries and veins for cannulation. In addition, the child's cardiac reserve is limited.[91] Thus a child's rapid heart rate demands a flexible but sensitive cardiac monitor that will not record movement and other artifacts but will accurately document changes in the child's heart rate or rhythm.

Quantitatively smaller systolic, diastolic, and mean arterial blood pressures in children must be measured by accurate monitoring devices, since quantitatively smaller changes in these parameters can indicate qualitatively greater changes in the child's cardiovascular function.

The relatively small stroke volumes of young children are generally near the maximum that can be achieved by their small ventricles.[91] For this reason a child's cardiac output is more dependent on heart rate than stroke volume.

Cardiac output measurements obtained by thermodilution may be influenced by the child's rapid heart rate. Therefore if a computer has a slow response, the calculated cardiac output may be erroneously high because the computer is measuring the dilution produced by several heart beats (or ventricular ejections).

Respiratory characteristics. The upper airway of the child is smaller and of a different shape than that of the adult. Thus endotracheal and tracheostomy tubes used for children must be smaller,[91] and they are generally uncuffed.

Smaller tidal volumes, rapid respiratory rates, and resultant shorter inspiratory times in children require that the mechanical ventilators used be able to accurately deliver small tidal volumes in a short time and at low pressure.

The increased compliance of the thoracic wall in young children also has important clinical consequences. First, the young child is not able to generate large negative intrathoracic pressures; thus his ability to increase tidal volume is minimal. Therefore the major compensatory mechanism for the child with respiratory distress is tachypnea.[42,91] Respiratory monitoring equipment must be capable of accurately measuring these rapid respiratory rates even when chest movement is minimal. Second, the child's compliant chest wall makes it more difficult to maintain sufficient end-expiratory pressure during periods of respiratory distress. This characteristic may cause an increased tendency for alveolar collapse[42,91] unless continuous positive airway pressure (CPAP) or positive end-expiratory pressure (PEEP) can be provided by pediatric respiratory assist devices. Finally, since the infant's chest wall provides little or no resistance to movement, it supplies no significant resistance to hyperventilation of the infant's lungs when hand or mechanical ventilation is performed. Unless pressure manometers are used with all types of inspiratory assist devices, this lack of resistance may increase the infant's risk of pneumothorax.

Respiratory work normally accounts for 2% to 6% of the child's total oxygen consumption, but, in an infant with respiratory distress, the requirement may be nearly 25% to 30% of the total oxygen consumption.[42] The rapid respiratory rates observed in children cause increased heat and water loss through the respiratory system. Therefore all respiratory assist devices must provide heat and humidity for the child.

Neurologic characteristics. The fact that the skull of an infant is thin influences the type of intracranial pressure monitoring devices that may be used.[91,92] Also, the critically ill child is usually frightened and uncooperative because of inability to comprehend his illness or treatment. Because the child's movement can cause interruption or distortion of instrument function or measurements, monitoring devices must be able to differentiate between movement artifact and abnormalities in the child's clinical status.

Miscellaneous characteristics

Metabolic rates. Higher metabolic rates in children necessitate increased caloric intake per kilogram of body weight per day. Numerically small changes in the child's caloric intake may create significant changes in the ability to heal or in the energy available for physical development or motor activity. Also, rapid heat loss in the child may result in temperature instability requiring constant temperature monitoring. The infant's oxygen consumption may increase significantly with changes in the ambient temperature.[92]

Body fluids. Small children have an increased percentage of total body water and extracellular water.[91] Therefore, careful attention must always be given to the amounts and types of oral and parenteral fluids that the child receives. Devices used to regulate the child's IV fluid administration and measure urine output must be calibrated in small units. Infusion pumps must be factory tested and clinically evaluated to ensure that they are able to accurately deliver specific fluid volumes.

Immunologic immaturity. Children are more

susceptible to infections; thus invasive monitoring may be a greater threat to a child than to an adult.[92]

■ General complications of monitoring

Although it is customary to review complications and recommendations at the end of the chapter, the following comments are relevant to the discussions later in this chapter of specific monitoring equipment. Three errors commonly observed in the critical-care unit when electrical or mechanical equipment is in use are described here.

1. *Lack of working knowledge of the monitoring systems.* The nurse must understand the principles and components of each piece of equipment used in order to understand its usefulness and hazards. *If the nurse is unfamiliar with equipment, she must get instructions immediately!*
2. *False sense of security with alarm systems.* Alarms may be turned off or malfunction without the knowledge of the bedside nurse. This may allow a problem to progress to a critical state before the situation is recognized. Remember, if an alarm fails, the nurse is responsible for the consequences that may follow. *The nurse should always check alarm settings and functions at least at the beginning and end of every shift, and whenever vital signs are obtained.*
3. *Risk of infection.* Contamination is particularly troublesome when invasive equipment is used, but it can also be a problem with noninvasive equipment in some patients.

■ Instrument theory and safety

Since the function of an instrument is to either *measure* a physiologic parameter or *regulate* a substance administered to the patient, several generalizations about such equipment may be made. The functional units of an electrical or mechanical monitoring system usually include a sensor, a transducer, an amplifier, and meters or alarms (Fig. 9-1).[15] The nurse interfaces with the patient and monitor unit at the point where the device senses the signal or converts it (with the transducer) to an electrical signal. The nurse can also influence the amplifier and meter with specific instrument adjustments, such as the "gain" on an ECG monitor. The monitor alarm systems can be manually adjusted to fit the patient needs. Finally, filters, which eliminate electrical "noise," and "grounding" devices, which deflect current as a safety measure, are also important in a monitoring system. All these elements of bioinstrumentation are discussed in a later section.[29]

Definition of terms. Several terms are used in electrical theory to describe the properties of electrical energy. In order to understand equipment function one must understand these terms.[34]

Current. Current is the number of free electrons (the negatively charged ions) flowing through a conducting substance per unit of time from the area of greatest concentration to the lowest (i.e., negatively charged electrons at one point move to another where there are fewer electrons). In electrolyte solutions (such as water) the ions move toward ions of the opposite charge. Current, thus produced, is measured in amperes (amp).

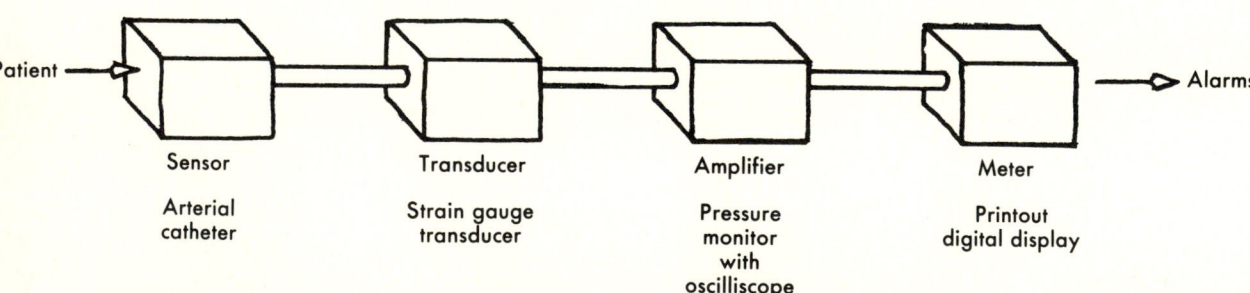

Fig. 9-1 Units of a bioinstrumentation system. Most instruments used to monitor critically ill patients require a sensor, a transducer, an amplifier, and a meter. If the instrument is used, for example, to monitor the child's arterial blood pressure, the arterial catheter obtains the signal (as the sensor), the strain-gauge transducer converts it to an electrical signal, the pressure monitor amplifies the signal, and a meter or digital monitor displays the signal.

Voltage. Voltage is the unit of potential difference in charge between two points (i.e., "gradient" or "potential"). Electrons carry a negative charge. An imbalance in electron concentration between two points creates a negative charge at one point and a positive charge (or a less negative charge) at a second point. This imbalance will create a flow of electrons from the negative to the positive point.

A ————————→ B
10 electrons   0 electrons
(−) charge   (+) charge
Electrical current will flow from A → B

Resistance. The opposition to the flow of electrons or electrical current inherent in any material is called resistance. The amount of resistance depends on the conducting property of the material. For example, silver conducts a flow of current with greater ease than glass; therefore glass provides a higher resistance to flow.

The relationship among these three terms—*current* (I), *voltage* (E), and *resistance* (R)—is described in the following equation and Fig. 9-2.[34]

$$\text{Voltage} = \text{Current} \times \text{Resistance}$$
$$E = I \times R$$

Power. Electrical power is the amount of work done per unit of time; it is measured in watts. When current flows through a conductor, a certain amount of energy is dissipated into the environment as heat or light (such as in a light bulb). The rate of energy dissipation is determined by resistance (R) and current (I); therefore the formula for calculating power (P) is[34]:

$$\text{Power} = \text{Current}^2 \times \text{Resistance}$$
$$\text{or}$$
$$P = I^2 \times R$$

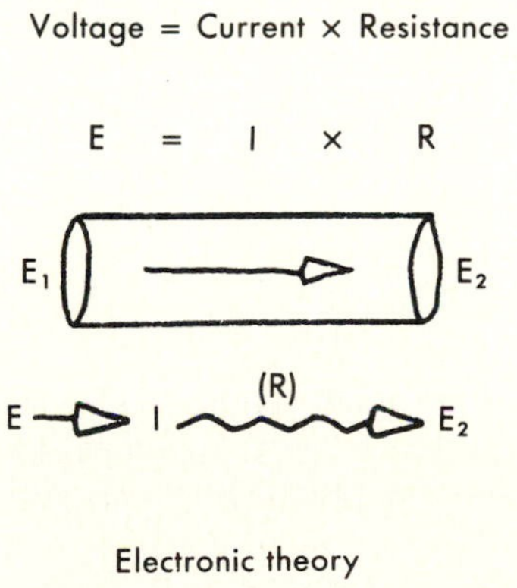

Voltage = Current × Resistance

$$E = I \times R$$

$$E_1 \qquad \longrightarrow \qquad E_2$$

$$E \multimap I \underset{(R)}{\sim\!\sim\!\sim} \multimap E_2$$

Electronic theory

Fig. 9-2 Electrical theory: voltage (E) is the product of current (I) and resistance (R). Voltage is the unit of potential difference in charge between two points (E_1 and E_2). Current flow is determined by voltage and resistance within the material.

Too much power may represent lost (or wasted) energy and may cause equipment to overheat.

Electrical theory, which explains the properties of electrical energy or power, also incorporates the following ideas.[34]
1. Flow occurs because of the electrical gradients (high to low).
2. There must be an energy source to sustain power (voltage).
3. There must be a closed electrical circuit, or loop, in order for current flow to be possible.

The cardiovascular system functions in a manner similar to that described by electrical theory just discussed. Understanding the physiologic system may provide a more familiar reference for understanding electrical principles. Comprehension of cardiovascular physiology requires knowledge of the terms flow (F), pressure (P), and resistance (R), and of their relationship, described in the following equation (see also Figs. 9-3 and 9-4).

$$\text{Pressure} = \text{Flow} \times \text{Resistance}$$
$$\text{or}$$
$$P = F \times R$$

There are several important parallels between electrical theory and the cardiovascular system.
1. There must be an electrical gradient between one point in an electrical system and the next for flow to occur. The direction of flow is from an area of high electron concentration to an area of low electron concentration.
2. There must be an energy source (current) to sustain power or voltage (or pressure in the cardiovascular system).
3. The system, either electrical or cardiovascular, must be a closed circuit or loop in order for the flow to be sustained (Fig. 9-5).
4. Power in the cardiovascular system generated by the heart represents the amount of work accomplished by a ventricle over a

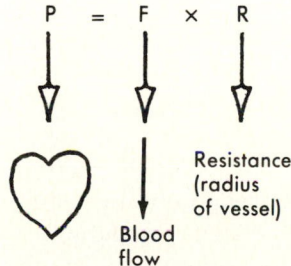

$$P = F \times R$$

Blood flow

Resistance (radius of vessel)

Fig. 9-3 Application of Ohm's law to the cardiovascular system. Pressure (P) is the product of blood flow (F) and resistance (R). Resistance to flow is largely determined by the radius of the vessels or areas through which the blood will flow.

Pressure = Flow × Resistance

$$P = F \times R$$

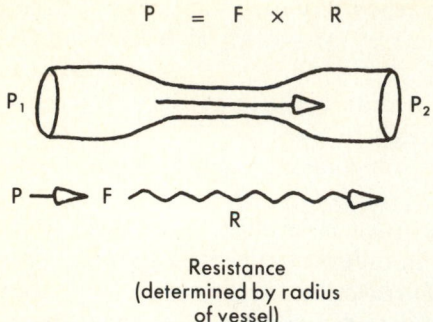

Resistance
(determined by radius
of vessel)

Fig. 9-4 Cardiovascular system: cardiovascular hemodynamic pressure (P) is the product of blood flow (F) and the resistance (R) to blood flow. For flow to occur, there must be a pressure difference between two points (P_1 and P_2). The amount of flow is determined by the pressure and the resistance to flow (compare Fig. 9-2).

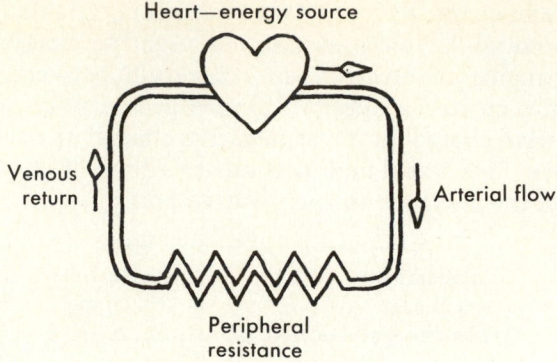

Fig. 9-5 Electrical system compared to the cardiovascular system. The cardiovascular system, like an electrical system, must have a power or pressure source (the heart). There must also be pressure gradients (blood flowing from areas of high pressure to areas of low pressure along the path of less resistance). Finally, the system must remain a closed loop for flow to be sustained.

given unit of time and may be calculated by the stroke work index or ventricular ejection fraction.

Although the electrical system is governed by voltage and resistance, it is the *current* that is the dimension of physiologic significance. If a current (measured in amperes) is passed through a human, limb to limb, it takes only 0.5 amp (500 milliamps [ma]) to cause ventricular fibrillation. However, if the current is directed at the myocardium, it takes as little as 0.2 amp (200 ma) to cause fibrillation[27] (Table 9-1). What is occurring, in either case, is that the person closes the electrical system loop so that current can travel from a source, through the person, and to another point (Fig. 9-6). This danger can be avoided by use of a mechanism called "grounding."

Grounding. A "ground" is simply a means of conducting electrical current to the earth or to some other object connected to the earth. Since the earth can accumulate electrical charge or give up charge without becoming charged itself, connecting an object to the earth *may* provide a safety feature. Current always travels along the path of least resistance, and, if a connection to the ground is available, grounding provides such a path. There are several methods of grounding used in the critical-care environment. They are circuit and system grounding, equipment grounding, and "isolated" system grounding.

Circuit and system grounding is accomplished by the grounding of major power distribution transformers that service entire areas with electrical power. When an individual piece of *equipment* is grounded, all metal parts of the equipment are connected

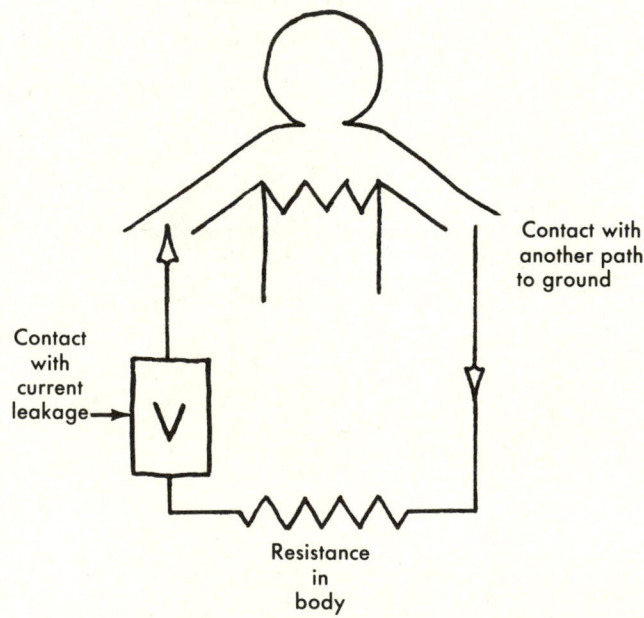

Fig. 9-6 Electrical dangers of ungrounded equipment. The patient may be included in a closed loop between a faulty piece of electrical equipment (with current leakage) and the ground or another person or object.

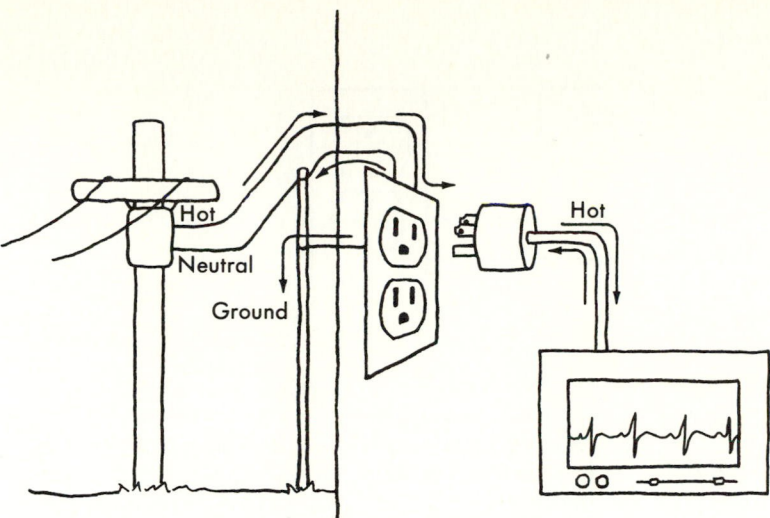

Fig. 9-7 "Grounding." Flow of current travels through a "hot" wire to the instrument and back out through a "neutral" or cold wire. A third, "ground," wire is added as a safety mechanism so that if stray current leaks in the instrument chassis, or, if the neutral wire is fractured, there is a low-resistance path for the current to ground.

Table 9-1   Physiologic effects of current leakage

Current	Effect	Comments
10 ma (0.01 amp)	Tingling sensations	Tingling when touching an electrical device indicates an impending hazard; unplug instrument and have it checked *immediately*
100 to 500 ma (0.1 to 0.5 amp)	"Can't let go" phenomena	*Do not touch* the victim or instrument; unplug device if possible; push victim out of contact with device with a broom or folded blanket, *or* throw your body against victim moving *away* from device
500-1500 ma (0.5 to 1.5 amp)	Cardiac fibrillation	See comment for 100 to 500 ma NOTE: These victims must receive cardiopulmonary resuscitation measures immediately

with a common wire to the ground (Fig. 9-7).

Unlike these systems, the type of system that is commonly set up in intensive care and operating room situations is an isolated system. The system grounding is removed by a special transformer, leaving the equipment "isolated" so that the current now seeks to flow only from one isolated line to another (see Fig. 9-8). In a totally isolated system, one could touch a water faucet (ground) with one hand and touch either of the two isolated lines, without receiv-

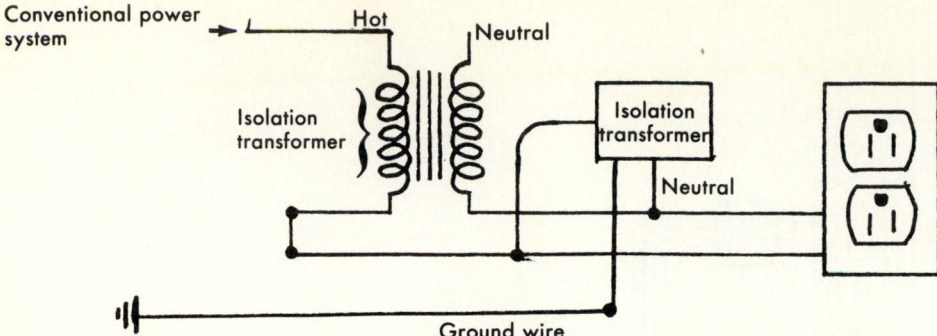

Fig. 9-8 An "isolated" grounding system. Current from a conventional power system is fed into the isolation transformer. Electrical flow enters an instrument by the hot wire and exits by the neutral wire to the transformer. Note that both sides of the circuit are isolated from ground (compare with Fig. 9-7). The isolation transformer represents the lowest potential in the system so that any stray current from the instrument will flow more readily toward the transformer than through the ground wire.

ing a shock. This system appears to offer a great advantage over other power systems but, in reality, it is impossible to construct a "perfect" isolation system (for further information refer to Mylrea[61] and Karselis[34]).

Electrical safety. Standards for electrical safety in each hospital should be based on an understanding of the principles of electrical theory. Daily instrument maintenance will prevent many equipment problems. Nurses should be responsible for the safety efforts listed here.[23,34,61]

1. Be alert to potential electrical hazards and make daily inspections of equipment and cords. Look for breaks in insulation of cords, broken prongs, or plugs that fall out of the wall outlet easily. Do not allow any wet surfaces to come into contact with the patient or equipment. Note inspection dates posted on equipment by the hospital bioengineers and notify them of expired inspections.

2. Always use three-prong plugs. Without a ground wire, there is the hazard of current leakage or a short circuit between the "hot" wire and the equipment housing, which may cause conduction of current through the patient to another grounded source. A similar problem will occur if a two-pronged extension cord is used as an adapter between the patient monitor and the wall or if a "cheater plug" (three-wire to two-wire) adapter is used.

3. Avoid using extension cords since they provide greater length of conduction material to leak current. Frequently, extension cords are placed in a space where they may be crushed by people or by machines that roll over them. Protect all cords from damage. Prevent ECG cables from becoming caught in side rails or bed mechanisms.

4. Make sure that any equipment leads connected to the patient (e.g., ECG leads) are insulated and isolated from possible contact with stray current or a "hot" wire.

5. Avoid 60-cycle (60-Hertz) interference, which reflects an interesting property of electricity. When two conductive surfaces (such as the human body and a monitor) are close to each other, they hold and transmit alternating current (AC) between them and can transmit current to other conductive surfaces. This is termed "capacitance," or the property of "holding" electrical energy. This capacitance between the patient and the monitor system, which is also surrounded by other conductors (e.g., apnea monitors or IV pumps), is observed as "fuzzy" baseline tracings on the ECG and can be minimized or dispersed by several methods[61]:

   a. Keep ECG leads as close together as possible (e.g., with tape) to avoid exposure of individual leads to environmental capacitance.

   b. Apply electrodes with scrupulous technique to decrease skin resistance caused by oils and loose skin cells; scrub the skin with alcohol and dry it with gauze.

   c. Move the ground (or reference) electrode to a point closer to other electrodes.

   d. Change all electrode wires and patches if interference continues.

6. Recognize special precautions for patients who have invasive heart lines in place, and

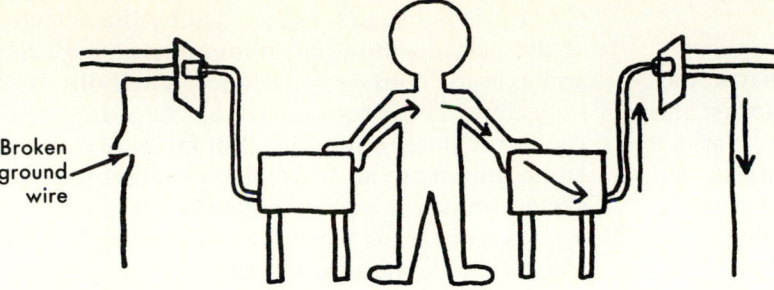

Fig. 9-9 Electrical hazards nurses should be aware of. The nurse should never touch two electrical units at the same time. If the ground wire is fractured on one unit and a stray current is present, the current will not follow the ground wire but will follow the other path to the ground, which, in this case, is the nurse.

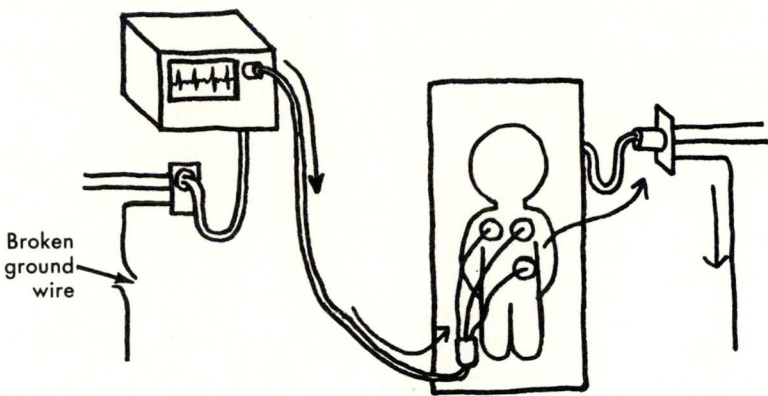

Fig. 9-10 Electrical hazards for the patient. The patient's bed should never be grounded. If the ground wire of the monitor is fractured and if the patient is grounded, stray current from the monitor will follow any other available path to ground, which, in this case, is the bed.

be certain that these lines are not in direct contact with electrical equipment (e.g., ECG leads).

7. Pay particular attention to those patients who are in high humidity environments (e.g., croup tent) or those whose skin resistance is circumvented by invasive catheters (e.g., dialysis catheters). Water is an electrolyte solution and will rapidly conduct current.

8. Do not place any instruments on metal carts/shelves or near water. Water and metal are highly conductive materials and may conduct stray current.

9. Never touch both the patient and an electrical device simultaneously or a path may be provided for stray current to travel from the device to the patient (see the previous section on grounding). Further, the nurse should never touch two electrical devices simultaneously. If there is a current leak, she may become a path to the ground from the broken instrument (Fig. 9-9).

10. *Never ground the patient.* Always use grounded *equipment*, but do not use a grounded bed (which grounds the patient). Stray current from a defective instrument will seek the path of least resistance leading to ground. If the patient (bed) is not grounded, the possibility of conducting current through the patient is eliminated (Fig. 9-10).

■ HEMODYNAMIC MONITORING

The most significant advances in pediatric bio-instrumentation have occurred in cardiovascular monitoring, including electrocardiography, various forms of hemodynamic monitoring, pacemakers, and invasive cardiac assist devices. The nurse must be familiar with basic cardiovascular physiology (see Chapter 3) in order to interpret cardiovascular measurements in an accurate way.

■ Electrocardiography

The ECG provides simple yet valuable information about cardiac electrical activity—specifically, the absolute heart rate, relative changes in rate, and the sequence of intracardiac conduction. The electrical activity of the heart can be easily monitored at the skin surface, and a recorder provides a graphic representation of the summation of electrical events (Fig. 9-11). Each waveform represents a summation of depolarization and conduction through specific areas of the heart. It is important to remember that the ECG waveforms indicate myocardial *electrical activity* and not necessarily the quality of *myocardial contractility*.

Electrodes that are frequently employed for recording ECGs are of two major types: (1) the direct contact electrode, involving needle leads placed under the skin or metal electrode surfaces that are directly applied to the skin or (2) the "floating" electrode, which rides on a layer of electrolytic jelly, interspaced between the skin and metal. The choice of

electrodes is usually determined by the activity level of the patient, duration of monitoring requirements, and existing contact impedance. The bulk of contact impedance is the result of oil on the skin surface plus the horny outer epithelial skin layer. Because infants and children are so active, they require a monitoring system that minimizes movement artifact.

Needle leads placed under the skin provide the most reliable monitoring system for patients who have a high activity level or who exhibit excessive perspiration or thickened skin. The invasive nature of needle leads, however, should limit their use except as the last resort in an attempt to obtain a stable ECG monitoring system. As with any invasive procedure, the placement of these leads requires skin preparation with a vigorous povidone-iodine (Betadine) scrub followed by a sterile gauze rub (until dry). The leads should be replaced every 24 hours. The risk of skin infection is the most common concern and is greatest in neonates. The puncture sites from the electrodes may heal with a scar, particularly if the patient is prone to keloid formation.

Most pediatric patients are easily monitored with the "floating" adhesive electrodes, which are manufactured in different sizes. The small metal electrode rides on a layer of jelly, which is mounted in a small cup, surrounded by an adhesive ring. In order to attain stable contact and minimize impedance, it is recommended that the skin at the electrode site be first rubbed with an alcohol swab to minimize the skin oil and to eliminate the dry layer of epithelium. Some irritation almost always occurs under an electrode, and for this reason the electrodes should be

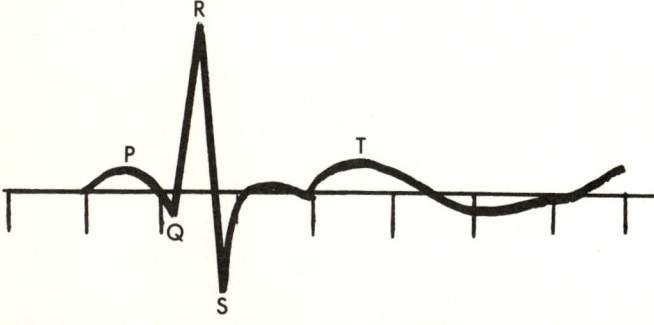

Fig. 9-11 Normal components of an electrocardiogram (ECG). The P wave represents atrial depolarization, the QRS complex represents ventricular depolarization, and the T wave represents ventricular repolarization. The light black vertical lines on ECG paper each represent a time segment of 0.04 sec (at a paper speed of 25 min/sec), and each heavy black vertical line on ECG paper represents a time period of 0.2 sec.

moved at 24-hour intervals. In small infants, however, the nurse may elect to leave the electrode patches in place as long as possible to avoid skin breakdown from pulling adhesive off the chest wall.

Limb-lead electrodes may consist of four metal plates (or the floating adhesive electrodes), secured on each limb. An electrode jelly or alcohol swab is placed between the metal plate and the skin to provide better conductance. Limb-lead ECG monitoring is usually used for obtaining recordings of each of the six *limb leads*, designated I, II, III, AVR, AVL, and AVF. The information obtained from these limb leads reflects the sequence of depolarization and repolarization through the conduction system (from the sinoatrial node to the atrioventricular node to the Purkinje fibers). Each of the six leads captures a recording of the conduction from a different vantage point. In all patients, including children, these limb leads lie in the frontal plane of dimension, and they reflect the direction of movement of the electrical current, which flows from the negative to the positive (Fig. 9-12).

The amount of artifact imposed by muscle movements limits the use of the four-limb monitoring system to short-term (diagnostic) purposes; it is usually not practical for continuous ECG recording. However, in patients who are immobile as a result of coma or cardiac arrest or because of paralyzing agents such as pancuronium bromide (Pavulon), the limb-lead system should be considered a potentially valuable monitoring technique. In addition to the limb leads, six precordial lead recordings may be obtained by the use of a small suction bulb attached to a metal cup that holds electrode jelly at the skin surface. The bulb is manually moved to six standard positions on the chest wall; the resultant strip recordings demonstrate conductive activity in the horizontal plane (anteroposterior). Recordings made from these exploring precordial leads allow qualification and quantification of cardiac electrical activity at specific points. Observations and measurements of the rate and magnitude of ventricular depolarization or repolarization can provide information about cardiac hypertrophy, myocardial strain, or infarction.

Adhesive chest electrodes are the most common form of long-term ECG monitoring and can provide recordings of the limb leads I, II, and III (Fig. 9-13) depending on the type of cable and monitor being employed. Use of chest leads I, II, and III offers enough information about the conduction system to be useful on a long-term basis. Some of the patients in the pediatric ICU may be very small and may require cumbersome dressings and tubes that cover much of the skin surface; therefore modifications in electrode placement may necessitate subaxillary or posterior lead placement. For this reason, interpretation of rhythm strips obtained from bedside monitors must be cautious because the relative *changes* in the ECG waveform may be of more importance than any isolated waveform interpretation.

The use of the modified chest leads (MCL) is another variation in placement available to the nurse, making chest lead monitoring possible for use in the identification of aberrant rhythms and blocks. The MCL sites produce simulated precordial lead tracing; for example MCL$_1$ approximates V$_1$. In the modified chest lead, the negative electrode (often indicated on the cable by "RA") is placed at the outer section of the left clavicle, and the ground is located on the right shoulder. The positive lead (usually indicated by left arm [LA] or left leg [LL] on the cables) can be placed at the fourth intercostal space (ICS) on the right sternal border (RSB), or at the fourth ICS at the left sternal border (LSB) for MCL$_1$ or MCL$_2$ leads, respectively (Fig. 9-14).

ECG monitors. The choice of electrocardiographic bedside monitors is vast. Many monitors are capable of tracing several parameters, such as ECG recordings, arterial or venous pressures, respiratory rate, and temperature. The desired specifications for each type of monitoring will be discussed for each individual system.

The ECG device consists of a sensor system (electrodes), an amplifier and filter, and a recorder (see Fig. 9-1). The selection of a good monitor depends on the quality and characteristics of each of these components. The recommendations presented here are based on personal experience as well as on data collected from other nurses at pediatric critical-care centers.

Amplifiers. Amplifier units magnify the signal into a more easily recognizable form and should include the specifications presented here.

ADEQUATE FILTERING UNITS. The amplifier must reject all electrical potentials except the one being investigated. Filters help to minimize interference such as muscle artifact and 60-cycle interference.[27]

COMMON-MODE REJECTION UNITS. The most common type of amplifier (a differential amplifier) may have the specific ability to cancel out signals common to all input points. An amplifier with good common-mode rejection will be capable of minimizing 60-cycle interference.[13]

"Gain" units. "Gain" indicates the degree of amplification of the signal, which is dependent on the voltage of the P wave and the QRS complex. The ability of the monitor to sense voltage may be altered by ECG lead placement and cardiac pathology.

FIXED GAIN. Diagnostic ECG recordings are fre-

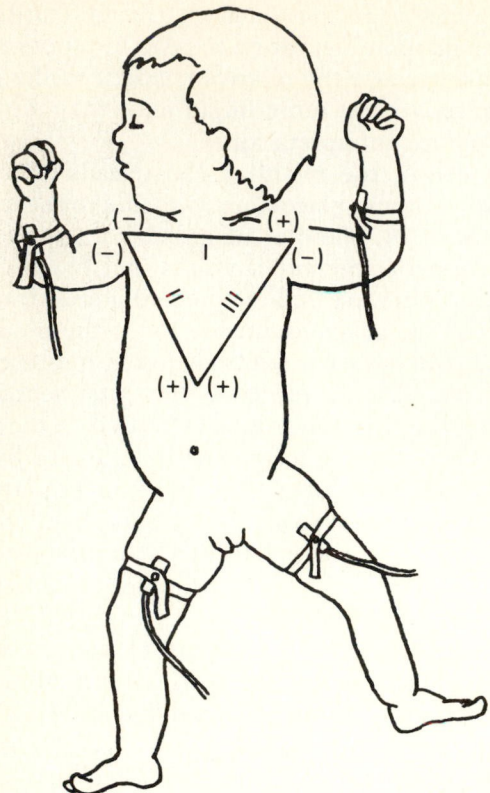

Fig. 9-12 Electrode placements and limb leads. A six-lead ECG recording may be accomplished by limb leads placed on all four extremities; or leads I, II, and III may be obtained with electrode patches placed on the chest surface. The triangular symbol represents the conduction path that is being monitored by the ECG. Each lead is in a different direction ([−] to [+]), so that the resulting waveform represents electrical activity in selected areas of the heart. On standard ECG cables, the negative (−) electrode is usually designated *RA* (right arm), and the positive electrode is designated either *LA* (left arm) or *LL* (left leg).

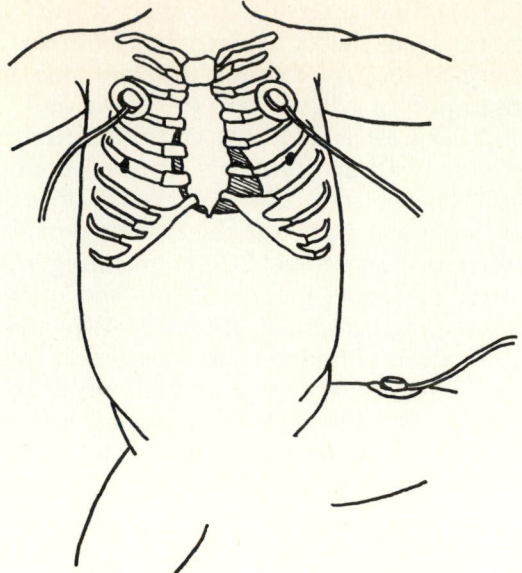

Fig. 9-13 Electrode placement for standard chest lead I ECG recordings. The *negative* electrode (often labeled *RA* on standard ECG cables) is placed at the second intercostal space, in the *right* midclavicular line. The *positive* electrode (often labeled *LA* or *LL* on standard ECG cables) is placed at the second intercostal space, in the *left* midclavicular line. A ground electrode can be placed on the lower abdomen or on either leg (it is shown here on the infant's left leg).

quently performed with fixed gain recorders since they record true voltage without interference.[28] As a result, changes in amplitude recorded with "fixed gain" recorders are usually clinically significant.

AUTOMATIC GAIN VERSUS ADJUSTABLE GAIN. Some monitors may have an "automatic" gain mechanism that will internally adjust the amplitude of the ECG complex to maintain a standard amplitude for the tracing. Other monitors have a gain adjustment to enable the operator to adjust the amplitude of the ECG complex. This is a necessary feature for continuous monitoring since the monitor must also count the child's heart rate. To calculate heart rate, the R-R interval is measured. In order to recognize the R wave, newer monitors are programmed to sense a

QRS complex of a given minimal slope. If the voltage of the child's QRS complex is low, it is possible the tachometer may not sense the R wave, and the heart rate will not be calculated accurately.[28] In this case the nurse can adjust the gain or change lead placement so that each QRS complex is recognized by the tachometer.

Recorders. Recording units compute the heart rate and provide a display of this rate.

TACHOMETER. This device senses a trigger point—usually the QRS complex—and computes the heart rate. Usually the trigger point is a QRS complex with a specific minimal slope. As a result, signals such as pacer spikes should be ignored (they will not be used to calculate the heart rate). Many monitors compute the rate by averaging the QRS frequency over several (3 to 4) seconds. The normal beat-to-beat variation in the child's heart rate (sinus arrhythmia) will cause inaccuracies in the heart rate reported by the monitor if the QRS frequency is averaged during a time when the heart rate is unusually rapid or slow. When noting the child's heart rate on a flow sheet, it is important that the nurse verify the rate over a 1-minute period. It is helpful if the rate meter is able to

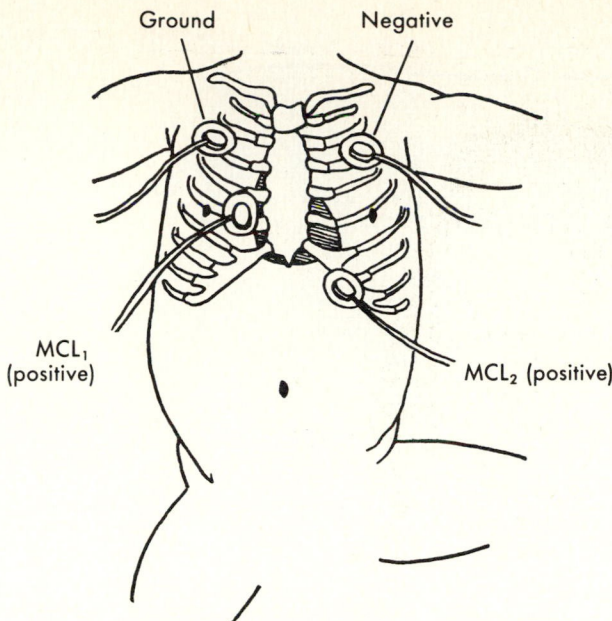

Fig. 9-14 Electrode placement for modified chest leads (MCL₁ and MCL₂). For MCL₁: the positive electrode is placed over the right fourth interspace. This lead helps to distinguish premature ventricular contractions from aberrant ventricular conduction. A disadvantage in interpreting this lead is that the sinus and retrograde P waves may appear either upright, biphasic, or inverted; thus P-wave polarity is of little diagnostic value. For MCL₂: the positive electrode is placed below the left costal margin, and the monitor is placed on lead III to correct the polarity of the electrodes. This lead is most useful for identifying retrograde P waves.

exclude artifacts produced by a pacemaker impulse so that the low heart rate alarms can still be triggered in the event that the pacemaker fails to capture or the ventricle fails to respond to a paced impulse. Many new monitors are programmed to sense only an impulse with the same QRS slope that has been calculated from a sample strip stored in memory. However, the nurse should always be aware that pacemaker spikes may be included in the computation of the heart rate.

ANALOG VERSUS DIGITAL READOUT METERS.   Although the experienced nurse may be able to glance at an oscilloscope and estimate the child's heart rate, it is preferable to have a continuous, visual, numerical display of the rate. Digital displays are perhaps more easily used for precise measurements since analog meters frequently are calibrated in 5 to 10 unit measures and are more difficult to read from a distance. The nurse should be aware that there is usually a 2- to 5-second lag through the amplifier between the signal

and the readout device. As the nurse is auscultating the child's heart rate, she may observe this discrepancy and should record the auscultated rate as the more current and accurate of the two. *Note* that the presence of a readout device does *not* eliminate the need for direct auscultation of the heart rate and palpation of peripheral pulses at regular intervals.

OSCILLOSCOPE.   The "scope" is a screen that continuously displays the ECG signal. The image displayed on an oscilloscope is created by a cathode-ray vacuum tube that projects an electron beam on to a phosphorescent coated screen.[34] There are several characteristics that should be considered when choosing an oscilloscope. The *size* of the screen required depends on the area in which it will be used. For bedside monitoring in an area in which the nurse is close to the monitor, the smaller screens are satisfactory. In a larger area, obviously, a larger screen provides greater visibility. The *intensity* (or brightness) of the display is usually determined by the type of phosphorescent chemical used to coat the screen. Many monitors also have brightness adjustment dials to enable the nurse to alter the brightness. When evaluating an oscilloscope, it is often helpful to place the monitor in the actual area in which it will be used so that the brightness can be evaluated in the desired working space.

The *trace speed* is the rate (measured in millimeters per second) that the electrocardiographic pattern moves across the screen (or recording paper). This may vary from 1 mm/second to 100 mm/second; however, the standard trace speed is 25 mm/second. It is desirable to have the option of at least two trace speeds on a monitor—the 25-mm sweep and a faster sweep, such as a 50-mm sweep. The faster sweep appears to spread out the signal so the P waves and other signals may be more readily identified (Fig. 9-15).

A *freeze* mechanism enables the nurse to freeze patterns on the scope for the purpose of analyzing waveforms. This is an important option in a pediatric critical-care unit where there is a high incidence of unexpected dysrhythmias. It is usually safest to use a half-screen freeze or to store the "frozen" strip above or below the continuous ECG display so that "real-time" ECG monitoring and display can continue even though a rhythm strip is retained on display.

STRIP RECORDERS.   Strip recorders are recording units that permanently record the patient's ECG on coated paper with a heated stylus, light beam, or ink stylus. In most cases, if a patient requires ECG monitoring, facilities for paper recording should be available to document ECG variations for future analysis and reference. A central recorder, *automatically* triggered by alarms or *manually* triggered from either

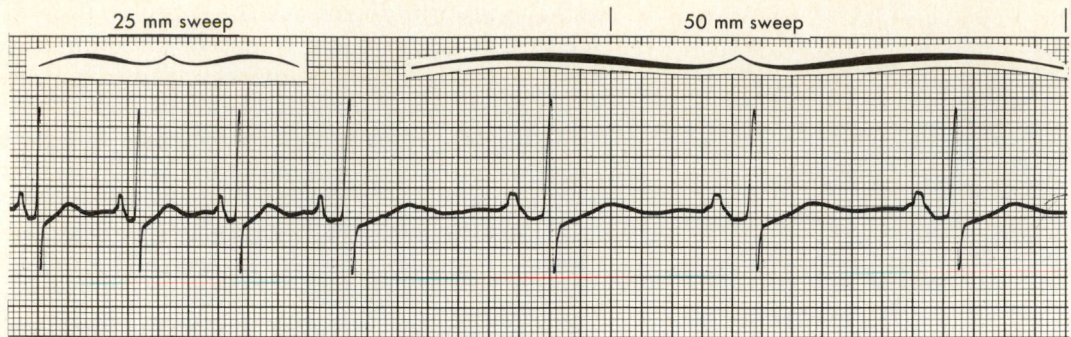

25 mm sweep   50 mm sweep

Fig. 9-15 Effect of varying paper speeds. The same patient's electrocardiogram has been recorded using paper speeds of 25 and 50 mm/sec. Note how much more easily P waves are identified when the 50 mm/sec sweep is used.

the bedside or central station, is usually most economical. Several types of recorders are available, but any recording system should have the capability of labeling each strip with date, time, and patient bed.

With strip chart recording, a hot stylus is used to record a tracing on moving paper. The heated edge of the stylus melts the white coating on the paper, which exposes the black underlayer. Strip chart recording provides a dry copy that can be handled but that may be scratched. Previously it was useful only for low-frequency parameters, but recent models show satisfactory adaptability for pediatric monitoring.[23,28,34]

In optical strip recorders, a moving light beam, which is directed by a mirror, is beamed on photographic or light-sensitive paper. Ultraviolet, light-sensitive paper allows immediate development of the tracing, providing either wet or dry copy. The problem with this system is that it must be protected from constant light exposure, making it impractical for daily ICU use. However, it is an excellent device for recording high-frequency parameters.[23,28,34]

With ink strip recorders, a hollow stylus is employed to deposit ink on moving paper. It provides a dry copy of the image. An advantage of ink over the hot stylus method is that the ink trace thickness remains uniform despite stylus motion or paper speed. It is a low-frequency response recorder.[23,28,34]

High-pressure ink-strip recorders squirt ink onto the recording paper through a nozzle and a pressurized sytem. They are flexible, they allow a very high-frequency response, and they work well in a pediatric setting, where the physiologic variables may change rapidly.[23,28,34]

The magnetic tape recording system records and stores monitored information on tapes. Voice monitoring may also be included, if desired. It is useful for lengthy monitoring and will record at low trace speeds (1 and 5 mm/sec). The data can be played back at any time on an oscilloscope, paper recorder, or computer.

GUIDELINES. Whenever a rhythm strip is obtained from a patient, the following guidelines may be useful for standardizing the recording and optimizing the quality of the tracing.

1. Trace speed should be 25 mm/second, and the sensitivity setting should be set at "1." The sensitivity device allows the clinician to compare the patient's signal voltage with the internal standard. When the sensitivity knob is set at "1," 1 millivolt (mv) produces a 10-mm deflection on the strip.
2. Lead selector should be set on "standard."
3. The power switch should be turned from "on" to "run."
4. The 1-mv standard marker should be depressed, and the standardization should be exactly ten small boxes—two large boxes—high. This standard marker should be displayed as each lead is recorded. If the 1-mv marker does not produce exactly a 10-mm deflection, the nurse should adjust the sensitivity control setting until it does so.
5. For accurate representation of the overall ECG, a rhythm strip should include at least 10 to 12 QRS complexes. Each entire QRS complex should be recorded on the strip (it should not "run off" the edge of the paper).
6. If the entire QRS complex does not fit on the paper or if the nurse notes a change in the QRS voltage,

the sensitivity setting may be adjusted to record a smaller or larger image. If the sensitivity is set at "½," large complexes are made smaller. At a sensitivity of "½," a 1-mv impulse creates only a 5-mm deflection on the strip recording. If the sensitivity is set at "2," smaller complexes are made twice as large. At a sensitivity of "2," a 1-mv impulse creates a 20-mm deflection on the strip recording. It is essential that the 1-mv standard marker is depressed at the beginning of each strip recording so that the standard is known when QRS voltage is calculated. If another sensitivity is used, the sensitivity should also be written on the strip.

7. The quality of the lines inscribed by the stylus should be inspected. Extremes of lightness and heaviness must be avoided in order for subtle changes in voltages to be recognized. On strip chart recorders the "heat" knob controls the stylus temperature and thus the intensity of the image.

8. It is often valuable to have a multichannel recording device, so that the ECG may be recorded simultaneously with other physiologic data. A two-channel recorder is sufficient in most cases.

9. Some recorders have a manual-delay mechanism that reproduces information that appeared on the scope several seconds before the actual recording. This is convenient when one wishes to more closely inspect an abnormal ECG waveform which passed across the screen so rapidly that the nurse was unable to record it in "real" time.

Alarms. Alarm limits should be available at the bedside monitor and displayed at the central station, with alarm reset buttons in both places. High– and low–heart rate limits need to be established and verified during each work shift for every child and for each parameter being monitored.

Troubleshooting: sources of error in ECG monitoring. The nurse is accountable for the accuracy and safety of the ECG monitoring system. Sources of error must be identified and rectified.

Mechanical "noise." This is artifact that results from vibration of the monitor or physical impact. Monitors permanently mounted above the bed out of patient reach are the most stable.

Electrical "noise." Failure of the monitor to reject outside artifact (poor filter or 60-cycle interference) may be alleviated by a change in electrode placement, by a change of electrode patches, or by a change in the electrode wires, and cables. A good investment for an ICU is an electrode wire test unit that will verify the function of any electrode wire immediately. Many new monitors incorporate a "lead-fault" component that serves this purpose. (If 60-cycle interference occurs, see the discussion of this problem at the

beginning of the chapter.) If the electrodes, wires, and cables have all been checked or changed and the problem persists, the cause may be an inadequate filter in the amplifier.

Biologic variations. Interrupted waveform reproduction may occur as a result of physiologic changes, such as edema or changes in patient position. The nurse must diligently test various lead placements and adjust the sensitivity control on the monitor. Sometimes the cable itself may be positioned in such a way that it pulls the electrode away from the chest wall. A common source of patient interference is shivering, which may cause muscle artifact. The problem is usually self-limited in nature.

Because patient movement is impossible to control in pediatrics, a certain amount of movement interference must be expected. However, inadequate ECG monitoring should not be tolerated for long periods of time, particularly if a child is at risk for the development of cardiac arrhythmias. For such a child, the nurse must combine her ingenuity with restraints, distractions, or sedation to achieve optimum monitoring.

■ **Vascular pressure monitoring**

Critically ill pediatric patients frequently have rapid fluctuations in vascular pressures that may precede or accompany the development of life-threatening crises. These fluctuations may be the result of arrhythmias, decreased cardiac function, altered peripheral vascular resistance, pulmonary vascular disease, or respiratory disease. In children the use of indwelling vascular catheters may also be indicated if continuous display of hemodynamic characteristics are desired or if frequent blood sampling is necessary.

Cuff blood pressure measurements are often difficult to obtain in children because their absolute stroke volumes and arterial pressures are normally low. In the seriously ill child, these parameters may be further diminished, causing a concurrent decrease in the quality of the child's pulses. In addition, many children have increased fat tissue in their arms and legs that diminishes the intensity of Korotkoff sounds during auscultation of cuff pressures.[91,92]

Venous or arterial sampling may be difficult in a child because adipose tissue obscures vessels or because the child is unable to cooperate during arterial or venous puncture. These patients may benefit by placement of arterial or venous lines for sampling.

Transducers for vascular pressure monitoring. Direct measurement of vascular pressures requires a system that senses the pressure from the arterial or venous catheter and transforms this mechanical energy into an electrical signal, which is then measured in millimeters of mercury. The most common transducer used in critical-care units operates on the principle of a "strain gauge." It employs four strain-sensitive resistance wires on the rear surface of the diaphragm. As positive pressure is applied to the diaphragm, there is a change in length (and therefore diameter) of the wires, stretching two of the wires and relaxing the other two. The change in the diameter of the wires alters their electrical resistance so that current flowing through them is changed; it is this electrical change that is measured and reflected as an electrical signal[23,34] (Fig. 9-16). Recently, disposable transducers have become available that use a silicone chip rather than a strain gauge for measurement. Because they are new on the market, evaluations must be completed to verify their accuracy and to establish other factors such as infection control and cost effectiveness.

When vascular pressure catheters are required, the nurse must assist in the initial catheter placement, ensure accuracy of measurement and calibra-

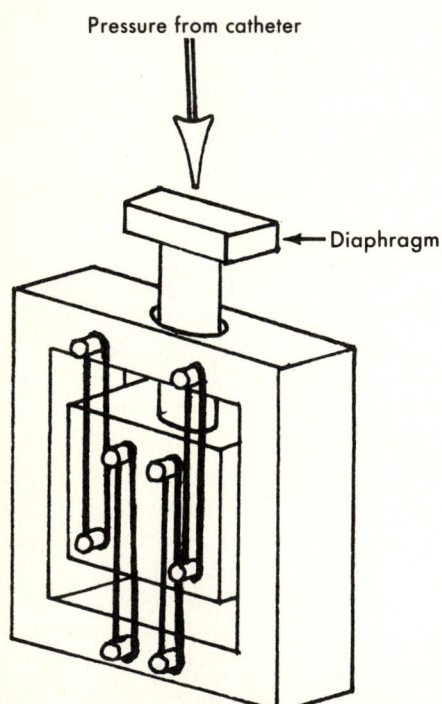

Pressure from catheter

← Diaphragm

Fig. 9-16 Strain-gauge transducer. As pressure is applied to the diaphragm, the center rod bears down on the core where four wires are placed. As the rod pushes down, two wires are stretched and two are relaxed. The electrical mechanism within these wires (called a "wheatstone bridge") measures the mechanical stretching/relaxing of these wires and converts it to an electrical signal.

tion of the transducer, and maintain sterility of the system. Once the catheter is in place, the nurse must be certain that it is maintained in its appropriate position, that the entrance site is protected, and that the catheter and transducer system are functioning properly.

The components of a vascular pressure monitoring system include the monitor, transducer, source for continuous pressurized infusion, ports for line access, low-compliance tubing, and a device to achieve simultaneous monitoring and constant fluid infusion.[37,88]

Basic components of the monitoring system

MONITOR AND TRANSDUCER. These provide the basis for hemodynamic monitoring. Frequently, one may choose to use a monitor from one manufacturer and a transducer from another because the desired specifications of each may not be met by one company. Thus inquiry should be made, when purchasing either, whether the selected devices may be used together. Most often, adapters can be made to join equipment from different manufacturers.

SOURCE FOR CONTINUOUS INFUSION. A fluid "flush" must be applied in-line to prevent blood backup into the monitoring system and to keep the line patent. This flush may be provided by a high-pressure bag or a continuous infusion pump. If the source of the infusion fluid is a plastic IV container enclosed in a high-pressure bag, the infusion pressure (indicated by a gauge attached to the pressure bag) must be greater than the vascular pressure being monitored (Fig. 9-17).

PORTS. These should be located both close to the catheter insertion site (for blood sampling and calibration) and at the transducer dome to allow access to the transducer chamber.

IV TUBING. Low-compliance ("high-pressure" or "arterial" tubing) will prevent pressure loss because the tubing will not stretch despite the high pressures generated by arterial pulsations. Invalid measurements or back-flow of blood may result if regular, compliant tubing is used. Thus the shortest practical length of tubing is required to minimize distortion of pressures.[71] In addition, small-bore tubing may also distort the signal and should be avoided.

CONTINUOUS INFUSION DEVICE. This device allows constant IV infusion and simultaneous monitoring without signal distortion. It contains a one-way valve that allows fluid to be infused under high pressure. This device is not needed if an infusion pump joins the transducer through a four-way stopcock (usually two or three such stopcocks are mounted on a manifold). The infusion pump then provides the constant infusion while the transducer senses the pressure in the line. The infusion pressure provided by the pump should not interfere with the pressure measurements as long as the infusion rate is low (1 to 3 cc/hour).

Variations in the basic monitoring system. Variations of the basic transducer setup depend on the vessel or pressure being monitored and on the specific equipment used; these variations include miniature transducers, intermittent monitoring, and pediatric monitoring systems.

MINIATURE STRAIN-GAUGE TRANSDUCER.   Miniature transducers may be used because of their convenience and small size. They require a smaller volume displacement than a standard transducer so that they can be connected close to the catheter insertion site (Fig. 9-18), and they are perhaps most useful for measuring pressures such as central venous pressure (CVP) and intracranial pressure. As with other transducer systems, a constant infusion valve may be in-

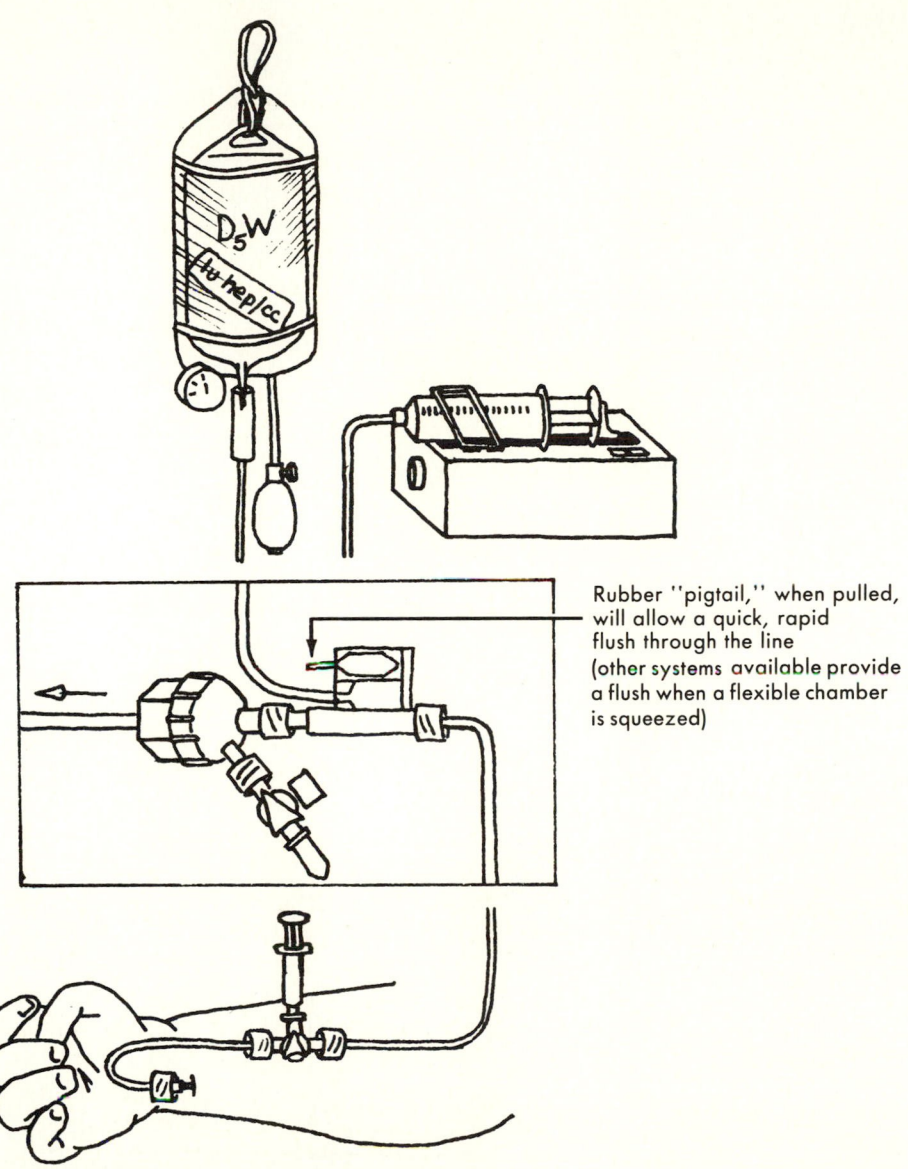

Rubber "pigtail," when pulled,
will allow a quick, rapid
flush through the line
(other systems available provide
a flush when a flexible chamber
is squeezed)

Fig. 9-17 Vascular monitoring equipment with continuous infusion mechanism. The source of infusion may be a high-pressure bag or a syringe or infusion pump. The infusion system is connected to a constant infusion valve that allows continuous infusion as well as pressure monitoring. A filter is added between the constant infusion valve and the infusion system to screen for air bubbles.

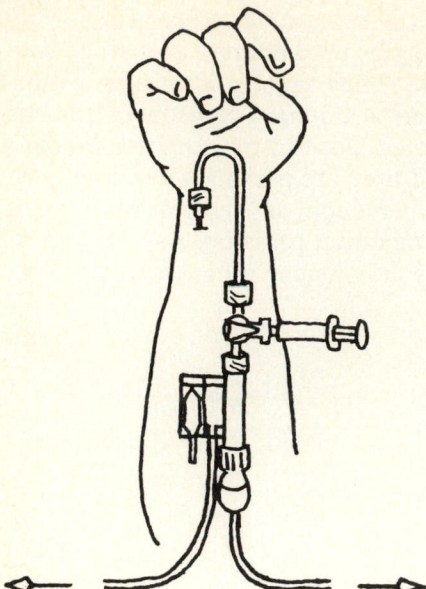

Fig. 9-18   Miniature strain gauge in a miniature transducer.

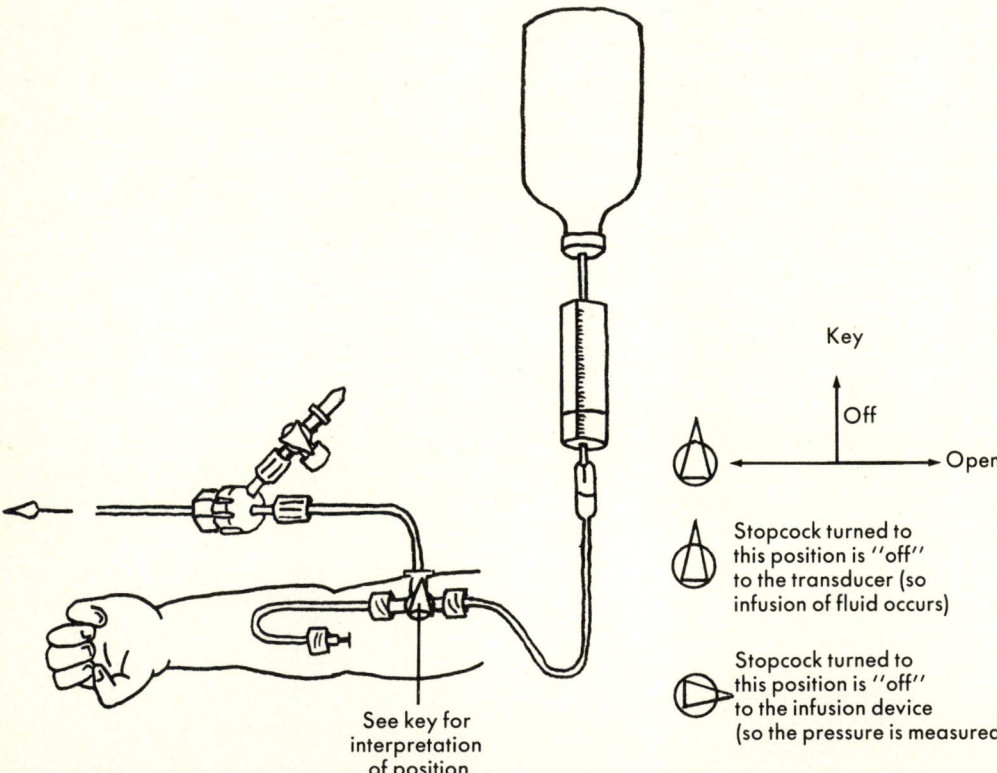

Key

Off

Open

Stopcock turned to this position is ''off'' to the transducer (so infusion of fluid occurs)

Stopcock turned to this position is ''off'' to the infusion device (so the pressure is measured)

See key for interpretation of position

Fig. 9-19   A system for intermittent measurement of vascular pressure. An intraflow device is not used. Continuous infusion is provided by a standard IV setup. To obtain a reading, the stopcock closest to the insertion site is turned *off* to the IV and *on* to the transducer (see key on illustration).

corporated to provide simultaneous pressure display and infusion. One disadvantage of this kind of transducer is that defibrillation may irreparably damage the transducer if it is not electrically isolated. Therefore the patient must be disconnected from the transducer before defibrillating or cardioverting is performed.[71]

INTERMITTENT MONITORING SYSTEMS. Some vascular lines, such as CVP lines, may be prepared using both an IV infusion line and pressure bag infusion set joined at a stopcock. With this setup, no constant infusion valve is used. The vascular line is then used primarily for IV infusions. Pressure measurements may be obtained intermittently by using the stopcock. When measurements are desired, the stopcock is turned so that the continuous infusion is interrupted and so that the stopcock port is open to the transducer (Fig. 9-19). Intermittent measurement systems of this type are not used with arterial lines.

PRECAUTIONS. Since vascular catheters may easily migrate, pressure waveforms must be frequently checked for evidence of catheter migration. The specific frequency with which they should be checked is often best determined by hospital policy or unit standards. If the waveform is continuously displayed, it should be checked constantly. If the waveform is only intermittently displayed, however, hospital policies or standards are particularly needed.

I recommend that pulmonary artery catheters never be placed on an intermittent display system since the complications of pulmonary catheter migration and arterial occlusion can be serious.[30,56,71] CVP lines might be better choices for intermittent measurements and waveform display.

PEDIATRIC MONITORING SYSTEMS. Fluid restriction is important in pediatric care, and many children cannot tolerate as much infusion fluid as may be administered if a standard constant infusion device is used with each monitoring line. Because the one-way valve in the constant infusion device is not always intact, greater volumes of fluid may be delivered than intended. Most continuous infusion devices are designed to deliver a 3-ml/hour infusion, although pediatric models are now available that manufacturers report deliver 2 ml/hour. Even if the continuous infusion valve is intact in the constant infusion device the hand-flush "pigtail" in the device may allow rapid infusion of a large but unknown quantity of fluid. Frequent manual "flushes" with this device may cause fluid overload in the child.

As an alternative to the standard system, the pediatric system uses a syringe pump in place of the high-pressure bag (see Fig. 9-17). The quantity of fluid injected hourly and with flushes can be readily

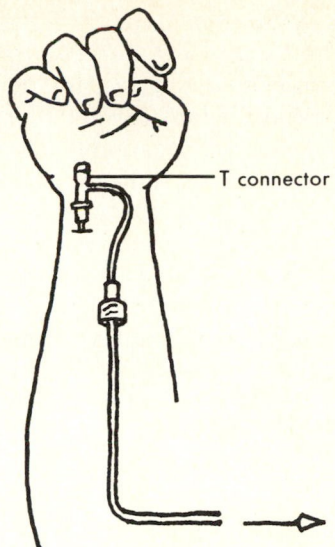

Fig. 9-20 Vascular infusion system with **T** connector. The **T** connector can be used to withdraw blood.

verified by marking the syringe. A 1-ml/hour infusion rate works well with most pressure lines exposed to pressures less than 60 mm Hg. However, for the higher pressure arterial lines, it may be necessary to infuse 2 ml/hour to ensure continued patency of the line.

LOW-PRESSURE MONITORING SYSTEMS. Right atrial (RA), central venous, and pulmonary artery (PA) pressures are measured by another variation to the standard setup, which dispenses with the continuous infusion device and pressure bag and places a four-way stopcock in-line to allow simultaneous fluid infusion and pressure monitoring. "Dampening" of the pressure waveforms can occur, however, because of dispersion of the patient's pressure at the two open ports of the stopcock.

T CONNECTORS. Galvis[21] proposes a system that eliminates stopcocks and places a T connector tube at (or close to) the catheter insertion site (Fig. 9-20). Galvis' proposed purpose is to control infection and decrease the number of manual (high-pressure) flushes pushed through the catheter. In order to draw blood, a clamp is placed on the infusion line, distal to the T connector, and a 25-gauge needle is inserted into the connector injection port. Three or four drops of fluid are allowed to drip out of the line; then a syringe is attached to withdraw the desired amount of blood. The pressure buildup within the infusion tubing during the clamping of the connector is sufficient to flush the line after the clamp is released. Therefore no fluids (in addition to the hourly infusion) are administered. Blood, however, may collect within the rubber port and may pose risk of infection.

Regardless of the system used, the flush connection should probably be located as far away from the patient as possible in order to avoid injuring the vessel endothelium by a rapid flush at the catheter tip.

Blood sampling. Since any catheter acts as a foreign body in the vessel, fibrin and other material will accumulate in or around the catheter, creating the risk of thromboembolic formation. For this reason, when drawing blood, it may be wise to withdraw and discard approximately 0.5 to 1.0 ml of blood in a separate syringe. This will allow aspiration and disposal of old blood and small emboli. Following this initial aspiration, another 2 to 3 ml of blood (depending on volume of the line) may be withdrawn to clear the line before drawing blood for laboratory work. After the laboratory sample is obtained, the blood drawn to *clear* the line (the second, 2 to 3 ml aspirate) can be reinfused. The longevity of small vessel lines (such as a radial artery line) may be greatly increased if any drawing-flushing procedures are minimized.[91] Therefore blood may be reinfused through a central line rather than through the small vessel catheter. This should minimize vessel spasm and rupture.

Note that in small infants, the initial discard may be limited to 0.5 ml of blood. With infants less than 1 year of age (or less than 10-kg body weight), a recording of blood withdrawn should be maintained on a flow sheet to alert the medical personnel of

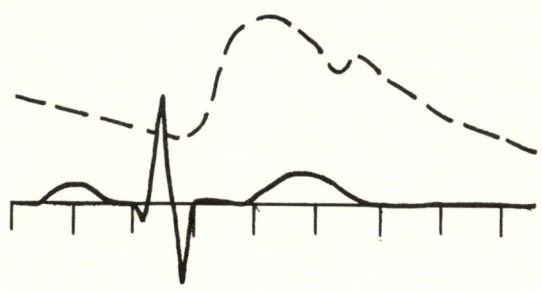

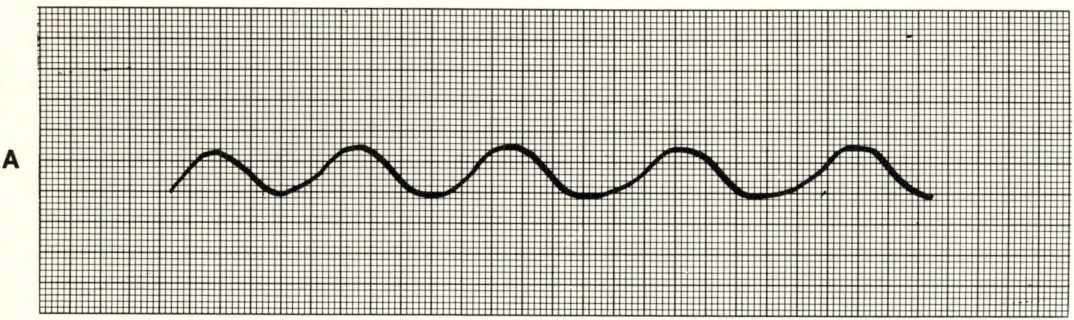

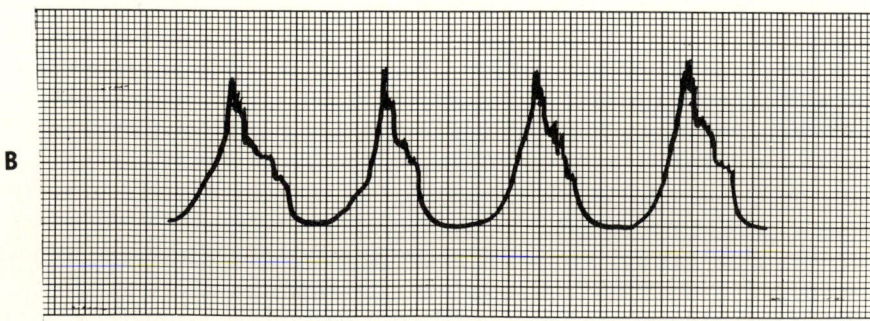

Fig. 9-21 Arterial waveforms shown in ECG cycle. **A,** A "dampened" waveform. **B,** The effects of "catheter fling" on the arterial waveform.

cumulative whole blood loss. A 7% loss (6 ml/kg) and/or a concurrent decrease in hematocrit should be brought to the attention of the physician.

Arterial pressure monitoring. Normal arterial pressure is represented by a waveform that reflects systole, valve closure, and diastole. The systolic pressure is the initial upstroke of the waveform, which occurs just after the QRS complex of the ECG. The downstroke of the waveform, beginning at the dicrotic notch, represents the diastolic time, and the dicrotic notch is thought to represent the closure of the aortic valve (Fig. 9-21). Valuable information may be gained from analysis of the arterial waveform,[37,41,63,71] as well as from the absolute systolic and diastolic blood pressure. The normal wave should have a sharp upstroke, clear dicrotic notch, and a definite end diastole. Mechanical causes of altered arterial waveform include a "dampened" tracing, which is caused by partial occlusion of the catheter, or catheter "fling," which is caused by the tip of the catheter "flinging" inside the vessel (see Fig. 9-21).

Catheter placement and maintenance of the arterial system. Several arterial line insertion sites are commonly used in children. The most frequently used arteries are the radial, temporal, femoral, and dorsalis pedis. Frequently, the catheter can be placed by percutaneous puncture using one of several techniques. (See Levin[41] and Adams[2] or the previous section on maintenance of vascular lines with transducers.)

One special precaution: *nothing* should ever be infused through an arterial line except heparinized/unheparinized IV flush solution that is isotonic or hypotonic.[91] In some hospitals, umbilical artery catheters (UACs) are handled as normal IV lines, and blood, drugs, and various IV solutions are infused through the line. Individual hospitals *must* establish specific policies regarding umbilical artery catheter care.

It is considered good practice to check the arterial pressure against a cuff measurement, but agreement between the two is *not* a criterion for ensuring accuracy of the arterial pressure monitor. Ordinarily, an intraarterial measurement is expected to be slightly higher than the cuff pressure if the intraarterial measurement is taken from a vessel more *distal* to the heart than the cuff since the resistance of distal vessels is higher. However, vasomotor changes or vascular obstruction may cause a wide or inverse disparity between the cuff pressure and the arterial line measurement. Also, the cuff pressure is determined by the quality of the Korotkoff sounds, which are diminished or lost in low cardiac output states or increased in the presence of mild to moderate vasoconstriction. Therefore, as with any other physiologic measurement, the clinical appearance of the child should always be given as much consideration as any single measurement.[13,71] Troubleshooting of arterial lines is outlined in Table 9-2.

Table 9-2 Troubleshooting: problems with arterial catheters and measurements*

Problems	Causes	Treatment	Prevention
"Dampened" tracing	Occlusion of tip by a clot NOTE: An early indication of a clot may be ability to flush a line but inability to aspirate blood	Attempt to aspirate clot; use 2 ml heparinized flush and *lightly* bounce plunger to loosen clot; aspirate with new syringe of flush; *never* forcefully flush catheter if great resistance is met	Ensure constant flush infusion Check pressure measurement system for leaks every hour with vital sign measurements Be sure flush solution is heparinized with 1 U heparin/ml fluid (or per hospital policy)

*Note: It is assumed that the nurse will first evaluate the patient's clinical condition, including blood pressure cuff measurements, to verify that the patient is stable before proceeding to troubleshoot the instruments.

Continued.

Table 9-2 Troubleshooting: problems with arterial catheters and measurements—cont'd

Problems	Causes	Treatment	Prevention
"Dampened" tracing—cont'd		Use different sizes (diameters) of syringes to aspirate clot since increased amount of suction applied with smaller syringes may successfully aspirate clot	
	Catheter tip against vessel wall	Reposition by rotating or withdrawing catheter	Check dressing and tape frequently, and secure tape so that catheter cannot be moved or rotated; benzoin may help tape adhere more securely
		Reposition patient or catheterized extremity	
	Clots or bubbles in pressure tubing or transducer	Flush entire system with stopcock port closed to patient	Examine entire line at least every 2 hr for cracks and bubbles
		Determine if entire flush system needs changing	Use clear stopcocks whenever possible to allow visualization of all connections
			Check connectors frequently to be sure they are tight and not cracked
Abnormally high or low readings	Catheter "fling"	Reposition catheter	Use no more than 3 ft of tubing between arterial catheter and transducer to minimize distortion of pressures[71]
		Minimize length of pressure tubing[71] between patient and transducer	
		Use small bore tubing between catheter and transducer. *Note* that this may affect pressure reading slightly, and transducer should be recalibrated	
	Change in level (position) of transducer	Check position of patient; head of bed should be elevated ≤45 degrees; transducer should be at level of left atrium	Check that the position of patient is consistent every time pressures are recorded; note this position in nursing-care plan
		Realign patient extremity	
		Check all connections to ensure sealed system	
		Recalibrate transducer	

Table 9-2 Troubleshooting: problems with arterial catheters and measurements—cont'd

Problems	Causes	Treatment	Prevention
Abnormally high or low readings—cont'd	Transducer no longer balanced	Recalibrate transducer	Recalibrate transducer every 2-4 hours (or per standard of care)
Bleeding at puncture site	Removal or dislodgement of catheter	Apply firm pressure to catheter insertion site for 5-15 min	Be sure that tape is *secure* Request periodic coagulation studies to identify coagulopathies
	Enlarged puncture in artery because hub of catheter has been pushed in and out of catheter insertion site	Check stability of catheter; take off all tape/dressing and inspect Determine if stitch around catheter may be required Check pulse/capillary refill distal to catheter to ensure adequate extremity perfusion	Tape catheter securely, and mount patient's extremity on armboard to minimize catheter movement
Change in circulation distal to puncture (decreased pulse, blanched color, or cyanosis)	Spasm of artery	Apply heat to extremity distal to puncture site Inject local vasodilator, such as lidocaine or phentolamine methanesulfonate (Regitine), if ordered by a physician Apply heat to the contralateral extremity (this may produce reflex vasodilation to the involved extremity)	Ensure prevention by clean insertion technique, *gentle* flushing—*never* flush forcefully—and general maintenance with heparinized flush
No waveform visible on oscilloscope	Incorrect gain setting (see also "dampened" tracing)	Check monitor to see whether gain is set too low	Anticipate the expected pressure ranges when setting up system and use the appropriate gain setting
	Damaged transducer or amplifier	Use a different transducer Use a different monitor	When in doubt, check arterial pressure against a cuff pressure or verify other monitored vascular pressure with a water manometer (1 mm Hg = 1.36 cm water)

Continued.

Table 9-2 Troubleshooting: problems with arterial catheters and measurements—cont'd

Problems	Causes	Treatment	Prevention
No waveform visible on oscilloscope—cont'd	Newer monitors with a mechanism to provide a "mean waveform," which may appear as a "dampened" or absent tracing	Check monitor for this mechanism	Be knowledgeable about equipment mechanisms
	Electrical failure	Check all electrical connections	Be sure equipment is mounted properly and has not been jolted or bumped
		Call engineer	Ensure regular maintenance
Cuff pressure differs from direct arterial pressure recording (arterial recording is usually 5-10 mm Hg higher)	Hypotension (the direct pressure is more accurate[32])	See Chapter 3 for treatment of low cardiac output	See Chapter 3
	Low cardiac output or increased systemic resistance, which make Korotkoff sounds more difficult to hear*		
60-cycle interference in tracings (electrical "noise")	A nonisolated transducer, artifact, or other environmental causes (other equipment) may cause dysfunction		Use isolated transducers
	Moisture accumulation in the back of isolated transducers	Use another transducer Inspect transducer and cable for cracks To remove moisture: 1. Place transducer through the aeration cycle of a gas-sterilizing chamber (unless manufacturer specifications recommend against gas sterilization) 2. Allow transducer to sit unused at room temperature for several days 3. Apply heat according to manufacturer's recommendations	Before using a transducer, inspect for cracks in the cable Plug transducer into amplifier; if 60-cycle interference persists, use another transducer Investigate aeration procedures for sterilizing transducers

*Direct pressure measurement is generally a more accurate representation of blood pressure and should be the preferred measurement; the discrepancy between the two, however, may provide a qualitative reflection of the systemic vascular resistance; markedly increased resistance may cause wide variants between the cuff and catheter pressures.

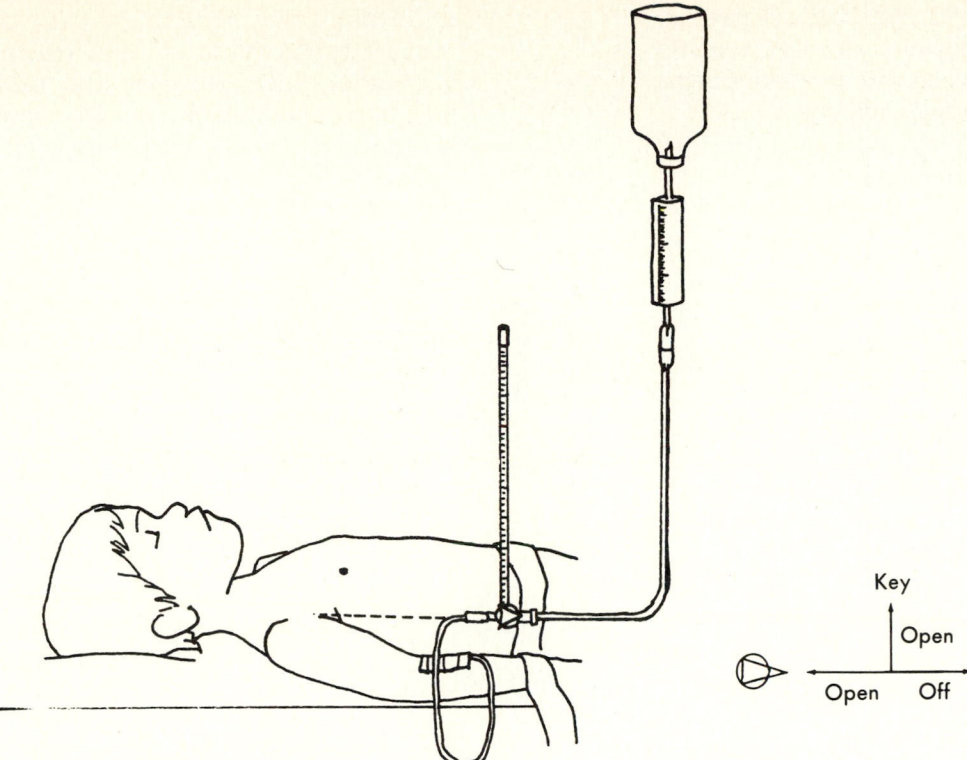

Fig. 9-22 Measurement with manometer of central venous pressure. The zero mark on water manometer should be placed at the level of the phlebostatic axis, which corresponds with the level of the right atrium.

Venous pressure monitoring. Indications for use of CVP lines in children include the following[40]: (1) monitoring of right heart pressures for the purpose of assessing blood volume and venous return, evaluating right ventricular function, or obtaining indirect information about the pulmonary vascular system, (2) infusion of vasoactive drugs, (3) infusion of hypertonic solutions, and (4) infusion of large volumes of fluid.

CVP lines may be inserted percutaneously or by cutdown through several sites, although the external jugular and subclavian veins are usually preferred. The CVP may be measured by either a transducer and monitor, as described earlier or by use of a water manometer (Fig. 9-22). The conversion value from the mercury (mm Hg) reading to centimeters of water is:

$$1 \text{ mm Hg} = 1.36 \text{ cm water}$$

For example:

CVP of 10 mm Hg = 13.6 cm water (10 mm × 1.36 = 13.6)

Normal CVP values = 4-8 mm Hg or 6-11 cm water

The water manometer measurement is accomplished in the following manner.

1. Determine a single position of the patient to be used for all measurements. Previously, it was thought that the patient must be flat to obtain an accurate measurement. Recently it has been demonstrated that the patient may be elevated up to 45 degrees as long as the *same* position is used for every measurement.[59] The "phlebostatic axis," the reference point for CVP measurement, may be determined by several landmarks:
   a. Using the midclavicle as a guide, locate the fourth intercostal space and follow this space across the chest wall to the midaxillary line.
   b. Mark this site with an "X" so that all CVP readings will be measured at a consistent point.
   c. Align this site with zero on the CVP manometer when taking measurements. This reference on the water manometer should correspond with the level of the right atrium.
2. Connect the water manometer to the stopcock port in the infusion line as illustrated in Fig. 9-22.

a. The patient's head may be elevated up to 45 degrees without error in measurement,[97] as long as consistent positioning is used with every measurement.

b. Ensure catheter patency by flushing CVP line before measurement.

c. Turn the stopcock so that the manometer fills with fluid (and stopcock port to patient is turned off).

d. Turn the stopcock so that the port is open between the patient and manometer.

e. The fluid column in the manometer will fall with fluctuations in patient inspiration and expiration. Once the fluid level has stabilized, the height of the fluid column at the peak of the respiratory oscillations corresponds to the patient's CVP measurement in centimeters of water. *Note* that respiratory oscillations *should be* present; if they are absent, the line may be partially occluded.

f. Turn stopcock to resume IV infusion.

g. Note that CVP measurements are most accurate if they are obtained when the patient is breathing spontaneously. If patient is on a ventilator, it is best to disconnect the ventilator momentarily if the patient can tolerate it, since the positive pressure ventilator may alter the CVP by decreasing venous return. If the patient cannot tolerate brief separation from mechanical ventilation, indicate that the measurements are made during positive pressure ventilation. Again, consistency of technique is the most important aspect in guaranteeing accuracy of measurement.

Blood samples may be obtained from a CVP line. To prevent air from entering the line during sampling, whenever the stopcock port is open, it *must* be held below the level of the right atrium. In some hospitals, a physician's order is required before blood samples may be withdrawn from CVP lines. As with other lines, the CVP line should be cleared of IV fluid before blood sampling so that erroneous laboratory results are avoided. Care must be taken to observe for air or clots in the line since these can be flushed into the heart. In order to preserve the patency of a CVP line that is being used for both measurement and sampling, heparinization of the line may be desirable. The physician should be consulted regarding this. Troubleshooting of CVP lines is outlined in Table 9-3.

Pulmonary and left-heart filling pressures. The progress in cardiovascular research has been supported by the development of techniques to measure intracardiac and pulmonary pressures. This was made possible in the late 1960s by development of the flow-directed–balloon-tipped ("Swan-Ganz") catheter.

Table 9-3 Troubleshooting: problems with CVP lines*

Problems	Causes	Treatment	Prevention
"Dampened" waveform or poor fluid fluctuation in CVP manometer	Partial clotting of venous line	Attempt to aspirate clots; always discard this blood	Ensure that flush solution is administered continuously
		Irrigate line but do not forcibly flush	Consider heparinizing CVP lines if this problem occurs (some hospitals do not recommend this; consult with physician)
			Flush with *heparinized* flush before blood sampling to help avoid fibrin or clot buildup on the line
	Kinked catheter	Straighten extremity at CVP insertion site	Secure catheter with tape/benzoin during daily dressing change

*See Table 9-2 for troubleshooting other line problems.

Table 9-3 Troubleshooting: problems with CVP lines—cont'd

Problems	Causes	Treatment	Prevention
"Dampened" waveform or poor fluid fluctuation in CVP manometer—cont'd		Remove dressing and check for kinking of catheter at insertion Check length of tubing between catheter and transducer/manometer for kinking and occlusion	
Inflammation or pain at catheter insertion site	Mechanical irritation or infection	Secure tape to minimize catheter movement Apply warm, dry heat Observe for signs of infection Administer antibiotics as indicated	Perform daily dressing changes using aseptic technique and antibiotic ointment[47] Change all tubing and solutions daily
Falsely low or high readings	Incorrectly leveled transducer or manometer	Correlate water manometer measurement with transducer reading to verify accuracy of instruments Check level of transducer or "0" level on water manometer for correct level	Determine position of patient to be used for all measurements and record in nursing care plan
	Valsalva's maneuver: patient coughing or "bearing down"	Provide measures to eliminate Valsalva's maneuver	*Do not* make measurements when patient is performing Valsalva's maneuver (NOTE: Infants and children may perform Valsalva's maneuver during defecation or forceful cry)
	Positive or negative pressure ventilation	If patient can tolerate it, remove from ventilator briefly during measurement	Determine whether measurements will be made with patient on or off ventilator (consult the physician) and do so consistently
	Partial line occlusion	Note quality of backflow in line (ease of blood withdrawal) and respiratory oscillations in the water manometer; decreased backflow may indicate partial occlusion of line, causing falsely high readings; after aspirating line for emboli, flush line and repeat measurement	Maintain constant flush infusion as ordered

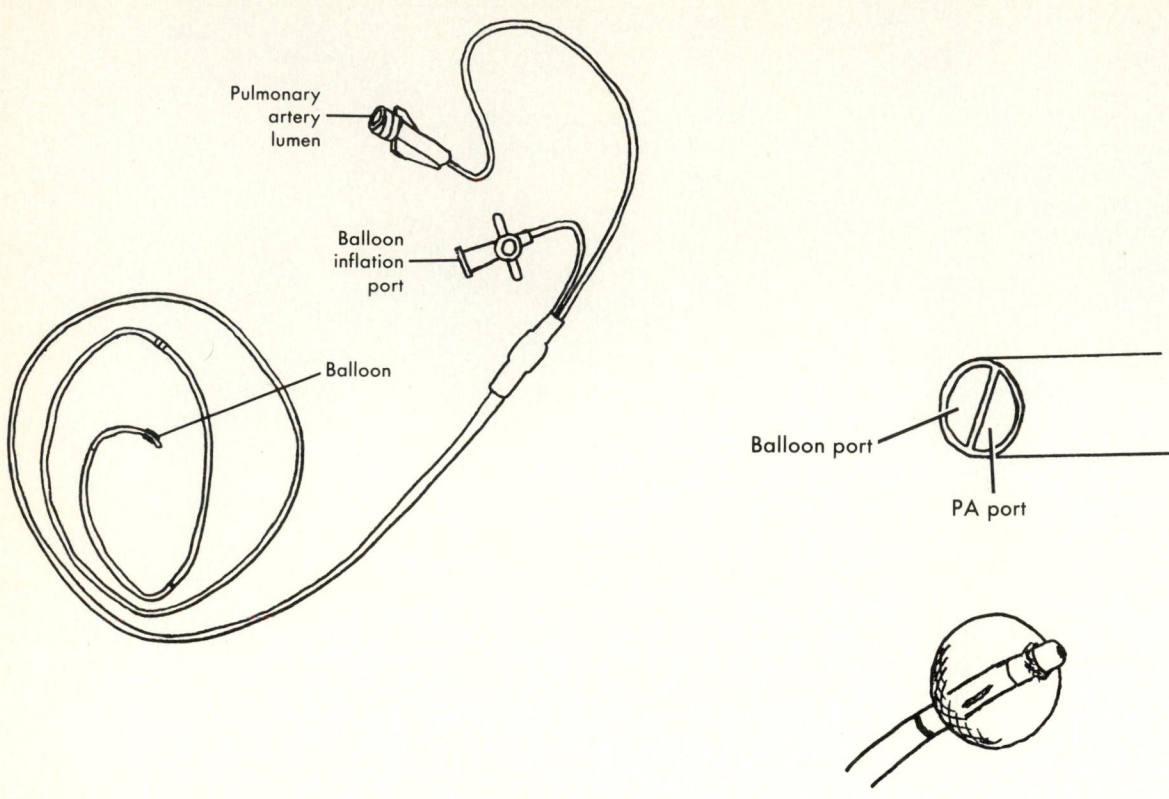

Fig. 9-23 Double lumen Swan-Ganz catheter. This catheter is used PAP and PAW or PCW pressures. Pulmonary artery blood samples may also be withdrawn for analysis of mixed venous oxygen ($P\overline{v}O_2$) tension.

This catheter allows bedside measurements of the right atrial (RA), pulmonary artery (PA), and pulmonary artery wedge (PAW or PCW) pressures, as well as the determination of cardiac output and mixed venous oxygen ($P\overline{v}O_2$) tension. Previously, these measurements were only possible by the placement of separate lines in the respective chambers or vessels at the time of open-heart surgery or through insertion of these lines under fluoroscopy.

Indications for Swan-Ganz monitoring.[27,52,55] Indications for Swan-Ganz monitoring include the following: (1) Assessment of right ventricular function as reflected by pulmonary artery systolic pressure and the CVP, (2) assessment of flow and resistance in the pulmonary vascular bed, (3) assessment of heart function on the left side, including adequacy of the mitral valve, (4) measurement of cardiac output, which also allows calculation of systemic vascu-

lar resistance, and (5) measurement of mixed venous oxygen tension ($P\overline{v}O_2$) (Figs. 9-23 and 9-24).

When Swan-Ganz catheters are used, transducer(s) are connected to the RA and PA ports. These ports are kept patent with use of the flush systems previously described. Continuous monitoring is then possible for the RA and PA pressures. When the balloon is inflated and wedged in a pulmonary arteriole, the PAW or PCW pressure will be demonstrated. Additionally, cardiac output measurements may be obtained by the thermodilution technique, with the use of the PA port for injection and a PA thermistor lumen for temperature measurement.

Insertion of Swan-Ganz catheter. The Swan-Ganz catheter is inserted percutaneously or through a cutdown under aseptic conditions. Fluoroscopy may be used to guide the placement of the catheter. More commonly, however, waveform analysis is used to

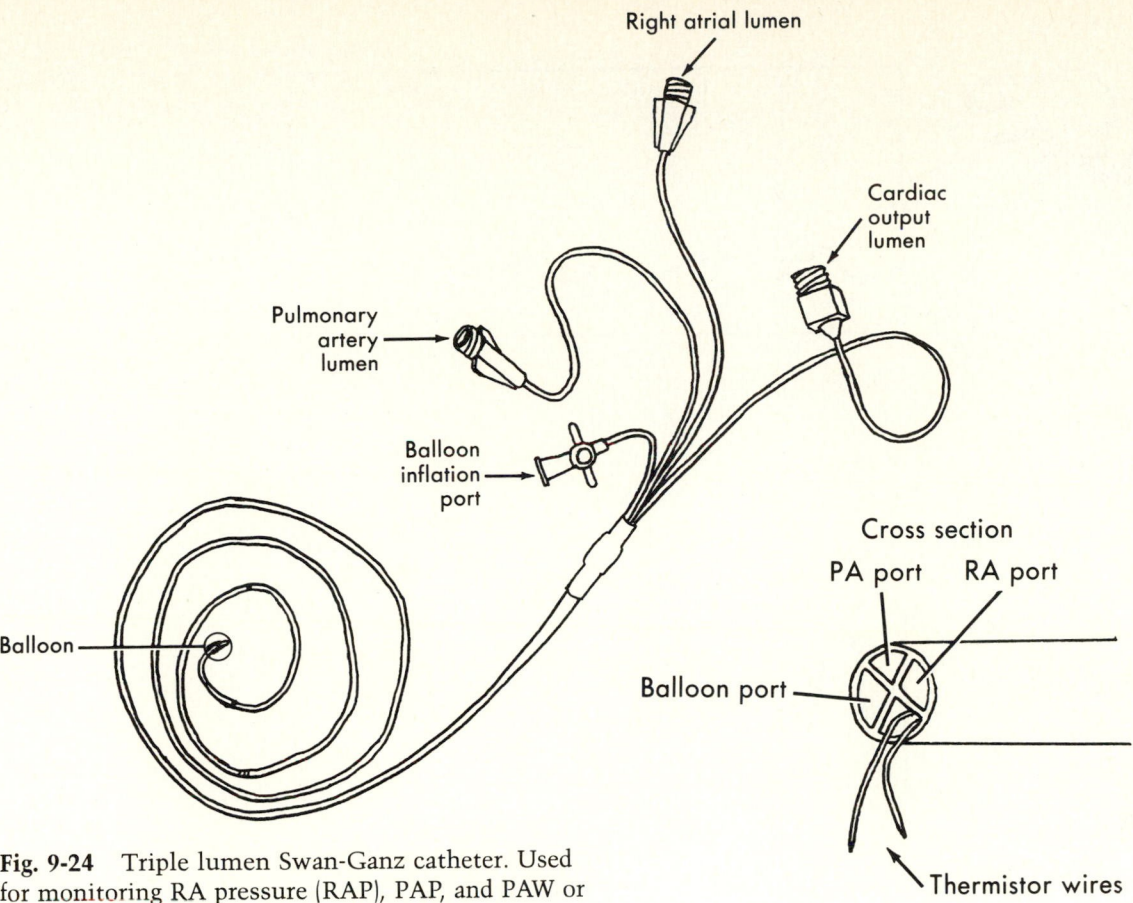

Fig. 9-24 Triple lumen Swan-Ganz catheter. Used for monitoring RA pressure (RAP), PAP, and PAW or PCW pressure. Also used for monitoring thermodilution cardiac output. Blood samples may be withdrawn from pulmonary artery port for analysis of mixed venous oxygen ($P\overline{v}O_2$) tension.

determine the position as the catheter passes from the right atrium to the pulmonary artery. As the catheter is advanced into the right atrium, as evidenced by the RA tracing, the balloon is inflated so that blood flow will propel the catheter through the tricuspid valve, through the right ventricle, past the pulmonic valve and into the pulmonary artery, as illustrated in Fig. 9-25. When a PAW tracing is observed, the *balloon is deflated* and the catheter sutured into position.

Nursing considerations

SETUP AND INSERTION. The nurse must explain the procedure to the family and patient (as age-appropriate). Continuous ECG monitoring is required, a defibrillator is on standby, the catheter must be checked, and appropriate insertion equipment must be assembled.

Steps for insertion of the catheter include the following.

1. Assemble and prepare equipment.
   a. Pressure lines and flush system
   b. Transducers (NOTE: Some transducers require a "warm-up" time of 15 to 30 minutes. This should be allowed whenever possible, to ensure accuracy of measurements.)
   c. Defibrillator
   d. Gloves, mask, gowns, cutdown tray and/or percutaneous line insertion tray, Betadine, Swan-Ganz catheter, 0.5% xylocaine solution, sterile water, 4 × 4 gauze pads
2. Prepare cutdown (or line insertion) tray; place sterile items needed on tray *(use sterile technique)*.
3. Check and record the integrity of the balloon before insertion. Integrity is checked by inflating the balloon under sterile water, using sterile technique. If bubbles appear in the water, the balloon has a leak and another catheter must be obtained.

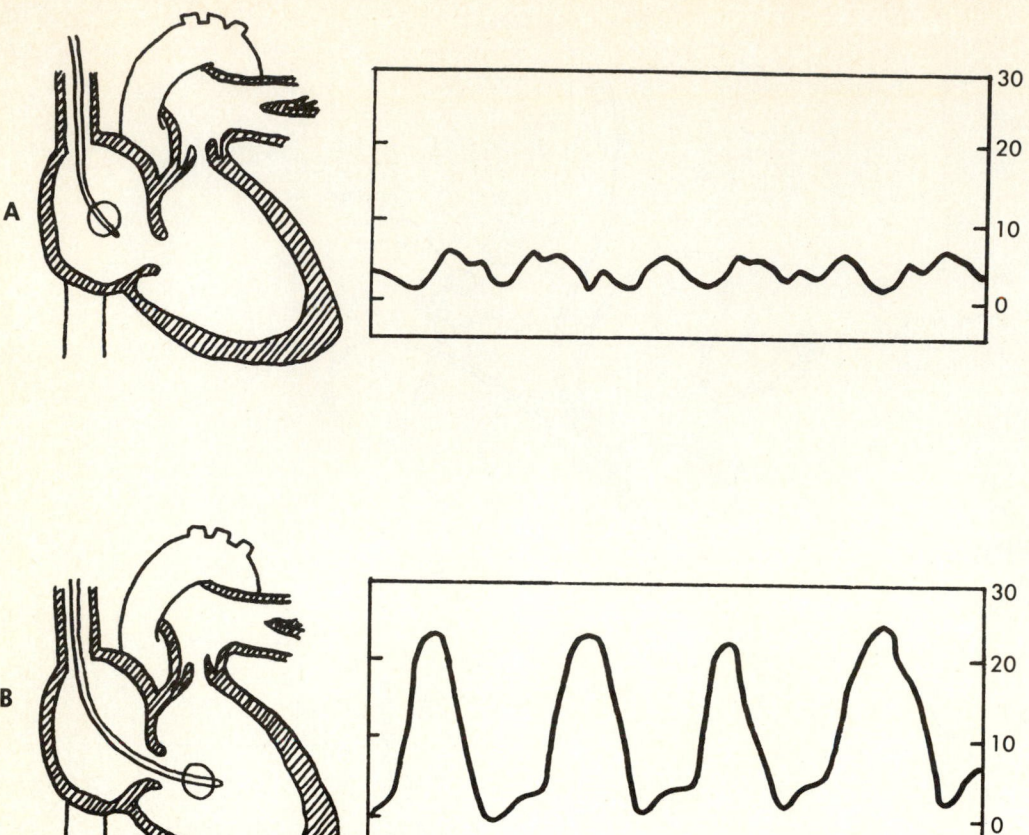

Fig. 9-25 **A,** RA position and waveform during Swan-Ganz catheter insertion (normal mean pressure = 0 to 5 mm Hg). **B,** Right ventricular position and waveform during Swan-Ganz catheter insertion (normal pressure = systolic <30 mm Hg and diastolic <5 mm Hg).

(Defective catheters can usually be returned to the manufacturer.)

4. Connect (using sterile technique) PA port of the catheter to the pressure monitoring system and flush the catheter. During insertion of the catheter, observe the progression and appearance of the pressure waveform and inform physician of progress.
5. Observe for any rhythm disturbances and inform physician. Watch closely for premature ventricular contractions and heart block as the catheter passes through the right ventricle.
6. If fluroscopy has not been used during the insertion procedure, a chest radiograph must be obtained following insertion to verify catheter position.*

*References 3, 4, 22, 43, 47, 54, 58.

MAINTENANCE.   One of the most critical aspects of the maintenance of a balloon-tipped catheter is verification of proper position of the catheter tip. This is accomplished through continuous monitoring of the PA waveform. If the catheter flows forward and "wedges" in a smaller PA branch (causing a PAW tracing), a pulmonary infarction may occur.[6,37,62,71] Therefore the nurse must be able to accurately identify the pressure tracings of the various chambers and recognize PA and PAW tracings (see Fig. 9-25).

The PA port of the catheter should be connected to a standard transducer system with heparinized flush, and the same may be done for the RA port. It is also possible to place both ports on one transducer, using the pulmonary artery pressure for continuous display and the right atrial pressure for intermittent display.

Additional observations must be made by the

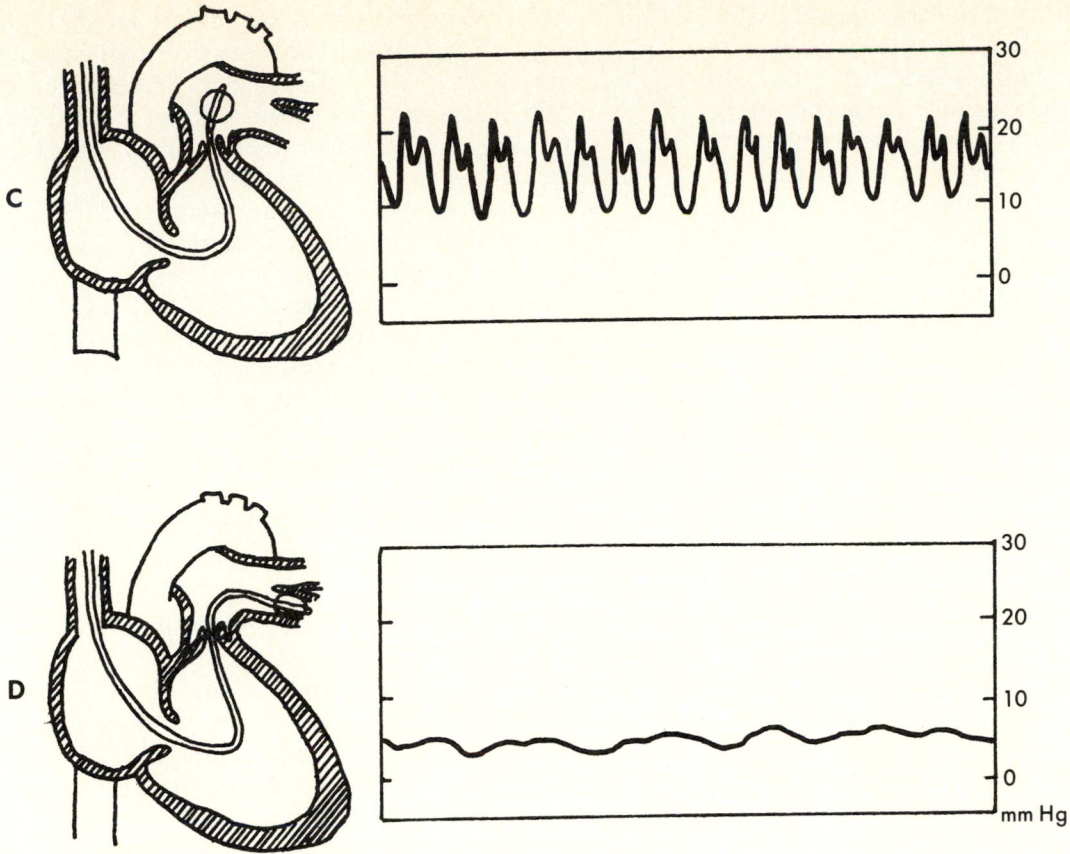

Fig. 9-25, cont'd **C,** Pulmonary artery position and waveform during Swan-Ganz catheter insertion (normal pressures = 20 to 25 mm Hg systolic pressure and 5 to 15 mm Hg diastolic pressure). **D,** PAW position and waveform during Swan-Ganz catheter insertion (normal mean pressure = 5 to 15 mm Hg).

nurse and recorded in the nursing notes. The nurse should:

1. Document the PA waveform with a strip recording (while balloon is deflated) at least every 8 hours.
2. Aspirate blood from the PA port at regular intervals, and flush the line to determine and/or maintain line patency. (NOTE: As with other vascular lines, it is prudent to discard the initial aspirate of blood, which may contain small emboli.)
3. Inflate the balloon and obtain a strip recording of the PAW tracing every 2 to 4 hours as indicated. The positive pressure in the thoracic cavity during positive pressure ventilation may alter venous return and pulmonary vascular tone and may affect pulmonary artery pressure. The nurse must record measurements and tracings in a consistent fashion (e.g., with or without positive pressure ventilation) to avoid inaccurate or uninterpretable measurements.
4. The patient does not need to be in the supine position for PA or PAW measurements, according to recent literature,[97] as long as the patient's head is not elevated more than 45 degrees and as long as the transducer is zeroed while the patient is in the new position. Always maintain consistency in patient positioning for measurements.
5. Check the line and all stopcocks for air bubbles every 2 hours.
6. Recalibrate transducers every 2 hours or according to manufacturer's recommendations.

INFLATION OF BALLOON. Extra caution is required during balloon inflation and deflation to prevent complications and maximize balloon/catheter longevity.

1. Carbon dioxide is the ideal gas to use for balloon inflation since it is highly soluble in blood (20 times more soluble than in air). Many hospitals, however, do routinely use room air. Particular care should be exercised when using an air-inflated balloon during catheter insertion in patients with right-to-left intracardiac shunts (e.g., children with cyanotic congenital defects). Balloon rupture during passage of the catheter through the right heart of these children may cause passage of air into the arterial system with resultant myocardial or cerebral infarction.

2. Fluids, such as a saline solution, are not recommended for balloon inflation since the viscosity and capillary action of these fluids will prevent complete balloon deflation.

3. Flush the PA lumen before inflating balloon.

4. The typical volume of air required for balloon inflation is:
   a. No. 7 French: 1.5 cc
   b. No. 5 French: 0.8 cc
   c. No. 4 French: 0.35 cc
   Use a tuberculin syringe for accurate volume inflation. Check the package insert of each catheter for the precise balloon inflation volume.

5. Watch the pressure tracing as the balloon is slowly inflated, and stop when the PAW pressure is achieved. (NOTE: Over-inflation may cause the balloon to rupture or may damage the pulmonary vessel.) *Never* leave the balloon inflated for more than 2 minutes.[40,62] Note any changes from previous inflations that may indicate catheter migration.

6. Be gentle with inflation technique; the balloons are fragile and may begin disintegrating within 48 hours after insertion.[27]

7. Deflation of the balloon may be accomplished by either of two methods.
   a. The balloon can be passively deflated by disconnecting the syringe from balloon port while the port is open to air. It is argued, however, that if there is a balloon rupture, this method may allow air to enter the pulmonary artery. However, if deflation time is limited to a few seconds and if the pulmonary port is held at or below heart level, the risk of air entry is minimal. Pulmonary air embolus from this source has not been reported in the literature.
   b. Active deflation by withdrawing the injected air with a syringe was originally suggested by Dr. Swan. A possible problem with this method is that the negative pressure applied by the syringe may cause more rapid deterioration of the elasticity of the balloon, thus decreasing its longevity. It is also believed that active deflation may cause the port of the balloon to be drawn up over the tip of the catheter; this has not been clearly documented, however.

A standard of care must be established by each hospital specifying the techniques to be used for inflation and deflation of the balloon.

8. If balloon rupture is suspected, insert a glass syringe in the balloon port and check to see if the syringe plunger will spring back when it is released. Balloon rupture is very probable if the plunger does not spring back, but further assessment must be made (see Table 9-4 on troubleshooting).

9. Change dressing daily and observe for signs of inflammation, such as heat, erythema, discharge, and odor.

Swan-Ganz catheterization in the critically ill infant

INDICATIONS. Some indications for use of the Swan-Ganz catheter are specific to problems occurring in infancy. These indications include (1) differentiation of respiratory from congenital heart disease, particularly if cyanosis or pulmonary hypertension is present in the neonatal period, (2) management of respiratory failure (particularly respiratory distress syndrome), and (3) management of the unstable infant in whom careful hemodynamic measurements and fluid therapy are required (e.g., the infant with shock, sepsis, or disseminated intravascular coagulation [DIC]).

TECHNIQUES. Size no. 5 French Swan-Ganz catheters are usually suitable for use in the newborn, if they are inserted through a large vein such as the femoral, subclavian, or right external jugular vein. Small peripheral veins in older infants and children may allow only the passage of the size no. 4 French catheter. The insertion procedure is the same as that discussed in the previous section.

NURSING CONSIDERATIONS. All of the nursing responsibilities for care of the patient with a Swan-Ganz catheter previously discussed are applicable. However, there are several additional considerations when the Swan-Ganz catheter is inserted in the infant.

1. Be certain that the balloon is checked before insertion, particularly in children with right-to-left intracardiac shunt defects. Balloon rupture (or leak) in these children may result in an air embolus to the left heart causing an

embolus to the coronary or cerebral vessels.

2. Monitor the infant's blood loss during insertion, and replace the blood loss as indicated by the physician.

3. The amount of fluid infused through this line must be regulated meticulously; this is especially important in infants. Organize the flush system, as well as the cardiac output measurements so that fluid overload is avoided, yet the lines have an adequate heparinized flush to maintain patency.

4. Since the balloon volume is so small, the nurse must increase her sensitivity to the resistance normally encountered during balloon inflation. By appreciating the resistance in relation to the normal volume required, as well as recognizing normal waveform changes, the nurse should quickly detect evidence of balloon rupture or increased resistance to inflation caused by catheter migration. It is helpful for the nurse to inflate the balloon before insertion so that she might have the benefit of a visual demonstration while getting a "feel" for inflation resistance.

Complications of Swan-Ganz catheterization in children. Although the use of Swan-Ganz catheters in critically ill pediatric patients is increasing, the literature remains sparse on the subject. Infection (including sepsis and thrombophlebitis) remains the most frequent complication in children.[24] Several pediatric centers now recommend removal or replacement of the Swan-Ganz catheter after 72 hours of use since it is believed that the risk of infection and the probability of balloon rupture are increased after this time.[49,61]

Wetzel[91] has reported Swan-Ganz balloon obstruction of the right ventricular outflow tract at the level of the pulmonary valve. If the balloon does obstruct the pulmonary outflow tract for more than a few seconds, the child may rapidly develop hypoxemia, bradycardia, and hypotension. Although this complication is not common, if it is not recognized immediately, the child may die. Immediate deflation of the balloon and/or withdrawal or advancement of the catheter should alleviate the obstruction.

The most frequently cited complications of Swan-Ganz catheterization include infection, arrhythmias, balloon rupture, knotting of the catheter, pulmonary infarction, pulmonary artery rupture, and pulmonary embolism. Each of these is discussed in the following section. Troubleshooting of the Swan-Ganz catheter is outlined in Table 9-4.

Table 9-4 Troubleshooting: problems with the Swan-Ganz catheters*

Problems	Causes	Treatment	Prevention
Dampening or absence of waveforms	Loose connections in line	Methodically check entire line from insertion site to flush system for loose connections	Check connections every 2 hr; watch for backflow of blood in line that might indicate a loose connection
		Check stopcocks for correct positions of stopcock valves	
		Flush air out of system (with stopcock port closed to patient)	
	Clots in line	Attempt to aspirate blood from each port and discard; do not flush line if unable to aspirate	Maintain continuous flush

*See Table 9-2 for other troubleshooting measures related to vascular lines.

Continued.

Table 9-4 Troubleshooting: problems with the Swan-Ganz catheters—cont'd

Problems	Causes	Treatment	Prevention
Dampening or absence of waveforms—cont'd			Manually flush every time blood samples are drawn
			If line is difficult to aspirate but easy to flush, this may be an early sign of partial clotting of line (notify physician)
	Decreased pressure in flush pressure bag	Reinflate bag to appropriate pressure, watch for leaks; replace bag or clamp tubing to inflation bulb	Check bag before using it in the infusion-line system
	Faulty transducer	Check transducer against manometer for accuracy	Check function of transducer before placing infusion line
Dampened RA tracing	Gradual occlusion by clots	Aspirate blood from line and discard; flush line with heparinized flush	Manually flush catheter after each blood sample is drawn
	Stopcock port not completely turned open to transducer		Check stopcock ports routinely; keep them free of clotted blood
Dampened PA tracing	Catheter tip lodged against vessel wall. NOTE: PAW pressure may be mistaken for "dampened" tracing	Check balloon—ensure that it is deflated. Reposition catheter or change patient position. See Dampening or absence of waveforms	Check daily chest films to verify position of catheter
Continuous PAW waveform	Balloon left inflated	Deflate balloon	Ensure balloon deflation after each PAW measurement
	Catheter advanced into a more peripheral branch of PA	Reposition patient; rotate extremity of catheter insertion site. Physician may need to pull back catheter; verify position with chest film, and call physician immediately	Since the injection ports are not clearly labeled, tag each port with large adhesive tags labeled "RA," "PA," and "balloon" for balloon port; in addition, tag may be marked with a red arrow indicating direction of valve movement required to open port

Table 9-4 Troubleshooting: problems with the Swan-Ganz catheters—cont'd

Problems	Causes	Treatment	Prevention
PAW pressure achieved by balloon inflation with smaller amount of air than balloon capacity	May be caused by catheter advance distally into a smaller vessel (so it takes less volume to "wedge" balloon)	Catheter may need to be pulled back; call physician immediately If satisfactory PA tracing is observed on balloon deflation and if wedge tracing is also satisfactory, physician may elect to not change catheter position	Do not inflate balloon more than is necessary; this predisposes catheter to migrate forward, and it decreases balloon longevity Note in nursing care plan exact amount of air that is needed for balloon inflation before insertion
PA waveform is normal but unable to obtain PAW with balloon inflation (CAUTION: Inability to obtain wedge tracing with injection of normal balloon inflation volume may indicate *balloon rupture*)	Catheter not far enough forward in PA for balloon to occlude lumen	Compare current PA waveform with earlier tracings Catheter may require repositioning—notify physician	Check daily chest film to verify catheter position
	Insufficient air injected for balloon inflation	Deflate balloon, then reinflate with the exact volume required	Check balloon to note exact air capacity before insertion
	Balloon rupture: no resistance felt when inflation is attempted; blood may be observed in balloon inflation port; this may be the result of overly vigorous inflation or inflating so frequently as to decrease longevity of the balloon	Clamp balloon inflation port and notify physician	Minimize number of balloon inflations performed in order to increase longevity of balloon; if PA diastolic pressure closely matches wedge pressure, balloon longevity may be dramatically reduced. NOTE: Correlate PA diastolic pressure with PAW pressure at least every 6-8 hr or more often if clinical condition indicates
Significant changes in PA or PAW waveforms or measurements	Air or blood in line	Methodically check entire line for loose connections, bubbles, or blood Aspirate and flush lines	Maintain constant flush of line as ordered
	Level of transducer changed	Check (and adjust as needed) transducer level	Standardize level of transducer for measurements and note that level in nursing-care plan

Continued.

Table 9-4 Troubleshooting: problems with the Swan-Ganz catheters—cont'd

Problems	Causes	Treatment	Prevention
Significant changes in PA or PAW waveforms or measurements—cont'd	Transducer calibration incorrect	Recalibrate/relevel transducer	
	Amplified waveform may indicate the catheter has drifted into right ventricle	Notify physician of need for repositioning catheter	
		Check diastolic pressure; right ventricular diastolic pressure is normally ≤ 4 torr, or $\leq$ RA mean	
		Get x-ray film to verify position; right ventricular position may cause arrhythmias	
		Have lidocaine ready at bedside (1 mg/kg per IV bolus is usual pediatric dose for treatment of ventricular arrhythmias)	

INFECTIONS. Infections seem to be generally more common in children.[24] Thrombi formation on the catheter may render the patient more susceptible to thrombotic endocarditis with the initial infection occurring most often at the venous cutdown site. Strict aseptic technique during insertion and daily dressing changes, with daily applications of topical bacteriocidal ointment, will minimize the incidence of this problem. When infection does occur, the catheter must be removed, blood cultures drawn, and parenteral antibiotics ordered.[62,66]

ARRHYTHMIAS. Ventricular arrhythmias may occur during catheter insertion as the catheter is moved through the right ventricle. After catheter placement, the distal tip may slip back into the right ventricle, causing arrhythmias. The best treatment for the arrhythmia is immediate repositioning of the catheter. The extremity in which the catheter is placed is repositioned to attempt to move the catheter tip into the pulmonary artery. The balloon is then inflated and allowed to be carried into the pulmonary artery. With the physician's order, the catheter can be pulled into the right atrium with the balloon inflated to 50% of its capacity. Xylocaine (Lidocaine) administration

may be necessary until the catheter is repositioned, and a defibrillator should be at the bedside.[4,14,36]

BALLOON RUPTURE. The latex membrane of the balloon can absorb some of the blood lipoproteins and lose elasticity, making it more susceptible to rupture. Injection of the normal balloon inflation volume of air into the ruptured balloon should not pose a major problem as long as the air enters only the right heart or pulmonary arterial circulation. However, if the air enters the left side of the heart,[6,62] a coronary or cerebral air embolus can occur. A fragment of the ruptured balloon may occlude a pulmonary vessel, causing cyanosis, possible loss of consciousness, and cardiovascular collapse. It is important that the nurse follow the prescribed guidelines for the care of the Swan-Ganz catheter in order to minimize the possibility of this complication.[6,27,62]

KNOTTING OF THE CATHETER. Knotting may occur during insertion or if the catheter tip slips back into the right ventricle. The waveform should reflect the position of the catheter tip unless the catheter is kinked, occluding the lumen and thus causing a "dampened" waveform. The physician will have to attempt to pull the catheter back under fluroscopy (a second, "snare," catheter may be used). However, if this is unsuccessful, the patient will require surgery (with use of cardiopulmonary bypass) in order to remove the catheter. The knotted line in the right ventricle may cause ventricular arrhythmias requiring treatment with lidocaine.[62]

PULMONARY INFARCTION.   An infarction may occur at the time of catheter insertion or during the monitoring period, particularly if the catheter migrates into a more peripheral pulmonary vessel and occludes it. If the PA tracing spontaneously becomes a PAW-pressure tracing (or a "dampened" tracing), the catheter may be withdrawn approximately 1 cm. The nurse should aspirate to check for clots and then *gently* flush the pulmonary port. Note that a rapid flush may damage the intima of the pulmonary vessel and aggravate the condition. A pulmonary infarction usually does not produce symptoms, but on occasion it may cause pleural pain, dyspnea, syncope, or total consolidation of the lung field on the chest film. The physician must be notified immediately if pulmonary infarction is suspected[6,27,62] or if the catheter remains in the wedge position despite maneuvers to dislodge it.

PULMONARY ARTERY RUPTURE.   This complication may occur when the catheter migrates distally into a small vessel so that when the balloon is inflated the vessel ruptures. It also may occur when fluid is flushed under high pressure through the PA port. The patient may exhibit hemoptysis, coughing, or rales on auscultation. Because this complication is serious, it has been recommended by Swan and Ganz that a balloon-tipped catheter not be left in place longer than 48 hours. A nurse needs to be very sensitive to the amount of resistance that is normal for balloon inflation and investigate any deviations. If the patient has developed increased pulmonary vascular resistance, the nurse must check with the physician before proceeding with further balloon inflations.[6,27,62] For this reason Swan-Ganz catheters should be inserted and maintained only with caution in patients with pulmonary hypertension.

PULMONARY EMBOLISM.   Although this is not a frequent problem with flow-directed catheters, thrombi can readily form on the balloon and shaft of the catheter. Patients in ICU are especially susceptible to the development of thromboemboli because of decreased activity and possibly decreased pulmonary blood flow. The patient with pulmonary embolism may exhibit pleuritic pain, cough, hemoptysis, substernal chest pain, syncope, shock, and death.[4,14,36]

Cardiac output measurements. Cardiac output defines the volume of blood pumped by the heart per unit of time (liters/per minute). This reflects myocardial function. Cardiac output measurements may be required for children who have had heart surgery, who have unstable cardiorespiratory function or fluid balance (such as observed in septic shock), who exhibit signs of low cardiac output refractory to usual treatment, and who are being ventilated with high-continuous airway pressures that may cause decreased cardiac output.[7]

The cardiac output measurements may be made with the use of a triple-lumen Swan-Ganz catheter or with the use of a single right atrial line with a separate thermistor probe placed in the pulmonary artery. Common approaches for cardiac output measurement use the principle of measuring the time course of an indicator as it circulates from one point to the next. The Fick method measures changes in oxygen content. The dye dilution method measures changes in dye concentration; thermodilution uses a cold solution as the indicator (see p. 92).

The thermodilution method is often preferable because it does not use toxic materials, it does not require blood withdrawal and reinfusion, it uses an inexpensive indicator (usually glucose [D_5W]), and it will not produce significant cardiovascular changes. The thermodilution method requires the rapid injection into the right atrium of a known quantity of solution at a known temperature; the solution mixes with the blood and flows from the right atrium into the right ventricle and then into the pulmonary artery where the thermistor measures the time course and degree of the temperature change.[71]

Cardiac output is computed by the average between the peak change in temperature and the exponential return to body temperature. This average indicates the volume of blood that is required to dilute the injected solution to the point where it produces changes in temperature detected by the thermistor:

$$\frac{\text{Amount of solution injected}}{\text{Mean temp of solution} \times \text{Duration of first circulation}} = \text{Cardiac output}$$

The specific technique of cardiac output measurement and the instrumentation warrant a brief discussion in order to ensure accurate measurements.

Cardiac output instrumentation.   Several manufacturers make thermodilution cardiac output computers, and some important features should be considered in selecting a cardiac output computer for use with critically ill children. The computation of the cardiac output volume contains a constant factor (K) that incorporates the variables of injectate volume, length and gauge of the right atrial catheter ("dead space"), and the distance between the tip of the RA catheter and the pulmonary artery thermistor. All of these variables must be known and programmed into the cardiac output computer. The injectate volume and temperature must also be entered into the calculations.

If the computer has a mechanism to manually adjust the K factor, several different catheters from various manufacturers may be used with the same computer and the K factor adjusted accordingly. Manual calculation of the K factor is a simple procedure.

$$K = \frac{V_I - V_D}{9.3} \times \frac{T_B - T_I}{T_B} \times 0.825^*$$

Where V_I is the volume of injectate, V_D is the volume of dead space, T_B is the patient's core temperature, and T_I is the injectate temperature.

The volume of injectate needed for each cardiac output calculation will vary from one machine and catheter to another. Since fluid requirements are small in children and since cardiac output measurements may be required frequently, the cardiac output computers (and catheters) used in the care of children should require injectate boluses of no more than 3 ml.

The temperature of the injectate is extremely important. With older models the injectate had to be exactly 0° C, requiring that it not be exposed to room air for longer than 15 seconds before injection. Current units now incorporate an internal sensor mechanism or a probe placed in the RA line through which the injectate is pushed. The sensor measures the temperature of the injectate and feeds the information into the computer. Thus the problem of maintaining an exact temperature is eliminated. One must note, however, that the lower the injectate temperature, the smaller the machine error (because the difference between the injectate temperature and patient blood temperature will be large). Therefore it is best to keep the injectate iced, although the *exact* temperature will not matter if the computer has an internal temperature sensor. However, frequent injections of iced saline can be a source of tremendous heat loss in small infants. Many units are now available that make accurate cardiac output computations with room temperature injectates. Regardless of the unit selected, the operator's manual should be read thoroughly to discover what the standard error will be with injectates of varying temperatures.

*Manual for Instrumentation Laboratory cardiac output computer, Instrumentation Laboratory, Lexington, MA 02173.

The thermistor position in the pulmonary artery must be verified by a chest film, a waveform if a Swan-Ganz catheter is used, or a comparison of strip recordings of the thermodilution tracings from one time to another (Fig. 9-26).

Reliability of cardiac output measurements is improved if multiple measurements are obtained with averaging of the results. Averaging three to five determinations is optimal but frequently not possible because of the fluid restrictions in small children. If a computer is capable of calculating an average with less than 3 ml injectate boluses, it may enable the

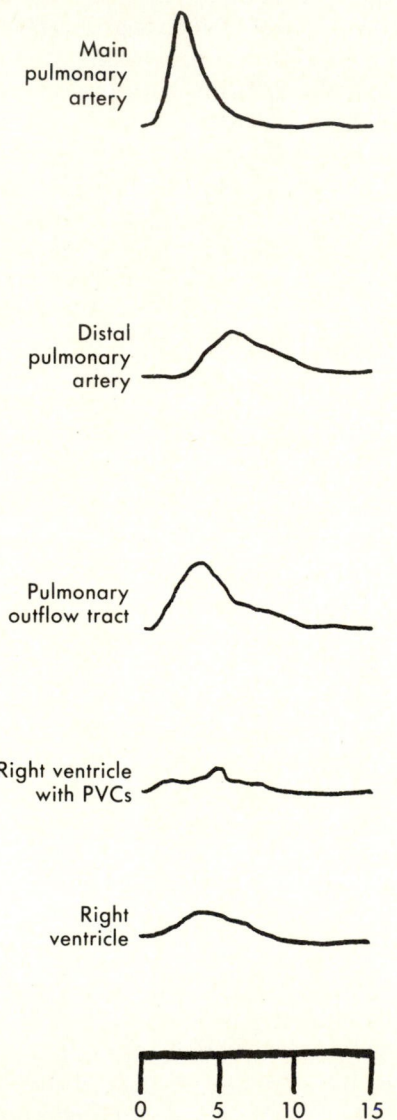

Fig. 9-26 Thermodilution tracings from various catheter (thermistor) positions.

Modified from Colgan, F.J., and Stewart, S.: Crit. Care Med. **5:**224, 1977.

clinician to make more than a single measurement. Every effort should be made to allow at least two to three injections per determination to ensure accuracy.

Precision and reliability of cardiac output measurements are dependent on the clinician who is making the measurement. The K factor must be identified (if it is manually adjustable), the technique of injectate bolusing must be rapid (less than 2 seconds) and identical from measurement to measurement (this can be verified by comparing the thermodilution curves), the child must be in a quiet state, the machine should be checked (instrument-tested per manufacturer's recommendation) every 8 hours, and appropriate attention to clean or sterile technique must be given to the entire system.

Nursing considerations. A child who requires cardiac output measurement is usually very ill and needs excellent nursing care. In addition to careful assessment of the child's systemic perfusion, recording of vital signs, monitoring of fluid intake and output, and maintenance of adequate mechanical ventilation, the nurse must care for all of the monitoring equipment and calculate and administer medications and electrolyte solutions. Unfortunately, because the child's care is so complex, proper maintenance of catheters and equipment is often the nurse's lowest priority; yet this equipment is essential to the care of the child.

Please refer to earlier discussions of nursing responsibilities regarding use of venous catheters (see also Table 9-3). Additional nursing responsibilities for use of a cardiac output computer/catheter follow.[13,71]

1. Be completely familiar with the cardiac output computer. Do not perform measurements if there is any uncertainty about the function of the machine or the technique of measurement.
2. Always run the manufacturer's specified "instrument test" at regular intervals to verify machine accuracy.
3. Verify the thermistor position of the Swan-Ganz catheter with analysis of the PA waveform before making measurements. If using a separate RA line, verify RA position by waveform. The distance between the RA lumen and the thermistor tip must remain constant.
4. There are many methods for cooling the in-

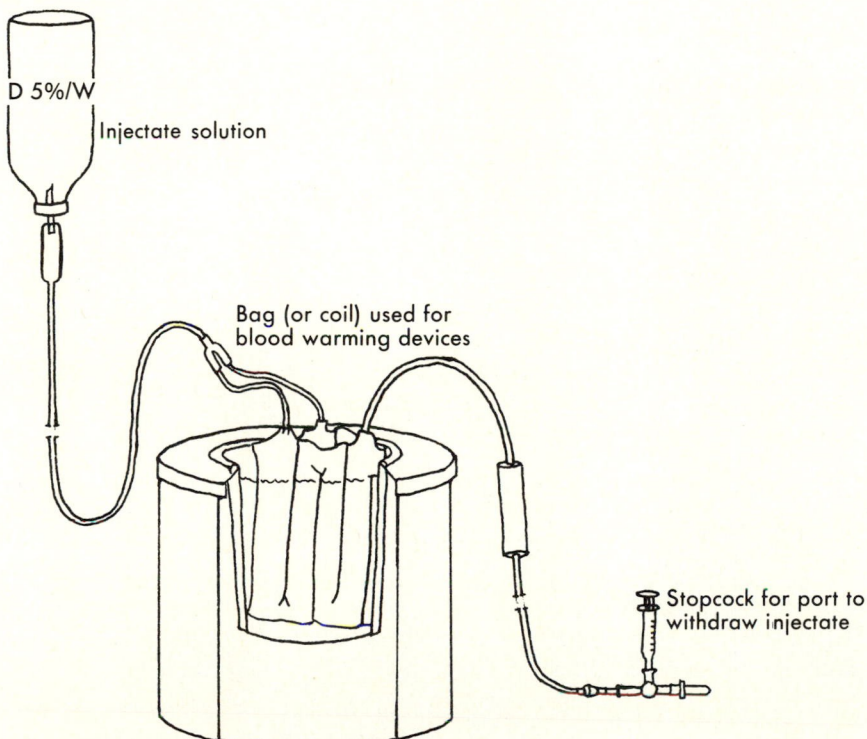

Fig. 9-27 Closed system for cooling injectate to be used in thermodilution cardiac output measurements.

jectate if a 0° C injectate is desired. Fig. 9-27 illustrates one system that avoids preparation of preloaded syringes, which are easily contaminated if they are immersed in the iced solution without being sealed within another container. (Using preloaded syringes is also expensive and time consuming.)

Establishment of individual "heart" lines following open-heart surgery. Individual lines may be placed directly into specific chambers of the heart or vessels (RA, PA, LA) through tiny needle punctures made during cardiovascular surgery. Each monitoring line is brought directly from the heart or vessel out through the chest wall. Although the principles for care and maintenance of each line are exactly the same as for the Swan-Ganz catheter, a brief discussion of each is presented here.

Left atrial line. The LA line allows measurement of left ventricular end-diastolic (filling) pressure and indirect assessment of left ventricular compliance (filling pressure required for satisfactory cardiac output). Pulmonary vascular resistance (right ventricular afterload) may be calculated, using the cardiac index, the mean left atrial (L$\overline{A}$) pressure, and the mean pulmonary artery (P$\overline{A}$) pressure, as follows:

$$\text{Pulmonary vascular resistance in units} = \frac{P\overline{A} - L\overline{A}}{\text{Cardiac index}}$$

If the child has a competent mitral valve and no pulmonary hypertension, the PA diastolic pressure and the PAW pressure (obtained with a Swan-Ganz catheter) should equal the mean LA pressure. If the child does have pulmonary hypertension, pulmonary artery diastolic and wedge pressures do not necessarily reflect the LA pressure. In such children, direct measurement of LA pressure (with an LA line) is the only means of obtaining left ventricular end-diastolic pressure. (Fig. 9-28 indicates the normal appearance of an LA waveform.)

LA lines are generally inserted during open-heart surgery if left ventricular function is poor or if left ventricular or mitral valve function is thought to be jeopardized during surgery (e.g., if a left ventricular cardiotomy incision was required to close muscular ventricular septal defects). Assessment and treatment of the child with low cardiac output is discussed thoroughly in Chapter 3.

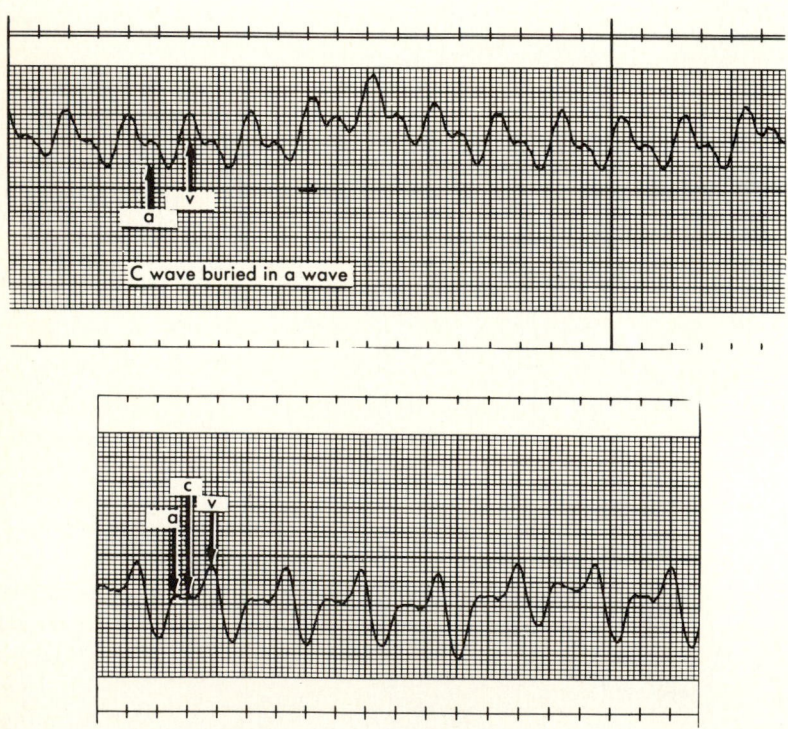

Fig. 9-28 Normal LA pressure waveforms: "a" wave: atrial systole; "c" wave: movement of the AV valve toward atrium during AV valve closure; "v" wave: atrial filling with AV valve closed (isovolumetric time period).

There are several important points to remember when caring for a child with an LA line:

1. The infusion line should be prepared with a standard transducer system.
2. The line should *never* be used to infuse medications or fluids of any kind. It exists solely for LA measurements.[55,91]
3. The line should be checked hourly for air bubbles or other emboli. If air or other emboli are seen in the line, the stopcock port nearest the patient should be immediately *closed* ("off" to the patient) and the line should be rapidly flushed.
4. If "dampening" of the waveform occurs, the nurse may attempt to aspirate the line, but she *should not flush the LA line* without a physician's order. If the doctor has requested the nurse to flush the line, it should *always* be aspirated first! Be sure to discard the aspirate (1 to 2 ml), which may contain emboli. The danger in flushing the line, of course, is that an air or blood embolus may be pushed into the coronary vessels or cerebral vessels and cause an infarction.

Pulmonary artery line.   A catheter inserted directly into the pulmonary artery during open-heart surgery will offer nearly the same information as that obtained with a Swan-Ganz catheter. However, since the catheter is inserted directly through the chest during surgery, it is probably not balloon tipped and such direct PA lines cannot measure PAW pressures. Nevertheless, the PA waveform should be the same as that obtained with a Swan-Ganz catheter (see the previous section on Swan-Ganz catheters).

PA lines inserted during surgery require the same care as a Swan-Ganz catheter. Some specific considerations for maintenance of these lines include extra care in perfusion and the flushing techniques presented here.[52,55,96]

Since the catheter is placed into a small pulmonary vessel with high flow and moderately low pressures (lower pressures than a peripheral arterial line), the maintenance infusion rate may be decreased to 1 to 2 ml/hour.

With frequent pulmonary arterial blood sampling (to obtain mixed venous samples for analysis of oxygen tension), the pulmonary vessel may be exposed to frequent manual flushing. In order to minimize damage to the vessel intima, the following steps may be taken: (1) flush from the furthest port possible, and (2) consider using a T connector in place of a stopcock for sampling. (Refer to section on transducer systems.)

Right atrial line.   The RA catheter provides the same data as the RA port of a Swan-Ganz catheter. It is used for right-sided heart pressure measurements, as a port for thermodilution cardiac output injection, and as a line for infusion of fluids and medications. The RA waveform should appear the same as that obtained from the RA port of the Swan-Ganz catheter.

Systemic vascular resistance may be calculated with the RA line, using the cardiac index, the mean RA pressure ($\overline{RA}$) and the mean arterial pressure as follows:

$$\text{Systemic vascular resistance in units} = \frac{\text{Mean arterial pressure} - \overline{RA}}{\text{Cardiac index}}$$

If the child has an RA line, nursing responsibilities include those discussed previously (see the section on venous measurements). Specific additional recommendations follow.

If a child has a cardiac septal defect, great care must be exercised to avoid infusion of *any* air or other thrombotic material through the RA line. Such material may easily cross to the left side of the heart and enter either the coronary or cerebral vasculature.

The RA line may be used for injecting medication or fluid since the catheter tip is located in the right atrium where there is a larger volume and faster flow of blood than in peripheral veins.

Since this is a low-pressure line, there is satisfactory maintenance of RA lines with infusion rates as low as 1 ml/hour.

■ Pacemakers

Pacemaker therapy is indicated in children who have developed or who have the potential to develop atrioventricular (AV) conduction block that may cause low cardiac output. Most commonly these children have required open-heart surgery, although cardiomyopathies or congenital or idiopathic AV block may also have created the need for a pacemaker. This discussion will be limited to the use of temporary external pacemakers (see p. 114 for further information).

Function.   The function of a pacemaker is to provide an external electrical stimulus to generate intracardiac electrical activity when the heart's own electrical system is failing.

Pacemaker unit.   This device consists of an energy source (the pacemaker pack or pulse generator) and two terminals: one ground (+) and one output (−) terminal (Fig. 9-29).

Types of pacemakers commonly used.[54,95] *Fixed rate* (asynchronous) pacemakers pace the heart

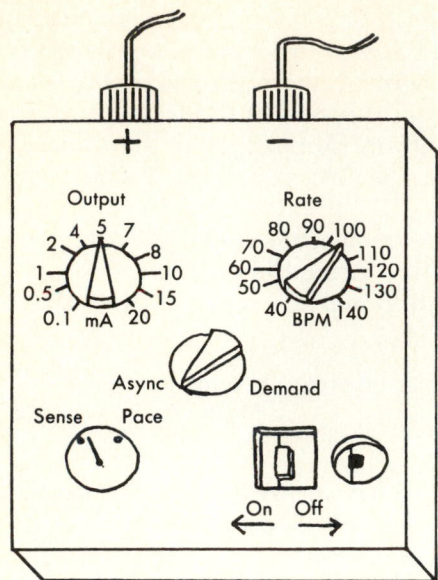

Fig. 9-29 External pacemaker unit: (+) terminal = ground wire; (−) terminal = myocardial wire.

at a set rate without regard for the patient's rate. *Demand* pacemakers fire only when the patient's own ventricular rate falls below a preset limit. *AV sequential* pacemakers are demand or control pacemakers that can provide both atrial and ventricular impulses in sequence. This pacemaker has a ventricular (and, recently, an atrial) *sensing* component, as well as ventricular and atrial *stimulators. Transvenous versus epicardial pacing:* transvenous pacemaker wires may be placed by threading them through a large vein (e.g., through the brachial vein) to the heart. Epicardial pacing wires are inserted directly through the anterior chest wall to the epicardium.

Components of a demand pacemaker

Output control (stimulation threshold). The output control adjusts the amount of current delivered to the myocardium by the pacemaker generator. The amount of current flow is measured in milliamperes (ma). The correct setting for this control is one that maintains consistent capture of the heart at the lowest possible output (ma). The patient's myocardial or epicardial threshold may change because of fibrosis around the leads or because of edema or electrolyte changes. The pacemaker should be maintained at the lowest possible output because it is delivering an electrical current to a local area, which may hasten the onset of edema or fibrosis. Also, pacemaker batteries are more quickly depleted at higher outputs.[54,95]

Rate control. This control adjusts the pacing rate up to 800 pulses/minute depending on the pace-

maker model being used. In the fixed rate (asynchronous mode) the physician will often set the rate above the patient's intrinsic rate ("overdriving" the patient's inherent rhythm). If *demand* pacing is desired as a backup, the rate is determined by the physician, who must consider the lowest possible heart rate that will provide adequate cardiac output.

Sensitivity control. This defines the *minimum* patient ECG signal that will inhibit a pacemaker impulse or initiate pacemaker firing. In most cases this "signal" is an R wave (from the QRS complex) of a given slope and amplitude.[54]

When the sensitivity dial is set fully clockwise, the pacemaker is functioning in the *demand* range so that maximum sensitivity to the patient's R-wave signal is attained. As the sensitivity dial is turned in the counter-clockwise direction, a progressively larger patient R-wave signal is required to inhibit pacer firing. If the sensitivity dial is set fully counterclockwise in the *asynchronous* range, the pacer operates at a fixed rate regardless of the patient's intrinsic heart rate. The patient's R-wave signal, in this case, will not inhibit pacer firing.[54]

The *sensitivity threshold*, then, is the point at which the pacemaker consistently senses every R-wave signal of the patient. Once this point is determined, it might be prudent to turn the control (clockwise) just a little beyond that point to ensure that optimum sensitivity to patient rhythm is obtained.

Sense-pace indicator. Pacemakers usually have a gauge or a light that will indicate whether the pacemaker is sensing patient R waves or generating an electrical impulse (pacing). The same or a similar gauge or light will reveal low battery voltage. Since low battery voltage causes pacemaker malfunction, it is important that batteries for each patient be kept functional.

Batteries. Battery replacement is recommended every 3 to 7 days or as indicated by the amount of use. When batteries are replaced, a label should be placed on the pacemaker with the date of change and the nurse's initials.

Pacemaker malfunctions

Competition

PROBLEM. The *demand* or *asynchronous* pacemaker may fire in competition with the patient's rhythm (Fig. 9-30). This often occurs when the patient's rate and the pacemaker rate are nearly the same. This is dangerous because the pacing spike may occur during the vulnerable period of the cardiac cycle or during cardiac repolarization (represented by the T wave), and it may cause patient ventricular fibrillation. The electrical impulse required to pace a ventricle is significantly less than that required to produce fibrillation. Usually the fibrillation threshold

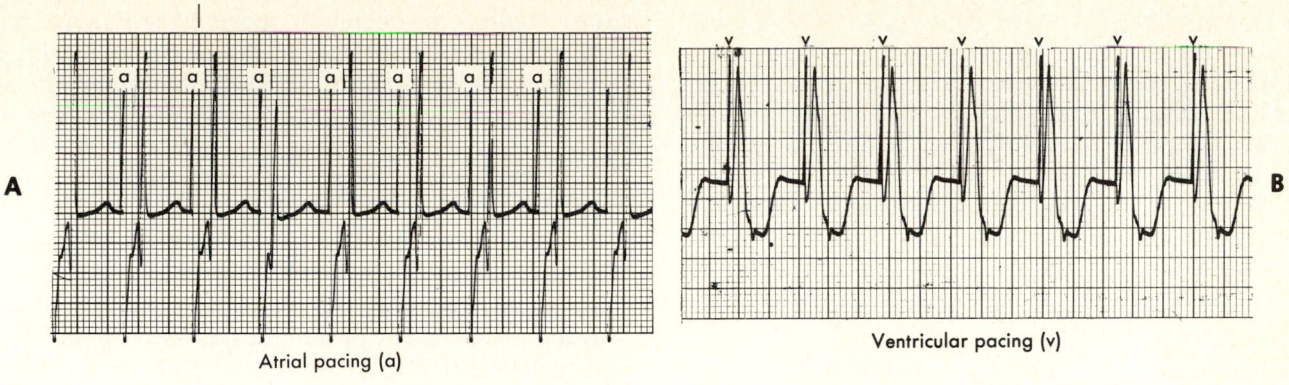

Atrial pacing (a)

Ventricular pacing (v)

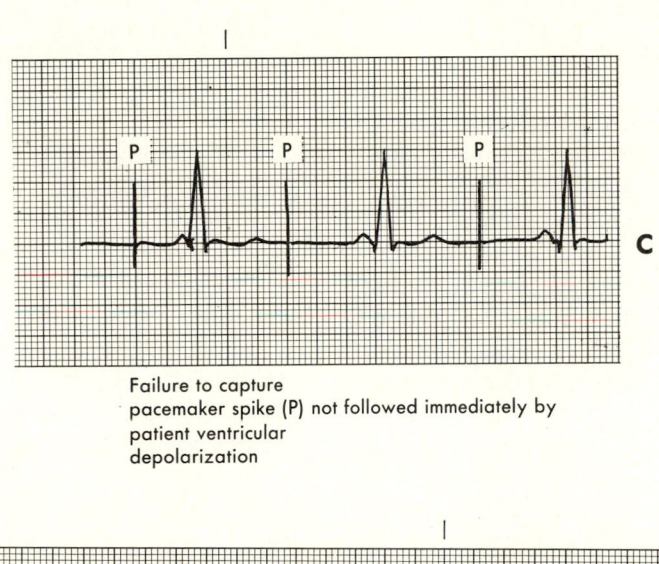

Failure to capture
pacemaker spike (P) not followed immediately by
patient ventricular
depolarization

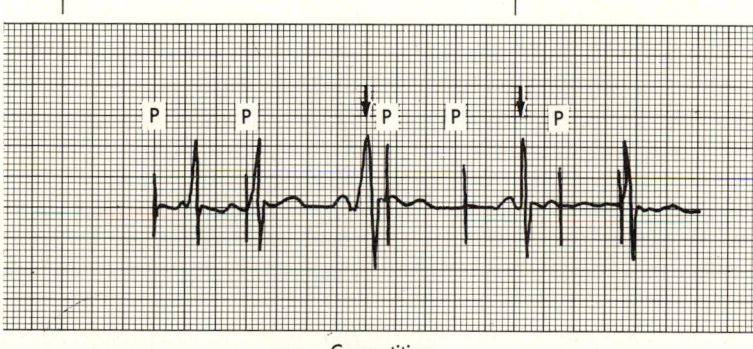

Competition

Fig. 9-30 Atrial and ventricular pacing. **A,** Atrial pacing. **B,** Ventricular pacing. **C,** Pacemaker failure to capture. Pacemaker spikes (P) are not followed by ventricular responses (QRS). **D,** Competition and failure to capture. Pacemaker spike (P) is not inhibited by patient ventricular depolarization (↓), and pacemaker spike (P) is not consistently producing ventricular depolarization (see first and third pacemaker spikes). Pacemaker activity is "competing" with the patient's intrinsic rhythm.

of the ventricle is 10 to 30 times greater than the pacemaker output. The ventricular fibrillation threshold, however, can be lowered in the presence of increased myocardial irritability caused by myocardial infarction, hypoxia, electrolyte imbalance, acidosis, alkalosis, drugs, or other factors.[67,95]

If the pacer is in the *fixed rate* mode, competition between the child's intrinsic cardiac electrical activity and the pacemaker is more likely. The nurse must recognize the danger of fibrillation that is present during fixed-rate pacing.

If the pacer is in the *demand* mode, competition may occur if the pacemaker's ability to sense the patient's R waves is lost. The pacemaker may be firing even though the patient's rate is greater than the demand pacemaker rate.

INTERVENTIONS. Whenever competition is occurring, the nurse should turn the pacer sensitivity control clockwise to the maximum sensitivity position in an attempt to improve the pacemaker's sensing function. The settings on the pacemaker unit should always be doublechecked whenever a problem arises. Once the nurse ensures the accuracy of the pacer unit settings, the integrity of the external system, including the pacer unit and the cables, must be checked. First, the external cables should be changed for a fresh set (this should be done as rapidly and carefully as possible, so that the pacing is not significantly interrupted). If the competition continues, a new pacer unit (with identical settings and a new battery) should be substituted. The nurse should also remove the dressings over the wire insertion sites to make sure that one of the wires (usually the ground wire) has not fallen out. If none of these measures succeeds, the internal pacemaker wires may require replacement by the physician. These wires may no longer work if the wire tip is surrounded by edematous or fibrotic tissue or if the wire is fractured. (The fracture can often be seen on the child's chest film.)

If a child's intrinsic heart rate is adequate to maintain cardiac output, the pacemaker may be turned off to eliminate competition, and the physician should be notified immediately. If the child's intrinsic rate is *not* sufficient to maintain cardiac output, the pacemaker rate may be increased until it surpasses and supresses the patient's rate and controls the rhythm. A physician and defibrillator should be present when the pacemaker rate is increased in this fashion.

Failure to "capture"

PROBLEM. There may be inadequate pacer stimulus to the heart.[30,67,95] Causes of a pacemaker not attaining "capture" of the patient's ventricle include the following: battery failure (the most common cause), faulty connections in the system, wire fracture, malposition of wires in the heart, increased patient stimulation threshold as a result of fibrosis or edema, or severe myocardial dysfunction (see Fig. 9-30).

INTERVENTIONS. Interventions should include immediate replacement of the pacemaker unit, especially if the patient is pacer-dependent. Additional measures are to (1) check the connections at the terminals and wire insertion sites, (2) turn up the output; then turn up the pacemaker sensitivity, (3) check and replace batteries as indicated and reposition the patient, (4) switch the wires in the terminals if more than one myocardial wire is in place, (5) obtain a chest film to check for wire fracture, and (6) evaluate electrolytes for any indications that electrolyte imbalance may be causing myocardial dysfunction. If the problem persists, prepare for insertion of a new wire.[30,67,95]

If one wire is defective, the system may be reinstituted by placement of another cardiac wire (either transvenous or transthoracic) or a subcutaneous ground wire, ordered by the physician, as indicated.

Complications of pacemaker therapy. There are some significant complications that may occur in a child who requires pacemaker therapy. A discussion of these complications follows.[66,94]

Premature ventricular contractions (PVC) and other arrhythmias may result from myocardial injury caused by the wires. If a pacemaker stimulus occurs during the vulnerable period of the QRS complex, ventricular tachycardia or ventricular fibrillation may result. *Pulmonary emboli* may be caused by dislodged thrombi at the tip of transvenous pacer wires. *Perforation* of the right ventricle may result (usually within the first 48 hours) when a transvenous wire is used. *Infection* may occur. *Shocks* may occur at the skin site of wire insertion if the milliamp output of the pacer is too high. *Hiccups* may result if pacer output is too high or if the pacemaker wire stimulates the phrenic nerve. *Defective leads* and continuously high output may shorten lead life. *Pacemaker wire fracture* may also occur.

If pacing is abruptly discontinued, a period of asystole may occur until the patient's intrinsic pacemaker resumes activity. In general, the higher the pacemaker rate was before discontinuance, the longer will be the period of asystole. If the pacemaker must be turned off, it is advisable to gradually reduce the pacemaker rate before turning the unit off. The patient's blood pressure and other indicators of cardiac output should be monitored as the pacemaker rate is reduced. (See Chapter 3 for further discussion of pacemaker therapy.)

Emergency pacing and defibrillation

Emergency pacing. To establish emergency pacing, two methods of implanting cardiac wires are commonly used. In the *transthoracic* method, a needle is introduced through the anterior chest wall to the heart, and a pacing wire is inserted through the needle. In the *transvenous* method, a wire guide is passed through the brachial, femoral, or jugular veins to the superior or inferior vena cavae. A pacer wire is then threaded along the guide wire to the right side of the heart. Recently, balloon-tipped, flow-directed catheters have become available with pacer wires included. In all cases a subcutaneous wire should also be placed as a ground. Temporary pacing may also be instituted using esophageal pacing catheters. Since this is less commonly performed, it is not discussed further here.

The transthoracic method of wire insertion is quick but has more potential risks. Transvenous wires are generally thought to be safer, but they are not easily placed in small vessels and may present problems with early wire fracture if the child's extremity is not adequately restrained.

Emergency defibrillation. If the patient requires defibrillation, the pacemaker should be turned off first. If time allows, the wires should be disconnected from their terminals.

Electrical hazards. Exposed metal wire tips can provide low-resistance pathways for otherwise harmless current leakage directly to the heart. Many pacemakers have built-in shielding, and with the use of bipolar leads, most external interference will not affect pacemaker operation. If interference is too strong (e.g., during electrocautery), the pacemaker output will be suppressed.[67,95]

Nursing considerations.[67,95] All patients who are being paced should be on an ECG monitor. The nurse should ensure optimum ECG recording for best pacemaker function.

The pacemaker settings—rate, mode, and output—should be checked against the physician's orders and charted every 8 hours. Additionally, the sensitivity threshold must be checked every 8 to 24 hours per hospital policy or physician's order. If the child is pacer-dependent, pacemaker function should be checked hourly, and the ICU nurse should observe for competition, failure to capture, or pacemaker failure. ECG and strip recording should be included in the nurses' notes at least every 8 hours to verify proper pacemaker function.

Steps should be taken to ensure that pacemaker equipment is used safely. The wires and pacemaker should be covered with a rubber glove or other rubber material to protect them from moisture (especially during baths) or to prevent stray current leakage. The wires near the insertion site should be secured to prevent accidental dislodgment. The wire and cable connection at the pacer terminals should be checked to verify that the wires are held securely by the pacemaker clamps. In addition, the child should be restrained or the pacemaker unit and wires situated so that the patient cannot damage or alter the pacemaker system. Children with pacemaker wires require frequent chest films to determine if there have been wire fractures or fraying.[67,95] The external pacer unit should always have a "child-proof" cover so that the child will be unable to change the pacer settings.

∎ Defibrillation

Defibrillation is a technique used to deliver a single source of electrical depolarization to the myocardium to interrupt disorganized electrical activity and restore the automatic nature of cardiac impulses. This is achieved with two metal-plated contacts (paddles or adhesive patches) placed on the chest wall or directly on the heart.

Electrical circuitry of the defibrillator and paddles. Most defibrillators in use today have what is termed "output isolation," which means that the paddles have no connection with other grounded electrical circuitry inside the same instrument.[28] The electrical current, then, cannot travel through other conductive points. For example, a nurse who is touching a patient during the defibrillation or who is touching the defibrillator itself should not receive a shock (Fig. 9-31).

"Input isolation" is another valuable feature offered on most defibrillator models. An electrical "input," such as the patient cable to the monitor-defibrillator, is isolated from any circuits that lead back to ground so that stray electrical current will not flow through the patient.[28]

Defibrillator paddles usually come in two sizes—adult and pediatric—and many models have internal as well as external paddles. It is safest and most convenient to have an ECG monitor unit (including cable and electrodes) that comes equipped with a defibrillator or the option of a "quick-look" feature, in which paddles, when placed on the chest wall, will display an immediate ECG pattern on the scope.

A *synchronization* control allows cardioversion to be achieved. *Cardioversion* delivers an electrical impulse in synchrony with the patient's rhythm during early systole.[28] This is often used in attempting to convert a potentially threatening arrhythmia, such as

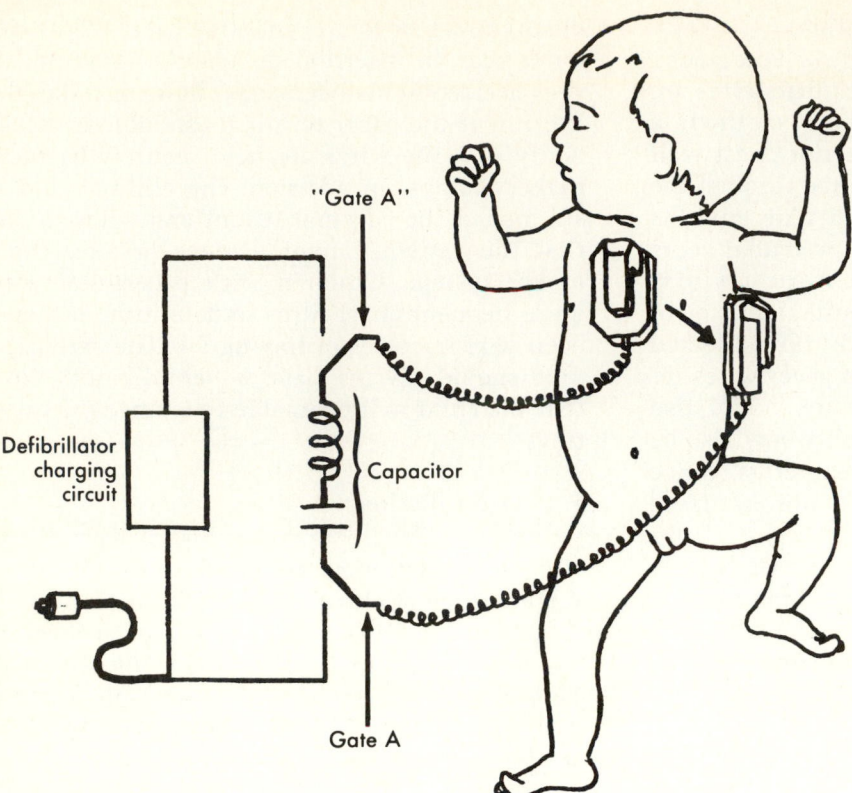

Fig. 9-31 Defibrillator circuit with output isolation. The defibrillator capacitor charges with "gate A" closed or *in line* with defibrillator. When the defibrillator is discharged, the gates swing forward (as shown) completing a circuit between the capacitor, cables, and patient. In this case there is no longer a connection with the charging circuit in the defibrillator. Therefore the current does not have an alternative pathway back to the defibrillator or ground, even if a nurse is touching the bed or instrument.

Modified from Higgins, S.: Defibrillation: what you should know, Redmond, Wash., 1978, Physio-Control Corp., p. 5. Drawing courtesy Physio-Control Corp.

atrial fibrillation or ventricular tachycardia, to a more normal rhythm.

Some units have a specific discharge control for the internal paddles, which is used for direct cardiac defibrillation during open thoracotomy. ICU nurses must be familiar with the use of this option so that they can respond quickly, should the need arise.

The energy select control on a defibrillator varies from unit to unit, usually within a range of 0 to 400 watt-seconds (or joules). For pediatric purposes, it is desirable to have energy selection available in small increments at the lower energy levels (e.g., 1-5-10-15-20-25-35-50-75-90 watt-seconds) to allow the operator to select the lowest but most effective defibrillator energy levels for small patients. The energy level most often recommended by the American Heart Association and others[58] for defibrillation of children is 2 watt-seconds/kg of body weight.

Factors determining success of defibrillation/ cardioversion. For cardioversion, ECG monitoring should always be done through the patient cable and electrodes and not through the "quick-look" paddles. The paddles may cause artifact, even with slight movements, which could be sensed by the monitor/

defibrillator and cause the defibrillator unit to discharge.

Some authorities discourage the use of gel or paste with defibrillator paddles in pediatric patients, but they recommend use of saline-damp 2×2 gauze pads. Since the child's chest is small, it is thought that paddles may slide with the gel as pressure on the paddles is applied to the chest wall. This, in turn, can cause potential "bridging" between the two paddles so that the current will flow from paddle to paddle. Skin burn may result, and the desired energy level may not be delivered to the myocardium. This concern supports the use of the new defibrillator pads (adhesive, pregelled patches) which, once applied, should provide a stable contact for defibrillation paddles.

Another difficulty in performing successful defibrillation occurs because of chest impedance. Chest impedance (resistance) to electrical current decreases with successive countershocks. If the same energy output from the defibrillator is maintained, the current delivered to the patient will increase slightly with each defibrillator discharge; the greatest increase occurs with the second shock. Therefore it is advisable to avoid increasing the selected defibrillator output too rapidly.[33]

The nurse should also be aware that if the patient's myocardium is ischemic or acidotic, it will not easily defibrillate. The patient should be adequately ventilated, chest massage must be performed perfectly (maintaining good perfusion), and adequate amounts of sodium bicarbonate must be given (if needed) before attempting defibrillation.

Patients receiving digitalis require adjustment of defibrillation and cardioversion joules. One recent study[32] suggests that digitalized cells demonstrate increased sensitivity to electrical stimulus. Cellular fibrillation occurs in circumstances when neither the electrical energy output of the defibrillator nor the serum digitalis levels would normally be expected to cause fibrillation. This suggests that extreme caution must be exercised if a digitalized patient requires cardioversion or defibrillation and that low electrical-shock energies should be used initially.

■ **Circulatory assist: the use of the intraaortic balloon pump**

Description. Technologic developments have recently enabled the use of the intraaortic balloon pump (IABP) in infants and children. Balloons ranging from 1 to 20 cc in volume are used (adult balloon capacity is 40 cc). The use of the intraaortic balloon

pump is not a common technique, but it is employed in a few major centers where pediatric open-heart surgery is done frequently.[65] The primary indication for use of this device in children is for support of left ventricular function that may be temporarily depressed following intracardiac surgery and for children with myocardiopathies. The balloon is placed in the aorta through a femoral artery cutdown. A sheath is patched from the skin to the artery, and the balloon catheter is then passed through this sheath.

Two specific effects of the intraaortic balloon pump are reduction of systemic afterload and augmentation of perfusion during diastole. Afterload reduction is accomplished by balloon deflation just before ventricular ejection; this leaves low volume space in the aorta. Because less left ventricular work is required to eject blood into an area of low blood volume, the ventricle should be more efficient. Diastolic augmentation is achieved because the balloon inflates during diastole displacing blood in the aorta. This blood is then forced back into the aortic root to augment coronary perfusion and into the systemic vessels to augment diastolic perfusion. (For detailed discussion of the physiologic basis of this device, refer to Schroeder.[71])

The problems of counterpulsation in children relate to their physiologic characteristics. Instrumentation is more difficult to accomplish because children have small vessels and because balloon sizes are not always predictable. Selection of the proper balloon size not only should be determined by the *diameter* of the vessel but by the *length* of the balloon within the aorta. If the balloon is too long, it may occlude the renal or mesenteric vessels that arise from the descending aorta.

Children exhibit greater aortic compliance than adults, and this may diminish the degree of augmentation achieved. Preliminary studies[86] have shown that diastolic augmentation may not be the essential effect of balloon-pumping in children and that afterload reduction may be the principal effect.

Increased heart rates in children necessitate a console with a sensitive mechanism that allows a "trigger" to be achieved from a rapid QRS signal. Additionally, the rapid heart rate demands a quick response gas flow in order to maximally inflate and deflate the balloon. Occasionally helium, rather than carbon dioxide, may inflate the balloon more effectively since it is a lighter gas. Preliminary work with the intraaortic balloon pump in children indicates that effective pumping is not achieved if the child's heart rate is faster than 150 to 160 beats/minute.[86]

Finally, the volume of gas needed for balloon

inflation in children is very small compared to adult models. Therefore the balloon console must be modified with a volume-limiting device placed between the console and the patient.

Potential complications. As with other invasive instrumentation, complications are observed that must be anticipated by the nurse caring for a child with an intraaortic balloon pump.[65,71] *Circulatory insufficiency* may occur in the catherized limb. This is the most frequent complication observed in children. *Platelet reduction* (up to 50%) is a frequent finding because of the mechanical action of the balloon as the blood flows around it. *Emboli* from the balloon, catheter, or graft may occur. Rare complications include *balloon rupture* and resultant gas (carbon dioxide or helium) embolism, *aortic damage* such as intimal lacerations or hematomas, and *hemolysis* caused by the mechanical action of the balloon.[71] *Infections* are also encountered with use of this device.

Nursing considerations. Specific responsibilities of the nurse caring for a child on an intraaortic balloon pump include:

1. Complete familiarity with the instrument and technique, including the ability to interpret cardiovascular measurements and the ability to maintain the console
2. Evaluation of the patient for the following complications: circulatory insufficiency in the catheterized limb, platelet reduction, emboli (gas or cell), aortic damage, hemolysis, or infections.
3. Documentation of counterpulsation waveform every 4 to 8 hours. The strip recorder should be run with the patient at a 1:3 (or less) balloon inflation frequency to patient QRS ratio, in order to be able to compare the augmented pulse pressure with the patient's inherent arterial waveform.
4. Attention to aseptic technique and possible sources of contamination. Dressing changes for the balloon insertion site should be performed daily. White blood cell counts should also be evaluated daily.
5. Maximum restraint of the child's catheterized leg. In order to avoid kinking the balloon catheter, the extremity must not be flexed.
6. Daily chest film for evaluation of placement of the balloon. The balloon should be located *below* the left subclavian artery but *above* the renal/mesenteric arteries.
7. Maintenance of anticoagulant protocol. Some balloons are composed of material that enhances fibrin formation. Therefore anticoagulation procedures may be recommended.

8. Provision of routine care, which should include the following:
   a. Respiratory therapy, including coughing/deep breathing, incentive spirometry, and chest percussion since immobilization may increase the risk of atelectasis or pneumonia
   b. IVs and fluid therapy, as indicated by hemodynamic and daily weight measurements
   c. Foley catheter care to minimize the risk of urinary tract infection
   d. Bed rest. Move patient by log rolling only, using measures such as sheepskin or air mattress to prevent bedsores.
   e. Daily blood sampling for laboratory analysis, including coagulation studies, cardiac enzymes, complete blood count with differential, electrolytes, urine and serum osmolality (to assess hydration), and blood gases as indicated

■ Contamination of vascular monitoring systems

A significant complication of invasive instrumentation is the risk of nosocomial infections. A recent report cites that 45% of all nosocomial infections are related to invasive lines and that one fourth of these may be attributed to infusion fluids, IV catheters (plastic), and monitoring devices. Donowitz[15] reports that 18% of the ICU population (n = 2441) develop nosocomial infections; this is in contrast to a 6% case rate in the non-ICU hospital population. In a recent study of 56 patients, Maki[49] concluded that 11.8% of 102 arterial infusion systems were contaminated and that 7.8% of these caused a bacteremia.

Most reports reveal a similar bacteriology profile. The bacteremias that result from invasive instrumentation are gram-negative rods, most notably *Pseudomonas* species (53.5%) and Seratia (27.9%), with gram-negative bacilli in the remaining cases.[75]

Risk factors for development of nosocomial infections include:

1. Plastic IV catheters. These are implicated in 8% of all bacteremias.[46,48] (Scalp vein needles are implicated less frequently.)
2. Cutdown versus percutaneous insertions. Cutdown insertion is associated with a higher incidence of infection.
3. Duration of time the IV remains in one site. After 2 to 3 days in the same site, there is an increased chance the IV will cause bacteremia.[20,46,48]
4. Failure to conform to aseptic technique during insertion.
5. Failure to clean and redress insertion sites with iodine ointment (this ointment may reduce rate of local infection).[36]

6. Motion of the catheter. This motion causes a shearing of the endothelium with fibrin clot formation. This is thought to be a significant factor in the pathogenesis of catheter-related phlebitis.[16]

7. IV fluids and lines. These are a recognized source of infection, and most notably support the growth of *Klebsiella* and *Pseudomonas* species. Acidic solutions such as glucose in water are more likely to cause phlebitis,[16] which seems to increase the risk of septicemia. Conflicting reports[10,14] about the efficacy of using 0.45 μg and 0.22 μg filters in-line to prevent phlebitis have led to a trend of eliminating filters except in situations where particulate matter could potentially be present.[22]

8. Transducer systems. These are a potential source of infection even with the recent use of disposable domes.[7] Walrath[90] reported a stopcock contamination rate of 48% (n = 46); however, bacteremias were infrequently associated with the stopcock contamination.

Precautions against infections with vascular monitoring. The risk of nosocomial infection is great with invasive monitoring, but measures may be taken to help reduce the incidence of such infections.

1. All administration sets and tubing of venous lines, including stopcocks and connectors, should be changed every 24 to 48 hours.[7,48]

2. More practically, all arterial and "heart" lines can be changed every 48 hours. (NOTE: Follow hospital standards regarding the changing of LA lines. The process of replacing new tubing may, in itself, increase the risk of an air embolus.)

3. Stopcocks should be cleaned with alcohol or Betadine every day to remove blood (blood in stopcocks provides a good medium for bacterial growth).

4. Because the use of glucose solutions in monitoring lines is associated with increased risk of some infections,[16,46] a 0.9% saline solution should be used for flushing whenever possible. However, since this may present a high sodium load to small children, one-half or one-quarter saline is an equally safe alternative. An added advantage of using saline in children's lines is that with saline monitoring, lines will not be contaminated with glucose so that accurate serum glucose samples can be obtained from the lines and repeated fingersticks or venipunctures may be avoided.

5. Pressure-monitoring systems should be stored empty rather than filled with flush solutions.

6. The space between the transducer head and dome should be filled with saline or bacteriostatic water, *never* with glucose-containing solutions

(some manufacturers recommend *only* the use of one or the other).

7. Elimination of stopcocks is desirable whenever possible. Stopcocks may be replaced with tubing or a T connector that has a rubber diaphragm sampling port for injection. This sampling port should be wiped with a Betadine swab and dry sterile gauze before sampling.

8. All IV insertion sites should be cleaned daily with the application of an antimicrobial or iodophor ointment and sterile dressing.[47]

9. After use, all transducers should be cleaned and disinfected with a chemical agent (or gas sterilized) and stored in a manner to prevent recontamination.

10. The hospital infection-control staff should evaluate the use of monitoring lines and IVs and periodically spot-check the ICU, obtaining cultures of the patients, the lines, and the staff. An ICU infection control nurse should periodically observe techniques of line insertion and catheter care. She can offer immediate feedback at this time and perhaps identify potential sources of contamination.

■ RESPIRATORY MONITORING

Respiratory monitoring is an important means of detecting respiratory distress and thus may avert the progression of distress to a critical state. The use of respiratory instrumentation warrants explicit discussion in order to enable the nurse to determine how to incorporate the monitoring system(s) within the scope of nursing care and how to use the devices safely.

■ Impedance pneumography

A common mode of respiratory surveillance uses impedance pneumography, a technique that monitors chest wall movement. This method records the changes in resistance of an electrical field (impedance) that occur with variations in thoracic volume. Impedance is measured by placing two electrodes on each side of the patient's chest. Most monitors have adequate filters that allow simultaneous ECG and respiratory monitoring with the same pair of electrodes (plus a "ground" electrode added for the ECG).[36,58] When the child's respiratory rate is monitored, a high and low rate alarm system is mandatory with an option of 10-, 15-, or 20-second apnea alarm intervals. Although there may be a high incidence of false-positive alarms, if the nurse readjusts electrode placement for maximum sensitivity to both ECG and respiratory pattern, the number of false-positive alarms should be diminished.

The primary problem with these monitors is that *all* chest movement activity is sensed by the device. If airway obstruction should occur, the child's (struggling) respiratory movements will continue to be demonstrated by the monitor even though air flow is significantly reduced. If a child requires close monitoring of his respiratory status, the nurse should never rely on this monitor alone for determination of effective respiratory function. Monitoring in this case should be augmented with expired or skin-surface (transcutaneous) CO_2 monitoring.

Another respiratory sensing device occasionally used is the "apnea mattress." This consists of an Isolette-size mattress or a small flat pad placed under the child's thoracic cavity. The pad senses respiratory movement in one of several ways: wire mesh in the pad measures the capacitance change caused by shifts in weight across the pad; air displacement in the mattress, caused by shifting movement, is sensed and transformed into an electrical signal; or voltage alterations, occurring in a coil inside the mattress are monitored.[42] All of these monitoring methods recognize artifact caused by excessive motion of the child. However, such motion will, in some models, trigger an alarm and frighten parents and visitors. If nurses must frequently respond to false alarms, they may develop a less vigilant attitude toward the alarm and patient. It is important to emphasize that many types of respiratory monitors indicate only the presence or absence of thoracic movement and will not provide the nurse with a reliable early warning of respiratory insufficiency.

■ **Spirometry**

Measurement of lung volume characteristics is accomplished by the use of spirometers. The limitations of spirometry in the pediatric population are related to either the device itself, which may not be able to measure the small lung volumes in infants, or to the measurement technique, which is effort-dependent, requiring a cooperative child who will follow instructions. In addition, the physical condition or mental attitude of the child may distort the measurements.

In the pediatric critical-care setting, spirometry is most frequently used to measure exhaled volumes of intubated children or of children on ventilators or to measure vital capacity of children with restrictive lung disease (such as Guillian-Barré Syndrome). How-

ever, spirometers that are used to measure "average" tidal volumes of intubated patients may provide falsely high data because of inherent limitations in most flow-measuring devices.[53]

Measurement of negative inspiratory-force pressures may be useful if respiratory muscle weakness is suspected; the expiratory pressure is specifically useful for providing quantitative data on the effective strength of a patient's cough reflex. These negative inspiratory-force pressures may be measured on school-age children who can cooperate by achieving their best maximum inspiratory effort (after an exhalation to a near residual volume) and their best maximum expiratory effort (exerted after a deep inhalation). A simple manometer or pressure gauge that can read both positive and negative pressures to about 100 to 150 mm Hg is required for these measurements. School-age children should be able to generate at least 30 mm Hg pressure on either inspiration or expiration.[43]

Other measurements, such as forced vital capacity, may be taken to assess and monitor pulmonary reserve. (The interested clinician is referred to Wade[87] and Lough[43] for further information.)

■ **Transcutaneous (skin surface)
oxygen pressure monitoring**

Definition. Transcutaneous (tc) oxygen pressure—$P_{tc}O_2$ or "skin surface"—monitoring is a noninvasive means of assessing the adequacy of tissue oxygenation and may yield more information about oxygen transport than the patient's arterial oxygen tension (PaO_2) or cardiac index alone. In pediatrics, measurement of mixed venous oxygen tension ($P\bar{v}O_2$) or cardiac output are not routinely performed (except in patients after open-heart surgery), so other means of assessing oxygenation must be used. The $P_{tc}O_2$ is measured by a heated electrode that is placed on the skin surface. The heat increases the capillary blood flow to the area, thus "arterializing" blood flow in the area. The sensor measures oxygen by one of two mechanisms[45]: measurement of oxygen that diffuses from the capillaries through the skin or measurement of oxygen at the skin surface itself.[45] The heat ranges of the electrodes vary (most commonly between 40° to 45° C), but the normal temperature is approximately 44° C.

A high correlation between PaO_2 and $P_{tc}O_2$ has been verified by many studies,* particularly when the

---

*References 8, 18, 19, 39, 45, 50.

range of Pa_{O_2} is 30 to 100 torr. These studies have also shown that patients may suffer significant periods of hypoxemia that are reflected by a fall in $P_{tc}O_2$ but are not demonstrated by intermittent Pa_{O_2} sampling. Frequently, these hypoxic episodes are related to nursing measures such as turning of the patient, vital signs measurement, dressing changes, suctioning, and chest physiotherapy.

Thick skin reduces the accuracy of the $P_{tc}O_2$ because it has fewer deep capillaries beneath a given site for a skin sensor. Therefore it offers more resistance to oxygen diffusion, and it has a high oxygen consumption; thus the sensor will receive less oxygen, and a deceivingly low $P_{tc}O_2$ measurement will result. Consequently, the transcutaneous electrodes should not be applied over areas of thickened skin (such as large scars or calluses). Additionally, the trunk is generally a better site than the extremities because vasoconstriction so commonly occurs in the limbs. The patient should never be positioned on top of a sensor since this may decrease local blood flow.

Although a reliable correlation between Pa_{O_2} and $P_{tc}O_2$ may seem dependent on adequate skin surface blood flow, recent studies[69,80,82,83] indicate that $P_{tc}O_2$ may indeed be a useful assessment tool for oxygen delivery in even low-flow states. A transcutaneous sensor measures the P_{O_2} through or at the cutaneous tissue and thus reflects the tissue P_{O_2} at that point. Since a shock state is characterized by low tissue oxygen levels because of hypoperfusion, one might expect a significant fall in $P_{tc}O_2$ while the Pa_{O_2} initially remains stable (the typical trend in shock).

In fact the relationship between $P_{tc}O_2$, Pa_{O_2}, and cardiac output have been documented in a somewhat predictive pattern: the $P_{tc}O_2$ no longer has a linear correlation with the Pa_{O_2} when the cardiac output falls to 65% of the control value.[81] Tremper et al.[82] report a high correlation between the Pa_{O_2} and $P_{tc}O_2$ levels when the cardiac index is greater than 1.54 L/minute.

Machine performance considerations. The electrodes must be replaced and moved to a new location on the child's trunk or extremities at regular intervals to avoid skin irritation and decreased electrode performance. Electrode performance is compromised by heat-induced edema or other changes at the electrode site. Microelectrodes, when heated to 44° C may require changing only every 6 hours, whereas large cathode electrodes require repositioning every 2 to 3 hours.[39]

Erythematous marks may occur at the electrode site, resulting from heat produced by the electrodes. Although these lesions may disturb the family and

staff, actual blisters (second-degree burns) seldom develop if the electrodes are changed as recommended. The erythematous sites usually disappear in several days to several weeks.

Unit calibration and skin-warming time varies from 7 to 25 minutes for each new position of the electrode. The nurse should consult the operator's manual for factory recommendations applicable to the specific unit.

Nursing considerations. Knowledge about the transcutaneous monitoring system is essential. The nurse should be especially aware of the following:
1. The correlation of measurements with the clinical condition of the patient
2. The calibration of the unit
3. The technique of skin preparation and electrode placement and the timing of electrode replacement
4. Recognition of electrical drift or other sources of machine error
5. Alarm systems
6. The procedures for troubleshooting

■ **Arterial oximetry**

Arterial oximetry is another method of measuring arterial oxygenation. An intraarterial electrode is threaded through an arterial line to the tip of the catheter. Clinical trials have showed the polarographic electrode to be accurate and effective, although a high incidence of electrode failure has been reported.[18] LeSoeuf et al.[39] compared the indwelling oximeter with a $P_{tc}O_2$ measuring device and reported moderately high correlations between the two. However, they did not verify the accuracy of the arterial oximetry with Pa_{O_2} measured by direct blood sampling using a conventional blood-gas machine.

The *advantages* of arterial oximetry include direct, continuous measurement of Pa_{O_2}, which is preferable to intermittent measurement. The indwelling electrode does not require repositioning.

The *disadvantages* of arterial oximetry include small vessel size in children; the possibility that the catheter may lodge against the arterial wall; the possibility of fibrin clots forming at the catheter tip; hemodilution of the patient (with hematocrits <30%), which may result in erroneous oxygen saturation measurements; and electrode failure to activate.

Further studies must evaluate the incidence of infection, thromboembolic events, and other potential complications of the indwelling arterial oximeter. Currently it is not a common monitoring mode since more research is required to verify the efficacy of the technique.

■ Transcutaneous (skin surface) carbon-dioxide pressure monitoring

Measurement of skin surface or transcutaneous carbon dioxide tension ($P_{tc}CO_2$ monitoring) may be a useful adjunct to the nursing care of children with acute or chronic respiratory disease. Several studies have verified high correlations between $P_{tc}CO_2$ and $PaCO_2$, with a predictable gradient between the two in children.[26,38,57]

Instrumentation. The $P_{tc}CO_2$ electrode, which is similar to the one used in standard blood gas machines, has the appearance of a small skin electrode. The sensor is often heated to 39° to 44° C to increase capillary blood flow, thus "arterializing" the blood flow beneath the electrode. Recent studies have showed, however, that the heat seems to be less essential for $P_{tc}CO_2$ than for $P_{tc}O_2$ monitoring.[8] The heat, in fact, is responsible for a predictable gradient between the $P_{tc}CO_2$ and $PaCO_2$ ($P_{tc}CO_2 > PaCO_2$) readings.[84] This gradient appears because CO_2 production (in the tissue) is increased by the heat, because heating the capillary blood beneath the sensor elevates the CO_2 (anaerobic temperature coefficient), and because a counter-current CO_2 exchange mechanism in the dermal loop maintains a higher PCO_2 at the tip of the loop (where the sensor lies).[45,84]

The schedule for rotation of electrode sites in skin surface PCO_2 monitoring should be strictly maintained. The erythematous marks caused by an electrode may last for hours or days after electrode removal but rarely leave scars. Many studies recommend a maximum 3 to 4 hour interval for each electrode placement,[38,84] but the nurse should check the manufacturer's recommendations for each electrode used.

Consistently good correlations between $PaCO_2$ and $P_{tc}CO_2$ make the transcutaneous carbon dioxide monitoring instrument a potentially invaluable tool in the pediatric ICU setting. It can reduce the number of arterial blood samples required and offers the distinct benefit of a continuous measurement during the course of all procedures and in response to all variables that could alter $PaCO_2$. The CO_2 electrode seems to be a reliable indicator of shock states (hypotension and decreased cardiac output). In Hansen's study[26] the correlation between $P_{tc}CO_2$ and $PaCO_2$ remained good in two infants who were acutely hypotensive with mean arterial pressures as low as 20 torr. Tremper et al.[84] reported similar findings in patients with poor systemic perfusion.

Predictive formulas have been developed that define the difference (gradient) between the $P_{tc}CO_2$ measurement and the $PaCO_2$. As stated earlier, the $P_{tc}CO_2$ will always be higher than the $PaCO_2$. Tremper[84] defines the gradient in stable patients as: $\Delta CO_2 = 23 \pm 2.7$ torr. This means that a patient with a $P_{tc}CO_2$ sensor in place, reading "64 mm Hg" probably has an $PaCO_2$ of $64 - 23 = 41 \pm 2.7$ torr.

Cabal et al.[8] report an even closer correlation and smaller $P_{tc}CO_2/PaCO_2$ gradient. In their study, using an unheated electrode in 25 newborns, the $P_{tc}CO_2$ was 9 torr higher than the $PaCO_2$ in normotensive infants. The clinician, then, can predict with confidence that if the $P_{tc}CO_2$ monitor reading is 50 torr, the $PaCO_2$ is 41 torr. Although further investigation is needed, it would seem that the unheated electrodes may provide a more stable reading of carbon dioxide than the heated sensors.

Nursing considerations. In some hospital units, nurses are required to draw an arterial sample for blood gas analysis after every electrode change, to compare the child's $PaCO_2$ with the concurrent $P_{tc}CO_2$. The nurse is then able, with the specific electrode and monitor, to estimate the gradient for that particular patient and monitoring system. In other hospitals these correlations are performed during clinical trials of equipment so that repeated clinical correlations are not required for every patient.

The nurse must be knowledgeable about the following aspects of the $P_{tc}CO_2$ monitor: procedure for machine calibration, technique of skin preparation and application of electrodes, recognition of signs of electrical drift or machine error, interpretation of measurements, procedures for troubleshooting, and alarm systems. One *disadvantage* of the instrument is that it is more delicate than the $P_{tc}O_2$ monitor and must be handled with greater care. Maintenance should include frequent observation of the fluid space in the sensor. Gain or loss of fluid will result in an erroneous $P_{tc}O_2$ measurement.

■ Monitoring of end-expiratory or end-tidal CO_2 ($P_{et}CO_2$)

Another indirect method for evaluating trends in $PaCO_2$ in an intubated child is with a device incorporated within the ventilator tubing that constantly measures carbon dioxide at end-expiration. End-expiratory, or $P_{et}CO_2$, may be measured by the use of a mass spectrometer or an infrared radiation module. The correct use of a $P_{et}CO_2$ device requires an evaluation of the patient's alveolar-arterial (A-a) CO_2 gradient. Studies performed on normal newborns demon-

Text continued on p. 703.

Table 9-5 Oxygen delivery systems[43,53]

Delivery system	Indications	Description	Advantages	Disadvantages
Aerosol tents ("croup" tents or mist tents)	Useful for children who do not require high or precise inspired O_2 concentrations but who need cool or warm aerosol	Clear plastic tent draped over frame that covers top portion of bed	Best used for *active* toddlers or children Some intubated children with tracheostomies, who do not tolerate a **T** piece connected to their tube, may tolerate the tent, but *they must be securely restrained to prevent extubation* (tongue-blade arm jackets, mittens, or other restraints may be used)	Difficult to establish and maintain specific inspired O_2 concentrations Can not reliably provide FIo_2 >0.4-0.5, although O_2 hoses may be placed inside the tent to "bleed in" more O_2 Difficult access to patient without interruption of O_2 delivery Patient may be difficult to see if humidification level in the tent is high A cool mist may cause markedly decreased body temperature, which increases the child's O_2 requirement
Isolette	Useful for smaller infants with temperature instability, who do not require precise inspired O_2 concentrations	O_2 piped into Isolette through the air-flow system	Frequently allows better visibility of *entire* patient than tents or hoods Stricter control of environmental temperature is possible if Isolette is not entered frequently	It is difficult to maintain uniform FIo_2 throughout Isolette because of air-current patterns and frequency of entering the Isolette If humidity is provided, microorganisms tend to develop in the Isolette—most notably *Pseudomonas*
Nasal prongs or cannula	Useful in children who require O_2 concentrations up to 0.50 and who are capable of nasal breathing	Vinyl catheter with two short prongs; one prong fits into each anterior nares; O_2 gas flow and humidity enter through each prong Maximum O_2 flow should not exceed 4-5 L/min	More comfortable than masks for many children Patient can eat and talk without altering FIo_2	If O_2 flow is too high, burning and drying of nasal mucosa can occur

Continued.

Table 9-5 Oxygen delivery systems—cont'd

Delivery system	Indications	Description	Advantages	Disadvantages
Nasal prongs or cannula—cont'd				Admixture may occur at different flow rates depending on patient's minute volume and mixing of O_2 with inspired room air in oropharynx Children who have upper respiratory disease may be mouth-breathing, which reduces effectiveness of this system
Head hood	Useful for an infant or small child who is too small for (or who will not tolerate) a mask	Clear Lucite or Plexiglass box placed over patient's head A removable lid or sliding ports provide quick access to patient Requires enough gas flow (7-12 L) to maintain O_2 concentrations and to flush CO_2 from hood through a port on cover FIo_2 may be >0.90	Provides easy visibility of and access to patient Allows quick recovery time of FIo_2 Hood provides large enough volume of replenished O_2 so that patient's entire tidal volume is taken from within hood Can be used in Isolettes, cribs, or open-warmers FIo_2 may be continuously monitored with an O_2 sensor placed inside hood	If aerosol is providing near 100% humidity in hood, child's face may be difficult to visualize, so assessment of color or respiratory effort may be impossible Loss of body heat can be significant in small infants if cool aerosol is used Extremely moist environment may cause skin irritation
Aerosol mask (connected to aerosol generator)	Useful for children who require an FIo_2 >0.40 and who are too large for a head hood	Simple vinyl face mask fits over nose and mouth Two open ports on each side of mask allow exhalation of CO_2 Patient may also draw in room air through ports if gas flow into mask does not meet peak inspiratory flow	Fairly comfortable for older children unless patient is acutely air hungry and struggling	Masks in general have the following disadvantages: Child cannot eat or drink without interrupting O_2 delivery If child vomits, this may not be easily seen through a mask and child may aspirate vomitus

Table 9-5 Oxygen delivery systems—cont'd

Delivery system	Indications	Description	Advantages	Disadvantages
Aerosol mask (connected to aerosol generator)—cont'd		Sufficient flow of gas must enter mask to prevent CO_2 accumulation Can be used to deliver almost any FIo_2 (see disadvantages)		FIo_2 is limited by child's minute ventilation (also tidal volume) Some children dislike masks and remove them repeatedly, making O_2 delivery inconsistent
Partial rebreather mask	Useful as above, depending on the child's size and tidal volume, since an FIo_2 of 0.60 or greater may be achieved The smaller the child's tidal volume, the higher the FIo_2 that can be achieved	Although the facepiece appears similar to a simple aerosol mask; a reservoir bag is added to mask O_2 is directed into the bag Child inhales gas from bag and may pull in room air through ports on the side of mask On exhalation, a certain percentage of exhaled gas (amount depends on size and tidal volume of child) goes back into reservoir bag; this initial exhalation gas represents the portion of tidal volume that remains in upper airway (dead-space ventilation) and is rich in oxygen and low in CO_2 This gas mixes with gas in reservoir bag and is inhaled on next breath Gas flow must be adjusted so that bag does not collapse during inspiration by more than a third of its volume	Can deliver higher FIo_2 concentrations in smaller children	As above FIo_2 may be variable if child's tidal volume changes

Continued.

Table 9-5 Oxygen delivery systems—cont'd

Delivery system	Indications	Description	Advantages	Disadvantages
Nonrebreathing mask	Useful as above Also for patients who require high FIo_2 concentrations	Face mask with reservoir bag attached Two valves are used: first valve, between the mask and bag, allows one-way gas flow from bag into the mask and prevents exhaled gas from flowing back into the bag; second valve, located at exhalation ports, is positioned so that when child inhales, valves are closed to prevent entrainment of room air On exhalation ports open to allow escape of exhaled air O_2 flow rate must be determined by patient's inspiratory demand	Can deliver an FIo_2 of 0.90 or more if mask fits snugly and gas flow is adjusted so that bag never collapses with inhalation	If mask fits very snugly, which it must do to achieve desired high FIo_2, patient can *only* breathe from bag (with a one-way gas flow); therefore nurse must prevent kinking of O_2 source tubing or disconnection of O_2 source tube Additionally, when a patient receives an $FIo_2 > 0.90$, he may develop atelectasis from alveolar nitrogen washout; thus patient should be encouraged to breathe deeply and cough frequently
Venturi mask (high air-flow O_2 enrichment)	Useful when very precise inspired oxygen concentration must be delivered	Vinyl face mask with an attached wide-bore cone containing an inner "jet" orifice *Diameter* of inner orifice, through which O_2 flows, may be altered to increase or decrease O_2 flow Air entrainment occurs on either side of this jet orifice to provide dilution (blending) of O_2 Venturi jets may be adjusted to deliver precise O_2 concentrations	Delivers a precise O_2 concentration Only rarely will FIo_2 delivered exceed amount intended (see disadvantages) These masks are good for those patients who require exact O_2 titration, such as those with chronic lung disease	Air entrainment ports can be occluded by bed linen, gowns, or patient position changes Patient can neither eat nor talk while wearing mask

Table 9-5 Oxygen delivery systems—cont'd

Delivery system	Indications	Description	Advantages	Disadvantages
Venturi mask (high air-flow O_2 enrichment)—cont'd		Flow rates associated with the most commonly required inspired oxygen concentrations are listed below (in approximate ranges)[5]:		

FI_{O_2}	O_2 FLOW
0.28	4-5 L
0.31	6 L
0.35	8 L
0.40	8 L
0.60	10 L

strate no significant difference between arterial and end-tidal CO_2 measurements. This is to be expected because normal newborns should demonstrate no significant A-aCO_2 gradient. Carbon dioxide in pulmonary capillaries should freely diffuse into the alveoli to be exhaled and measured as $P_{et}CO_2$. However, when newborns with hyaline membrane disease are tested,[64] a significant gradient of 13 torr was present between end-tidal and arterial CO_2 tensions. This gradient represents an A-aCO_2 gradient that results from impairment of CO_2 diffusion (from the blood into the alveoli) so that blood CO_2 tension is higher than alveolar or $P_{et}CO_2$ tension. Therefore $P_{et}CO_2$ measurements accurately reflect the patient's absolute Pa_{CO_2} only if no A-aCO_2 gradient is present. However, even if a gradient is present, $P_{et}CO_2$ measurements may still be useful as indicators of *trends* in the patient's Pa_{CO_2}.

The $P_{et}CO_2$ measuring device with an infrared radiation module may be purchased as part of the ventilator system or as a separate module. This analyzer measures expired CO_2 concentration, and thus alveolar ventilation may be estimated. Since carbon dioxide absorbs infrared radiation of specific wavelengths, as the rays are passed through the expiratory gas, a detector may then register the intensity of the radiation in the gas as a measurement of the CO_2 concentration.

Finer's study[19] of the use of the infrared analyzer in ten neonates demonstrated a high correlation between the Pa_{CO_2} and $P_{et}CO_2$. The correlation was best in infants who received muscle relaxants during mechanical ventilation.

When a constant $P_{et}CO_2$ analyzer is in use, the nurse must be aware of the principles of its operation. She must also be able to interpret the data produced, which requires an awareness of the relationship between the patient's alveolar or end-tidal and arterial CO_2 tensions. The nurse must be able to correlate results with the clinical status of the patient, she must be able to calibrate the instrument, and she must be aware of sources of instrument error. The *absolute value* of the CO_2 volume measured by the analyzer is usually not as important as the *trends* documented by this equipment.

∎ **Oxygen administration systems**

Oxygen is a commonly used and often overlooked therapy. Although oxygen may be administered in a variety of ways, it should always be treated as a drug, and dosage and patient response must be carefully documented. Table 9-5 is designed for the pediatric clinician who must assess and manage a child requiring supplemental oxygen. It describes types of oxygen delivery systems and their advantages and disadvantages (see also Fig. 9-32).

The nurse caring for the child receiving oxygen must monitor the oxygen delivery system as well as the child's response to therapy.

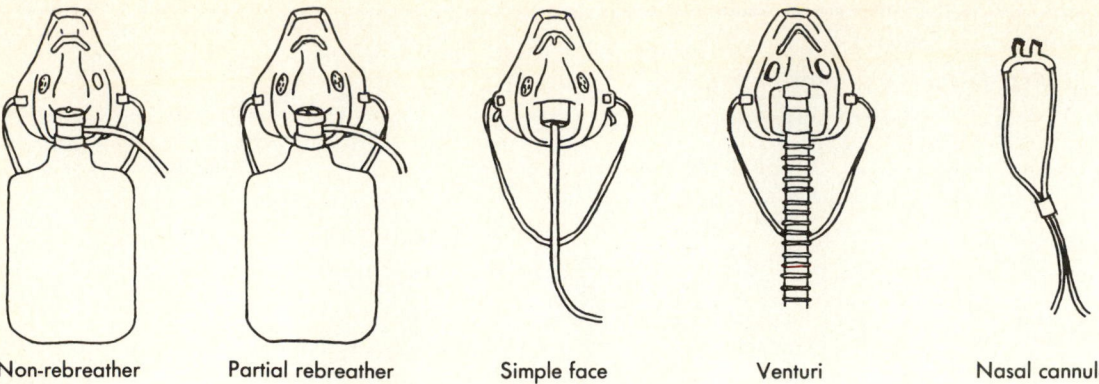

| Non-rebreather | Partial rebreather | Simple face | Venturi | Nasal cannula |

Fig. 9-32 Types of oxygen delivery masks. (See also Table 9-5 for description of each.)

Table 9-6   Examples of oxygen and air flow rates* required to blend specific inspired oxygen concentrations[53]

Total flow	Desired FIo$_2$	O$_2$ (LPM†)	Air (LPM)
20 LPM	0.25	1.25	18.75
	0.35	3.75	16.25
	0.45	6.25	13.75
	0.6	10.0	10.0
	0.8	15.0	5.0
15 LPM	0.25	0.93	14.0
	0.35	2.8	12.2
	0.45	4.7	10.3
	0.6	7.5	7.5
	0.8	11.25	3.75
10 LPM	0.25	0.6	9.4
	0.35	1.9	8.1
	0.45	3.1	6.9
	0.6	5.0	5.0
	0.8	7.5	2.5

*Formula for calculating flow rates: O$_2$ Flow $= \dfrac{\text{Total flow} \times (\text{FIo}_2 - 0.21)}{0.8}$
†LPM, Liters per minute.

Nursing considerations

1. Analyze inspired oxygen (FIO_2) frequently (many hospitals require continuous or hourly analysis). If O_2 drift is a problem, continuous analysis of the inspired concentration is usually indicated. (Table 9-6 provides a formula for calculation of inspired oxygen concentrations.)

2. Obtain blood gas analysis to document effectiveness of O_2 therapy, and verify with the physician the desired frequency of blood gas sampling for the particular child. Blood gas samples should be obtained 15 to 20 minutes after any change in FIO_2 has occurred.

3. Observe for changes in respiratory rate, effort, or color of the patient, and document these observations. Notify the physician of any clinical changes.

4. Ensure that the inspired oxygen is humidified and warmed unless otherwise directed by the physician.

5. Ensure that any tubing associated with the O_2 delivery system is changed daily to minimize the risk of nosocomial infection.

6. Keep infants and children dry. Frequent clothing and linen changes may be necessary. Monitor the child's temperature closely, particularly immediately after O_2 therapy has been initiated or if heated or cooled aerosol is used.

7. Assess for potential complications of oxygen therapy.[43,87]

   a. *Respiratory depression* may occur in the sedated patient or in the child with chronic lung disease in whom the basic respiratory drive may be hypoxia.

   b. *Atelectasis* may occur, particularly when 1.00 FIO_2 (100% O_2) concentration is being used. The alveoli are filled with oxygen and nitrogen is subsequently washed out. As oxygen is absorbed from the alveoli, atelectasis can develop.[5,87]

   c. *Substernal pain* occurs in patients who receive 1.00 FIO_2 for 6 hours, or 0.6 FIO_2 for 36 hours. The mechanism is not well understood but may be related to pulmonary endothelial damage.[5,87]

   d. *Pulmonary toxicity* tends to occur in patients who have received more than 0.5 FIO_2 for longer than several days and/or are receiving positive-pressure ventilation. Endothelial damage and alveolar epithelial damage occur and lead to fibrotic scarring and chronic lung disease.[5,87]

   e. *Retrolental fibroplasia* occurs in newborns and most frequently in the premature infant in whom retinal vessels are not fully developed. The initial effect of high PaO_2 is retinal vasoconstriction. New vessels, which grow into the vitreous, may then proliferate. These unusually permeable vessels may hemorrhage into the vitreous producing traction on the retina that may result in blindness.[5] Risk of retrolental fibroplasia is increased if high PaO_2 (>100 torr) is maintained during the newborn period.

■ Mechanical ventilation

Assisted ventilation is indicated for patients who are unable to maintain adequate oxygenation or normocapnia. These patients will generally exhibit clinical signs of respiratory failure (see Chapter 4).

Positive versus negative pressure ventilation. Two basic types of ventilation are used today—positive pressure ventilation or, more rarely, negative pressure ventilation.

Negative pressure ventilation. Negative pressure ventilation is an infrequently used technique that uses negative pressure around the child's chest to cause inspiration. This form of respiratory assistance may be the best mode of therapy in a few specific situations (e.g., when the child's lungs are normal but the respiratory effort is diminished, or for a child with respiratory failure caused by a neuromuscular disorder such as muscular dystrophy or Werdnig-Hoffmann disease). Previously, body-enclosing tanks, which sealed around the patient's neck, were used. More recently, however, smaller "shells," which are placed around the patient's anterior thorax, are available that offer much better patient accessibility and visibility.

The tank or shell that surrounds the thoracic area creates a negative force (with a vacuum unit) that "pulls" the thoracic cage outward, creating a pressure gradient between the mouth (atmospheric pressure) and the intrathoracic space that causes air to flow into the lungs. Expiration occurs passively when the vacuum cycles off. Negative pressures, typically of up to -60 cm H_2O, may be achieved with the tank.

Although these ventilators have the *advantage* of providing ventilatory support without patient intubation, there are some distinct *disadvantages* that limit their use: the tanks are cumbersome for the patient and caretakers, and they render the child virtually immobile. "Shell" devices must also be precisely the right size for the child's thorax in order to obtain a good seal. Another problem is that it is frequently difficult to achieve a good seal with either a tank or shell. This diminishes the effectiveness of the machine. Further, patients using a tank ventilator may suffer exaggerated dilation of the thoracic great vessels and diminished cardiac output. In addition, there is the possibility of venous pooling in the legs from the effects of negative pressure.

In spite of these problems, negative pressure ventilators are definitely useful for chronically ill patients and should be considered as a response to peculiar ventilatory problems that are refractory to more conventional management. Patients who are faced with chronic ventilator therapy at home may benefit because the quality of their daily lives can be improved by the elimination of the tracheostomy or endotracheal (ET) tube.

Positive pressure ventilation. Positive pressure ventilation is achieved by the use of a unit that delivers a gas flow (oxygen/air mix) to the patient's proximal airway. Normally, spontaneous inspiration occurs because negative pressure (relative to atmospheric pressure) is created when the thoracic cage expands, causing air to flow down the airways. It is as if a "vacuum" effect is occurring within the lungs to

---

CHARACTERISTICS OF AN IDEAL PEDIATRIC VENTILATOR[51,94]

Specifications

Volume or time cycled

Assist/control, control, IMV (intermittent mandatory ventilation), and spontaneous modes

Tidal volume range of 20-450 ml/breath (minute ventilation of 0.4-6 L/min)

Respiratory rate of 1-100/min (high-frequency ventilation capability is also desirable)

Variable inspiratory flow of 0.5-40 L/min

Variable inspiratory/expiratory flow ratios

Adjustable peak inspiratory pressure of 10-80 cm H_2O

Adequate humidification (with temperature Servo control)

Provision for PEEP/CPAP with minimal adjustments

Alarms

High and low pressure

Apnea

Loss of PEEP

Power failure/disconnect

Loss of air/O_2

High temperature

Failure to cycle

(Output jacks to allow ventilator alarms to be connected to a remote alarm in nursing station)

Visual indicators

Proximal airway pressure (measured at patient airway)

Proximal airway temperature (measured at patient airway)

F_{IO_2}

Inspiratory/expiratory times

Inspiratory to expiratory ratio

Flow rate (L/min)

Tidal volume

"pull" the air down into the alveoli. Expiration in this case is, normally, a passive process. Positive pressure ventilation reverses the physics of ventilation so that gas is forced down the airway with positive pressure from the machine, creating *positive* pressure within the thoracic cage during inspiration (see Chapter 4 for a more detailed discussion of ventilatory physics).

The types of ventilatory units available may be classified according to their inspiratory cycling mechanism—specifically, by the manner in which inspiration is *terminated*. *Volume-cycled* ventilators are preset to deliver a specific tidal volume during inspiration. Once this volume is delivered, the ventilator cycles off, allowing exhalation. *Pressure cycled* ventilators use a preset peak-inspiratory pressure (PIP) during inspiration, without regard for the amount of volume delivered. *Time-cycled* ventilators are preset for a specific inspiratory time, without regard for the volume delivered or the peak pressure achieved.

Most ventilators use a combination of cycling mechanisms; for example, the Babybird* or Bourns BP200 are *time cycled* and *pressure limited*. Many volume ventilators, such as the BEAR II (Bourns†) incorporate pressure limiting and timing mechanisms.

Most pediatric patients requiring ventilatory assistance are placed on positive pressure ventilators. Selection of the appropriate ventilator should take into consideration the following factors[51,94]:

1. The size of the child and minute ventilation required
2. Lung compliance. If the patient requires high-inspiratory pressures (>40 cm H_2O), specific pressure ventilators may be required.
3. Rapidly changing lung compliance. Such changes in compliance may demand a volume cycled ventilator (or a combination volume/time cycle) for optimum ventilation.
4. Flail chest or median sternotomy incision complications. If a child has an unstable chest wall as a result of these conditions, volume cycled ventilators may be most appropriate.

The box opposite presents three categories of criteria for selection of the ideal ventilator for pediatric use. Frequently, hospitals find themselves in the dilemma of choosing ventilators that are appropriate for the greatest number of patients rather than buying a large number of different ventilators, each of which is suitable for only a small group of patients. When

*Bird Corp., Palm Springs, CA 92262.
†Bourns, Inc. Life Systems Division, Riverside, CA 92503.

considering the selection of ventilators for the pediatric ICU, the following information may be useful.

Many adult volume ventilators may not be capable of providing a tidal volume of ≤100 cc without generating high peak inspiratory pressures because of a wide inherent range of machine flow rates available, high internal equipment resistance to a flow, and large apparatus dead space. On the other hand, neonatal time- or pressure-cycled ventilators may not provide a high enough flow rate to deliver adequate tidal volume and minute ventilation to the larger infant or child. Manufacturer's specifications and recommendations and clinical trials should be used to determine the maximum size of a child to be satisfactorily ventilated with each specific neonatal ventilator (the patient size limit for use of neonatal ventilators is generally 12 to 15 kg body weight).

The clinical condition of the patient will indicate which specific ventilator functions are needed to provide optimum ventilation. Table 9-7 offers comparative specifications on current, standard ventilators. Since there is not enough space in the table to incorporate all available ventilator specifications and models, the units included will provide a model of information that is important in the selection of any ventilator.

The clinician must not fail to maintain a vigilant attitude toward the respiratory assessment of the child just because the child is receiving mechanical ventilation. Constant monitoring of the ventilator settings and the adequacy of the child's ventilation is necessary. *When ventilatory function is in doubt, the child should be manually ventilated with a hand-resuscitator bag*. Table 9-8 offers a troubleshooting guide for the nurse to use when there are problems with the patient's mechanical ventilator. It is intended to address *equipment* problems that may be manifested by clinical signs in the child. (For further related information refer to Chapter 4.)

■ **Endotracheal tubes**

ET intubation may be necessary to manage the child with a variety of respiratory disorders such as those discussed in Chapter 4.

Cuffed versus uncuffed tubes. Tubes used in children up to 8 years of age should generally be uncuffed since the cricoid diameter of a child is quite narrow and will provide a natural seal. Cuffed tubes in these children may produce pressure on the tracheal wall, causing tissue damage.[42] Occasionally a child will require administration of high inspiratory pressures and will need a low-pressure cuffed tube.

Text continued on p. 721.

Table 9-7 Comparison of ventilator specifications[51,53,60]

Parameter	Time-cycled ventilators (Pressure-limited)			
	Babybird	**Siemens Servo 900B**	**Bourns BP200 infant**	
Patient-ventilator modes	IMV; spontaneous (CPAP); control	Assist, IMV (with f*/2, f/5, f/10, and 0 setting for spontaneous breathing)	IPPB/IMV, off-alarm test, CPAP inspiratory plateau	
Rate	0-100 variable (depends on I:E ratio)	6-60 breaths/min on assist or control mode (divide by 2, 5, or 10 on IMV mode)	Rate setting available from 1-60 breaths/min	
Volume	Variable (depends on inspiratory time and flow)	Preset inspiratory minute ventilation (V_E) 0.5-30 L; tidal volume = V_E/Rate	Variable	
Inspiratory time	0-3 sec	Five possible fixed inspiratory times—15%, 20%, 25%, 33%, and 50%—set as a percentage of the total respiratory cycle in conjunction with pause time	0.2-5.0 sec	
Expiratory time	0.4-10 sec	Dependent on preset inspiratory time and pause time	Internally preset minimum 0.45-0.55 sec for exhalation	
I:E ratio	Variable	Set by inspiratory time control at 4:1-1:6 (must use both inspiratory time control and pause time control to achieve the inverse ratio)	4:1-1:10	
Peak inspiratory flow	0-30 L/min	Inspiratory flow (constant flow pattern) is calculated by the formula: inspiratory minute volume/inspiratory time percentage (accelerating, decelerating, and constant flow patterns are possible)	0-20 L/min	
FIo₂	0.21-1.00 (±.3)	0.21-1.00 (±.3)	0.21-1.00 (±.3)	
PEEP/CPAP	0-20 cm H_2O	Maximum of 20 cm H_2O (but another option is available to achieve a PEEP of 50 cm H_2O)	0-20 cm H_2O (depending on flows used)	

Information on this table was derived from individual manufacturer's specifications: Martz,[51] McPherson[53], and Mushin.[60]
*f, Frequency per minute.

Volume-cycled ventilators		Mixed volume-cycled and pressure-cycled ventilator
Bennett MA-1	**BEAR II**	**Bourns LS104-150 infant**
Control, assist, IMV, CPAP assist/control	Control, assist/control, IMV, CPAP, SIMV	Assist, control, assist/control, IMV, assist control ÷ 10
On IMV mode 1 breath/3 min to 60 breaths/min (on assist/control)	5-60; (or 0.5-6 with ÷ 10 switch)	5-80 breaths/min (or 1 breath/2 min up to 8 breaths/min with a ÷ 10 mode)
Preset to 2200 ml	100-2000 ml	5-150 ml
Can be calculated	Can be calculated	Can be calculated
Can be calculated	Can be calculated	Can be calculated
Visible alarm if <1:1 ratio; the I:E ratio is a function of rate, volume, and peak flow	On-off selection: if "on," 1:1 ratio is set and inspiratory phase will stop when half of cycle time (set by rate) is reached; when "off," any I:E ratio may be achieved	Variable
10-100 L/min at 0 cm H_2O pressure (0-75 L/min at 40 cm H_2O + inspiratory pressure)	20-120 L/min	CPAP and IMV: 0-20 L/min; assist/control: 25-200 ml/sec
0.21-1.00 (±.3)	0.21-1.00 (±.3)	0.21-1.00 (±.3)
0-15 cm H_2O (Negative end-expiratory pressure [NEEP] is also available for generating pressures to −9 cm H_2O)	0-30 cm H_2O	0-20 cm H_2O

Continued.

Table 9-7 Comparison of ventilator specifications—cont'd

Parameter	Time-cycled ventilators (Pressure-limited)		
	Babybird	**Siemens Servo 900B**	**Bourns BP200 infant**
Inspiratory-pressure–control relief valve	Yes—preset by operator	Can be set at 10-100 cm H_2O	Can be set at 10-80 cm H_2O
Inspiratory time limit control	0.4-2.5 sec	Inspiratory time is limited to a *maximum* of 80% of the respiratory cycle (inspiration + pause) when the machine cycles off	0.2-5 sec
Inspiratory hold	Inspiratory plateau	Pause-time control is an end-inspiratory pause or "inflation hold" (the time is 0%-30% of the total respiratory cycle)	Plateau duration is affected by inspiratory time (breathing rate and I:E ratio controls) and flow rate
Sigh	No	On-Off selection: when "on," a double tidal volume is delivered every 100 breaths	No
Expiratory retard	Not listed	2-100 L/min retard on expiratory flow; if patient expiratory flow is lower than preset limit, expiratory valve will be fully open	Not listed
Adjustable sensitivity (patient-assist effort)	No	−20-+45 cm H_2O (if patient on PEEP, sensitivity must be adjusted to the positive range)	No
Manual ventilatory override	No (a bag that can be used for manual ventilation is incorporated within the circuitry)	No	Only in CPAP mode
Humidification	Continuous, controllable nebulization	Humidifier and Servo-controlled temperature monitor available options	Does not provide continuous nebulization but does provide continuous heated humidifier

Volume-cycled ventilators		Mixed volume-cycled and pressure-cycled ventilator
Bennett MA-1	**BEAR II**	**Bourns LS104-150 infant**
Can be set at 20-80 cm H_2O (a backup relief valve is also incorporated, which opens at 85 cm H_2O)	Can be set at 0-100 cm H_2O	Can be set at 0-100 cm H_2O, adjustable by either the high-pressure alarm (pop-off) or positive-pressure limit
No	No	Can be calculated
Can give a plateau by manipulating the expiratory retard button	0-2 sec	0-2 sec
100-2200 ml; 1, 2, or 3 sighs at 4-15 times/hr	150-3000 ml; 0-100 cm H_2O pressure; 1, 2, or 3 sighs at 2-60 times/hr	A sigh at 1-9 times/min at 2 times the tidal volume or "off"
Yes	No	No
0.1-10 cm H_2O	"Less to more": with range of 50 msec response time, patient displaces 10 ml gas creating -1 cm H_2O pressure, or patient displaces 50 ml gas creating -6 cm H_2O pressure	-0.05 cm H_2O to -1 cm H_2O
Manual sigh and manual normal (breath) buttons	Single (normal) breath or single sigh buttons	In assist mode, the single sigh button may be pushed to initiate a respiratory cycle
Heated humidifier, with no Servo-control present for inspired air temperature	Nebulizer with on-off selection, heated, with bacteria filter	Heated humidification or continuous controllable nebulization

Continued.

Table 9-7 Comparison of ventilator specifications—cont'd

| Parameter | Time-cycled ventilators (Pressure-limited) | | |
	Babybird	Siemens Servo 900B	Bourns BP200 infant
Alarms	(No built-in alarm system—must be added) Low-pressure alarm for (1) operating pressure < preset value or (2) pressure in O_2 blender <45 psi Inspiratory time limit control to back up inspiratory time function if a low operating pressure occurs—spontaneous mode results Overpressure/obstruction alarm	Lower expired minute ventilation limit, which serves as a disconnect, pressure failure, and apnea alarm (if spontaneous breathing mode is selected) and is functional in all modes Upper expired minute ventilation limit, which warns that minute volume has exceeded preset limit 2-min reset alarm, which silences lower and upper limit alarms for 2 min (to allow for suctioning) but permits visual indicator to continue to flash High airway pressure alarm, adjustable from 15-100 cm H_2O Electrical power disconnect alarm	Power failure or disconnect alarm Low-pressure alarm (air or O_2) High temperature electrical shutoff alarm (not integral to ventilator but optional accessory)
Visual indicators	Operating pressure gauge Proximal airway pressure gauge Flow rate gauge No visual indicators for respiratory rate or I:E ratio	*Lights:* IMV, airway pressure, trigger level, 2-min reset, power, upper and lower volume alarm limits with 2-min reset *Gauges:* airway pressure, expired minute volume, working pressure, minute ventilation—controls are all visible on front of ventilator *Additional features:* other monitors available to calculate lung mechanics such as compliance or inspiratory resistance (Servo 940); CO_2 analysis of expired gases as well as CO_2 measurements also options, central monitoring capability with alarms (available with unit 910) for monitoring volumes on patients Battery option for transport is available	*Lights:* power pilot light Insufficient expiratory time light that indicates incompatible ventilator settings, which do not allow an exhalation phase of at least 0.5 sec; inspiratory time light, which indicates the inspiratory time limit has been reached Airway temperature (≥104° F) light (not integral to ventilator but available as an accessory) *Gauges:* air inlet pressure gauge, O_2 inlet pressure gauge, proximal airway pressure gauge

Volume-cycled ventilators		Mixed volume-cycled and pressure-cycled ventilator
Bennett MA-1	**BEAR II**	**Bourns LS104-150 infant**
Low-volume and low-rate alarm on spirometer	Low inspiratory pressure alarm	High- and low-pressure
Rate alarm	Minimum exhaled volume alarm	Patient apnea alarm (if unit is in *assist* mode); however, if rate meter falls to 60% of the rate control setting for 10 sec, the unit converts to the *control* mode for 5 sec and then reverts to the assist mode unless unit alarm recurs
O_2 supply	PEEP alarm	
Power disconnection	Apnea alarm (machine and patient)	Airway temperature ($\geq 104°$ F) alarm (not integral to ventilation but optional accessory)
High-pressure/pressure relief alarm	Ventilator inoperative alarm	
Lights: assist, sigh, inadequate oxygen supply pressure	*Gauge:* proximal airway pressure gauge	Gauges: air-inlet pressure gauge, O_2-inlet pressure gauge, proximal airway pressure gauge, flow control, rate meter, volume-selected meter
High proximal airway pressure indicator	*Digital monitors:* minute ventilation, exhaled volume, rate, I:E ratio (if *flashing* means the I:E is >1:10)	
	Lights: power on, standby, alarm silence; nebulizer "on"; mode-control: assist, control, SIMV, CPAP; rate ÷ 10; inspiratory source (mode), i.e., spontaneous, control-assisted, sigh	

Continued.

Table 9-7 Comparison of ventilator specifications—cont'd

| Parameter | Time-cycled ventilators (Pressure-limited) | | |
	Babybird	Siemens Servo 900B	Bourns BP200 infant
Disadvantages	Complicated system with many components and many potential sites for inadvertent disconnections and air leaks; can only be used for respiratory rates up to 100; ventilator may not be capable of ventilating children larger than 12-15 kg, depending on the required flow rates; no digital readouts to check ventilator settings unless Bourns alarm adaptor is added; humidification system is not heated	Costly; minute ventilation must always be changed when respiratory rate is altered if tidal volume is to remain the same	Electrically driven—possible problem in the event of a power failure; no emergency manual resuscitator; does not provide continuous nebulization; with high flows may be difficult to avoid creation of PEEP

Table 9-8 Troubleshooting guide for problems with mechanical ventilators*

Machine observation	Patient observation	Causes	Treatment
High peak pressures observed on gauge; high airway pressure indicated by alarm sounds	Agitation/fighting ventilator, anxiety Sudden change in clinical appearance, particularly development of pallor or cyanosis	Displacement of ET tube by extubation or movement to a mainstem bronchus (If child can phonate around tube, it is no longer in place)	Manually bag-ventilate patient; assess chest movement, auscultate breath sounds, and assess lung compliance Suction patient Notify physician if patient does not immediately improve or if abnormal findings are noted, such as decreased breath sounds

*Although this table is designed to troubleshoot machine problems, the reader should note the "Patient observation" column and refer to other chapters for more detailed information on patient (clinical) problems. In all cases, if a sudden change is observed in the ventilator or in the appearance of the patient, the nurse should immediately remove the patient from the ventilator, manually bag-ventilate the patient, and *call for help!* Do not further compromise the patient by ignoring him while investigating the equipment problem. NOTE: With many ventilator problems, the nurse will note that the corresponding "Patient observation" is "agitation," "anxiety," or "restlessness." These signs require a *thorough* investigation of the cause of such restlessness. Frequently, it is erroneously assumed that the child needs restraints and/or sedation. Hypoxia or changes in the Paco$_2$ may cause such symptoms, and the source of the clinical problem may be the ventilator system.

Volume-cycled ventilators		Mixed volume-cycled and pressure-cycled ventilator
Bennett MA-1	**BEAR II**	**Bourns LS104-150 infant**
Inspiratory and expiratory times cannot be set; frequently difficult to establish ventilation on infants/small children because the flow rate cannot be decreased enough to fix the correct tidal volume; spirometer must be used to measure exhaled volume	Exhaled volume indicator is not accurate when using an uncuffed ET tube (a spirometer must be used to measure exhaled volume); may be difficult to use on small infants or children since the flow may not be low enough to accommodate the smaller tidal volume/min ventilation required by small patients	Difficult to wean sensitive patients because the rate increments are in groups of 5 breaths/min; pressure relief popoff valve is placed in back of unit, PEEP/CPAP are controlled from back (pressure bleedoff in back); many costly accessories are necessary; humidifier awkward to fill

Table 9-8 Troubleshooting guide for problems with mechanical ventilators—cont'd

Machine observation	Patient observation	Causes	Treatment
High peak pressures observed on gauge; high airway pressure indicated by alarm sounds—cont'd			If unilateral diminished breath sounds are noted, the following steps should be taken: 1. While one person *slowly* withdraws ET tube (0.5-1 cm), another listens for improvement of breath sounds (if hospital policy permits) 2. If breath sounds improve retape tube in new position 3. Order stat chest radiograph and obtain arterial blood gases per physician order or unit policy

Continued.

Table 9-8   Troubleshooting guide for problems with mechanical ventilators—cont'd

Machine observation	Patient observation	Causes	Treatment
High peak pressures observed on gauge; high airway pressure indicated by alarm sounds—cont'd		Pneumothorax	Manually bag-ventilate patient, assessing breath sounds and symmetry of chest excursion (watch for improvement in color with manual ventilation)
			If arterial line is in place, observe for pulsus paradoxus on the oscilloscope
			Order stat chest radiograph and call physician if no improvement occurs (per unit policy)
			Transilluminate infants to check for free air in chest
			Prepare for chest tube insertion or needle aspiration of air
		Ventilator support inappropriate (e.g., tidal volume, O_2 flow supply, I:E ratio) or patient's lung compliance may have changed (requiring changes in ventilatory support)	Manually bag-ventilate patient, and reassess patient thoroughly
			Recheck ventilator settings, and observe inspiratory times, flow rates, volumes, etc.
			Notify physician if clinical status does not improve when patient is manually ventilated or if deterioration occurs when child is placed back on ventilator (call physician also to reevaluate ventilator settings)
			Obtain arterial blood gases per physician order or unit policy
		Coughing or plugged ET tube, thick secretions (may be present as a result of inadequate humidification of inspired air)	Manually ventilate patient and suction
			Assess chest expansion, lung aeration, lung compliance

Table 9-8 Troubleshooting guide for problems with mechanical ventilators—cont'd

Machine observation	Patient observation	Causes	Treatment
High peak pressures observed on gauge; high airway pressure indicated by alarm sounds—cont'd			If breath sounds are diminished, if suctioning and bagging do not help, if chest excursion is diminished, and if pneumothorax is *not* suspected, pull ET tube, and mask-ventilate patient
			Notify physician *immediately*
			Check humidification system if other problems are ruled out
		Ventilator tubing kinked or obstructed	Manually ventilate patient
			Check all tubing for water collection and/or kinking
		Inadequate humidity or irritation of airways	Manually ventilate patient
			Assess patient; if other, more serious, problems are ruled out (e.g., extubation), check ventilator settings and humidification system
		Patient anxiety	Manually ventilate patient
			Reassess patient as above including assessment of arterial blood gases
			Reassure patient and maintain good verbal contact
			With older children, use of picture boards, alphabet boards, or grease boards for writing may increase the child's ability to communicate, thus alleviating some anxiety
			Sedation may be necessary if optimum ventilation cannot be achieved and if hypoxia is ruled out as cause of anxiety

Continued.

Table 9-8 Troubleshooting guide for problems with mechanical ventilators—cont'd

Machine observation	Patient observation	Causes	Treatment
High peak pressures observed on gauge; high airway pressure indicated by alarm sounds—cont'd	Patient's respiratory effort not synchronized with the ventilator (there may be a deterioration in patient's arterial blood gases)	Obstructed ET tube Pneumothorax Inadequate ventilatory support (e.g., inappropriate flow rate, I:E ratio) Patient anxiety Change in blood gases (e.g., low Pao_2 or high $Paco_2$) may increase the patient's respiratory drive	Manually ventilate patient Assess patient carefully (chest expansion, aeration, etc.) Recheck ventilator settings Notify physician of change in patient's clinical condition Check arterial blood gases (and possibly, chest radiograph) per unit policy
Decreased peak inspiratory pressure	Deterioration in patient's clinical appearance: poor color, decreased chest excursion, audible leak around ET tube	Altered ventilator settings Disconnected tube in the ventilator-patient circuit Extubation Leak around ET tube caused by improper tube size, inadequate cuff inflation, or malposition of tube (children <8-10 yr require an ET tube without a cuff because of airway anatomy) NOTE: A *mild* leak around the tube when peak inspiratory pressure is ≥30 cm H_2O verifies that the tube size is not too large for the child's airway Leak in exhalation tubing	Manually ventilate patient Assess respiratory status, including chest movement, aeration, lung compliance; observe for leak around ET tube during peak inspiration; check ET tube cuff pressure Check ventilator system for flow rate, peak inspiratory pressure setting, I:E ratio, tidal volume provided by ventilator, sensitivity, adequate humidification Call physician if patient has not improved with manual ventilation Consider obtaining arterial blood gases (and, possibly, chest radiograph) if patient does not immediately improve with manual bag-ventilation.
	Improved patient condition—color pink, chest excursion improved, breath sounds clearer	Lung compliance improved with resolution of medical problem	No treatment

Table 9-8 Troubleshooting guide for problems with mechanical ventilators—cont'd

Machine observation	Patient observation	Causes	Treatment
Decreased tidal volume delivered by ventilator	Decreased chest excursion A change (deterioration) in patient's clinical appearance such as pallor, cyanosis, decreased level of consciousness	Altered ventilator settings, including decreased volume, flow rate, PIP limit, and I:E ratio (see pneumothorax earlier in table)	Manually ventilate patient Assess respiratory status as described above Notify physician of observed abnormalities or changes in patient's condition Evaluate ventilator system
Increased tidal volume delivered by ventilator	There may or may not be change in chest expansion, depending on lung compliance (C_L): if there is increased C_L, chest excursion will be noticeably increased; if there is decreased C_L, chest excursion may not change Change in respiratory rate With hyperventilation, a decreased Pa_{CO_2} (and increased pH) may be observed; with severe hyperventilation (and severe hypocapnia), twitching, tetany and carpopedal spasm may occur	Increased C_L may mean lung function is improving	Check all ventilator settings Evaluate patient's ventilatory requirements, and readjust machine accordingly Obtain blood gases (per unit policy) NOTE: If tidal volume delivered by ventilator has increased markedly with a concurrent increase in patient's chest excursion and aeration, it might be prudent to manually ventilate patient in order to minimize risk of a pneumothorax
Change in the PEEP/CPAP delivered	Patient may be agitated Patient's spontaneous respiratory rate may exceed the ventilator rate Patient's own inspiratory pressure may be strong enough to override the PEEP with each breath	Change in lung compliance or tidal volume (if there is inadequate ventilatory support, patient may demonstrate spontaneous respiration since a rise in patient Pa_{CO_2} increases respiratory drive) If an external CPAP device is used evaporation of H_2O may decrease CPAP provided by the system; disconnection of tubing may also cause loss of CPAP Accidental change in PEEP/CPAP settings	Check all ventilator settings and ventilator system Reassess patient and note respiratory rate, chest excursion, aeration, breath sounds Consider increasing machine gas flow rate to maintain level of PEEP (if PEEP is too low) Patient may better tolerate the IMV mode Check humidification system

Continued.

Table 9-8   Troubleshooting guide for problems with mechanical ventilators—cont'd

Machine observation	Patient observation	Causes	Treatment
Change in the PEEP/CPAP delivered—cont'd		Increase or decrease in condensation of H_2O within tubing	
I:E ratio alarm (frequently associated with high-pressure alarm)	Patient may be fighting or anxious Clinical condition may or may not change	Inadequate inspiratory flow provided by ventilator Accidental change of ventilator settings Inappropriate ventilator sensitivity to patient's respiratory effort Increased airway secretions Subtle leaks in system	Manually ventilate patient Assess patient chest excursion, lung aeration, and color, and notify physician of deterioration in clinical condition Check all ventilator settings including flow rate, respiratory rate, and tidal volume Suction ET tube Obtain arterial blood gases if patient's condition warrants
Drift in inspired oxygen (FIo_2) provided by ventilator	Patient may or may not exhibit clinical changes (e.g., in color, respiratory rate, general mental alertness)	O_2 analyzer error Blender error O_2 source error O_2 reservoir leak	If patient has deteriorated, manually ventilate and ensure tube patency Calibrate O_2 analyzer Check O_2 systems and correct dysfunction
Increased or decreased condensation in ventilator tubing—water flows to patient rather than H_2O trap (if water collection is significant PEEP/CPAP may increase)	Patient may have thick secretions (with rising peak respiratory pressure) Patient may exhibit copious, thin secretions, requiring frequent suctioning	Too much or too little H_2O in humidifier Ventilator tubing arranged so that the H_2O traps are *elevated* rather than in a *dependent* position Temperature of inspired air may be inappropriate Tubing may be resting on cooling mattress (resulting in condensation of H_2O caused by cooling)	Check humidifier system and temperature Reposition ventilator tubing so water traps are at lowest point in tubing system Check temperature of inspired air Lift tubing off cooling mattress using pad or linen roll
Inspired gas temperature inappropriate	Patient's temperature may be increased or decreased Patient may be agitated	Addition of cold water to humidifier Thermostat failure Altered thermostat settings	Check temperature of infant and treat accordingly Wait for humidifier water to warm if child can tolerate the delay

Table 9-8 Troubleshooting guide for problems with mechanical ventilators—cont'd

Machine observation	Patient observation	Causes	Treatment
Inspired gas temperature inappropriate—cont'd	Secretions may be too thick or copious or too thin	Warming or cooling of inspiratory ventilator tubing by radiant warmers, heating mattress, or cooling blanket	Replace heater Correct thermostat settings Prevent inspiratory tubing from direct contact with or exposure to heating or cooling equipment

The ET tube is the appropriate size if it easily passes through the vocal cords and if a small, audible air leak is present when inspiratory pressures of approximately 30 cm H_2O are reached. This small leak indicates to the nurse that the tube is probably small enough to avoid undue pressure on the trachea.

Position markings. All ET tubes should have radiopaque markings to allow radiographic verification of the tube position. In addition, the tube should have markings at 1 cm intervals from end to end so that once appropriate placement is established and correlated with the distance of insertion, the nurse can regularly check the tube insertion point to prevent tube displacement. (This should be done whenever vital signs are recorded.)

Shape of the tube. Some ET tubes have a sharp curvature designed to enable a quick intubation to the point of curvature. When the patient requires intubation for more than a few hours, however, curved tubes are undesirable because it is difficult to pass a suction catheter through the tube. Further, these tubes are not easily placed nasotracheally.

With all critically ill children, the nurse must keep emergency airway and ventilation equipment (O_2 source, bag, and mask) at the bedside. Intubation equipment should be nearby (refer to the box that lists essential equipment for an intubation tray).

■ **Resuscitation bags for hand ventilation**

There are a variety of manual resuscitator bags available, each with several distinctive features from which to choose. In general, there are two main types of bags: the self-inflating bag and the uninflated bag, which requires air flow to fill it before manual ventilation can begin.

Self-inflating bags. Self-inflating bags may be used with or without an oxygen source (Fig. 9-33). They are called "self-inflating" because they will inflate, as a result of the recoil of the bag, without an oxygen (or other gas) supply. When this occurs, room air is drawn into the bag and administered to the patient. The *advantages* of using this bag include[43,53]

Essential equipment for endotracheal intubation tray

Laryngoscope handles

Laryngoscope blades—five sizes

1. Premature and term newborns—no. 0 straight blade

2. Infant to 2½ years—no. 1 straight blade

3. 2½ to 5 years—no. 2 curved and no. 2 straight blade

4. Older than 5 years—no. 3 curved blade

Endotracheal tubes (two of each size from 2.5 to 8.0 mm)

Other requirements

Stylets (two or three sizes)

Magill forceps (two sizes)

Lidocaine gel

Lidocaine spray

Tape and benzoin with applicators

Extra laryngoscope bulbs and batteries for the handle

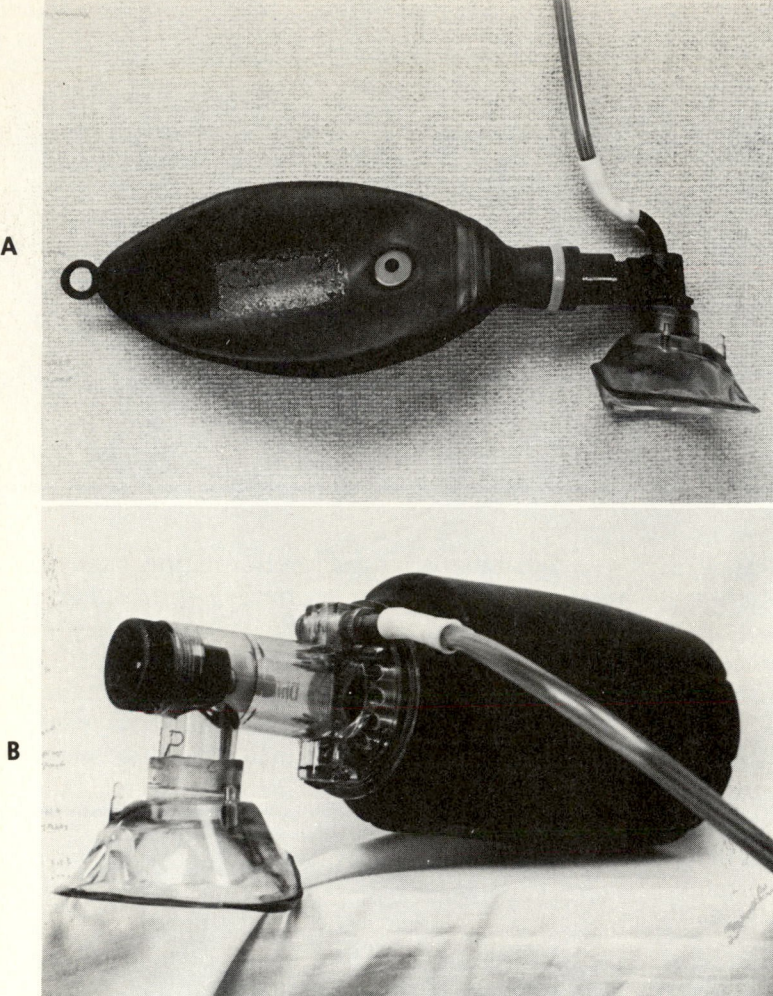

Fig. 9-33 Manual resuscitation bags. **A,** Uninflated manual resuscitation bag (requires gas source for inflation). **B,** Self-inflated manual resuscitation bag (does not require gas source for inflation).

ease of operation for those who are not skilled in manual ventilation (there are no valves for the operator to maneuver, only the bag to squeeze) and ability to ventilate, using room air, before oxygen or air flow meters are set up. Although the child receives only room air, he is at least manually *ventilated* for the moment. The ½ to 1 L bags will ventilate children up to 8 to 10 years of age. The larger 1½ L bags may be used for adolescents.

There are several *disadvantages* of the self-inflating bags.[43,53] There must be a reservoir of some kind in order to obtain an FIO_2 greater than 0.60. This reservoir is not a standard part of the bag and must be added if needed. As inspiratory pop-off valve (frequently set at approximately 40 mm Hg to prevent the delivery of high inflation pressures) may also prevent delivery of adequate tidal volumes during mask ventilation. The operator must be familiar with appropriate manual ventilation technique. A quick, snapping motion on inspiration should be avoided since the pressure at which the pop-off valve can be triggered will be quickly reached and inadequate tidal volume may be delivered. Spontaneous patient inspiration may not be possible unless a low-resistance valve is in place that allows the patient to draw in room air between manually delivered breaths. Otherwise, the valve between the mask-adapter and the bag is opened only with the force of bag compression. The volume and oxygen concentration delivered during manual ventilation may be variable and will depend on the speed and force of bag compression, and on patient lung compliance.

Self-inflated resuscitation bags are particularly useful (1) on resuscitation carts, where often the first people to initiate cardiopulmonary resuscitation (CPR) are not skilled in mask-bagging, and (2) for patient transport (either within or outside the hospital), when it is frequently impossible to predict how much air/oxygen to carry. If the supply runs out, the self-inflated bags may still be used to ventilate the patient with room air, whereas uninflated bags are dependent on gas flow.

Uninflated bags. These bags are so named because they are collapsed at rest and reinflate only if a continuous oxygen (gas) source is available (Fig. 9-33). This gas source must be equal to at least three to five times the patient's minute volume requirements in order to adequately fill the bag between breaths. The *advantages* of this type of bag are that FIO_2 of 1.0 can be provided without addition of a reservoir; that there are no *internal* valves which might dysfunction; that patients can breathe spontaneously between manual breaths since O_2 is continuously flowing to the patient's airway; that CPAP/PEEP can easily be established with an adapter; and that the patient's proximal airway pressure and lung compliance are more readily assessed, using a pressure gauge that is attached to the system with a T piece.[53]

The *disadvantages* of uninflated bags are that they require a gas source at all times and that the technique of bagging is difficult for the inexperienced person and can be dangerous to the patient if incorrectly done. The minute volume may be inadequate or high peak-inspiratory pressures may be delivered, causing a pneumothorax.[53]

■ **Chest tube systems**

Chest tubes are inserted for the purpose of evacuating air or fluid from the intrapleural or mediastinal spaces. Since intrapleural pressure is normally subatmospheric, drainage of this space requires a special collection system using an underwater seal. The following discussion refers, specifically, to those systems used for intrapleural drainage.

For drainage to occur, there must be a pressure gradient between the intrapleural space and the collection chamber. (Pressure must always be lower in the collection chamber than in the pleural or mediastinal space.) Two evacuation systems may be used: gravity drainage or a system that applies suction through the collection chamber[11] (Fig. 9-34). Either system may be created with a series of bottles or with a single disposable plastic unit.

While the bottle drainage system may seem inconvenient and perhaps more complicated than the disposable system, there are several *advantages* to this system. In pediatric patients large volumes of

drainage fluid are not usually collected, so that use of small (100 ml) bottles with single unit calibrations can make hourly drainage measurement easier. A two-bottle system consisting of a single bottle for both water seal and collection chamber and a second bottle for bubble suction system often works adequately. However, as drainage accumulates in the bottle, the water seal tube must be constantly adjusted or the bottle emptied and releveled at a 2-cm depth to prevent an increase in the height of the water seal. (The taller the column of fluid in the water seal, the more difficult it becomes to evacuate fluid from the pleural cavity.) One might easily understand this effect by the analogy of a soda straw placed first in a glass half-filled with liquid—noting the amount of pressure that must be exerted to push air through the straw and, then, comparing this with the amount of pressure required if the straw is placed in a glass that is full. The more deeply the straw is immersed in the fluid or the higher the level of fluid above the bottom of the straw (the water seal), the greater the force that will be required to produce flow through the straw. Therefore, if large quantities of fluid drainage are expected, a three-bottle drainage system may be more convenient.

A three-bottle system uses three bottles connected in series. Each bottle is used for a specific purpose: the bottle nearest the patient is used to collect and measure drainage; the middle bottle serves as the underwater seal; and the third bottle may be used as the suction control chamber (see Fig. 9-34). The chief *advantage* of the bottle system is that it is *much* less expensive than the disposable units, and components can be resterilized and reused. The major *disadvantages* are (1) the need for emptying or releveling the drainage bottle or underwater seal if significant drainage occurs and (2) the danger of spillage from careless placement of bottles on the floor. The second disadvantage can be alleviated by the use of thick wooden blocks (8 × 8 × 2 inches) with holes cut to fit the bottles. Such blocks can successfully secure the bottles on the floor.

For those who prefer disposable suction systems, the operating principles are the same as for the three-bottle system,[11] but the units are housed within a single container (Fig. 9-35). There are several *advantages* of a disposable, one-unit system. It is a self-contained, three-chambered unit, providing water seal, collection, and bubble suction chambers suitable for all purposes. Also, a large accumulation of fluid drainage can be accommodated before the system requires changing or emptying, thus minimizing the risk of infection and reducing maintenance. Further, the disposable system may be attached to the

Components of water-seal suction

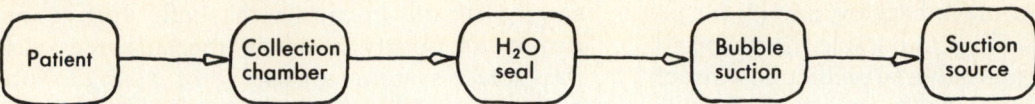

Gravity drainage: one-bottle system

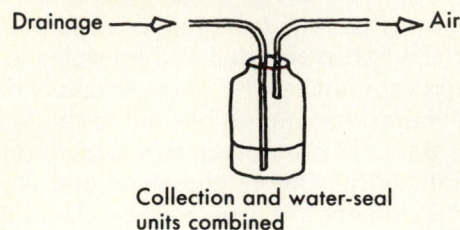

Two-bottle system

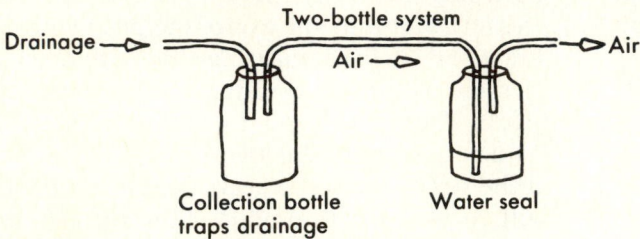

Suction and drainage two-bottle system

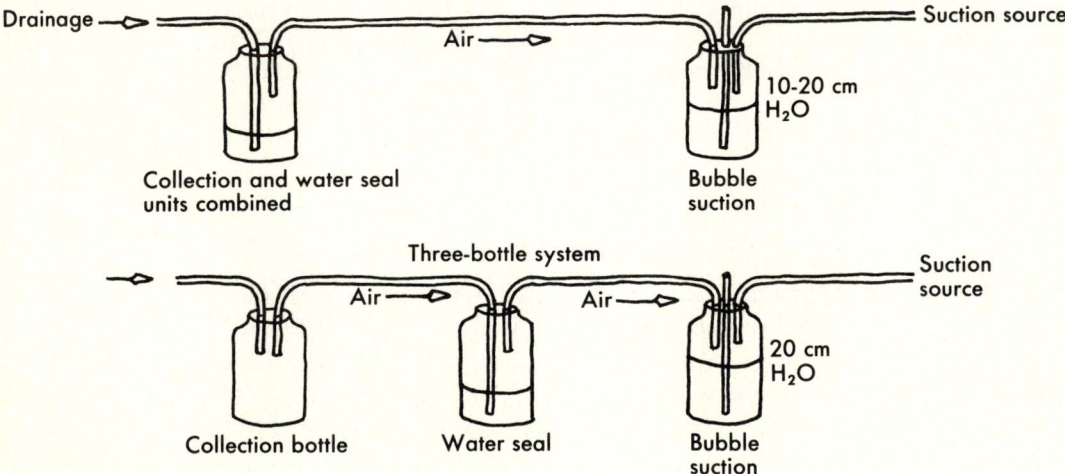

Fig. 9-34 Components of a chest-tube system. The top row represents individual components that may comprise a system. All systems have a collection chamber and a water seal. Each specific system has its respective components aligned (vertically) under the figures in each row.

bed frame, minimizing the risk of spillage, and it renders the patient more mobile since the single unit is easier and safer to carry with a patient than several glass bottles. The *disadvantages* of the system are the cost and the fact that some collection chambers are calibrated in only 10 ml increments.

Normal function of the chest tube system. The "normally functioning" pleural drainage system demonstrates these characteristics.[11] Fluid fluctuations with respirations or silent, intermittent, placid bubbling should be present in the water seal compartment. *Note* that if bubbling is present in the water

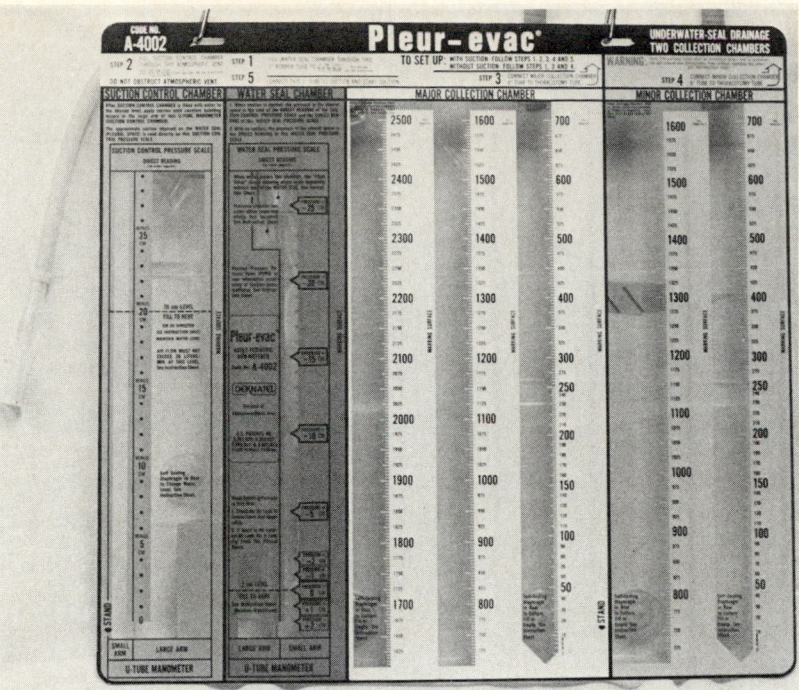

Fig. 9-35   Disposable chest-tube collection and suction unit (Pleur-evac).

seal when the suction is eliminated, this usually indicates the presence of an "air leak" (a result of a leak in the system or drainage of air from the pleural cavity). Continuous audible bubbling in the suction control chamber is evident in some models when suction is applied. Other systems indicate the suction applied with a visible fluid level.

When describing bubbling in the water seal chamber, the terms "silent versus noisy," "placid versus turbulent," and "intermittent versus continuous" can be used.[11,35] Note that the first term of each pair is the *normal* status. If fluid is being evacuated, respiratory fluctuations of the fluid in the chest tube itself (between insertion site and collection chamber) will be seen.

When assessing the pleural drainage system, the nurse should always remember to *look at the patient first!* Determine if respiratory distress is present and if it is increasing. Then observe the water seal chamber and the suction control chamber for bubbling. Assessment of these three factors can be used to detect problems discussed in Table 9-9. This table is intended for troubleshooting *equipment* malfunction, which may be manifested by a change in the patient's condition. (See Chapter 4 for discussion of respiratory pathophysiology and management of clinical problems.)

■ NEUROLOGIC MONITORING
■ Intracranial pressure monitoring

Monitoring of intracranial hypertension in the pediatric ICU has become a relatively common technique (see Chapter 6). The methods of intracranial monitoring are described briefly here.

Fontograms.   Noninvasive monitoring of intracranial pressure (ICP) is accomplished by use of the fontogram, which is produced by placing a transducer over the infant's fontanelle. The transducer has a spring-loaded rod centered in a base plate. Displacement of the rod will occur when increased pressure is transmitted across the fontanelle.[68] This generates a signal.

The transducer must be securely fixed in place over the infant's anterior fontanelle. Stretch gauze (Fig. 9-36) may provide the best method of securing the transducer. (Artifact will occur if the transducer is manually held in place.) The transducer must be centered exactly over the fontanelle—if it is not, the central piston of the transducer will come into contact with bone, giving a falsely high reading. Measurements should be consistently taken with the infant in the supine position. The transducer must be recalibrated every 2 to 4 hours. It is believed that the ap-

Text continued on p. 731.

Table 9-9 Troubleshooting guide for chest tube system

| Condition | Observations | | Causes | Intervention |
	Patient	Chest tube		
Evacuation of intrapleural air[11,35]				
Increasing respiratory distress	Increased respiratory rate: Pallor/cyanosis Use of accessory muscles Deterioration in arterial blood gases Increased respiratory effort	Continuous, noisy, turbulent bubbling in water seal chamber	A leak in the system; if the bubbling stops when the tube is clamped *briefly* at the skin insertion site, then the bubbling probably results from a patient air leak or drainage of air from the pleural space Loose tubing connections or leak in the chest tube	Check all connections immediately; if leak is not apparent, then clamp tube at skin insertion site (if hospital policy permits), while observing water seal for cessation of turbulent bubbling. If bubbling does not stop, reclamp every few inches along tubing down to the bottle in an attempt to isolate the site of the air leak. The point of the air leak is just above that point where clamping of the pleural or drainage tube eliminates water seal bubbling* Call physician for unresolved distress or for persistent bubbling in water seal
		Absence of respiratory fluctuations in water seal compartment (with a short-term tube obstruction, fluid in suction control chamber will bubble)	Obstruction of tube (caused by clot or accumulation of fibrin)	Check entire length of tubing for kinking, clamping, or compression such as by a crib rail "Milk" tubing in an attempt to dislodge a clot Check suction unit and all tubing connections
		No bubbling in suction control chamber NOTE: This indicates appropriate function of some units	Defect in suction unit Kinking or compression of suction tube	If problem is not *quickly* identified or if patient appears to be distressed (from accumulation of air in chest), call physician immediately, and prepare for insertion of new tube

*If patient is rapidly deteriorating, or in marked distress, the nurse must be reasonable in the time spent with clamping/unclamping chest tubes for air leak identification. Call physician immediately, and be prepared for insertion of new tube.

Table 9-9   Troubleshooting guide for chest tube system—cont'd

Condition	Observation		Causes	Intervention
	Patient	**Chest tube**		
Evacuation of intrapleural air—cont'd				
Decreasing respiratory distress	Normal respiratory rate and effort	Continuous, silent, turbulent bubbling in water seal	Small patient air leak or unit leak	Check as in first intervention
	No cyanosis or pallor			Patient may tolerate a small leak in tubing system without development of a pneumothorax as long as suction is applied; however, the system should be completely replaced as soon as possible for safety
	Normal or improved blood gases			
		No bubbling in water seal	Normal, if there is little or no air in the intrapleural space and no system leak	None needed
		Intermittent, silent, placid bubbling in water seal with no bubbling in suction control chamber NOTE: Absence of bubbling in suction control chamber is normal in some units	Recent kink in suction tube	Check all tubing and connections
			Leak distal to water seal	Consider replacing suction tubes or units
			Disconnection in suction tube	
Evacuation of intrapleural (or mediastinal) fluid[11,35]				
Increasing respiratory distress	Increased respiratory rate	No disconnection or dependent loops present in tubing	Breakdown in suction unit	Check for kinks in suction tube
	Pallor/cyanosis	Water seal normal	Kink (long-standing) in tube	Check suction unit
	Use of accessory muscles	Suction control has no bubbling NOTE: Bubbling is no longer expected in all units		
	Increased respiratory effort			
	Deterioration in arterial blood gases			
		No fluctuations in chest tube fluid or water seal with respirations	Clot in internal or external portion of chest tube	Check for kinks in, or compression of, chest tube

Continued.

Table 9-9 Troubleshooting guide for chest tube system—cont'd

Condition	Observation		Causes	Intervention
	Patient	Chest tube		
Evacuation of intrapleural (or mediastinal) fluid—cont'd				
Increasing respiratory distress— cont'd			Kink in chest tube Compression of chest tube	"Milk" chest tube; if clot is successfully removed, fluctuations should resume in water seal or chest tube fluid
				If clot is not removed and obstruction of chest tube is suspected, notify physician. If clot is visible, the chest tube may require direct suctioning with a tracheal suction catheter. This is performed (with physician present or with physician order) using *aseptic* technique, with the chest tube clamped at skin insertion site (if it is a *pleural* tube)
				If a clot is not visible but is thought to be at insertion site or in the intrapleural portion of the tube, "back-stripping" the tube may dislodge clot (a physician order may be needed)
				If the tube remains obstructed and significant intrapleural (or mediastinal) fluid accumulates, the physician may directly suction the chest tube or may insert a new tube immediately
	Turbulent bubbling in water seal; normal bubbling in suction control	Leak proximal to underwater seal	Check for leaks in system	
	Decrease in chest tube drainage	Dependent loops in chest tube	Strip tube and reposition so no dependent loops are present, or add suction if needed to ensure drainage	

Table 9-9   Troubleshooting guide for chest tube system—cont'd

Condition	Observation		Causes	Intervention
	Patient	**Chest tube**		
Evacuation of intrapleural (or mediastinal) fluid—cont'd				
Increasing respiratory distress— cont'd				Suction (with physician order) inside of chest tube (see intervention for first problem)
			Partial or complete clotting of tube, which may lead to a tension hemothorax (if tube is in pleural space and pleural blood is present) or cardiac tamponade (if tube is in mediastinum and mediastinal blood is present)	
			Decreased amount of drainage	No intervention needed
Decreasing respiratory distress	Normal respiratory rate and effort	Continuous, noisy and turbulent bubbling in water seal	Leak in system proximal to underwater seal	Check all connections and tubing (see intervention for first problem)
	No cyanosis Improvement in arterial blood gases	Water seal has continuous, *silent* bubbling	Small leak proximal to water seal	See first intervention
		Suction control is bubbling (fluctuations in the fluid within the chest tube and water seal are present with respirations)	Normal status with no fluid/air left in intrapleural space	Patient's condition should be confirmed by clinical assessment and (at some point) chest film
		No bubbling in suction control (of unit that *normally* has bubbling in suction control)	Malfunction of suction unit Kink in suction tubing Leak in system distal to water seal Suction tubing disconnected	Check entire unit, including tubing (see intervention for first problem)

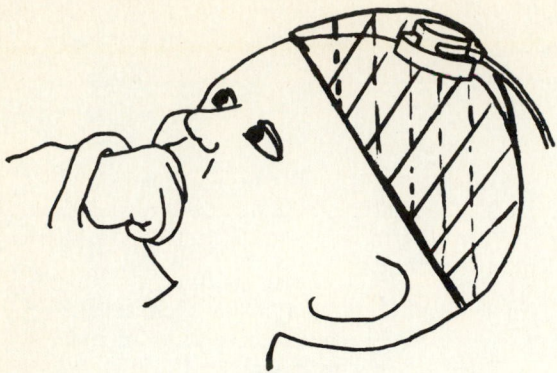

Fig. 9-36 Securing of fontogram with stretch gauze. The fontogram is held in place (over the infant's fontanelle) using stretch gauze. The transducer head must not be in contact with bone.

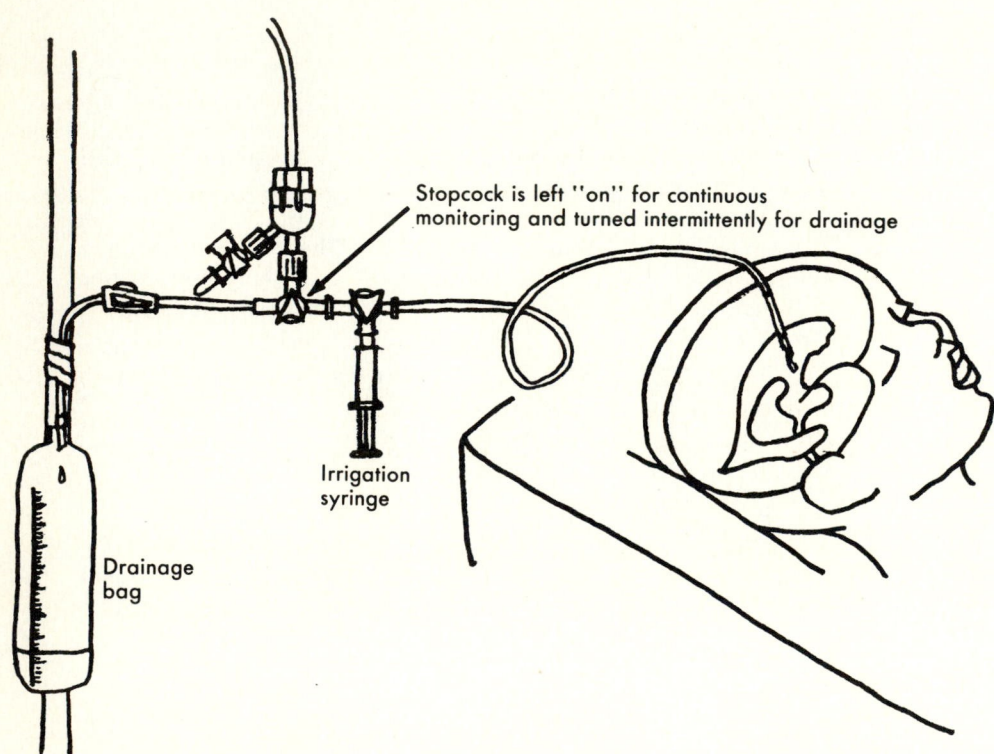

Stopcock is left "on" for continuous monitoring and turned intermittently for drainage

Irrigation syringe

Drainage bag

Fig. 9-37 Intraventricular monitoring and drainage system. Both the transducer head and the tip of the drainage catheter within the bag should be at the level of the child's lateral ventricle. Taping the transducer to the child's head at this level is one way of maintaining this alignment.

paratus may not be useful if the infant's fontanelle is markedly depressed, but this limitation has not been specifically indicated by the manufacturer or confirmed by clinical trials.[68]

The "normal" fontogram pressure is about 3 to 10 mm Hg. Some studies have reported good correlations between the fontogram and invasive pressure monitoring, but research with this device is not abundant.[68]

Invasive intracranial pressure monitoring. Several methods of invasive intracranial pressure monitoring are currently in use: the intraventricular cannula, the subarachnoid bolt, and the epidural monitor.

Intraventricular cannula.[13,74] This cannula is inserted through a burr hole in the skull and directed into one of the lateral ventricles. The cannula is then attached to a two-port system, which will allow simultaneous intracranial pressure monitoring (with a standard transducer) and drainage of cerebrospinal fluid (CSF)[25] (Fig. 9-37).

The *advantages* of this method of monitoring are that pressure measurements are taken directly from the CSF space and there is access to cerebrospinal fluid for sampling or for drainage (as a relief measure when intracranial pressure increases to dangerous levels).

There are several disadvantages to this method.

The physician may be unable to locate a lateral ventricle with the cannula because of diffuse cerebral edema or a midline brain shift caused by edema or intracranial mass lesions. There is an increased risk of hemorrhage (subdural bleeding) caused by tearing of the pia vessels or bridging veins. There is also an increased risk of intraparenchymal hemorrhage during cannula insertion. Finally, there is a risk of infection ranging from 1% to 5% among patients with cannulas.[13,74]

Subarachnoid bolt.[13,30,31,74] The subarachnoid bolt was first used in 1973. It provides clinical information that allows early recognition of increased intracranial pressure. A hollow metal bolt or screw is inserted into the subarachnoid space through a burr hole made in the skull (Fig. 9-38). This insertion may be accomplished in the ICU. The bolt is then connected to a transducer for continuous pressure monitoring (Fig. 9-39). Subarachnoid bolts cannot be used in infants less than approximately 8 to 10 months of age because their skull is thin and will not support the heavy bolt. The bone, in fact, may develop "shattered glass" cracks around the insertion site.[89] Some physicians[89] have had success in using plastic stopcocks in place of the heavy metal bolt in infants.

Among the advantages of the subarachnoid bolt is that it allows direct measurement of intracranial pressure from cerebrospinal fluid. In addition, the

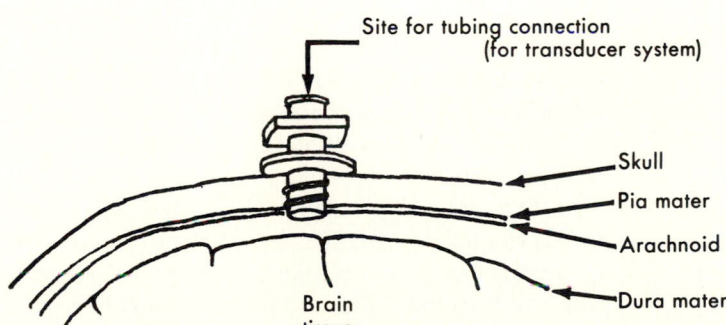

Fig. 9-38 Subarachnoid bolt. The bolt is placed in either the right or left frontal area through a burr hole. A short piece of noncompliant tubing is connected to the bolt for the transducer system.

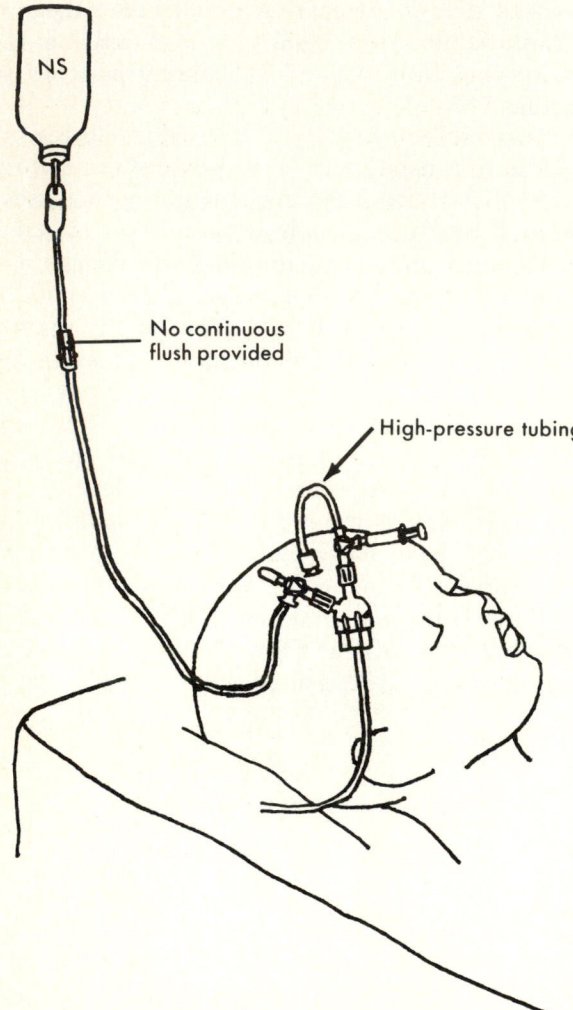

NS

No continuous
flush provided

High-pressure tubing

Fig. 9-39 Intracranial pressure monitoring through subarachnoid bolt. (*Note* that there is *not* continuous flush!) Transducer is taped to side of head at level of ventricle. A syringe is in place for irrigation, and normal saline flush is placed in the system so that there is a low incidence of needing to "break into the line" to flush, thus decreasing risk of contamination. Some hospitals may choose to delete the IV bottle.

technique does not require invasive penetration of brain tissue.[30,31,74]

Disadvantages of the subarachnoid bolt include the fact that the bolt cannot be used on young infants and that the risk of infection is nearly comparable to that occurring with the intraventricular technique.[13]

Epidural monitoring.[13] This technique involves the placement of a device, such as a fiberoptic transducer, between the skull and the dura. The device is inserted through a burr hole and is connected to a stopcock assembly and a transducer, which provides a digital readout of the epidural pressure.

The advantages of the epidural system are provided here. It is a less invasive technique than intraventricular cannulae and bolts; therefore the risk of infection is lessened. The transducer is not subject to environment interference; thus "drift" is minimized. Problems with the cannula or bolt, such as obstruction, are avoided.

The disadvantages of the epidural device include inconsistent correlations between epidural measurements and pressure readings of the subarachnoid bolt or intraventricular cannula. In addition, recalibration and checking of the transducer are impossible. Further, determination of volume-pressure responses are not feasible as they are with the other monitoring devices.

Equipment maintenance. The transducers for both ventricular and subarachnoid monitoring should be set up *without* the use of a flush device.[74] These cannulae do not need continuous flush to remain patent, and, further, the child's intracranial pressure may elevate to dangerous levels when even the slightest amount of fluid is injected. If a flush is required, it is preferable not to flush with greater than 0.1 ml normal saline solution. The nurse should then carefully observe the volume-pressure response in the patient to the flush. However, even if the patient's intracranial compliance is low, a volume increase of even 0.1 to 0.2 ml may cause an increase in intracranial pressure.[25]

Intracranial pressure tracings obtained with either the bolt or intraventricular cannula may appear as a series of soft, undulating waves or sharp rhythmic oscillations[25] (Fig. 9-40). As with other transducers, these intracranial monitoring devices should be zeroed and calibrated every 2 to 4 hours. Any leaks that occur in these systems are not only potential sources of infection but may also allow spinal fluid to rise up through the bolt or cannula. If the intracranial pressure is high, brain tissue may herniate into the bolt or cannula, causing "dampening" of the waveform and potential brain damage. Therefore all connections should be checked every 4 hours to ensure a tight seal.[25,31] (For more information regarding pathophysiologic changes resulting from increased intracranial pressure in the pediatric patient, refer to Chapter 6.)

■ **Continuous monitoring of cerebral electrical function in the ICU**

A modified electroencephalogram (EEG) device, with a single channel, bipolar monitor, is used for continuous monitoring. It is used most frequently to monitor patients who are placed in barbiturate comas, thus ensuring the presence of minimal brain activity during periods of increased intracranial pressure.[77]

The modified, bipolar EEG device uses two disc or needle electrodes. One electrode disc is usually placed over one eye and the corresponding parietal area, and the other, a grounding disc, is placed on the same side, below the ear. Changes in electrical potential between the two discs are amplified and passed over filters to screen 60-cycle interference and selectively amplify higher frequency signals.

The tracing obtained is not that of a conventional EEG but is rather a plot of peak-to-peak amplitudes, which are compressed by the slow speed of the recorder, thus appearing as a thick band on the recording strip[77] (Fig. 9-41). The desired EEG pattern for a child in a barbiturate coma is described as a burst suppression tracing. As with other needle electrodes, these leads should be replaced every 24 hours, and the skin should always be scrubbed with a Betadine skin preparation before electrode insertion.

The disadvantages of continuous EEG recordings include those described here. The recording is

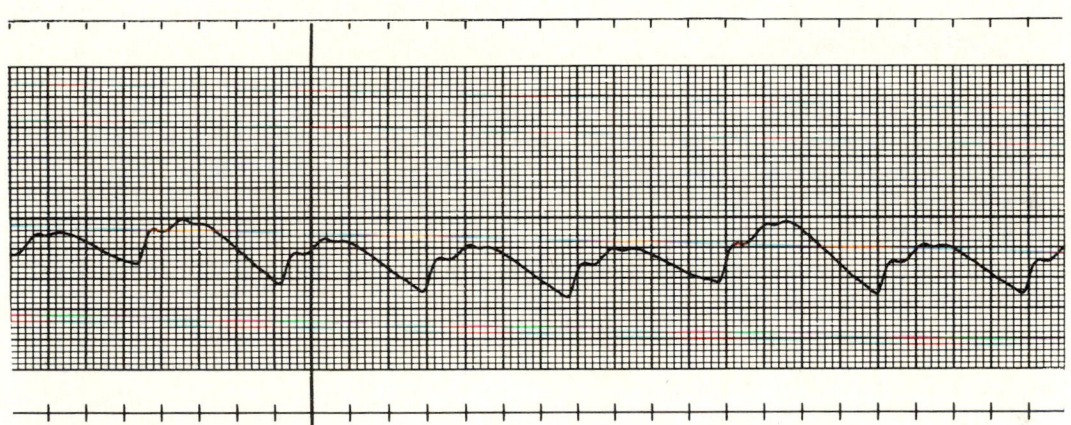

Fig. 9-40 Intracranial pressure waveform. Paper speed is 50 mm/sec. Note the oscillations in the pressure tracing.

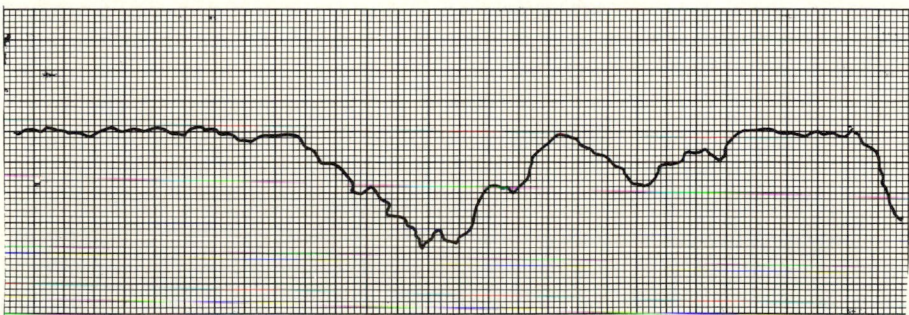

Fig. 9-41 Continuous (bipolar) EEG monitoring. This tracing demonstrates the "burst suppression" pattern that is desirable when titrating barbiturate coma.

useful only in conditions of diffuse cerebral cortical dysfunction. Localized dysfunctional activity such as seizures may not be detected unless the needle lead placement is specifically guided using full-channel EEG localization of the seizure focus.[40,77] In addition, the tracing reflects a composite of EEG frequency and amplitude; therefore information cannot be ascertained about either parameter separately.[48,77]

One advantage of continuous EEG monitoring is its use for patients who are electively paralyzed with a nondepolarizing neuromuscular blocking agent. There is evidence which suggests that untreated seizure activity in paralyzed animals may have serious consequences on brain metabolism.[77] Many critically ill patients may require paralysis for various reasons such as ventilator management; therefore continuous EEG monitoring would offer more sensitive detection of localized seizure activity in these patients and would thus allow prompt treatment of status epilepticus.

■ THERMOREGULATION DEVICES

Monitoring of environmental and patient temperatures in the pediatric ICU is extremely important. Small children have a large body surface area in proportion to their body mass and may lose heat very rapidly by convection. Cold stress can cause increased oxygen consumption, which may compromise the cardiorespiratory function of the critically ill child.

■ Temperature-sensing devices

Temperature-sensing devices may be of two types. The first is the *thermo-expansive thermometer*—the standard mercury thermometer—which most commonly measures temperatures in the range of 34° C to 44° C (thermometers are available that measure lower temperatures). The second is the *thermo-resistive thermometers*, or *thermistor tips*, which contain heavy metals that respond to changes in electrical resistance with small changes in temperature. Electronic thermometers are frequently thermoresistive thermometers.

Thermoresistive thermometers have a rapid response time, which may be an important consideration in pediatrics. Although most thermistors record the standard range of temperatures, some are available for recording lower temperatures, which would be useful for patients who are hypothermic.

In the pediatric ICU setting, safety, speed of measurement, and convenience are the most important considerations in the selection of temperature

devices. Skin or rectal probes (thermistor tips) and electronic thermometers fit these criteria satisfactorily. (For specific information about brand testing of several electronic thermometers, refer to Abbey.[1])

If temperature instability is a potential problem, the child's environmental temperature can be maintained at an appropriate level through the use of an Isolette or an over-bed radiant warmer.

■ Closed warmers (Isolettes)

The *advantages* of Isolettes for sick newborns are that they provide humidity and temperature control through recirculation of warm air. Oxygen may also be added to the Isolette.

The *disadvantages* of Isolettes include impaired access to the infant, loss of heat (and oxygen) when the doors are opened, and wide variance of ambient temperature within some Isolettes because of erratic airflow patterns. Specific device evaluations for these considerations should be checked before purchasing the unit.

Temperature variance may be minimized by using a Servo control device with temperature probe so that the heating mechanism is adjusted according to the infant's skin temperature. In addition, if the baby is extremely unstable, the nurse may wish to place an additional thermistor probe a few inches above the infant to monitor the temperature of the air directly around the infant. A small, Plexiglass shield (tent) may also be placed over the infant inside the Isolette to minimize radiant heat loss to the cool walls of the Isolette unit.

■ Open radiant warmers

Open radiant warmers heat the air above the patient. The radiant warmer may be purchased as a free-standing over-bed unit, or as an open bed with a radiant warmer fixed 80 to 100 cm above the patient's mattress. Most models offer both the Servo control and non-Servo modes of heating. If the non-Servo heating mode is used, the infant's temperature must be monitored continuously.

It is important to note that when the infant's body temperature is low, perfusion to the skin is diminished. If a radiant warmer is placed over a cold patient with poor skin perfusion, the normal dissipation of heat by surface blood vessels will be diminished or absent. Therefore burns may occur much more easily since the unit will continue warming the infant since the skin temperature probe is still measuring a low temperature.

The *advantages*[17] of open-bed warmers include

quick access to, and complete visibility of, the patient and surrounding equipment, rapid patient warming time, stable ambient temperatures (since the radiated area is fairly insensitive to drafts) and a Servo-control mechanism, which delivers heat output that is based on the infant's measured skin temperature, similar to the Servo-control mechanism in closed Isolettes. The heater turns on when the infant's measured skin temperature falls below a preset level and turns off when the infant's skin temperature rises to within the preset range. Alarms are frequently available for indicting when the infant's temperature has exceeded the preset range.

Disadvantages of open-bed warmers include possible risk of infection (health care personnel often forget to wash hands before and after patient contact (since the infant is so readily accessible), increased insensible water loss (when infants are nursed under open-bed warmers rather than when they are nursed in Isolettes), and increased heat loss by convection, especially if the room is subject to drafts.

In selecting a warming device, the following features should be considered.

1. High and low temperature alarms (including 15-minute continuous-heat alarms)
2. A high-heat limit set at less than 45° C for radiant warmers (to minimize direct patient–tissue damage that could occur)
3. An alarm to indicate a damaged probe, a probe open to air, or heater malfunction
4. Manual (non-Servo) and automatic (Servo control) modes
5. A mattress that is adjustable to various heights and angles
6. Adequate mattress size to provide work space around the infant
7. Adequate space between bilateral radiant warmers for x-ray machines, phototherapy lights, and hanging IV racks
8. Electrical safety measures: maximum leakage of current from probe-to-ground of 500 microamperes[28,52]

■ Nursing considerations

Even if Servo control is used, the infant's core temperature should be checked at least every 2 hours for comparison of skin temperature and core temperature. It is important to note that if the child has decreased skin perfusion (such as occurs with low cardiac output), the skin probe will sense a low temperature, causing the Servo-control warmer to increase heat output, even though the infant's core temperature may be normal or elevated. Therefore assessment of capillary perfusion should be routinely performed by the nurse.

It is necessary that radiant warming devices be at least 80 cm above the patient. The child who is extremely cold is more susceptible to burns from radiant heaters. It may be advisable to wrap a cold child in a single, warmed blanket and then place the radiant heater over the youngster to maintain warmth.

Infants cared for in open-bed radiant warmers will have increased water loss (an average of 20%) because of evaporation. The nurse must recognize this, routinely assess the hydration of the infant, and ensure the continuous administration of appropriate fluids, according to physician's orders. (Calculate maintenance rate plus approximately 20%.)

Infants who are cared for in open-bed radiant warmers are potentially more vulnerable to infection because their accessibility allows people to handle them without a reminder to wash their hands. Closed Isolettes, on the other hand, provide a barrier (and therefore a reminder) to wash hands. The nurse must devise a means of monitoring handwashing by hospital personnel when infants are nursed in open warmer beds.

If a closed Isolette is used, the portholes rather than the doors should be used to gain access to infants. This minimizes heat loss when the Isolette is entered. If the infant must be exposed for procedures, a radiant warmer should be placed 80 cm over the infant, with a skin probe in place for continuous monitoring.

■ CONCLUSIONS

There are an enormous number of devices used in the pediatric ICU setting. This chapter has attempted to provide principles for the selection and use of the most common instruments employed in the ICU.

In addition, there is a publication, *Health Devices*, available in many medical-center libraries—an invaluable resource that may be helpful when major pieces of equipment must be purchased. *Health Devices* is published by a private institution (with subscription by private donation to the institution) that acts as a consumer-rating center to evaluate and report on available medical equipment.

In the final analysis, the equipment necessary for the safe and precise care of the critically ill child should allow more efficient use of nursing hours, and it should improve the quality of care. The child, and not the equipment, must be the focus of the nurse's attention.

REFERENCES

1. Abbey, J.C., and others: How long is that thermometer accurate? Am. J. Nurs. **78**(8):1375, 1978.
2. Adams, J.N., and Rudolph, A.J.: The use of indwelling radial artery catheters in neonates, Pediatrics **55**(2):261, 1975.
3. Adams, N.R.: Reducing the perils of intracardiac monitoring, Nursing 76 **6**:66, 1976.
4. Bair, J.N., and Peterson, R.V.: Surface characteristics of plastic intravenous catheters, Am. J. Hosp. Pharm. **36**(12):1707, 1979.
5. Bushnell, S.S.: Respiratory intensive care nursing, Boston, 1973, Little, Brown & Co.
6. Bolognini, V.: The Swan-Ganz pulmonary catheter: implications for nursing, Heart Lung **3**(6):976, 1974.
7. Buxton, A.E., and others: Failure of disposable domes to prevent septicemia acquired from contaminated pressure transducers, Chest **74**(5):508, 1978.
8. Cabal, L., and others: Factors affecting heated transcutaneous Po_2 and unheated transcutaneous Pco_2 in preterm infants, Crit. Care Med. **9**(4):298, 1981.
9. Calgan, F.J., and Stewart, S.: An assessment of cardiac output by thermodilution in infants and children following cardiac surgery, Crit. Care Med. **5**(5):220, 1977.
10. Chamberland, M.E., Lyons, R.W., and Brock, S.M.: Effect of in-line filtration of intravenous infusions on the incidence of thrombophlebitis, Am. J. Hosp. Pharm. **34**(10):1068, 1977.
11. Cohen, S.: How to work with chest tubes: programmed instruction, Am. J. Nurs. **80**(4):685, 1980.
12. Cromwell, L., and others: Medical instrumentation for health care, New Jersey, 1976, Prentice-Hall, Inc.
13. deAsla, R.A., and Smith, R.N.: The critical care environment: instrumentation. In McKinney, M., and others, editors: AACN's clinical reference for critical care nursing, New York, 1981, McGraw Hill, Inc.
14. Deluca, P.P., and others: Filtration and infusion phlebitis: a double blind prospective study, Am. J. Hosp. Pharm. **32**(10):100, 1975.
15. Donowitz, L.G., and others: High risk of hospital-acquired infection in the ICU patient, Crit. Care Med. **10**(6):355, 1982.
16. Elving, G., and Saikky, K.: Effect of pH on the incidence of infusion thrombophlebitis, Lancet **1**:953, 1966.
17. Evaluation: infant radiant warmers, Health Devices **4**:128, 1975.
18. Finer, N.N.: Newer trends in continuous monitoring of critically ill infants and children, Pediatr. Clin. North Am. **27**(3):553, 1980.
19. Finer, N.N., and Stewart, A.R.: Continuous transcutaneous oxygen monitoring in the critically ill neonate, Crit. Care Med. **8**(6):319, 1980.
20. Freeman, R., and King, B.: Analysis of results of catheter tip cultures in open-heart surgery patients, Thorax **30**(1):26, 1975.
21. Galvis, A.G., and others: An improved technique for prolonged arterial catheterization in infants and children, Crit. Care Med. **4**(3):166, 1976.
22. Garvan, J.M., and Gunner, B.W.: The harmful effects of particles in intravenous fluids, Med. J. Aust. **2**:1, July 1964.
23. Geddes, L.A., and Baker, L.E.: Principles of applied biomedical instrumentation, ed. 2, New York, 1975, John Wiley & Sons.
24. Goldberg, A., and Fadigran, M.: The Swan-Ganz catheter in pediatrics, Grand Rounds Presentation, Chicago, April 25, 1979, Children's Memorial Hospital.
25. Hanlon, K.: Description and uses of intracranial pressure monitoring, Heart Lung **5**(2):277, 1976.
26. Hansen, T.N., and Tooley, W.H.: Skin surface carbon dioxide tension in sick infants, Pediatrics **64**(6):942, 1979.
27. Hathaway, R.: The Swan-Ganz catheter: a review, Nurs. Clin. North Am. **13**(3):389, 1978.
28. Hill, D.W., and Dolan, A.M.: Intensive care instrumentation, New York, 1976, Grune & Stratton.
29. Jacobs, M.K.: Sources of measurement error in noninvasive electronic instrumentation, Nurs. Clin. North Am. **13**(4):573, 1978.
30. Johanson, B.C., and others: Standards for critical care, St. Louis, 1981, The C.V. Mosby Co.
31. Johnson, M., and Quinn, J.: The subarachnoid screw, Am. J. Nurs. **77**(3):448, 1977.
32. Jones, J.L., and Jones, R.E.: Postcountershock fibrillation in digitalized myocardial cells in vitro, Crit. Care Med. **8**(3):172, 1980.
33. Jones, J.L., and Jones, R.E.: Postshock arrhythmias—a possible cause of unsuccessful defibrillation, Crit. Care Med. **8**(3):167, 1980.
34. Karselis, T.C.: Descriptive medical electronics and instrumentation, Thorofare, N.J., 1973, Charles B. Slack, Inc.
35. Kersten, L.: Chest tube drainage system, Heart Lung **3**(1):97, 1974.
36. Kramer, L.I.: Rapid, accurate electrocardiogram and apnea monitoring, J. Pediatr. **87**(1):107, 1975.
37. Lantiegne, K.C., and Ciretta, J.M.: A system for maintaining invasive pressure monitoring, Heart Lung **7**(4):610, 1978.
38. Laptook, A., and Oh, W.: Transcutaneous carbon dioxide monitoring in the newborn period, Crit. Care Med. **9**(10):759, 1981.
39. La Souef, P.N., and others: Comparison of transcutaneous oxygen tension with arterial oxygen tension in newborn infants with severe respiratory illnesses, Pediatrics **62**(4):692, 1978.
40. Levin, D.L., and Lesh, D.: Venous catheters. In Levin, D.L., Morriss, F.C., Moore, G.C., editors: A practical guide to pediatric intensive care, ed. 2, St. Louis, 1984, The C.V. Mosby Co.
41. Levin, D.L., and Mast, C.P.: Arterial catheters. In Levin, D.L., Morriss, F.C., Moore, G.C., editors: A practical guide to pediatric intensive care, ed. 2, St. Louis, 1984, The C.V. Mosby Co.
42. Levin, R.M.: Pediatric respiratory intensive care, New York, 1976, Medical Examination Publishing Co.
43. Lough, M.D., Doershuk, C.F., and Stern, P.C.: Pediatric respiratory therapy, Chicago, 1974, Year Book Medical Publishers, Inc.

44. Lough, M.D., Williams, T.J. and Rawson, J.E., editors: Newborn respiratory care, Chicago, 1979, Year Book Medical Publishers, Inc.

45. Lubbers, D.W.: Theoretical basis of the transcutaneous blood gas measurements, Crit. Care Med. **9**(10):721, 1981.

46. Maki, D.G., Anderson, R.L., and Shulman, J.A.: In-use contamination of intravenous infusion fluid, Appl. Microbiol. **28**:778, 1974.

47. Maki, D.G., and Band, J.D.: A comparative study of polyantibiotic and iodophor ointments in prevention of vascular catheter-related infection, Am. J. Med. **70**:739, 1981.

48. Maki, D.G., Goldman, D.A., and Rhame, F.S.: Infection control in intravenous therapy, Ann. Int. Med. **79**:867, 1973.

49. Maki, D.G., and Hassemer, C.A.: Endemic rate of fluid contamination and related septicemia in arterial pressure monitoring, Am. J. Med. **70**:733, 1981.

50. Martin, R.J., Herrell, N., and Pultusker, M.: Transcutaneous measurement of carbon dioxide tension: effect of sleep state in term infants, Pediatrics **67**(5):622, 1981.

51. Martz, K.V., Joiner, J., and Shepherd, R.M.: Management of the patient-ventilator system, St. Louis, 1979, The C.V. Mosby Co.

52. McHugh, T.J., and others: Pulmonary vascular congestion in acute myocardial infarction: hemodynamic and radiologic correlations, Ann. Int. Med. **76**(1):29, 1972.

53. McPherson, S.P.: Respiratory therapy equipment, ed. 2, St. Louis, 1981, The C.V. Mosby Co.

54. Medtronic: Model demand external pacemaker—operators manual, Minneapolis, 1978, Medtronic, Inc.

55. Mills, L.J.: Left atrial catheters. In Levin, D.L., Morriss, F.C., Moore G.C., editors: A practical guide to pediatric intensive care, ed. 2, St. Louis, 1984, The C.V. Mosby Co.

56. Mills, L.J.: Pulmonary artery catheters. In Levin, D.L., Morriss, F.C., Moore, G.C., editors: A practical guide to pediatric intensive care, ed. 2, St. Louis, 1984, The C.V. Mosby Co.

57. Monaco, F., and McQuitty, J.C.: Transcutaneous measurements of carbon dioxide partial pressure in sick neonates, Crit. Care Med. **9**(10):756, 1981.

58. Morriss, F.C., Carew, J., and Mast, C.P.: Cardiopulmonary arrest. In Levin, D.L., Morriss, F.C., Moore, G.C., editors: A practical guide to pediatric intensive care, ed. 2, St. Louis, 1984, The C.V. Mosby Co.

59. Morriss, F.C., and Patz, J.: Electrocardiographic and respiratory monitors. In Levin, D.L., Morriss, F.C., Moore, G.C., editors: A practical guide to pediatric intensive care, ed. 2, St. Louis, 1984, The C.V. Mosby Co.

60. Mushin, W.W., and others: Automatic ventilation of the lungs, Oxford, 1979, Blackwell Scientific Publications.

61. Mylrea, K.C., and O'Neal, L.B.: Electricity and electrical safety in the hospital, Nursing 76 **6**(1):52, 1976.

62. Nichols, W.W., Nichols, M.A., and Barbour, H.: Complications associated with balloon-tipped, flow-directed catheters, Heart Lung **8**(3):503, 1979.

63. Nielson, M.A.: Intraarterial monitoring of blood pressure, Am. J. Nurs. **74**(1):48, 1974.

64. Parehk, A., and others: Arterial-alveolar CO_2 gradients as a prognostic indicator in the premature neonate with IRDS, Pediatr. Res. (abstract) **13**:502, 1979.

65. Pollock, J.C., and others: Intra-aortic balloon pumping in children, Ann. Thorac. Surg. **29**(6):522, 1980.

66. Prachar, H., and others: Bacterial contamination of pulmonary artery catheters, Intensive Care Med. **4**:79, 1978.

67. Proctor, D., Fletcher, R.D., and DeInegro, A.: Temporary cardiac pacing, Nurs. Clin. North Am. **13**(3):409, 1978.

68. Robinson, R.O., Rolfe, P., and Sutton, P.: Noninvasive method for measuring intracranial pressure in normal newborn infants, Dev. Med. Child Neurol. **19**(3):305, 1977.

69. Rowe, M.I., and Weinberg, G.: Transcutaneous oxygen monitoring in shock and resuscitation, J. Pediatr. Surg. **14**:773, 1979.

70. Salmon, J.H., Hajjar, W., and Bada, H.: The fontogram: a non-invasive intracranial pressure monitor, Pediatrics **60**(5):721, 1977.

71. Schroeder, J.S., and Daley, E.K.: Techniques in bedside hemodynamic monitoring, St. Louis, 1976, The C.V. Mosby Co.

72. Severinghaus, J.W., Dafford, M., and Bradley, A.F.: $tcPCO_2$ electrode design, calibration and temperature gradient problems, Acta Anaesthesiol. Scand. **68** (Suppl.):68, 1978.

73. Siemen-Elema Co.: Servo ventilator 900B and the Servo ventilator concept, product information book, New Jersey, 1979, Sieman Co.

74. Sklar, F.H., Patz, J., and Stein, P.: Intracranial pressure measurements and ventricular taps. In Levin, D.L., Morriss, F.C., Moore, G.C., editors: A practical guide to pediatric intensive care, ed. 2, St. Louis, 1984, The C.V. Mosby Co.

75. Spaccavento, L.J., and Hawley, H.B.: Infections associated with intra-arterial lines, Heart Lung **11**(2):118, 1982.

76. Stanger, P., and others: Use of the Swan-Ganz catheter in cardiac catheterization of infants and children, Am. Heart J. **83**:749, 1972.

77. Stidham, G.L., Nugent, S.K., and Rogers, M.C.: Monitoring cerebral function in the ICU, Crit. Care Med. **8**(9):519, 1980.

78. Stillman, R.M., and others: Etiology of catheter associated sepsis, Arch. Surg. **112**:1497, 1977.

79. Todres, I.D., and others: Swan-Ganz catheterization in the critically ill newborn, Crit. Care Med. **7**(8):330, 1979.

80. Tremper, K.K., and Shoemaker, W.C.: Transcutaneous oxygen monitoring of critically ill adults, with and without low flow shock, Crit. Care Med. **9**(10):706, 1981.

81. Tremper, K.K., and Shoemaker, W.C.: Transcutaneous PO_2 monitoring useful in adults, too, Crit. Care Monitor **1**(1):1, 1981.

82. Tremper, K.K., Waxman, K., and Shoemaker, W.C.: Effects of hypoxia and shock on transcutaneous P_{CO_2} values in dogs, Crit. Care Med. **1**(12):526, 1981.

83. Tremper, K.K., and others: Continuous transcutaneous O_2 monitoring during respiratory failure, cardiac decompensation, cardiac arrest and CPR, Crit. Care Med. **8**(7):377, 1980.

84. Tremper, K.K., and others: Transcutaneous PCO_2 monitoring on adult patients in the ICU and operating room, Crit. Care Med. **9**(10):752, 1981.

85. Vallbona, C.: Physiologic monitoring in children. In Ray, C.D., editor: Medical engineering, Chicago, 1974, Year Book Medical Publishers, Inc.

86. Veasy, G.L., and others: Intra-aortic balloon pumping in infants and children, Circulation **68**:1095, 1983.

87. Wade, J.: Respiratory nursing care, St. Louis, 1973, The C.V. Mosby Co.

88. Walinsky, P.: Acute hemodynamic monitoring, Heart Lung **6**(5):838, 1977.

89. Walker, M.L.: Personal communication, 1980.

90. Walrath, J.B., and others: Stopcock: bacterial contamination in invasive monitoring systems, Heart Lung **8**(1):100, 1979.

91. Wetzel, R.C., and Rodgers, M.C.: Pediatric hemodynamic monitoring, Manuscript submitted for publication, 1984.

92. Whaley, L.F., and Wong, D.F.: Nursing care of infants, ed. 2, St. Louis, 1983, The C.V. Mosby Co.

93. Williams, J.K., and Lancaster, J.: Thermoregulation of the newborn, J. Matern. Child Nurs. **1**(6):355, 1976.

94. Williams, T.J.: Mechanical ventilators. In Lough, M.D., Williams, T.J., and Rawson, J.E., editors: Newborn respiratory care, Chicago, 1979, Year Book Medical Publishers, Inc.

95. Winslow, E.H.: Temporary cardiac pacemakers, Am. J. Nurs. **75**(4):586, 1975.

96. Woods, S.L.: Monitoring pulmonary artery pressures, Am. J. Nurs. **76**(6):58, 1976.

97. Woods, S.L., and Mansfield, L.W.: Effect of body position upon pulmonary artery and pulmonary capillary wedge pressure in non-critically ill patients, Heart Lung **5**(1):83, 1976.

98. Zeidelman, C.: Increased intracranial pressure in the pediatric patient, nursing assessment and intervention, J. Neurosurg. Nurs. **12**(1):7, 1980.

Appendixes

Initial Management of the Injured Child

■ PEDIATRIC TRAUMA

Trauma accounts for approximately 50% of all children's deaths and is the major health hazard in the pediatric age group. Motor vehicle accidents are the most common cause of death followed by thermal injuries and falls.

The initial treatment priorities are to clear the airway and establish effective ventilation. Simultaneously one should support circulation, arrest bleeding, and treat shock.

This booklet will briefly describe the recommendations of the staff of the Primary Children's Medical Center and the faculty of University of Utah College of Medicine Departments of Surgery and Pediatrics regarding the initial management of the child with multiple injuries. Emphasis will be placed on treatment priorities and the sequence of evaluation of the child with multiple injuries. The treatment suggestions are applicable to the scene of the accident, during transportation, and in the emergency room.

Michael E. Matlak, M.D.
Pediatric Surgeon, Primary Children's Medical Center
Assistant Professor of Surgery and Pediatrics
University of Utah College of Medicine

Dale G. Johnson, M.D.
Chief of Surgery, Primary Children's Medical Center
Professor of Surgery and Pediatrics
University of Utah College of Medicine

Marion L. Walker, M.D.
Chairman, Division of Neurological Surgery
Primary Children's Medical Center
Medical Director, Trauma Transport Team
Clinical Assistant Professor of Surgery (Pediatric Neurosurgery)
University of Utah College of Medicine

Wm. Martin Palmer, M.D.
Medical Director of Ambulatory Services
Primary Children's Medical Center
Associate Professor of Pediatrics
University of Utah College of Medicine

Peter M. Stevens, M.D.
Pediatric Orthopedic Surgeon
Primary Children's Medical Center
Clinical Instructor
University of Utah College of Medicine

■ TABLE OF CONTENTS

Reproduced with permission from Matlak, M.E., Initial management of the injured child (pamphlet), Salt Lake City, 1980, Primary Children's Medical Center.

742   ■ *Appendixes*

■ Phase 1

■ LIFE SAVING MEASURES
■ Airway and ventilation

Establishment of an **unobstructed airway** with **adequate ventilation** is the first priority in the management of the injured child. Direct injury to the larynx and trachea is unusual. Thus, emergency tracheostomy or cricothyroidotomy is rarely necessary. Oral-facial injuries are quite common, however, and these may result in accumulation of foreign matter within the oral cavity. **Foreign matter** should be quickly removed by finger sweep or suction. Head and neck injuries frequently accompany major trauma, especially when the child is unconscious. In an unconscious state the mandible is relaxed and posterior displacement of the tongue will result in airway obstruction. A simple plastic oral airway usually reestablishes airway patency. Next, the child's head should be in the **"sniffing position"** for optimal ventilation as demonstrated in Fig. A-1. Ventilation and oxygenation are supplied by the most readily available means, usually first by mouth-to-mouth resuscitation or by a ventilating bag and mask. For infants and small children, the rescuer covers both the mouth and nose of the child with his mouth and uses small puffs of breath to inflate the lungs. The chest wall should expand with each breath to insure adequate ventilation. Only after these simple measures have been applied should the use of an endotracheal tube or an esophageal obturator airway be considered. The proper size endotracheal tube may be selected by picking a tube which would fit comfortably into the child's nostril. Pediatric esophageal obturator airways are not currently available, but in the near future they will probably replace the endotracheal tube for the initial management of the airway at the scene of the accident.

The child should be ventilated according to his age:

	Breaths per minute
Infants	40
Preschool aged child	30
School aged child	20

■ Circulation and cardiac arrest

Once ventilation is assured circulation becomes the next consideration. Cardiac arrest is treated by massaging the heart at 80 to 100 beats per minute. The ventricles of infants and small children lie higher in the chest. Thus, in infants and small children cardiac massage is effectively given by compressing the **midsternum** one-half to three-fourths of an inch toward the spine as demonstrated in Fig. A-2. Older children require three-fourths to one-and-a-half inches of sternal compression. The danger of lacerating the liver is considerable because of the pliability of the ribs and the higher position of the liver. Good pulses should be palpable

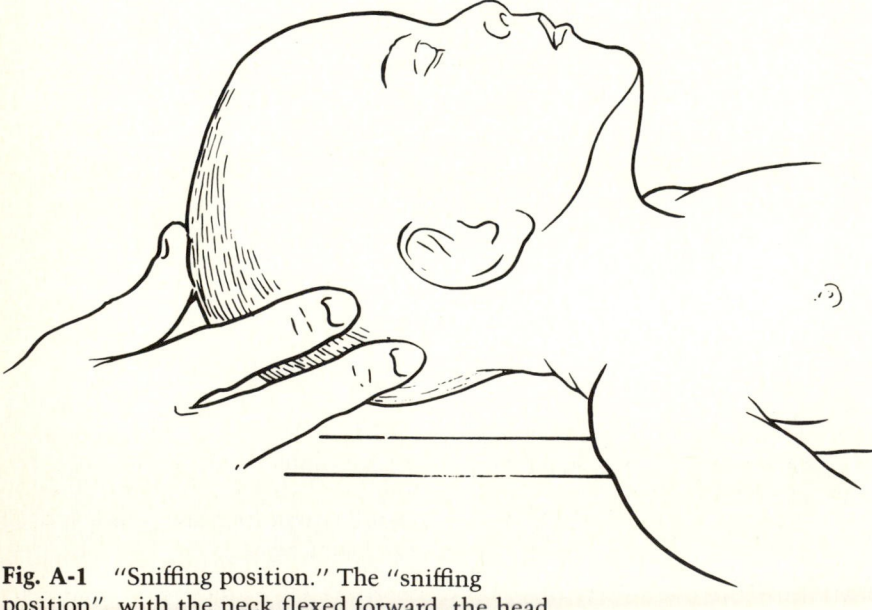

Fig. A-1 "Sniffing position." The "sniffing position", with the neck flexed forward, the head extended on the neck, and the jaw held forward is required for effective ventilation.

in the neck, groin or antecubital fossa with each massage. Breaths should be delivered as quickly as possible between sternal compressions.

A dependable IV should be started through which 2 mEq per kg of sodium bicarbonate are injected followed by 0.1 cc per kg of epinephrine diluted 1:10,000 (see Table A-1). Epinephrine is inactive in alkaline solution, and, thus, the bicarbonate should be well-flushed into the vein or given through a separate intravenous site. If bleeding is the obvious cause of the cardiac arrest, then 20 cc per kg of Ringer's lactate solution should be rapidly administered.

Check EKG

A. Asystole. If the electrocardiogram reveals asystole then ventilation and massage should be continued for two minutes. One or more sharp blows (sternal thumps) should be applied to the midsternum using only two fingers in infants, but the whole fist in the older child. Sodium bicarbonate and epinephrine should be repeated, and if asystole persists, 10% calcium chloride should be diluted to 1% and given **slowly** in a dose of 20 mg per kg or 2 cc per kg.

If it is impossible to administer the emergency medications intravenously, then epinephrine can be administered either by intramuscular injection into the base of the tongue, or by instillation of the drug through an endo-tra-

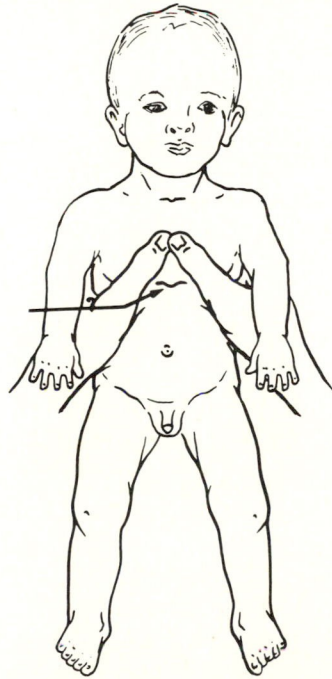

Fig. A-2 Cardiac massage. In infants and small children cardiac massage is given by compressing the mid-sternum one-half to three-fourths of an inch toward the spine. The thumbs or fingertips should be placed exactly on the midline of the sternum in order to avoid fracture-dislocation of the ribs. Compression of the lower third of the sternum may result in laceration of the liver or ineffective cardiac massage.

Table A-1 Emergency medications and pediatric dosages*

Medication	IV dosage
Ampicillin	<40 kg, 100 to 200 mg/kg/day
Atropine	0.01 mg/kg/dose
Calcium chloride (1%)	20 mg (2cc)/kg/dose (give slowly)
Dexamethasone (Decadron)	1.5 mg/kg push for brain swelling then 1.5 mg/kg/day
Diazepam (Valium)	0.1 to 0.25 mg/kg/dose (respiratory depressant, give slowly)
Dilantin	10 to 20 mg/kg/dose for traumatic seizure, then 5 to 10 mg/kg/day
Dopamine	5 to 20 micrograms/ kg/minute
Epinephrine 1:10,000	0.1 cc/kg/dose
Gentamicin	Infant—6 mg/kg/day Child—3 to 5 mg/ kg/day
Isoproterenol	0.1 to 0.5 micrograms/ kg/minute
Mannitol	1 gm/kg/dose
Morphine	0.1 mg/kg/dose
Naloxone (Narcan)	0.01 mg/kg/dose
Phenobarbital	2 to 3.5 mg/kg/day
Sodium bicarbonate	2 mEq (2cc)/kg/dose
Staphcillin	100 to 200 mg/kg/day
Xylocaine Spray (4%)	2 mg/kg for vocal cords
Xylocaine	0.75 to 1.5 mg/kg/dose for arrhythmias

*Editor's note. Some of these dosages differ from most recent recommendations (especially, e.g., mannitol). Therefore the reader is referred to Appendix B for current drug dosages.

cheal tube. If these routes of administration are unsuccessful, then epinephrine and if necessary, sodium bicarbonate, can be administered directly into the heart. The intracardiac injection can be given either from the precordial or subxiphoid route. The needle is inserted midway between the sternum and the mid-clavicular line, i.e. about 2 cm away from the sternum in the fourth intercostal space, or the needle can be inserted from the subxiphoid region and aimed up towards the left shoulder. Blood should aspirate as the needle is inserted to insure that the needle is inside the heart. Generally, calcium should not be administered directly into the heart since it produces asystole.

B. Fibrillation. Ventricular fibrillation is treated by continued ventilation and massage followed by repeated doses of sodium bicarbonate. The heart should be shocked once with a current of 2 to 5 watt-seconds per kg. If the weight is not known, then the defibrillation current should be 25 to 50 watt-seconds in infants; 50 to 100 watt-seconds in older children; and 100 to 300 watt-seconds in adults. If fibrillation persists after 20 seconds of ventilation, then cardiac massage should be resumed. After 2 minutes sodium bicarbonate and epinephrine should be repeated followed by the slow administration of calcium chloride. Epinephrine and/or bicarbonate can be given by intracardiac injection but only if no other route of administration is available. Defibrillation should be attempted again with a higher current level. If a defibrillator is not available, then one or more sharp blows (sternal thumps) to the midsternum should be applied.

C. Low cardiac output. If a regular beat returns but remains weak, the circulation should be supported with an intravenous drip containing isoproterenol or dopamine. Isoproterenol is given at 0.1 to 0.5 micrograms per kg per minute and dopamine at 5-20 micrograms per kg per minute. The Rule of Six (see Table A-2) can be used to prepare the solution*:

ISOPROTERENOL. The weight of the patient in kilograms is multiplied by **0.6.** This amount in milligrams is placed in IV fluid to equal 100 cc of fluid. The cc per hour infusion rate on the intravenous pump is the amount of isoproterenol given in 0.1 micrograms per kg per minute.

DOPAMINE. The weight of the patient in kilograms is multiplied by **6.0.** The amount in milligrams is placed in IV fluid to equal 100 cc of fluid. The cc per hour infusion rate on the intravenous pump is the amount of dopamine given in micrograms per kg per minute.

D. Bradycardia. Marked bradycardia should initially be treated with epinephrine. However, if bradycardia persists give 0.01 mg per kg of atropine. Always remember that if the arrest is caused by exsanguination, 20 cc per kg of 0 negative low-titer uncross-matched blood, plasma, or Ringer's lactate should be **rapidly** infused by pump.

■ **External bleeding**

Hemorrhage should be arrested by **direct pressure** over the wound. **Elevation** may greatly reduce the blood

*See Appendix C for continuous infusion dosage charts ("drip charts").

Table A-2   Rule of six

Calculations used to prepare solutions of vasopressors are confusing, time-consuming, and fraught with error. When the Rule of Six is applied, the calculations are quick and simple. The patient's weight in kg is multiplied by **0.6** or **6.0** for isoproterenol or dopamine, respectively. This amount in **milligrams** is added to IV fluid to equal 100 cc of fluid. When administered in cc/hour, this solution supplies 0.1 micrograms/kg/minute of isoproterenol or 1.0 micrograms/kg/minute of dopamine. For example, if the child needs **10** micrograms/kg/minute of dopamine to maintain an adequate cardiac output, then the infusion pump is set at **10** cc/hour.

---

loss, and this is particularly true with massive bleeding from scalp wounds. On occasion, spurting vessels may be clamped with hemostats, but only if the bleeding points are clearly visible. Remember that nerves are generally adjacent to vessels, especially in the extremities and the face. The only blood vessels that may be clamped without significant risk of nerve injury are those of the scalp. Bleeding from the extremities may be **controlled temporarily** by **tourniquets.** Blood pressure cuffs serve as useful tourniquets under these conditions. The tourniquet must be tight enough to obliterate the distal pulses or else blood loss will be promoted. Ischemic pain usually becomes unbearable within 15 to 20 minutes after application of the tourniquet and ischemic damage may be present within 30 to 45 minutes of tourniquet application. Within a few minutes the tourniquet should be replaced by sterile pressure dressings over the wound to avoid ischemic damage and pain.

■ **Shock**

Shock in the trauma patient is caused by hypoxia or blood loss. The keys to the management of hemorrhagic shock are recognition, replacement, and arrest of further bleeding. **An injured child is in shock if tachycardia and cool, pale extremities accompany a systolic pressure below 70 mm Hg.** If inadequate tissue perfusion is allowed to continue, a very simple problem may eventually result in a fatality.

The estimated blood volume is 80 cc per kg regardless of age or size. The upper limits of normal for pulse rate vary with age:

	Beats per minute
Infants	160
Preschool aged child	140
School aged child	120

The normal systolic blood pressure in mm of Hg for children from one year to 20 years is 80 plus twice their age in years. Normal minimal urine output averages 2 cc per kg per hour in small children and 1 cc per kg per hour in children over two years of age. A summary of these important physiologic parameters is presented in Table A-3.

A previously healthy child who is in shock after an injury has lost at least one-fourth and usually not more than one-half of his normal blood volume. Thus, children in hemorrhagic shock have lost between 20 to 40 cc per kg of blood. A dependable intravenous line should be started. Initially, percutaneous placement of the IV should be attempted, but if this is unsuccessful a cutdown should be performed. Venous access can usually be achieved by using the greater saphenous or external jugular veins. The details of a saphenous venous cutdown are shown in Fig. A-3. If a saphenous or external jugular vein cutdown is unsuccessful, the antecubital fossa should be explored. One should not forget that a vein is very often present on the dorsum of the hand between the fourth and fifth fingers. Ideally two IV routes should be started, one above and one below the diaphragm, and, if possible, avoid placement of an IV in an

Table A-3 Physiologic parameters in infants and children

Ventilation	Breaths per minute
Infants	40
Preschool-aged child	30
School-aged child	20

Circulation	Beats per minute
Infants	160
Preschool-aged child	140
School-aged child	120

Estimated blood volume

80 cc per kg

Systolic blood pressure

80 mm Hg plus twice the age in years

Urine output

Infants	2 cc per kg per hour
Children over 2 years	1 cc per kg per per hour

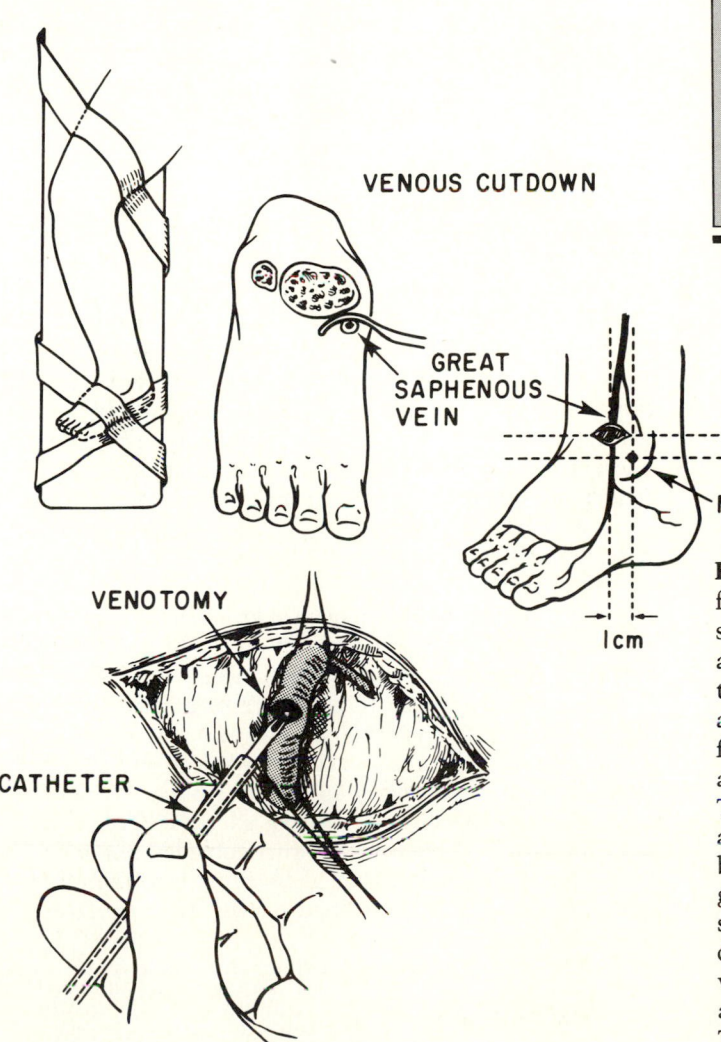

VENOUS CUTDOWN

GREAT SAPHENOUS VEIN

1cm

MALLEOLUS

1cm

VENOTOMY

CATHETER

Fig. A-3 Saphenous vein cutdown. The leg and foot are taped to a padded board with the medial side up. Betadine is used to prep the skin and a local anesthetic is injected intradermally. A 3-5 mm transverse incision is made one centimeter above and in front of the tip of the medial malleolus. A fine, curved hemostat is inserted into the posterior aspect of the incision until the tibia is encountered. The tip of the hemostat is then scraped forward against the bone and all the tissue is scooped up and brought out through the incision. The hemostat is gently teased open until the vein is freed from the surrounding tissue and nerve. The vein is tied distally with 4-0 Dexon. Direct cannulation of the vessel with an angiocatheter is easily accomplished although at times a transverse venotomy is helpful. The catheter is anchored to the vein with a 4-0 Dexon. Careful skin closure completes the cutdown.

injured extremity. We would strongly discourage routine use of percutaneous subclavian or internal jugular venapunctures in children less than four to five years of age as these procedures are hazardous in this age group even when attempted by experienced personnel.

Military antishock trousers (**MAST trousers**) are now available in pediatric sizes. Trousers will probably be an important adjunct to the treatment of shock in selected pediatric patients. However, extensive experience with this relatively new tool is still lacking. If the trousers are applied they should be removed in the operating room only after adequate resuscitation. Refer to Appendix A-1 for details regarding the use of MAST trousers.

Initial treatment of hemorrhagic shock consists of placement in the Trendelenberg position, prevention of heat loss, and the rapid administration of a bolus of 20 cc per kg of Ringer's lactate. If the blood pressure returns to normal the IV may be maintained at 5 cc per kg per hour. If the pulse rate remains elevated and the blood pressure is below 70 mm Hg, then a second bolus of Ringer's lactate is given. The need for this second bolus implies that blood transfusion will be needed and strongly suggests that the child may still be bleeding. The detection of continuing bleeding is much easier if solutions are administered as a bolus rather than a constant rate. **Comparison of pre- and postinfusion parameters are important in detecting hemodynamic instability.** If the child remains hypotensive the freshest whole blood available should be rapidly administered in a bolus of 20 cc per kg over a short period of time. Type specific blood should be given when available. However, O negative low titer uncross-matched blood is acceptable. Blood, colloid, or crystalloid solutions should be administered until the blood pressure is at least 70 mm Hg.

Recognition of occult blood loss may require a much longer observation period. Fractures of the pelvis or major long bones, scalp lacerations, and renal injuries may be associated with loss of more than one-fourth of the total blood volume. Significant occult bleeding is usually intra-abdominal but occasionally is within the thoracic cavity.

■ Phase 2

■ EVALUATION OF REGIONAL TRAUMA

Following the initial cardiopulmonary support and treatment of shock a brief physical examination of the injured child is appropriate. A nasogastric tube is always inserted and consideration should be given to an indwelling urethral catheter. The order in which the regions of the body are evaluated will vary with the nature of the injury. The child's care may be individualized, but the following list roughly parallels the descending order of urgency with which the usual injuries of children must be managed: 1) thorax, 2) abdomen, 3) head and neck, 4) genitourinary, and 5) orthopedic injuries.

■ Thorax*

Injuries of the thorax may affect ventilation and circulation and are thus of prime importance. The rib cage of children is quite pliable and does not afford great protection to the underlying organs. Unlike adults, fractured ribs in children do not usually accompany thoracic injury but when present one should assume that the child is at risk to a major injury. All children with fractured ribs should, therefore, be admitted to the hospital for 24 to 48 hours of observation.

The goals of management of thoracic trauma are as follows:

To control hemorrhage and life-threatening infection by prompt recognition and surgical closure of rents in the heart, major vessels, and esophagus.

To evacuate the pleural cavities, mediastinum, and pericardium of air, blood, or fluid.

To re-expand collapsed lungs with closure of tears in the trachea or major bronchi when necessary.

To guard against recurrent pulmonary collapse or accumulation of air, blood, or fluid.

Airway obstruction. Foreign matter, such as blood or stomach content, may contaminate the entire tracheobronchial tree. All foreign debris should be quickly removed from the oropharynx. Repeated gentle suctioning via an endotracheal tube is usually adequate to clear the airway. Insertion of a nasogastric tube will prevent further aspiration of gastric contents.

Tension pneumothorax. Tension pneumothorax is a very common cause of impaired ventilation in the injured child. The involved hemithorax is hyper-resonant with diminished breath sounds. The trachea and mediastinum are shifted toward the opposite side. If a pneumothorax is suspected a large needle attached to a syringe or Heimlich valve should be inserted into the chest in the anterior axillary line. Aspiration of as little as 50 cc of air may be lifesaving. Consideration should be given to insertion of a chest tube in order to remove reaccumulated air. The details of chest tube insertion are reviewed in Fig. A-4.

Hemothorax. Significant hemothorax produces dullness, diminished or absent breath sounds, and a shift of the mediastinal structures to the opposite side. Most injuries in children are accompanied by a combined hemopneumothorax. The management depends on the amount of blood in the chest and the rapidity with which it accumulates. A large needle attached to a syringe or a Heimlich valve should be inserted into the chest in the posterior axillary line. A large chest tube is usually required and should be inserted in the midaxillary line. The amount of blood removed is recorded. If the blood loss exceeds 30 cc per kg in the first eight hours following injury consideration for operation is indicated. As a rule, if bleeding into the chest is sufficient to cause hemorrhagic shock, then operation is urgently needed.

Cardiac tamponade. Cardiac tamponade, a rare cause

---

* See also Chapters 3 and 4.

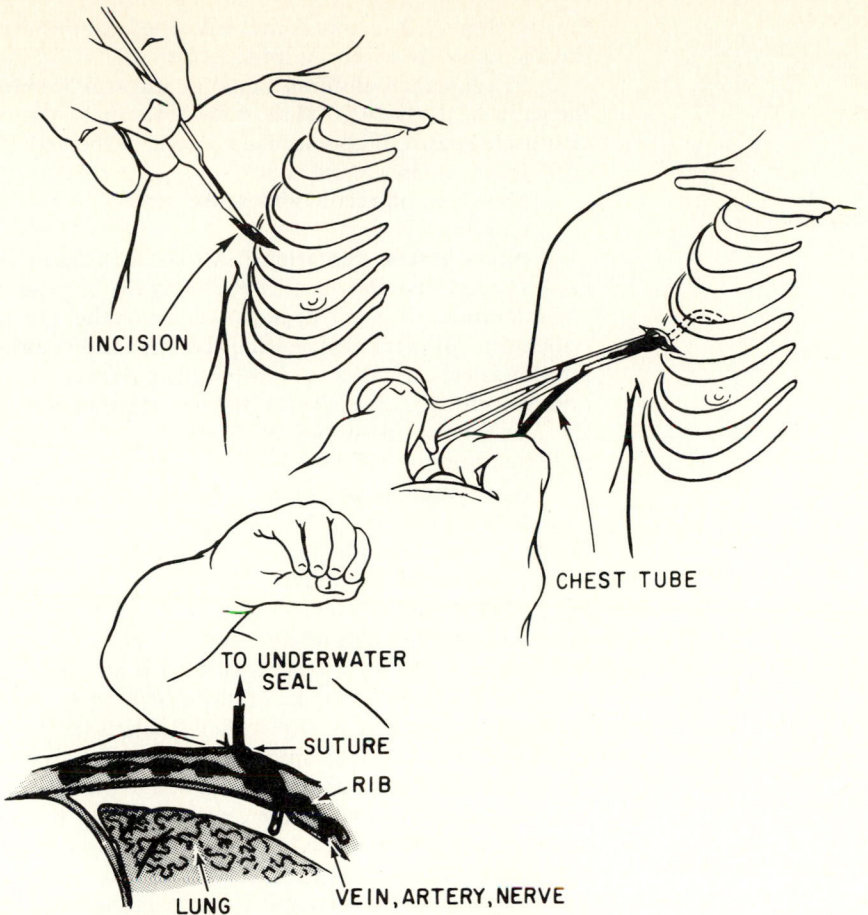

INCISION

CHEST TUBE

TO UNDERWATER
SEAL

SUTURE

RIB

LUNG

VEIN, ARTERY, NERVE

Fig. A-4 Chest tube insertion. The upper arm is elevated to expose the axilla. Betadine is used to prep the skin and a local anesthetic is injected intradermally, subcutaneously, and into the muscles of the chest wall. A 1-1.5 cm transverse skin incision is made in the mid-axillary line just above the level of the nipple (4th or 5th intercostal space). A curved hemostat is used to dissect an oblique narrow tract from the skin site to the next higher intercostal space. The hemostat is then passed bluntly thru the intercostal space just above the rib to avoid injury to the intercostal bundle. The chest tube is inserted into the pleural space along the "Z-shaped" tract. Should accidental dislodgement of the chest tube occur, it is unlikely that a significant volume of air will enter the pleural cavity with the described tunnelling technique. The incision is closed snuggly around the chest tube to avoid an air or fluid leak. The chest tube should be carefully anchored to the skin with sutures and tape. Vaseline gauze and a small dressing are placed around the tube to insure an airtight seal. Attach the chest tube to an underwater seal or Heimlich valve depending upon availability.

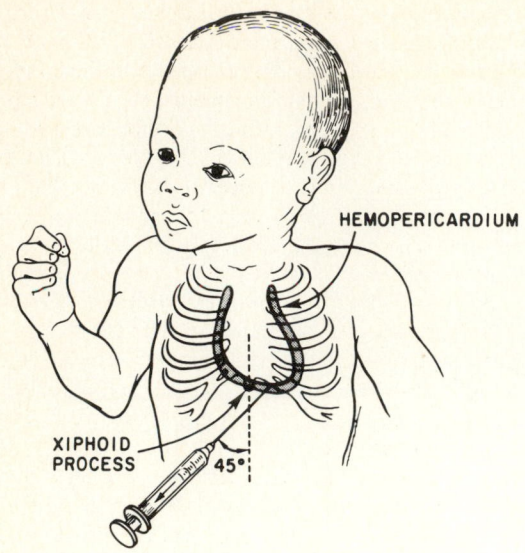

Fig. A-5 Pericardiocentesis. Cardiac tamponade can be relieved by aspiration of a small volume of fluid from the pericardial space. An 18 gauge needle is inserted below and to the left-side of the xiphoid process. The tip of the needle is aimed at the left scapula, 45° laterally and 45° upward. Aspirate the syringe while advancing the needle to avoid injury to the myocardium. Blood in the pericardial space will not clot. However, if the heart chamber is entered, this blood will clot.

of circulatory insufficiency, results from accumulation of blood within the pericardium. It is usually caused by a penetrating wound of the heart. The condition is characterized by hypotension, tachycardia, a narrow pulse pressure, and a high central venous pressure suggested by the finding of distended neck veins. The emergency treatment consists of the **rapid** administration of a bolus of Ringer's lactate followed by pericardiocentesis. The needle is inserted below the xiphoid and aimed at the left scapula, 45° upward and 45° lateral to the point of entrance. Fig. A-5 demonstrates the appropriate technique for pericardiocentesis.

Open wound and flail chest. Open chest wounds should be covered with large, air-tight dressings. Ventilation of a flail chest is improved by external splinting or preferably with placement of an endotracheal tube.

◼ Abdomen*

In abdominal trauma bleeding is the major threat to life. Eighty percent of abdominal injuries are blunt, and 20% are penetrating injuries. The usual abdominal injuries are rupture of the spleen, liver, or intestine. Less common are injuries of the pancreas or major vessels. Often more than one organ is injured. Rupture of the spleen or liver produces bleeding while rupture of the bowel produces peri-

*See also Chapter 8.

tonitis. Repeated, careful, and unhurried examinations of the abdomen are essential for diagnosis.

In conscious children blood or intestinal content in the peritoneal cavity produces pain, tenderness, distention, or muscle spasm. If abdominal injury is suspected:

Insert a nasogastric tube
Measure and record abdominal girth
Crossmatch

Acute gastric dilatation. Air swallowing frequently causes abdominal distention which may result in acute gastric dilatation. The left upper quadrant of the abdomen is tympanitic. In extreme cases the abdomen is distended, respiration is embarrassed, and the child appears to be in hemorrhagic shock. A nasogastric tube establishes the diagnosis, reduces the likelihood of aspiration, and offers definitive treatment.

Abdominal lavage. The decision for abdominal lavage should be made by the consulting surgeon. Abdominal lavage is performed liberally in patients with head injuries, fractures of the ribs or pelvis, and in those with hematuria. Prior to an abdominal tap, abdominal films should be taken to evaluate the patient for free air or fluid, masses, or fractures. The procedure is performed with an angiocatheter through which 20 cc per kg of buffered Ringer's lactate or dialysis fluid is injected. One liter of Ringer's lactate should be buffered with a 50 cc ampule of sodium bicarbonate (44 mEq) in order to decrease the likelihood of peritoneal irritation from the solution. The preferred sites for catheter insertion are just below the umbilicus in the midline, or lateral to the rectus sheath. A red blood cell count of over 100,000 per mm³ or the inability to read newsprint through a test tube full of the effluent is significant.

Serial evaluation of the abdomen is difficult following abdominal lavage as abdominal pain, tenderness and spasm can be expected for 24 to 48 hours.

Penetrating wounds. In general, children with penetrating wounds of the abdomen are not subjected to laparotomy unless the abdomen is tender. This nonoperative policy demands repeated observation for detection of developing signs of intraabdominal injury. Most gunshot wounds require exploration because of obvious abdominal pain, tenderness, or blood loss. In doubtful situations a catheter can be sutured into the wound through which water-soluble contrast material is injected. Abdominal films are checked for evidence of dye in the peritoneum. Exploration is advised for positive or equivocal radiologic findings.

Amylase. Rapid rise of serum amylase levels to more than 4 to 6 times normal signifies either an injury to the pancreas or perforation of the duodenum or jejunum. Usually these children have clear evidence of peritoneal irritation demanding abdominal exploration.

Evisceration. Eviscerated abdominal contents should be covered with moist, clean (sterile) dressings. The organs should not be replaced into the abdomen and they should not be allowed to twist or kink. Acceptable dressing materials are clean sheets and towels, aluminum foil and plastic wrap. One should not use any material that clings or loses its structure when wet, such as absorbent cotton, paper towels, or Kleenex tissue.

■ **Head and neck***

In children with head injuries and multiple trauma, the usual mistakes in caring for the child often center around failure to support ventilation and circulation and failure to detect additional injuries in other parts of the body. If the child is in shock, it must be assumed that there are additional injuries to account for that shock. Shock is rarely attributable entirely to a head injury. Once ventilation and circulation have been restored or are being supported artificially and once other regional injuries have been stabilized so as not to cause further deterioration, there is rarely need for heroic speed except to stop uncontrolled hemorrhage or to decompress a rapidly expanding intracranial hematoma.

A decision regarding the urgency of neurosurgical care can often be made during the first few moments of the initial emergency room evaluation. Information obtained from the history is vitally important. Efforts should be made to determine the time of the injury and the time that has transpired during transport to the emergency care facility. Witnesses can often provide reliable information as to the patient's condition at the scene of the accident, and a determination of deterioration can often be made by comparing that condition with the patient's present condition while in the emergency room. Documented neurological deterioration associated with focal neurological abnormalities, i.e. a dilated and fixed pupil, hemiplegia, and abnormal respiration identify the need for urgent neurosurgical care.

Emergency surgery is usually necessary for uncontrolled hemorrhage or rapidly expanding intracranial hematomas. Other injuries requiring urgent care include uncontrolled hemorrhage from the scalp and bleeding from the dural sinuses through open-skull fractures. Treatment of these conditions will be discussed in the appropriate parts of this text.

A mini-neurological examination (Table A-4) is quite important in assessing the patient's neurological status at different points in time. Decisions regarding the urgency of surgical intervention and/or transportation to neurosurgical centers are often based upon information obtained from the mini-neurological examination.

Aside from surgery to decompress expanding intracranial hematomas and repair of dural sinus lacerations, other neurosurgical procedures may be indicated, but usually not with such urgency. Other injuries which frequently require surgical treatment are more slowly expanding intracranial hematomas, open depressed skull fractures, and closed depressed skull fractures if the fragment is depressed more than the thickness of the skull. Operation is usually not indicated for cerebral concussions and contusions, closed depressed skull fractures with minimal depressed fragments, and unconscious patients who show no evidence of deterioration and who subsequently are shown not to have an intracranial mass lesion.

Scalp bleeding. Scalp lacerations can be the source

*See also Chapter 6.

of large amounts of blood loss in children. It is not rare for a child to exsanguinate from a scalp laceration without other serious injury. Bleeding from the scalp should be controlled with direct pressure and with appropriately placed hemastats on scalp arteries. Do not underestimate the amount of bleeding that may occur in a child from a scalp laceration.

Skull fractures. Skull fractures may often be detected by feeling over the head and palpating for asymmetry. Localized areas of scalp hematomas may suggest the presence of depressed fractures, but a diagnosis of depressed fracture should not be made without verification on skull x-ray or visualization through a scalp laceration.

Before suturing any scalp laceration, the underlying skull should be explored for fractures and for depression. If the fragment is depressed more than the thickness of the skull, then operation is usually indicated.

Linear fractures of the skull rarely require specific treatment. Linear fractures located in certain areas, i.e., the middle cranial fossa or the posterior cranial fossa, alert the physician to the possibility of epidural hematomas in these areas. These patients should be closely observed for signs of increasing intracranial pressure.

Basilar skull fractures are rarely seen on plain skull films. Their presence is documented by the presence of blood and CSF coming from either the ear or the nose. A basal fracture through the anterior cranial fossa may be manifest by periorbital bleeding and lateral scleral hemorrhage. Care should be taken when NG tubes are inserted if the patient has a known fracture in the anterior fossa. It is not wise to use instrumentation to clean out the ears when basilar fractures are present in this area. Initially, our preference is to withhold antibiotics for basilar skull fractures.

Open depressed skull fractures will require a neurosurgical procedure as a part of their treatment. The area should be covered with sterile saline soaked sponges. The patient should be started on antibiotics as early as possible following the injury. If brain is found to be coming from the wound, the patient should also be started on anticonvulsants. Our preference is Dilantin.

Closed depressed skull fractures may or may not require a neurosurgical procedure. These do not usually require antibiotics prior to the time of surgery.

Uncontrolled hemorrhage through open scalp lacerations may be associated with skull fractures and tears in the dural venous sinuses. Rapid exsanguination can occur in such circumstances. Emergency treatment should consist of elevating the head approximately 90 degrees, even if the child is in profound shock. This maneuver, however, is not without danger. Great care should be taken to cover the entire exposed cranium with sterile dressings so that massive air embolism does not occur through the skull fractures into the open venous sinuses. Large bore intravenous catheters are necessary for blood and fluid resuscitation in these patients. Elevation of the head has often been helpful since the bleeding is venous, not arterial, and may stop with simple head elevation and scalp dressings. Sometimes an emergency craniotomy is necessary to control the hemorrhage from torn venous sinuses. This decision cannot be undertaken lightly and should be attempted only when ap-

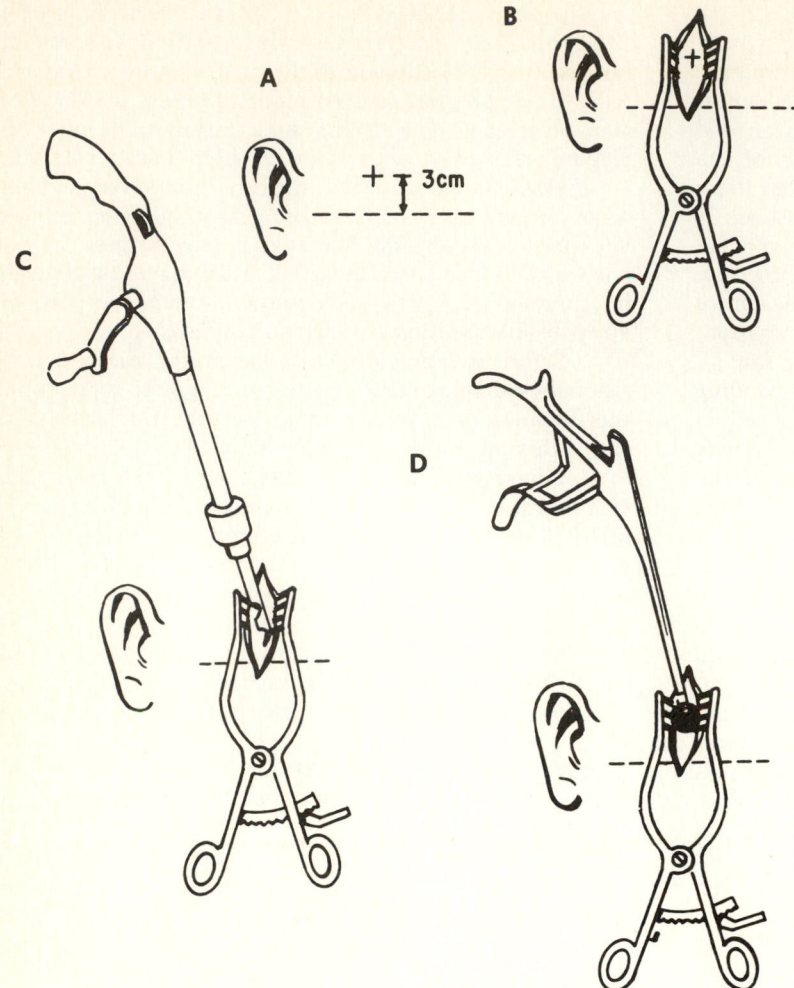

Fig. A-6 Techniques of placing burr holes.

A, Appropriate location for temporal burr hole.

B, Scalp and temporalis muscle are retracted with a self-retaining retractor, exposing the temporal bone.

C, A hole is made through the temporal bone using either a twist drill or a cranial perforator.

D, If a twist is used, enlarge the opening with a small bone rongeur.

propriate personnel and facilities are available.

It is best to stabilize the patient and have the skull x-rays made in the x-ray department if possible. This results in a better quality film and a more accurate assessment of the patient's x-rays.

Intracranial hematomas. Rapidly expanding intracranial hematomas are associated with neurological deterioration. This can usually best be diagnosed by frequent documentation of the patient's neurological status. As previously noted, frequent mini-neurological examinations (Table A-4) are an important part of the ongoing evaluation of the patient's neurological status.

It is also important to be aware of the patient's neurological status prior to the time of arrival in the emergency treatment center. Paramedical personnel can frequently give excellent status reports of the patient's condition at the scene of the accident and during transportation.

A. Epidural hematomas

Epidural hematomas usually represent arterial bleeding and may show rapid neurological deterioration. Epidural hematomas can be rapidly fatal. These hematomas are often associated with low velocity injuries to the skull, i.e., patient hit by a rock, fall from a bike, etc. A period of unconsciousness followed by consciousness (a lucid interval) followed by rapid deterioration, hemiparesis, and unilateral dilated pupil strongly suggests the evolution of an epidural hematoma. If these signs are present, rapid decompression is imperative.

Initial treatment for a rapidly expanding epidural hematoma would be mannitol. This should be given as a rapid infusion intravenously at 1 gram per kilogram.* Be sure that the patient has an indwelling Foley catheter in place

---

*This dose of mannitol has recently been reevaluated. See Appendix B for further information.

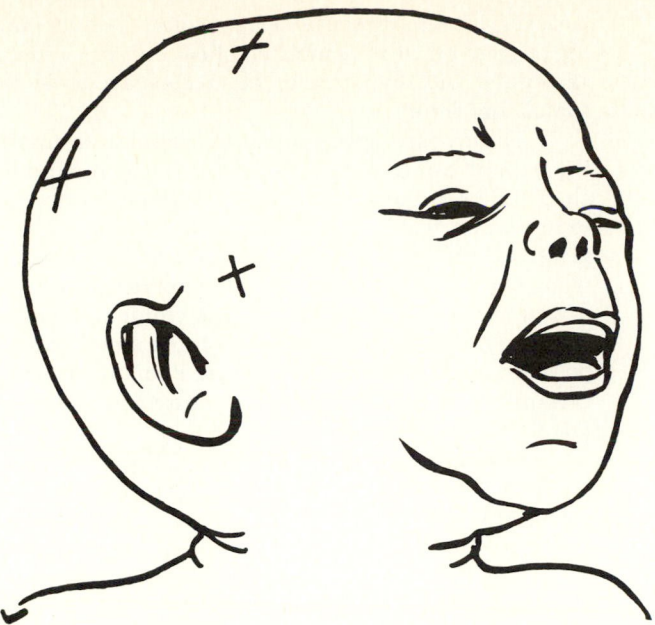

Fig. A-7 Locations for placement of burr holes.

when the mannitol is given. The mannitol may actually provide enough brain shrinkage that referral for appropriate neurosurgical care can be accomplished. However, if the patient continues to deteriorate, strong consideration for surgical intervention should be given. A burr hole placed in the emergency room or more appropriately, in the operating room, carries far less risk to the child than does helpless inactivity. However, every attempt should be made to transfer the patient to the care of a neurosurgeon. Placement of a burr hole should be done only after neurosurgical consultation.

If a decision to place burr holes is made, it is extremely important that they are placed in the appropriate positions. A short vertical incision should be made just above the zygomatic process in front of and above the ear as shown in Fig. A-6. The scalp and temporalis muscle should be held with a self-retaining retractor. The hole in the skull can be made with a twist drill or with a cranial perforator. If a twist drill is used, it should be enlarged to approximately the size of a five cent piece. If no blood is found in the epidural space, then the dura mater should be opened to check for the presence of a subdural hematoma. If no blood is found in this area, then burr holes should be placed in the posterior frontal and posterior parietal regions as illustrated in Fig. A-7. If there is still no subdural or epidural hematoma to be found, the procedure should be repeated on the opposite side.

B. Subdural hematomas
Subdural hematomas occur more frequently in children, especially smaller children, than do epidural hematomas. Subdural hematomas are often associated with high velocity injuries and often are associated with more serious

brain injury than are epidural hematomas. Diffuse brain injury, brain lacerations, and severe brain swelling are often accompaniments of subdural hematomas.

Occasionally the symptoms of subdural hematoma can be much less dramatic than those of an epidural hematoma because the bleeding is often venous and expansion of the intracranial hematoma may be slower to evolve. Baseline neurological observations are extremely important so that clinical deterioration can be documented.

It should be stressed that the decision to place burr holes in a patient prior to definitive neurosurgical care requires careful consideration. This maneuver can certainly be life saving when the child is acutely deteriorating on the basis of an expanding intracranial hematoma and time allows no further delay. However, mannitol will frequently provide extra time and appropriate help can then be obtained. Only under the most unusual circumstances should consideration be given to placing the burr hole prior to neurosurgical consultation.

Foreign bodies in the brain. Occasionally a patient will present with a foreign body in the brain. If this foreign body is visibly protruding from the skull, there is sometimes the tendency to remove it. It should not be removed! Removal of foreign bodies should be attempted only under controlled circumstances. The patient is usually in the operating room with the procedure ready to begin when foreign bodies are removed. There is a high incidence of foreign bodies producing a tamponade of blood vessels. Since removal of the foreign body may release this tamponade, serious intracranial hemorrhage may occur.

Evaluation of brain injuries
A. LEVEL OF CONSCIOUSNESS
It is important to describe the patient's neurological status. Such words as comatose, stuporous, and lethargic may have different meanings to different people. It is more

important to describe the patient's responses to such things as answering questions, obeying commands, and response to painful stimuli. The following is an appropriate way of describing the patient's response, but it should be remembered when using these terms, always describe the patient's responses in addition to using the terms.

1. ALERT

The patient is awake and remains awake. He may or may not be fully oriented and may or may not have amnesia for the event surrounding the injury.

2. LETHARGIC

The patient tends to sleep, but can be aroused with stimulation to follow commands and give appropriate responses. He tends to sleep when not stimulated.

3. STUPOROUS

The patient cannot be aroused to follow commands or give appropriate responses. The patient remains in an unconscious state. When given painful stimulation, he may thrash about and withdraw, but does not awaken to follow any commands.

4. SEMI-COMATOSE

The patient has only reflex responses to painful stimulation. This includes decerebrate and decorticate posturing.

5. COMATOSE

The patient has no response to pain. The patient is completely unresponsive.

B. LOCALIZED NEUROLOGICAL DEFICIT

1. HEMIPARESIS

Check for weakness in a conscious child by asking for appropriate responses. If a patient is uncooperative or if he is unresponsive, give a deep, painful stimulus and record the appropriateness of the response. Responses are generally classified as purposeful, semi-purposeful, or reflex such as decerebrate or decorticate. Another way to classify the motor response might be, as listed in the Glasgow Coma Scale (Table A-5), localizes, withdraws, flexion, extension, or no response.

2. EYES

Check for obvious injuries to the globe. Are the eyes spontaneously roving and moving together (conjugate) or roving and not moving together (dysconjugate)? If the patient is awake, check for appropriate eye movements if he will cooperate.

Are the pupils equal, and do they react directly to light? Are both pupils widely dilated and fixed? If so, check again for cardiac arrest.

One of the more common causes of fixed dilated pupils is injury to the head in the region of the forehead or eye resulting in traumatic iridoplegia. One pupil dilated, deviated outward, with ptosis of the same eyelid suggests a third nerve paresis and a localized intracranial hematoma.

C. VITAL SIGNS

Slowing of the pulse and rising blood pressure suggest increasing intracranial pressure. The Cushing response (slowing pulse and rising blood pressure) is often a late sign in head injuries. Do not wait for this response before seeking neurosurgical consultation. A rapid pulse and hypoten-

sion suggest the presence of hypovolemic shock and thus the suggestion to remember to check for other injuries. A slow pulse with hypotension in a responsive child suggests spinal cord injury.

These observations can form a baseline against which the patient can be compared. It should be remembered to check all of the parameters listed in the mini-neurological examination (Table A-4). Those children who do show progressive improvement in their level of consciousness or who remain the same without deterioration rarely require urgent surgical intervention. Those children who do show deterioration often have increased intracranial pressure and possibly an expanding intracranial hematoma. They will certainly require intensive medical care and probably intracranial pressure monitoring.

GLASGOW COMA SCALE. The Glasgow Coma Scale (Table A-5) is an aide in categorizing the seriousness of neurological injury as well as helping us to offer some prediction regarding eventual outcome. Every patient should be graded according to the scale. It simply requires recording the patient's best response to verbal command, eye opening, and motor response. The patient is scored according to the numerical value assigned to the level of his response.

Treatment of brain injury. Most children with brain injuries do not require surgery. Treatment is aimed at supporting vital functions, minimizing secondary complications from the injury and maintenance of an environment to allow the patient's brain injury to recover.

A. BRAIN SWELLING

If the child is not in shock, the head should be elevated approximately 30 degrees. Although there is no strong evidence at present that Decadron is helpful in the acute management of head injuries, it remains a very commonly used medication. A dose of 1.5 mg per kg is given as an initial intravenous bolus. Subsequently the patient is maintained on dexamethasone at a dose of 1.5 mg per kg per day divided every 4 to 6 hours.

Mannitol should be used only for documented neurological deterioration or after neurosurgical consultation has been obtained. Mannitol may aggravate intracranial bleeding, may aggravate early intracranial hyperemia (frequently seen in head injuries in children), and may mask a neurological deterioration because of brain shrinkage. If mannitol is given, the child must have an indwelling urinary catheter. Rupture of the urinary bladder may occur when a catheter is not inserted.

Hypothermia is not a standard part of our emergency management for head injuries, but a high fever should receive appropriate management because it tends to increase intracranial pressure.

Normovolemia does not increase intracranial pressure, and more problems arise from the child being hypovolemic than from trying to maintain normal intravenous fluids. We recommend maintenance of IV fluids between three-fourths and normal maintenance unless there are other reasons to give more or less fluid. In the treatment of hypovolemic shock, appropriate fluid therapy for the shock should be given without concern for the head injury.

Table A-4   The mini-neurological examination

A. History

Document time of injury, mechanism, neurological status at the time patient was first seen post-injury, elapsed time from injury to arrival in hospital, any neurological change which may have occurred.

B. Level of consciousness

1. Awake—may be disoriented or confused but still awake
2. Lethargic—can be aroused to follow commands
3. Stuporous—cannot be aroused to follow commands—purposeful withdrawal to deep painful stimuli
4. Semi-comatose—only reflex responses to pain, i.e. decorticate or decerebrate
5. Comatose—no response to pain

C. Pupils

Size, reaction

D. Response to pain

1. Purposeful
2. Semi-purposeful
3. Decorticate
4. Decerebrate
5. No response

E. Movement of extremities

Describe the movement seen spontaneously and in response to pain

F. Plantar responses

Upgoing, downgoing, or equivocal

G. Facial movements

Central or peripheral weakness may be present

H. Fundi

Describe hemorrhages—rare to see papilledema prior to 12-24 hours post-injury

I. CSF otorrhea/rhinorrhea

Usually blood with or without CSF in acute phase

J. Vital signs

Obtain baseline, monitor closely

Table A-5   The Glasgow Coma Scale

Eye opening
4 Spontaneous
3 To Speech
2 To Pain
1 None

Best verbal response
5 Oriented
4 Confused
3 Inappropriate
2 Incomprehensible
1 None

Best motor response
6 Obeys commands
5 Localizes pain
4 Withdraws
3 Flexion to pain
2 Extension to pain
1 None

B. CONVULSIONS

An impact seizure, a seizure occurring at the time of injury or very shortly thereafter, is relatively common with head injuries in children. A detailed history will often elicit that a seizure did occur near the time of impact. This does not statistically predispose the child to seizures in the future, and is usually not treated with anticonvulsant medication unless seizures continue.

When seizures persist, the initial anticonvulsant management of seizures should begin with Dilantin. Dilantin should be given intravenously in the dose of 10 milligrams per kilogram and this dose may be repeated in 30 minutes if the seizures continue. The daily maintenance dose of Dilantin is 5 mg per kg. This drug should not be given intramuscularly. It must be given mixed with normal saline and should be given slowly.

If Dilantin is not successful in controlling the seizures, diazepam may be given slowly over a 3 minute period of time in a dose not to exceed 0.25 mg per kg.

Phenobarbital should be avoided in the initial management of head injury children because of its cardio-respiratory depressive affects.

C. ANTIBIOTICS

Antibiotics are not indicated for basilar skull fractures except in patients with documented middle ear infections. Patients with open depressed skull fractures should receive antibiotics as early as possible following the injury. We recommend ampicillin in doses of 100 to 200 mg per kg per day, and methicillin 100 to 200 mg per kg per day, if not allergic.

Neck

Children who complain of pain in the neck following multiple trauma should be suspected of having cervical spine injuries and appropriate care given.

Fortunately, it is much less common to have associated cervical spine injuries in multiple trauma with young children than it is with adults. Nevertheless, spine injuries do occur in association with head injuries. If the neurological evaluation suggests a spinal cord injury, then steroids should be administered as early as possible. All spinal cord injuries should be considered reversible and emergency neurosurgical consultation is mandatory.

Penetrating injuries of the neck are a potentially hazardous problem and exploration of these injuries is best accomplished in the operating room by those experienced with such explorations. Penetrating injuries of the neck should not be probed.

Transportation of children with suspected spine injuries should not be undertaken until the head is immobilized by taping the head and the upper part of the thorax to a backboard. A KED splint, if available, is ideal for transporting suspected spinal injury patients.

■ Genitourinary system

Genitourinary and pelvic injuries are common and easily overlooked. A pelvic fracture should be suspected if pain is elicited during compression of the wings of the ilium or with abduction of the legs. Do not insert a urethral catheter if the pelvis is fractured, if a urethral injury is suspected, or if there is resistance to attempted passage of a catheter. Microscopic hematuria (5-6 red cells/HPF) usually warrants an early rapid bolus pyelogram.

Renal injury. Renal injuries are characterized by flank pain, tenderness, and hematuria. The amount of blood in the urine does not correlate well with the severity of the injury. If the child cannot void after a reasonable time, a catheter should be gently and carefully inserted into the bladder. If the catheter meets resistence, do not force it in as this may indicate a ruptured urethra. When a urethral injury or a pelvic fracture is suspected, a catheter should **not** be inserted until a urethrogram is performed. An infusion pyelogram should be obtained as soon after initial stabilization as possible.

Renal contusions, with or without perirenal hematoma, account for about 75% of renal injuries. They require no specific treatment. Renal lacerations permitting marked extravasation of urine are best treated by early elective debridement, repair, and drainage. Renal pedicle injuries are uncommon, but require emergency management if the kidney is to be salvaged. An isolated renal injury may permit enough blood loss to produce shock but usually not enough to cause exsanguination. An expanding, pulsatile renal hematoma may require surgical exploration. Remember, about 40% of renal injuries are accompanied by injuries to other organs.

Ureteral injuries. Ureteral injuries are very rare in children, and most are due to penetrating injuries.

Bladder injury. Rupture of the bladder frequently accompanies pelvic fractures, although a distended bladder may rupture in the absence of a pelvic fracture. This injury may be suspected when lower abdominal pain and tenderness are associated with hematuria. A cystogram will establish the diagnosis and operative repair is indicated.

Urethral injury. Urethral injuries are easily overlooked. The hallmarks are perineal swelling and the presence of a drop of blood at the urethral meatus. Retrograde urethrography using contrast material injected via the tip of the penis will demonstrate the point of disruption. Passage of a urethral catheter should not be attempted if the urethral injury is suspected because it may transform an incomplete urethral tear to a complete urethral disruption. The bladder may be decompressed temporarily by inserting a percutaneous suprapubic polyethylene catheter.

■ Orthopedic injuries

Except for cervical and displaced pelvic fractures, orthopedic trauma is rarely life-threatening. Thus it is appropriate to assess and stabilize injuries to the head, chest and abdomen before evaluating the extremities. However, one should not underestimate the importance of peripheral injuries; initial mismanagement can result in serious sequelae such as infection, growth disturbance, paralysis and even amputation.

Axial trauma. Fractures or dislocations of the axial skeleton (spine, pelvis) are frequently unrecognized, especially when accompanied by shock or unconsciousness. Physical signs such as tenderness, swelling or ecchymosis may be subtle or absent; accurate diagnosis requires x-ray studies. A high index of suspicion and careful transport of the patient are essential. Any significant craniofacial trauma warrants x-rays of the cervical spine, including the odontoid. Fractures of the thoracolumbar spine in children are exceedingly rare.

Regarding transport, a papoose board or KED splint is recommended, in conjunction with straps or sandbags. This combination minimizes forces of flexion and rotation which would tend to displace an unstable injury. Following x-ray confirmation of a spinal injury, definitive stabilization with traction, casting or surgery is instituted.

Pelvis. High energy trauma to the torso or lower extremities should alert one to the possibility of significant pelvic trauma. Once again, physical signs are unreliable. Unless an x-ray of the pelvis is taken in each multiple trauma case, fractures and dislocation of the hip or pelvis can easily be missed, with disastrous consequences.

Fracture or dislocation of the hip is an orthopedic emergency requiring anatomic reduction and stabilization. Displaced pelvic fractures are usually accompanied by shock. A large volume of blood may accumulate in the retroperitoneal space, causing ileus and mimicking intraperitoneal trauma. Peritoneal lavage, ultrasonography, or CAT scan are helpful in establishing the diagnosis.

One should resist the temptation to explore a retroperitoneal hematoma; exsanguination and death may result. Successful treatment requires resuscitation with fluids and adequate transfusion. Inflatable trousers are useful as a temporary measure. If available, selective angiography and embolization of arterial bleeder(s) can be lifesaving.

One must also rule out the possibility of a ruptured viscus, most commonly the bladder. Bone fragments may lacerate the rectum or vagina, leading to aerobic and anaerobic infection.

Peripheral injuries. Peripheral skeletal injuries are more easily diagnosed. Sterile dressings should be applied to wounds, utilizing direct compression to control bleeding. Avoid insertion of intravenous lines into injured extremities. Tourniquets are not recommended except as a desperation maneuver; they potentiate the effects of swelling and ischemia and have contributed to many unnecessary amputations.

Prior to moving or splinting an extremity, it is advisable to assess and record the neurovascular status. Sensation and circulation should be noted. Active motion is usually compromised by pain or deformity.

Sprains are rare in children; a swollen joint represents a fracture until proven otherwise. This is because the growth plate is weaker than the adjoining ligaments and is more apt to yield under stress. The true nature and prognosis of an epiphyseal fracture can only be determined by x-rays.

There are two indications for an attempt at reducing an obvious limb deformity:

1. Inadequate distal perfusion

Irreversible damage to muscles and nerves occurs after six hours of ischemia. One occasionally encounters a child with a cold, pulseless, anesthetic limb distal to an angular deformity. If there is any anticipated delay in transport or treatment, an attempt at realignment is warranted.

2. Impending skin necrosis

Sometimes bone fragments blanch the overlying skin, threatening to penetrate and convert a closed fracture into an open one. In this situation, it is advisable to reposition the limb in order to alleviate skin pressure.

A single, gentle effort at reduction is reasonably safe; repeated attempts, however, are dangerous and rarely successful. Interposition of soft tissue, including neurovascular structures may prevent satisfactory reduction.

Splints. It is imperative that all injured limbs are properly splinted in order to:

1. Decrease blood loss and shock
2. Decrease wound contamination
3. Decrease pain and muscle spasm
4. Reduce the risk of further soft tissue damage

A confusing array of splints is now available. The type selected is not as critical as its proper application in achieving the goals enumerated.

Traction splints (Thomas, Hare) are most useful in stabilizing femoral fractures for transport. Excessive traction is unnecessary and may cause skin sloughing around the foot and ankle.

A variety of rigid splints (wood, metal, plastic, cardboard) can be used to protect forearm and leg fractures. The fastening straps should be snug but not constricting. Inflatable splints are popular; one should avoid overinflation

which could compromise limb perfusion. A pillow taped around a wrist or ankle can be an extremely safe and comfortable means of protecting distal fractures. Injuries of the humerus and shoulder are most effectively immobilized with a sling and swath.

Infection. There are several determinants of infection in an open musculoskeletal injury:

1. Mechanism of injury
2. Degree and type of wound contamination
3. Extent of soft tissue necrosis
4. Presence of foreign bodies
5. Elapsed time between injury and treatment
6. Host immune defenses

Sterile compression dressings are the recommended initial treatment. Wound cultures should be obtained prior to commencing antibiotics. Meticulous debridement and copious irrigation of wounds is best performed under an anesthetic with tourniquet control. Primary wound closure is generally not recommended.

Tetanus is a rare but devastating complication which must be considered. Most American children have received adequate active immunization. If more than five years have elapsed since the last tetanus shot, another booster is recommended. Any wound with gross contamination or extensive soft tissue damage warrants passive immunization with human immune globulin (Hypertet), along with a tetanus toxoid booster. Of course, adequate wound debridement is mandatory.

Gas gangrene (clostridial myonecrosis) may complicate any penetrating wound or open fracture. Prophylactic penicillin is of unproven benefit and may promote a false sense of security. Wound management as previously discussed represents the best means of preventing this lethal disease.

The principles of initial management of orthopedic trauma have been outlined. By observing these guidelines one can reduce the risk of serious and disabling complications. Suspect fractures and splint accordingly until x-ray confirmation and definitive treatment are available.

■ **TRAUMA AND CHILD ABUSE**

One might wonder why a specific section on child abuse (non-accidental or inflicted injury) should be included in a manual on pediatric trauma. The necessity of directing some consideration to child abuse as a specific entity is brought into focus when one considers that the major serious causes for injury and death in child abuse and neglect involve those areas which are often dealt with in pediatric trauma. By far the leading cause of death and significant debilitation in association with child abuse is head injury. Prominent in these areas are subdural hematomas, cerebral contusion, subarachnoid hemorrhage, and intracerebral hemorrhage. These may occur either with or without skull fractures. The presence of a skull fracture, particularly if it seems out of magnitude with the history of the trauma, should always alert one to the possibility of inflicted injury. The second most common cause of death and debility in child abuse is abdominal injury. This usually involves rupture of an organ such as the liver, the most commonly injured organ, or the kidney or spleen, or it involves traumatic perforation of the intestine or bladder.

Since these injuries are commonly seen in legitimate childhood trauma, the professional staff evaluating an injured child must always be sure that the **injury is consistent with the history** which has been obtained surrounding the injury. This is particularly true when there is no known major traumatic event such as an auto-auto, auto-pedestrian, or other high velocity accident in association with the trauma. In addition the professional staff must be carefully observant as to the appropriateness of the parents' concern, their need to place blame on someone else, and their interaction with the professional staff. If the child is conscious, pay attention to the remarks which he makes in response to the direct questioning regarding the circumstances of the injury. Often children may be very helpful in raising concern regarding the possibility of the non-accidental or inflicted nature of the injury.

An important facet of the evaluation of pediatric trauma should be a careful examination of the child for other signs which might suggest the possibility of non-accidental or inflicted injury. Some of these signs include perioral ecchymosis in the absence of an appropriate injury. This is of concern because of the association of subdural hematoma and vigorous shaking or jarring of the infant's head. The general nutritional and groomed state of the victim may be a clue which might suggest non-accidental causes for the child's injury. Others include more obvious visible diagnostic signs such as cigarette burns, unusual bruising, or other cutaneous markings which might suggest unusual objects as causative in the injury; and in any child where the circumstances seem not clearly defined as causative in the injury, a careful examination of the genitalia and anal areas should be part of the evaluation of the injured child.

As has been mentioned in the other sections of this manual, the most important considerations are those which deal with the stabilization, diagnosis, and the appropriate management of the injured area. However, once these ABCs of management have been fulfilled, then it is essential to carefully consider the factors which might suggest that non-accidental or inflicted injury should be a consideration in the cause of the child's injury.

At the hospital or facility of origin of the child, as well as at the Medical Center, there may well be an organized and functioning Child Protection Team. If non-accidental injury is raised as a legitimate consideration in the etiology of the child's injury, the members of the Child Protection Team may be able to play a valuable role in clarifying the circumstances surrounding the injury.

■ Appendix A-1*

■ OBSERVATIONS ON THE USE OF THE PNEUMATIC COUNTER-PRESSURE DEVICE

The Committee on Trauma reviewed its list of "Essential Equipment for Ambulances" at a meeting in Anaheim in 1977 and published an updated version in the September 1977 issue of the *Bulletin*. A major addition to the list was the pneumatic counter-pressure device, or antishock (MAST) trousers, an item found to be of value for emergency medical technicians treating shock in the field. **The device shunts blood from the abdomen and legs to the heart, brain, and lung circulations. This instant transfusion of up to 30 percent of the patient's total blood volume is an effective noninvasive management of hypotension.** Studies have continued to demonstrate the usefulness of the garment and the fact that it can be used with minimal complications.

The indications for the use of MAST trousers have been enlarged to include all types of shock. **The only contraindication is pulmonary edema.** Thoracic injuries are no longer contraindications in the prehospital phase because use of the device constitutes an effective means of combating hypotension from blood loss as well as the possibility of adult respiratory distress syndrome and capillary leak. **There is no question that hypertension and overcirculation are detrimental in head injuries.** When associated injuries can produce hypotension, usually from hemorrhage, the pneumatic compression device is beneficial because it alleviates shock and returns cerebral circulation to normal. When cerebral circulation is compromised and edema has begun to develop, ischemia can make the edema worse. From a theoretical standpoint, therefore, use of the garment should help to prevent cerebral edema.

For several years, emergency medical technician training programs have included indications and instructions for use of pneumatic trousers. Technicians who are inadequately familiar with the timing and technique of removal have been a problem. For this reason, the Committee on Trauma felt that it was appropriate to develop a poster on the subject for use in emergency departments.

If any hazard exists in the use of this device, it results from inappropriate or too rapid removal of the garment in the emergency department, not in the field. The trousers are inflated and deflated in response to the patient's blood pres-

*Norman E. McSwain, Jr., MD, FACS, New Orleans, A.C.S.: Bulletin 9, **64**(10), Oct. 1979.

sure. Deflation is allowed to occur gradually while monitoring the patient's blood pressure closely. Any time the blood pressure drops 5 mm Hg systolic, deflation should be discontinued. Fluids, either crystalloid or blood, are then infused until the patient's blood pressure returns to acceptable limits. Just as rapid inflation can produce the effect of a transfusion of up to 30 percent of the patient's total blood volume, rapid deflation can simulate an acute blood loss of a similar amount. This amount may well be enhanced if peripheral vasodilatation exists.

As with any medical device, appropriate indications, contraindications, and procedures should be recognized. Problems with both application and removal may develop if the trouser is used incorrectly. The physician whose EMS system utilizes these pneumatic compression devices should certainly be aware of their advantages and shortcomings.

■ Pneumatic Counter-Pressure Device

■ THEORY

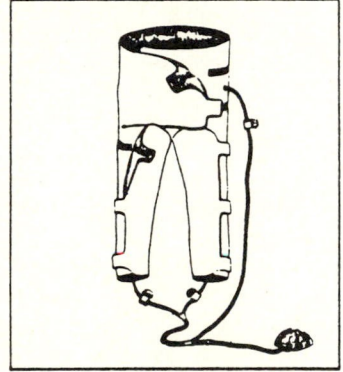

Theory

Just as leg elevation is effective in resuscitating simple fainting, and the G-Suit is effective in preventing blackout from centrifugal force in high-performance aircraft, so pneumatic counter-pressure trousers can mobilize blood from the lower extremities and abdomen and return it to the heart-brain-lung circulation for temporary resuscitation without excessive crystalloid replacement. Since 80% of blood is located in the capillary and venous circulation, approximately 30% of cardiovascular volume can be mobilized and used.

Indications

1. Systolic blood pressure below 100 when shock-like state exists.*
2. Hemorrhage control from fractured pelvis or intra-abdominal bleeding.
3. Stabilization of fractured pelvis or femur.

CAUTION

1. During later stages of pregnancy, only the leg segment is inflated.
2. Deflation must be done gradually and carefully. Rapid deflation can return the patient to shock.

CONTRAINDICATIONS

Pulmonary edema

Summary

Application of the pneumatic compression device on the abdomen and legs transfers a significant volume of blood into the heart-brain-lung circulation. Although the lower extremities and abdomen may be partially deprived of blood supply, for this short period of time (less than two hours), no detrimental effect has been shown.

The major complication that has arisen with the application of a pneumatic compression device is its too rapid removal in the emergency room without proper volume replacement.

Deflation must be slow and gradual. Rapid deflation reduces the blood volume in the heart-brain-lung circulation, and can return the patient to a shock-like state.

Important aspects during inflation, then, are monitoring of the blood pressure and inflating only as necessary to return the pressure to within adaptable limits. On deflation, the hallmark again is blood pressure monitoring to prevent recurrence of shock. *Blood pressure* is the single most important factor in the use of pneumatic pressure device for treating patients in shock.

---

*Systolic blood pressure below 70 in children when shock-like state exists.

■ **APPLICATION**

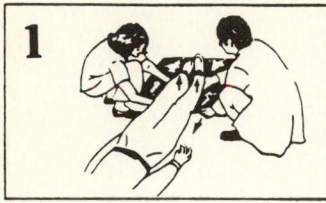

Slide open trousers beneath raised feet . . .

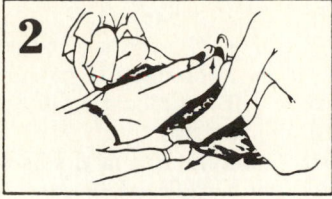

. . . to the buttocks.

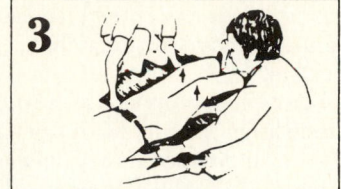

Elevate buttocks and bring trousers up to rib cage.

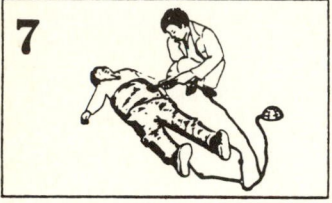

Open stopcocks.

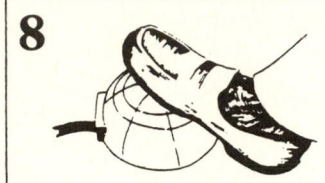

Inflate with foot pump.

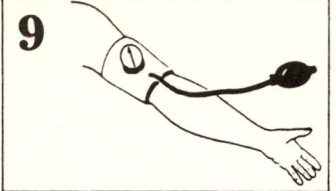

Check blood pressure. Stop inflation at 100 mm Hg (70 mm Hg in children).

■ **GRADUAL DEFLATION**

Warning: Rapid deflation can return patient to shock.

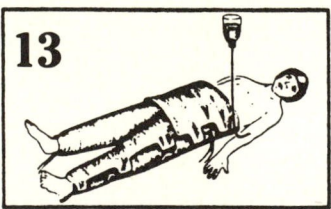

Intravenous lines are established and operating room is readied.

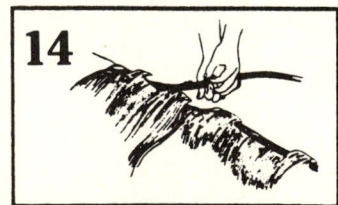

Open stopcock on abdominal section.

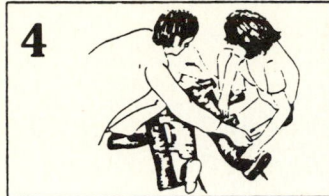

Enclose left leg and close Velcro.

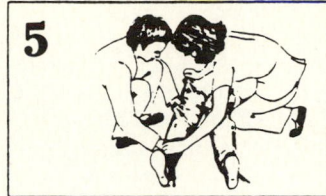

Enclose right leg and close Velcro.

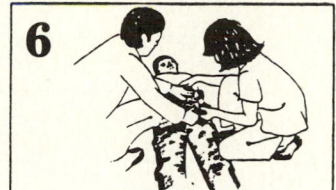

Enclose abdomen and close Velcro.

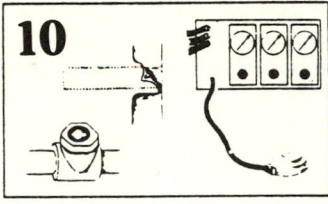

Velcro straps, pop-off valves, or gauges prevent overinflation.

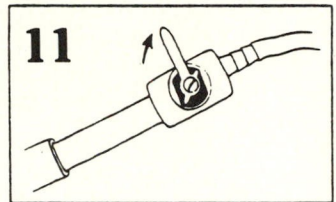

Close stopcocks.

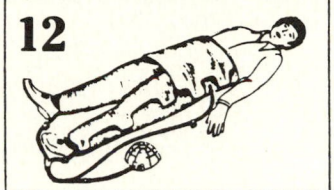

The device can be left in place fully inflated for two hours if necessary. If a longer period of inflation is necessary, alterations and additions should be considered.

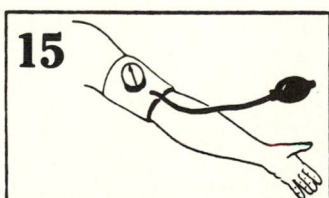

Stop deflation if blood pressure drops 5 mm Hg.

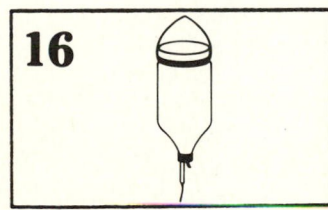

Administer intravenous fluid to restore blood pressure.

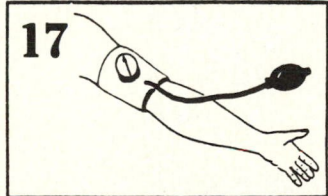

Deflation can continue while blood pressure is closely monitored. Patient can be taken to the operating room with the device inflated, if necessary.

■   **Appendix A-2**
Pediatric Trauma Algorithm

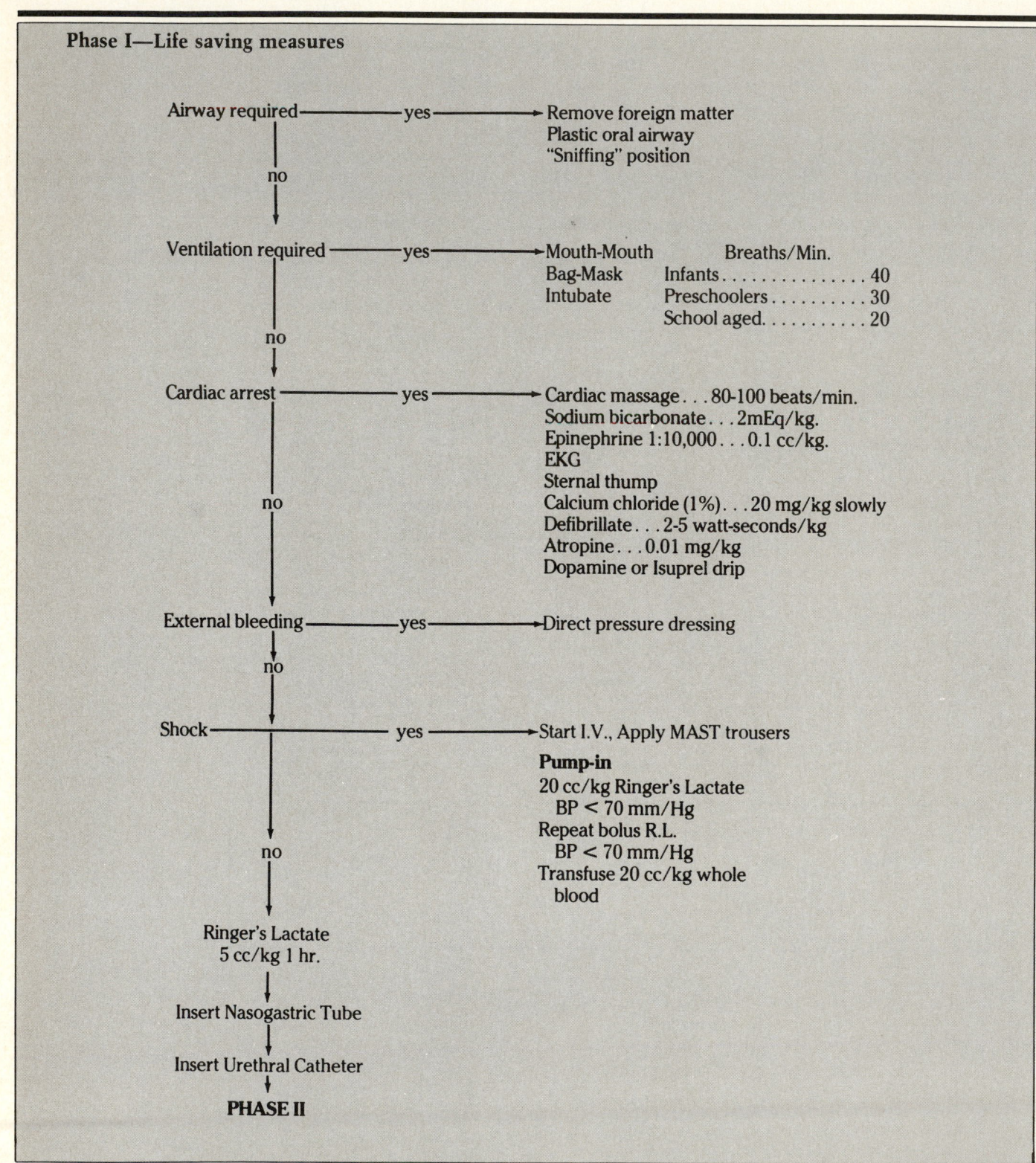

Phase I—Life saving measures

Airway required ——————— yes ——————→ Remove foreign matter
                                                        Plastic oral airway
                                                        "Sniffing" position

no

Ventilation required ——————— yes ——————→ Mouth-Mouth   Breaths/Min.
                                                         Bag-Mask   Infants 40
                                                         Intubate   Preschoolers 30
                                                                         School aged. 20

no

Cardiac arrest ——————— yes ——————→ Cardiac massage . . . 80-100 beats/min.
                                                        Sodium bicarbonate . . . 2mEq/kg.
                                                        Epinephrine 1:10,000 . . . 0.1 cc/kg.
                                                        EKG
                                                        Sternal thump
                                                        Calcium chloride (1%) . . . 20 mg/kg slowly
                                                        Defibrillate . . . 2-5 watt-seconds/kg
                                                        Atropine . . . 0.01 mg/kg
                                                        Dopamine or Isuprel drip

no

External bleeding ——————— yes ——————→ Direct pressure dressing

no

Shock ——————— yes ——————→ Start I.V., Apply MAST trousers

                                                        Pump-in
                                                        20 cc/kg Ringer's Lactate
                                                            BP < 70 mm/Hg
                                                        Repeat bolus R.L.
                                                            BP < 70 mm/Hg
                                                        Transfuse 20 cc/kg whole
                                                            blood

no

Ringer's Lactate
5 cc/kg 1 hr.

Insert Nasogastric Tube

Insert Urethral Catheter

PHASE II

Phase II—Evaluation of regional trauma

Body region and injury	Initial treatment	Hospital evaluation
Thorax		
Pneumothorax ⎤ Hemothorax ⎦ →	Needle aspiration Heimlich valve Chest tube Bolus Ringer's lactate	Chest x-ray EKG Crossmatch
Cardiac tamponade ⟶	Pericardiocentesis	
Flail chest ⟶	External splint or intubate	
Abdomen		
Bleeding ⎤ Perforation ⎦ →	Nasogastric tube Measure abdominal girth Bolus Ringer's lactate	Crossmatch Abdominal films Lavage Amylase
Evisceration ⟶	Cover with moistened dressing	
Head and neck		
Scalp or dural sinus laceration ⟶	Stop bleeding Elevate head Cover lacerations to prevent air emboli	Crossmatch Skull and neck films
Epidural/subdural hematoma ⟶	Mannitol [Only after Burr holes Neurosurgical consultation]	CAT scan
Brain swelling ⟶	Elevate head 30° Decadron Restrict fluids to ¾ maintenance Mannitol	
Convulsions ⟶	Dilantin	
Antibiotics ⟶	Ampicillin and Staphcillin	
Cervical spine injury ⟶	Immobilize cervical spine Decadron for spinal cord injury Do not probe neck wounds	
Genitourinary		
Pelvic fracture or ⟶ Urethral injury	No urethral catheter	Crossmatch I.V.P. Cystogram
Renal injury (Hematuria) ⟶	Bolus Ringer's lacate	Urethrogram
Orthopedic injuries		
Fractures ⟶	Stop bleeding Splint	X-rays

Repeat vital signs every 15 minutes

■ Appendix A-3
Summary of Pediatric Trauma Protocol

PHASE I—LIFE SAVINGS MEASURES
I. Airway and ventilation
A. Unobstructed airway
  1. Remove foreign matter
  2. Plastic oral airway
  3. "Sniffing" position
B. Ventilation
  1. Mouth to mouth
  2. Bag and mask
  3. Intubation
  4. Ventilation rate

	Breaths/min.
Infants	40
Preschool	30
School age	20

  5. Check for chest expansion

II. Circulation and cardiac arrest
A. Circulation
  1. Cardiac massage 80 to 100 beats/min.
  2. Midsternal compression: ½ to ¾ inch infants
       ¾ to 1½ inch older children.
  3. Check pulses.
  4. Start a dependable IV
B. Cardiac arrest
  1. Sodium bicarbonate — 2 cc (mEq) per kg
  2. Epinephrine 1:10,000 — 0.1 cc per kg
  3. If bleeding, **pump in** — 20 cc per kg Ringer's lactate (R/L)
  4. EKG
    a. Asystole
       Sternal "thump"
       Continue ventilation and massage for 2 minutes.
       Repeat sodium bicarbonate and epinephrine.
       Slowly give 20 mg per kg calcium chloride (1%).
    b. Fibrillation
       Repeat sodium bicarbonate and prepare to defibrillate.
       Shock heart once with 2-5 watt-seconds/kg.
       Ventilate for 20 seconds.
       If fibrillation persists, resume massage.
       After 2 minutes, repeat sodium bicarbonate.
       Shock again with a higher current.
       Sternal "thump."
    c. Low cardiac output
       Support the circulation with isoproterenol (0.1 to 0.5 μg/kg/min) or dopamine (5 to 20 μg/kg/min).
       Use Rule of Six to prepare solutions.
    d. Bradycardia
       Treat initially with epinephrine, but if bradycardia persists, give 0.01 mg/kg Atropine.

III. Stop external bleeding
IV. Shock
Start IV, apply MAST trousers.
Pump-in 20 cc per kg R/L.
If BP normal, give 5 cc per kg per hr R/L.
If BP below 70 mm Hg, **pump-in** second bolus R/L.
If BP still below 70 mm Hg, **pump-in** 20 cc/kg whole blood or colloid.
Keep on pumping blood, plasma or R/L until BP at least 70 mm Hg.
Insert nasogasric tube.
Insert urethral catheter.

PHASE II—EVALUATION OF REGIONAL TRAUMA
I. Thorax
Relieve airway obstruction.
Tension pneumothorax
  Needle aspiration with syringe or Heimlich valve in anterior axillary line, followed by chest tube if necessary.
Hemothorax
  Needle aspiration with syringe or Heimlich valve in posterior axillary line, followed by chest tube. Bolus R/L.
Cardiac tamponade
  Bolus R/L.
  Pericardiocentesis.
Open wound
  Cover it.
Flail chest
  External splint or intubate.

II. Abdomen
In all unconscious children, or when pain, tenderness, distention, or spasm are present:
  Insert nasogastric tube and aspirate.
  Measure and record abdominal girth.
  Crossmatch.
  Cover evisceration with moistened, sterile dressing.

III. Head and neck
HEAD
  Continue to support circulation and ventilation.
  Control scalp bleeding with pressure or hemostats.
  For massive scalp or brain bleeding, elevate the head even if child is in shock.
  Cover all open fractures.
  Epidural hematoma may require emergency burr holes.
  Serially evaluate level of consciousness, localizing neurologic deficit and vital signs.
  Grade all patients according to Glasgow Coma Scale.
Brain swelling
Elevate head 30° if child not in shock.
  Decadron 1.5 mg/kg IV push, followed by 1.5 mg/kg/day.
  Mannitol used for documented deterioration, but only after neurosurgical consultation if possible.
  Restrict fluids to 3/4 maintenance unless child in shock.
  Insert Foley catheter if mannitol is used.

Convulsions

Dilantin 10 mg/kg IV, repeat if necessary.

Do not treat single seizure within 30 minutes of injury.

Antibiotics

Ampicillin and Staphcillin 200 mg/kg/day for open depressed skull fracture.

NECK

All children with neck pain or head injury should have neck immobilized.

Check arm and leg movement, ask for pain or paresthesias.

All penetrating neck wounds are explored in the OR; do not probe!

Spinal shock is manifested by hypotension and bradycardia in an awake patient. Treat with a bolus of R/L followed by maintenance fluids.

If weakness suggests spinal cord injury, give Decadron 1.5 mg IV push.

IV. **Genitourinary system**

Inspect genitalia and perineum, and check for pelvic fracture.

Do not insert a Foley catheter if pelvis is fractured, or a urethral injury is suspected.

V. **Orthopedic injuries**

Control bleeding with direct pressure.

Splint fractures before moving patient.

Compound fractures, dislocations, and other fractures which impair blood flow require urgent treatment.

BIBLIOGRAPHY

1. Care for the Injured Child. Baltimore, Williams and Wilkins Co., 1975.
2. Kempe, C.H., and Helfer, R.E.: Helping the Battered Child and His Family. Philadelphia, J.B. Lippincott Co., 1972.
3. Ravitch, M.M., Welch, K.J., et. al.: Pediatric Surgery (Ed. 3). Chicago, Year Book Med. Publ. Inc., 1979.
4. Touloukian, Robert J.: Pediatric Trauma. New York, Wiley Med. Publ., 1978.
5. Randolph, J.G., Ravitch, M.M., et.al.: The Injured Child, Surgical Management. Chicago, Year Book Med. Publ. Inc., 1979.
6. Grosfeld, Jay L.: Symposium on Childhood Trauma. Pediatric Clinics of North America **22**:269-511, 1975.
7. Alpert, Joel J.: Symposium on Pediatric Emergencies. Pediatric Clinics of North America **26**:707-941, 1979.
8. Marshall, Lawrence F., M.D. and Bowers, Sharon A., B.S.N.: Head Injury: Medical Management; Contemporary neurosurgery, Vol. 2, #7, March 25, 1980, pp. 1-6.
9. Bruce, Derek A., M.D., and Schut, Luis, M.D.: Management of Acute Craniocerebral Trauma in Children; Contemporary neurosurgery, 10, pp. 1-6.
10. Marshall, Lawrence F., M.D., Smith, Randall W., M.D., and Shapiro, Harvey M., M.D. The Outcome with Aggressive Treatment in Severe Head Injuries Part I: The Significance of Intracranial Pressure Monitoring; J. Neurosurg, Vol. 50, Jan, 1979, pp. 20-25.

Pediatric Medication Dosages

Pediatric medication dosages*

Drug name (trade name)	General type	Dosage	Cautions	Metabolism/excretion
Acetaminophen (Tylenol)	Antipyretic	Oral: 60 mg/yr of age *or* 5-10 mg/kg/dose q 4-6 hr Maximum oral dose: 650 mg Rectal: (over 1 yr); 100 mg/yr of age *or* 5-10 mg/kg/dose q 4-6 hr Maximum rectal dose: 1200 mg	Overdose may produce hepatotoxicity; skin rash or fever may also develop	Hepatic metabolism with urinary excretion of metabolites
Acetazolamide (Diamox)	Carbonic anhydrase inhibitor (diuretic and anticonvulsant)	Diuretic: 5 mg/kg/day as single dose IV or IM Anticonvulsant: 10-15 mg/kg/day in single dose or 2-3 doses orally	May produce increased urine potassium losses; can result in paresthesias	Renal excretion: eliminated unchanged in urine

Amikacin (Amikin)	Antibiotic	Neonates: 15/mg/kg/day given in divided doses q 12 hr IM or IV
		
		Infants or children: 15-22.8 mg/kg/day given in divided doses q 8 hr IM or IV *or* 420 mg/M² body surface area/day given q 12 hr IV or IM
		
		Therapeutic serum levels:
		    Peak—20-30 mg/L
		    Trough—4-8 mg/L
		    Toxic—35 mg/L
			Give IV dose *slowly*; may produce ototoxicity, nephrotoxicity, eosinophilia, or rash	Renal excretion

*Please note that the dosages listed in this table represent approximate dosages used for children. These dosages must always be modified according to patient condition and response to therapy.

Pediatric medication dosages—cont'd

Drug name (trade name)	General type	Dosage	Cautions	Metabolism/excretion

Aminophylline (Aminodur, Cardophyllin, Diophyllin, Methophyllin, Somophyllin)	Bronchodilator	For status asthmaticus: 4-7 mg/kg IV over 15-20 min, then 1.0 mg/kg/hr as continuous infusion
		
		For bronchodilation:
		  Oral maintenance: 5-7 mg/kg/dose given q 6 hr
		  Rectal dose: 5 mg/kg given q 6 hr
		Maximum dose for bronchodilation: 20 mg/kg/day
		For prevention of apnea: 1-2 mg/kg/oral dose, given q 6-8 hr
		Therapeutic serum levels (theophylline levels are assayed):
		  For bronchodilation: 10-20 mg/L
		  For apnea: 5-12 mg/L
			Potentiates epinephrine; incompatible with ACTH, potassium, penicillin, chloramphenicol, methicillin, erythromycin, tetracycline, meperidine, pressor amines, and phenytoin	Primarily hepatic metabolism with 10% excreted unchanged in urine

Amoxicillin— see penicillins				
Ampicillin— see penicillins				
Antacids— see Table 8-22				
Atropine	Anticholinergic	0.01-0.02 mg/kg/IV dose (this dose may also be given subcutaneously) Maximum dose: 0.4 mg	May produce tachycardia, or AV dissociation; hyperpyrexia may also occur	Distributed throughout body, then excreted through urine
Benzathine penicillin—see penicillins				

Continued.

Pediatric medication dosages—cont'd

Drug name (trade name)	General type	Dosage	Cautions	Metabolism/excretion
Calcium chloride (27% calcium, usually administered as a 10% solution containing 1 gm/10 cc)	Electrolyte replacement	IV supplement: 20-50 mg/kg/dose (this dose may also be given orally) Maximum dose: 1 gm	May produce bradycardia if infused rapidly; administer at a rate *no faster* than 100 mg/min; may produce vascular irritation so monitor infusion site	Used throughout the body
Calcium gluconate (9.4% calcium, usually administered as a 10% solution containing 1 gm/10 cc)	Electrolyte replacement	IV supplement: 100-200 mg/kg/dose (this dose may also be given orally) Maximum dose: 2 gm	Monitor for bradycardia during infusion; maximum infusion rate: 100 mg/min	Used throughout the body
Carbenicillin—see penicillins				
Cephalexin (Keflex)	Antibiotic	25-100 mg/kg/day given in divided doses q 4-6 hr orally Maximum dose: 4 gm/day	Patients with penicillin sensitivity may have cross-sensitivity reaction; risk of nephrotoxicity may be enhanced if administered concurrently with aminoglycoside antibiotic	Renal excretion
Cephalothin (Keflin)	Antibiotic	50-100 mg/kg/day given in divided doses q 4-6 hr IV or deep IM Maximum dose: 12 gm/day	May produce vascular irritation (see also Cephalexin)	Renal excretion
Chloral hydrate (Noctec)	Sedative and hypnotic	1-30 mg/kg/dose, orally or rectally Maximum dose: 2 gm/dose or 50 mg/kg/day	Administer with caution if hepatic disease is present	Hepatic metabolism

Pediatric medication dosages—cont'd

Drug name (trade name)	General type	Dosage	Cautions	Metabolism/excretion
Chloramphenicol (Chloromycetin)	Antibiotic	Loading dose for severe infections: 20 mg/kg IV or po Maintenance dose: Neonates—25-50 mg/kg/day, given in divided doses q 6 hr IV or po Infants and children—50-100 mg/kg/day given in divided doses q 6 hr IV or po Therapeutic serum levels: Peak—20 mg/L Range—10-20 mg/L Toxic level—>25 mg/L	Monitoring of blood levels is *essential*; bone marrow suppression can occur; administer with caution if hepatic or renal dysfunction is present	Hepatic inactivation with urinary excretion of metabolites
Chlorothiazide (Diuril)	Diuretic	20-40 mg/kg/day orally (given in 1 or 2 doses)	May cause hyperbilirubinemia, hypokalemia, hyperglycemia, or metabolic alkalosis	Renal excretion
Cimetidine (Tagamet)	Antacid	20-40 mg/kg/day, given in divided doses q 6-8 hr IV or po Maximum dose: 2400 mg/day	May produce diarrhea, rash, neutropenia, myalgia, or gynecomastia	Renal excretion
Clindamycin (Cleocin)	Antibiotic	Oral: 8-25 mg/kg/day given in divided doses q 6-8 hr Parenteral: 15-40 mg/kg/day IV or IM given in divided doses q 6-8 hr Maximum dose: 4.8 gm/day	Use with caution if hepatic or renal disease is present	Hepatic metabolism
Cloxacillin— see Penicillins				

Continued.

Pediatric medication dosages—cont'd

Drug name (trade name)	General type	Dosage	Cautions	Metabolism/excretion
Codeine	Analgesic	0.5-1.0 mg/kg/ dose, given po or subcutaneously q 4-6 hr Maximum dose: 3 mg/kg/day	May produce cardiorespiratory. depression (but less depression than occurs with morphine or meperidine)	Hepatic metabolism with inactive forms excreted in the urine
d-Tubocurarine—see Tubocurarine				
Dexamethasone (Decadron)	Adrenocortical steroid	For increased intracranial pressure: 0.5-1.0 mg/kg IV or IM for loading dose then 0.25-0.5 mg/kg/day For treatment of asthma or upper airway obstruction: 0.25-0.5 mg/kg/day given in divided doses q 6 hr	If chronic therapy is discontinued, dose must be tapered before discontinuation to prevent adrenal insufficiency; this drug may interfere with the action of phenytoin sodium (Dilantin); steroid therapy may produce gastrointestinal bleeding, delayed wound healing, or increased susceptibility to infection	Renal excretion
Diazepam (Valium)	Anticonvulsant, muscle relaxant	For status epilepticus: 0.1-0.5 mg/kg/ IV dose Maximum dose: 10 mg Relaxant: 0.1-0.8 mg/kg/day given orally in divided doses *or* 0.1-0.3 mg/kg/dose IV or IM	May produce hypotension or respiratory depression	Hepatic metabolism
Dicloxacillin—see Penicillins				

Pediatric medication dosages—cont'd

Drug name (trade name)	General type	Dosage	Cautions	Metabolism/excretion
Digoxin (Lanoxin)	Cardiac glycoside	Oral digitalizing dose (given in divided doses over 18-24 hr): Preterm neonate—0.025-0.050 mg/kg Term neonate—0.04-0.08 mg/kg 2 wk-2 yr—0.06-0.08 mg/kg 2 yr-10 yr—0.5-1.0 mg Intravenous digitalizing dose: calculated at two-thirds oral dose Maintenance dose: calculated at one-eighth digitalizing dose given q 12 hr Therapeutic serum level: <1 yr up to 3.0-3.5 ng/ml >1 yr 0.6-2.5 ng/ml	May produce arrhythmias	Renal excretion (60% to 75%)
Diphenylan— see Phenytoin				
Dobutamine (Inotrex)	Beta-adrenergic agonist	For treatment of low cardiac output as continuous infusion: 2-10 μg/kg/min; dosages and effects in neonates may be different	May produce tachyarrhythmias, hypotension	Rapidly inactivated in the body

Continued.

Pediatric medication dosages—cont'd

Drug name (trade name)	General type	Dosage	Cautions	Metabolism/excretion
Dopamine (Intropin)	Beta-adrenergic agonist	For the treatment of low cardiac output as continuous infusion: 1-5 μg/kg/min produces "dopaminergic" effects (especially increased renal blood flow and glomerular filration rate) 5-10 μg/kg/min produces primarily beta$_1$ effects, especially increased cardiac contractility and cardiac output Dosages >10 μg/kg/min produce primarily alpha-adrenergic effects (especially peripheral vasoconstriction) Dosages and effects in neonates may be different	May result in increased pulmonary artery pressure; renal blood flow is probably reduced once the dosage exceeds approximately 10 μg/kg/min; may produce tachyarrhythmias	Rapidly inactivated in the body
Doxycycline (Vibramycin)	Antibiotic	Initial dose: <45 kg: 4.4-5 mg/kg/day, given in divided doses q 12 hr IV or po >45 kg: 200 mg/day given in divided doses q 12 hr IV or po Maintenance dose: <45 kg: 2.2-2.5 mg/kg/day, given in divided doses q 12 hr IV or po >45 kg: 100 mg/day as single dose or 2 doses divided q 12 hr IV or po	Can produce vasculitis and subcutaneous burn so monitor infusion site; give with caution if renal or hepatic disease is present	Renal excretion (20%-60%) and fecal excretion NOTE: There is greater elimination of this drug in the feces than other tetracyclines, making this one of the safest tetracyclines to administer to the patient with renal failure

Pediatric medication dosages—cont'd

Drug name (trade name)	General type	Dosage	Cautions	Metabolism/excretion
Epinephrine (Adrenalin)—see also Racemic epinephrine	Alpha- and beta-adrenergic agonist	Aerosol: 1:100 solution nebulized for 1 min; *not to be confused with 1:1000 solution* For status asthmaticus: 0.01 ml/kg/dose subcutaneously (of 1:1000 aqueous solution) Maximum dose: 0.5 ml As a vasopressor: 0.01 ml/kg/dose (of 1:1000) *or* 0.05-1.0 μg/kg/min as continuous infusion	May produce tachyarrhythmias, nausea, vomiting, headaches, or hypertension; this drug increases myocardial oxygen consumption, often increases systemic vascular resistance or pulmonary artery pressure, and may reduce renal blood flow	Hepatic metabolism with urinary excretion of metabolites
Erythromycin (Erythrocin, Pediamycin, Ilosone, E-Mycin)	Antibiotic	Oral dose: 30-100 mg/kg/day given in divided doses q 6-8 hr Intravenous dose: 10-30 mg/kg/day given in divided doses q 4-6 hr	Do not give intramuscularly; use with caution in patients with liver disease; gastrointestinal side effects are common	Concentrated and/or inactivated in the liver with biliary excretion; renal excretion (10%-15%) may be present
Ethacrynic acid (Edecrin)	Diuretic	1.0 mg/kg/IV dose *or* 2-3 mg/kg/oral dose	Causes increased potassium loss in the urine	Renal excretion (66%) and hepatic metabolism (33%)
Furosemide (Lasix)	Diuretic	For treatment of congestive heart failure: 1.0-2.0 mg/kg/dose IV, IM, or orally; up to 4 mg/kg/dose may be administered orally For treatment of renal failure: 2.0-6.0 mg/kg/dose IV (may be repeated)	Produces potassium and chloride loss in the urine; may produce a hypochloremic metabolic alkalosis; ototoxicity has been reported	Renal excretion (and a small amount is excreted in feces)

Continued.

Pediatric medication dosages—cont'd

Drug name (trade name)	General type	Dosage	Cautions	Metabolism/excretion

Gentamicin (Garamycin)	Antibiotic	3.0-7.5 mg/kg/day, IV or IM given in divided doses q 8 hr
		
		Therapeutic serum level:
		  Peak—6-8 mg/L (or μg/ml)
		  Trough—1-2 mg/L
			Has been reported to cause renal and ototoxicity, especially when peak concentrations exceed 10 mg/L or trough concentrations exceed 2 mg/L; infuse over a minimum of 15-30 min	Primarily renal excretion

Glucose solutions	Electrolyte replacement	D_{25}: 1-2 ml/kg/dose D_{50}: 0.5-1.0 ml/kg/dose Should be diluted before administration in peripheral IV	May produce vascular irritation or burn	Used throughout the body; may also be excreted in the urine
Glucose and insulin	For treatment of hyperkalemia	Acute treatment of hyperkalemia: 0.5-1.0 ml D_{50}/kg *plus* 0.1 unit regular insulin/8-12 gm dextrose infused *or* 0.5-1.0 ml D_{50}/kg *plus* 0.02-0.04 units regular insulin/kg	Give lower range of insulin dose for premature infants	Used throughout the body; may also be excreted in the urine
Glycerin (Glyrol)	Osmotic diuretic	0.5-1.5 gm/kg/day orally (titrated to control increased intracranial pressure)	May produce increased serum osmolality resulting in rebound cerebral edema and increased intracranial pressure; may also produce hyperglycemia and glycosuria	Used in the body and excreted in the urine
Hydrochlorothiazide + spironolactone (Aldactazide)	Diuretic	1.65-3.3 mg/kg/day given orally	See cautions of spironolactone	Renal excretion

Pediatric medication dosages—cont'd

Drug name (trade name)	General type	Dosage	Cautions	Metabolism/excretion
Hydrocortisone (Cortef, Hydrocortisone, Solu-Cortef)	Adrenocortical steroid	Gram-negative shock: 50 mg/kg IV then 50-70 mg/kg/day given in divided doses Status asthmaticus: 10 mg/kg/day IV given in divided doses q 6 hr Physiologic replacement: 12.5-15 mg/m²/day IV or IM in one dose *or* 25.0 mg/m²/day po in 3 doses	May produce Cushing's syndrome (including hypertension, weight gain, muscle atrophy, fluid retention, psychiatric disturbances, or osteoporosis), impaired immunologic status and/or wound healing, steroid dependence, nausea, vomiting, hyperglycemia, or gastrointestinal ulceration; if patient has received chronic therapy, dosage should be tapered before discontinuation, to prevent adrenal insufficiency	Renal excretion (cortisol metabolites are excreted as 17-hydroxycorticosteroid)
Isoetharine hydrochloride (Bronkosol)	Beta$_2$ adrenergic agonist (bronchodilator inhalant)	0.25-0.5 ml is usually diluted with 3 ml normal saline and given in an oxygen aerosol; 3-7 inhalations are usually administered q 4 hr	May produce tachycardia, headache, or hypertension	Hepatic metabolism
Isoproterenol (Isuprel, Aludrine)	Beta-adrenergic agonist	For bradycardia: 0.05-0.1 μg/kg/min IV continuous infusion For hypotension: 0.05-0.5 μg/kg/min For bronchodilation: 1-2 inhalations q 4-6 hr (1:500 mesometer)	May produce tachyarrhythmias at even low doses; patient may feel anxious, nauseated, or dizzy, or the patient may complain of headache; inhalation overdose may produce ventricular arrhythmias	Hepatic metabolism

Continued.

Pediatric medication dosages—cont'd

Drug name (trade name)	General type	Dosage	Cautions	Metabolism/excretion
Lidocaine (Xylocaine)	Antiarrhythmic	1 mg/kg/IV bolus dose Maximum dose: 5 mg/kg Continuous infusion: 10-20 μg/kg/min	May produce seizures in toxic doses	Hepatic metabolism and renal excretion
Mannitol 10%-20% (Osmitrol)	Osmotic diuretic	Increased intracranial pressure: 0.15-0.3 gm/kg/q 1-2 hr *or* continuous infusion of 0.05-0.15 gm/kg/hr; may be titrated to maintain serum osmolality of 310 mOsm/L If necessary, up to 0.25-2.0 gm/kg/day may be administered to control increased intracranial pressure	May produce increased serum osmolality resulting in rebound cerebral edema and increased intracranial pressure; monitor serum and urine osmolality and serum electrolyte concentration	Renal excretion
Meperidine (Demerol)	Analgesic narcotic	1 mg/kg/dose IV Maximum dose: 100 mg	May produce respiratory depression, or decreased gastrointestinal motility; may produce excitation, hyperpyrexia, or delirium in patients receiving monamine oxidase (MAO) inhibitors	Hepatic metabolism
Metaproterenol sulfate (Alupent, Metaprel)	Beta$_2$ adrenergic agonist	Inhalant: (0.65 mg or approximately 0.2 ml in 3 ml saline) 2-3 inhalations Syrup or tablet: 1.3-2.6 mg/kg/day given in 3 doses	Adverse reactions include tachycardia, hypertension, palpitations, nervousness, nausea, and vomiting	Renal excretion

Pediatric medication dosages—cont'd

Drug name (trade name)	General type	Dosage	Cautions	Metabolism/excretion
Morphine sulfate	Analgesic narcotic	For analgesia: 0.1 mg/kg/dose IV or subcutaneously For hypercyanotic spells ("Tet" spells): 0.1-0.2 mg/kg/dose IV or subcutaneously Continuous IV infusion: 100 μg/kg/hr Maximum dose: 15 mg	May produce respiratory depression; chronic administration can produce addiction; also may produce decreased gastrointestinal motility or nausea; administer naloxone for reversal of morphine (see naloxone)	Conjugated throughout the body, then excreted in the urine; free morphine may accumulate in kidneys, lungs, liver, and spleen for hours after administration
Moxalactam	Antibiotic	50-75 mg/kg/day, given in divided doses q 8 hr For treatment of meningitis or other severe infections: 100 mg/kg/day, given in divided doses q 8 hr	See cephalothin	Renal excretion
Nafcillin—see Penicillin				
Naloxone (Narcan)	Opioid antagonist	0.005-0.010 mg/kg/dose IV or IM	May stimulate respirations and may enhance pain perception	Hepatic metabolism
Nitroglycerin	Vasodilator	Continuous infusion IV dose: 1-25 μg/kg/min (NOTE: maximal dose reserved for patients with severe pulmonary hypertension) Topical ointment (2%): 0.5-1.5 cm reapplied q ½-6 hr, or long-acting disks changed q 12 hr	Produces hypotension in the hypovolemic patient; may require simultaneous volume infusion; may also produce severe headache; since IV nitroglycerine is adsorbed by polyvinyl chloride tubing and buretrols, special IV administration equipment is necessary	Hepatic metabolism

Continued.

Pediatric medication dosages—cont'd

Drug name (trade name)	General type	Dosage	Cautions	Metabolism/excretion
Nitroprus-side—see Sodium nitroprusside				
Oxacillin—see Penicillins				
Pancuronium (Pavulon)	Paralyzing (nondepolarizing) agent	Intermittent IV dose: Neonates: 0.02 mg/kg Older infants and children: 0.1-0.15 mg/kg for loading dose, then 0.1 mg/kg/q 30-60 min Continuous infusion: 0.1 mg/kg/hr IV	Drug effect can be accentuated by hypothermia, acidosis, some anesthetics, decreased renal function, and aminoglycoside antibiotics; may produce tachycardia and venous pooling	Hepatic metabolism and renal excretion
Paraldehyde	Anticonvulsant	For status epilepticus: 0.15 mg/kg IV (may be repeated) *or* 0.3 ml/kg rectally	Intravenous dose must be administered using a glass syringe and special tubing	Depolymerized in the liver and ultimately excreted in the urine or exhaled
The penicillins				
Penicillin G (Pentids, Pfizerpen G)	Antibiotic	Newborn <7 days: 50,000-100,000 U/kg/day, given in 2 doses IV or IM Newborns >7 days: 100,000-200,000 U/kg/day, given in divided doses IV or IM q 6-8 hr Child: 25,000-300,000 U/kg/day, given in divided doses IV, IM, or po q 4-6 hr	Monitor for sensitivity reaction or rash NOTE: Potassium penicillin contains 1.68 mEq potassium ion per 1 million units; sodium penicillin contains 1.68 mEq sodium ions per 1 million units	Primarily renal excretion (60%-90%) with small amount excreted in bile

Pediatric medication dosages—cont'd

Drug name (trade name)	General type	Dosage	Cautions	Metabolism/excretion
The penicillins—cont'd				
Amoxicillin (Amoxil, Larotic, Poly-mox)	Antibiotic	Under 20 kg: 20-40 mg/kg/day orally, given in divided doses q 8 hr Greater than 20 kg: 200-500 mg/kg/day orally, given in divided doses q 8 hr	May produce diarrhea (although this occurs less frequently than with ampicillin); monitor for sensitivity reaction or rash; may be taken with meals	Primarily renal excretion (70%) within 6 hr
Ampicillin (Amcill, Omnipen, Polycillin)	Antibiotic	Neonate <7 days: 50-100 mg/kg/day, given in divided doses q 8 hr IV or po Beyond the first week: 100-200 mg/kg/day, given in divided doses q 8 hr IV or po Severe infections (IV or IM): <40 kg: 200-400 mg/kg/day given in divided doses IV or IM q 4-6 hr; >40 kg: 8-12 gm/day, given in divided doses IV or IM q 4-6 hr Maximum dose: 1.2 gm/day	May produce diarrhea; monitor for sensitivity reaction or rash; less complete absorption occurs if oral dose taken with meals	Primarily renal excretion (70%) within 6 hr
Benzathine penicillin (Bicillin, Permapen)	Antibiotic	0.3-1.2 million U/single (deep) IM dose	Monitor for sensitivity reaction or rash	Primarily renal excretion (70%)
Carbenicillin (Geopen, Pyopen)	Antibiotic	50-200 mg/kg/day, given in divided IV doses q 6-8 hr NOTE: Oral administration not recommended since the drug is poorly absorbed in the gastrointestinal tract Severe infections: 400-600 mg/kg/day, given in divided doses, q 4-6 hr Maximum dose: 40 gm/day	May produce thrombocytopenia or anaphylaxis; may interact with gentamicin; this drug produces large urinary potassium losses; contains large amounts of sodium ion (4.7 mEq sodium/gm); give with caution if renal impairment is present	Hepatic metabolism and renal excretion

Continued.

Pediatric medication dosages—cont'd

Drug name (trade name)	General type	Dosage	Cautions	Metabolism/excretion
The penicillins—cont'd				
Cloxacillin (Cloxapen, Tegopen)	Antibiotic	Under 20 kg: 50-100 mg/kg/day, given orally in divided doses q 6 hr Greater than 20 kg: 1-2 gm/day, given orally in divided doses q 6 hr Maximum doses: 4 gm/day	Monitor for sensitivity reaction or rash	Primarily renal excretion with significant hepatic metabolism
Dicloxacillin (Dycill, Dynapen, Veracillin)	Antibiotic	Under 40 kg: 12.5-25 mg/kg/day, given orally in divided doses q 6 hr Greater than 40 kg: 0.5-1.0 gm/day, given orally in divided doses q 6 hr	Administer 1-2 hr before meals to maximize absorption; monitor for sensitivity reaction or rash	Primarily renal excretion with significant hepatic elimination
Nafcillin (Unipen)	Antibiotic	Newborn: <7 days—40 mg/kg/day, given in 2 doses; >7 days—60 mg/kg/day, given in divided doses q 6-8 hr Older infants and children: 50-100 mg/kg/day, given orally *or* 100-200 mg/kg/day given IM (in 2 doses) or IV (in divided doses q 4-6 hr) NOTE: Oral administration is not recommended since the drug is poorly absorbed in the gastrointestinal tract	May produce sensitivity reaction or rash	Primarily hepatic metabolism with small amount (10%) excreted unchanged in the urine
Oxacillin (Bactocill, Prostaphlin)	Antibiotic	50-100 mg/kg/day, given in divided doses q 4-6 hr IV	May produce hematuria or nephritis; monitor for sensitivity reaction or rash	Primarily renal excretion with significant hepatic elimination

Pediatric medication dosages—cont'd

Drug name (trade name)	General type	Dosage	Cautions	Metabolism/excretion
The penicillins—cont'd				
Procaine penicillin (Bicillin, Crysticillin, Duracillin, Wycillin)	Antibiotic	0.3-1.2 million U as single IM injection NOTE: The procaine provides a slight anesthetic effect —each 300,000 U contains approximately 120 mg procaine	Monitor for sensitivity reaction or rash	Primarily renal excretion (60%-70%) with small amount excreted in bile
Pentobarbitol (Nembutol)	Barbiturate Sedative	For sedation: 2-3 mg/kg/dose orally For barbiturate coma: loading dose: 2-5 mg/kg IV; then additional doses provided as needed to maintain serum pentobarbitol level of 20-40 μg/ml (or 2.0-4.0 mg/dl)— usually 0.5-3.0 mg/kg/hr are required	May produce hypotension or arrhythmias (see discussion in Chapter 6)	Hepatic and renal excretion
Phenobarbitol	Barbiturate Anticonvulsant	For status epilepticus: 5 mg/kg/IV dose—may give as many as 3 doses For chronic anticonvulsant: 4-6 mg/kg/day, given orally in 2 doses Therapeutic serum level: 15-40 μg/ml	May produce drowsiness and respiratory depression	Hepatic metabolism with renal excretion (25%)
Phenytoin (Dilantin)	Anticonvulsant antiarrhythmic	For status epilepticus: 10-15 mg/kg/IV dose Maximum dose: 1250 mg Maintenance anticonvulsant: 5-8 mg/kg/day Antiarrhythmic: 2-4 mg/kg/IV dose *or* 2-8 mg/kg/day given orally Therapeutic serum level: 10-25 μg/ml	May produce bradycardia, decreased myocardial contractility, hypotension, or ventricular fibrillation; may produce central nervous system depression	Primarily hepatic metabolism

Continued.

Pediatric medication dosages—cont'd

Drug name (trade name)	General type	Dosage	Cautions	Metabolism/excretion
Potassium chloride	Electrolyte replacement	Intravenous supplement: 0.5-1 mEq/kg/dose, given over 1-2 hr; concentration of KCl in peripheral IV should not exceed equivalent of 40 mEq/L, to prevent vascular irritation Oral supplement: 2-4 mEq/kg/day	Intravenous infusion tubing should be labeled carefully to prevent inadvertent bolus infusion; rapid infusions can produce arrhythmias or cardiac arrest; administer with caution if renal failure is present	Used throughout the body, and excreted by the kidneys
Prednisone	Adrenocortical steroid	1.5-2.0 mg/kg/day, given orally, in a single or several divided doses	Chronic therapy can produce growth retardation; chronic therapy dose should be tapered before drug is discontinued to prevent adrenal insufficiency; steroid therapy can cause gastrointestinal bleeding, delayed wound healing, or increased susceptibility to infection	Renal excretion
Procaineamide (Pronestyl)	Antiarrhythmic	IV bolus: 3-10 mg/kg/dose, given over 5 min Maximum bolus dose: 500 mg Continuous infusion: 20-50 μg/kg/min Oral dose: 15-50 mg/kg/day Therapeutic serum level: 4-8 mg/L	May depress cardiac contractility or produce thrombocytopenia; toxic effects include AV dissociation	Hepatic metabolism

Pediatric medication dosages—cont'd

Drug name (trade name)	General type	Dosage	Cautions	Metabolism/excretion
Propranolol (Inderal)	Antiarrhythmic, beta-adrenergic blocker	For treatment of arrhythmias: 0.01-0.1 mg/kg, given IV over 10 min For treatment of hypercyanotic ("tet") spells: 0.15-0.25 mg/kg, given slowly IV For treatment of hypertension: 0.5-1 mg/kg/day, given in divided IV doses Oral dose: 0.2-8 mg/kg/day, given in divided doses	May produce severe bradycardia, AV conduction disturbances, and decreased cardiac contractility; also known to cause hypotension, nausea, and vomiting	Hepatic metabolism
Quinidine	Antiarrhythmic	Oral dose: 15-60 mg/kg/day, given in divided doses	May depress myocardial contractility; may also produce a rise in serum digoxin levels if these drugs are given concurrently	Hepatic metabolism
Racemic epinephrine (Vaponefrin, Micronefrin)	Bronchodilator	0.125-0.25 ml of 2.25% solution diluted to 3 ml with normal saline and administered by nebulizer; occasionally, a dose of 0.05 ml/kg/dose is calculated and diluted to 3 ml with normal saline and administered by nebulizer	If administered in conjunction with a beta-adrenergic blocker, the racemic epinephrine can potentiate existing bronchospasm; may also produce tachyarrhythmias, headache, nausea, or palpitations	Hepatic metabolism
Sodium bicarbonate	Electrolyte replacement	1-2 (or 1-4 if acidosis severe) mEq/kg/dose or kg wt × base excess × 0.3 = _____ mEq $NaHCO_3$ needed to correct the calculated base deficit Maximum dose: 8 mEq/kg/24 hr	Metabolism of bicarbonate produces carbon dioxide so that ventilation must be adequate to prevent the development of hypercapnia; may produce vascular irritation if administered through a peripheral IV	Used throughout the body

Continued.

Pediatric medication dosages—cont'd

Drug name (trade name)	General type	Dosage	Cautions	Metabolism/excretion
Sodium nitroprusside (Nipride)	Vasodilator	0.1-8 μg/kg/min, given as continuous infusion Toxic thiocyanate levels: >10 mg/dl	Will produce hypotension in hypovolemic patients; may require simultaneous volume infusion; may produce headaches NOTE: Metabolism of this drug results in the formation of *cyanide* and *thiocyanate,* so levels of thiocyanate should be checked if therapy continues for 48 hr (check sooner if hepatic dysfunction is present)	Hepatic metabolism
Spironolactone (Aldactone)	Diuretic	1.5-3.3 mg/kg/day orally	Since this drug enhances renal potassium reabsorption, hyperkalemia can result; this drug is often administered in conjunction with a "potassium wasting" diuretic such as furosemide; may potentiate ganglionic blocking agents	Hepatic metabolism with renal excretion of metabolites
Streptomycin	Antibiotic	Infants: 15-40 mg/kg/day, in divided doses IM q 12 hr Children: 40 mg/kg/day, given in divided doses IM q 12 hr Maximum dose: 2 gm/day	May produce central nervous system depression or ototoxicity; reduce dosage in the presence of renal insufficiency	Primarily renal excretion

Pediatric medication dosages—cont'd

Drug name (trade name)	General type	Dosage	Cautions	Metabolism/excretion
Succinylcholine (Anectine)	Paralyzing (neuromuscular blocking) agent	1-2 mg/kg/IV dose	Effects may last 10 min; must be able to intubate immediately to prevent respiratory insufficiency; side effects include bradycardia, hypotension, and arrhythmias	Hydrolyzed by pseudocholinesterase in the liver and plasma
Terbutaline (Brethine)	Beta$_2$ adrenergic agonist (bronchodilator)	For treatment of status asthmaticus: 7-10 μg/kg/min, given subcutaneously Oral dose: 75 μg/kg/dose (usually, 10 times the effective subcutaneous dose is given orally)	Side effects include tachycardia, palpitations, headaches, nervousness, tremors, drowsiness, nausea, vomiting, and sweating	Renal excretion (60%), and hepatic metabolism (40% conjugated in the liver), with some (3%) biliary excretion

Tetracycline (Achromycil)	Antibiotic	Older infants and children:
		  Oral: 25-50 mg/kg/day, given in divided doses q 6 hr
		  Intravenous: 10-15 mg/kg/day, given in divided doses q 12 hr
		  Intramuscular: 10-25 mg/kg/day, given in divided doses q 8-12 hr
		Children >40 kg:
		  Oral: 1-2 mg/day, given in divided doses q 6 hr
		  Parenteral: 10-20 mg/kg/day, given IM or IV in divided doses
			Recommended for use in children *only when other antibiotics are not suitable*; may produce increased intracranial pressure, tooth staining, and decreased bone growth; oral dose should be taken 1 hr before meals, and should never be taken in conjunction with oral calcium supplements	Primarily excreted in the urine and feces

Continued.

Pediatric medication dosages—cont'd

Drug name (trade name)	General type	Dosage	Cautions	Metabolism/excretion

Theophylline (Accurbron, Aerolate, Aqualin supprettes, Bronkodyl, Elixophyllin, Lanophyllin, Oralphyllin, Theo-II, and Theolair)	Bronchodilator	5-8 mg/kg/dose, given orally or IV q 6 hr (rectal administration also possible)
		
		For treatment of apnea: 1-2 mg/kg/oral dose, given q 6 hr
		
		Therapeutic serum levels:
		  Bronchodilation—10-20 mg/L
		  For treatment of apnea—5-12 mg/L
		  Toxic levels—>20 mg/L
			May produce palpitations, tachyarrhythmias, anorexia, nausea, vomiting, anxiety, irritability, insomnia, dizziness, hypokalemia, alkalosis, or seizures
			NOTE: This drug antagonizes propranolol; concurrent administration of phenothiazides will antagonize the chronotropic effect of the theophylline; erythromycin administration will inhibit the clearance of theophylline
				Primarily hepatic metabolism, a small amount (10%) is recovered unchanged in the urine

Tobramycin (Nebcin)	Antibiotic	5-7.5 mg/kg/day, given in divided doses q 8-12 hr
		
		Therapeutic serum levels:
		  Peak—6-8 mg/L
		  Trough—1-2 mg/L
			May produce nephrotoxicity or ototoxicity	Primarily renal excretion

Tocainide	Antiarrhythmic	Adult dosages range from 1200-2400 mg/day Pediatric dosages not yet determined	Monitor heart rate, rhythm, and systemic perfusion Toxic effects include nausea and neuropathies	Hepatic metabolism and renal excretion

Pediatric medication dosages—cont'd

Drug name (trade name)	General type	Dosage	Cautions	Metabolism/excretion
Trimethoprim (TMP) or sulfamethoxazole (SMZ) (Bactrim, Septra)	Antibiotic	Minor infections: 8-10 mg/kg/day TMP *or* 40-50 mg/kg/day SMZ given in divided doses q 12 hr For treatment of *Pneumocystis carinii* pneumonia: 20 mg/kg/day TMP *or* 100 mg/kg/day SMZ given in divided doses q 6 hr	Reduce dosage if renal failure is present; may produce bone marrow depression	Primarily renal excretion
d-Tubocurarine (Curare)	Paralyzing (neuromuscular blocking) agent	Neonates: 0.3 mg/kg initially, then 0.15 mg/kg/dose Infants and children: 0.2-0.4 mg/kg initially, then 0.04-0.2 mg/kg/dose	Drug effects are enhanced if gentamicin or related antibiotics are administered simultaneously; this drug may produce heart rate and blood pressure lability; *patient ventilatory support must be adequate*	Primarily renal excretion (33%-75%) with some biliary excretion (11%)
Urea	Osmotic diuretic	1 gm/kg, given q 4-6 hr, titrated to control intracranial hypertension	May produce increased serum osmolality and rebound cerebral edema and further increase in intracranial pressure; monitor serum and urine osmolality and serum electrolyte concentrations	Renal excretion
Vancomycin (Vancocin)	Antibiotic	Neonates: 30-45 mg/kg/day, given in divided doses q 8-12 hr Infants and children: 40 mg/kg/day, given IV q 6 hr	May produce nephrotoxicity or phlebitis	Primarily renal excretion

Continued.

Pediatric medication dosages—cont'd

Drug name (trade name)	General type	Dosage	Cautions	Metabolism/excretion
Vasopressin (Pitressin)	Antidiuretic hormone	Aqueous: 1-3 ml/day, given subcutaneously in 3 divided doses Tannate in oil: 0.2 ml/dose IM q 1-3 days Nose drops: 1-2 gtts in each nostril q 4-6 hr prn	May produce arrhythmias when given intravenously	Rapidly inactivated by body enzymes
Verapamil (Cordilox)	Antiarrhythmic	Intravenous: 0.15-0.25 mg/kg/dose Oral: 20-80 mg/dose q 6-8 hr	May produce decreased cardiac contractility resulting in hypotension; can also produce decreased renal clearance of digoxin (if these drugs are given concurrently) causing digoxin levels to rise	Hepatic metabolism (80%)

□ These drug dosages and cautions have been verified whenever possible with the following sources: Biller, J.A., and Yaeger, A.M., editors: The Harriet Lane handbook, ed. 9, Chicago, 1981, Year Book Medical Publishers, Inc.; Gilman, A.G., Goodman, L.S., and Gilman, A., editors: Goodman and Gilman's The pharmacological basis of therapeutics, ed. 6, New York, 1982, Macmillan Publishing Co.; Waring, W.W., and Jeansonne, L.O., editors: Practical manual of pediatrics, ed. 2, St. Louis, 1982, The C.V. Mosby Co.

Continuous Infusion Dosage Charts ("drip charts")

NOTE: The following charts enable determination of the exact μg/kg/minute given by continuous infusion of drugs concentrated as 1, 50, or 100 mg/100 ml. If standard drug concentrations are not used, a formula may be used to make a medication concentration that will allow administration of **1 μg/kg/minute** for **each ml/hour** administered of the drug (e.g., if 3 ml/hour of the drug are administered, the patient is receiving 3 μg/kg/minute). This formula would require a drug concentration that varies with the weight of the child as follows:

Patient's weight (kg) $\times$ 6 = mg of medication/100 ml

For example, a 7 kg child receiving dopamine would have a dopamine concentration of 7 $\times$ 6 or 42 mg/100 ml. Then, if the infusion rate is 5 ml/hour, that child receives 5 μg/kg/minute of dopamine. If the infusion rate is changed to 10 ml/hour, the child receives 10 μg/kg/minute of dopamine. This calculation is also useful for continuous infusion of drugs such as dobutamine, nitroprusside, and nitroglycerine.

If isoproterenol will be administered, it may be desirable to prepare a medication concentration that will allow administration of **0.1 μg/kg/minute** for each **ml/hour** of the drug that is administered. In this case the drug concentration will vary with the weight of the child as follows:

Patient's weight (kg) $\times$ **0.6** = mg of medication/100 ml

Pediatric continuous infusion rates* (Dosage concentration 1 mg/100 cc)

Flow rate—ml/hr	Weight in kg											
	2	3	4	5	6	7	8	9	10	11	12	13
1	.08	.055	.042	.033	.028	.024	.021	.019	.017	.015	.014	.013
2	.16	.11	.084	.066	.056	.05	.042	.04	.034	.03	.028	.026
3	.24	.165	.126	.1	.08	.07	.06	.057	.051	.045	.042	.038
4	.32	.22	.17	.13	.11	.1	.08	.076	.068	.06	.056	.052
5	.40	.275	.21	.165	.14	.12	.11	.10	.09	.08	.07	.065
6	.48	.33	.25	.2	.17	.14	.13	.11	.10	.09	.08	.078
7	.56	.385	.29	.23	.19	.17	.15	.13	.12	.11	.10	.09
8	.64	.44	.34	.26	.22	.19	.17	.15	.136	.12	.11	.10
9	.72	.495	.38	.297	.25	.22	.19	.17	.15	.135	.126	.12
10	.8	.55	.42	.33	.28	.24	.21	.19	.17	.15	.14	.13
11	.88	.6	.46	.36	.31	.26	.23	.21	.187	.165	.15	.14
12	.96	.66	.5	.4	.33	.29	.25	.23	.2	.18	.17	.16
13	1.04	.715	.55	.43	.36	.31	.27	.25	.22	.195	.18	.17
14	1.12	.77	.59	.46	.39	.34	.29	.27	.24	.21	.2	.18
15	1.2	.825	.63	.495	.42	.36	.315	.29	.26	.22	.21	.195

* Values expressed represent μg/kg/minute.

Weight in kg

14	15	16	17	18	19	20	21	22	23	24	25	
.012	.011	.01	.009	.009	.009	.008	.008	.008	.007	.007	.007	1
.024	.02	.02	.018	.018	.017	.017	.016	.015	.015	.014	.013	2
.036	.03	.03	.029	.028	.026	.025	.023	.023	.022	.02	.019	3
.05	.04	.04	.039	.037	.035	.033	.032	.03	.03	.028	.027	4
.06	.055	.05	.049	.046	.044	.042	.040	.038	.036	.035	.033	5
.07	.066	.06	.058	.055	.053	.05	.048	.046	.044	.042	.04	6
.083	.077	.07	.068	.064	.06	.058	.056	.053	.051	.049	.047	7
.096	.09	.08	.078	.074	.07	.067	.064	.06	.058	.056	.053	8
.11	.1	.09	.088	.083	.08	.075	.07	.068	.065	.063	.06	9
.12	.11	.1	.098	.092	.09	.084	.08	.076	.073	.07	.067	10
.13	.12	.11	.107	.10	.097	.09	.087	.084	.08	.077	.073	11
.14	.13	.12	.118	.11	.106	.10	.095	.09	.087	.083	.08	12
.16	.14	.13	.127	.12	.114	.11	.10	.1	.094	.09	.087	13
.17	.15	.14	.137	.13	.12	.117	.11	.106	.10	.097	.094	14
.18	.165	.15	.147	.14	.132	.125	.12	.114	.11	.104	.1	15

Flow rate—ml/hr

Pediatric continuous infusion rates* (Dosage concentration 50 mg/100 cc)

						Weight in kg							
	2	**3**	**4**	**5**	**6**	**7**	**8**	**9**	**10**	**11**	**12**	**13**	
1	4.2	2.8	2.0	1.7	1.4	1.2	1.0	0.93	0.83	0.76	0.69	0.64	
2	8.3	5.6	4.2	3.3	2.8	2.4	2.1	1.85	1.7	1.5	1.4	1.3	
3	12.5	8.3	6.2	5.0	4.2	3.6	3.1	2.8	2.5	2.3	2.0	1.9	
4	16.7	11.0	8.3	6.7	5.6	4.8	4.2	3.7	3.3	3.0	2.8	2.6	
5	20.8	13.9	10.4	8.3	6.9	6.0	5.2	4.6	4.2	3.8	3.5	3.2	
6	25.0	16.7	12.5	10.0	8.3	7.0	6.3	5.6	5.0	4.5	4.2	3.8	
7	29.0	19.4	14.6	11.7	9.7	8.3	7.3	6.5	5.8	5.3	4.9	4.5	
8	33.0	22.0	16.7	13.3	11.0	9.5	8.3	7.4	6.7	6.0	5.6	5.1	
9	37.5	25.0	18.7	15.0	12.5	10.7	9.4	8.3	7.5	6.8	6.2	5.8	
10	41.7	27.8	20.8	16.7	13.9	11.9	10.4	9.3	8.3	7.6	6.9	6.4	
11	45.8	30.6	22.9	18.3	15.3	13.1	11.5	10.2	9.2	8.3	7.6	7.0	
12	50.0	33.3	25.0	20.0	16.7	14.3	12.5	11.0	10.0	9.0	8.3	7.7	
13	54.0	36.0	27.0	21.7	18.0	15.5	13.5	12.0	10.8	9.8	9.0	8.3	
14	58.3	38.9	29.0	23.3	19.4	16.7	14.6	13.0	11.7	10.6	9.7	9.0	
15	62.5	41.7	31.0	25.0	20.8	17.9	15.6	13.9	12.5	13.4	10.4	9.6	

Flow rate—ml/hr

*Values expressed represent μg/kg/minute.

					Weight in kg								
14	**15**	**16**	**17**	**18**	**19**	**20**	**21**	**22**	**23**	**24**	**25**		
0.6	0.56	0.52	0.49	0.46	0.44	0.42	0.40	0.38	0.36	0.35	0.33	**1**	
1.2	1.1	1.0	0.98	0.93	0.88	0.83	0.79	0.76	0.72	0.69	0.67	**2**	
1.8	1.7	1.6	1.5	1.4	1.3	1.25	1.2	1.1	1.09	1.04	1.0	**3**	
2.4	2.2	2.1	2.0	1.9	1.8	1.7	1.6	1.5	1.4	1.38	1.3	**4**	
3.0	2.8	2.6	2.5	2.3	2.2	2.1	2.0	1.9	1.8	1.7	1.67	**5**	
3.6	3.3	3.1	2.9	2.8	2.6	2.5	2.4	2.3	2.2	2.1	2.0	**6**	
4.2	3.9	3.6	3.4	3.2	3.1	2.9	2.8	2.7	2.5	2.4	2.3	**7**	Flow rate—ml/hr
4.8	4.4	4.2	3.9	3.7	3.5	3.3	3.2	3.0	2.9	2.8	2.7	**8**	
5.4	5.0	4.7	4.4	4.2	3.9	3.8	3.6	3.4	3.3	3.1	3.0	**9**	
6.0	5.6	5.2	4.9	4.6	4.4	4.2	4.0	3.8	3.6	3.5	3.3	**10**	
6.5	6.1	5.7	5.4	5.1	4.8	4.6	4.4	4.2	4.0	3.8	3.7	**11**	
7.1	6.7	6.2	5.9	5.6	5.3	5.0	4.8	4.5	4.3	4.2	4.0	**12**	
7.7	7.2	6.8	6.4	6.0	5.7	5.4	5.2	4.9	4.7	4.5	4.3	**13**	
8.3	7.8	7.3	6.7	6.5	6.1	5.8	5.6	5.3	5.0	4.9	4.7	**14**	
8.9	8.3	7.8	7.3	7.0	6.6	6.3	6.0	5.7	5.4	5.2	5.0	**15**	

Pediatric continuous infusion rates* (Dosage concentration 100 mg/100 cc)

						Weight in kg						
	2	**3**	**4**	**5**	**6**	**7**	**8**	**9**	**10**	**11**	**12**	**13**
1	8.33	5.56	4.17	3.33	2.8	2.4	2.1	1.85	1.67	1.5	1.39	1.3
2	16.67	11.1	8.30	6.67	5.56	4.8	4.2	3.7	3.3	3.0	2.8	2.6
3	24.9	16.7	12.5	10.0	8.3	7.1	6.2	5.6	5.0	4.5	4.2	3.8
4	33.3	22.2	16.7	13.3	11.1	9.5	8.3	7.4	6.7	6.0	5.6	5.1
5	41.7	27.8	20.9	16.7	13.9	11.9	10.4	9.3	8.3	7.6	6.9	6.4
6	50.0	33.3	25.0	20.0	16.7	14.3	12.5	11.0	10.0	9.0	8.3	7.7
7	58.3	38.9	29.0	23.3	19.4	16.7	14.6	13.0	11.7	10.6	9.7	9.0
8	66.6	44.4	33.3	26.7	22.2	19.0	16.7	14.8	13.3	12.0	11.1	10.3
9	75.0	50.0	37.5	30.0	25.0	21.0	18.7	16.7	15.0	13.6	12.5	11.5
10	83.3	55.6	41.7	33.3	27.8	23.8	20.8	18.5	16.7	15.0	13.9	12.8
11	91.6	61.0	45.9	36.7	30.6	26.2	22.9	20.4	18.3	16.7	15.3	14.0
12	100.0	66.7	50.0	40.0	33.3	28.6	25.0	22.0	20.0	18.2	16.7	15.4
13	108.0	72.0	54.0	43.0	36.0	31.0	27.0	24.0	21.7	19.7	18.0	16.7
14	116.6	77.8	58.4	46.7	38.9	33.3	29.0	25.9	23.3	21.0	19.4	17.9
15	125.0	83.4	62.5	50.0	41.7	35.7	31.0	27.8	25.0	22.7	20.8	19.2

Flow rate—ml/hr

*Values expressed represent μg/kg/minute.

Weight in kg

14	15	16	17	18	19	20	21	22	23	24	25	
1.2	1.1	1.0	0.98	0.93	0.88	0.83	0.79	0.76	0.72	0.69	0.67	**1**
2.4	2.3	2.1	1.96	1.85	1.75	1.7	1.6	1.5	1.4	1.39	1.33	**2**
3.6	3.3	3.1	2.9	2.8	2.6	2.5	2.4	2.3	2.2	2.1	2.0	**3**
4.8	4.4	4.2	3.9	3.7	3.5	3.3	3.2	3.0	2.9	2.8	2.7	**4**
6.0	5.5	5.2	4.9	4.6	4.4	4.2	4.0	3.8	3.6	3.5	3.3	**5**
7.0	6.6	6.3	5.9	5.5	5.3	5.0	4.8	4.5	4.3	4.2	4.0	**6**
8.3	7.7	7.3	6.9	6.5	6.1	5.8	5.6	5.3	5.1	4.9	4.7	**7**
9.5	8.8	8.3	7.8	7.4	7.0	6.7	6.4	6.1	5.8	5.6	5.3	**8**
10.7	9.9	9.4	8.8	8.3	7.9	7.5	7.0	6.8	6.5	6.2	6.0	**9**
11.9	11.1	10.4	9.8	9.3	8.8	8.3	7.9	7.6	7.2	6.9	6.7	**10**
13.0	12.2	11.5	10.8	10.2	9.6	9.2	8.7	8.3	8.0	7.6	7.3	**11**
14.3	13.3	12.5	11.8	11.0	10.5	10.0	9.5	9.1	8.7	8.3	8.0	**12**
15.5	14.4	13.5	12.7	12.0	11.4	10.8	10.3	9.9	9.4	9.0	8.7	**13**
16.7	15.6	14.6	13.7	13.0	12.3	11.7	11.0	10.6	10.0	9.7	9.3	**14**
17.9	16.7	15.6	14.7	13.9	13.2	12.5	12.0	11.4	10.9	10.4	10.0	**15**

Flow rate—ml/hr

I. Content of Infant Formulas

II. Content of Formulas for Nasogastric or Gastrostomy Feedings

III. Content of Tube Feedings and Oral Supplements

I. Content of infant formulas

Formulas	Calories per ounce	Percentage of total calories from each specific source			mg/dl			mOsm/kg	Description/indications
		Carbohydrate	Protein	Fat	Fe	Ca	Na (mEq)		
Full term									
Breast milk	22	33% Lactose	6% 60:40*	56% Human milk fat	0.15	34	16	300	Healthy, full-term infants
Enfamil	20	41% Lactose	9% Cow's milk	50% Soy oil 20% Coconut oil	0.15	55	28	290	Healthy, full-term infants
Enfamil with iron	20	41% Lactose	9% Cow's milk	50% Soy oil 20% Coconut oil	1.3	55	28	290	Healthy, full-term infants
Similac	20	43% Lactose	9% Cow's milk	48% Coconut oil 40% Soy oil	0.1	50	24	290	Healthy, full-term infants
Similac with iron	20	43% Lactose	9% Cow's milk	48% Coconut oil 40% Soy oil	1.2	50	24	290	Healthy, full-term infants
Premature									
Premature Enfamil	20, 24	44% 60% Corn syrup solids 40% Lactose	12% 60:40*	44% 40% MCT oil 40% Corn oil 20% Coconut oil	0.13	95	32	300	Premature infants with immature gastro-intestinal tract
Low-Birth Weight Enfamil	24	42% 50% Lactose 50% Corn syrup solids	11% Cow's milk	47% 50% MCT oil 30% Corn oil 20% Coconut oil	0.30	73	37	290	Premature infants with immature gastro-intestinal tract
Similac Special Care	20, 24, 27	42% 50% Lactose 50% Corn syrup solids	11% 60:40*	47% 50% MCT oil 30% Corn oil 20% Coconut oil	0.30	144	35	275	Premature infants with immature gastro-intestinal tracts

*Demineralized whey:casein ratio.

Continued.

I. Content of infant formulas—cont'd

Formulas	Calories per ounce	Percentage of total calories from each specific source			Fe (mg/dl)	Ca (mg/dl)	Na (mEq)	mOsm/kg	Description/indications
		Carbohydrate	Protein	Fat					
Low Na and low renal solute load									
S-M-A	20, 24, 27	43% Lactose	9% 60:40*	48% Oleo 33% Coconut oil 27% Oleic 25% Soy 15%	1.3	44	15	300	Infants with renal dysfunction; ascites; CHF
Similac PM 60/40	20	41% Lactose	9% 60:40*	50% Coconut oil 60% Corn oil 40%	0.26	40	16	265	Infants with renal dysfunction; ascites; CHF
Lactose-free with modified protein source									
Nutramigen	20	52% Sucrose 72% Modified 28% tapioca starch	13% Casein hydrolysate	35% Corn oil	1.3	63	32	443	Hypoallergenic protein hydrolysate for easy protein digestion
Pregestimil	20	54% Corn syrup solids 85% Modified 15% tapioca starch	11% Casein hydrolysate	35% Corn oil 60% MCT oil 40%	1.3	63	32	338	Easy protein digestion, plus MCT oil for patients with fat malabsorption; good for infants with short bowel syndrome where absorptive area is decreased
Lactose-free with soy protein source									
Isomil	20	40% Sucrose and corn syrup solids	12% Soy isolate	48% Coconut oil 60% Soy oil 40%	1.2	70	30	250	Full-term infants requiring soy protein base

Soyalac	20	39% Sucrose and corn syrup solids	12% Soybean extract	49% Soybean oil	1.6	63	35	N/A†	Full-term infants requiring soy protein base
Prosobee (sucrose-free)	20	40% Corn syrup solids	12% Soy isolate	48% 80% Soy oil 20% Coconut oil	1.3	63	29	160	Full-term infants requiring both sucrose and lactose-free formula, and soy protein base
Nursoy	20	40% Sucrose	12% Soy isolate	48% Oleo, coconut, oleic, soy	1.2	63	20	N/A†	Full-term infants requiring soy protein base and corn-free formula
Neo-mull-soy	20	40% Sucrose	11% Soy protein isolate	49% Soybean oil	1.0	83	36	270	Full-term infants requiring soy protein base and corn-free formula
i-Soyalac	20	39% Sucrose tapioca dextrin	12% Soy protein isolate	49% Soybean oil	1.6	63	44	N/A†	Full-term infants requiring soy protein base and corn-free formula
CHO-free	20	41% (This source must be added)	11% Soy protein isolate	48% Soybean oil	1.0	83	36	N/A†	Permits modified carbohydrate source (may use lactose)
Modified fat source								
Portagen	20	44% 25% Sucrose 75% Corn syrup solids	14% Sodium caseinate	42% 86% MCT oil 14% Corn oil	1.3	63	32	236	Infants with fat malabsorption or liver disease with impaired bile excretion

* Demineralized whey : casein ratio.
† N/A, Not available.

II. Formulas for nasogastric or gastrostomy feedings

Formulas	Calories per ounce	Percentage of total calories from each specific source			mg/dl		Na (mEq)	mOsm/kg	Description/indications
		Carbohydrate	Protein	Fat	Fe	Ca			
Complete diet; lactose-containing									
Complete B	30	48% Hydrolyzed cereal solids Maltodextrin Vegetables, fruits, orange juice	16% Beef Nonfat milk	36% Corn oil	1.1	62	5.2	390	Blenderized; moderate residue; for eventual progression to home blenderizing with normal proportions of meat, vegetables, fruit, and milk
Complete diet; lactose-free									
Isocal	30	50% Glucose Oligosaccharidase	13% 80% Calcium and sodium caseinate 20% Soy protein isolate	37% 80% Soy oil 20% MCT oil	0.94	62	2.2	300	Normal protein and fat absorption present; low residue
Osmolite	30	55% Corn syrup solids	14% 88% Sodium and calcium caseinate 12% Soy protein isolate	31% 50% MCT oil 40% Corn oil 10% Soy oil	0.92	54	2.4	300	Useful with infants who have mild to moderate degree of fat malabsorption
Vipep	30	68% 57% Corn syrup solids 6% Sucrose 2% K gluconate 2% Cornstarch 1% tapioca	10% Hydrolyzed fish protein	22%	0.90	60	3.2	520	More elemental protein source; contraindicated in conditions not tolerant of high-gut osmotic load

III. Tube feedings and oral supplements

Formulas	Calories per ounce	Percentage of total calories from each specific source			mg/dl		Na (mEq)	mOsm/kg	Description/indications
		Carbohydrate	Protein	Fat	Fe	Ca			

Complete diet; lactose-free

Formulas	Calories per ounce	Carbohydrate	Protein	Fat	Fe	Ca	Na (mEq)	mOsm/kg	Description/indications
Portagen	30	46% 73% Corn syrup solids 25% Sucrose	14% Na caseinate	40% 86% MCT oil 12% Corn oil	1.9	94	2.0	354	Infants with decreased fat absorption secondary to decreased bile or pancreatic enzymes (obstructive liver disease)
Precision Isotonic (Vanilla, orange)	30	60% 75% Glucose Oligosaccharides 25% Sucrose	12% Eggwhite solids Sodium caseinate	28% Soy oil Monoglycerides and Diglycerides	1.2	68	3.5	300	Flavorable, palatable; for infants with inflammation of small bowel and/or colon
Precision LR (Orange, lime, cherry, lemon)	33	89% 93% Maltodextrins 7% Sucrose	9.5% Eggwhite solids	1.5% MCT oil Soy oil	1.0	58	3.0	530	Low residue; useful for infants with severe small bowel inflammation; contraindicated in conditions not tolerant of high-gut osmotic load
Ensure (Vanilla, chocolate)	30	54% 74% Corn syrup solids 26% Sucrose	14% 88% Na and Ca caseinate 12% Soy isolate	32% Corn oil	0.94	54	3.3	450	Somewhat less palatable because of straight amino acids as protein source; for infants with inflammation of small bowel or colon

Continued.

III. Tube feedings and oral supplements—cont'd

Formulas	Calories per ounce	Percentage of total calories from each specific source			mg/dl			mOsm/kg	Description/indications
		Carbohydrate	Protein	Fat	Fe	Ca	Na (mEq)		
Complete diet; lactose-free—cont'd									
Ensure Plus (Vanilla, cherry, orange, lemon, strawberry, chocolate)	35	53% 74% Corn syrup solids 26% Sucrose	15% 88% Na and Ca caseinate 12% Soy isolate	32% Corn oil	1.4	62	4.5	610	Higher caloric density; useful when po volume is limited
Sustacal Liquid (Vanilla, chocolate, eggnog)	30	55% 70% Sucrose 30% Corn syrup solids	24% Ca caseinate Soy isolate	21% Soy Oil	1.7	100	4.0	610	Palatable; high-protein with lower-fat concentration; useful for patients with cystic fibrosis and other fat malabsorptive problems
Oral supplements; lactose-containing									
Sustacal pudding (Vanilla, chocolate, butterscotch)	51	53% Sucrose Lactose Modified food starch	11% Nonfat milk	36% Partially hydrogenated soy oil	1.9	157	3.7	N/A*	Palatable supplement when decreased caloric intake is primary problem

Oral supplements; lactose-free

Citrotein (Grape, orange)	20	74% Maltodextrins sucrose	24% Egg white solids	2% Monoglyceride and diglyceride Partially hydrogenated soy oil	3.8	104	2.9	500	Considered a clear liquid; useful following gastrointestinal surgery before progression to solid foods; also used for patients with chylothorax

Oral supplements; special therapeutic considerations

Amin aid	60	75% Maltodextrins sucrose	4% Amino acids	21% Partially hydrogenated soybean oil Lecithin Monoglycerides and diglycerides	—	—	<5	500	A limited amount of essential amino acids in high-caloric density with high-osmotic load for patients with acute or chronic renal failure; vitamins must be added; start in small amounts initially to prevent gastrointestinal upset
Hepatic aid	48	70% Maltodextrins sucrose	10% Amino acids	20% 96% Partially hydrogenated soybean oil 1.5% Lecithin 0.7% Monoglycerides and diglycerides	—	—	<5	495	Amino acid combination prevents added protein metabolism problems in acute or chronic liver disease; vitamins must be added; start in small amounts to prevent gastrointestinal upset

*NA, Not available.

Daily Nutritional Requirements

Recommended dietary allowances, USA Food and Nutrition Board, National Academy of Sciences,

Age and sex group	Protein	Fat-soluble vitamins			Water-soluble vitamins			
		Vitamin A	Vitamin D	Vitamin E	Vitamin C	Thiamin	Ribo-flavin	Niacin
	g	μgR.E.[b]	μg[c]	mgαT.E.[d]	mg	mg	mg	mgN.E.[e]
Infants								
0.0-0.5 yr	kg × 2.2	420	10	3	35	0.3	0.4	6
0.5-1.0 yr	kg × 2.0	400	10	4	35	0.5	0.6	8
Children								
1-3 yr	23	400	10	5	45	0.7	0.8	9
4-6 yr	30	500	10	6	45	0.9	1.0	11
7-10 yr	34	700	10	7	45	1.2	1.4	16
Males								
11-14 yr	45	1,000	10	8	50	1.4	1.6	18
15-18 yr	56	1,000	10	10	60	1.4	1.7	18
19-22 yr	56	1,000	7.5	10	60	1.5	1.7	19
23-50 yr	56	1,000	5	10	60	1.4	1.6	18
51 + yr	56	1,000	5	10	60	1.2	1.4	16
Females								
11-14 yr	46	800	10	8	50	1.1	1.3	15
15-18 yr	46	800	10	8	60	1.1	1.3	14
19-22 yr	44	800	7.5	8	60	1.1	1.3	14
23-50 yr	44	800	5	8	60	1.0	1.2	13
51 + yr	44	800	5	8	60	1.0	1.2	13
Pregnancy	+30	+200	+5	+2	+20	+0.4	+0.3	+2
Lactation	+20	+400	+5	+3	+40	+0.5	+0.5	+5

[b]Retinol equivalents: 1 retinol equivalent = 1 μg retinol or 6 μg β-carotene.
[c]As cholecalciferol: 10 μg cholecalciferol = 400 I.U. vitamin D.
[d]αtocopherol equivalents: 1 mg d-α-tocopherol = 1 αT.E.
[e]1 N.E. (niacin equivalent) = 1 mg niacin or 60 mg dietary tryptophan.

National Research Council

Water-soluble vitamins			Minerals					
Vitamin B$_6$	Folacin	Vitamin B$_{12}$	Calcium	Phos-phorus	Mag-nesium	Iron	Zinc	Iodine
mg	μg	μg	mg	mg	mg	mg	mg	μg
0.3	30	0.5	360	240	50	10	3	40
0.6	45	1.5	540	360	70	15	5	50
0.9	100	2.0	800	800	150	15	10	70
1.3	200	2.5	800	800	200	10	10	90
1.6	300	3.0	800	800	250	10	10	120
1.8	400	3.0	1,200	1,200	350	18	15	150
2.0	400	3.0	1,200	1,200	400	18	15	150
2.2	400	3.0	800	800	350	10	15	150
2.2	400	3.0	800	800	350	10	15	150
2.2	400	3.0	800	800	350	10	15	150
1.8	400	3.0	1,200	1,200	300	18	15	150
2.0	400	3.0	1,200	1,200	300	18	15	150
2.0	400	3.0	800	800	300	18	15	150
2.0	400	3.0	800	800	300	18	15	150
2.0	400	3.0	800	800	300	10	15	150
+0.6	+400	+1.0	+400	+400	+150		+5	+25
+0.5	+100	+1.0	+400	+400	+150		+10	+50

Isolation Precautions for the Patient Hospitalized with Viral Hepatitis

■ GENERAL PRECAUTIONS

The care of patients hospitalized with a diagnosis of viral hepatitis A, B, or non-A, non-B or hepatitis of unspecified type should emphasize blood precautions. The same precautions that should be used when handling feces, urine, and excretions from all other hospitalized patients should be used for patients admitted with a diagnosis of viral hepatitis. These guidelines pertain to all patients hospitalized with a diagnosis of viral hepatitis B regardless of HBeAg status.

■ SPECIFIC PRECAUTIONS

Private room. A patient need not be put in a private room unless he or she is fecally incontinent, as with small children, and the type of hepatitis is unknown or has been shown to be non-B hepatitis. Because the continence of young children is especially difficult to ensure and because their toys and books can become soiled with feces, consideration should be given to isolating all young children with viral hepatitis in a private room.

Gloves. Persons having direct contact with the patient's feces or blood or articles contaminated with blood or feces or using instruments for vascular access must wear gloves. Persons who have dermatitis should wear gloves for all patient contact.

Hands. Hands must be washed before and after direct contact with a patient or with items in contact with a patient's blood or feces.

Gowns. Persons should wear gowns when they have contact with a patient's blood or feces, are carrying out procedures in which excessive blood spills or spatters may occur, or are using instruments on a patient in such a manner that excessive fecal or blood contamination can be expected, such as proctoscopy.

Masks. Masks are not needed for normal patient contact including venipuncture. However, if a patient is being treated or is undergoing instrumentation in such a manner that blood or feces may be spattered, masks should be worn.

Articles such as books, magazines, and toys. These items require no special precautions unless they are contaminated visibly with feces or blood. Infected children should not share toys. Contaminated articles should be wiped clean with a detergent and wiped with a disinfectant.

Sphygmomanometer and stethoscope. These items require no special precautions unless visibly contaminated with feces, blood, or other body fluids contaminated with blood. If contaminated, the articles should be cleaned with a detergent solution and wiped with a disinfectant.

Thermometers. The thermometer, its container, and a suitable disinfectant such as 0.2% iodine in 70% to 90% alcohol should remain in the patient's room, and the disinfectant should be changed every 3 d. Oral thermometers may be kept dry; before and after each use, they should be washed with soap and water, rinsed, and wiped dry.

Needles and syringes. Special precautions should be taken when blood is collected from patients with hepatitis. Disposable needles and syringes should be used. They must not be reused. Used needles should not be recapped; they should be placed in a prominently labeled, impervious, puncture-resistant container designated for this purpose. Needles should not be purposely bent or broken by hand, since accidental needle puncture may occur. Used syringes should be placed in an impervious bag. Both of these containers should be incinerated, or autoclaved before discarding. Reusable syringes should be rinsed thoroughly in cold water by a person wearing gloves and should be wrapped using the double-bag technique. The outer bag should be labeled "hepatitis," and the syringes should remain bagged until they have been decontaminated or sterilized.

Dressings and tissues. These items should be placed in an impervious plastic or paper bag; it should be closed securely. The bag should be discarded in the room in a wastebasket lined with an impervious plastic bag. On removal, the wastebasket liner should be sealed and then dis-

Reproduced with permission from Favero, M., et al.: Guidelines for the care of patients hospitalized with viral hepatitis, Ann. Intern. Med. **91:**874-876, 1979.

posed of properly. Local regulations may call for incineration or disposal in an authorized sanitary landfill without being opened. Impervious bags should be readily available at the patient's bedside.

Urine and feces. The usual precautions practiced with urine and feces of all other hospitalized patients should be used with those of hepatitis patients. For example, when directly handling urine and feces or containers with urine or feces, personnel should wear gloves, and urine and feces should be flushed directly down the toilet. Utensils should be cleaned and replaced at bedside. Each patient should be assigned a bedpan, and after the patient is discharged from the hospital, the bedpan should be cleaned and disinfected or sterilized. Unless they have fecal incontinence or behavioral problems, patients with hepatitis may share a toilet facility with other patients. Each patient must wash his or her hands after using toilet facilities.

Special instruments. For instruments such as endoscopes, cystoscopes, proctoscopes, colonoscopes, bronchoscopes, nebulizers, and intermittent positive-pressure breathing machines, no special precautions are required except for instruments used for vascular access, or those that may be contaminated with blood or that may become visibly contaminated with feces. After use, these should be cleaned thoroughly and sterilized or disinfected with an appropriate high-level disinfectant.

Linen. No special precautions are needed with linens unless they are visibly contaminated with feces or blood, in which case they should be put in a laundry bag in the patient's room. A hot-water-soluble bag is preferable. The water-soluble bags containing contaminated linen should be placed unopened in hospital washing machines. Bags that are insoluble must be opened and the contents carefully dumped into washing machines without being sorted; the bags must also be washed or discarded. For incontinent patients, mattresses and pillows should be covered with impervious plastic. This covering should be cleaned with a germicidal detergent solution or removed with the linens and laundered when the room is disinfected after the patient no longer occupies it.

Dishes. No special precautions are needed with dishes.

Drinking water. No special precautions are needed with drinking water.

Clothing and personal effects. No special precautions are needed for these items unless there is visible contamination with feces or blood, in which case clothing should be treated as linen and personal effects as articles (see above).

Laboratory specimens. Specimens (urine, sputum, feces, and blood) should be put in sterile, labeled containers with the lid securely closed. Containers should be prominently labeled "hepatitis" so that the ward transport and laboratory personnel can take necessary precautions while handling and processing them.

Patient's chart. No special precautions are required for the patient's chart.

Visitors. No special precautions are required for visitors.

Transporting patients. There are no special precautions required for transporting patients except that clean sheets and pajamas should be used for fecally incontinent patients.

Concurrent cleaning. Routine daily cleaning procedures that are used in the rest of the hospital ward can be used for rooms housing hepatitis patients. Special attention should be given to areas or items grossly contaminated with feces or blood. Cleaning personnel must be alerted to the potential hazards associated with feces, blood, and serum contamination from hepatitis patients. Floors and other environmental surfaces contaminated visibly with blood or feces should be thoroughly cleaned with a detergent disinfectant. Gloves should be worn by cleaning personnel doing these duties.

Terminal disinfection. There are no special precautions for disinfection after a room is no longer occupied by a hepatitis patient except for those described under "concurrent cleaning."

APPENDIX G

Neutral Thermal Environment (Scopes' Chart)

Neutral thermal environmental temperatures (Scopes' Chart)*†

Age and weight	Starting temperature (°C)	Range temperature (°C)
0-6 Hours		
Under 1200 gm	35.0	34.0-35.4
1200-1500 gm	34.1	33.9-34.4
1501-2500 gm	33.4	32.8-33.8
Over 2500 (and >36 weeks)	32.9	32.0-33.8
6-12 Hours		
Under 1200 gm	35.0	34.0-35.4
1200-1500 gm	34.0	33.5-34.4
1501-2500 gm	33.1	32.2-33.8
Over 2500 (and >36 weeks)	32.8	31.4-33.8
12-24 Hours		
Under 1200 gm	34.0	34.0-35.4
1200-1500 gm	33.8	33.3-34.3
1501-2500 gm	32.8	31.8-33.8
Over 2500 (and >36 weeks)	32.4	31.0-33.7
24-36 Hours		
Under 1200 gm	34.0	34.0-35.0
1200-1500 gm	33.6	33.1-34.2
1501-2500 gm	32.6	31.6-33.6
Over 2500 (and >36 weeks)	32.1	30.7-33.5

Reproduced with permission from Klaus, M.H., et al.: The physical environment. In Klaus, M.H., and Fanaroff, A.A., editors: *Care of the high-risk neonate,* ed. 2, Philadelphia, 1979, W.B. Saunders Company.
*Adapted from Scopes and Ahmed. For his table, Scopes had the walls of the incubator 1° to 2° warmer than the ambient air temperatures.
†Generally speaking, the smaller infants in each weight group will require a temperature in the higher portion of the temperature range. Within each time range, the younger the infant, the higher the temperature required.

Neutral thermal environmental temperatures (Scopes' Chart)—cont'd

Age and weight	Starting temperature (°C)	Range of temperature (°C)
36-48 Hours		
Under 1200 gm	34.0	34.0-35.0
1200-1500 gm	33.5	33.0-34.1
1501-2500 gm	32.5	31.4-33.5
Over 2500 (and >36 weeks)	31.9	30.5-33.3
48-72 Hours		
Under 1200 gm	34.0	34.0-35.0
1200-1500 gm	33.5	33.0-34.0
1501-2500 gm	32.3	31.2-33.4
Over 2500 (and >36 weeks)	31.7	30.1-33.2
72-96 Hours		
Under 1200 gm	34.0	34.0-35.0
1200-1500 gm	33.5	33.0-34.0
1501-2500 gm	32.2	31.1-33.2
Over 2500 (and >36 weeks)	31.3	29.8-32.8
4-12 Days		
Under 1500 gm	33.5	33.0-34.0
1501-2500 gm	32.1	31.0-33.2
Over 2500 (and >36 weeks)		
4-5 days	31.0	29.5-32.6
5-6 days	30.9	29.4-32.3
6-8 days	30.6	29.0-32.2
8-10 days	30.3	29.0-31.8
10-12 days	30.1	29.0-31.4
12-14 Days		
Under 1500 gm	33.5	32.6-34.0
1501-2500 gm	32.1	31.0-33.2
Over 2500 (and >36 weeks)	29.8	29.0-30.8
2-3 Weeks		
Under 1500 gm	33.1	32.2-34.0
1501-2500 gm	31.7	30.5-33.0
3-4 Weeks		
Under 1500 gm	32.6	31.6-33.6
1501-2500 gm	31.4	30.0-32.7
4-5 Weeks		
Under 1500 gm	32.0	31.2-33.0
1501-2500 gm	30.9	29.5-32.2
5-6 Weeks		
Under 1500 gm	31.4	30.6-32.3
1501-2500 gm	30.4	29.0-31.8

Conversion Factors to Système International (SI) Units

Conversion factors to SI units for some biochemical components of blood*

Component	Normal range in units as customarily reported	Conversion factor	Normal range in SI units, molecular units, international units, or decimal fractions
Acetoacetic acid (S)	0.2-1.0 mg/dL	98	19.6-98.0 μmol/L
Acetone (S)	0.3-2.0 mg/dL	172	51.6-344.0 μmol/L
Albumin (S)	3.2-4.5 g/dL	10	32-45 g/L
Ammonia (P)	20-120 μg/dL	0.588	11.7-70.5 μmol/L
Amylase (S)	60-160 Somogyi units/dL	1.85	111-296 U/L
Base, total (S)	145-160 mEq/L	1	145-160 mmol/L
Bicarbonate (P)	21-28 mEq/L	1	21-28 mmol/L
Bile acids (S)	0.3-3.0 mg/dL	10	3-30 mg/L
		2.547	0.8-7.6 μmol/L
Bilirubin, direct (S)	Up to 0.3 mg/dL	17.1	Up to 5.1 μmol/L
Bilirubin, indirect (S)	0.1-1.0 mg/dL	17.1	1.7-17.1 μmol/L
Blood gases (B)			
P_{CO_2} arterial	35-40 mm Hg	0.133	4.66-5.32 kPa
P_{O_2}	95-100 mm Hg	0.133	12.64-13.30 kPa
Calcium (S)	8.5-10.5 mg/dL	0.25	2.1-2.6 mmol/L
Chloride (S)	95-103 mEq/L	1	95-103 mmol/L
Creatine (S)	0.1-0.4 mg/dL	76.3	7.6-30.5 μmol/L
Creatinine (S)	0.6-1.2 mg/dL	88.4	53-106 μmol/L
Creatinine clearance (P)	107-139 mL/min	0.0167	1.78-2.32 mL/s
Fatty acids (total) (S)	8-20 mg/dL	0.01	0.08-2.00 mg/L
Fibrinogen (P)	200-400 mg/dL	0.01	2.00-4.00 g/L
Gamma globulin (S)	0.5-1.6 g/dL	10	5-16 g/L
Globulins (total) (S)	2.3-3.5 g/dL	10	23-35 g/L
Glucose (fasting) (S)	70-110 mg/dL	0.055	3.85-6.05 mmol/L
Insulin (radioimmuno-assay) (P)	4.24 μIU/mL	0.0417	0.17-1.00 μg/L
	0.20-0.84 μg/L	172.2	35-145 pmol/L

*This is a selected (not a complete) list of biochemical components. The ranges listed may differ from those accepted in some laboratories and are shown to illustrate the conversion factor and the method of expression in SI molecular units. From Tilkian, S.M., Conover, M.B., and Tilkian, A.G.: Clinical implications of laboratory tests, ed. 3, St. Louis, 1983, The C.V. Mosby Co., pp. 491 and 492. Modified from Henry, J.B., editor: Todd-Sanford-Davidsohn clinical diagnosis and management by laboratory methods, ed. 16, Philadelphia, W.B. Saunders Co.

Conversion factors to SI units for some biochemical components of blood—cont'd

Component	Normal range in units as customarily reported	Conversion factor	Normal range in SI units, molecular units, international units, or decimal fractions
Iodine, BEI (S)	3.5-6.5 μg/dL	0.079	0.28-0.51 μmol/L
Iodine, PBI (S)	4.0-8.0 μg/dL	0.079	0.32-0.63 μmol/L
Iron, total (S)	60-150 μg/dL	0.179	11-27 μmol/L
Iron-binding capacity (S)	300-360 μg/dL	0.179	54-64 μmol/L
17-Ketosteroids (P)	25-125 μg/dL	0.01	0.25-1.25 mg/L
Lactic dehydrogenase (S)	80-120 units at 30 °C	0.48	38-62 U/L at 30 °C
	Lactate → pyruvate		
	100-190 U/L at 37 °C	1	100-190 U/L at 37 °C
Lipase (S)	0-1.5 U/mL	278	0-417 U/L
	(Cherry-Crandall)		
Lipids (total) (S)	400-800 mg/dL	0.01	4.00-8.00 g/L
Cholesterol	150-250 mg/dL	0.026	3.9-6.5 mmol/L
Triglycerides	75-165 mg/dL	0.0114	0.85-1.89 mmol/L
Phospholipids	150-380 mg/dL	0.01	1.50-3.80 g/L
Free fatty acids	9.0-15.0 mM/L	1	9.0-15.0 mmol/L
Nonprotein nitrogen (S)	20-35 mg/dL	0.714	14.3-25.0 mmol/L
Phosphatase (P)			
Acid (unit/dL)	Cherry-Crandall	2.77	0-5.5 U/L
	King-Armstrong	1.77	0-5.5U/L
	Bodansky	5.37	0-5.5 U/L
Alkaline (units/dL)	King-Armstrong	1.77	30-120 U/L
	Bodansky	5.37	30-120 U/L
	Bessey-Lowry-Brock	16.67	30-120 U/L
Phosphorus inorganic (S)	3.0-4.5 mg/dL	0.323	0.97-1.45 mmol/L
Potassium (P)	3.8-5.0 mEq/L	1	3.8-5.0 mmol/L
Proteins, total (S)	6.0-7.8 g/dL	10	60-78 g/L
Albumin	3.2-4.5 g/dL	10	32-45 g/L
Globulin	2.3-3.5 g/dL	10	23-35 g/L
Sodium (P)	136-142 mEq/L	1	136-142 mmol/L
Testosterone: Male (S)	300-1,200 ng/dL	0.035	10.5-42.0 nmol/L
Female	30-95 ng/dL	0.035	1.0-3.3 nmol/L
Thyroid tests (S)			
Thyroxine (T_4)	4-11 μg/dL	12.87	51-142 nmol/L
T_4 expressed as iodine	3.2-7.2 μg/dL	79.0	253-569 nmol/L
T_3 resin uptake	25%-38% relative uptake	0.01	0.25%-0.38% relative uptake
TSH (S)	10 μU/mL	1	$<10^{-3}$ IU/L
Urea nitrogen (S)	8-23 mg/dL	0.357	2.9-8.2 mmol/L
Uric acid (S)	2.6 mg/dL	59.5	0.120-0.360 mmol/L
Vitamin B_{12} (S)	160-950 pg/mL	0.74	118-703 pmol/L

Equivalent values of kPa and mm Hg units*

kPa	0.1	0.2	0.3	0.4	0.5	0.6	0.7	0.8	0.9
mm Hg	0.750	1.50	2.25	3.00	3.75	4.50	5.25	6.00	6.75

kPa	mm Hg	kPa	mm Hg
1	7.50	21	158
2	15.0	22	165
3	22.5	23	172
4	30.0	24	180
5	37.5	25	188
6	45.0	26	195
7	52.5	27	202
8	60.0	28	210
9	67.5	29	218
10	75.0	30	225
11	82.5	31	232
12	90.0	32	240
13	97.5	33	248
14	105	34	255
15	112	35	262
16	120	36	270
17	128	37	278
18	135	38	285
19	142	39	292
20	150	40	300

*From World Health Organization: The SI for the health professions, Geneva, 1977, The Organization, p. 40.

Some hematology values*

Component	Normal range in units as customarily reported	Conversion factor	Normal range in SI units, molecular units, international units, or decimal fractions
Red cell volume (male)	25-35 mL/kg body weight	0.001	0.025-0.035 L/kg body weight
Hematocrit	40%-50%	0.01	0.40-0.50
Hemoglobin	13.5-18.0 g/dl	10	135-180 g/L
Hemoglobin	13.5-18.0 g/dl	0.155	2.09-2.79 mmol/L
RBC count	$4.5-6 \times 10^6/\mu L$	1	$4.6-6 \times 10^{12}/L$
WBC count	$4.5-10 \times 10^3/\mu L$	1	$4.5-10 \times 10^9/L$
Mean corpuscular volume	$80-96 \mu m^3$	1	80-96 fL

*The International Committee for Standardization in Hematology recommends that the numbers remain the same but that the units change, so that hemoglobin is expressed as grams per deciliter (g/dL) even though other measurements are expressed as units per liter (U/L).

Index